Walter and Miller's

TEXTBOOK OF RADIOTHERAPY

RADIATION PHYSICS, THERAPY AND ONCOLOGY

Ninth Edition

Walter and Miller's TEXTBOOK OF RADIOTHERAPY

RADIATION PHYSICS, THERAPY AND ONCOLOGY

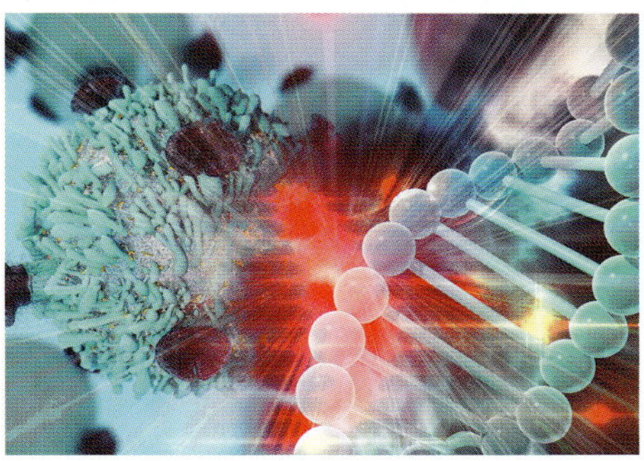

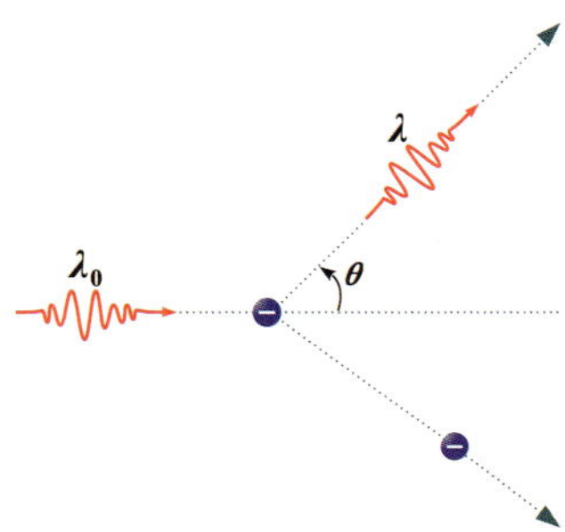

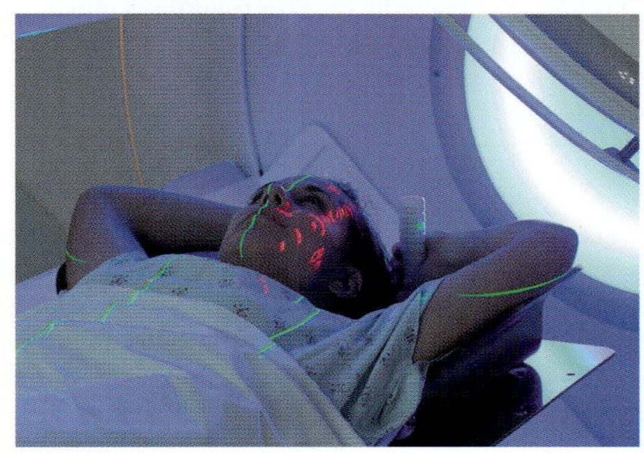

Edited by

Thankamma V. Ajithkumar, MD, FRCP, FRCR, MBA
Consultant Clinical Oncologist
Department of Oncology
Cambridge University Hospital
Cambridge, United Kingdom

John A. Mills, PhD, MIPEM, CPhys
Quality Control Provider
Megavoltage Acceptance and Commissioning Service (MACS)
Leicestershire, United Kingdom

Pete Bridge, PhD, MSc, BSc Hons, BSc SFHEA
Senior Lecturer (Radiotherapy)
School of Allied Health Professions and Nursing
Institute of Population Health
University of Liverpool
Liverpool, United Kingdom

ANNIVERSARY EDITION 75 YEARS

ELSEVIER

For accessibility purposes, images in electronic versions of this book are accompanied by alt text descriptions provided by Elsevier. For more information, see https://www.elsevier.com/about/accessibility.

Books and Journals published by Elsevier comply with applicable product safety requirements. For any product safety concerns or queries, please contact our authorised representative, Elsevier B.V., at productsafety@elsevier.com.

Publisher's note: *Elsevier* takes a neutral position with respect to territorial disputes or jurisdictional claims in its published content, including in maps and institutional affiliations.

First edition 1950
Second edition 1959
Third edition 1979
Fourth edition 1979
Fifth edition 1993
Sixth edition 2003
Seventh edition 2012
Eighth edition 2019

Notice

Practitioners and researchers must always rely on their own experience and knowledge in evaluating and using any information, methods, compounds or experiments described herein. Because of rapid advances in the medical sciences, in particular, independent verification of diagnoses and drug dosages should be made. To the fullest extent of the law, no responsibility is assumed by Elsevier, authors, editors or contributors for any injury and/or damage to persons or property as a matter of product liability, negligence or otherwise, or from any use or operation of any methods, products, instructions, or ideas contained in the material herein.

ISBN: 978-0-4431-1978-1

Content Strategist: Trinity Hutton
Content Project Manager: Arpita Paul
Design: Christian Bilbow
Illustration Manager: Akshaya Mohan
Marketing Manager: Deborah Watkins

Printed in India
Thomson Press India Private Ltd.
18/35, Delhi-Mathura Road, Faridabad - 121007, Haryana

Last digit is the print number: 9 8 7 6 5 4 3

CONTENTS

PREFACE

As we celebrate the 75th anniversary of *Walter and Miller's Textbook of Radiotherapy*, we reflect on the long journey of this seminal work and its pivotal role in shaping the field of radiotherapy. It was first published in 1950 with the primary objective of being a text for student technicians working for the examinations of the Society of Radiographers, especially in radiotherapy. It was also hoped to 'serve as a bird's-eye view for doctors and others, who would be repelled by longer or more technical works'. Since then, this textbook has been a treasured text for oncologists, medical physicists, therapeutic radiographers and other healthcare professionals dedicated to cancer treatment. Its enduring presence in the medical community is a testament to its foundational value, comprehensive coverage and adaptability to the rapidly evolving technological and procedural landscape of radiotherapy.

The origins of *Walter and Miller's Textbook of Radiotherapy* can be traced back to when radiotherapy was in its nascent stages and clinical guidelines were still developing. The textbook became renowned for setting a benchmark for quality in radiotherapy education. Over the decades, each edition of this textbook has documented the remarkable advancements in technology and clinical practice. The evolution from the rudimentary orthovoltage and giant gantry systems of the early 20th century to today's sophisticated image-guided linear accelerators is meticulously chronicled within these pages (Fig. 1). Recent editions have introduced readers to multileaf collimation (MLC), intensity-modulated radiotherapy (IMRT), image-guided radiotherapy (IGRT), stereotactic body radiotherapy (SBRT) and proton therapy. This 75th-anniversary edition continues this tradition with a focus on evidence-based best practices, clinical trials and experimental technologies, ensuring that it remains an indispensable resource for seasoned practitioners and those new to the field (Fig. 2).

Joseph Walter (1910–1979) and Harold Miller (1909–1995) became colleagues at the Sheffield National Centre for Radiotherapy in 1942 when Miller was appointed physicist following his unwillingness as a pacifist to undertake military work. Walter had been appointed assistant medical officer to the Sheffield Radium Centre in 1940 and became the deputy director of the Sheffield National Centre for Radiotherapy in 1943. Both were very active with development and teaching. Walter, from Salford, Lancashire, had won a scholarship and studied at Oxford and then Kings College, London. At Sheffield, he gave himself wholeheartedly to the improvement of cancer treatment, not only with radiation but also by chemotherapy, becoming one of the first true oncologists. Miller, from Staveley, Derbyshire, also obtained a scholarship and studied at Cambridge, obtaining his PhD at the Cavendish Laboratory, supervised by Chadwick, who discovered the neutron. Medical and scientific advances in Sheffield were wide-ranging, and technical developments included the installation of a 2MeV Van de Graaf X-ray generator from the United States in 1946.

Teaching demands were high for medical, nursing, radiography and technical staff training. Walter and Miller understood the learning requirements of students at all levels, and *A Short Textbook of Radiotherapy*, written jointly based on a series of lectures, was an instant success when it appeared in 1950.

One of the defining strengths of *Walter and Miller's Textbook of Radiotherapy* is its holistic approach to radiotherapy. It addresses the technical and biological aspects of radiation therapy and emphasises the importance of patient-centred care. Integrating psychosocial considerations, patient safety and quality-of-life issues underscores the textbook's commitment to comprehensive cancer care. This edition places a renewed focus on personalised radiotherapy treatment and care, exploring how image guidance, biological optimisation and adaptive radiotherapy are delivering individualised treatment while patient-reported outcomes are enhancing survivorship in our patients.

As we celebrate this milestone, we honour the countless professionals, especially the editors and authors of the previous editions, who have contributed to the textbook's success. Their dedication to advancing the science and practice of radiotherapy is reflected in the depth and breadth of this edition. This collective effort ensures that *Walter and Miller's Textbook of Radiotherapy* remains at the forefront of educational resources, continuing to inspire and educate future healthcare providers.

In the second edition (1959), in his foreword, J L A Grout, a former vice president of the Faculty of Radiologists, wrote, 'His book will do much to allay those fears which the very names Physics and Radiotechnics engender in the hearts of those preparing for examinations in Radiotherapy'. As a postgraduate trainee in clinical oncology, one

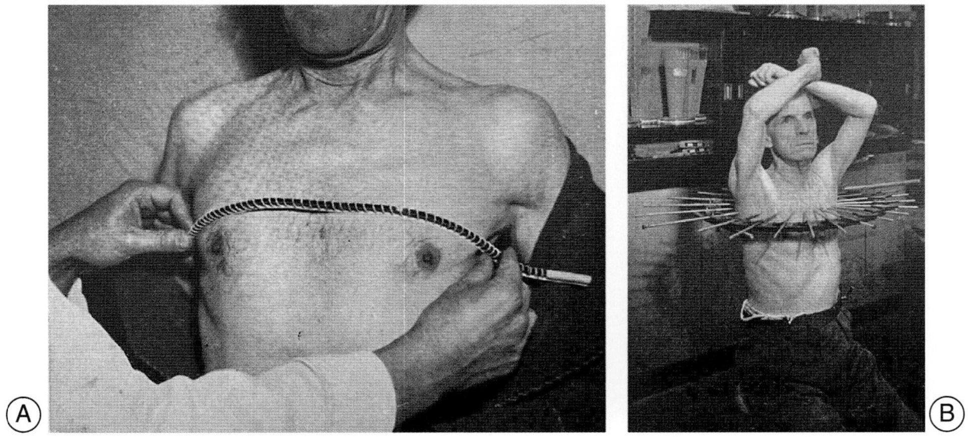

Fig. 1 *Field planning for oesophageal radiotherapy using a malleable lead strip to transfer a cross-section of the patient onto drawing paper (A) or using a contouring device with adjustable spokes (B) (from the second edition of* A Short Textbook of Radiotherapy*).*

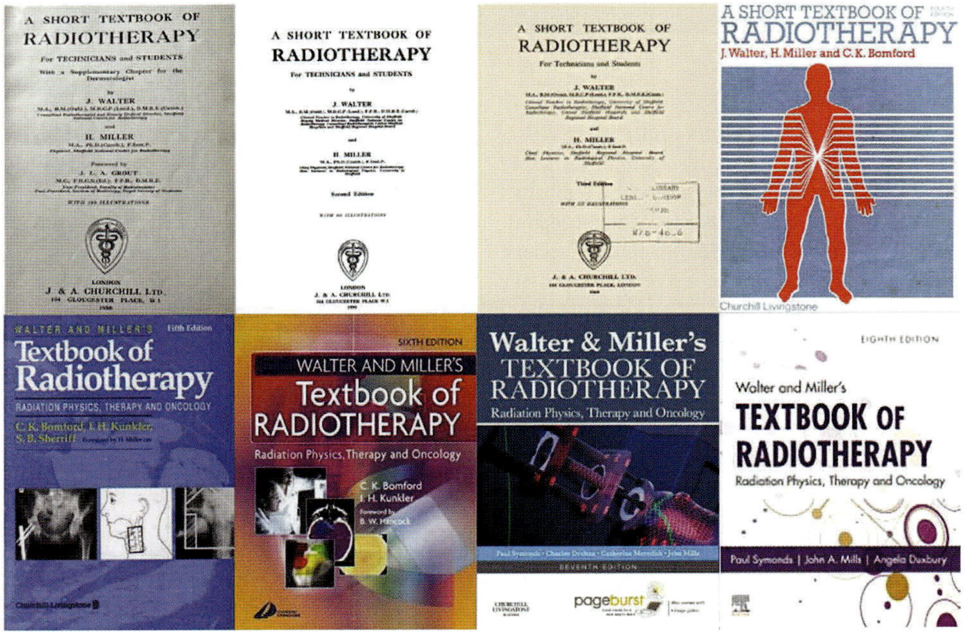

Fig. 2 *Front/cover pages of the last eight editions of* Textbook of Radiotherapy.

of the editors of this edition started using this book in 1995, initially for two radiotherapy examinations abroad and, subsequently, for the FRCR examination in the United Kingdom. On all these occasions, different editions of this textbook served as a revision and helped to alleviate the anxiety as predicted. Numerous trainees during the past 75 years could relate to this experience. We hope this textbook continues to ease the fears of those preparing for radiotherapy examinations.

The 75th-anniversary edition of *Walter and Miller's Textbook of Radiotherapy* stands as a testament to the enduring legacy of its founders and the continuous advancements in cancer treatment. It is more than just a textbook; it is a beacon of knowledge, innovation and hope in the ongoing fight against cancer. We hope this edition will serve as a valuable guide and inspiration for all those dedicated to the noble cause of cancer treatment and patient care.

Thankamma V. Ajithkumar
John A. Mills
Pete Bridge

CONTRIBUTORS

Thankamma V. Ajithkumar, MD, FRCR, FRCP
Consultant Clinical Oncologist
Cambridge University Hospitals NHS Trust
Cambridge, United Kingdom

Oyeyemi O. Akala, MD, BSc, MRCP
Clinical Research Fellow
Leicester Cancer Research Centre
University of Leicester
Leicester, United Kingdom

Matthew Aldridge, PhD
Consultant Clinical Scientist
Nuclear Medicine Physics
King's College Hospital NHS Foundation Trust
London, United Kingdom

Sarah Aldridge, BSc(Hons), MSc, MIPEM, MInstP, CSci, CMgr
Consultant Clinical Scientist
Department of Medical Physics & Clinical Engineering
Guy's and St. Thomas' NHS Foundation Trust
London, United Kingdom

Richard A. Amos, BSc(Hons), MSc, CPhys, CSci, MInstP, FIPEM
Associate Professor of Proton Therapy Physics
University College London
London, United Kingdom

Maria Mania Aspradakis, PhD
Head of Radiotherapy Physics
Clinic of Radiation Oncology
Kantonsspital Winterthur
Winterthur, Switzerland

Sarah Bacon, MSc
Medical Physicist (MRI)
Medical Physics Department
St. James's University Hospital
Leeds, United Kingdom

Helen Baines, MSc
Quality System Manager
Department of Radiotherapy Physics
St. James University Hospital
Leeds, United Kingdom

Laura Beaton, MBBS, BSc, MRCP, FRCR
Consultant Clinical Oncologist
Barts Health NHS Trust
London, United Kingdom

Douglas Brand, PhD, MB, BChir, FRCR, MRCP
Consultant Clinical Oncologist
University College London Hospitals
London, United Kingdom
University College London
London, United Kingdom

Pete Bridge, PhD, MSc, BSc Hons, BSc SFHEA
Senior Lecturer (Radiotherapy)
School of Health Sciences
Institute of Population Health
University of Liverpool
Liverpool, United Kingdom

Emilia Bruton, MB BChir, MRCP, FRCR
Consultant Clinical Oncologist
Royal Berkshire Hospital
Reading, United Kingdom

Amy Colori, MRCP, MSc, FRCR
Speciality Registrar in Clinical Oncology
University College London Hospitals NHS Foundation Trust
London, United Kingdom

Cathryn Crockett, MB, BCH, MRCP (UK), FRCR
Consultant in Clinical Oncology
Northern Ireland Cancer Centre
Belfast Health and Social Care Trust
Belfast, Northern Ireland, United Kingdom

Elizabeth Davies, DClinSci, MIPEM
Head of Leicester Radiation Safety Services
University Hospitals of Leicester NHS Trust
Leicester, United Kingdom

Jody Deacon-Viney, BSc
Quality Assurance Radiographer
Arden Cancer Centre
University Hospitals Coventry and Warwickshire NHS Trust
Coventry, United Kingdom

Charles Deehan, PhD, BSc, MinstP, MIPEM, CPhys
Former Head of Radiotherapy Physics
Guy's and St Thomas' NHS Foundation Trust and Kings College
London, United Kingdom

Adrian Franklin, MRCP, FRCR
Consultant Clinical Oncologist in Gynae-Oncology
Royal Surrey NHS Foundation Trust
Surrey, United Kingdom

Jenny Gains, MBBS, MRCP, FRCR, MD
Consultant Clinical Oncologist
University College London Hospitals NHS Foundation Trust
London, United Kingdom

Pinelopi Gkogkou, MD, MSc, PhD
Consultant Clinical Oncologist
Norfolk and Norwich University Hospital NHS Trust
Norwich, United Kingdom

John R. Goepel, MB, ChB, FRCPath
Clinical Associate Professor and Consultant Histopathologist
University of Nottingham
Royal Hallamshire Hospital
Sheffield, United Kingdom

Gerard G. Hanna, MB, PhD, MRCP (UK), FRCR, FFRRCSI (Hons)
Marie Curie Chair of Clinical Oncology
Trinity College
University of Dublin
Dublin, Ireland
Consultant in Radiation Oncology
St. Luke's Radiation Oncology Network
Dublin, Ireland

Fiona Harris, MBChB, MRCP, FRCR
Consultant Clinical Oncologist
Cambridge University Hospitals NHS Trust
Cambridge, United Kingdom

Maria A. Hawkins, MD, MRCP, FRCR
Professor in Radiation Oncology
University College London
London, United Kingdom

Paul Hinton, MSc, CSci, MIPEM
Consultant Clinical Scientist
Nuclear Medicine Physics
Royal Surrey County Hospital
Guildford, United Kingdom

Gail Horan, FRCR
Consultant Clinical Oncologist
Cambridge University Hospitals NHS Trust
Cambridge, United Kingdom

Steve Hunt, PhD
Clinical Radiation Technologist (Retired)
Department of Medical Physics
University Hospitals Leicester
Leicester, United Kingdom

Shakardokht Jafari, PhD, FIPEM
Clinical Scientist
Radiotherapy Physics
Portsmouth Hospitals University NHS Trust
Portsmouth, United Kingdom

Kamalram Thippu Jayaprakash, MBBS, MSc, MD RT, MD, MRCP (UK), FRCR
Consultant Clinical Oncologist
Cambridge University Hospitals NHS Foundation Trust
Cambridge, United Kingdom
Affiliated Assistant Professor
University of Cambridge
Cambridge, United Kingdom

Sarah J. Jefferies, PhD, FRCP, FRCR
Consultant Clinical Oncologist
Cambridge University Hospitals NHS Trust
Cambridge, United Kingdom

Andrzej Kacperek, PhD, BSc, FIPEM
Honorary Professor
Department of Medical Physics and Biomedical Engineering
University College London
London, United Kingdom

Ian Kunkler, MA, DMRT, FRCPE, FRCR
Professor of Clinical Oncology
MRC Institute of Genetics and Cancer
University of Edinburgh
Edinburgh, United Kingdom

Daniel Leach, BSc, PGDip
Pre-Treatment Team Lead Radiographer
Radiotherapy Department
Raigmore Hospital
Inverness, United Kingdom

Sofia Michopoulou, PhD
Consultant Clinical Scientist
Nuclear Medicine Physics
University Hospital Southampton NHS Foundation Trust
Southampton, United Kingdom

John A. Mills, PhD, MIPEM, CPhys
Physicist
Megavoltage Acceptance and Commissioning Service
James Watt House
Hinckley, United Kingdom

Abhik Mukherjee, MBBS, DMRT, MSc, PhD, FRCPath
Clinical Associate Professor and Consultant Histopathologist
University of Nottingham and Nottingham University Hospital NHS Trust
Nottingham, United Kingdom

Somnath Mukherjee, MD, FRCR, FRCP
Associate Professor and Consultant Oncologist
University of Oxford
Oxford, United Kingdom

Alan E. Nahum, PhD, FIPEM
Visiting Professor
Physics Department
University of Liverpool
Liverpool, United Kingdom

Amit Nautiyal, PhD
Clinical Scientist
Nuclear Medicine Physics
University Hospital Southampton NHS Foundation Trust
Southampton, United Kingdom

Elizabeth Parvin, BSc, PhD, FInstP, MIPEM
Honorary Associate
School of Physical Sciences
Open University
Milton Keynes, United Kingdom

Hersha Patel, MRCOG, PhD
Consultant Surgeon in Gynaecological Oncology
Royal Surrey NHS Foundation Trust
Honorary Senior Lecturer
University of Surrey
Surrey, United Kingdom

Sarah Prewett, MRCP, FRCR
Consultant Clinical Oncologist
Cambridge University Hospitals NHS Trust
Cambridge, United Kingdom

Kiran Purushothaman, MD, FRCR
Consultant Clinical Oncologist
Cambridge University Hospitals NHS Trust
Cambridge, United Kingdom

Richard Raynor, MSc
Principal Clinical Scientist
Leicester Radiation Safety Services
University Hospitals of Leicester NHS Trust
Leicester, United Kingdom

Heather Reid, BSc (Hons)
Information and Support Advanced Practitioner
NHS Greater Glasgow and Clyde
Glasgow, United Kingdom

John Rodgers, MSc
Senior Clinical Officer
UK Health Security Agency
Didcot, United Kingdom

John Sage, BSc, MSc, PhD
Senior Research Scientist
Mirada Medical Ltd.
Oxford, United Kingdom

Giuseppe Schettino, PhD, FInstP, FIPEM
Fellow
Radiotherapy and Radiation Dosimetry Group
National Physical Laboratory
Teddington, United Kingdom

Christopher D. Scrase, MA, MB, FRCP, FRCR
Consultant Clinical Oncologist
North Wales Cancer Treatment Centre
Senior Clinical Lecturer in Medical Education
North Wales Medical School
North Wales, United Kingdom

Phil Sharpe, MSc, MIPEM, CSci
Principal Clinical Scientist
Radiotherapy Physics
University Hospitals Coventry and Warwickshire NHS Trust
Coventry, United Kingdom

Aspazia Spyrou, MB, BCh, BAO, MSc
Specialist Registrar in Clinical Oncology
Royal Surrey Hospital
Guildford, United Kingdom

Alexandra Stewart, DM, MRCP, FRCR, FBIR
Consultant Clinical Oncologist
Royal Surrey NHS Foundation Trust
Honorary Senior Lecturer
University of Surrey
Surrey, United Kingdom

Aravindhan Sundaramurthy, MBBS, FRCR, FRCP
Consultant Clinical Oncologist
Edinburgh Cancer Centre
NHS Lothian
Edinburgh, United Kingdom

Robin Taylor, MPhys, MSc
Radiotherapy Physicist
Radiotherapy Department
Raigmore Hospital
Inverness, United Kingdom

Carl Tiivas, BSc, MSc
Former Head of Vascular Ultrasound
Department of Clinical Physics
University Hospital Coventry
Coventry, United Kingdom

Jonathan Wadsley, MA, MRCP, FRCR
Consultant Clinical Oncologist
Weston Park Cancer Centre
Sheffield, United Kingdom

Karen Waite, DCR(T)
Quality Management and Governance Radiographer
Nottingham Radiotherapy Centre
Nottingham University Hospitals NHS Trust
Nottingham, United Kingdom

Harriet S. Walter, MBChB, MSc, PhD
Associate Professor of Medical Oncology
Director of Hope Cancer Trials Centre
Leicester Cancer Research Centre
University of Leicester
Leicester, United Kingdom

Tim Wood, PhD
Principal Medical Physicist
Radiation Protection and Radiology Physics
Hull University Teaching Hospitals NHS Trust
Hull, United Kingdom

Kevin Young, PhD, MIPEM, CSci
Principal Clinical Scientist
Radiotherapy Physics
University Hospitals Coventry and Warwickshire NHS Trust
Coventry, United Kingdom

INTERNATIONAL SYSTEM OF UNITS AND PREFIXES FOR PHYSICAL QUANTITIES

There are seven international system (SI) base units:

Physical Quantity	Unit	Symbol for Unit
Length	Metre	m
Mass	Kilogram	kg
Time	Second	s
Electric current	Ampere	A
Temperature	Kelvin	K
Amount of substance	Mole	mol
Luminous intensity	Candela	cd

There is also a large number of derived units, some of which are listed here:

Quantity	Derived Unit	Conversion
Speed	$m\ s^{-1}$	—
Acceleration	$m\ s^{-2}$	—
Angular frequency	s^{-1}	—
Angular speed	$rad\ s^{-1}$	—
Angular acceleration	$rad\ s^{-2}$	—
Linear momentum	$kg\ m\ s^{-1}$	—
Angular momentum	$kg\ m^2\ s^{-1}$	—
Force	newton (N)	$1\ N = 1\ kg\ m\ s^{-2}$
Energy	joule (J)	$1\ J = 1\ N\ m = 1\ kg\ m^2\ s^{-2}$
Torque	N m	—
Power	watt (W)	$1\ W = 1\ J\ s^{-1}$
Pressure	pascal (Pa)	$1\ Pa = 1\ N\ m^{-2}$
Frequency	hertz (Hz)	$1\ Hz = 1\ s^{-1}$
Charge	coulomb (C)	$1\ C = 1\ A\ s$
Potential difference	volt (V)	$1\ V = 1\ J\ C^{-1}$
Electric field	$N\ C^{-1}$	$1\ N\ C^{-1} = 1\ V\ m^{-1}$
Radioactivity	Becquerel (Bq)	$1\ Bq = 1\ s^{-1}$
Resistance	ohm (Ω)	$1\ \Omega = 1\ V\ A^{-1}$
Capacitance	farad (F)	$1\ F = 1\ A\ s\ V^{-1}$
Inductance	henry (H)	$1\ H = 1\ V\ s\ A^{-1}$
Magnetic field	tesla (T)	$1\ T = 1\ N\ s\ m^{-1}\ C^{-1} = 1\ kg\ s^{-2}\ A^{-1}$
Physical dose	gray (Gy); see Chapter 2	$1\ Gy = 1\ J\ kg^{-1}$
Biological dose	sievert (Sv); see Chapter 4	$1\ Sv = 1\ J\ kg^{-1}$

Following are the most common multiples and submultiples:

Multiple	Prefix	Symbol for Prefix
10^{12}	tera	T
10^{9}	giga	G
10^{6}	mega	M
10^{3}	kilo	k
10^{0}	—	—
10^{-3}	milli	m
10^{-6}	micro	μ
10^{-9}	nano	n
10^{-12}	pico	p
10^{-15}	femto	f

Online references: http://www.npl.co.uk/reference/measurement-units/

SECTION 1

1

Atoms, Nuclei and Radioactivity

Elizabeth Parvin

CHAPTER OUTLINE

INTRODUCTION

The aim of this chapter is to lay some of the foundations of the physics of radiotherapy. It starts by looking at the main subatomic particles and the forces that hold them together in the atom. This leads to an examination of the different types of nuclei, with an emphasis on some of the important ones used in medical physics. The behaviour of charged particles in electric and magnetic fields, central to much of the physics of radiotherapy, is covered in the 'Particles in Electric and Magnetic Fields' section. Waves, including the electromagnetic spectrum, and the basics of radioactive decay are introduced in the remaining sections.

For some readers, this chapter will be a reminder of previous knowledge; for others it will be new territory. For the latter, the references should provide additional in-depth material that was not possible to include here. For convenience, SI units are listed in the 'Physical Units and Constants' section.

ATOMIC STRUCTURE

Particles

Most readers will be familiar with the idea that molecules are composed of atoms chemically bonded together. Perhaps the most familiar example is the water molecule, which consists of two hydrogen atoms bonded to one oxygen atom to give the well-known molecular formula H_2O. In radiotherapy, we are often more interested in the particles that make up the atom—these are known as *subatomic particles.*

Table 1.1 lists the properties of the subatomic particles of most relevance to radiotherapy: the *proton*, *neutron*, *electron*, *positron*, *neutrino* and *antineutrino*. Strictly speaking, only the electron, positron and neutrino are fundamental particles; the proton and neutron are composed of *quarks*. Charges are, as is customary in physics, given as multiples of the electronic charge, e, which is 1.602×10^{-19} C. The proton and positron have charges of $+e$ and the electron has a charge of $-e$; all the other particles listed are neutral. The fourth column gives the masses in kilograms, but in nuclear physics it is a common practice to express the mass of a particle not in kilograms but in terms of its *rest mass energy*. This is based on Einstein's famous equation, which gives the equivalence of mass and energy:

$$E = mc^2 \quad \textbf{(1.1)}$$

where m is the mass of the particle, c is the speed of light in a vacuum (2.998×10^8 m s^{-1}) and E is the energy. For an electron, the rest mass energy associated with a mass of 9.109×10^{-31} kg is 8.187×10^{-14} joules (J). It is more convenient to express this very small magnitude of energy in units of the *electron volt* (eV), where:

$$1\text{eV} = 1.602 \times 10^{-19}\,\text{J} \quad \textbf{(1.2)}$$

The electron volt is the amount of energy acquired by an electron when it is accelerated through a voltage of 1 volt (see the 'Electric Fields' section), hence the name *electron volt.* Using this conversion, we arrive at the values given in the last column in Table 1.1. Note that the proton and neutron (known collectively as *nucleons*) are much more massive than the electron and positron, and the neutrino has almost zero mass—the exact value is still the subject of experiment.

The positron is the antiparticle of the electron, having the same mass but the opposite charge; it is emitted during β^+ decay (see the 'Beta Decay' section) and is important in positron emission tomography (PET) (see Chapter 7). Neutrinos play a role in β decay (see the

TABLE 1.1 Properties of the Subatomic Particles of Most Relevance to Radiotherapy

Particle	Symbol	Charge, e^a	Mass (kg)	Rest Mass Energy (MeV)
Proton	p	+1	1.673×10^{-27}	938
Neutron	n	0	1.675×10^{-27}	940
Electron	e^-	−1	9.109×10^{-31}	0.511
Positron	e	+1	9.109×10^{-31}	0.511
Neutrino	ν_e	0	>0	>0
Antineutrino	$\bar{\nu}_e$	0	>0	>0
Photon	γ	0	0	

[a] e is the charge on an electron.

'Beta Decay' section). The photon is the particle associated with electromagnetic radiation (see the 'Waves' section).

The Atom and the Nucleus

The *atom* is the smallest identifiable amount of an element. Each atom consists of a central *nucleus*, made up of protons and neutrons, which is surrounded by a 'cloud' of electrons. The diameters of an atom and nucleus are typically 10^{-10} m and 10^{-14} m, respectively. To put these dimensions into a more accessible perspective, if the atomic nucleus is represented by the point of a pencil (diameter approximately 0.5 mm) held in the centre of a medium-sized room (say 5 m × 5 m), the electron cloud surrounding the nucleus would extend to the walls of the room.

It is the number of protons in a nucleus that determines the type of element. Because the protons in the nucleus are positively charged and the electrons are negatively charged, a neutral atom must contain equal numbers of protons and electrons. It is the electrons, which surround the nucleus and are often described as orbiting it, that interact with electrons from other atoms, thereby determining the chemical behaviour of the atom.

For example, a hydrogen atom has one proton in the nucleus, helium has two, carbon has six and so on. This number is known as the *atomic number*, *Z*, of the element. The elements listed in order of increasing atomic number form the periodic table of the elements.[1]

As shown in Table 1.1, the neutrons in the nucleus carry no charge but do have a similar mass to the protons. The electrons have a very small mass, so the mass of an atom is almost entirely due to the mass of the protons and neutrons. The sum of the number of neutrons (N) and protons in a nucleus is known as the *atomic mass number*, A, and $A = Z + N$. Because both A and Z are needed to identify a nucleus, the notation used is of the form:

$$^{A}_{Z}\mathrm{X} \tag{1.3}$$

The symbol shown here as X is the chemical symbol for the element—H for hydrogen, He for helium, C for carbon and so on—and A and Z are the mass and atomic numbers. Because Z determines the chemistry and therefore the element, strictly speaking, it is not necessary to have the value of Z shown. For example, $^{12}_{6}\mathrm{C}$ represents a carbon nucleus with six protons and six neutrons, but it could be written simply as $^{12}\mathrm{C}$, or even as carbon-12, because carbon always has six protons. However, to avoid confusion, it is often easier to include both atomic and mass numbers.

For any one element, the number of protons is always the same, but the number of neutrons, and hence A, can vary. For example, carbon can exist as $^{11}_{6}\mathrm{C}$, $^{12}_{6}\mathrm{C}$, $^{13}_{6}\mathrm{C}$ or $^{14}_{6}\mathrm{C}$. These have five, six, seven and eight neutrons, respectively, and are known as the *isotopes* of carbon. For many elements, some of the isotopes are radioactive (see the 'Radioactive Decay' section), and this fact can be very useful in clinical investigations because the chemical behaviour of all the isotopes is the same. For example, radioactive $^{15}_{8}\mathrm{O}$ is taken up by the body in the same way as the stable (i.e. nonradioactive) isotope $^{16}_{8}\mathrm{O}$ so it can be used in PET; the radioactive iodine isotope $^{131}_{58}\mathrm{I}$ is taken up by the thyroid gland in the same way as the stable isotope $^{127}_{58}\mathrm{I}$, so it can be used to treat thyroid cancer.

The Forces

The next point to address is the question of what holds the atoms together. The protons in the nucleus are positively charged and the electrons surrounding the nucleus are negatively charged, so there is an attractive force between them. This electrostatic or *Coulomb force* depends on the product of the charges and is inversely proportional to the square of the distance between them. For one electron (charge $-e$) and a nucleus (charge Z), the magnitude of the force (F_{el}) is given by the equation:

$$F_{el} = k\frac{Ze^2}{r^2} \tag{1.4}$$

where k is a constant and r is the distance between the electron and the nucleus. This inverse-square relationship is analogous to the gravitational force between two masses, and we could use the rules of classical physics to calculate the orbits of the electrons around the nucleus (analogous to the orbits of the planets around the sun). However, there is one big difference between the planetary orbits and the orbits of the electrons around the nucleus; in the planetary case, it is possible to have any value of the radius (and therefore energy), whereas in the atomic case, quantum theory only allows certain permitted orbits. This gives rise to *electron energy levels* (or shells), which are the subject of the section titled Electron Energy Levels.

For like charges, the Coulomb force is repulsive, so, because the protons in the nucleus are all positively charged, it might be expected that the Coulomb force would cause the nucleus to fly apart. However, there is another force that acts on both protons and neutrons: the *strong force*. This force acts on protons and neutrons and other heavy particles, called *hadrons*; it is independent of charge and is always attractive but only at very short range. Fig. 1.1 shows the way in which the energy of a proton varies depending on how far away it is from the nucleus. As a proton approaches the nucleus, it experiences a repulsive force, but if it has enough energy to overcome this 'Coulomb barrier' and gets

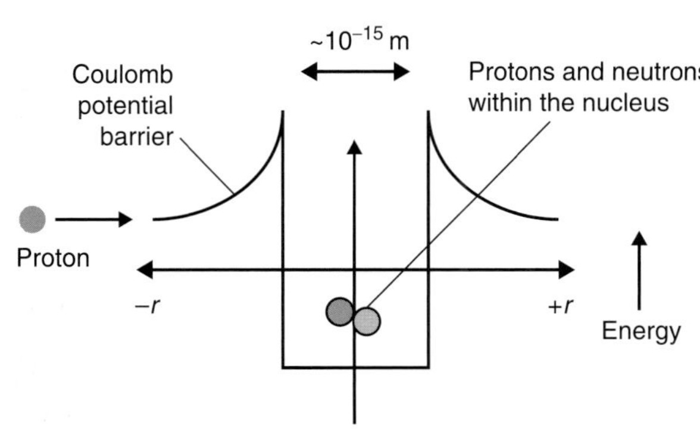

Fig. 1.1 Schematic illustration of the energy of a proton as a function of its distance, *r*, from the centre of the nucleus. As the proton approaches the nucleus, the repulsive Coulomb force increases, but close to the nucleus, this repulsion is overcome by the attractive strong force, so the energy is reduced and the nucleons are held together in the nucleus.

within the range at which the strong force works, it has a much lower energy in the nucleus and stays there. An energy diagram like this is known as a *potential well.*

Electron Energy Levels

As mentioned in the section titled 'The Forces', planetary orbits around the sun and electron orbits around the nucleus differ in that, in the case of the electrons, quantum theory predicts that only certain orbits are allowed. This means that only certain orbit energies can occur—these different values of energy are referred to as *energy levels* or shells and were first hypothesised by Niels Bohr in 1913.

A free electron, which is outside the nucleus, is said to have zero energy; any electrons in levels closer to the nucleus have a lower and therefore negative energy. Fig. 1.2 shows the possible energy levels for the simplest element, hydrogen. No energy is lost or gained while an electron occupies a particular shell, and only discrete amounts of energy can be gained or lost by electrons when they move between shells. You can see from Fig. 1.2 that the lowest energy state for hydrogen is –13.6 eV. Therefore the amount of energy that would be required to remove this electron from the atom is 13.6 eV. This is the *ionisation energy* of the hydrogen atom. The energy required to raise an electron from the lowest energy state to the second lowest energy state is equal to the difference between the energies of the two states, that is, (13.6 – 3.40) = 10.2 eV, and so on for all other pairs of energy levels.

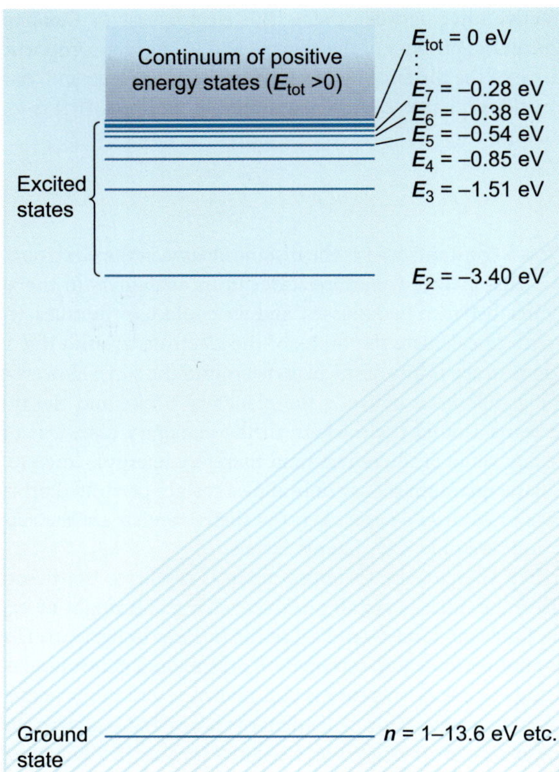

Fig. 1.2 The possible energy levels of the electron in the hydrogen atom. Note that when the electron is bound in the atom, the energy is negative and can only take certain values. Outside the atom, the energy of the unbound electron is zero. The energy levels are numbered—n = 1, 2 and so on—from the inside outwards.

Large atoms have more complicated arrangements of electron energy levels. The energy levels are numbered according to the *principal quantum number*, n (n = 1, 2, 3 etc.), and are subdivided into other energy levels, sometimes known as *suborbitals*, with more quantum numbers relating to angular momentum and spin. These quantum numbers also dictate the number of electrons which can be in each shell. Historically, the principal quantum number may also be represented by the letters K (n = 1), L (n = 2), M (n = 3) and so on, so the shells are often referred to as the *K-, L-, M-shells* and so on. If all the electrons in an atom are in the lowest possible energy states allowed by the rules, the atom is said to be in the *ground state*. For example, a hydrogen atom in the ground state has the electron in the state with energy –13.6 eV.

Band Theory of Solids

In individual atoms, outer electrons occupy specific energy levels. When atoms are brought together, as occurs in solid materials, interactions between atoms broaden these specific energy levels into 'energy bands'. Electrons may occupy energy states only within these bands, between which are forbidden zones that normally do not have energy states for electrons to occupy, as illustrated in Fig. 1.3.

The outermost energy bands within the solid material are termed the *valence band* and the *conduction band*. Electrons within the valence band are considered linked to the chemical bonds between individual atoms and are therefore bound in place, although the term *bound* is used loosely because at normal temperatures such bonds may continually be broken and re-formed. At an energy level slightly above the valence band is the conduction band. Electrons within this band are surplus to any requirements for chemical bonding. At normal temperatures, these electrons are not associated with specific atoms and chemical bonds but migrate readily through the material. In some materials, there are insufficient electrons to fill the available energy levels of the valence band, so the conduction band is empty. Where a large forbidden zone exists, these materials are classed as nonconductors or insulators (see Fig. 1.3A). Other materials may have more outer electrons than the valence band

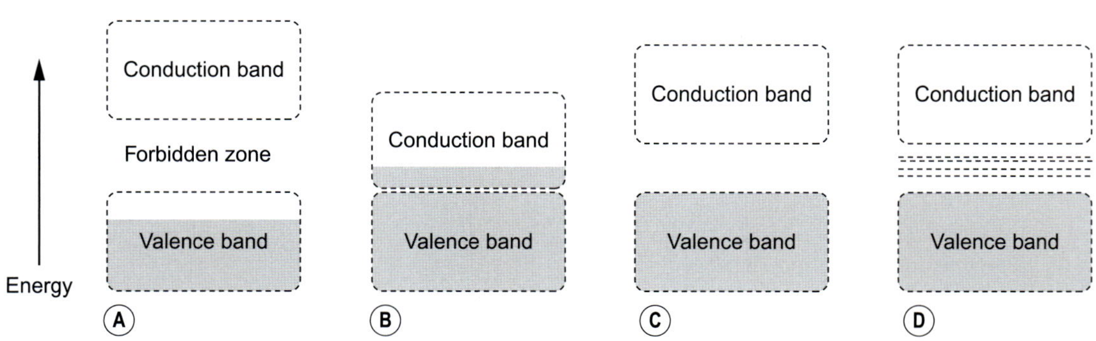

Fig. 1.3 Simplified energy level diagram for solid materials: the shaded regions show those levels that are normally occupied by electrons for (A) an insulator; (B) a conductor; (C) a semiconductor (undoped); and (D) material with impurity levels within the forbidden zone.

can accommodate so that the lower levels of the conduction band are also occupied. In these materials the conduction band overlaps with the valence band and the forbidden zone disappears, as shown in Fig. 1.3B. These materials will generally be good conductors of electricity. There are some materials in which just the valence band is filled, the conduction band is effectively empty and a small but significant forbidden zone exists. These materials are classed as *semiconductors* and are illustrated in Fig. 1.3C. Any charges injected into a semiconductor will be free to travel through the material. It is to be stressed that this description is overly simplistic but serves as a basis for understanding the principles of solid-state dosimeters discussed in Chapter 3.

Impurity Bands

The introduction of impurities at low concentrations can alter the structure of the energy bands and may create energy bands that are located between the valence and conduction bands and within the forbidden zone, as shown in Fig. 1.3D. The properties of the material so formed will depend upon (1) whether these extra bands are normally occupied or empty of electrons and (2) their actual energy levels. The addition of impurities is critical to the formation of active semiconductor devices (see Chapter 3) and to the development and functioning of both scintillator and thermoluminescent materials (see Chapter 3).

PARTICLES IN ELECTRIC AND MAGNETIC FIELDS

Electric Fields

As already explained, a single charge exerts either an attractive or a repulsive force on another charge. A collection of charges will also exert a force on another charged particle. This force can be written as:

$$F = qE \tag{1.5}$$

where F is the force on the charge q and the quantity E is known as the *electric field* (caused by other charges in the vicinity). The direction of the electric field is the direction in which a free positive charge would move; a free negative charge would move in the opposite direction, so the force on a particle in an electric field is always parallel or antiparallel to the field.

Magnetic Fields

The force on a charged particle in a magnetic field is more complicated. There is no force at all if the particle is not moving; if it is moving, the force is, like the force in an electric field, dependent on the charge, q, but it is perpendicular to the direction of both the magnetic field, B, and the velocity, v, of the particle and depends on the angle between them. Fig. 1.4 shows some examples.

The largest force occurs when the velocity of the particle is perpendicular to the magnetic field. As the angle θ between B and v decreases, the force decreases; when the velocity and field are parallel, $\theta = 0$ and there is no force. In fact, the magnitude of the force is given by:

$$F = qvB\sin\theta \tag{1.6}$$

So, when v and B are perpendicular, $\theta = 90^\circ$ and $F = q\,v\,B$.

The Lorentz Equation

The forces on a moving charged particle, which is subject to both an electric field and a magnetic field, are complicated and are best dealt with using the mathematics of vectors, which is beyond the scope of this book. However, for the simple case where the magnetic field is perpendicular to the velocity of the charged particle, we can write:

$$F = (qE + qvB) \tag{1.7}$$

The electric component of the force (qE) and the magnetic component (qvB) are not necessarily in the same direction. This equation is known as *the Lorentz equation*, after the Dutch physicist Hendrik A. Lorentz, and is an extremely important equation in many areas of physics. In radiotherapy, it is useful when considering the behaviour of electrons in a linear accelerator and of charged particles in a cyclotron or synchrotron.

WAVES

Transverse and Longitudinal Waves

Energy in the form of light, heat or sound may be transmitted from place to place by waves. The direction of propagation of a wave is the direction in which the energy is transported. However, the particles in the medium do not change their overall position; they simply vibrate about an average position. We can distinguish two types of wave: *longitudinal* and *transverse*.

In a transverse wave (Fig. 1.5A), the oscillations are perpendicular to the direction of propagation of the wave. Water waves, or waves on a string, are good examples of transverse waves.

In the case of longitudinal waves (Fig. 1.5B), the particles in the medium move backwards and forwards in a direction parallel to the direction of propagation, although their mean position stays the same. A good example is a sound wave; the particles of the medium (e.g. air) oscillate parallel to the direction of the sound wave, and this gives rise to changes in pressure along the wave.

Fig. 1.5 shows the *wavelength*, λ, of the wave—the distance between two adjacent peaks (or two adjacent troughs). Another important parameter is the *frequency*, f, which is the number of peaks that pass a point per second. In all cases, the speed of the wave, c, is related to the wavelength and frequency by the equation:

$$c = f\lambda \tag{1.8}$$

This means that for a wave with constant speed, a larger wavelength corresponds to a lower frequency, and vice versa. Wavelength is measured in units of metres (m) and frequency in hertz (Hz).

Longitudinal sound waves are important in ultrasound imaging (see Chapter 6), but for radiotherapy applications, we are mostly concerned

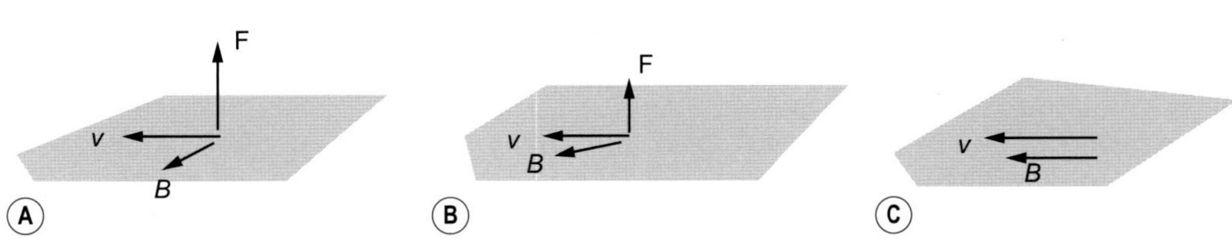

Fig. 1.4 The force on a moving charge (positive in this case) in a magnetic field depends on the relative directions of the velocity *(v)* and the magnetic field *(B)*. In (A), both *v* and *B* are perpendicular to each other. The force *(F)* is large and perpendicular to both *v* and *B*. In (B), the angle between *v* and *B* is less than 90 degrees and the force is less but still perpendicular to both. In (C), both *v* and *B* are parallel: there is no force.

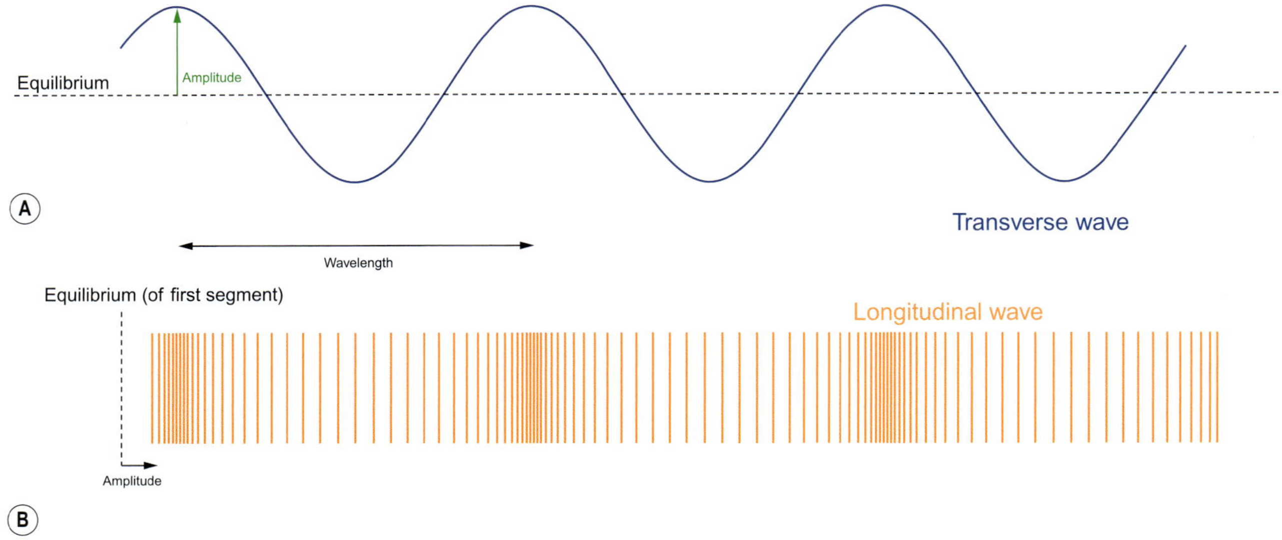

Fig. 1.5 (A) Transverse and (B) longitudinal waves. Note that the wavelength is the distance between two maxima.

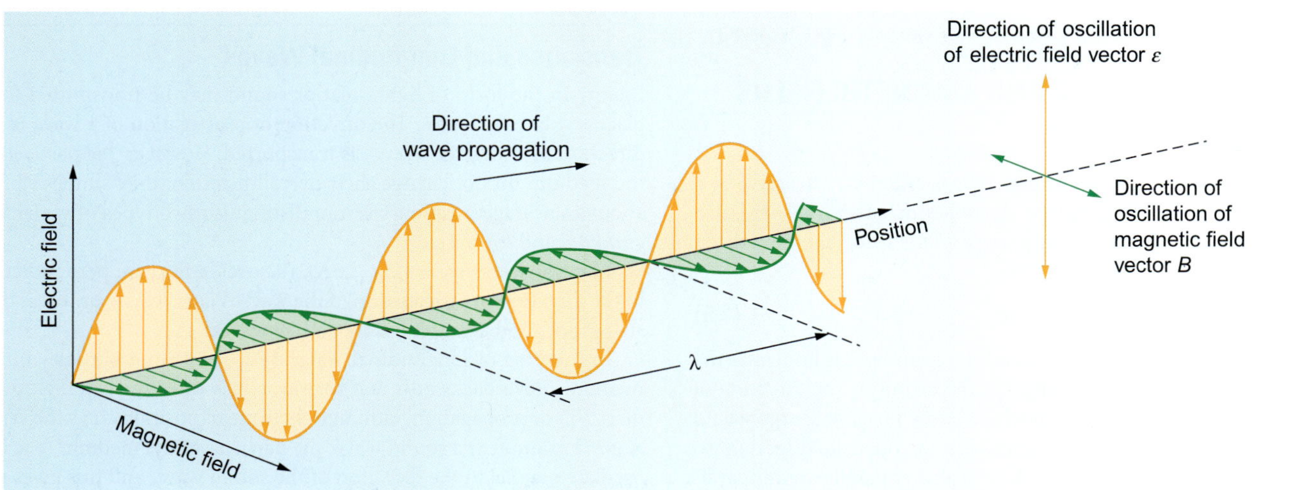

Fig. 1.6 The oscillations of electric and magnetic fields in an electromagnetic wave.

with the transverse waves of *electromagnetic radiation*, which is the subject of the next section.

Electromagnetic Radiation

Electromagnetic radiation is so called because it can be described as waves in which the quantities that oscillate are electric and magnetic fields. Fig. 1.6 shows how the fields in these electromagnetic waves oscillate at right angles to one another.

Because electromagnetic waves depend only on electric and magnetic fields, they can travel through any medium, including a vacuum. In a vacuum, all electromagnetic waves travel at a speed of approximately 3×10^8 m s^{-1} (often known rather loosely as *the speed of light in a vacuum*), but the properties of the radiation vary greatly with wavelength and frequency. Fig. 1.7 shows the vast range of the electromagnetic spectrum; note that as the frequency increases, the wavelength decreases according to Eq. (1.8). Radiotherapy physics is mostly concerned with the high-frequency/small-wavelength end of the spectrum, although radio waves are important in radiotherapy, as they are used to accelerate the electron beam in a linear accelerator.

By the end of the 19th century, physicists were aware that all the different types of radiation shown in Fig. 1.7 were electromagnetic waves and could be explained in terms of wave physics. However, the beginning of the 20th century saw the development of quantum physics. Several key experiments, including the investigation of Compton scattering, an important process in radiotherapy (see Chapter 2), showed that when electromagnetic radiation interacts with matter, wave physics does not always predict the correct result. Instead, the radiation behaves as particles known as *photons*. A photon is a small 'packet' or quantum of energy, and each one has an energy given by:

$$E = hf \tag{1.9}$$

where E is the energy, f is the frequency of the electromagnetic wave and h is a constant, known as *Planck's constant* and equal to 6.626×10^{-34} J s.

As with the masses in the 'Atomic Structure' section, it is more usual to give these energy values in electron volts (eV), where 1 eV = 1.602×10^{-19} J. This has the advantage of allowing an easy comparison between the energy of a photon and the mass energy of a particle, and it is especially useful when considering the transfer of energy between a photon and a particle or the conversion of particles into radiation (annihilation radiation) or radiation into particles (pair production) (see Chapter 2). Fig. 1.7 shows the energies in eV in addition to the wavelengths and frequencies.

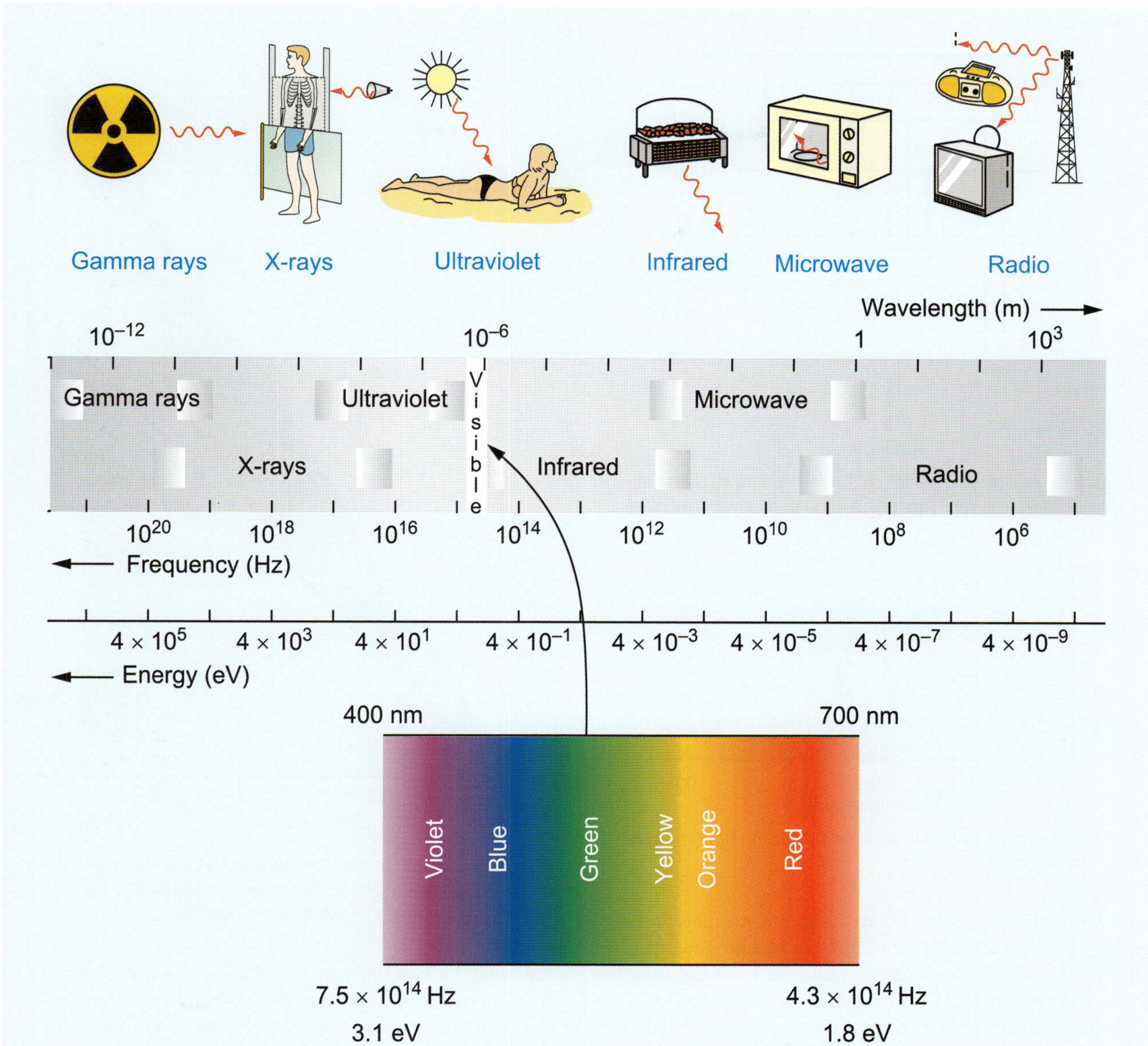

Fig. 1.7 The different types of radiation that form the electromagnetic spectrum. The visible spectrum covers a very small range of wavelength values and is expanded below the spectrum.

Continuous Spectra and Characteristic Radiation

In the 'Electron Energy Levels' section, we described the way in which the electrons in atoms can only be in specific energy states, defined by their quantum numbers. The energies of these states are different for each element; for example, Fig. 1.8 shows the main energy levels for tungsten, which is an element commonly used for the target in x-ray production, such as x-ray tubes and linear accelerators (see Chapters 2, 9 and 10).

As previously described, to raise an electron from one energy level to another, the energy required is equal to the difference in energy of the two states. If an atom is excited above its ground state by absorbing energy from incoming particles (e.g. photons or electrons), some electrons can be moved up into allowable but normally empty energy levels. This happens, for example, in an x-ray tube (see Chapters 6 and 9). This leaves the atom in an excited state—that is, with a higher total energy than in the ground state. After a period of time, the atom will return to the ground state as the excited electrons drop from the higher levels back to vacant lower-energy states. When this happens, the excess electron energy is carried away as a photon of electromagnetic radiation. Thus, if we have two states with energies E_1 and E_2, the energy of the photon (E_X) is the difference between E_1 and E_2. Using Eq. (1.9) to relate the energy of the photon to its frequency, we arrive at:

$$E_1 - E_2 = E_X = hf \qquad \textbf{(1.10)}$$

The energy of photons produced is therefore dictated by the differences in energy between electron shells of the particular atom from which they are emitted. The spectrum of photons produced by an element is termed the *characteristic radiation* and will be different for each element. Fig. 1.8 shows the possible electron transitions leading to the production of characteristic photons for tungsten. Distinctions are made between electron transitions originating from different shells to the same destination shell by denoting the transition (and characteristic photon) with the final shell letter (K, L etc.) and adding a Greek letter suffix to indicate the originating shell, as shown in Fig. 1.8.

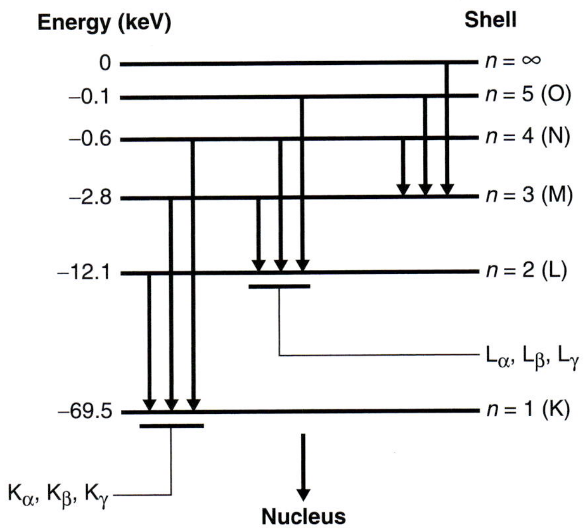

Fig. 1.8 Electron energy levels and transitions leading to characteristic photons for tungsten. The main transitions into each shell are marked.

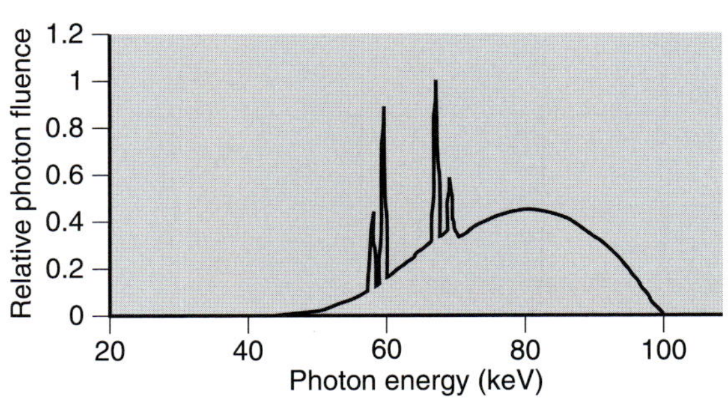

Fig. 1.9 Characteristic spectral lines from tungsten superimposed on the continuous spectrum.

If the electrons in tungsten are excited, as in an x-ray tube, the emitted photons will be a mixture of the continuous background spectrum (see Chapter 2) and the characteristic radiation from the tungsten atoms. This is shown in Fig. 1.9. The energy differences between the levels in heavy elements tend to be much larger than for lighter elements: note that for tungsten (see Fig. 1.8), the photon energies of the two main spectral lines are in the x-ray region at around 60 keV, which is in the x-ray range. They correspond to the transition from L to K and the transition from free electron to K. Contrast this with the energy of the largest possible transition in hydrogen, which is 13.6 eV, and in the ultraviolet region (see Fig. 1.7).

RADIOACTIVE DECAY

Stable and Unstable Isotopes

In the section titled 'The Atom and the Nucleus', we explained that although the atomic number, Z, of a particular element is always the same, the atomic mass number, A, can vary so that each element can have several different isotopes. Some of them will be stable, meaning they will not decay; others will be unstable and will undergo radioactive decay. It is instructive to plot a graph which shows the number of neutrons (A–Z) against the number of protons (Z) for stable and unstable nuclei (Fig. 1.10). This figure shows the stable nuclei in black, which is known as the *stability line*. It also shows the solid line corresponding to equal numbers of protons and neutrons. We see that for low-atomic-number nuclei, an equal number of protons and neutrons is favoured, whereas a greater proportion of neutrons is needed to provide stability for large nuclei.

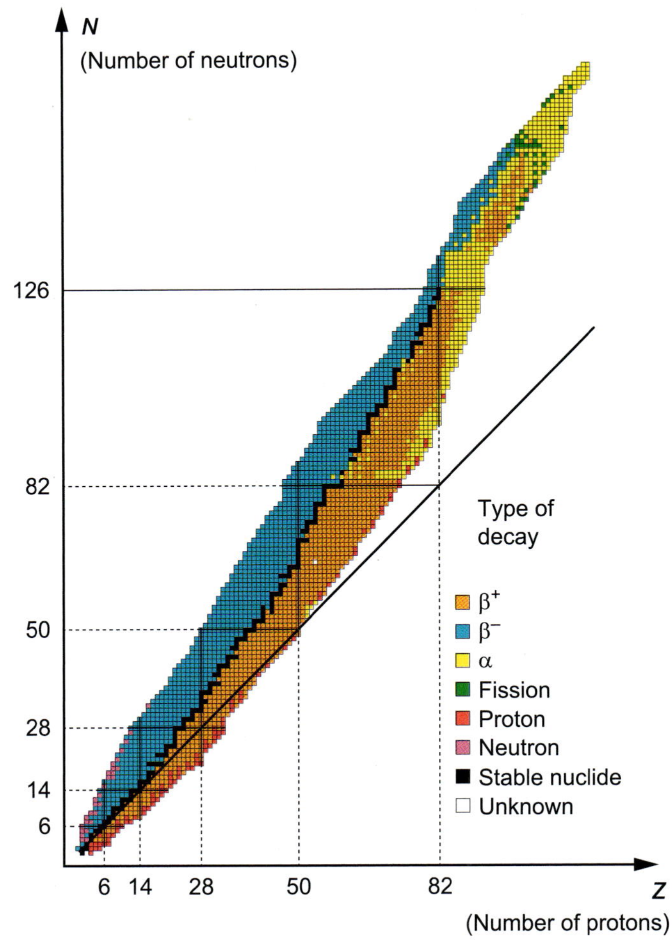

Fig. 1.10 A graph of neutron number *(A–Z)* plotted against proton number *(Z)*. The stable isotopes are shown in *black*, and the *solid line* represents equal numbers of protons and neutrons.

This may be explained by considering the increasing electrostatic force of repulsion between protons in the nucleus as the number of protons is increased. The Colourful Nuclide Chart is a more detailed, interactive diagram which allows you to look up individual nuclei.[2]

Evidence suggests that protons and neutrons within a nucleus adopt a shell-like structure analogous to electron orbits and show particular stability when the number of protons or neutrons, or both, corresponds to a *magic number* (2, 8, 20, 28, 50, 82, 126). The strength of the strong force that holds the nucleons together is associated with a *nuclear binding energy* that must be overcome to break the nucleus apart. Essentially, the mass of a given nucleus is less than the sum of its constituent protons and neutrons; this is known as the *mass defect*. Representing this in terms of energy, using $E = mc^2$, gives the nuclear binding energy. Nuclei with an even number of protons or an even number of neutrons are more stable than those with an odd number of one or both.

A nucleus lying off the stability line shown in Fig. 1.10 is unstable and decays by rearranging its nucleon numbers. This is achieved by releasing particles, by changing a proton to a neutron (or vice versa), or by absorbing nearby particles. The activity of an unstable, or radioactive, isotope is the rate at which its nuclei decay, expressed in *becquerels* (Bq). One becquerel corresponds to one decay or disintegration per second. The becquerel is a very small unit, so the activity of sources used in medicine is generally represented in MBq (1×10^6 disintegrations per second) or GBq (1×10^9 disintegrations per second). (You may also occasionally come across the old unit of activity, the curie (Ci); 1 Ci = 37 000 MBq.) Nuclei that undergo radioactive decay are known as *radionuclides*.

In the construction of practical radioactive sources, we are also interested in the amount of material that is needed to manufacture a source with a required activity, determined by the *specific activity*, or the activity per unit mass (MBq kg^{-1}).

Half-life

Radionuclides decay at very different rates, so it is important to have some way of quantifying the rate of decay. If we have a collection of identical nuclei, it is impossible to know exactly which one will decay next; one can only predict the probability of decay. The number of nuclei, *dN*, which decay in a short time, *dt*, will depend on two factors: the decay constant, λ, which is essentially the probability of decay; and *N*, the number of nuclei present at the start. This is expressed by the equation:

$$dN = -\lambda N dt \quad \textbf{(1.11)}$$

This equation can be rearranged and integrated to give:

$$N(t) = N_o e^{-\lambda t} \quad \textbf{(1.12)}$$

where N_o is the number of nuclei present at $t = 0$, $N(t)$ is the number of nuclei present at time *t* and *e* is the exponential function. A graph of $N(t)$ plotted against time gives an exponential decay curve similar to that shown in Fig. 1.11.

The interesting thing about an exponential decay is that the length of time it takes for the number of undecayed nuclei to halve is always the same. In Fig. 1.11, this time is shown as 2 (arbitrary) time units. This time is known as the *half-life*, $T_{½}$, and it is related to the decay constant, λ, by the equation:

$$T_{1/2} = \frac{\ln 2}{\lambda} = \frac{0.693}{\lambda} \quad \textbf{(1.13)}$$

where the term ln represents the logarithm to base *e*; if $y = e^x$, then $x = \ln y$.

Half-lives can vary enormously—for example, the half-life of uranium-238 (not used for medical purposes!) is approximately the same as the age of Earth, 4.5 billion years; the half-life of krypton-81, used in nuclear medicine, is 13 s, and others are even shorter. The length of the half-life is an important consideration when choosing a radionuclide for medical use; if the half-life is too long, the patient may be radioactive for the rest of their life; if it is too short, the activity will decay too quickly for it to be useful.

When radioactivity was first discovered at the end of the 19th century, three different types of emitted particle were identified and were labelled alpha (α), beta (β) and gamma (γ) radiation. These names have remained, although there are now a few variants of them; the next three sections will cover these different types of decay.

Alpha Decay

Alpha (α) decay occurs most often from the unstable nuclei of heavy elements, such as uranium, radium or plutonium. The nucleus emits an alpha particle, which is actually a nucleus of helium, $^{4}_{2}He$. Having an equal number of protons and neutrons (both of which are magic numbers), the helium nucleus is very stable. The *parent* nucleus (X) decreases its atomic number by 2 and its mass number by 4, so the general equation is:

$$^{A}_{Z}X \rightarrow \, ^{A-4}_{Z-2}Y + \, ^{4}_{2}He \quad \textbf{(1.14)}$$

where Y is the *daughter* nucleus. For example, radium ($^{226}_{88}Ra$) decays to radon ($^{222}_{86}Rn$) and an alpha particle. Energy must be conserved in the transformation, so any difference, *Q*, between the nuclear binding energies of the parent and daughter nuclei is shared between the emitted alpha particle, (in the form of kinetic energy), and any photons that are produced (see the 'Gamma Decay' section). Alpha particles are typically emitted with kinetic energies on the order of several MeV.

Being relatively heavy (approximately 4 × the mass of a proton) and highly charged (containing two protons), α particles are readily stopped in matter. For example, the 4.79-MeV α particle emitted from radium has a range of less than 4 cm in air and less than 0.04 mm in tissue. This means that α particles can be very useful for radiotherapy, but only if they can be released very close to the tumour tissue. Radium-226 was used in some very early external radiotherapy treatments but has the

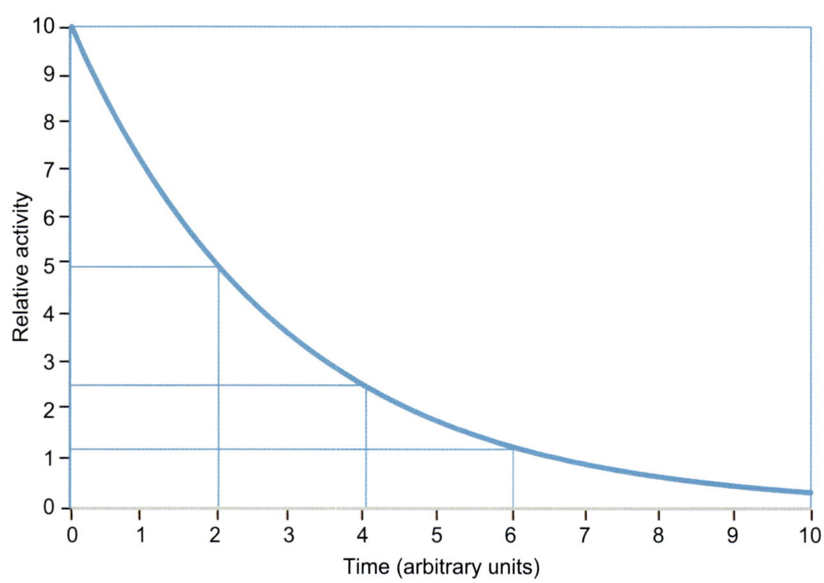

Fig. 1.11 Exponential decay of radioactivity with time. Note that the half-life is the time taken to drop to one-half of the original value and is the same as the time taken to halve again to one-fourth and again to one-eighth.

big disadvantage that the daughter product, radon, is a radioactive gas. More recently, radium-223 is used as an unsealed source of treatment for bone metastases.

Beta Decay

There are now known to be two types of beta decay. Beta minus (β^-) decay occurs frequently in naturally occurring radionuclides and involves the emission of an electron; beta plus (β^+) decay occurs mainly in artificially produced radionuclides, and the particle emitted is a positron.

A nucleus lying above the stability line in Fig. 1.10 is neutron rich and, by emitting an electron, can convert a neutron to a proton, thereby approaching the stability line. An example is iodine-131, which undergoes β^- decay to become xenon-131:

$$^{131}_{53}\mathrm{I} \rightarrow {}^{131}_{54}\mathrm{Xe} \qquad (1.15)$$

Note that, because the total number of nucleons has not changed, the mass number stays the same, but because a neutron has been converted into a proton, the atomic number increases by 1. The emitted β^- particle is a high-energy electron from the nucleus and should not be confused with the orbiting electrons in the atom.

By contrast, a nucleus lying below the stability line of Fig. 1.10 is proton rich and therefore decays by converting a proton into a neutron. As with β^- decay, the mass number does not change, but in this case, because a proton is converted into a neutron, the atomic number decreases by 1. The emitted β^+ particle is a positron, the antimatter equivalent of the electron. A good example, which is widely used in PET imaging, is fluorine-18:

$$^{18}_{9}\mathrm{F} \rightarrow {}^{18}_{8}\mathrm{O} \qquad (1.16)$$

Observation that the β particles produced display a spectrum of kinetic energies, rather than the discrete energy difference between parent and daughter nuclei, indicates that a further particle must be involved. For β^+ decay, this particle is the neutrino, ν_e; for β^- decay, it is its antiparticle, $\bar{\nu}_e$. The processes for iodine-131 and fluorine-18 are therefore:

$$^{131}_{53}\mathrm{I} \rightarrow {}^{131}_{54}\mathrm{Xe} + {}^{0}_{-1}\beta + \bar{\nu}_e \quad \text{and}$$

$$^{18}_{9}\mathrm{F} \rightarrow {}^{18}_{8}\mathrm{O} + {}^{0}_{+1}\beta + \nu_e \qquad (1.17)$$

The energy arising from the difference in masses of the initial and final particles is carried away as kinetic energy of the beta particle and the neutrino. The total energy of the two particles is always the same, but the individual energies of the beta particle and neutrino may vary. The energies quoted for beta particles in Table 1.2 are therefore averages.

The range of a β^- particle is larger than that of an α particle, as it is much lighter. However, whereas the heavy alpha particles will travel along a straight path, the beta particles will follow a much more erratic path as they interact with atomic electrons. The range of a beta particle in tissue is only on the order of a few millimetres and will depend on the energy with which it was emitted.

An emitted positron (β^+) travels through matter, rapidly losing kinetic energy through interactions with atomic electrons. When it collides with an electron, which is its antiparticle, both particles are annihilated and their energy is converted into electromagnetic radiation. Using Einstein's mass-energy equivalence equation, $E = mc^2$, the total energy of the radiation must be 2 × 0.511 MeV (see Table 1.1). Conservation of momentum demands that two photons, each with energy 0.511 MeV, are produced in opposite directions. This is the basis of PET (see Chapter 7).

Depending on its energy, a positron will be stopped within a very short distance of the site of emission in tissue. The annihilation photons, on the other hand, at 0.511 MeV each, can pass relatively easily through tissue. Detection of these coincident photons following administration of a positron-emitting radionuclide, such as fluorine-18, to a patient therefore reveals where the annihilation event occurred and hence where the radionuclide was taken up within the body.

Gamma Decay

In the 'Electron Energy Levels' section, we showed that the electrons in atoms could only occupy certain allowed energy levels. In an analogous way, each nucleus can only have certain discrete energies, and transitions between two levels involve the emission or absorption of photons of electromagnetic radiation. As with electron transitions, the energy values of the levels are different for different elements; however, in the nuclear case, the differences are much larger, so the photons produced are generally of much higher energy. Following an α or β decay, the daughter nucleus is often left in an excited state. It will then reach its ground state by emitting a photon with an energy corresponding to the difference between the two energy levels. These photons are known as *gamma (γ) rays.* Fig. 1.12 shows the decay scheme for cobalt-60, which is an isotope formerly widely used for external beam therapy and now used in the Gamma Knife; see Chapter 9.

In most cases the emission of gamma rays occurs immediately after the alpha or beta decay, but occasionally the nucleus remains in an excited state and decays with a measurable half-life. Such an excited state is known as a *metastable* energy state and is denoted by the addition of an 'm' to the mass number. There is no change in Z or A during the transition from the excited state of the metastable nucleus to the ground state, so this is known as an *isomeric transition.* One important example, widely used in nuclear medicine, is technetium-99m (Fig. 1.13). This is a useful radionuclide because it produces only gamma rays, with an energy of 140 keV, which can be used for imaging, and no short-range α or β particles, which would only damage tissue.

Note that both gamma rays and x-rays are electromagnetic radiation at the top end of the spectrum (see Fig. 1.7); the energy ranges overlap, and indeed both are used in radiotherapy. They are only distinguished by their origin: gamma rays coming from the nucleus and x-rays from the atomic electrons (see Chapter 2).

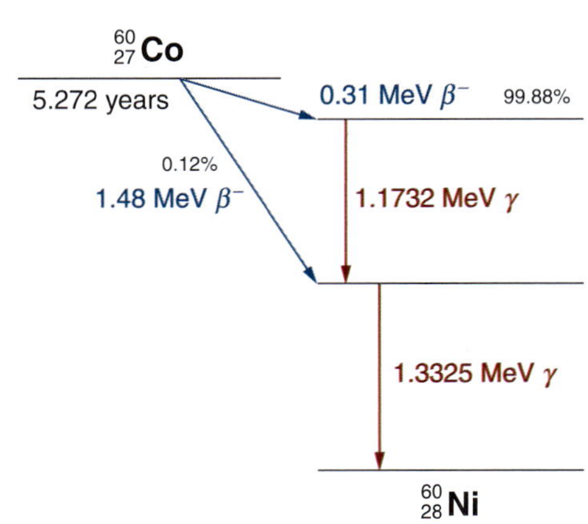

Fig. 1.12 Cobalt-60 decays via beta decay to give nickel-60. The nickel nucleus is in an excited state and decays via the scheme shown, giving gamma rays with energies 1.1732 and 1.3325 MeV.

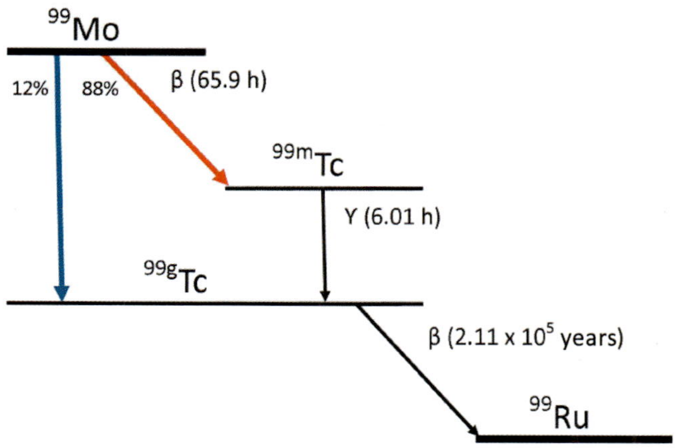

Fig. 1.13 Technetium-99m is produced from molybdenum-99 by beta decay and then decays to the ground state (Tc-99g) via an isomeric transition with a half-life of 6 hours. The ground state technetium eventually decays to stable ruthenium-99, but with an extremely long half-life and therefore very low activity.

Electron Capture and Internal Conversion

As an alternative to positron emission (β^+ decay), the nucleus of a proton-rich atom may capture one of its own inner shell electrons via *electron capture (EC)*. The captured electron combines with a proton in the nucleus to produce a neutron and a neutrino, the latter being emitted from the nucleus carrying kinetic energy equal to the difference in nuclear binding energy between the parent and daughter nuclei. As with β^+ decay, the mass number does not change, but the atomic number decreases by 1. Nuclei that decay by this method can be useful because there is no particulate emission. An example of a nuclide that decays by EC is iodine-125; it emits gamma rays of up to 35 keV, which can be used for brachytherapy (see Chapter 9).

Another possible mode of decay is *internal conversion (IC)*. An excited nucleus may de-excite by emitting a single photon, which interacts with the inner shell electron so that the electron is ejected from the atom. In contrast to beta decay, the emitted electron will have a single kinetic energy equal to the excitation energy of the nucleus minus the electron binding energy. The vacancy in the atomic shells left by the emitted electron will be filled by outer electrons, giving rise to characteristic radiation (see the 'Continuous Spectra and Characteristic Radiation' section).

Radioactive Decay Series

There are many cases of radioactive nuclei that decay to give daughter nuclei which are themselves radioactive and so on. This gives rise to a decay series. Fig. 1.14 shows the decay series of uranium-238, a naturally occurring radionuclide. At each stage, the α or β decay leads to a new nucleus which itself decays, the final product in this case being a stable isotope of lead. At each decay, the rate of growth of the activity of the daughter nuclide depends on the relative values of the decay constants (λ) of the parent and the daughter. Another example, of much more clinical importance, is the decay of molybdenum-99 (see Fig. 1.13) to technetium-99m, which is widely used for imaging.

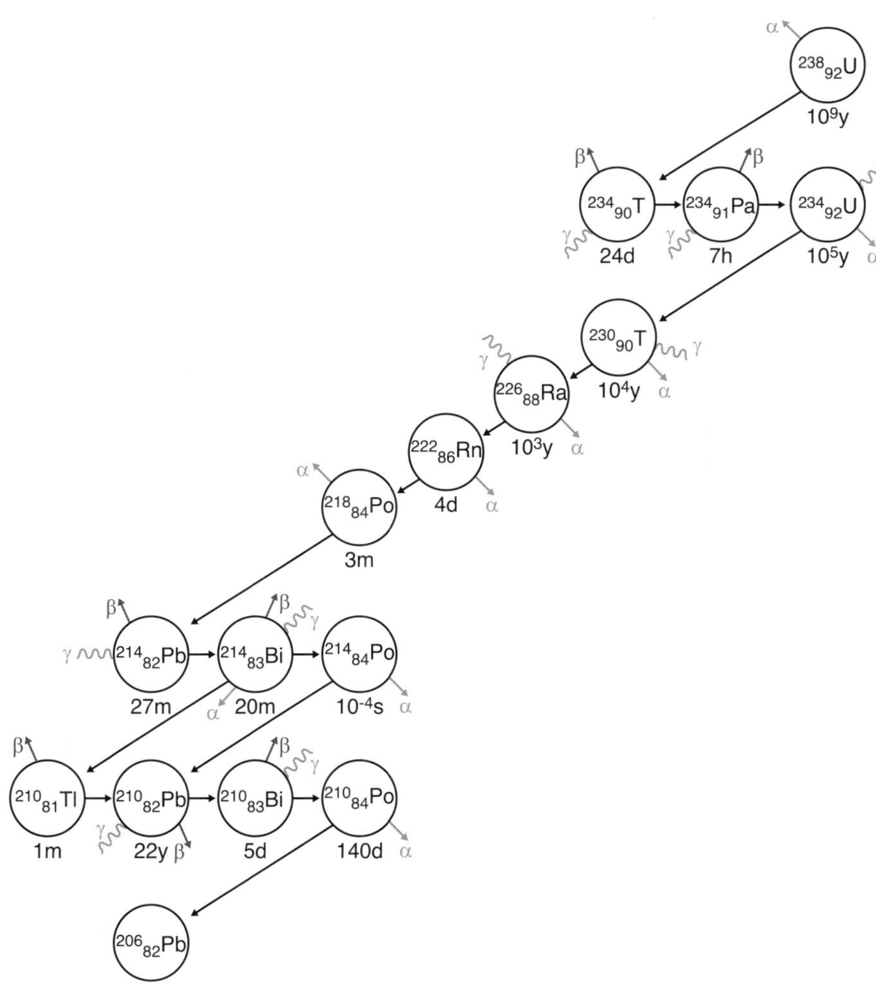

Fig. 1.14 Decay series for $^{238}_{92}U$. Half-lives are indicated in seconds (*s*), minutes (*m*), hours (*h*) and years (*y*).

If we assume that there is no daughter present at time $t = 0$ and that all the disintegrations of the parent lead to the required daughter product, the activity of the daughter at time t, $A_2(t)$, is given by:

$$A_2(t) = \frac{\lambda_2}{\lambda_2 - \lambda_1} A_1(0)\left(e^{-\lambda_1 t} - e^{-\lambda_2 t}\right) \quad \textbf{(1.18)}$$

where $A_1(0)$ is the initial activity of the parent at time $t = 0$ and λ_1 and λ_2 are the decay constants of parent and daughter, respectively. Eq. (1.18) is of relevance to radionuclide generators, as it allows calculation of the optimum time between elutions of the daughter radionuclide.

If the decay of the parent is much slower than that of the daughter, that is, if $\lambda_2 >> \lambda_1$, Eq. (1.18) reduces to:

$$A_2(t) = A_1(0)\left(e^{-\lambda_1 t} - e^{-\lambda_2 t}\right) \quad \textbf{(1.19)}$$

This is the situation for ionisation chamber consistency check devices containing a strontium-90 source. Strontium-90 undergoes beta decay with a half-life of 28.7 years to yttrium-90, which itself decays via beta decay with a half-life of 64 hours. The activity of the long-lived strontium parent determines and maintains the activity of the short-lived yttrium daughter.

RADIONUCLIDES OF MEDICAL INTEREST

The isotopes listed in Table 1.2 are just some of those used in radiotherapy and nuclear medicine. There are many others that readers may encounter, but the basic principles remain the same. The choice of isotope for a particular application is based on decay product type (γ, β^+, β^- or α), the energy of the products, the half-life, the specific activity (activity per unit mass) and availability. The α particles, which are heavy helium nuclei, have a very short range in tissue, so they will deposit energy close to the site at which a radionuclide is taken up in the body; β^- particles (electrons) have a slightly longer but still small range. If the site of disease can be preferentially targeted by these emissions, this leads to significant sparing of surrounding normal tissues in therapeutic applications. If greater penetration is required, of the order of centimetres for brachytherapy, photons (γ) would be the choice. Or if imaging of radioactivity uptake through external detection is required, photons (γ) or β^+ emissions will be the product of choice.

TABLE 1.2 Characteristics of Some Radionuclides Used in Radiotherapy as Either Unsealed Sources or Sealed Sources

Isotope	Decay Mechanism (energy[a])	Half-Life	Clinical Application
Unsealed Sources			
^{11}C	β^+ (385 keV)	20 m	PET imaging
^{13}N	β^+ (492 keV)	10 m	PET imaging
^{15}O	β^+ (735 keV)	122 s	PET imaging
^{18}F	β^+ (250 keV)	109 m	PET imaging
^{32}P	β^- (695 keV)	14.3 d	Polycythaemia vera
^{64}Cu	β^+ (278 keV)	12.7 h	PET imaging
^{68}Ga	β^+ (836 keV)	68 m	PET imaging
^{89}Sr	β^- (587 keV)	50.5 d	Bone metastases (palliation)
^{90}Y	β^- (933 keV)	2.7 d	SIRT[b] liver therapy
^{99m}Tc	γ (143 keV)	6.0 h	Gamma camera imaging
^{131}I	β^- (191 keV) γ (364 keV)	8.1 d	Thyrotoxicosis and thyroid cancer
^{177}Lu	β^- (148 keV) γ (208, 113 keV)	6.7 d	NETs[c] and prostate (PSMA)[d]
^{223}Ra	α (5.7 MeV)	11.4 d	Bone metastases
^{225}Ac	α (5.83 MeV)	9.9 d	NETs and prostate (PSMA)
Sealed Sources			
^{60}Co	β^- (96 keV), γ (1.17, 1.33 MeV)	5.26 y	External beam units and gamma knife
^{103}Pd	EC, γ (20 keV)	17 d	Brachytherapy (seeds)
^{125}I	EC, γ (27–36 keV)	60 d	Brachytherapy (seeds)
^{137}Cs	β^- (174 keV), γ (662 keV)	30 y	Brachytherapy (pellets)
^{192}Ir	β^- (179 keV), γ (300–400 keV)	74 d	Brachytherapy

[a]Energies given for beta particles are average; energies for gamma are those of the dominant emission/s.
[b]SIRT = Selective internal radiation therapy.
[c]NET = Neuro-endocrine tumours.
[d]PSMA = Prostate-specific membrane antigen.

REFERENCES

1. Interactive Periodic Table, Royal Society of Chemistry, http://www.rsc.org/periodic-table/.
2. Colourful nuclide chart, http://people.physics.anu.edu.au/~ecs103/chart/. (Note that this plots Z against N—the opposite of Fig. 1.10. Both versions are commonly used.)

FURTHER READING

Dendy PP, Heaton B. *Physics for diagnostic radiology*. 3rd ed. CRC Press; 2012.

Grant IS, Phillips WR. *The elements of physics*. Oxford University Press; 2001.

2

Interactions of Ionising Radiation With Matter

Giuseppe Schettino

CHAPTER OUTLINE

INTRODUCTION

In this chapter, we are mostly concerned with the interactions of electrons and photons with matter, as these are most commonly used in radiotherapy.

The Effect of Electrical Charge

Electrons carry a charge of -1.6×10^{-19} C and readily interact via the Coulomb force with other charged particles in the matter they traverse, predominantly with atomic electrons and, to a lesser extent, with protons in atomic nuclei. Photons, by contrast, carry no charge and interact relatively rarely with matter. The use of clinical proton beams for radiotherapy is increasing as new facilities are constructed worldwide. As charged particles ($+1.6 \times 10^{-19}$ C), proton beams passing through matter behave in a similar way to electrons: that is, they readily undergo interactions with atomic electrons. The difference between proton and electron interactions lies in the proton having a mass of 1.67×10^{-27} kg, which is roughly 2000 times greater than the electron mass of 9.11×10^{-31} kg. The characteristics of proton energy loss in matter make protons highly attractive for radiotherapy, and protons offer distinct advantages over photons and electrons, as will be discussed later. Neutron beams are less often selected as the beam of choice for radiotherapy at the present time; however, they also offer advantages over photon beams for some tumours because of their biological effect on tissue. Being uncharged, neutrons interact in a similar manner to photons and produce very similar depth-dose characteristics.

It should be remembered that radiotherapy is not restricted to these particles alone. Ion beams consisting of atomic nuclei stripped of their electrons may also be used. A proton can be thought of as a hydrogen atom without its orbital electron. Carbon ions, in particular, have been used to treat a number of cancers in what is presently a small number of facilities worldwide, and their characteristics are being actively researched. Negative pions (π^-) were also, at one time, thought to have great potential for radiotherapy because of the nature of their interactions and their energy loss at the end of their range. Clinical studies on the use of pions have not demonstrated this advantage to date.

Excitation and Ionisation

Ionising radiation, by definition, has sufficient energy to ionise matter. That is, it has sufficient energy to overcome the binding energy of atomic electrons. Radiation of energy below the binding energy of a particular electron shell may still interact with an electron by raising it to a higher, vacant shell (see Chapter 1). As a result of this interaction, the atom has gained energy and is left in an excited state (Fig. 2.1A). It will eventually lose this excess energy to return to its lowest energy state, or ground state. An electron occupying an outer shell relative to the vacancy may achieve a lower-energy state by filling the vacancy (see Fig. 2.1C). The excess energy is released as a characteristic photon (i.e. with an energy equal to the difference in shell binding energies). If this electron is also in an inner shell, it too will leave behind a vacancy which an outer electron can again occupy (see Fig. 2.1C), again losing energy in the form of a characteristic photon. This process results in a cascade of electrons moving between shells and a corresponding set of characteristic photons, which eventually return the atom to its ground state.

Even if its own kinetic energy exceeds the atomic electron's binding energy, an incoming electron or photon may transfer part of its kinetic energy to an atomic electron to produce excitation. Where the

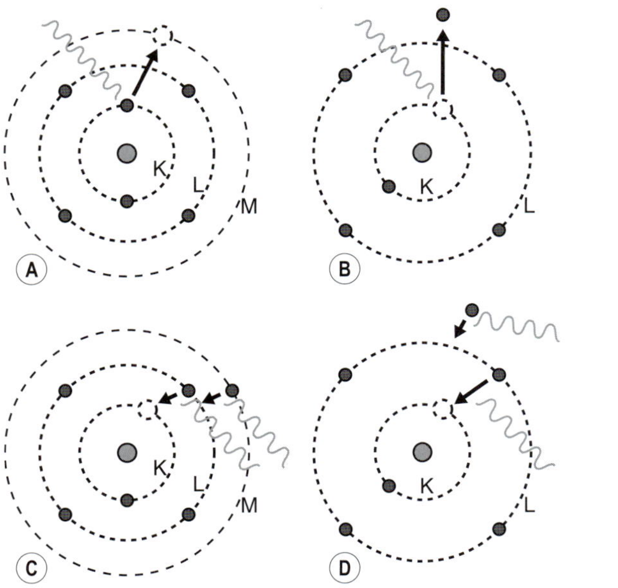

Fig. 2.1 (A) Excitation for a carbon atom. An incoming photon raises an inner shell electron to a vacant orbit; the electron has gained energy. As a result, the atom is left in an excited state. (B) Ionisation for a carbon atom. An incoming photon ejects a K shell electron from the atom; the atom is ionised, having an overall positive charge. As no scattered photon was produced, the emitted electron has acquired kinetic energy equal to the energy of the incoming photon minus the electron's binding energy. (C) De-excitation: an L-shell electron drops into the vacancy in the K shell, emitting a characteristic photon; the L-shell vacancy is filled by the electron involved in the original interaction. (D) De-excitation: an L-shell electron fills the K shell vacancy, and a free electron from the medium is captured to the L-shell.

incoming electron or photon transfers more than the binding energy of an atomic electron to the atom, the excited electron is ejected from the atom, with kinetic energy equal to the total energy transferred minus the binding energy. As a result of losing an electron, the atom has been ionised (see Fig. 2.1B). The positive ion will seek an electron from its surroundings to return to its uncharged state and so be chemically reactive. In addition, the ejected electron will leave a vacancy behind, which represents an excited state. The cascade process will then follow as described earlier, as de-excitation takes place (see Fig. 2.1D).

ELECTRON INTERACTIONS

Collisional and Radiative Energy Loss

The preceding section was concerned with the dominant interaction that a beam of electrons undergoes when travelling through matter: that of collisions with atomic electrons in the energy range of interest to radiotherapy. These interactions lead to excitation and ionisation of the medium traversed, as represented schematically in Fig. 2.2. More rarely, electrons from an incident clinical beam will pass near to and interact with the atomic nucleus, again as a result of the Coulomb force of attraction between a negatively charged electron and positively charged nucleus. The path and momentum of the incident electron are changed under the influence of the nucleus, resulting in a loss of electron energy. This loss of energy is the radiative energy loss resulting in a radiated photon, or x-ray. The term *bremsstrahlung* (braking radiation) is a helpful descriptive name given to this process, which is shown schematically in Fig. 2.3. The probability of this interaction occurring is inversely proportional to the square of the incident particle's mass. As a result, bremsstrahlung is only significant for electrons. This important

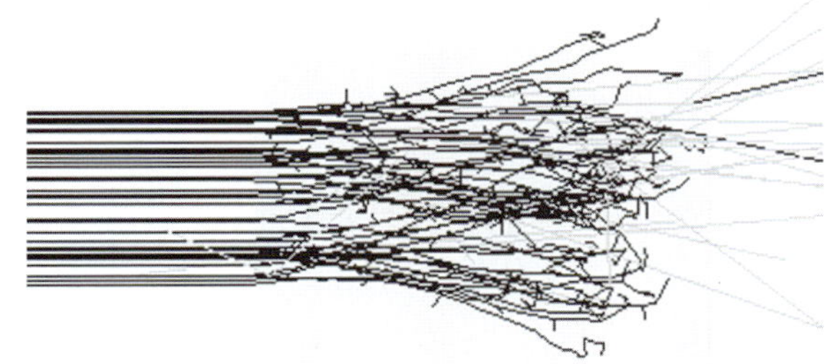

Fig. 2.2 Illustration of the frequent interactions, scattering and finite range of electrons traversing matter. A beam of 10-MeV electrons *(black)* strikes a slab of water from the left. Incident electrons readily scatter, losing energy through collisions with electrons in the medium. Occasionally, energy is lost through x-ray production (bremsstrahlung, indicated by *light grey lines*). Note that no primary electrons escape the slab, as it exceeds the finite range of these electrons (x-ray photons and secondary electrons generated by these photons may leave the slab, however), and that the total distance travelled by an incident electron (path length) is greater than the maximum depth reached (range).

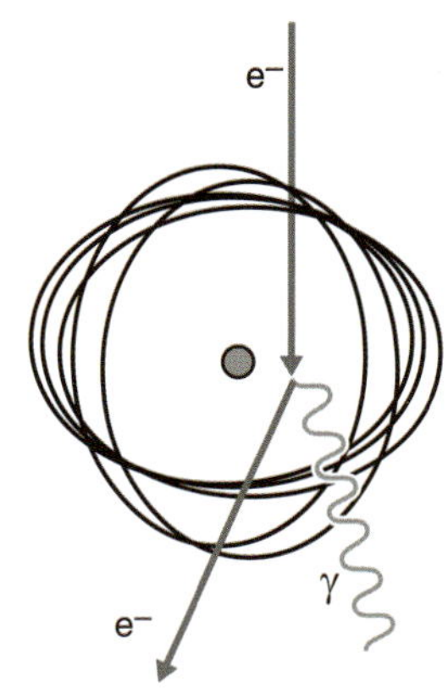

Fig. 2.3 Schematic representation of photon production by electrons (bremsstrahlung). An incident electron deflected by the nuclear Coulomb field loses energy, which appears in the form of an emitted photon.

process by which x-ray photons can be produced is described in the following section.

X-ray Production

The conversion of electron kinetic energy into photons as a beam of electrons striking a target is decelerated in the nuclear Coulomb field (bremsstrahlung) is the primary method for obtaining clinical photon beams. As suggested earlier, however, for the normal range of energies considered for diagnostic imaging and radiotherapy (20 keV to 25 MeV), electrons are far more likely to interact through collisions with atomic electrons. The efficiency of this process is therefore generally low. The likelihood of bremsstrahlung depends on the atomic number of the material traversed, Z (the total charge of the nucleus), and the energy of the incident electron, E, according to:

$$\text{Probability} \sim ZE \quad \textbf{(2.1)}$$

The energy of the electron beam is dictated by the maximum photon energy required. The use of high-atomic-number materials gives the best yield of photons. Table 2.1 presents the proportion of electron beam kinetic energy converted to photons for a tungsten target. The

TABLE 2.1 Percentage of Incident Electron Beam Energy Appearing as Bremsstrahlung for Electrons Incident on a Tungsten Target

Electron Energy (MeV)	Photon Yield (%)
0.05	0.5
0.25	2
1	6
10	30
50	63

Data calculated using the ESTAR program.[1]

remainder of the incident electron's kinetic energy is lost through collisions with atomic electrons in the target, causing excitation and ionisation. A large amount of this energy is eventually released in the form of heat, requiring the target to be cooled.

In the bremsstrahlung process, an electron may lose any amount of energy, up to its total kinetic energy. Rather than discrete photon energies, as are observed during de-excitation of atoms, a continuous spectrum of photon energies is produced. An example of the photon spectra produced when electrons are used to generate a 100-kV and 6-MV photon beam is shown in Fig. 2.4.

Photon spectra are commonly designated by kilovoltage (kV) or megavoltage (MV) to indicate the nominal potential used to accelerate the electrons that created the spectrum. For example, a potential difference of 100 kV between cathode and anode in an x-ray tube will result in electrons with an energy of 100 keV striking the target, producing a 100-kV photon spectrum. Although there is no lower limit on the energy of photons produced, the low-energy components of the spectrum are preferentially removed by photon attenuation within the target and other machine components so that the peak in the spectrum occurs at approximately one-third of the maximum photon energy.

For electrons striking a thin target, photons are produced in all directions. The intensity (or number) in a particular direction depends on the energy of the incident electrons and the atomic number of the target. For low electron energies (up to 100 keV), the intensity is almost equal in all directions, and as the electron energy increases, the photons produced become more forwards directed. This variation in photon intensity with incident electron energy is illustrated in Fig. 2.5, where electrons (indicated by the dashed line) are incident from the left. In this figure, bremsstrahlung production is simulated for a number of incident electrons, with the emitted photon energy and direction sampled from known probabilities (cross sections). Some 2000 photon tracks are represented in each figure, projected from a three-dimensional distribution into a two-dimensional plane. The length and shade of each photon track are representative of the individual photon energy. Note that higher-energy photons (lightly shaded, long tracks) appear predominantly in the forwards direction. This is one of the reasons for the average photon energy emitted from a linear accelerator target being lower at angles off the beam's central axis.

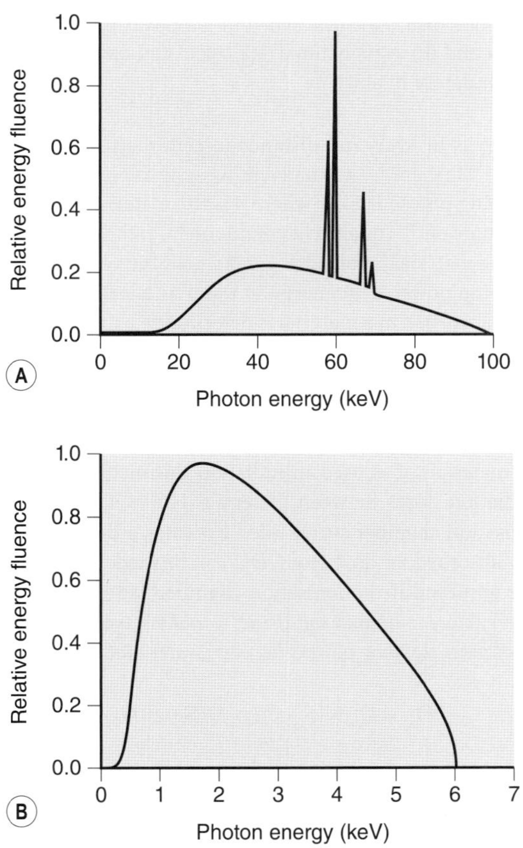

Fig. 2.4 X-ray spectra. (A) A 100-kV diagnostic spectrum; a bremsstrahlung (continuous) spectrum with superimposed discrete characteristic tungsten x-rays. (B) The 6-MV photon spectra from an Elekta SL25 linear accelerator. ((A) from IPEM (Institute of Physics and Engineering in Medicine)[2]; (B) from Baker and Peck.[3])

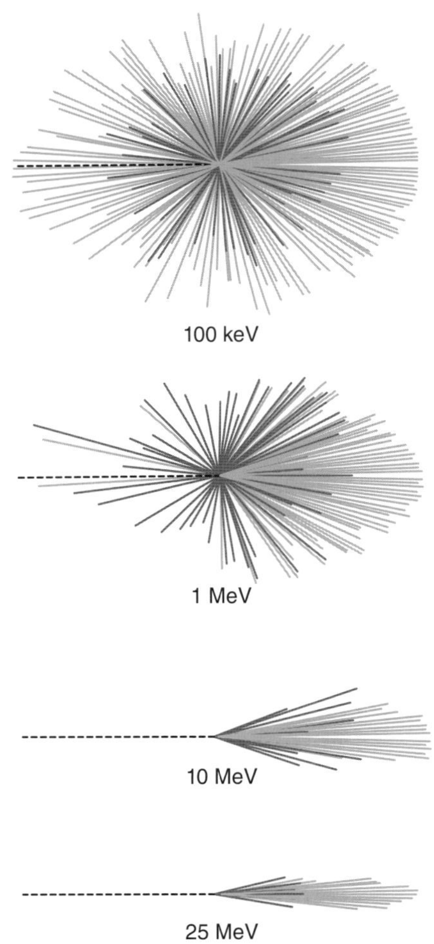

Fig. 2.5 Spatial and energy variation of bremsstrahlung produced by electrons incident on a thin target. Electrons are incident from the left *(dashed line)*; bremsstrahlung photon energy is indicated by track length and shade (short/dark = low energy). In each case, 2000 bremsstrahlung interactions are simulated from known probabilities.

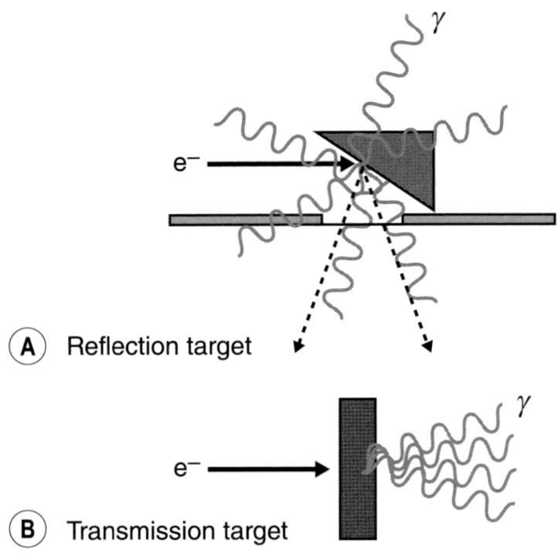

Fig. 2.6 Reflection and transmission targets for the production of x-rays. (A) represents the production of a kilovoltage therapy beam and (B) represents the production of a megavoltage beam.

The observed variation in spatial intensity of bremsstrahlung photons affects the design of x-ray targets. At kilovoltage energies, a reflection target is generally used, where photons produced at right angles to the direction of incident electrons are extracted for use. At megavoltage energies, a transmission target is required as photons are mostly travelling approximately parallel to the incident electron beam. This is shown schematically in Fig. 2.6.

Characteristic X-rays and Auger Electrons

Discrete spectral lines can be seen superimposed on the continuous 100-kV spectrum in Fig. 2.4. These are as a result of characteristic photons being produced during de-excitation of tungsten atoms after inner shell electrons have been excited or ejected through collisions with the incident electron beam. The energies of these characteristic photons correspond to the difference between the binding energies of the inner shell vacancy and the outer shell electron that fills the vacancy. The difference between electron binding energies depends on the atomic number of the target. For tungsten, with a K shell binding energy of 69 keV and an L-shell binding energy of 12 keV, it follows that the minimum energy of a characteristic photon produced by filling an electron vacancy in the K shell is 57 keV. The same characteristic photons are not observed in the 6-MV spectrum, as they now represent very low energies within this spectrum and are preferentially removed by photon attenuation.

In some instances the characteristic x-ray does not escape the atom but excites an outer electron sufficiently for the electron to leave the atom. These electrons are referred to as *Auger electrons* after the physicist who identified the process.

Stopping Power and Linear Energy Transfer

The rate at which energy from an incident beam of charged particles is lost as it passes through a material is described by the *stopping power*. If an electron of energy, E, loses a small amount of energy, dE, in a small thickness, dx, of material, the stopping power, $S(E)$, is defined by:

$$S(E) = \mathrm{d}E/\mathrm{d}x \ [\mathrm{MeV\,cm^{-1}}] \qquad \textbf{(2.2)}$$

If the energy loss is separated into that lost in collisions, S_{coll}, with atomic electrons and that lost through bremsstrahlung (or radiative loss), S_{rad}, the stopping power is defined by:

$$S(E) = S_{coll}(E) + S_{rad}(E) \qquad \textbf{(2.3)}$$

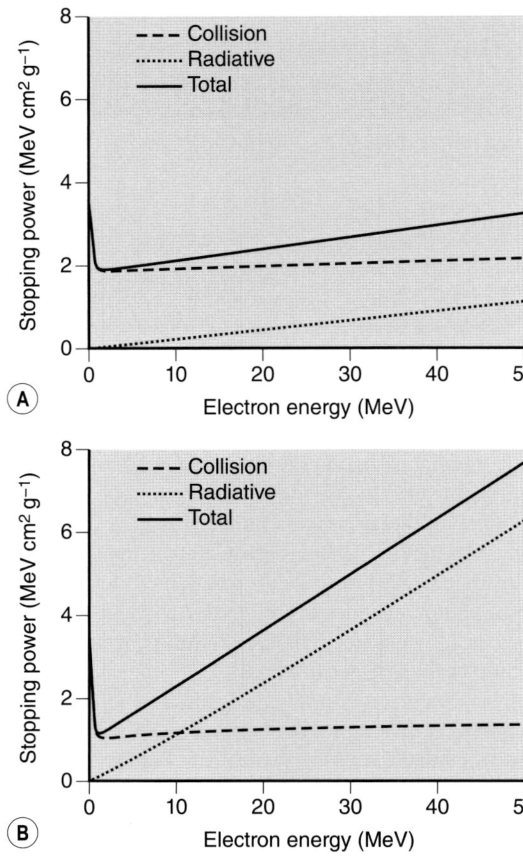

Fig. 2.7 Collisional, radiative and total stopping power for electrons (A) in water and (B) in tungsten. Data calculated using the ESTAR program. (From Berger et al.[1])

If energy is in MeV and distance in centimetres, stopping power has units of MeV cm^{-1}. Alternatively, we may express this in terms of mass stopping power, $S(E)/\rho$, where ρ is the material density (g cm^{-3}). The magnitude of this quantity depends on both the energy of the electron and the material involved. Fig. 2.7 shows the variation of electron mass stopping power with energy in water and lead. Measurement of the energy absorbed in a material is determined using stopping power, and the energy absorbed per unit mass is referred to as the *absorbed dose*. Its units are J/kg, and given the special unit gray, its symbol is Gy.

Because stopping power reflects the difference in energy absorption between materials, it is used in radiation dosimetry to convert measured radiation doses between materials. For example, using an air-filled ionisation chamber surrounded by water, a direct measurement of energy absorbed, or dose to air, D_{air}, can be made. The dose, D_w, that would be absorbed if the ionisation chamber were *replaced by water, which is very close to human soft tissue, would be given by multiplying by the ratio of mass stopping powers between water and air:*

$$D_w = D_{air} \times (S_w(E)/\rho_w)/(S_{air}(E)/\rho_{air}) \qquad \textbf{(2.4)}$$

where ρ_w and ρ_{air} are the densities of water and air, respectively. Strictly speaking, the stopping power used in Eq. (2.4) must be restricted to energy absorbed within the ionisation chamber volume and must exclude any energy that is lost from the beam but travels beyond the chamber (site of interaction). An example is energy lost in the form of bremsstrahlung, or collisions in which a large amount of the incident electron's energy is transferred to an atomic electron such that it travels beyond the chamber.

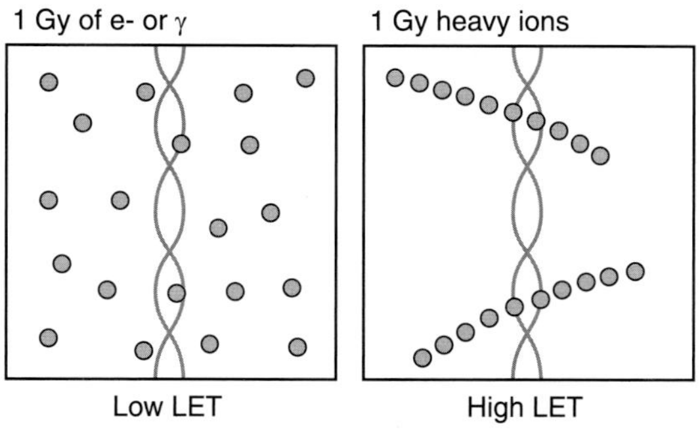

Fig. 2.8 Comparison of dose deposition and biological effect for low and high linear energy transfer (LET) beams. *Circles* refer to ionising events. The increased track density of ionisation events occurring for the higher LET beam leads to greater biological (DNA) damage. This increase in biological damage in comparison to low LET radiation (e.g. photons) can be expressed as a relative biological effectiveness (RBE), defined as the ratio of radiation doses required to produce the same degree of biological damage. For example, if an RBE of 1.1 is assumed for protons, a prescribed proton dose of 70 Gy would achieve the same biological effect as a dose of 77 Gy delivered by photons.

Linear energy transfer (LET) also refers to the amount of energy deposited by ionising radiation in matter. Units are also energy per unit length, often expressed in keV μm^{-1}. The LET is commonly used to distinguish between types of ionising radiation. Photons and electrons have a lower LET than protons and alpha particles. The terms *low LET* and *high LET* are often used in radiobiological descriptions. The smaller length units (μm) for LET reflect its application to energy deposition over subcellular dimensions. Fig. 2.8 shows a schematic comparison between energy deposition for high and low LET beams in relation to radiobiology.

Range and Path Length

Electrons have a negative charge and a relatively small mass. As a result, electron transport through matter is characterised by a large number of interactions through which generally a small amount of energy is lost in each interaction and a high degree of scattering occurs (Fig. 2.2). Because of these frequent interactions, it can often be assumed that electrons lose energy continuously as they traverse matter, and to a good approximation the energy loss can be assumed to be at a constant rate. It follows that if electrons or any other particles lose energy continuously, they must have a finite range. This is true of all charged particles. Calculated ranges for charged particles can be obtained using this continuous slowing down approximation (CSDA), resulting in the *CSDA range*. If a beam of monoenergetic electrons is incident on a given material and we assume continuous energy loss, the total distance travelled, or path length, must be the same for all electrons in the beam. The depth of penetration, or range, will vary because of the different paths traversed by individual electrons, as indicated in Fig. 2.2. This range straggling leads to a slope in the measured depth-dose curve, as illustrated in Fig. 2.9A. The steepness of this slope decreases as electron energy is increased, as shown in Fig. 2.9B. Note that the dose does not fall to zero immediately beyond the steep region of dose falloff, because of bremsstrahlung photons being produced. The intersection between the slope as a result of range straggling and the bremsstrahlung tail gives the practical range of the electron beam, R_p. As a guide, for clinical electron beams produced by linear accelerators (approximately 4–20 MeV), the range of electrons in water (or tissue) can be approximated by:

$$\text{Electron range (cm)} \approx \text{Beam energy (MeV)}/2 \quad \textbf{(2.5)}$$

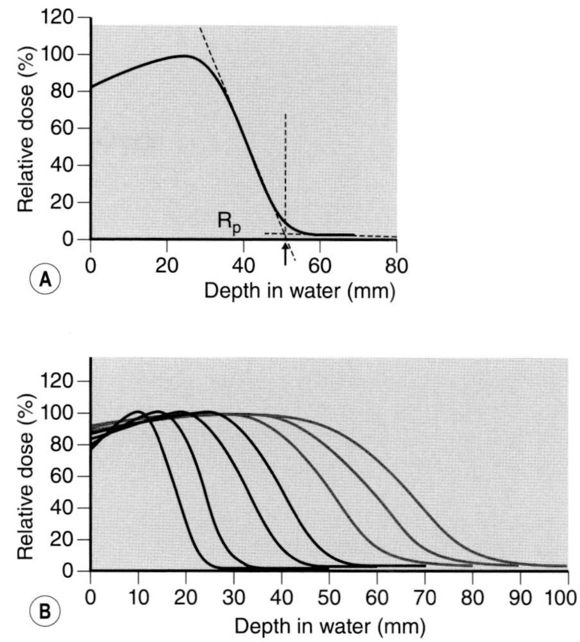

Fig. 2.9 Electron depth-dose distribution in water. (A) A 10-MeV electron beam, indicating practical range, Rp. (B) Variation of depth dose with beam energy for (from left to right) 4-, 6-, 8-, 10-, 12-, 15- and 18-MeV beams. (From the Clatterbridge Centre for Oncology NHS Foundation Trust: Douglas Cyclotron. With permission.)

TABLE 2.2 Electron Continuous Slowing Down Approximation Ranges in Water

Electron Beam Energy (MeV)	Continuous Slowing Down Approximation Range (cm)
0.1	0.01
0.25	0.06
0.5	0.18
1	0.44
5	2.55
10	4.98
25	11.3
50	19.8

Data evaluated using the ESTAR program.[1]

An indication of the accuracy of the aforementioned expression can be made by comparison with electron CSDA ranges in water, given in Table 2.2.

PHOTON INTERACTIONS

In the photon energy range of interest for radiotherapy, three major interactions can occur as a beam of photons passes through matter: photoelectric, Compton and pair production.

The Photoelectric Effect

This interaction, shown schematically in Fig. 2.10, occurs between an incident photon and atomic electron, generally assumed to be an inner shell electron. If the photon has sufficient energy to overcome the shell binding energy of the electron, it may disappear by transferring all its energy to the electron. The electron is then emitted from the atom,

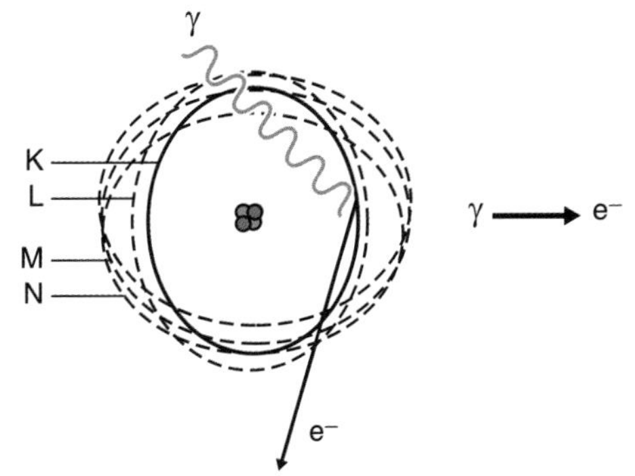

Fig. 2.10 Schematic representation of the photoelectric effect. An incoming photon transfers all its energy to an inner shell electron, ejecting the electron with a kinetic energy equal to the photon energy minus the electron binding energy. Electron shells K to N are indicated.

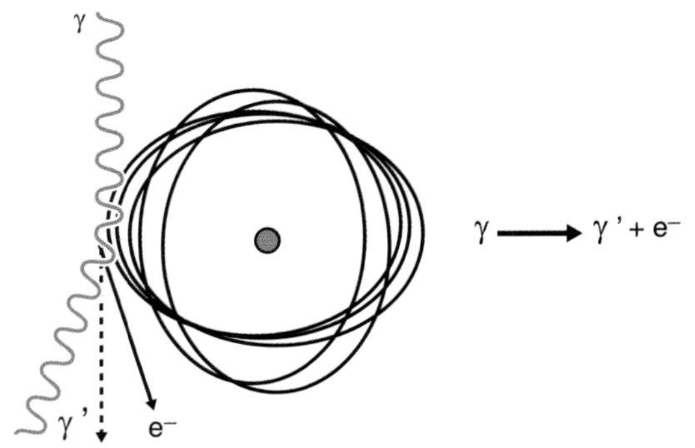

Fig. 2.11 Schematic representation of the Compton effect. An incident photon, γ, transfers part of its energy to an electron, and a lower-energy, scattered photon, γ′, is produced.

with kinetic energy, k.e., equal to the energy of the incident photon, E_γ, minus the electron binding energy, b.e.:

$$\text{k.e.} = E_\gamma - \text{b.e.} \quad \textbf{(2.6)}$$

As a consequence of this interaction, the atom is ionised and in an excited state. De-excitation then occurs, releasing characteristic photons, in the same manner as described in the 'Characteristic X-rays and Auger Electrons' section after ionisation or excitation by electron interactions. The probability of the photoelectric effect occurring is strongly dependent on the atomic number, *Z*, of the material traversed and on the energy, *E*, of the incident photon:

$$\text{Probability} \approx Z^3 / E^3 \quad \textbf{(2.7)}$$

This strong dependence on the atomic number is put to considerable use in diagnostic imaging because it provides clear differentiation between tissues with different atomic numbers as well as, or in the absence of, differences in physical density. For example, a 70-kV beam of photons passing through a human pelvis is much more likely to interact and be absorbed when passing through bone, with an atomic number of approximately 13, than it is when passing through adjacent soft tissue, with an approximate atomic number of 7. The photon intensity transmitted through the patient therefore clearly distinguishes between bone and soft tissue, providing a high-contrast x-ray image.

The Compton Effect

The Compton effect dominates in water between 100 keV and 20 MeV and is therefore the dominant interaction in tissue throughout the radiotherapy energy range of interest for photons. This interaction involves an incident photon interacting with an atomic electron, overcoming the electron binding energy, and transferring some of its energy to the electron in the form of kinetic energy and the remainder as a lower-energy photon. Unlike the photoelectric effect, no resonance effect is observed, and the interaction is likely to occur with outer shell electrons with binding energies far lower than the energy of the incoming photon. As a result, this interaction is often referred to as occurring with free electrons. The interaction is shown schematically in Fig. 2.11.

The probability of the Compton interaction depends on the density of electrons in a material, which varies as *Z*/*A*, a ratio of the atomic number *Z* and mass number *A*. This ratio is almost constant for elements above hydrogen. As a result, the Compton effect can be considered to be independent of the atomic number of the material the photons pass through and is dependent only on the physical density. It is for this reason that medical imaging with megavoltage photons leads to poorer contrast than imaging with kilovoltage photon beams. This represents a benefit for radiotherapy to soft-tissue tumours, however, as a significant dependence on atomic number would lead to a higher absorbed dose being delivered to bone than to soft tissue.

The average proportion of the incident photon's energy transferred to the electron depends on the incident photon energy. For a 100-keV incident photon, on average, approximately 10% of its energy, 10 keV, is passed to the electron, whereas the scattered photon retains 90 keV. As the incident photon energy increases, however, a higher proportion of its energy is transferred to the electron; a 10-MeV photon transfers an average of approximately 70%, 7 MeV, to the electron and the scattered photon retains 3 MeV. The variation of average energy transferred to the electron via the Compton effect is illustrated in Fig. 2.12. These characteristics of the Compton effect have implications for radiotherapy and radiation dosimetry. For kilovoltage photon beams, electrons set in motion through Compton interactions can be assumed to deposit their energy very close to the site of interaction, whereas for megavoltage photons, these interactions produce high-energy secondary electrons that will travel a significant distance. The latter results in the observed skin-sparing effect of absorbed dose deposition in tissue by megavoltage photon beams, as electrons set in motion near the skin surface deposit their energy over a significant depth. For example, a 3-MeV photon (approximately the average photon energy in a 10-MV photon spectrum) will provide an electron with an average energy of 1.8 MeV (60%), which will deposit energy over a distance of approximately 1 cm in tissue. The angular distribution of electrons set in motion by the Compton effect is also of interest. For kilovoltage photons, the secondary electrons set in motion are emitted over a wide range of angles

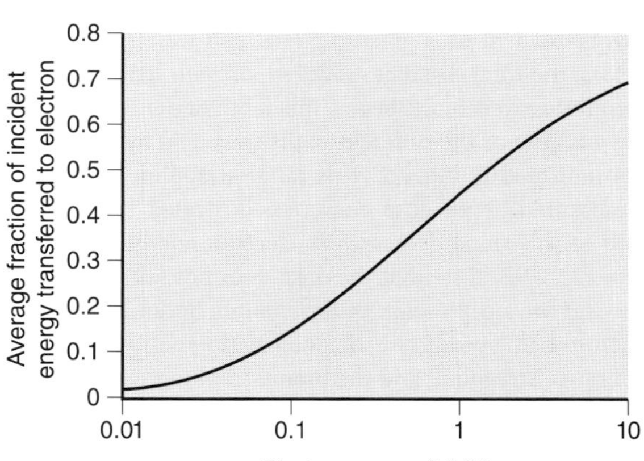

Fig. 2.12 Average proportion of photon energy transferred to secondary electrons during the Compton effect. (From Attix.[4])

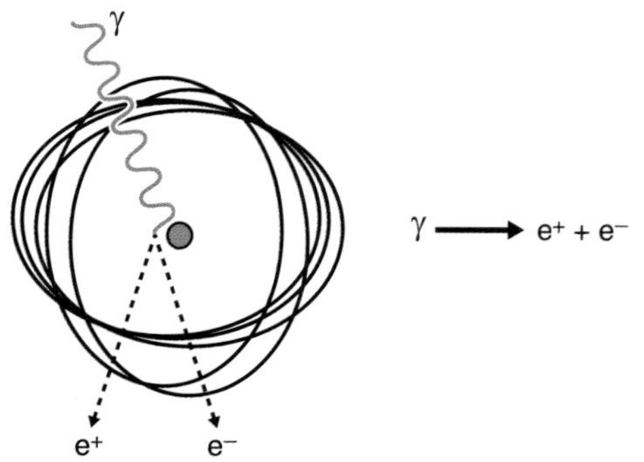

Fig. 2.13 Schematic representation of pair production in the nuclear Coulomb field.

from the direction of the incident photon. As the incident photon energy is increased, this distribution of electrons becomes more forwards directed.

Pair Production

Above a few mega electron volts (MeV), photons may interact with the nuclear Coulomb field to produce an electron–positron pair, shown schematically in Fig. 2.13. In this interaction, the photon vanishes, and all its energy is transferred to the rest mass and kinetic energy of the electron, k.e.(e^-), and positron, k.e.(e^+). For an incident photon of energy E, conservation of energy demands that:

$$E = 1.022 + \text{k.e.}(e^+) + \text{k.e.}(e^-)[\text{MeV}] \quad \textbf{(2.8)}$$

Hence the incoming photon must have a minimum energy of 1.022 MeV for the interaction to occur. The probability of a photon being attenuated by pair production is proportional to the atomic number of the material traversed and, for the energy range of interest to radiotherapy, increases gradually with the incoming photon's energy:

$$\text{Probability} \quad ZE \; (E > 1.022\,\text{MeV}) \quad \textbf{(2.9)}$$

In water and soft tissue, pair production only becomes significant at photon energies above approximately 10 MeV, so it accounts for very little of the absorbed dose to a patient undergoing radiotherapy. With higher atomic number materials, pair production becomes significant at lower energies, for example at approximately 3 MeV for lead.

The electron and positron produced will lose energy in the medium traversed, mainly through interactions (collisions) with atomic electrons, as discussed earlier. The positron eventually annihilates with a local electron, releasing the remaining positron kinetic energy and rest mass of the positron and electron in the form of photons. This annihilation event becomes more likely as the positron slows down. If it occurs at rest, that is, when the positron has lost all of its kinetic energy, the energy of each photon is equal to 0.511 MeV, the electron (and positron) rest mass. To conserve momentum, these two photons must travel in opposite directions. This feature of positron–electron annihilation is the key to positron emission tomography (PET), as coincident detection of the two photons produced reveals information about the position of the annihilation event (see Chapter 7).

Photons may undergo a similar interaction to the nuclear pair production interaction described earlier in the Coulomb field of an electron. However, the probability of this is very low compared with the interaction in the nuclear Coulomb field.

Exponential Attenuation

An experimental arrangement is shown in Fig. 2.14 for measuring the number of photons that reach a detector as a filter, or attenuator, is placed in the beam path. We are interested in measuring how many

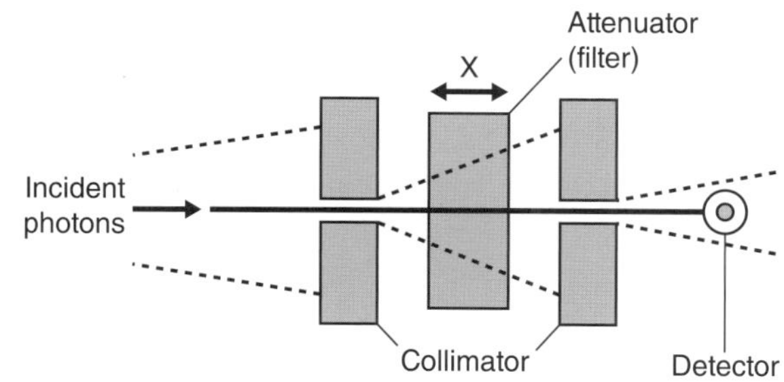

Fig. 2.14 Geometry for photon attenuation measurements. Collimators are present to prevent scattered photons from reaching the detector.

photons arrive at the detector without undergoing any interaction in the filter (i.e. how many photons are unattenuated). The purpose of the collimators is to prevent any scattered photons, resulting from an interaction in the filter, from reaching the detector and so causing us to overestimate the number of photons that have not interacted. If scattered photons are excluded, this arrangement is referred to as *narrow-beam geometry*. The detector records N photons arriving at the detector for a thickness, x, of filter. If the number of photons reaching the detector changes by an amount, dN, when a thin (infinitely thin) filter of thickness, dx, is placed in the beam, and we represent the relative change (dN/N) per unit thickness as μ, we have:

$$\mu dx = -dN / N \quad \textbf{(2.10)}$$

By integrating this expression and applying the condition that for zero filter thickness, N_0 photons are recorded at the detector, it is straightforward to show the number of photons, N, transmitted by the filter and reaching the detector when a filter of thickness x is placed in the beam:

$$N = N_0 e^{-\mu x} \quad \textbf{(2.11)}$$

Parameter, μ, is the linear attenuation coefficient (units of per-unit distance, e.g. cm^{-1}), and its value is dependent on the filter material and the energy of the photon beam. To compare the effect of varying atomic number on attenuation properties, it is convenient to remove the variation because of material density, ρ. This is achieved by defining the mass attenuation coefficient, μ/ρ. If μ is expressed in units of cm^{-1} and density in g cm^{-3}, the units of mass attenuation coefficient are $cm^2\,g^{-1}$; the corresponding thickness of the filter must then be expressed in terms of mass thickness (linear thickness × density), g cm^{-2}.

The interactions occurring in a slab of water when irradiated with a beam of 3-MeV photons are illustrated in Fig. 2.15. The mass attenuation coefficient is a macroscopic quantity that, in principle, can be measured relatively simply. It represents the total probability that a photon of a given energy will interact with matter, regardless of the type of interaction. The variation of mass attenuation coefficient with energy for water ($Z = 7$) and lead ($Z = 82$) is shown in Fig. 2.16. The reason for the particular shape of the attenuation curves for water and lead is explained by the varying probability with energy of the underlying photon interactions that combine to give the total interaction probability and hence attenuation coefficient. It can be seen that in water, the attenuation coefficient decreases monotonically as photon energy is increased, up to approximately 50 MeV, at which point it begins to increase.

In Fig. 2.17, the region of dominance for each interaction type is indicated as photon energy increases from the kilovoltage to megavoltage range. A summary of the energy ranges in which each interaction dominates is shown in Table 2.3. The photoelectric effect dominates in water or tissue for energies up to approximately 30 keV, and in lead for energies up to approximately 500 keV.

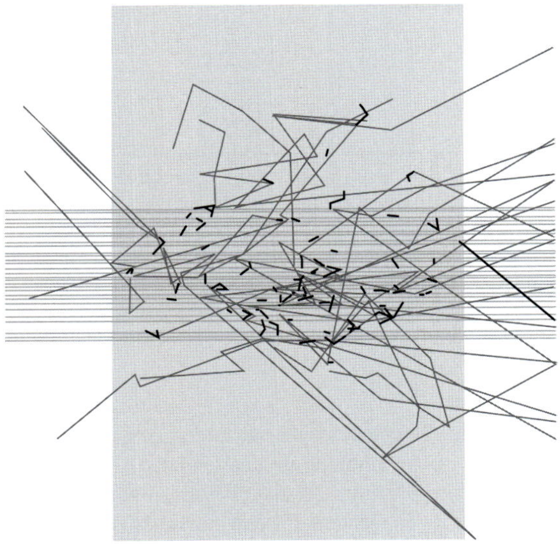

Fig. 2.15 Illustration of photon interactions. A beam of 3-MeV photons *(light grey)* is incident from the left on a 25-cm thick water slab. Photons may escape the slab without interacting; others interact in the water, generating secondary electrons (*black*), which cause further ionisation and may escape the slab if they are generated close to the exit face. Photons may be backscattered from the face of the slab, along with secondary electrons.

The large discontinuities observed at approximately 15 keV and 88 keV for the mass attenuation coefficient in lead, shown in Fig. 2.17B, are a result of incident photons having sufficient energy to overcome the binding energies of the lead L and K shells, respectively. This large increase in interaction probability around an electron binding energy suggests that a resonance effect is involved, whereby the probability of interaction is highest when the photon energy is close to that of the electron binding energy. This feature in the mass attenuation coefficient curve is referred to as an *absorption edge*. The lack of visible absorption edges in water (Fig. 2.17A) is caused by the lower probability of the photoelectric effect occurring in water relative to the Compton effect and the low binding energies of the K shell electrons for oxygen and hydrogen.

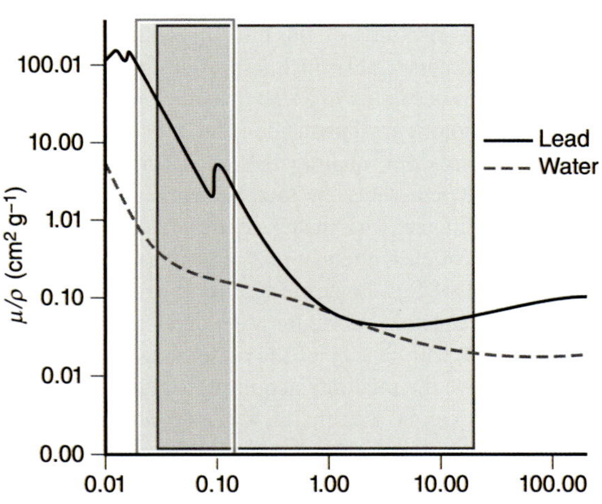

Fig. 2.16 Mass attenuation coefficient variation with photon energy in water and lead. The *light and dark shaded regions* indicate the approximate range of photon energies commonly used for diagnostic imaging and radiotherapy, respectively. (From Hubbell and Seltzer[5]; Berger et al.[6])

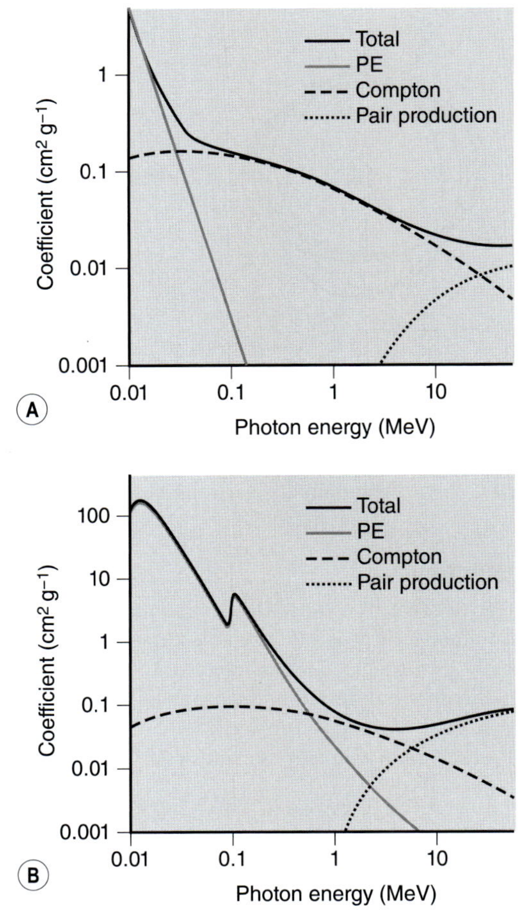

Fig. 2.17 Mass attenuation coefficients showing the relative contributions from the photoelectric effect *(PE)*, Compton effect and pair production in (A) water (effective $Z = 7$) and (B) lead ($Z = 82$). Note the large region of dominance for the Compton effect in water because of the lower effective atomic number *Z*. (From Hubbell and Seltzer[5]; Berger et al.[6])

For lead, the minimum attenuation occurs at a much lower energy of approximately 4 MeV compared with water, after which it begins to rise. It follows that the thickness of lead required to provide a chosen degree of attenuation would be greater for 4-MeV photons than it would be for 20-MeV photons. At higher energies, above approximately 8 MeV, photons may still undergo interactions directly with the atomic nucleus, releasing neutrons and forming radioactive isotopes.

Note that here we are considering monoenergetic photons (MeV), whereas in practice, clinical photon beams contain a spectrum of energies (denoted by *MV* to indicate this). The effective attenuation coefficients averaged over all energies in the spectra in lead for 6-MV and 15-MV beams are roughly equal. The mass attenuation coefficients of water and lead are approximately equal for 1-MeV photons.

TABLE 2.3 Energy Regions of Domination for Photoelectric, Compton and Pair Production Interactions

Interaction	Low *Z* (Water)	High *Z* (Lead)
Photoelectric	<30 keV	<500 keV
Compton	30 keV–25 MeV	0.5–5 MeV
Pair production	>25 MeV	>5 MeV

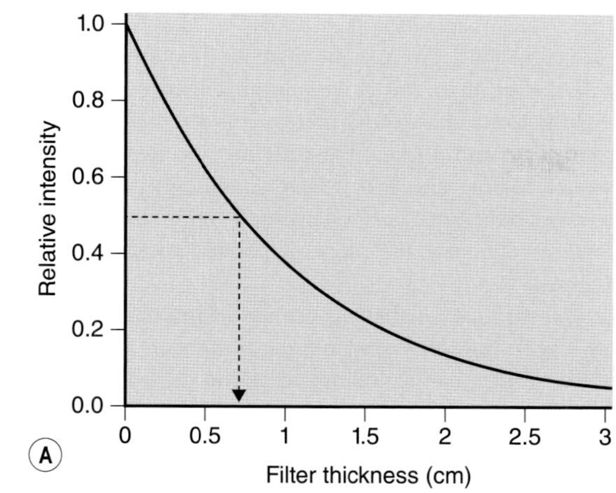

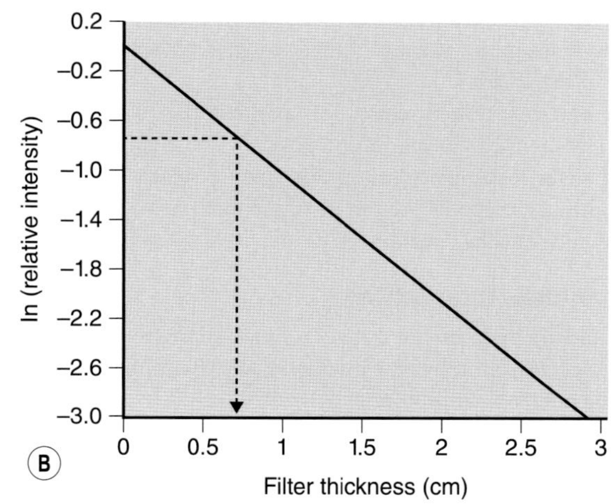

Fig. 2.18 Exponential attenuation of monoenergetic photons. (A) Relative transmission versus filter thickness and (B) ln (relative transmission) versus thickness. The half-value layer of 0.7 cm Al is indicated on each plot.

At 10 MeV the coefficient for lead is a little over twice that of water, whereas at 100 keV the coefficient for lead is over 30 times that of water.

The mathematical form of Eq. (2.12) is identical to that describing radioactive decay. For a chosen material and filter thickness placed in the path of a monoenergetic photon beam, adding filters of the same material and thickness will result in the same fraction of beam being transmitted; for example, if 1 cm of a filter results in the beam intensity falling to 70% of its original value, 2 cm will result in 49% of the original intensity being transmitted. Fig. 2.18A shows a plot of relative transmitted photon intensity ($N/N_0 = e^{-\mu x}$) for a monoenergetic beam of photons incident on aluminium filters. Taking natural logarithms of this equation yields a linear function, shown in Fig. 2.18B. The slope of the straight line is equal to $-\mu$. For a filter thickness that reduces the intensity to half the original value, we have:

$$N/N_0 = 0.5 = e^{-\mu t_{1/2}} \quad \textbf{(2.12)}$$

where $t_{1/2}$ is denoted the half-value layer (HVL) or half-value thickness. Rearranging this expression and taking natural logarithms gives:

$$t_{1/2} = \text{HVL} = \ln(2)/\mu \quad \textbf{(2.13)}$$

For a chosen filter material, the HVL of a beam of photons provides a measure of the beam's power of penetration. In the kilovoltage region, HVL is therefore used to represent the quality of a beam of photons, and it is generally reported in mm of aluminium or mm of copper. For a monoenergetic beam of photons, it follows that after one HVL, the intensity drops to 50%; after two HVLs, 25%; after three HVLs, 12.5% and so on. The presence of inherent filtration for a monoenergetic source of photons would therefore have no effect on the measured beam quality.

Attenuation of Photon Spectra

In practice, photon beams generated by fast-moving electrons striking a high-atomic-number target will have a spectrum of energies, as described earlier. We may expect the attenuation coefficient to decrease as photon energy is increased (i.e. higher-energy photons are more penetrating). As a photon spectrum (i.e. a polyenergetic beam) is filtered, lower-energy photons will be preferentially removed from the beam because of their larger attenuation coefficients. This results in the average energy of the beam increasing and the average attenuation coefficient decreasing. As a result of this changing attenuation coefficient, the measured transmission curve will no longer be a true exponential. This is represented in Fig. 2.19, where successive HVLs are no longer constant but depend on the amount of filtration already present in the beam.

Beam Hardening

In addition to the photon attenuation provided by the target and other machine components, referred to as the *inherent filtration*, additional filters may be placed in the path of the emerging photon beam (Fig. 2.14). This is used particularly in the kV radiotherapy beams as well as in the kV photon beams used for diagnostic imaging. The effect of this is to preferentially remove lower-energy components from the spectrum, as a result of their higher attenuation. This is a desirable effect, as these low-energy photons will reduce the penetration of a radiotherapy beam, and for x-ray imaging they contribute little to an x-ray image and result in unnecessary radiation doses. Adding filters in the path of the beam reduce beam intensity (number of photons) but increase the average energy of the beam, referred to as *hardening the beam*. Comparison of the first and second HVLs (HVL_1/HVL_2; Fig. 2.19) gives an indication of the degree of beam hardening occurring and is termed the *homogeneity coefficient*.

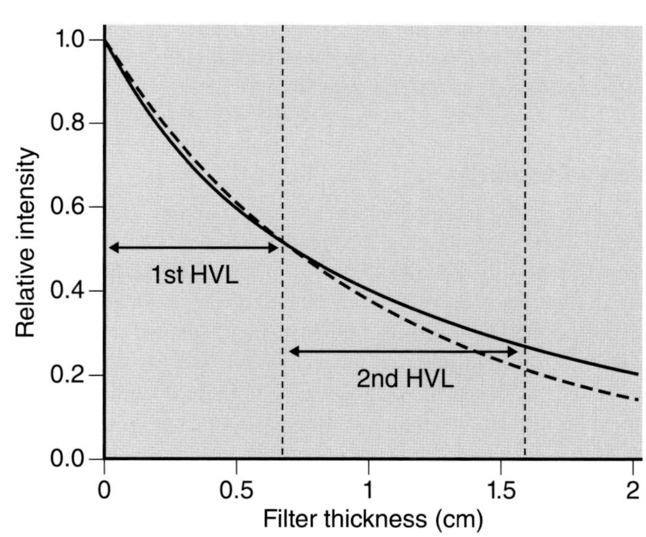

Fig. 2.19 Attenuation comparison between a 100-kV photon spectrum *(solid line)* and a monoenergetic beam *(dashed line)* of the same first half-value layer (HVL). The first and second HVLs (0.7- and 0.9-cm Al, respectively) for the spectrum are indicated. For the monoenergetic beam, the first and second HVLs would be equal, whereas for a spectrum of energies, the subsequent HVLs increase because of beam hardening, as indicated.

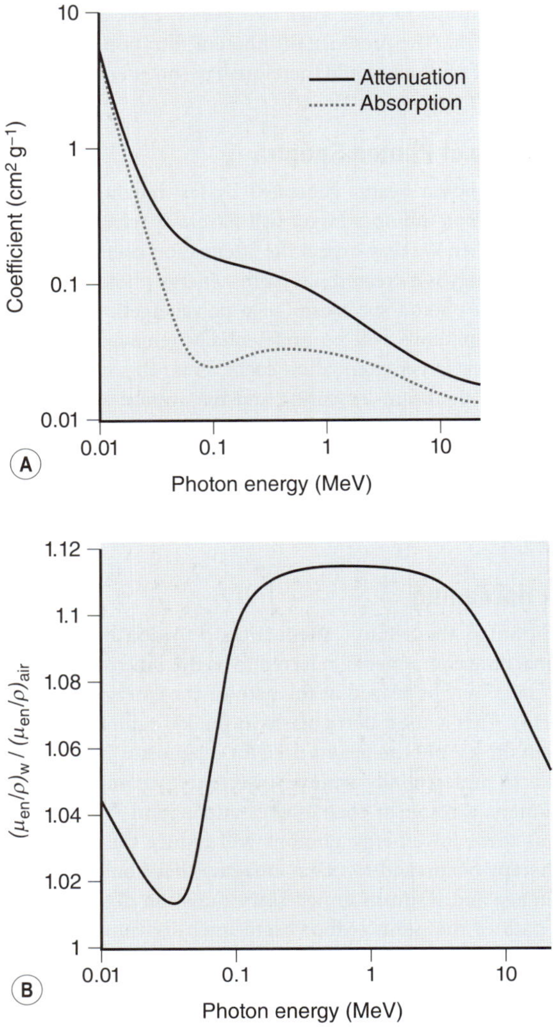

Fig. 2.20 (A) Comparison of photon mass attenuation and mass energy absorption coefficients in water. Note that the difference is largest where the Compton effect dominates because of energy being transported away from the site of interaction by Compton-scattered photons. (B) Ratio of water to air mass energy absorption coefficient. (From Hubbell and Seltzer[5]; Berger et al.[6])

Energy Absorption

As well as being interested in how many photons are transmitted without interacting in a filter (i.e. remain unattenuated), we may also be interested in the amount of energy absorbed in the filter, particularly if we replace the filter with biological tissue. This information is given by the energy absorption coefficient, denoted μ_{en}. In a similar approach to that followed for attenuation, we can also define the mass energy absorption coefficient, μ_{en}/ρ. These quantities have the same units as their attenuation counterparts. In terms of the geometry shown in Fig. 2.14, to determine energy absorption we must detect all unattenuated photons together with any other energy not absorbed locally. Assuming all charged particles are absorbed (stopped) locally, it is the energy transported away in the form of photons that must be accounted for: that is, all characteristic photons released from excited atoms following photoelectric interactions, scattered photons resulting from the Compton effect, bremsstrahlung photons produced by charged particles (e.g. Compton electrons) and finally photons arising from positron annihilation following pair production (if the incident photon energy is high enough). The geometry for this situation then represents broad-beam conditions. It follows that the attenuation coefficient for a given monoenergetic photon beam in a given material is larger than the corresponding energy absorption coefficient for the same energy and material, as attenuation accounts for both absorption and scatter. Practical measurement geometry will fall between narrow and broad-beam conditions. Fig. 2.20A compares mass attenuation coefficients and mass energy absorption coefficients in water for the range of photon energies of interest to radiotherapy.

Energy absorption coefficients are used in radiation dosimetry in a similar way to how electron stopping powers are used for electron beams, as described earlier. Taking again the example of an air-filled ionisation chamber in water, having determined the dose deposited by photons in the air cavity, D_{air}, the dose to the same region when filled with water, D_w, is given by:

$$D_w = D_{air} \times (\mu_{en}/\rho)_w/(\mu_{en}/\rho)_{air} \quad \textbf{(2.14)}$$

The variation in the ratio of mass energy absorption coefficients is shown in Fig. 2.20B.

The aforementioned expression assumes that all electrons set in motion by the incident photons deposit their energy within the chamber. This is a reasonable assumption for kV photon beams. For MV photon beams, however, the ranges of secondary electrons become significant and must be considered.

Photonuclear Interactions

At sufficiently high energies, that is, above approximately 8 MeV, or a 15-MV spectra, photons may interact directly with the atomic nucleus, releasing neutrons or protons:

$$\begin{aligned} \gamma + {}^{A}_{Z}X &\rightarrow {}^{A-1}_{Z}Y + n \\ \gamma + {}^{A}_{Z}X &\rightarrow {}^{A-1}_{Z-1}Y + p \end{aligned} \quad \textbf{(2.15)}$$

These interactions do not lead to a significant patient dose, but the production of neutrons can lead to additional shielding requirements for the treatment room. Activation of linear accelerator components, particularly the photon target, can also occur, which must be allowed to decay to acceptable levels before any intervention, such as machine servicing.

PHOTON DEPTH DOSE AND THE BUILDUP EFFECT

The transmission of photons decreases exponentially as the amount of matter traversed is increased, as shown in Fig. 2.18. The quantity we are generally more interested in, however, is the absorbed dose received at a depth in tissue and how this varies with depth. This quantity is commonly described as *percentage depth dose (PDD)*:

$$\text{PDD} = 100 \times D(d)/D(d_{max}) \quad \textbf{(2.16)}$$

where $D(d)$ is the measured dose at depth, d, and d_{max} is the depth of the maximum dose. Example PDD curves for megavoltage photon beams are shown in Fig. 2.21. An important feature of these curves is the fact that the maximum dose is not reached at the surface, but at a depth, d_{max}, which is dependent on the energy of the beam. This provides the skin-sparing effect of megavoltage photon beams.

The dose buildup effect is explained by considering the photon interactions taking place in tissue at the energies involved. Table 2.3 shows us that the Compton effect dominates in low atomic number materials, such as tissue, right across the MeV range of photon energies

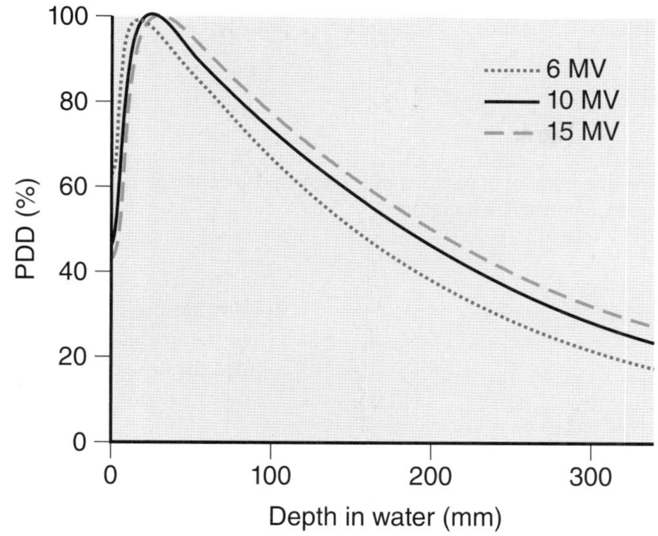

Fig. 2.21 Example percentage depth-dose *(PDD)* profiles for photon beams in water. (From the Clatterbridge Centre for Oncology NHS Foundation Trust: Douglas Cyclotron. With permission.)

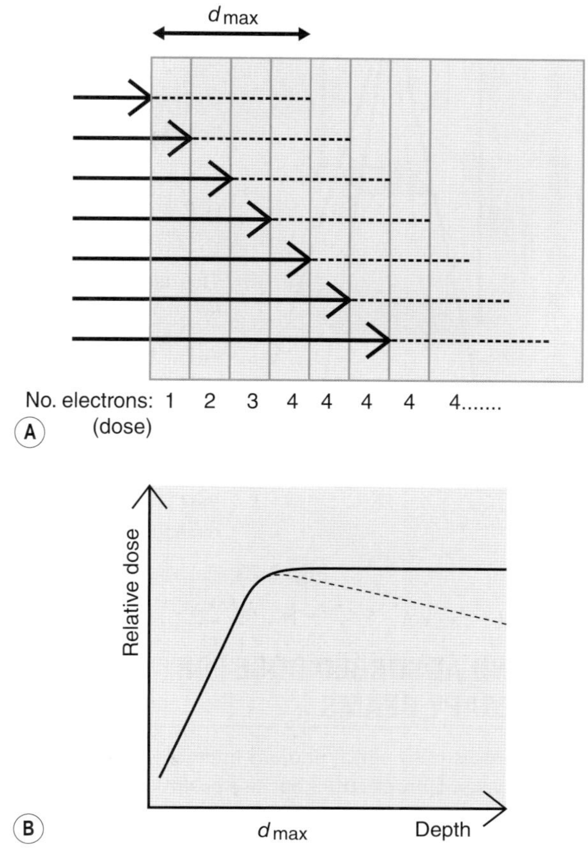

Fig. 2.22 Schematic illustration of dose buildup in MV photon beams. (A) Incident photons *(solid lines)* interact in each layer, liberating secondary electrons *(dashed lines)*. These electrons deposit their kinetic energy over their (finite) range, here corresponding to four layers. The total dose in each layer is proportional to the number of electrons crossing it (1 to 4). (B) The *solid line* indicates the buildup of dose in the absence of photon attenuation. The *dashed line* indicates the exponentially decreasing dose beyond d_{max} because of photon attenuation.

commonly used for radiotherapy. This interaction provides a scattered photon, which generally leaves the site of interaction, and a secondary electron, which has a finite range over which it deposits its energy. For an incident 1-MeV photon, Fig. 2.12 shows us that approximately 0.4 MeV, on average, is passed to the secondary electron, whereas for a 10-MeV incident photon, roughly 6.8 MeV on average would be passed on. This kinetic energy of the secondary electrons is not all deposited at the site of the Compton interaction, but rather, is spread out over the electron's range, which depends on the electron's energy, as shown in Table 2.2. Let us now consider the total absorbed dose from secondary electrons as we move between thin layers from the surface to the depth of d_{max}, in steps of some fraction of d_{max}. As illustrated in Fig. 2.22, some energy is deposited in the surface layer by secondary electrons set in motion within this layer, and some is transported along with the electrons to underlying layers. Taking a step deeper, we again have a dose from secondary electrons set in motion within this layer, and we have an additional dose contribution from secondary electrons entering from the surface layer (upstream)—that is, we now have contributions from two layers. At the next layer, we have three layers contributing: the one we are in and two upstream. At each successively deeper layer, the number of upstream layers contributing electrons increases, so the total absorbed dose rises, or builds up. This process continues until we are at a depth beyond the range of electrons set in motion in the surface layer, at which point we have reached full buildup, at d_{max}. The depth of d_{max}, then, corresponds to the average range of secondary electrons set in motion by the incident photon beam, which increases with photon beam energy, as shown in Fig. 2.21, in moving from 6 to 15 MV. In practice, this depth will also be influenced by the field size, by contaminant electrons generated in the head of the accelerator and in any beam-modifying devices in the path of the beam. If we assume that photon attenuation is negligible over a number of layers, then at d_{max} and beyond, the total number of electrons crossing each layer is constant; the number entering a given layer from upstream equals the number moving downstream (see Fig. 2.22). This condition is termed *charged-particle equilibrium* and is discussed further in the section titled Bragg-Gray Cavity Theory in Chapter 3. Note that for kilovoltage photon beams, the energies and ranges of secondary electrons will be very much reduced. For example, a 100-keV photon interacting by the Compton effect will produce, on average, a secondary electron of around 15 keV, which has a range of less than 1/100 mm. Secondary electrons generated by kilovoltage photon beams can therefore be assumed to deposit their energy at the site of interaction in tissue, and no dose buildup or skin sparing occurs.

For a phantom, or patient, irradiated at a fixed source to surface distance (SSD) with a diverging beam (e.g. that from a small or point source, such as a clinical linear accelerator or x-ray tube), the absorbed dose beyond the depth of d_{max} will decrease with depth because of both increasing attenuation of the incident photons and increasing distance of the point of interest from the source. This latter effect is known as the *inverse-square law*, as the dose from a point source, in the absence of any attenuating material, will decrease as $1/r^2$, where r is the distance from the source. The derivation of this law is given in Fig. 2.23. We can combine the effect of photon attenuation with the inverse-square reduction in photon intensity to approximate the PDD beyond d_{max} as:

$$\mathrm{PDD} \approx e^{-\mu_{eff}(d-d_{max})} \times (f + d_{max}/f + d)^2 \qquad \textbf{(2.17)}$$

where μ_{eff} is the effective attenuation coefficient for the beam. The term *effective attenuation coefficient* is used here, as our geometry does not exclude scattered radiation and is likely to represent an average over a photon spectrum. The μ_{eff} will therefore vary with field size and depth.

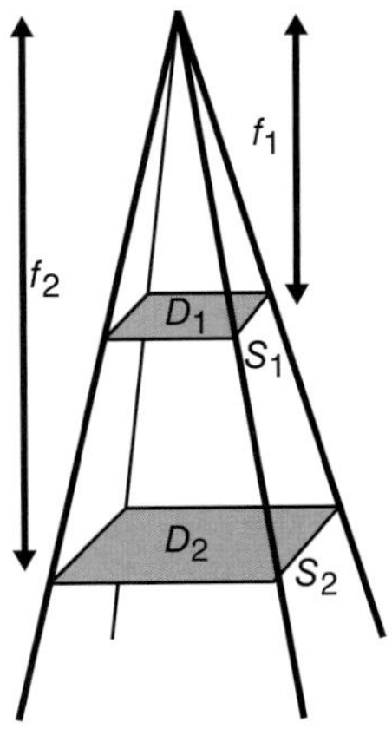

Given a square field of side s_1 at distance f_1, the size s_2 at distance f_2 is given by:
$s_2 = s_1 \times (f_2 / f_1)$ [1]

Field areas are related by:
$s_2^2 = s_1^2 \times (f_2 / f_1)^2$ [2]

In the absence of photon interactions, the number of photons over each field is constant (= n, say) and the number per unit area (intensity) is therefore:
$I_1 = n/s_1^2$ and $I_2 = n/s_2^2$

The ratio of intensities is therefore:
$I_2/I_1 = s_1^2/s_2^2$ [3]

From [2], we have:
$s_1^2/s_2^2 = (f_1 / f_2)^2$

So, [3] can be written as: $I_2/I_1 = (f_2 / f_1)^2$ [4]
As dose is proportional to intensity, we can replace Is by Ds in [4] to obtain:
$D_2 = D_1 \times (f_1 / f_2)^2$ or $D_2 \propto 1/f_2^2$.
This is the inverse-square law; dose, D_2, is *inversely proportional* to the *square* of the distance, f_2.

Fig. 2.23 Illustration of field size scaling and derivation of the inverse-square law.

KERMA AND ABSORBED DOSE FOR RADIOTHERAPY BEAMS

The various processes by which photons interact with matter produce charged particles, mainly electrons but also positrons which then travel through matter, losing energy by the collision processes of ionisation and excitation of atoms and through the radiative processes of production of bremsstrahlung, as illustrated in Fig. 2.24.

For photon beams, the transfer of energy from radiation to matter may be seen in two distinct stages:

- Transfer of energy from the radiation to emitted charged particles
- Deposition of energy by the emitted charged particles through collision processes

For charged particle beams, only stage 2 is relevant.

Stage 1 is governed by the interaction coefficients for photons in matter: photoelectric, Compton and pair production. Stage 2 is dependent upon the energies of the charged particles and their subsequent patterns of energy deposition as determined by their stopping powers. The deposition of energy is different from the transfer of energy by different amounts dependent upon the photon energies and materials.

Kerma

Kerma, a term for kinetic energy released per unit mass, is used to quantify the first of the aforementioned stages. It is defined by the International Commission on Radiation Units and Measurements (ICRU)[7] as:

$$K = \Delta E_{tr} / \Delta m \quad \textbf{(2.18)}$$

where ΔE_{tr} represents the energy transferred from photons to charged particles and is the sum of initial kinetic energies of all the charged particles liberated by uncharged ionising radiation from an amount of material of mass Δm.

It may be seen from Fig. 2.24 that for the Compton interaction illustrated:

- The energy of an incident photon is shared between a scattered photon and the ejected electron. The scattered photon carries its energy away from the immediate region of the interaction. The term *terma* represents the total energy removed from the beam per unit mass of matter, including that given to the charged particles and that scattered as photons. Terma is therefore always greater than kerma.
- The electron travels through matter, losing energy continually until its kinetic energy is exhausted.
- The travelling electron may lose some energy by bremsstrahlung, producing photons, which, like the scattered photon, carry energy away from the immediate vicinity. The term *collision kerma* refers to that proportion of kerma that is deposited via collision processes only. Kerma and collision kerma differ only in accounting for the energy that is reradiated. In body tissues, the energy reradiated is small, being less than 1%, so these two quantities are almost equal.

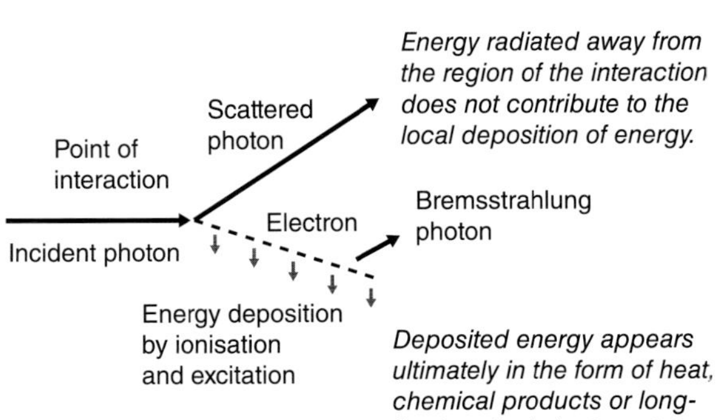

Fig. 2.24 Schematic diagram of energy deposition arising from Compton interaction on matter.

Absorbed Dose

The travelling electrons deposit energy in matter through which they pass, and so the energy deposited by these electrons is displaced in distance from the site of initial transfer of energy from the photon beam. The amount of energy deposited in a small mass of the material is termed the *absorbed dose*, which is defined by the ICRU[7] as:

$$D = \Delta E_{d} / \Delta m \quad \textbf{(2.19)}$$

where ΔE_d is the total energy deposited by these charged particles in a volume element of mass Δm.

The absorbed dose is similar in value to collision kerma but is displaced because of the motion of the secondary charged particles.

Absorbed dose equals collision kerma if one of the following conditions are met:

- The distance travelled by secondary charged particles is sufficiently small for it to be neglected, such that energy may be considered to be absorbed by the matter at the point where it is transferred from photons to the charged particles, a condition known as *point deposition of dose*. This occurs for low-energy photons, where the emitted electrons can travel only short distances, as detailed earlier.
- The energy lost from the region of initial transfer by the movement of charged particles away from that region is exactly compensated for by energy brought into the region by other travelling electrons produced elsewhere, a condition known as *energy equilibrium*, or more generally as *charged particle equilibrium*.

Units of Kerma and Dose

Both kerma and absorbed dose have units of energy per unit mass, the units for which are joules (J) and kilograms (kg), respectively. The unit gray (Gy) is used for both absorbed dose and kerma and is defined as:

$$1\ \text{Gy} = 1\ \text{J/kg} \quad \textbf{(2.20)}$$

Neither absorbed dose nor kerma is material specific and can therefore be related to any matter: a subscript is generally used to indicate the material. Hence K_a and K_w may be used to refer to air kerma and water kerma, respectively. Likewise for absorbed dose.

HEAVY PARTICLE INTERACTIONS

As mentioned in this chapter's Introduction section, the predominant radiation beams used in radiotherapy are x-ray photons and electrons. The other radiation beams which are used less frequently provide beam characteristics directly related to their interactions with matter.

Protons

Carrying the same magnitude but the opposite sign of charge to electrons, protons readily interact with atomic electrons, causing ionisation and excitation as they continuously lose energy passing through matter. The proton mass, being approximately 2000 times larger than that of an electron, results in protons undergoing far less lateral scattering. As bremsstrahlung losses are inversely proportional to the square of the incoming particle mass, such losses are negligible for protons. Rather than the approximately linear relationship between energy and range, as observed for electrons (where range ≈ MeV/2 cm), proton range scales roughly with the square of the proton energy. As protons lose energy far more rapidly than electrons when traversing matter, energies of up to approximately 250 MeV are required to treat deep-seated tumours. Table 2.4 lists proton ranges for a number of beam energies.

A key difference in the characteristics of energy deposition with depth for protons as opposed to electrons is the appearance of a Bragg peak, shown in Fig. 2.25. This results from a reduced amount of lateral scattering and a sharp increase in stopping power (dE/dx) as protons slow down in a material (see Fig. 2.25B). The Bragg peak is ideally suited to radiotherapy, as the high-dose region is concentrated at depth, protecting both overlying and underlying normal tissue. The Bragg peak is also a characteristic of other heavy charged particle beams, such as carbon ions and pions.

TABLE 2.4 Proton Range Variation With Energy

Energy (MeV)	Range (cm)
60	3.1
100	7.7
150	15.8
200	26.0
250	37.9

Quoted CSDA range calculated using the PSTAR program.[1]

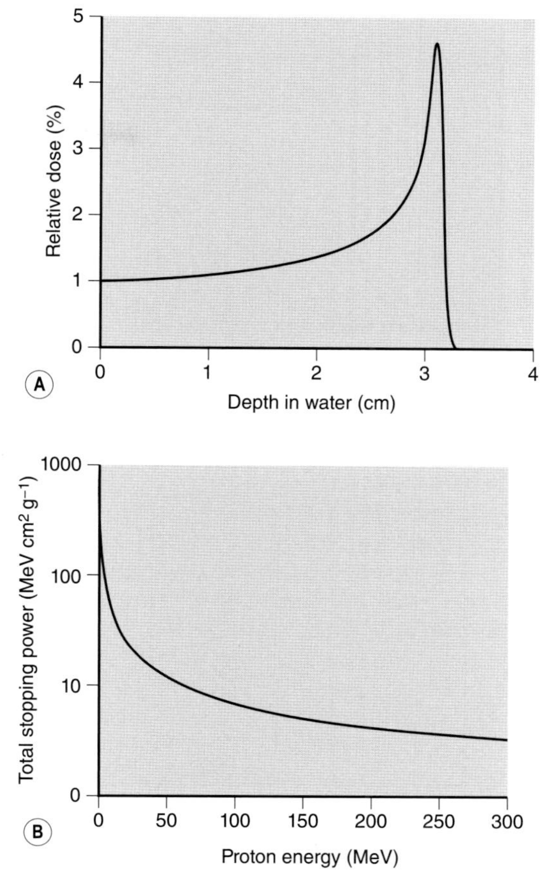

Fig. 2.25 (A) Bragg peak for 60-MeV protons in water, and (B) proton stopping power in water. Note how the shape of the stopping power curve is reflected in the observed depth-dose curve. (© Copyright by the U.S. Secretary of Commerce on behalf of the United States of America. All rights reserved. [From Berger et al.[1]])

Although interactions with atomic electrons is the dominant process by which clinical proton beams (50–250 MeV) lose energy and so deposit dose, an incident proton beam may also interact with the atomic nucleus through elastic or nonelastic scattering. In elastic scattering events, kinetic energy is passed from the incident proton, and the internal structure of the nucleus is unchanged. In nonelastic scattering, the nucleus may be fragmented or left in an excited state, in which case kinetic energy is not conserved. Charged particles such as secondary protons, which are alpha particles produced during these events, will deposit their energy close to the site of interaction, whereas neutrons and photons, being uncharged, may carry energy a significant distance away.

To deliver a required dose distribution over a defined target, the Bragg peak is spread out as described in Chapter 10.

Other Charged Particles

In addition to protons, heavier nuclei and other particles may offer potential advantages for radiotherapy because of the physical characteristics of their dose deposition in matter and their relative biological effectiveness (RBE). Beams of carbon ions and pions, in particular, have been applied clinically for radiotherapy.

To reach deep-seated tumours, the energies of heavy ion beams need to be significantly higher than those of protons. For example, although

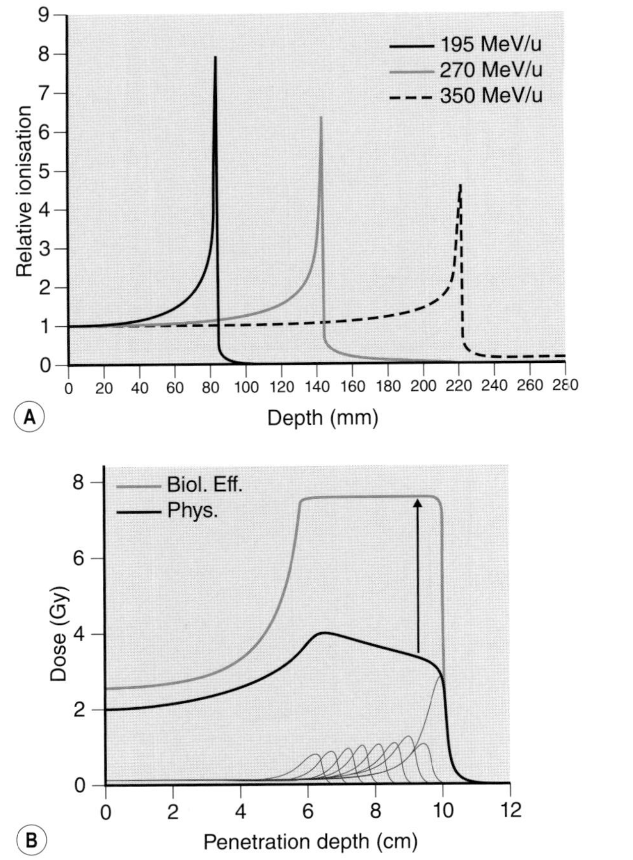

Fig. 2.26 (A) Monoenergetic Bragg peaks for carbon ions incident on water. Note the dose tail beyond the peak because of nuclear fragments. (B) Physical dose and biologically effective dose within a clinical target volume for 170-to-220-MeV carbon ions in water. Note the enhanced biological effect across the target region, resulting in preferential damage to tumour. (From M Krämer, GSI, Darmstadt. With permission.)

150-MeV protons have a range of approximately 16 cm in water, the same penetration depth for carbon ions requires a beam energy of close to 3600 MeV, or 300 MeV for each of the 12 nucleons in the ion.

Carbon ion beams have a significantly higher LET in the Bragg peak than in the plateau region. As with the clinical proton beams described in Chapter 10, the Bragg peak of carbon ion beams is spread out across the target, which leads to an increased radiobiological effect across the target region relative to the surrounding low-dose region. Hence, in addition to a lower physical dose, normal tissue is spared further because of a lower biological effect. The increased LET in the Bragg peak is a result of nuclear fragments being produced in collisions, which leads to a dose tail following the Bragg peak, illustrated in Fig. 2.26.

Emerging research into helium ion therapy is showing promise for deep-seated and complex tumours such as ependymomas.[8] Helium ions have higher mass and RBE than protons, and their reduced lateral scattering results in sharper dose gradients than protons. Although still in the early stages, initial findings indicate effectiveness of helium ion therapy against radioresistant tumours.

Pion beams have been used clinically to treat over 500 patients at a small number of centres worldwide. Pions are negatively charged particles with a mass approximately 15% that of a proton and a half-life of 26 ns (2.6×10^{-8} s). They can be produced by bombarding carbon or beryllium targets with protons. The potential advantage from these particles over alternatives is the star effect, which enhances the dose deposited in their Bragg peak as a result of their capture by atomic nuclei. This capture process causes the nucleus to become unstable and disintegrate into a number of fragments, each of which has a high LET and very short range in tissue.

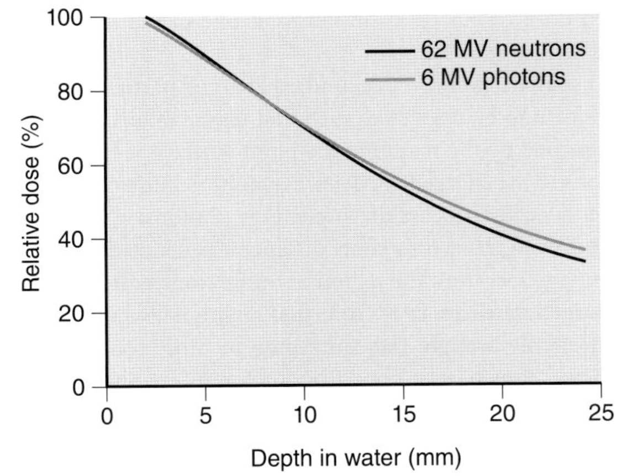

Fig. 2.27 Comparison of percentage depth dose in water at 150-cm source-to-surface distance for 62-MeV neutrons. (From the Clatterbridge Centre for Oncology NHS Foundation Trust: Douglas Cyclotron. With permission.)

Neutron Interactions

Clinical beams of fast neutrons, on the order of 60 MV, were the subject of particular interest during the 1970s and 1980s. Being uncharged, they show similar depth-dose characteristics to megavoltage photons (Fig. 2.27). However, they offer potential advantages for some tumours in causing a greater degree of irreparable DNA damage in targets, which have low oxygenation as a result of factors such as poor vascularity. Low-energy neutron beams, referred to as *thermal beams*, are of interest in their application to boron–neutron capture therapy. This treatment involves first depositing boron (^{10}B) in the tumour, using tumour-targeting compounds, and then applying an external beam of thermal neutrons. These neutrons are captured by boron nuclei within the tumour, creating ^{11}B, which subsequently disintegrates, releasing helium and lithium nuclei (^{4}He and ^{7}Li, respectively), with kinetic energies of 1.47 and 0.84 MeV, respectively. Being highly charged, these particles deposit their energy within a very short distance of the site of their release.

Aside from their therapeutic applications, fast neutrons are also produced in interactions involving high-energy photons and protons, as mentioned earlier. Fast neutrons lose energy primarily through elastic collisions with atomic nuclei. In the body, this readily produces knock-on protons through collisions with hydrogen, which travel only a short distance in tissue. The proportion of energy that neutrons lose through each collision decreases as the atomic number of the target material increases, with the average energy loss, *E*, being given by:

$$E/E_0 = 2\,mM/(m+M)^2 \qquad \textbf{(2.21)}$$

where E_0 is the incident neutron energy, m is the neutron mass (1.67×10^{-27} kg) and M is the mass of the target nucleus. Materials with a high hydrogen or other low atomic number content (e.g. lithium) are therefore the most effective in slowing down fast neutrons. Wall cladding with a high proportion of low atomic number material may be used in the maze of bunkers housing high-energy photon machines (≥15 MV) to rapidly slow fast neutrons produced by photon interactions (photonuclear interactions) in the photon target. Once thermalised, neutrons are captured by a nucleus (nonelastic interactions), for example:

$$\begin{aligned} n + {}^{1}H &\rightarrow {}^{2}H + \gamma[2.2\ \text{MeV}] \\ n + {}^{14}N &\rightarrow {}^{14}C + p[0.6\ \text{MeV}] \end{aligned} \qquad \textbf{(2.22)}$$

In the case of capture by hydrogen (^{1}H), this results in the release of a high-energy photon, which itself presents a potential radiation-shielding hazard.

REFERENCES

1. Berger M, Coursey J, Zucker A, Chang J. ESTAR, PSTAR, and ASTAR: computer programs for calculating stopping-power and range tables for electrons, protons, and helium ions (version 1.2.3). Gaithersburg, MD: National Institute of Standards and Technology; 2005. http://physics.nist.gov/Star.
2. IPEM (Institute of Physics and Engineering in Medicine). Catalogue of diagnostic x-ray spectra and other data. *IPEM report.* 1997;78.
3. Baker C, Peck K. Reconstruction of 6MV photon spectra from measured transmission including maximum energy estimation. *Phys Med Biol.* 1997;42:2041–2051.
4. Attix F. *Introduction to radiological physics and radiation dosimetry.* John Wiley & Sons Inc, London, UK; 1996.
5. Hubbell JH, Seltzer SM. Tables of x-ray mass attenuation coefficients and mass energy-absorption coefficients from 1keV to 20MeV for elements Z = 1 to 92 and 48 additional substances of dosimetric interest. *Natl Inst Stand Technol.* 1995. https://www.nist.gov/publications/tables-x-ray-mass-attenuation-coefficients-and-mass-energy-absorption-coefficients-1-0.
6. Berger MJ, Hubbell JH, Seltzer SM, et al. XCOM: photon cross sections database. *Natl Inst Stand Technol.* 2010. https://www.nist.gov/pml/xcom-photon-cross-sections-database.
7. *International Commission on Radiation Units and Measurements).* Washington, DC: ICRUICRU; 1980 Radiation quantities and units. ICRU Report No. 33.
8. Wickert R, Tessonnier T, Deng M, et al. Radiotherapy with helium ions has the potential to improve both endocrine and neurocognitive outcome in pediatric patients with ependymoma. *Cancers.* 2022; 14(23):5865.

FURTHER READING

Joint Working Party of the British Institute of Radiology and the Institution of Physics and Engineering in Medicine and Biology; Aird EGA, Burns JE, et al. Central axis depth dose data for use in radiotherapy: a survey of depth doses and related data measured in water or equivalent media. *Br J Radiol Suppl.* 1983;17:1–147.

Mayles P, Nahum A, Rosenwald J-C, eds. *Handbook of radiotherapy physics, theory and practice.* Taylor and Francis, Boca Raton, USA; 2007.

3

Radiation Detection and Measurement

Shakardokht Jafari

CHAPTER OUTLINE

INTRODUCTION

Detection of ionising radiation involves using the physical interaction between the radiation and the materials in a manner which renders the radiation perceptible through physical changes such as a temperature increase or decrease, an electrical current or charge release, colour changes or even biological and chemical changes.

Radiation is measured to quantify the energy released in the interaction and how much is deposited in the material. We refer to this as *absorbed dose*, and its measurement requires detailed knowledge of the physical interaction process which occurs between the radiation and the materials.

As with the measurement of any physical quantity, it is essential to have a standard unit of measurement so that measurement devices can be calibrated and so that measurements are consistent and accurate comparisons can be made.

In the first section of this chapter, two simple and widely used radiation detectors are described: the gas detector and the scintillation detector. Radiation dose measurement and standardisation is then described based upon the simple air cavity ionisation chamber.

Although the air-based ionisation chamber is the primary measurement technique, the advantages and disadvantages of quantifying absorbed dose with other detectors, including liquid-filled ionisation chambers, are also described. For effective radiotherapy, accurate measurement of absorbed dose under well-controlled conditions at a single point is essential. However, it is also essential to have in vivo dosimetry during treatment and, with the prevalence of dynamically produced radiotherapy delivery, to have patient-specific checks as part of treatment preparation. So lastly, devices for in vivo dose measurement and the distribution of radiation dose are described.

RADIATION DETECTION

Common types of devices that are used in the detection and measurement of radiation in radiotherapy are based upon gas and solid-state interactions. Doserates and dose levels vary considerably in radiotherapy, from low-level radiation protection doserates to high-doserate teletherapy beams. There are also a range of doserates in treatments using radioisotopes, and in many cases, the spatial resolution of the detector can be of significant importance where there are steep dose gradients, such as in electron and proton beams as well as brachytherapy dose distributions.

The basic principles behind gas and solid-state radiation detection can be appreciated by considering gas amplification devices and scintillation devices.

Gas Amplification Devices

In ionisation chambers filled with gas, including air, the ion pairs produced by particles crossing the air cavity are separated, collected and measured such that the charge collected equates to the number of ion pairs produced. A polarising voltage is placed across the electrodes of the chamber in a manner sufficient to separate the ions and direct them to the electrodes of the device. Any kinetic energy gained by ions as they move towards an electrode is continually removed by collision interactions with other air molecules, but the ions do not gain sufficient energy to create additional ionisation. If the polarising voltage is increased, the charge detected may rise slightly as ion recombination is overcome, but the level will rapidly reach saturation and no further increase in collected charge will occur, as shown in Fig. 3.1.

In gas amplification devices, air in the detector chamber is replaced by a gas, the pressure of which is greatly reduced, thereby allowing any ions produced in it to travel much farther before interacting with atoms of the gas. If the electric field across the device is sufficiently high, ions can gain sufficient energy themselves to cause further ionisation of the gas, producing additional ion pairs. This leads to an increase in the charge collected. As the polarising voltage is increased further, these additional ions may also gain sufficient energy to cause further ionisation, leading to a cascade effect that produces further increase or amplification of the charge, a process that can be repeated many times, as illustrated in Fig. 3.2A. The net result is that the detected pulse of the charge is proportional to the amount of ionisation produced by the radiation but is amplified many times. The size of the pulse is determined by both the number of ions initially generated by the radiation and the amount of amplification that takes place. This, in turn,

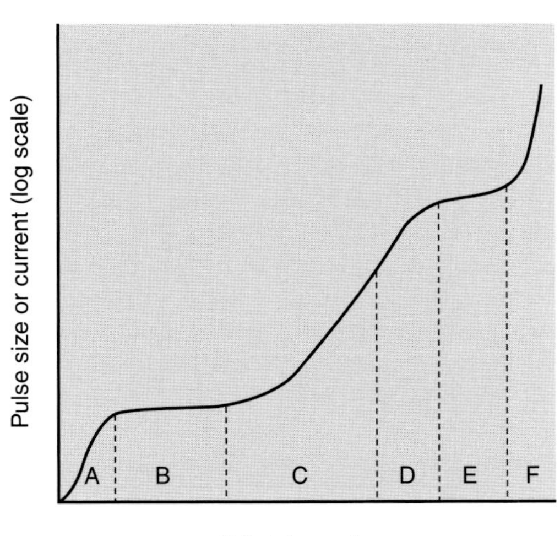

Fig. 3.1 Detector pulse size or current as a function of applied polarising potential. Region A is dominated by recombination of ions. Ionisation chambers operate in region B, proportional counters in region C and Geiger counters in region E. Region D represents transition between proportional and Geiger regions, and region F illustrates continuous discharge and electrical breakdown.

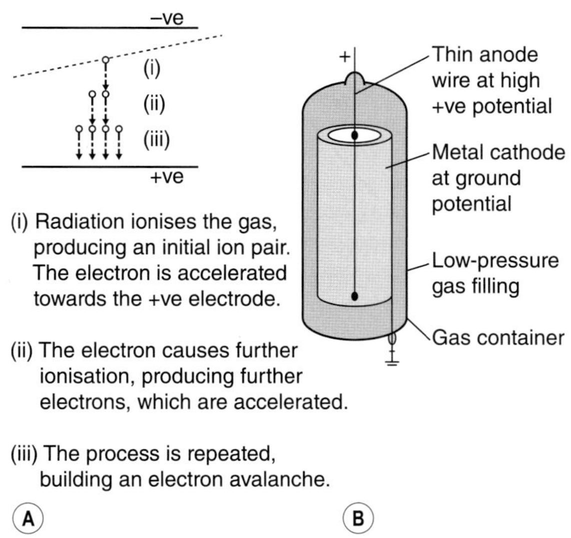

Fig. 3.2 Schematic diagrams showing (A) the gas amplification process and (B) a typical Geiger counter.

is dependent upon the applied voltage across the chamber, as shown in Fig. 3.1. Gains of many orders of magnitude are possible, and radiation detectors that use this principle are known as *proportional counters*.

If the voltage across the device is further increased, proportionality between the initial signal and pulse size starts to break down as the size of the charge avalanche increases. Eventually, the whole chamber volume becomes involved. Ions reaching the electrodes may interact and produce further ions which continue the process. The result is a charge pulse that is determined not by the number of ions initially created but by the design of the electronics of the detector. Each pulse is of the same height and causes a temporary discharge of the polarising voltage. This temporary reduction in voltage immediately after a pulse allows the counter to recover and any remaining ions in it to be absorbed. Introduction of special materials known as *quenching agents* into the gas speeds up this residual ion removal. Such detector devices are known as *Geiger counters*.

A typical Geiger counter detector is shown schematically in Fig. 3.2B and consists of a small, cylindrical metal tube that forms the negative electrode, with a thin-wire positive electrode running along the axis of the cylinder. The structure is sealed to enclose the low-pressure gas, typically a mixture of argon and ethanol or neon and chlorine. The structure can be designed as either a side-window device (i.e. where radiation enters through the side of the device) for general radiation detection or an end-window device (where radiation enters through the end cap of the device) for beta particle detection, the latter having a thin mica window to allow passage of beta particles. The efficiency of a Geiger counter is high for beta particles but is very low for x-rays and gamma rays where the reliance is upon interaction with the wall of the device to generate secondary electrons that pass into the chamber cavity.

Each detected event results in an electric pulse, the size of which is independent of the number of ions initially causing the event but which lasts for a few microseconds. The chamber then has to recover for a few tens of microseconds, a period known as the *dead time*, during which it will not respond to any further ionisation stimulus. Because the pulse size does not reflect the number of ions initiating the event, the counter cannot distinguish between different types of radiation. Further, the dead time has implications for use in high-intensity or pulsed radiation fields. As the radiation intensity increases, so does the rate of events and the chance of missing pulses

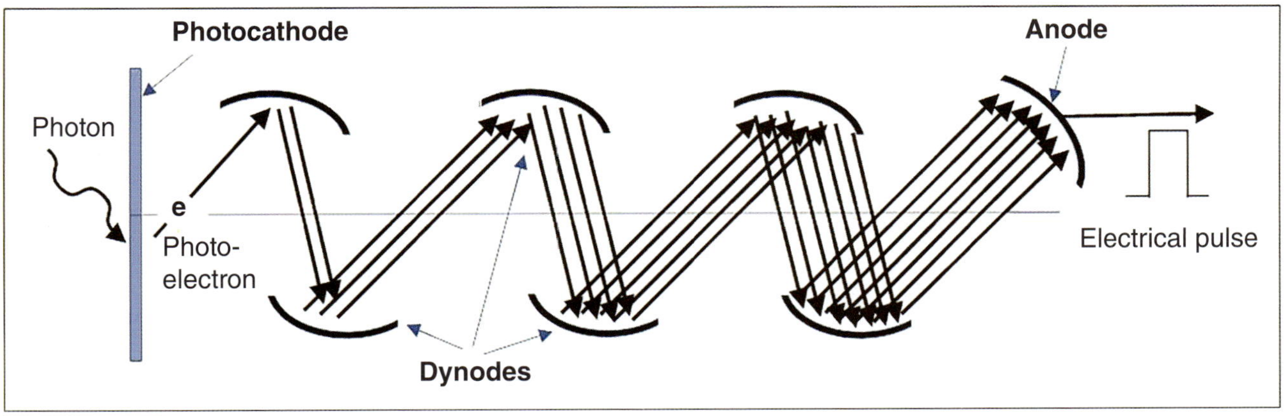

Fig. 3.3 The principles of a Photomultiplier Tube, demonstrating transformation of an incident photon into an electrical pulse.

because of the extended dead time, resulting in underrecording. Similarly, in the pulsed radiation field of a linear accelerator where the pulse lengths are less than the dead time of the detector, the most that a Geiger counter will record will be one count per pulse, regardless of the actual radiation intensity. Hence Geiger counters cannot be used to measure the intensity of a linear accelerator beam, and great care must be exercised when using them to monitor radiation levels around a linear accelerator installation.

The pulse height from a Geiger counter varies only slowly with increasing voltage, as shown in Fig. 3.1, making the device relatively insensitive to small changes. At higher voltages, however, the electric field strength can be sufficient in itself to ionise the gas, resulting in continued electrical discharge, or breakdown.

Scintillation Devices

Solid-state materials, such as thallium-doped sodium iodide, are known as *scintillator materials*, which are a form of fluorescent material that emits light when irradiated. Scintillator materials are transparent to the light emitted, and so photon interactions cause short flashes of light in the material. The amount of light emitted is proportional to the energy deposited in the crystal. These short flashes of light can be detected by a *photomultiplier tube*, a device that converts very low levels of light into measurable electrical pulses. Sodium iodide is hygroscopic and is housed within a container that encompasses the material, prevents ingress of water vapour and reflects light back into the crystal—the inner surface of the container being covered in a reflective coating of titanium dioxide or magnesium oxide. One surface is coupled onto the face of the photomultiplier tube either directly or via a specially constructed light guide. An optical coupling gel is used whenever two material faces are coupled together to reduce scattering caused by any tiny surface irregularities.

The inner surface of the front face of the photomultiplier tube, called the *photocathode*, has a material deposit that causes electrons to be emitted when subjected to visible light. These are called *photoelectrons*, and they are accelerated along a series of electrodes, called *dynodes*, by an electric field between each dynode (Fig. 3.3). When an electron hits a dynode, it causes emission of other electrons, which in turn are accelerated towards the next dynode. Eventually, the avalanche of electrons reaches the anode, from where an electrical pulse is extracted. The electrical pulse from the photomultiplier is proportional to the amount of light hitting the photocathode, which in turn is proportional to the energy deposited by the initial radiation interaction in the scintillator crystal. Thus a 300-keV gamma ray will, on average, produce a pulse that is twice as large as that produced by a 150-keV gamma ray, provided that in both cases the total energy of the gamma ray is absorbed in the crystal. The magnitude of the pulse is referred to as the *pulse height*.

A pulse-height analyser is a device that has a number of counters, each representing one channel. Each channel counts the pulses that occur within a narrow band of pulse heights. For example, the channel set to detect between 290 keV and 310 keV would detect the 300-keV gamma rays and not the 150-keV gamma rays.

Successive channels are set to count increasingly larger pulses. Hence small pulses will appear in the lower channels and large pulses will be counted in the higher channels. When a scintillation detector is connected to a pulse-height analyser, the counts per channel represent the spectrum of energies deposited in the scintillator crystal. When measuring monoenergetic radiation such as gamma rays, those interaction events that result in all the gamma ray energy being absorbed in the crystal will have similar pulse heights and will be counted together in a narrow series of channels that represent this photon energy level. This is referred to as the *photopeak*.

Interactions that result in less energy being deposited in the crystal—for example, the detection of Compton-scattered photons—will be counted in the wide range of channels below the photopeak channels, as shown in Fig. 3.4. Because the positions of peaks in the spectrum represent specific energy levels, scintillation counters are able to differentiate between different energies of incident photons. By matching measured energy levels and their rates of decay against

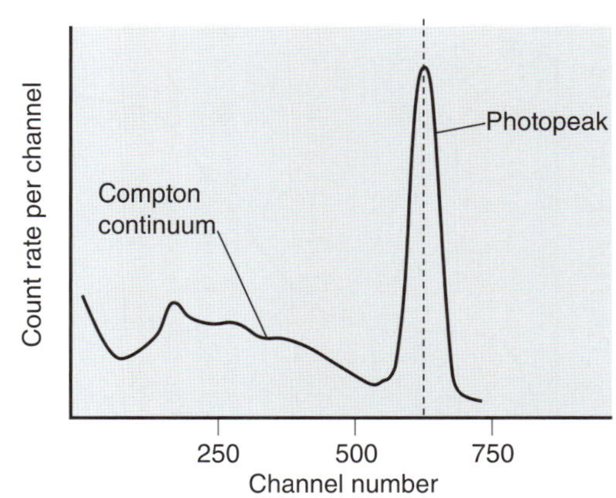

Fig. 3.4 Typical pulse-height spectrum from a gamma source that emits a single-energy gamma ray. The channel number equates to the energy deposited in the detector and the position of the photopeak is dependent on the energy of the emitted gamma ray. The width of the photopeak is dependent on the energy resolution of the detector system.

tabulated energies of emissions and half-lives of known radioactive materials, specific radioactive substances can be identified in any given sample. This process is called *gamma spectroscopy*.

The pulse from a sodium iodide/photomultiplier detector has a pulse length of a few microseconds. Additional signals that occur within this period combine and appear as an enlarged signal. These will fall outside the main photopeak channels. The chance of two interactions occurring within the short period will increase when the radiation intensity increases and thus the count rate increases. This results in an underestimate of the true radiation intensity. Some plastic scintillators can have much shorter pulse lengths and can be constructed with large surface areas. These can be used to measure higher radiation intensities or to detect and measure radiation distributed over a large area.

Also, small plastic scintillators can be connected to distant photomultiplier tubes via long fibre-optic light guides and used to measure dose distributions in radiotherapy.[1] The high sensitivity of the device allows the use of tiny detectors that are of particular use in the measurement of rapidly varying spatial intensities, such as in the penumbra of megavoltage beams or in the measurement of distributions from radioactive eye plaques.[2] More recently, tomographic reconstruction techniques have been applied to the optical signals from liquid scintillators to reconstruct full three-dimensional dose distribution maps around brachytherapy sources and eye plaques.[3]

Ideal Air Ionisation Chamber

The stable part of the gas amplification response, region B in Fig. 3.1, can be used for the collection of ion pairs. Air, as a readily available medium with its density only affected by pressure and temperature, which can be easily measured, made such a device very attractive and expedient to use for the measurement of dose, thus not only detecting the radiation but also quantifying it. The use of air ionisation is attributed to early work of Pierre Curie.[4]

The challenge of using air ionisation to measure dose is to know the interaction processes, to know the energy related to absorbed dose to the air, and to ensure that all the relevant electrons produced from the ionisation can be measured. The latter represents a physical challenge for the design of the ionisation chamber with which to make the measurement.

The essential aspects of such a physical device are illustrated in Fig. 3.5. In the following sections describing the accurate measurement of absorbed dose, all these aspects and how they are addressed are described.

Proton and Ion Beam Detection

In principle, the same detection systems that are used in x-ray and electron beams can be used for detection of proton fluence, charge or

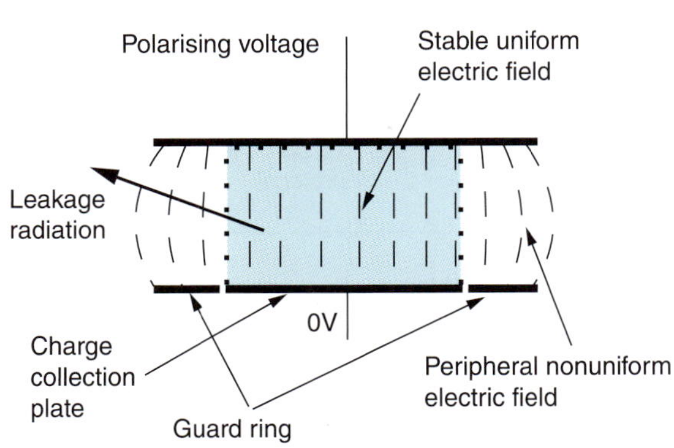

Fig. 3.5 Essential aspects of a free ionisation chamber.

proton dose, albeit with caution and knowledge of their limitations in proton and heavier clinical beams.

Certain instruments, such as scintillation counters or silicon- and germanium-based solid-state detectors, are single-particle detectors. These are count-rate limited and unable to measure the fluence required at clinical dose rates, which is around 10^9 protons per minute. Detection and measurement using ionisation provides a wide dynamic dose range suitable for most clinical conditions.

The energy dependence of dose measurement of protons and other heavy charged particles is known as *Bragg peak quenching* or simply *low-energy underresponse*. This is because of the intensely ionising proton tracks at low energy, which saturate detector response. The magnitude of the underresponse depends on the mechanism of measurement of a particular detector (e.g. film, thermoluminescent dosimeter (TLD), polymer gels, Fricke gels or solutions).

Ionisation chambers, usually air filled, are considered the gold standard in particle therapy relative measurements because they have considerable dose-rate range, insignificant change in response with particle energy and little degradation with accumulated radiation dose. Some solid-state detectors have been developed which demonstrate minimal underresponse, such as microdiamond detectors which are also used in heavy ion beams. Devices for rapid measurement of the spread-out Bragg peak (SOBP) (see Chapter 10), depth doses using multilayer ion chambers, or Faraday plates combined with absorbers or moveable parallel plate ion chambers in water tanks are commercially available.

The proton range, and hence energy, is affected by other absorbers, such as detector windows or casings, and these need to be compensated for by calculation or estimation from tables. The use of scintillation detectors for charged particles requires consideration of Birk's law, which describes a nonlinear response with proton energy and an energy threshold.

Atmospheric air in ionisation chambers is particularly fortuitous, as the stopping-power ratio between water and air is relatively constant over a large energy range and only deviates at very small energies which are not clinically relevant. For dose measurement, air ionisation devices require correction for the standard temperature, standard atmospheric pressure and air humidity. However, some centres have adopted nitrogen-filling gas for in-line beam monitors. Nitrogen, unlike air, is not electronegative, and free electrons are far less likely to attach to nitrogen molecules and thus will arrive at the chamber anode significantly quicker and more efficiently. This is particularly important when monitoring rapidly changing beam pulses from a synchrotron or synchrocyclotron.

FLASH proton therapy involves the delivery of large dose fractions, at ultrahigh dose rates (UHDRs) of >40 Gy/s, within a fraction of a second. This poses considerable challenges for conventional in-beam monitors and quality control devices. To reduce excessive recombination effects, ionisation chambers used in reference and daily dosimetry checks of proton fields are operated at much higher bias potentials. This provides a strong electric field with which to maintain collection efficiency. Parallel plate ion chambers with electrode gaps of less than 1 mm have been shown to require much smaller corrections than larger cylindrical chambers. However, operating at higher than recommended bias potentials may lead to charge multiplication and breakdown.

Nonionising devices, which are dose-rate independent and suitable for monitoring UHDRs, include Faraday cups, 'noninterceptive' resonator detectors and secondary emission monitors (SEMs). Faraday cups, measuring beam charge, have been used to calibrate in-beam monitor chambers. Calorimeters,[5] such as the graphite calorimeter at the UK National Physical Laboratory, can be used to provide absolute proton dosimetry and are used to cross-calibrate reference parallel plate ion chambers. Passive detectors such as TLDs, alanine and radiochromic films (see the 'Alternative Dose Measurement Systems' section) may also be used in UHDR measurements, mainly for periodic checks, with corrections for Bragg underresponse.

MEASUREMENT AND STANDARDISATION OF DOSE

The interaction of photons in matter results in energy transfer to matter via the emission of charged particles resulting in ionisation and the excitation of atoms. The energy manifests as heat or as some form of internal potential energy increase of electrons and atoms.

Systems detect radiation using parts of this energy pathway. Some systems seek to determine the energy deposited in matter by measuring the temperature rise, known as *calorimetry*. Other detection systems utilise the chemical changes generated, known as *chemical dosimetry*, or utilise long-lived excited electron states, such as in thermoluminescent dosimetry.

Still other systems utilise the ionisation produced by charged particles to measure the energy transferred to those particles, known as *ionisation dosimetry*.

This section describes the systems adopted for the measurement and standardisation of absorbed dose that underpin clinical practice. Later sections consider other methods of radiation detection and measurement, including other systems for measuring absorbed dose.

Dose Standards

It is of particular importance in radiotherapy to ensure that a dose of radiation delivered in any one treatment centre is consistent over time and with that delivered in other centres, this being a central part of ongoing quality control. It also allows direct comparison of treatment techniques and results between centres and is essential for multicentre clinical trials to be effective. Consistency of measurements on a national or international basis is achieved through a process of central standardisation, with all measurements being traceable to an accepted national or international standard. In the United Kingdom, the National Physical Laboratory (NPL) houses the instruments and radiation sources that are used to determine the national standard for absorbed dose measurement. These instruments are purely laboratory instruments that are impractical for routine use within radiotherapy departments. Great care has been taken to provide radiation sources with the comparable energy spectrum, doserate and intensities to clinical radiation beams and radioactivity sources. This includes utilising filtration and clinical treatment machines.

The UK national standard instruments for the standardisation of absorbed dose are of two types:

1. Calorimeters for megavoltage photon and electron beams. Calorimeters are used to provide direct determination of absorbed dose.[6]
2. Free air ionisation chambers for lower-energy photon beams from x-ray generators operating at up to 300 kV.[7,8] These provide a direct determination of air kerma from which the absorbed dose to water can be calculated.

Similar national standards laboratories exist in other countries.

Traceability of Measurement

To ensure consistency of dose measurement between centres, it is necessary for measurements to be traceable back to the appropriate national standard. This is achieved through a hierarchical arrangement, shown schematically in Fig. 3.6. Dose measuring instruments within individual hospitals, referred to as *field instruments*, are used routinely to measure the dose delivered by radiotherapy treatment units. In the United Kingdom, these are calibrated annually against a secondary standard instrument. The secondary standard instruments are reserved solely for this purpose and are not used to make routine dose measurements. Guidelines on the choice of dosimeter systems for use as secondary standard instruments have been produced by the Institute of Physics and Engineering in Medicine (IPEM).[9] In the United Kingdom, each secondary standard instrument is calibrated every three years by the NPL standards laboratory by comparing the response against the national reference-level instruments, which in turn are compared annually with the national standard instruments. The national standards are themselves compared at intervals with equivalent standard instruments developed by standards laboratories in other countries.

Radiotherapy treatment units, such as linear accelerators and kV therapy units, have in-built dose measuring instruments, known as

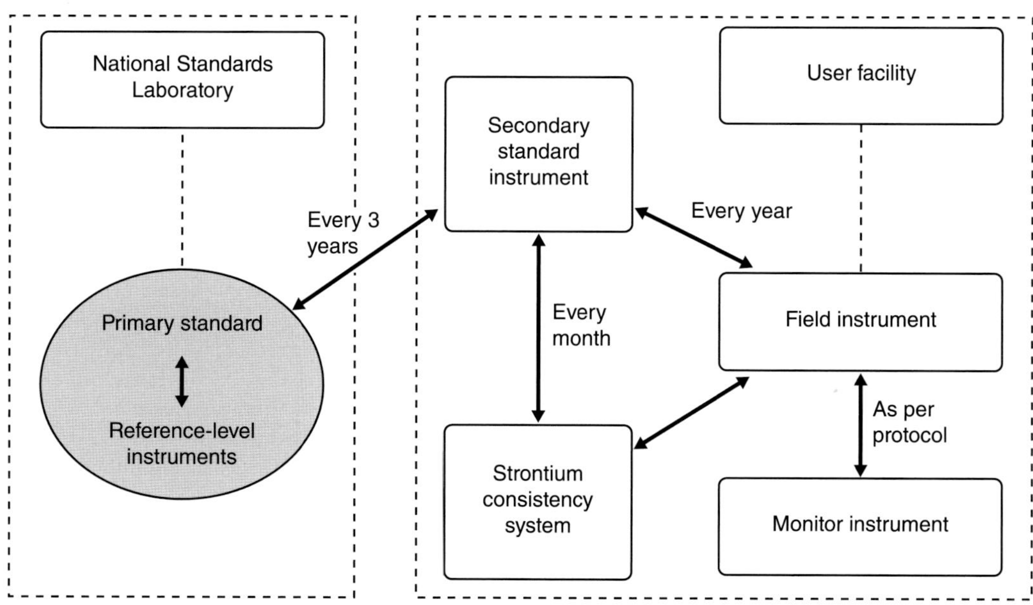

Fig. 3.6 Traceability to the national standard is assured through a chain of intercomparisons, some of which are carried out at the National Standards Laboratory and others in local radiation beams. Between intercomparisons, calibration is assured using a consistency system.

monitor chambers, that monitor and determine the amount of dose delivered. Field instruments are used to calibrate these monitor chambers so that each monitor unit delivers a known amount of radiation. These field instruments may be used to determine not only the amount of radiation delivered but also the pattern of deposition of energy within matter by measuring dose at different points within the matter. They may also be used to calibrate other dose measuring equipment designed for special-purpose measurements, such as in vivo dosimeters.

For the transfer of calibration from instrument to instrument down the chain to be reliable, the method of calibration must be strictly controlled. This is achieved by the adoption of calibration protocols which specify:

- The basis for the standard dose measurement
- The instrumentation and methods for transfer of dose to field instruments by a series of intercomparisons, including specification of any equipment used and any conditions that must exist for the intercomparison to be reliable
- Instructions for use of the calibrated dosimeter in routine practice

Each protocol is specific for an energy range and type of radiation. The protocols for calibration of field instruments are covered in a later section.

Standard Calorimeter

In situations where all the absorbed energy is manifest solely as heat (i.e. no energy is lost to form new chemicals or stored in excited electron states), the relationship between radiation dose and change in temperature is given by:

$$\text{Dose (Gy)} = C \times \delta T \tag{3.1}$$

where C is the specific heat of the irradiated matter (the amount of energy needed to raise the temperature of the unit mass of a substance through 1°C, expressed in units of J $kg^{-1}°C^{-1}$) and δT is the change in temperature in degrees Celsius. Eq. (3.1) assumes no loss of heat to the surrounding environment or structures. Note that the specific heat may also be expressed in calories rather than joules, in which case an additional numerical multiplier of 4.18 is necessary in the aforementioned equation.

The rise in temperature is extremely small (e.g. a beam of x-rays delivering a dose of 5 gray (Gy) to soft tissue causes a temperature rise of only 10^{-3}°C). Such a small rise in temperature is very difficult to measure accurately, and extreme precautions are necessary to prevent heat loss outside the irradiated vessel.

The national standard calorimeter is based on the irradiation of a known mass of graphite (the core of the NPL high-energy photon calorimeter measures approximately 20 mm in diameter by 3 mm in thickness) within a graphite phantom. The design of the calorimeter, a photograph and schematic drawing of which are shown in Fig. 3.7, has the core shielded by three jackets, each separated by a vacuum to minimise heat loss. Temperature measurements are carried out using thermistors embedded in the graphite core, the resistances of which change with temperature. In practice, because the amount of heat energy lost from the core to surrounding structures is not negligible and may be difficult to determine, the rise in temperature resulting from irradiation is compared with the rise in temperature produced by heating the core using a known amount of electrical energy, allowing absorbed dose to be determined directly instead of using Eq. (3.1).

Graphite has the advantage of having no chemical defect (i.e. all the absorbed energy appears as heat) and a specific heat that is one-fifth that of soft tissue or water, thereby producing greater changes in temperature per unit dose. The absorbed dose to water may be calculated from the absorbed dose to graphite using the correction factors determined by Nutbrown and colleagues.[10]

Measurement by calorimetry is largely independent of whether the radiation is delivered continuously or in pulses and of the pulse intensity. It is therefore ideal for measuring radiation from

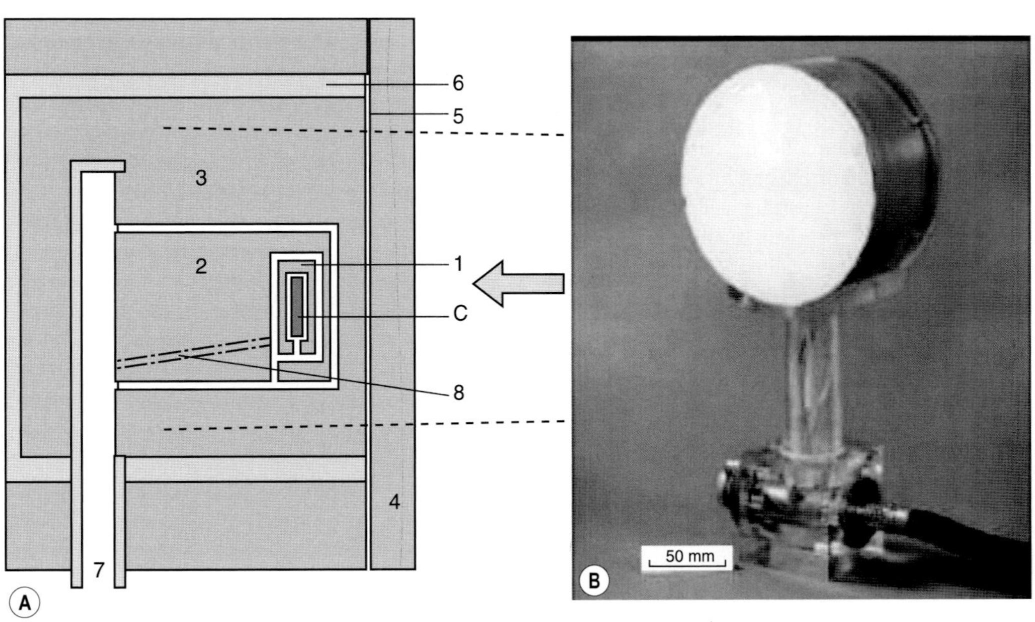

Fig. 3.7 Simplified schematic drawing (A) and photograph (B) of the national standard high-energy photon calorimeter, showing the graphite core *(C)* surrounded by three insulating graphite jackets *(1, 2, and 3)*. The entire device is housed within a Perspex evacuation vessel *(6)* which has a thin aluminised mylar front window *(5)* and which is evacuated via a port *(7)*. A plate *(4)* suitable for the energy to be measured can be added to the front face. Electrical connections to the core pass through the device *(8)*. (Modified from DuSautoy AR. The UK primary standard calorimeter for photon beam absorbed dose measurement. *Phys Med Biol.* 1996;41:137–151.)

TABLE 3.1 Photon Beam Qualities, Used for Therapy-Level Absorbed Dose to Water Calibrations

Beam Quality ($TPR_{20/10}$)	Equivalent Beam Energy	Reference Depth (cm)
0.568	60 Co	5
0.621	4 MV	5
0.670	6 MV	5
0.717	8 MV	5
0.746	10 MV	5
0.758	12 MV	7
0.779	16 MV	7
0.790	19 MV	7

The quantity $TPR_{20/10}$ is the tissue-to-phantom ratio at depths of 20 cm and 10 cm, respectively, used by standards laboratories as the specifier of beam quality. A number of standards laboratories have developed water calorimeters that directly measure the rise in temperature of a known mass of water. These avoid uncertainties with the national standard instrument in moving from a graphite phantom to a water phantom. Such instruments have been used to confirm doses specified using other systems of dosimetry for photon and charged particle beams and are being increasingly developed as national dosimetry standards.[11–15]

constant-output sources, such as cobalt units, as well as pulsed output from linear accelerators. The pattern of temperature rise (from irradiation) and fall (from leakage of heat away from the core) may be used to determine both the peak and mean dose rates for pulsed radiation sources.

Because the standard calorimeter cannot be used in a water tank, a number of specially constructed ionisation chambers termed *reference standard instruments* are calibrated annually against the graphite calorimeter in a common graphite phantom. These reference instruments are then used to calibrate the secondary standard instruments using a water phantom. The calibration factor provided for each secondary standard instrument is specific to a stated beam quality and depth of measurement, the latter being important as the spectral content of a radiation beam changes with depth. Table 3.1 shows those photon beam qualities at which calibration factors based on absorbed dose to water, as determined by the standard graphite calorimeter, are provided by the NPL.[16,17] When used as a basis for calibration in a radiation beam in the user's department, the beam quality for that beam must be determined and the appropriate calibration factor obtained by interpolating from the results provided by the standards laboratory. Calibrations in megavoltage photon beams are carried out at the depths shown in Table 3.1, which are beyond the range of contaminating electrons in the radiation beam that have been ejected from the head of the treatment machine.[18]

Free Air Chamber

The free air chamber is the primary standard instrument for kV beams and is shown schematically in Fig. 3.8. The free air chamber effectively determines the energy transferred to secondary electrons as a result of interactions of a photon beam within a defined mass of air (i.e. air kerma (k_a)).

A well-defined beam of radiation, confined by external collimators, is incident upon a volume of air located between metal plates that act as electrodes. The radiation causes ionisation of the air, resulting in electrons being ejected. These electrons, in turn, cause further excitation and ionisation as they interact with air molecules: the electrons lose kinetic energy with each interaction and will travel an irregular,

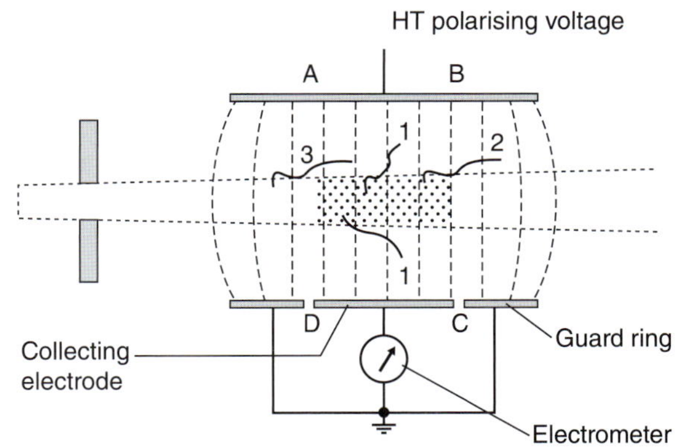

Fig. 3.8 The free air ionisation chamber. Irradiation of the mass of air shown shaded, defined by the cross-sectional area of the radiation beam and the length of the collecting electrode, results in emission of electrons that lose their kinetic energy by ionisation of air. Those ions created within the region ABCD are collected and measured.

tortuous path until they come to rest. Each ejected Compton electron or photoelectron can produce several hundred ion pairs. An essential requirement of the free air chamber is that the electrons produced by photon interactions lose all their kinetic energy in air and do not reach the metal electrodes. This requirement determines the minimum separation between the metal electrodes, and the overall size of the chamber. For example, measurement of x-rays generated at 200 kV will require a separation of at least 20 cm.

A potential difference, the polarising voltage, is applied between the metal electrodes. This causes positively and negatively charged ions produced in the air to separate, such that positive ions will move towards the negative potential plate while electrons will move towards the other positive plate. All ions of one charge sign are collected on one electrode, termed the *collecting electrode*. The charge reaching this electrode is measured; from this measurement, the number of ions produced may be calculated because the charge carried by each electron is constant (equal to 1.602×10^{-19} C). The average energy expended by electrons in creating an ion pair that is allowing for energy lost in exciting atoms as well as energy lost in ionising them is well determined from experimental work. Hence, because the number of ions may be determined using the free air chamber and the average energy necessary to produce each one is known, the total energy transferred to secondary electrons by photon interactions can be calculated.

Fig. 3.8 shows the physical arrangement. The metal plate that forms the electrode which carries the high-tension (HT) polarising voltage runs the full length of the chamber, whereas the other plate has the collector electrode as the central part only, separated and electrically isolated from adjacent metal plates called *guard rings*, which are held at the same electrical potential as the collector electrode. This arrangement ensures that the electric field within the region of the collector electrode is uniform and perpendicular to that electrode. Any ions produced in air within the region ABCD on the diagram will be collected on the collector electrode, whereas any ions produced outside this region will be collected on the guard rings and will not be included in the measurement.

Proton Beam Dose Standard

There is no UK code for the measurement of absorbed dose with proton beams, but at the time of this writing, an IPEM document, 'Code of Practice for Proton Dosimetry', is due to be published. Although mainly intended for scanned beams, it also includes passively scattered beams.

The primary standard will be a portable graphite calorimeter with a transfer ion chamber planned to be the Roos chamber, which is a parallel plate design, as shown in Figs. 3.10 and 3.13B, and which has the same dimensions as the calorimeter graphite measurement core. The measurement results will be converted to dose to water using stopping-power ratios and depth displacement factors.[5] In this way the resultant dose uncertainty will approach that achieved in clinical x-ray dosimetry.

Currently, the International Atomic Energy Agency (IAEA) TRS 398 Code of Practice,[19] which is a dose to water based on cobalt-60, is being used with factors for a particular ion chamber along with mean proton energy. This code provides correction factors for all commonly available thimble and parallel plate ion chambers at specified measurement depths in water. In the United Kingdom, the cobalt-60 calibrations are traced back to the NPL via the local secondary standard dose meter.

The code uses the most up-to-date data on proton interactions, such as stopping powers, the energy to produce ionisation in air and perturbation corrections. Some guidance is also offered on ion chamber recombination calculations assuming pulsed beams and polarity corrections. This code estimates that the combined uncertainty for proton and carbon beam measurements under reference conditions is 2.3% and 3.4%, respectively. For proton beams, this is approaching the uncertainty of 1.5% achieved with photon beams.

There is no international reference standard for absorbed dose. In the early days of proton therapy, it was a good practice to seek independent checks through dosimetry intercomparisons between new and existing clinical centres. This ensured uniformity of procedure if not absolute dose.

Usually, absolute or actual patient dose is measured in the middle of an SOBP (see Chapter 10). Although in most clinical cases the SOBP dose curve is quite uniform, there may be a slight ripple effect, and it is important to sample the average beam dose, avoiding the peaks and troughs. This is described in the provisional IPEM Code of Practice for scanned and passively scattered proton beams.

Absolute dosimetry for FLASH proton beams is also under development.[20]

PRACTICAL IONISATION CHAMBERS

The aforementioned primary standard instruments are complex, sophisticated and sensitive and are unsuitable for routine use within a hospital environment where small, relatively robust, simple instrumentation is needed.

One such instrument is the ionisation chamber.

Bragg-Gray Cavity Theory

The absorbed dose within any medium cannot generally be measured directly and so a surrogate has to be used. Ionisation chamber dosimetry is based upon replacing a small volume of the medium by an air cavity within which the ionisation of air by radiation can be measured and from which the dose to the medium can be determined.

When a medium is irradiated uniformly by electrons, the fluence of electrons (i.e. the energy carried across unit cross-sectional areas) will be the same at all points within the medium. If a small air cavity is introduced of a size such that it does not perturb the electron fluence (i.e. does not introduce changes to the energy spectrum or number of electrons), the fluence of electrons in the air is the same as in the medium, and the cavity is termed a *Bragg-Gray cavity*. Under these conditions the energy per unit mass (absorbed dose) imparted to the air (D_a) is given by:

$$D_a = J_a W \tag{3.2}$$

where J_a is the ionisation produced per unit mass of air and W is the average energy lost by the *electrons per ion pair formed in the air*. If the air is now to be replaced by the medium, *the energy* per unit mass imparted to the medium (D_m) would equal the absorbed dose to air multiplied by the electron mass stopping power for the medium divided by that for air $(S/\rho)^m_a$ (averaged over the energy spectrum of the electrons) and is given by:

$$D_m = J_a W (S/\rho)^m_a \tag{3.3}$$

This is the basic equation governing the use of ionisation chambers in the dosimetry of electron beams. For other charged particle beams, the stopping-power ratio for those particles must be used.

Where the medium is irradiated by a photon beam, photon interactions produce secondary electrons which cause ionisation within the air cavity. Provided that interactions of photons with air molecules are negligible such that all electrons crossing the air cavity arise as secondary electrons from within the medium, and provided that the aforementioned conditions relating to constancy of electron fluence are met, the air volume can be regarded as a Bragg-Gray cavity. The aforementioned Eq. (3.3) still holds.

In practice, when using ionisation chambers, the air volume is enclosed by a wall of material that differs slightly from both air and the medium. The construction of the chamber may introduce perturbations both to the fluence of electrons crossing the air cavity and to the photon beam itself. A wall of infinitesimally small thickness may be considered as having no impact on either, such that the chamber is effectively an air cavity within the medium. As the wall increases in thickness, an increasing percentage of secondary electrons crossing the air volume will be from the wall rather than the medium until, in the extreme, all electrons crossing the air volume originate from within the wall. In this situation the electron fluence across the air volume is the same as the fluence within the wall, and the dose to the wall (D_w) is given by:

$$D_w = J_a W (S/r)^w_a \tag{3.4}$$

Assuming the photon field is not perturbed by the presence of the chamber, the dose deposited by photons in the medium is related to that deposited in the chamber wall and is given by:

$$D_m = D_w (\mu/\rho)^m_w \tag{3.5}$$

where $(\mu/\rho)^m_w$ is the ratio of the mass absorption coefficient for the medium divided by that for the chamber wall.

The conditions for this equation to be strictly valid are not met in practice. For measurement of charged particle beams, the fluence of particles may vary with depth and the introduction of the chamber may cause perturbations to this fluence. In measurement of photon beams, the wall of the chamber may be insufficient to stop electrons from outside it reaching the air volume, and the wall of the chamber differs from the medium in its attenuation and scattering of photons. In the UK Codes of Practice used to measure absolute dose, correction factors are tabulated to be included in dose calculations. These can be energy dependent and account for differences in materials from water and the perturbation effect of chambers.

Dose Determination Based on Calibrated Instruments

The aforementioned correction factors are not necessary when ionisation chambers are used solely as instruments that are calibrated in terms of absorbed dose to water against a suitable primary standard where their effects are considered an intrinsic part of the calibration process. They are required where calibration is in terms of air kerma. Such calibrations are by a series of intercomparisons that are traceable directly to the aforementioned national standard instruments. The absorbed dose is determined using an instrument calibrated in terms of absorbed dose to water (the UK standard for megavoltage photon beams) and is given by:

$$D = R \cdot N_D \tag{3.6}$$

where D is the dose, R is the mean-corrected reading and N_D is the absorbed dose calibration factor.

For kV-energy photons in the United Kingdom, the chamber calibration (N_k) is in terms of air kerma. The factor $(\mu_{en}/\rho)w_{air}$, which is the ratio of mass energy absorption coefficients for water and air, needs to be included to calculate the dose to water, and a perturbation factor (k), as described earlier, needs to be applied. The equation becomes:

$$D = R \cdot N_K \cdot k \cdot [(\mu_{\varepsilon n}/\rho)w_{air}] \tag{3.7}$$

The nature and magnitude of the correction factor k depends on whether calibration is carried out in air (for low-energy x-rays) or in water. Similar expressions may be derived for other modalities of radiation.

Requirements for Practical Ionisation Chambers

Radiation dosimeters based upon ionisation chambers have two basic components: the detector chamber, which produces electrical charge when irradiated, and an associated electrometer, which is an electronic amplifier to which the chamber is connected that is designed specifically for the purpose of measuring charge. The response of the dosimeter represents the response of the chamber to radiation together with the accuracy and consistency of the electrometer in measuring the charge.

Practical instrumentation must have a well-determined, predictable and slowly varying response to different energies of radiation and be consistent over time.

In addition, other dosimeter requirements are necessary depending upon the type of radiation and the nature of the measurement being carried out.

Dosimeter chambers used within standards laboratories are specially constructed or selected. Materials used in their construction are fully investigated to determine chemical content, and each chamber is meticulously assessed in terms of its assembly and response to radiation. Electronic equipment used to measure the electrical charge is equally carefully designed, constructed and calibrated. The prime requirements here are the elimination of sources of inaccuracy in response and the consistency of that response. The overall accuracy of calibration of these instruments depends upon uncertainties in fundamental parameters being measured and to the extent that systematic uncertainties can be avoided. Overall consistency of calibration is between 0.5% and 1%.

Secondary standard instruments are constructed to less stringent standards but are required to operate over a range of beam energies and to remain consistent in response between recalibrations by the standards laboratories (i.e. 3 years). They must be fully transportable so that they can be used to transfer calibrations to other instruments in beams from different treatment machines or even across different hospital sites. These chambers maintain an accuracy of calibration of around 1%. Guidelines covering secondary standards instruments have been published.[9]

Field instruments are used in daily measurements within hospitals. Different types of instruments exist, depending upon the nature of those measurements. Thimble chambers, described in detail in the following section, are generally used for calibration of megavoltage photon beams. Chambers based upon the design of the Farmer chamber[21] feature an air cavity of about 0.6 cc, providing a reasonable balance between the response to radiation and smallness of size, and are adequate for measurements in relatively uniform radiation beams, with an accuracy of 1% to 2%. Chambers which have much smaller internal dimensions are used to measure variations in dose distributions, which can be very rapid at beam edges. Here, chambers of 0.1 cc or less may be used, with a trade-off between accuracy of response and spatial resolution. Where there is a rapid variation in dose deposited with depth, such as for measurements in the build-up region of photon beams or in the falloff region of electron beams, parallel plate chambers are used to ensure good depth resolution for the measurements.

Both thimble ionisation chambers and parallel plate ionisation chambers are used widely for routine beam calibration and radiation distribution measurements. Other types of detector systems are useful in particular circumstances and may be used as alternatives to ionisation chambers. In particular, in vivo measurements use systems that do not require the application of polarising voltages, thereby reducing electrical risks to the patient. These various forms of radiation detectors are described in the following sections. Some forms, such as TLDs, have no definitive, maintained calibration and are suitable only for comparative measurements of a radiation dose against a known radiation dose, whereas other forms do maintain a definitive calibration and can be used as absolute dosimeters.

THIMBLE IONISATION CHAMBER

Physical Description

The thimble chamber is an ionisation chamber that has a central electrode (the collector electrode) in a volume of air that is contained by a thimble-shaped cap that forms the HT electrode which fits closely onto a metallic stem. The central electrode passes through the inside of the stem and is insulated from the metallic stem by a suitable, high-quality insulator material such as amber or polythene. This is schematically shown in Fig. 3.9. The cap is generally made of a low-atomic-number, low-density material such as graphite, although various plastic materials have been used where the plastic has been manufactured to be conductive (e.g. Shonka plastic[22]) or has been coated with graphite to be conductive. The central electrode may be made of aluminium or conductive plastic.

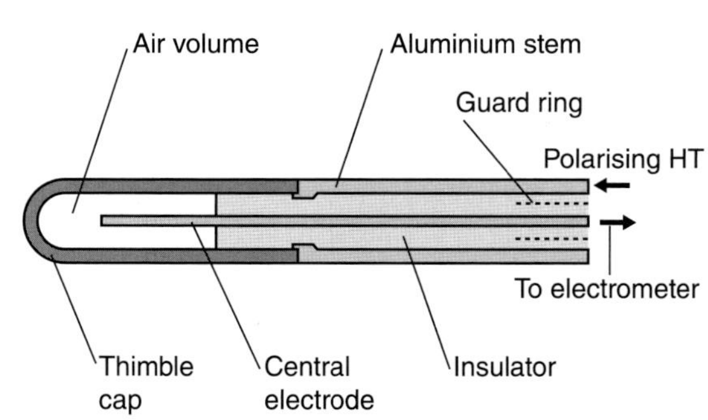

Fig. 3.9 Thimble ionisation chamber. Ionisation produced within the air volume in the thimble cap is collected by the central electrode. The aluminium stem transmits the polarising voltage to the thimble cap. The guard ring minimises charge leakage between the outer *(HT)* and the inner (signal) elements of the interconnecting cable. A thimble chamber of the Farmer type has the air volume linked to the atmosphere via a venting aperture (not shown). *HT,* High-tension.

A potential difference (the polarising voltage) applied between the outer cap and the inner electrode drives apart any ion pairs produced in the trapped air and prevents ion recombination, but it is insufficiently large to cause ionisation of the air itself so that in the absence of ionising radiation no current flows. A voltage gradient of a few hundred volts per millimetre is generally sufficient for this purpose. In the presence of ionising radiation, ionisation within the air results in the ion pairs being separated, with the ions of one sign (depending upon the polarity of the polarising voltage) being collected on the central electrode. The electrometer is generally floating, in that the input to it can be at any voltage level with respect to ground without this affecting the reading. In use, the aluminium stem is held at ground potential and the electrometer is floated to the level of the polarising voltage so that exposed conductive parts carry no electrical risk to operators. This arrangement allows easy reversal of polarising voltage as required.

When the chamber is introduced into a photon beam, photoelectric and Compton interactions in the walls of the chamber generate electrons that traverse the air cavity, causing ionisation of the air. The wall of the thimble must be sufficiently thick to ensure that all the electrons crossing the air cavity originate in the wall and not in the surrounding material. The wall must therefore be at least as thick as the range of the electrons produced by the photon interactions. However, the wall of the chamber will also attenuate the photon beam, and this attenuation will need to be considered. If the wall is thick, the attenuation will be large. Practical ionisation chambers, such as the Farmer chamber,[21] have a wall thickness of about 1 mm. This is sufficient to produce electronic equilibrium for photons generated at kV energies but is insufficient for megavoltage energies when an additional tight-fitting build-up cap is needed to increase the effective wall thickness. This is particularly important when measurements are made in a phantom constructed from a material that differs markedly from the wall material.

The calibration factor of a thimble chamber varies with photon energy. This calibration corrects for wall attenuation, differences in the mass attenuation coefficient between the wall material and water, and perturbations to the photon beam caused when the chamber (and its associated build-up cap, where applicable) is inserted into a water phantom, thereby displacing water. A typical calibration curve for such an instrument in terms of air kerma for photon beams of kV energies is shown in Fig. 3.10. The calibration factor rises sharply at low photon energies, which limits the lowest energy to which this type of instrument may be used, as small variations in photon energy spectrum for low-energy beams can give rise to considerable uncertainties in calibration factor.

The effective point of measurement for the instrument is taken within UK protocols for photon beam calibrations as the chamber centre. The effective point of measurement is forwards of the chamber centre for calibration of electron beams. Some international photon calibration protocols are derived for the effective point of measurement being displaced from the chamber centre.

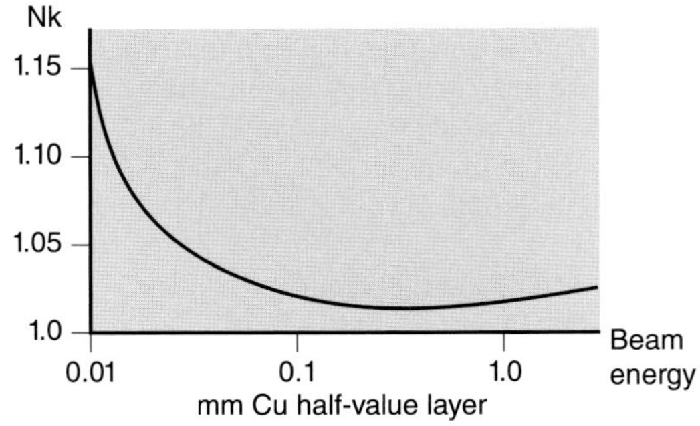

Fig. 3.10 Typical variation in air kerma calibration versus beam energy for a thimble chamber for photon beam energies within the kV range—expressed in terms of their half-value layer (see Chapter 2).

Ionisation of the air volume within the cap of a thimble chamber results in a flow of charge onto the collecting electrode. The rate of flow of charge will depend upon the mass of air within the cavity and on the radiation beam intensity. A balance must be made between the physical size of the chamber and the ability to measure the charge with sufficient accuracy. Chambers with large air volumes (200–2000 cc) must be used to measure the very low dose rates associated with radiation protection measurements. Chambers with volumes of 10 to 60 cc are available for measurement of diagnostic radiology beams. For measurement of radiotherapy beams, chambers of about 0.6 cc are used for calibration measurements, whereas chambers with smaller air volumes may be used for other measurements, as described earlier.

Measurement of Dose and Dose Rate

When an ionisation chamber is irradiated, a flow of ions is collected by the collecting electrode. The ions may be accumulated and the total charge determined by the electrometer. Such a measurement would be used to determine the radiation dose delivered over the course of the irradiation. The accumulation of charge is effectively achieved by collecting the charge in a capacitor: the voltage across the capacitor plates increases with the charge stored.

The rate at which the dose is delivered may be obtained by dividing the measured dose by the irradiation time. This will produce an average value for the dose rate over the irradiation time, although the actual dose rate may vary during the irradiation period. The actual dose rate at any time point within the irradiation period may be determined by measuring the rate of flow of charge. This is achieved by measuring the potential difference produced as the charge flows through a known high-value resistor.

The charge levels referred to previously are extremely small for typical radiotherapy doses, usually on the order of nanocoulombs, and dose rate measurements may involve currents of tens of picoamps. The electrometer instrument that measures them must be carefully designed to avoid introducing instrument-induced charges and voltage differences that may interfere with the measurements. Modern instruments are based on purpose-designed, high-impedance operational amplifiers with low noise levels that are able to measure either dose or dose rate and can operate over a range of current and charge levels.

PARALLEL PLATE IONISATION CHAMBER

Although the thimble chamber described earlier is suitable for many dosimetry situations, there are circumstances that require alternative chamber designs:

- For the measurement of low-energy photons, the wall of a thimble chamber causes too much attenuation such that the calibration factor is large and varies rapidly with energy. This may lead to considerable uncertainties in measurement of dose.
- The wall of a thimble chamber will also produce too much build-up for dose measurements close to the surface for megavoltage radiation.
- In measurement of electron beams, the cylindrical air volume of a thimble chamber causes significant perturbation of the beam that must be corrected for.

Each of these may be addressed by use of a different design of ionisation chamber. This design has two planar elements: one thin electrode (the HT electrode) forms the entry window for the beam, whereas a second element consists of the collector electrode surrounded by a guard ring. The air between the electrodes is trapped by insulating walls that form the sides of the chamber and which hold the electrodes apart.

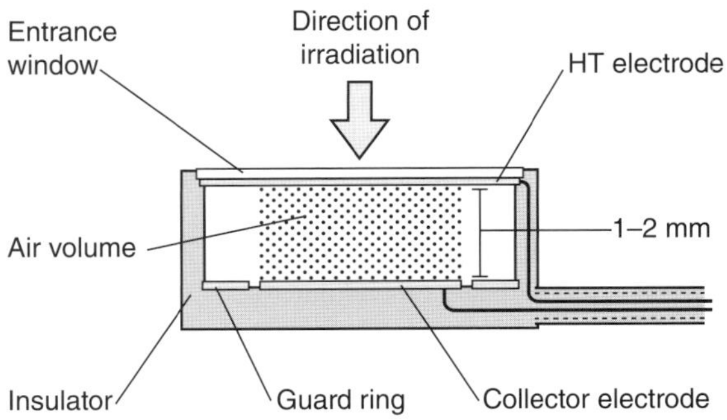

Fig. 3.11 Schematic diagram of a parallel plate ionisation chamber. Ionisation produced within the shaded volume of air is collected by the collector electrode. The guard rings minimise the effects of the chamber walls. The effective point of measurement is the inside surface of the entrance window. *HT*, High-tension.

The entry window of such a chamber can be made extremely thin—a few micrometres of plastic material on which a conductive surface (e.g. a graphite layer) has been deposited—but it must be sufficiently rigid so as to maintain chamber geometry. For accurate measurement of low-energy x-rays, it is important that the materials of the chamber have atomic numbers close to those of water to avoid undue perturbation of the beam. The measuring volume of the chamber, shown as the shaded region in Fig. 3.11, is defined by the cross-sectional area of the collecting electrode and the separation between the plates. Interactions with the lateral walls of the chamber generate ions primarily at the edges of the chamber which are collected by the guard ring and not by the collecting electrode.

BEAM MONITOR CHAMBER

Linear accelerators and higher-energy kV x-ray units have in-built ionisation chambers to monitor and control the amount of radiation being emitted. For these units, the amount of radiation emitted is specified in terms of monitor units, that is, by the quantity of radiation measured by the in-built monitor chamber. The sensitivity of these monitor chambers must be adjusted to give the correct amount of radiation dose per monitor unit, a process known as *calibration*.

Monitor chambers are forms of the parallel plate type that sample the entire radiation beam emitted from the treatment unit. In linear accelerators, each monitor chamber consists of at least two independent ionisation chambers to provide backup should problems develop with one chamber during patient treatment. One or both chambers may be segmented, having the collector electrode constructed of a number of different and electrically isolated segments, so that assessment of beam uniformity can be made by comparing the current flowing from the various segments. Some monitor chambers are manufactured as sealed units that require no correction for ambient temperature and pressure but which must be checked to ensure that they remain sealed. Others are manufactured as unsealed chambers that do need correction for temperature and pressure; some modern linear accelerators have in-built pressure and temperature transducers and perform this correction automatically, whereas others rely on manual adjustment. All monitor chambers must be calibrated regularly (e.g. daily) as specified in the calibration protocol being followed by the treatment centre or in radiation protection guidance.

In linear accelerators, the monitor chamber is situated below the primary collimator and flattening filter/scattering foil carousel, and before the adjustable collimators, as shown in Fig. 3.12. In this location, although the chamber is protected as far as practicable from backscatter that arises from the adjustable collimator jaws, it will still be subject to

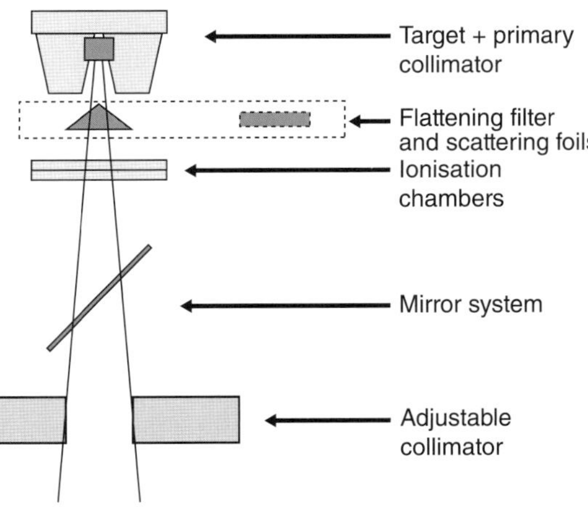

Fig. 3.12 Schematic diagram of a linear accelerator treatment head showing the location of the monitor (ionisation) chambers in relation to other components of the head.

some backscatter. The monitor chamber may also be subject to backscatter from any physical wedges placed in the beam. Variations in backscatter contribute to changes in output with field size and to the apparent effect of the wedge. In kV therapy units, the monitor chamber is located after the exit window of the tube housing and after any added beam filters so that it samples the final beam. However, the monitor chamber is susceptible to backscatter from the applicator plate, and this contributes to differences in output between different treatment applicators.

INTERCOMPARISONS WITH SECONDARY STANDARD INSTRUMENTS

Transfer of calibration from the primary standard instrument to the field instrument is achieved via a series of intercomparisons. The response of each field instrument is compared with that of a calibrated secondary standard instrument every 12 months (or following repair to the field instrument) at each beam energy and treatment modality at which it is to be used. Where a specific build-up cap was used in determining the relevant calibration factor of the secondary standard instrument, the same build-up cap should be fitted during intercomparison measurements, even when those measurements are to be carried out in a Perspex phantom.

Intercomparisons are carried out, wherever possible, by placing the field chamber and the secondary standard chamber side by side in the irradiation field and taking simultaneous readings. Several readings should be taken and averaged for each measurement, and the relative positions of the two chambers should be interchanged to minimise any effects should the radiation beam produce different dose rates at the positions of the two chambers. The relevant conditions (e.g. type of phantom, depth of measurement, field size) under which these intercomparison measurements and subsequent equipment calibration measurements are made are specified in the appropriate dosimetry protocol. In the United Kingdom, separate protocols have been produced by the IPEM or its forerunner organisations covering:

- X-ray beams below 300-kV generating potential[23,24]
- High-energy (megavoltage) x-ray beams[9,25]
- Electron beams of energy from 4 to 25 megaelectron volts (MeV)[26]

Because of the very different penetration properties of the beams concerned, the first of these is split into three separate sections covering different energy ranges. For very low-energy beams, such as HVL <1.0 mm aluminium (Al), measurements are specified for the surface of

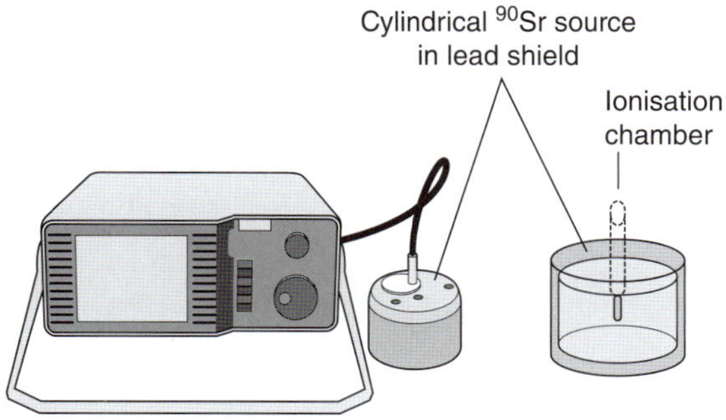

Fig. 3.13 Strontium checking device used to check the consistency of a thimble chamber, together with a schematic of the device showing the source wrapped around the chamber.

a phantom. For low-energy beams (HVL 1–8 mm Al), measurements are specified in air, with no phantom present. For medium-energy beams (HVL 0.5–1.0 mm Copper (Cu)), which are more penetrating, measurements are specified at a depth of 2 cm in a phantom.

STRONTIUM CONSISTENCY CHECK DEVICE

Between calibration sessions, the consistency of each instrument has to be checked using an appropriate consistency checking device.

One such device uses a strontium check source[27] and is illustrated in Fig. 3.13. A device of this type for thimble chambers has a ring-shaped source of ^{90}Sr housed within a fully shielded enclosure, into the centre of which the sensitive volume of the ionisation chamber can be accurately placed. The ^{90}Sr is a beta emitter and decays at a constant rate with a half-life of 28.7 years. The chamber response within the device is measured at the time at which intercomparison measurements are made. The response to be expected at any subsequent time can then be calculated simply by accounting for radioactive decay, on the proviso that repositioning of the ionisation chamber can be carried out with sufficient precision. Different source geometries may be used for different types of ionisation chamber; for example, planar ^{90}Sr sources may be used to check the consistency of response of parallel plate ionisation chambers.

Measurements are carried out periodically (e.g. every month). The chamber response is determined either by measuring the reading achieved for a defined period of measurement or by measuring the time for the chamber to reach a given reading once measurement has been initiated. These measurements ensure the consistency of operation of the measuring device but cannot be used for calibration of the measuring device, because the radiation from ^{90}Sr is not representative of the radiation beams in which the device will be used in clinical practice.

IONISATION CHAMBER CORRECTIONS

Whenever instruments that are based upon collection of ions produced in air are used to determine absorbed dose, a number of factors in addition to the calibration factor have to be considered.

Ion Recombination Losses

When the air volume of an ionisation chamber is irradiated, ion pairs generated as atoms become ionised. To determine the absorbed dose or air kerma accurately, it is necessary to ensure the collection of all the positive or negative ions (depending on polarity) by the collecting electrode. A potential difference is applied across the electrodes to drive the ion pairs apart. If the ion pairs are not driven apart by the applied electric field, they may recombine such that they are lost from collection and the charge is therefore reduced. When ions recombine, the positive and negative ions of an ion pair may recombine with each other (self-recombination), or the negative ion from one ion pair may recombine with the positive ion of a neighbouring ion pair (volume recombination). Both self-recombination and volume recombination result in a reduction in the measured charge. The likelihood of recombination is less where the ions are driven apart rapidly, such as when the polarising voltage is high.

Recombination is more likely to occur when ion pairs are created close together, both physically and in time. This occurs when measuring high dose rates, or when measuring in beams in which the radiation is delivered in pulses. The radiation from a ^{60}Co gamma-beam therapy unit is emitted continuously. The radiation from a modern kilovoltage therapy unit is also virtually continuous, although it does depend somewhat on the type of voltage generator used. For both of these radiation sources, polarising voltages across a thimble chamber of a few hundred volts are generally sufficient such that recombination losses are negligible at dose rates commonly used in radiotherapy. The radiation from a linear accelerator is strongly pulsed: a linear accelerator delivering a dose rate of 4 Gy/min will deliver the radiation in short pulses, each a few microseconds in duration, with the instantaneous dose rate within each pulse being about 40 Gy/s. Under these circumstances, accurate determination of dose requires knowledge of and correction for recombination losses. The amount of recombination may be determined by carrying out measurements using different levels of polarising voltage across the chamber, applying an empirically derived equation for the equipment being used, or applying the half-voltage technique.[28,29]

Correction for Atmospheric Conditions

It has been previously stated that the rate of flow of ions onto the collector electrode will depend on the amount of air enclosed within the thimble of the chamber, and examples have been given of different instrument sizes for measuring in dose rates at typical protection, radiodiagnostic and therapy radiation levels. It is, however, the mass of air within the thimble on which the response depends.

For a chamber that is sealed to trap air inside the thimble, variations in atmospheric temperature and pressure will have no impact upon the enclosed mass and will therefore not affect the chamber response. However, the condition of the air within such an instrument may change with time, perhaps because of vapours leaching from the walls of the cap or the surrounding materials. In addition, there is always potential for the seal to fail, allowing some flow of air between the chamber and the environment. If a chamber is unsealed, allowing free passage of air between the inside of the thimble and the general environment, the mass of air within the thimble will fluctuate with atmospheric temperature and pressure, and a correction to any reading will be required to compensate for these changes. As the temperature increases, the air density falls and the mass of air within the thimble will reduce, thereby reducing the chamber sensitivity. As atmospheric pressure rises, the density of air also increases, increasing the mass of gas within the thimble and thereby increasing the chamber sensitivity. If the assumption is made that air affected by temperature and pressure changes in the same way as an ideal gas, the ideal gas laws can be applied to determine the magnitude of variation in response. If measurements are made at a temperature of T degrees Celsius (°C) and a pressure of P kilopascal (kPa) using an unsealed instrument, the response may be corrected to what it would have been at a standard temperature of 20°C (293 K) and a pressure of 101.325 kPa by applying the correction factor:

$$\text{Correction} = (101.325/P) \times [(T+273)/293] \quad \textbf{(3.8)}$$

Most practical field instruments are designed and constructed to be unsealed. The design of such an instrument has to ensure that the thimble does not distort with changes in temperature or pressure so that the volume remains constant. Water vapour can affect the chamber response and the aforementioned correction for atmospheric conditions, producing a variation of about 0.7% for change in relative humidity from 10% to 90%. To minimise the impact of relative humidity changes, the secondary standard calibration factor is specified for a humidity value of 50%: variations in chamber response in normal use because of relative humidity changes may generally be ignored.

Chamber Stem Effect

If the stem of the ionisation chamber is within the radiation field, it may perturb the radiation beam and may generate scatter into the air volume of the chamber, thereby affecting the reading (termed the *stem effect*).

During absolute calibration, the chamber is irradiated with a specific field size, and a correction is applied for the stem effect with this field size. It is therefore considered whenever the calibration factor is applied. There is, however, potential for the effect to increase or decrease for other field sizes.

With well-designed ionisation chambers, such as the Farmer chamber, the stem effect is small, and variations in it can generally be ignored.

Polarity Effect

When an ionisation chamber is used to measure charged particles, some of the charged particles may come to rest on the collecting electrode. These will either add to or subtract from the ionisation charge being collected, depending upon the charge on the particle and on the direction of the polarising voltage (whether the collector electrode is collecting positive ions or electrons). The effect is particularly important when using parallel plate chambers to measure proton or electron beams and can be overcome by averaging measurements taken with both positive and negative polarising voltages.

A related problem is that if measurements are carried out in a solid insulating material such as polystyrene, particles stopped within the material will result in a build-up of charge there, which will perturb the radiation beam being measured. To avoid this, an insulating phantom should be made of thin sheets of material which allows charge built up in this way to leak away.

LIQUID-FILLED IONISATION CHAMBER

Air-filled ionisation chambers have provided a stable, well-characterised method of measuring dose. However, for the small fields and steep dose gradients prevalent in modern radiotherapy, the requirement for high spatial resolution has led to the development of small-volume, liquid-filled ionisation chambers. Used for relative and absolute dose measurements, organic liquids provide almost water-equivalent energy response and a high signal-to-noise ratio.[30] They suffer less radiation damage than solid-state detectors which can provide similar resolution (see the next section). However, there are significant recombination losses requiring stable polarisation voltage and temperature monitoring. Also, the purity of the organic liquid requires consideration for a robust and stable response. Overall, such chambers require careful design.[31]

ALTERNATIVE DOSE MEASUREMENT SYSTEMS

In the preceding sections, the primary processes for detection of radiation and measurement of dose centred on calorimetry and ionisation of air. National standard and secondary standard instruments are based on these processes, and field instruments of the thimble or parallel plate chamber design are recommended for routine measurement of radiation output from therapy machines. There are, however, other techniques that are suitable for measurement of dose or dose rate for different circumstances. These are briefly described in the following section, and a selection of such devices is represented schematically in Fig. 3.14.

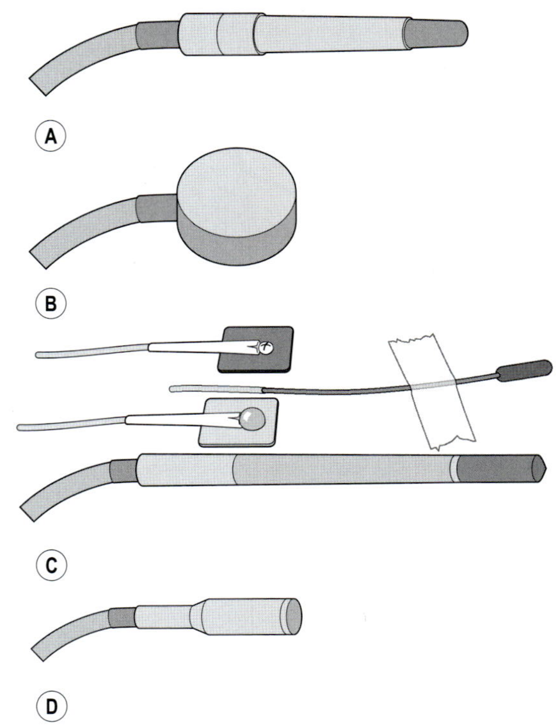

Fig. 3.14 Schematic diagram of radiation detectors showing (A) a Farmer chamber without an additional build-up cap; (B) a parallel plate chamber for electron measurements; (C) a selection of diode detectors for phantom and for in vivo measurements, together with a Farmer-type chamber for comparison; and (D) a diamond detector.

Film Dosimetry

Film has been a very long-standing system for detecting and measuring radiation in radiotherapy. It is particularly useful for measurement of radiation distributions, having applications in phantom measurement of simple and complex radiation beams, verification of field placements on individual patients, establishment of geometrical accuracy of light beams that delineate radiation beams, and determination of leakage patterns around the head of a treatment unit.

Standard Photographic Film

Photographic film consists essentially of a transparent polyester material (the base) on which is deposited a layer of silver bromide trapped in a gel (the emulsion). The emulsion may be deposited on one side or on both sides of the base. The emulsion is sensitive to light and so must be used in a light-tight packaging or housing. The silver bromide is in the form of small crystals, each crystal being formed as a lattice of negative bromide and positive silver ions. When irradiated, some lattice bonds are broken, and electrons are transferred from the bromine to the silver ions, neutralising those atoms. The presence of neutral silver atoms at key positions of the lattice within a crystal makes the whole crystal developable. In the subsequent development process, the silver ions of developable crystals are converted to atoms of silver. These are fixed in position on the film, and the rest of the emulsion, including any nondevelopable crystals, is removed. The deposited silver absorbs light, so these regions of the film appear black while the rest of the film appears transparent.

The degree of blackness depends on the relative concentration of deposited crystals which, in turn, depends upon the intensity of radiation at that location on the film. This is measured by shining light through the developed film and measuring the transmitted intensity. A logarithmic scale is used to define the optical density of the film and is given by:

$$\mathrm{OD} = \log_{10}(I_0/I) \quad (3.9)$$

where I_0 is the incident light intensity and I is the transmitted intensity. The resultant optical density has to be corrected for the intrinsic density of the developed film base. A graph of optical density against absorbed dose is known as the *dose response curve* and can be produced for any film. Accurate dosimetry requires full knowledge of the dose response curve. The response curve may be effectively linear over a restricted range of doses, and simple dose comparisons can be made within this range. Used in this way, film has high spatial resolution unmatched by other measuring systems and can provide a full two-dimensional display of dose distribution (such as variation in dose with depth and position across the beam). However, silver bromide has a high atomic number, and therefore the response to low-energy photons is greatly increased as a result of increased photoelectric interactions. This makes film unsuitable as an absolute dosimeter and makes accurate comparative measurements difficult in situations where the energy spectrum varies markedly. Although the areas of application of film dosimetry are steadily being reduced as other methods of measurement come to the fore, film dosimetry still has a vital role within radiotherapy. It also has a role in radiation protection dosimetry where the film badge has been the historical standard for personal dosimetry, although this is steadily being replaced by other forms of detector.

Radiochromic Film

Standard photographic film, as described earlier, is sensitive to both ionising radiation and visible light. When used for radiation measurements, it has to be kept in a light-free container and processed under controlled light conditions. In contrast to this, radiochromic reactions produce direct coloration of a substance by direct absorption of radiation, without the need for chemical processing.

Radiochromic films have been developed that have little or no sensitivity to visible light but which demonstrate a change in colour when subjected to ionising radiation.

These may be based upon release of leuco dyes within the material or upon the formation of coloured cross-linked polymers from otherwise colourless monomers. The degree of colour change is dependent upon absorbed dose and may be determined by measuring the attenuation of light of specific frequencies that relate to the colour change. Radiochromic films are commercially available which have good response for doses within the range of 0.5 to 25 Gy and have no high-atomic-number materials present. Such films therefore have uniform response across a wide range of photon energies. Materials of this type have been used to determine dose distributions for complex radiotherapy treatments and around brachytherapy sources. The most common type is the commercial GAF chromic film.[32] The principle of polymer cross-linkage is similar to that of polymer gels and is described in a later section.

Semiconductor Detectors

A number of different types of semiconductor-based radiation detectors have been developed. This text describes the principles of operation of semiconductor detectors: diode detectors, metal oxide semiconductor field effect transistors (MOSFETs), diamond detectors, TLDs and radiophotoluminescent detectors (RPLs).

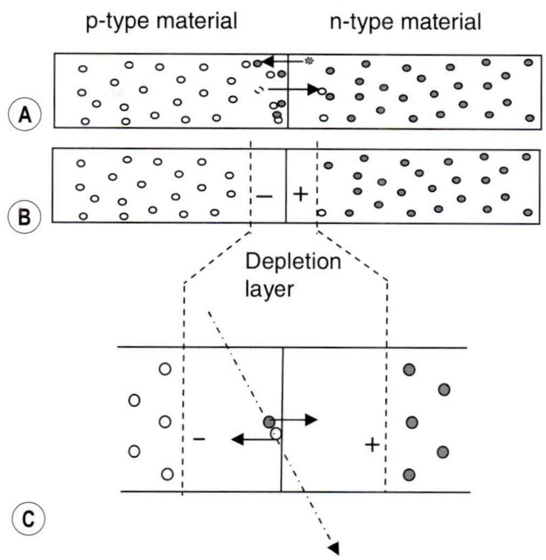

Fig. 3.15 Schematic diagram of a p–n junction diode detector. Electrons from the n-type material and holes from the p-type material diffuse across the junction (A), forming a depletion layer across which an internal potential difference forms (B). Electron–hole pairs formed in the depletion layer are pulled apart by the internal electric field (C).

The physical process which enables radiation detection and measurement to be achieved with these devices is based upon the way a material can be understood in terms of band structure (see Chapter 1).

These devices use semiconductor materials, the most common of which is silicon, to which specific impurities are added at very low concentrations, a process known as *doping*. Two types of doping are used. Doping by an electron donor results in n-type material. For example, arsenic and selenium introduce free electrons into the conduction band of silicon. Doping by an electron receptor produces p-type material. For example, aluminium and gallium effectively introduce additional vacant levels into the valence band of silicon. These unfilled levels are termed *holes*. If electrons are introduced into a p-type material, they will fill vacant holes and become trapped.

Diode Detector

When adjacent p-type and n-type doping occurs in a single crystal of silicon, a p–n junction is formed. Conduction electrons in the n-type region will diffuse into the p-type region and become trapped, as shown in Fig. 3.15. This results in:

- The region around the interface being devoid of free electrons and unfilled holes. This region is called the *depletion layer*.
- A transfer of electrons (and hence charge) from the n-type to the p-type side of the interface. This transfer of charge generates a small potential difference across the depletion layer.

When this depletion layer is irradiated, electrons are released by ionisation, creating electron–hole pairs as shown in Fig. 3.15C. These drift in opposite directions under the influence of the potential difference across the depletion layer. Electrons will be drawn towards the n-type material while holes will be drawn towards the p-type material, causing charge to flow through the circuit in which the diode is connected. The charge produced is proportional to the dose deposited in the depletion region, and the flow of charge can be measured by an electrometer.

The sensitive region of the diode is very thin, with the depletion layer being only a few micrometres in thickness and the cross-sectional area of the silicon crystal being only a few millimetres in thickness. However, the sensitivity to radiation is high, as the density of the material is over 1000 times that of air in an ionisation chamber and the mean energy to produce an electron–hole pair is about one-tenth of the energy to create an ion pair in air. Diodes can therefore produce measurable signals from extremely small, sensitive volumes that make them particularly suitable for measurements that require high spatial resolution. The absence of any applied polarising voltage makes diodes particularly useful for in vivo dosimetry.

Diodes have various inherent problems that must be addressed when they are used as radiation detectors. The size of the depletion layer, and hence the sensitivity of the device, strongly depends on temperature.[33] Diodes therefore need to be calibrated at the temperature at which they are to be used. They are constructed from materials with atomic numbers higher than water, making them overresponsive to low-energy photon radiation. Their response is therefore sensitive to variations in the energy spectrum of any radiation field such as may be caused by (1) changes in depth, radiation field size and position within the field, or (2) the energy setting of equipment being measured. In addition, the construction of the device can influence its angular sensitivity.[34,35] A further problem is that diodes may suffer radiation damage after receiving high doses of radiation which causes them to change their sensitivity. It has been shown that diodes formed using predominantly heavy p-type doping are less susceptible to sudden changes in sensitivity and have longer working lives than predominantly n-doped diodes.[36] The majority of commercial diodes are p-type.

Diodes are used widely in radiotherapy as:

- Individual detectors for measuring dose distributions (e.g. depth doses and profiles, particularly where high spatial resolution is required, such as in regions of high dose gradient) of radiotherapy beams during initial commissioning and subsequent quality control measurements
- Individual or groups of detectors for measuring radiation doses delivered to patients (in vivo dosimetry)
- Arrays of detectors for rapidly checking beam uniformity as part of a quality assurance program

Metal Oxide Semiconductor Field Effect Transistor Detector

The structure of a MOSFET is shown schematically in Fig. 3.16, which illustrates a device based upon p-doped silicon substrate material onto which layers of heavily n-doped material and SiO_2 are formed. There are three electrical contacts, which are termed the *source*, *gate* and *drain*. The source and drain regions may be considered p–n junctions, which are linked by the SiO_2 channel onto which the gate is deposited.

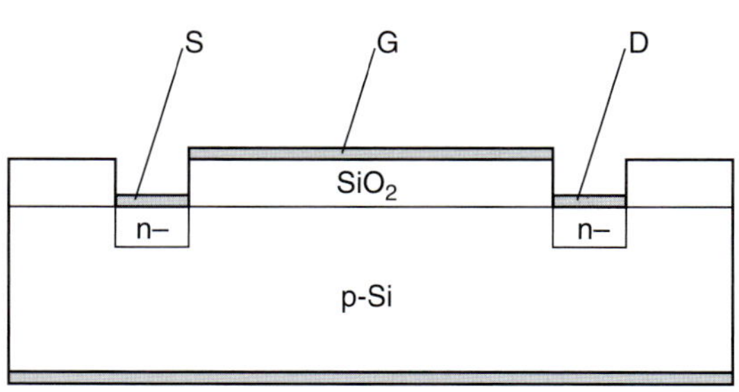

Fig. 3.16 Cross-sectional schematic of a metal oxide semiconductor field effect device. A conducting channel is formed through the oxide layer between the source *(S)* and the drain *(D)* when a voltage is applied to the gate *(G)*. The threshold voltage at which this channel is formed is reduced by the effects of radiation.

The device operates essentially like a voltage-controlled switch. If a small voltage is generated between the source and the gate, with the drain held at the same potential as the gate, no current flows initially between the source and drain until the applied voltage exceeds a specific value, known as the *threshold voltage*. At the threshold voltage, a current starts to flow between the source and the drain along a conduction channel.

When the device is irradiated, electron–hole pairs are generated and the holes become trapped at the oxide/silicone surface. These additional holes reduce the threshold voltage, and the reduction is almost linearly related to the radiation dose received by the device.

MOSFET devices are extremely small (<0.1 mm) and are easily fabricated in various shapes and geometries. They can be used for measurement of point doses or complex dose distributions. No electrical connections are necessary during irradiation, and the electronic equipment needed for readout is relatively simple, making these devices ideally suited to in vivo dosimetry. However, the specific response variation with radiation damage and temperature should be available from the manufacturer so that they are considered in the application.

Diamond Detector

Carbon in the form of diamond is an intrinsic semiconductor with a large energy gap between the conduction and valence bands (5.5 eV). At normal room temperatures, there are very few electrons in the conduction band. If a voltage is placed across a diamond crystal, a tiny current will flow because of these electrons, the magnitude of which is dependent for any given crystal on the applied voltage. The diamond therefore behaves as a resistor.

When irradiated, ion pairs generated within the material increase the number of carriers and so the resistance falls. The radiation-induced current increases with increasing dose rate. Certain impurities within the diamond can improve the linearity of response between current and dose rate, but the dose rate response has to be considered when using these devices.

A diamond detector consists of a diamond crystal onto which metal contacts have been deposited and to which a voltage of about 100 V is applied. The radiation-induced current is considerably larger than the natural current and so can be measured with precision. Under these conditions, the response is largely independent of temperature. The detector is not readily damaged by radiation, so the device has a long operational life. The diamond crystal may be selected from natural diamonds or grown using chemical vapor deposition processes. They are small detectors and so are useful in measuring high radiation gradients, with good angular response characteristics. Being composed of carbon, they are low-atomic-number devices with electron stopping-power values similar to those for water.[37]

Thermoluminescent Dosimetry

We have seen in the 'Band Theory of Solids' section in Chapter 1 that some materials have a normally empty conduction band. When such a material is irradiated, some electrons within the valence band may be given sufficient energy to excite them into the conduction band, leaving a 'hole' in the valence band. These electrons will eventually lose their extra energy and fall back to the valence band to fill the vacant energy level (hole) there. In doing this, the electron has to lose the energy difference between the two energy levels.

The energy lost in this transition may be a few electron volts. In some materials, this energy loss is in the form of emission of electromagnetic radiation, akin to the emission of characteristic x-rays from an x-ray target but at much lower energies. This process appears simple but involves complex energy-level changes for both the electron and the hole that are beyond the scope of this book. The result for some types of material is that it is transparent to the electromagnetic radiation released by these transitions, which is then emitted. The energy of the radiation emitted may be within the visible spectrum, in which case the irradiated material emits light. Materials of this type are said to be *luminescent* in general. When the electrons excited into the conduction band fall back and emit light immediately, the material is said to be *fluorescent*. Fluorescent screens are used to enhance the response of x-ray film to radiation and are used within some types of portal imaging devices. In luminescent processes, additional energy levels within the forbidden zone, as shown in Fig. 1.3A, formed either from impurities or as a result of discontinuities in the crystal structure, play a part both in trapping the excited electrons and in emitting light. Energy levels immediately below the conduction band form traps for some of the electrons from that band. Electrons falling into these traps may be held there until they gain sufficient energy to move back into the conduction band, from where they can decay back to the valence band. If the trap level is close to the conduction band, ongoing energy variations from thermal fluctuations will result in traps being emptied rapidly, producing fluorescence. The farther a trap is from the conduction band, the longer it will take for it to empty. Traps are therefore characterised by two related features: the distance from the conduction band (the trap depth) and the rate at which it empties (the trap half-life).

In some materials, such as metal-doped lithium fluoride (LiF; i.e. doped with magnesium or manganese), the trap levels are well below the conduction band. At normal room temperatures, these traps would empty exceedingly slowly. If, however, the temperature of the crystal is raised, the additional heat energy imparted may allow electrons to rapidly escape the traps. The light output from the crystal is dependent upon this supply of heat, and these materials are termed *thermoluminescent*.

When a thermoluminescent material is irradiated, electrons are transported into the conduction band. A small number, about 1%, of these electrons fall into the thermoluminescent traps. When the material is later heated to a temperature that allows the traps to empty, light is given off. This process is shown in Fig. 3.17. The amount of light is proportional to the number of electrons trapped and hence to the radiation dose delivered to the crystal material. Thermoluminescent dosimetry[38] uses a TLD reader that both heats the detector and simultaneously measures the amount of light emitted, as indicated in Fig. 3.18.

A material such as LiF, which is the most common TLD material in clinical use, will have a number of traps at differing depths. The light output from LiF as a function of the temperature of the crystal is known as a *glow curve*, and a typical glow curve is illustrated in Fig. 3.19. The traps closest to the conduction band empty first, producing the glow

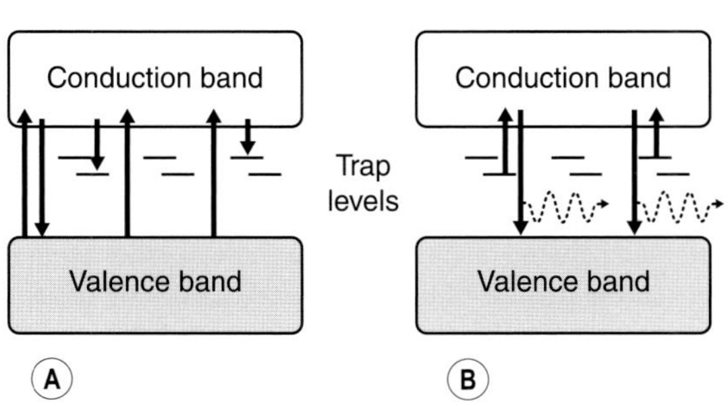

Fig. 3.17 Illustration of thermoluminescent dosimeter processes. Irradiation of the material raises electrons into the conduction band. Some of these fall back to the valence band while others become trapped in intervening energy levels, as shown in (A). When heat is applied, the electrons in the traps are raised back into the conduction band and subsequently fall back to the valence band, releasing visible photons, as shown in (B).

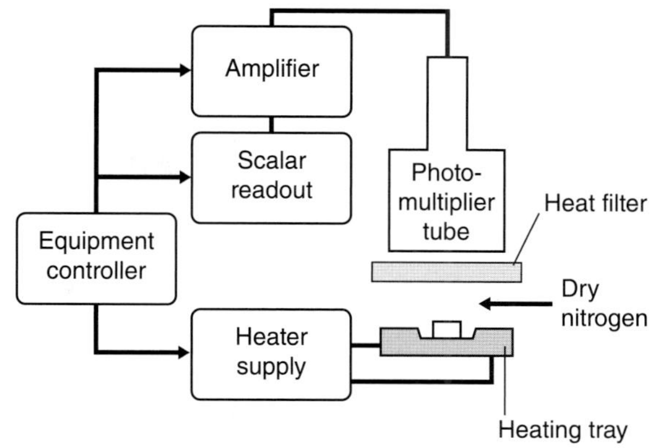

Fig. 3.18 Schematic diagram of a thermoluminescent dosimeter readout system. The heat filter protects the photomultiplier tube and reduces thermal counts. The dry nitrogen atmosphere prevents oxidation of the detector surface.

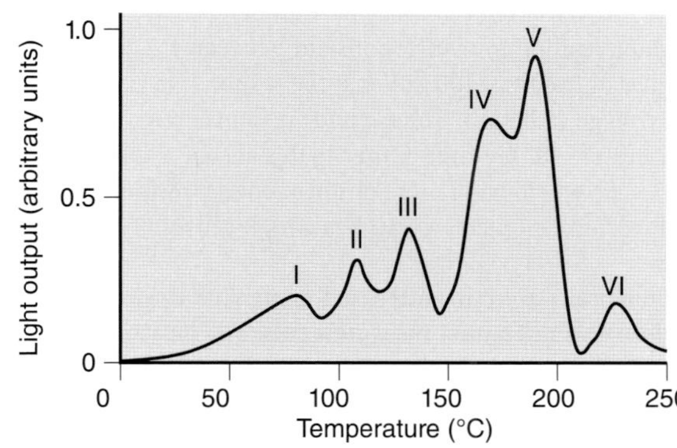

Fig. 3.19 Schematic illustration of the glow curve from LiF:Mg,Ti showing the six peaks representing different trap depths.

peaks labelled I to III. These traps have relatively short half-lives at room temperatures such that the signal falls too rapidly for reliable dose estimates, so the output from these bands is usually ignored. The signal from the higher-temperature peaks IV and V is from traps with half-lives measured in years, so that timing between irradiation and readout is not generally relevant—the light from these traps is measured to estimate the dose. After use, the material is thermally annealed, a process which resets the electron energy levels and traps occupancies to their initial values, after which the material may be reused.

The light output from a specific dosimeter will depend upon a number of factors:

- The amount of intrinsic thermoluminescent material.
- The nature and extent of the doping.
- The previous thermal history in general and the postanneal cooling in particular.
- The radiation history of the material. Radiation-induced damage may alter the energy band structure of the material.
- The surface condition of the crystalline material. Marks and scratches attenuate and scatter the light.
- The detailed nature of the readout cycle.

Some of the aforementioned cause differences in response between different dosimeters, whereas others cause differences in response of a single dosimeter from use to use. In addition, the response is not strictly linear with dose but increases with increased dose, a feature known as *supralinearity*. TLD is not used as an absolute dosimeter (i.e. where the calibration is stable and constant). To address these issues,

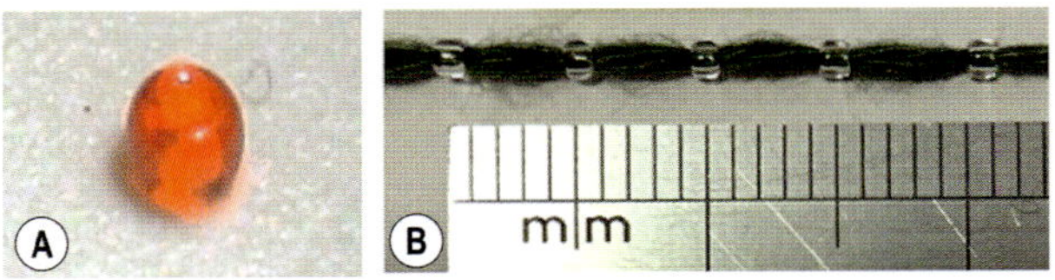

Fig. 3.20 (A) A magnified view of a microsilica bead thermoluminescent dosimeter (hollow, with 0.5-mm internal diameter). The bead is coloured for illustration only. (B) Microsilica beads arranged on a piece of cotton with 5-mm spacing distance.

TLD dosimeters are used in batches, where the dosimeters in each batch have the same handling and general history and where some are selected as measuring dosimeters and others are irradiated to known doses to calibrate the batch response in a traceable manner.

LiF is the most commonly used TLD material and is available in various forms that include powder; single-crystal chips (size 4 mm × 4 mm × 1 mm approximately) and rods (size 6 mm in length × 1 mm in diameter); sintered chips, disks and rods; and Teflon-embedded disks and rods. The effective atomic number is slightly greater than that of water, leading to overresponse of between 1.3 and 1.7 for photon energies of less than 100 keV, but the response is virtually uniform for megavoltage radiation. The detector response remains constant up to dose rates of 10^6 Gy/min. Other materials are available, including lithium borate, which has a more uniform energy response at low energies, and calcium sulphate, which has a high sensitivity to low-energy photons.

TLD materials are currently used as in vivo dosimeters for both surface dose and interstitial measurements. For measurements on the patient surface to estimate the maximum dose at the depth of dose, care must be taken to ensure that appropriate build-up is used both for patient measurement and for calibration irradiation. Despite the variations in response described earlier, TLD is used to provide a traceable postal calibration service to centres without access to a primary or secondary standards laboratory and to check on the accuracy of calibration across various centres as part of clinical trial quality control procedures.

Microsilica bead TLDs have recently been introduced as a high spatial resolution detector for use in complex high-gradient dose distribution measurements, such as advanced radiation therapy techniques.[39,40] These spherical, doughnut-shaped beads have an outer diameter measuring approximately 1.5 mm and are 1.0 mm thick (Fig. 3.20A). This physical shape allows for two-dimensional and three-dimensional arrangements (e.g. Fig. 3.20B, where bead TLDs are arranged on a cotton thread for a line profile of dose measurement). This, along with robustness and an inert nature, makes them an ideal passive in vivo dosimetry system when it is difficult to control environmental factors such as humidity and temperature inside the patient's body.

Although they can be read out using a conventional TLD reader, one might use a large number of bead TLDs for high-resolution measurements in complex two-dimensional and three-dimensional arrangements which require significant labour resources for readout and data analysis. In such occasions, use of a fully automated TLD reader and data processor that is introduced specifically for the readout process of bead TLDs seems to be a more practical approach.

The detector response does not vary with beam angle and dose rate. The effective atomic number of silica bead TLDs is almost two times greater than that of water, leading to a significant energy dependency, similar to that of bone, for beam energies of kV range where photoelectric effect is the main radiation interaction process. Being bone equivalent makes them a suitable detector if one wants to measure dose to the bone. However, when dose measurement to water or soft tissue is intended, a careful calibration using the same beam energy is required. Moreover, silica bead TLDs together with a soft tissue–equivalent detector can be used as a means of beam energy discrimination.

Radiophotoluminescence Detectors

Luminescence in the optical energy range features in several radiation detectors, and radiophotoluminescence (RPL) detectors have distinct characteristics and advantages compared with the others. Scintillation crystals emit light while being irradiated. To detect the radiation, photomultipliers are therefore required to transform the optical emission in the scintillation material into an electrical signal as the detector is irradiated. With TLD dosimeters, the detector is thermally stimulated to release the energy trapped in the detector in the form of light which is measured and is proportional to the dose the detector received.

In contrast, with RPL, the radiation alters the constituents of the detector material and makes it almost permanently luminescent. A reduction in luminescence of 5% per year has been reported for some RPL materials. The phenomenon was discovered in 1921, and subsequent development has led to dosimeters which provide sensitive, reliable and accurate dose measurements for personnel, accident and environmental monitoring.

The advantage of the RPL detector lies in its robust, long-term storage of the dose. With TLD and optically stimulated dosimeters (OLDs), problems in the reading cycle or detector handling could lead to a loss of information. The RPL can be cleared of the dose information by high temperature. However, despite a decay in the luminescence of RPL with time, it offers a more robust system if the decay rate is known.

Summary of Direct Reading Radiation Detectors

Of the various types of radiation detectors described in the previous sections, it can be seen that some can be used for direct measurement: ionisation chambers, diodes and diamond detectors. The others—film, MOSFET, TLD and RPL—while having specific advantages and the ability to measure accumulated dose, cannot be used for direct measurement as they have to be processed post irradiation.

Each type of detector has particular applications for which it is ideally suited. Cylindrical ionisation chambers (see Fig. 3.14A) are particularly useful as instruments for calibration of megavoltage photon beams. Parallel plate ionisation chambers (see Fig. 3.14B) are useful when measuring in regions of high dose gradient, such as in the dose falloff region of an electron beam. Diodes (see Fig. 3.14C) are useful for in vivo dosimetry. The small size of their detection region makes these devices also useful when measuring in small radiation fields or within beam penumbral regions. Cylindrical forms of these detectors, which include corrections within the design of the device for enhanced low-energy photon response, are readily available. Diamond detectors (see Fig. 3.14D) may be used as an alternative to diode detectors and are especially resistant to radiation damage.

Chemical and Biochemical Detectors

Energy deposited in matter may be manifest ultimately in various forms, one being altered chemistry. Radiotherapy relies upon this to a large extent in the process of damaging and destroying tissue cells. In some cells, direct interaction of the radiation with DNA causes irreparable damage, leading to the death of those cells. In others, radiation-induced chemical changes within the cells produce active free radicals that cause similar damage to DNA.

In some materials, the altered chemical makeup remains and can be detected. Where the effect is stable and proportional to dose, this may be used in chemical and biochemical dosimetry. If the chemical yield is known (number of chemical molecules formed per unit of energy absorbed), chemical dosimetry could be used as a primary standard.

Fricke dosimetry was used for a short period in the past in this way to provide a definitive calibration of electron beams for which the yield was well established.

Fricke Dosimetry

Fricke dosimetry is based upon conversion of ferrous sulphate ions (Fe^{2+}) to ferric ions in a weak sulphuric acid solution.[41] The concentration of ferric sulphate is determined by measuring the attenuation of light passing through the solution. Light of a particular wavelength (304 nm) is used as this is attenuated differentially by ferrous and ferric ions. The instrument used for accurate measurement of attenuation at a particular frequency of light is a *spectrophotometer*. The ferrous sulphate solution has to be carefully prepared and handled to avoid chemical contaminants that can affect the result.

The dose is given by:

$$D = k\Delta A/[\varepsilon\delta\rho G(Fe^{3+})] \tag{3.10}$$

where k is a constant, ΔA is the change in absorption (optical density), δ is the optical path length, ρ is the Fricke density, ε is the difference in molar extinction coefficient and $G(Fe^{3+})$ is the chemical yield.

This system is not very sensitive such that doses of greater than 10 Gy are required to produce sufficient concentration of ferric ions, but accuracies of better than 2% are readily achievable. The process is effectively insensitive to dose rate and can be used to determine doses up to 400 Gy. The detector is 96% water and is therefore essentially water equivalent. It can be used over a wide range of energies and modalities. Fricke dosimetry has been used in the past by standards laboratories to confirm measurements of absorbed dose using other dosimetric techniques.

Ceric Dosimetry

Similar to Fricke dosimetry, ceric dosimetry relies on the reduction by radiation of ceric ions (Ce^{4+}) to cerous ions (Ce^{3+}) in a mixture of ceric and cerous ions in 0.4-M sulphuric acid. The concentration of cerous ions is determined by spectrophotometry using light with a wavelength of 320 nm.

Gel Dosimetry

The techniques described previously are suitable for producing single-point measurements of dose (e.g. ionisation chambers) or measurements of two-dimensional distributions (e.g. film) and three-dimensional arrangement of bead TLDs with a limited number of measuring points. In contrast to these, gel dosimeters allow measurement of three-dimensional distributions. These are ideally suited to determination of distributions arising from complex treatments such as intensity-modulated radiotherapy. In addition, gel dosimetry is proving useful in situations where other forms of measurement are difficult, such as in dosimetry of very small radiation fields (e.g. stereotactic radiotherapy and proton beams) and measurements around brachytherapy sources where the radiation dose varies rapidly with position relative to the source. Phantoms to hold the gel material can be made to reflect anatomical shapes.

There are currently two forms of gel detectors in use: Fricke gel and polymer gel. For each, various ways of reading out the signal have been developed, the most common of which are magnetic resonance (MR) and optical computed tomography (CT). Gel detectors in general are insensitive to dose rates and effectively water equivalent, and the signal is relatively linear with dose. Overall accuracy is limited (typically around 5%), although spatial resolution is excellent.

Fricke Gels and FXG Gels

In 1984 Gore and colleagues proposed the use of MR techniques on Fricke solutions[42] and Fricke-infused gels in which ferrous ions are held within the gel matrix. When reduced by radiation to ferric ions, the spin–spin (T2) relaxation times of linked protein atoms change. This change in relaxation time in each small volume of the material can be measured using an MR scanner. Each measurement is accompanied by a test irradiation that is used to determine the sensitivity of each detector batch to different dose levels.

Although able to produce accurate dose distributions, the process has two main drawbacks. First, measurement is time consuming and requires ready access to an MR scanner. Second, the ferric ions migrate through the gel matrix with time, so measurements have to be undertaken shortly after irradiation.[43]

A development of this technique led to the introduction of xylenol orange into the gel mix.[44] This material is photochromic and has the property of changing colour from orange to purple when the mix is irradiated. This change in colour can be determined by measuring the optical attenuation of filtered light. A set of two-dimensional slice readouts can be obtained using an optical CT device.

Polymer Gels

Polymer gels are based upon the polymerisation of monomers embedded in the gel matrix which produces long polymer chains and cross-linkage of polymers.[45] These reduce the T2 relaxation time which can be determined using an MR scanner. A common polymer gel in current use is the commercial BANG gel of Maryanski and colleagues,[46] which is based upon polymerisation of the monomer acrylamide. This may be produced in forms that allow optical readout using an optical CT device, as radiation induces white opacity in an otherwise transparent material. Because cross-linkage of monomers stabilises the material, there is no migration away from irradiated areas, such that these devices are stable over time.

BANG gels have to be produced and sealed while under a nitrogen atmosphere to avoid oxygen-induced polymerisation affecting the results. This necessity has been removed in newer gel formulations in which oxygen in the gel is bound into a chemical matrix which prevents it from causing polymerisation, making the production of gels for dosimetry far simpler.[47]

Alanine-Electron Paramagnetic Resonance Dosimetry

Alanine is a polycrystalline amino acid which has the chemical formula $CH_3CH(NH_2)COOH$. When irradiated, stable free radicals are formed within the material. These radicals can exist unchanged for long periods, allowing separation of irradiation from the readout process.[48] Some of these free radicals have a single unpaired electron attached to one of the atoms of the radical. The single unpaired electron exists in one of two energy states. When subjected to a magnetic field, these energy states equate to what is referred to as *parallel* and *antiparallel spin states*, the difference in energy between them being proportional to the strength of the magnetic field.

The electron normally occupies the lower state, but it may be excited into the higher state by absorbing a specific resonant wavelength of electromagnetic radiation of photon energy ($h\nu$) equal to the energy separation between the two states, for magnetic field strengths of 300 mT and frequency of about 9 MHz, which is within the microwave part of the electromagnetic spectrum. The concentration of free radicals can be assessed by measuring the degree of absorption of this resonant radiation, a process known as *electron paramagnetic resonance* (or traditionally *electron spin resonance*).[49] A number of free radicals are involved, the most important one involving the loss of the NH_2 group.

Dosimeters are formed by mixing known quantities of alanine with one or more binding agents to produce a compact, solid detector which has both density and atomic number values that differ only slightly from water and which is suitably sensitive to radiation. The dose response is almost linear from 10 to 10^4 Gy and is largely independent of dose rate. Lower doses down to below 1 Gy can be measured, provided that the device is calibrated to account for nonlinearity of response at these dose levels. Accuracies of better than 2% are achievable under controlled conditions. The combination of accuracy and stability has led to them being used by a number of standards laboratories as a basis for a remote calibration service which rivals the use of thermoluminescent dosimetry. Alanine dosimetry systems are also available commercially. A number of research groups are currently investigating the development of two-dimensional and three-dimensional measurement systems based upon spatially distributed alanine. Other groups are investigating chemical variations of alanine (e.g. 2-methylalanine) to develop dosimeters more suited to lower dose ranges for in vivo dosimetry.[50]

Biological Dosimetry

The response of biological systems has been used as an indicator of the dose delivered since the very first applications of radiation for the treatment of human disease. Early dosimetry standards were based upon skin erythema levels, with the absorbed dose determined by the degree of reddening of the skin and on the resultant type of erythema produced. This system was very inaccurate and was abandoned in favour of other physical forms of radiation dosimetry long before the introduction of skin-sparing megavoltage treatments. There are, however, circumstances, such as accidental exposures, where other forms of dosimetry are not applicable and where doses have to be estimated on the basis of the biological responses. There are various possible biological indicators of absorbed dose based upon the response of different biological systems. These include effects on biological molecules and genetic structures, but also effects on cells and structures.

Biological Molecules

The process described earlier in relation to alanine dosimetry, in which the concentration of long-lived free radicals can be determined by using electron spin resonance, may also be applicable to estimate doses to specific tissues. This process is relatively insensitive but has been used to estimate doses received around sites of nuclear explosions and accidents.[51,52]

An alternative method to assess absorbed dose is based upon quantifying changes in the chemical composition of bodily fluids. The concentration of thymidine in blood serum has been shown to be a sensitive indicator of absorbed dose in mice[53] but is unfortunately less applicable to primates.

Genetic Structures

The most advanced and established method of biological dosimetry is based upon determining the concentration of chromosome aberrations by counting the number of dicentrics in human peripheral blood lymphocytes.[54] This form of dosimetry is able to estimate doses down to about 0.1 Gy and is used in cases of accidental overexposure.

An alternative method is based upon determining the concentration of micronuclei formed as a result of the radiation exposure. This method may possibly be developed to compete with dicentric concentration analysis.[55]

Cells and Biological Structures

The dose responses for various biological systems are well documented in the literature. Radiation inhibits the production of blood cells, inhibits the production of sperm in males and leads to the death of hair follicles—all of which may be used to estimate the absorbed dose shortly after exposure. For high doses of radiation, breakdown of other organs may be used where the absorbed dose exceeds tissue tolerance levels for those organs.

COMPOSITE DETECTORS AND ARRAYS

Measurement of radiation dose distributions has been important in radiotherapy, primarily to assess the uniformity of radiation beams and determine the size of the radiation beam. Radiographic film densitometry (see the 'Film Dosimetry' section) was extensively used for this, and it provided a high-resolution detector with uniform response. Film provided a simple, practical and easily assessed hard copy of the results with almost no data processing.

The alternative method used a single scanning ionisation chamber, or solid-state photon or electron detector which traversed the beam. Single-detector scanning and film techniques were time-consuming to undertake and to process. However, while treatment techniques remained simple, there was little impetus for greater measurement complexity. In addition, in the past, the consistency of detector production and performance was variable, and multiple detector arrays were problematic because of nonuniform performance.

This situation has changed dramatically with dynamic and intensity-modulated beam delivery. It is worth mentioning at this point that there have been two approaches to performing quality control measurements on volumetric modulated dose distribution such as those delivered by volumetric modulated arc therapy (VMAT). The first technique measures the two-dimensional distribution of fluence from a beam and compares it with the intended delivery. The second technique measures a distribution delivered to a regular phantom with the modulated beams intended for treatment. Both techniques are used; the first requires an area detector array, whereas the second needs a volumetric detector array.

Linear Detector Arrays

As mentioned earlier, single-detector scanners (Fig. 3.21) could provide measurement of the radiation distribution within the beam, and the use of a single detector ensured that the measurements were entirely consistent with each other and there were no inherent artefacts because of detector response variation. The first complication with the use of a single-detector scanner arose with the introduction of dynamic wedges (see Chapter 10).

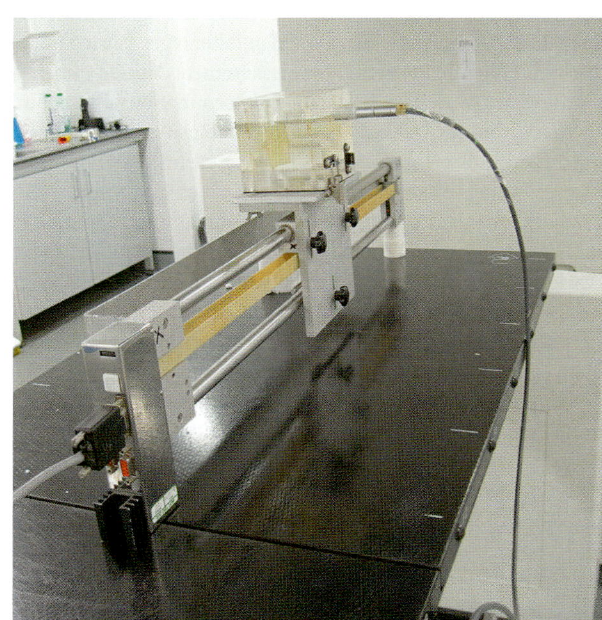

Fig. 3.21 One-dimensional single-detector scanner.

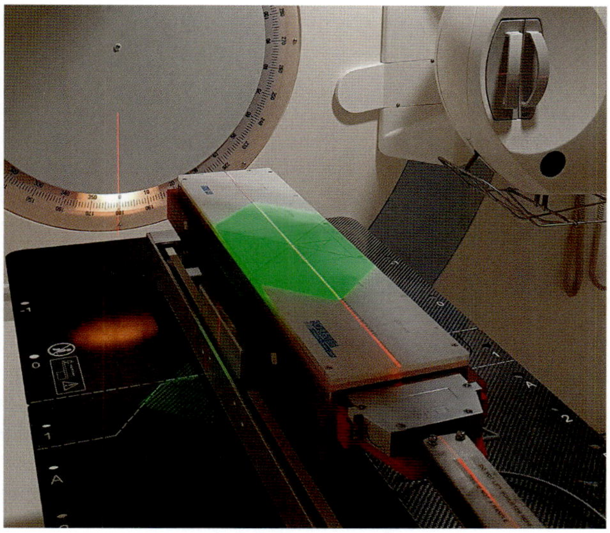

Fig. 3.22 Schuster array.

The variability in detector response was overcome in a linear array by checking and correcting the response of each detector on an individual basis before its practical use. Fig. 3.22 shows such a system, known as a Schuster array. An initial calibration of the array before its use would step through all 88 detectors in the array, placing each on the central axis of the radiation beam and determining calibration factors for each detector to provide a uniform response across the entire array. Following this calibration, the equipment users could confidently interpret the beam profiles and make adjustments to the radiotherapy beams as required.

Area Arrays

One of the earliest two-dimensional measurement devices used a radiofluorescent screen and imaging system which captured a digital image using a camera (Fig. 3.23). This enabled the beam fluence to be captured for analysis. The system was a logical extension of film to a measurement system which would effectively process the image data to assess the fluence distribution, the beam size and the field edges. The system was large and cumbersome and did not lend itself to easy use.

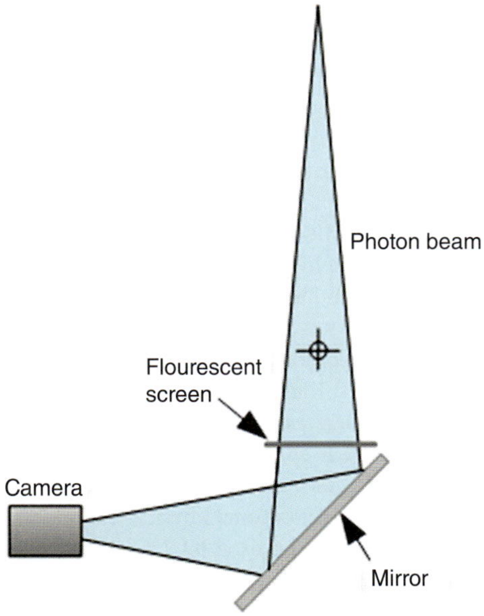

Fig. 3.23 The main components of a beam imaging system to measure fluence in two dimensions.

With improved consistency of detector production and electronic processing performance, detector arrays which could be used with confidence of insignificant inherent detector variation became practically feasible. Modern two-dimensional arrays are lightweight devices (Fig. 14.5) which can be used on couch tops or mounted to the radiation head of the machine. Detectors can be solid-state diodes or ion chambers, depending upon the manufacturer. They provide real-time monitoring of beam profiles along major axes and diagonal axes of the radiation beam. They also enable intensity-modulated beam fluences to be readily measured and assessed as part of patient-specific quality control (PSQC)—see Chapter 14.

Digital two-dimensional fluence measurements, whether from densitometered film or two-dimensional arrays, require analysis software to fully use the information acquired. Commercial software packages were developed for this and could be applied to any digital two-dimensional measurement.

Volume Detector Arrays

The introduction of intensity-modulated treatment delivery has meant that there is a need for patient-specific checks to be undertaken, often on an individual patient basis. With the widespread adoption of volumetric intensity-modulated treatment delivery, the need to rapidly assess a treatment delivery in three dimensions as part of patient pretreatment verification has made volumetric arrays essential. Although gel systems, as described earlier, can provide high-resolution three-dimensional measurements, the processes they use are time-consuming and lend themselves to research work and quality audit. For routine PSQC work, the consistent performance of modern radiation detectors has enabled reliable three-dimensional arrays to be developed (see Fig. 14.6).

ELECTRONIC PORTAL DOSIMETRY

From the start of developing megavoltage electronic portal imaging devices (EPIDs), it was envisaged that such an imaging system could be used to measure dose distribution within a patient by combining CT images of the patient with the beam fluence detected by the EPID. Initially, the CT data set was considered to be the planning data set. However, with cone beam CT routinely used to verify treatment setup, the CT data set acquired at treatment could now be used to improve accuracy. As has been seen in this chapter, physical radiation detectors need to be considered carefully and their performance understood to obtain accurate measurements. In addition, the beam model needs to be able to accurately model the dose distribution from the measured fluences. The value of portal dosimetry depends upon measurement accuracy. Currently, the best accuracy is to within ±5%, depending upon the physical situation with regard to the patient and beam delivery. This method of treatment verification is now used clinically (see Chapters 11 and 14).

ALTERNATIVE SYSTEMS FOR PROTON AND ION BEAM DOSE MEASUREMENT

There are three types of measurement to be considered in proton and carbon therapy clinical measurements:

- Relative dose measurements
- Reference dose measurements
- Absolute dose measurements

Relative measurements of proton beams refer to measurements proportional to dose but expressed in either units of percent or simple ratios. Because cyclotron beam intensity can vary, any measurements are referenced to the incoming primary beam. Relative measurements encompass lateral two-dimensional scans, and importantly, depth-dose scans of the pristine Bragg peak and of the prescribed depth dose or SOBP (see Chapter 10).

Many devices used in radiotherapy physics quality assurance are unsuitable for proton therapy purposes. X-ray film is rarely used, and Fricke and polymer gels and TLD detectors are categorised as one-hit detectors and exhibit significant underresponse in the low-energy Bragg peak region, where the proton tracks are highly ionising and therefore of high linear energy transfer (LET). These devices may be used where only measurements at a single energy or depth are being monitored. Radiochromic films such as GAF, based on density change brought about by radiation-induced polymerisation, show a much-reduced quenching effect, which has led to their wider adoption in proton therapy quality control of field area homogeneity, skew and aperture verification checks.

Measurement of the pristine Bragg peak at particular energies, and also the prescribed SOBP, is performed by central axis depth-dose scans as in photon and electron radiotherapy beams. The gold standard for proton and carbon ion beam depth-dose measurement is considered to be the use of a waterproof parallel plate ion chamber, moveable in a water tank. The ion chamber, if used at an appropriate bias potential, does not exhibit Bragg peak quenching, and there is no evidence of significant ion recombination effect changes with energy and clinical dose rates.

Early developments for rapid measurement have used flat silicon photodiodes in air, behind a rotating polymethacrylate (PMMA) wheel, which creates a variable depth. The latter has to be converted to water-equivalent depth by correcting with PMMA-to-water stopping-power ratios. It should be noted that in certain cases, semiconductor diodes can exhibit slight overresponse at the Bragg peak and a gradually reduced sensitivity induced by radiation damage. Of note is recent work with microdiamond detectors which are essentially carbon and close to being water equivalent. These have demonstrated excellent spatial resolution with both negligible quenching at the proton Bragg peak and negligible response fading with accumulated dose.

Water tank measurements, for Bragg peak, SOBP and range constancy checks, are time-consuming and suitable only for horizontal beam orientations. Vendors, such as IBA (with Zebra) and PTW (with Pathfinder), have provided sealed, in-water depth-dose scanners where a bellows reservoir acts as the variable absorber before a moving flat ion chamber. These provide fast scans and recording, at submillimetric resolution, at any orientation. In other configurations, devices such as the IBA Zebra offer even faster acquisition with an array of ion chambers sandwiched in a water-equivalent absorber, but with reduced spatial resolution.

Proton lateral fields for pencil beam scanning (PBS) beams (see Chapter 10) need to be measured for beam commissioning, beamlet characterisation, homogeneity, skewness and patient plan verification by two-dimensional detector arrays with fast readout. Vendors provide two-dimensional arrays; IBA with Matrix and PTW with Octavius, with more than 1000 vented miniature ion chambers which automatically analyse and store results. Typical chamber spacings are 2 mm, with fields up to 24×24 cm^2. Miniature ion chamber arrays avoid dose degradation and energy dependence issues. An alternative system by IBA, the Lynx PT, uses large plastic scintillation screens, up to 30×30 cm^2, with multiple CCD detectors with 0.5-mm spatial resolution; however, corrections are required.

Three-dimensional dose distributions are particularly problematic for measuring in the vicinity of high dose gradients in small or complex proton fields. This is because of the limited choice of detectors, whether semiconductor diodes or miniature ion chambers. Pinpoint thimble ion chambers with volumes less than 0.03 cm^3 have become available, with the PTW N31015®, offering excellent spatial resolution for higher energy proton beams, as does synthetic micro-diamond detectors such as the PTW 60019®. PRESSAGE radiochromic gels have also shown promise in small, complex, three-dimensional dose distributions, but they have a quenching underresponse at end of range which requires correction.

REFERENCES

1. Beddar AS, Mackie TR, Attix FH. Water-equivalent plastic scintillation detectors for high-energy beam dosimetry: 1. Physical characteristics and theoretical considerations. *Phys Med Biol.* 1992;37:1883–1900.
2. Fluhs D, Heintz M, Indenkampen F, Wieczorek C, Kolanoski H, Quast U. Direct reading measurement of absorbed dose with plastic scintillators: the general concept and applications to ophthalmic plaque dosimetry. *Med Phys.* 1996;23:427–434.
3. Kirov AS, Piao JZ, Mathur NK, et al. The three-dimensional scintillation dosimetry method: test for a ^{106}Ru eye plaque applicator. *Phys Med Biol.* 2005;50:3063–3081.
4. Marie and Pierre Curie, 'Quartz piezo electrometer', College of physicians of Philadelphia digital library. https://www.cppdigitallibrary.org/items/show/2593
5. Lourenco A, Lee N, Shipley D, et al. Application of a portable primary standard level graphite calorimeter for absolute dosimetry in a clinical low-energy passively scattered proton beam. *Phys Med Biol.* 2022;67(22):1–8. https://doi.org/10.1088/1361-6560/ac95f6.
6. DuSautoy AR. The UK primary standard calorimeter for photon beam absorbed dose measurement. *Phys Med Biol.* 1996;41: 137–151.
7. Marsh ARS, Williams TT. *50 kV Primary standard of exposure: design of free-air chamber. RS(Ext) 54.* 1982.
8. Palmer JA, Duane S, Shipley R, Moretti CJ. The design and construction of a new primary standard free air chamber for medium energy x-rays. *Med Biol Eng Comput.* 1997;35:1086.
9. Morgan AA, Aird EGA, Aukett RJ, et al. IPEM guidelines on dosimeter systems for use as transfer instruments between UK primary dosimetry standards laboratory (NPL) and radiotherapy centres. *Phys Med Biol.* 2000;45:2445–2457.
10. Nutbrown RF, Duane S, Shipley DR, Thomas RAS. Evaluation of factors to convert absorbed dose calibrations from graphite to water for the NPL high-energy photon calibration service. *Phys Med Biol.* 2002;47:441–454.
11. Damen P. *Design of a water calorimeter for medium energy x-rays: a status report. CCRI(I)/05-38.* The Netherlands: NMi Van Swinden Laboratorium; 2005. https://www.bipm.org/documents/20126/48195240/working-document-ID-1751/11e7219f-76b0-3bc8-449c-481d525349f5.
12. Krauss A. The PTB water calorimeter for the absolute determination of absorbed dose to water in 60Co radiation. *Metrologia.* 2006;43(3):259–272.
13. Palmans H, Seuntjens JP. Construction, correction factors and relative heat defect of a high purity 4° calorimeter for absorbed dose determinations in high-energy photon beams. *Proceedings of the NPL Calorimetry Workshop.* Teddington, Middlesex, UK: National Physical Laboratory; 1994.
14. Ross CK, Seuntjens JP, Klassen NV, Shortt KR. The NRC sealed water calorimeter: correction factors and performance. In: Williams AJ, Rosser KE, eds. *Proceedings of the NPL Workshop on Recent Advances in Calorimetric Absorbed Dose Standards.* Teddington, Middlesex, UK: National Physical Laboratory; 2000.
15. Williams AJ, Rosser KE, Thomson NJ, DuSautoy AR. Recent advances in water calorimetry at NPL. *Proceedings of the 22nd Annual EMBS International Conference.* Chicago; 2000.
16. Rosser KE, Owen B, DuSautoy AR, Pritchard DH, Stoker I, Brend CJ. The NPL absorbed dose to water calibration service for

high-energy photons. *Proceedings of the Symposium on Measurement Assurance in Dosimetry*. Vienna: IAEA; 1994:73–81 IAEA-SM-330/35.

17. NPL. *Practical Course in Reference Dosimetry*. United Kingdom: National Physical Laboratory; 2006.
18. Lillicrap SC, Owen B, Williams JR, Williams PC. Code of practice for high-energy photon therapy dosimetry based on the NPL absorbed dose calibration service. *Phys Med Biol*. 1990;35:1355–1360.
19. IAEA. *Absorbed Dose Determination in External Beam Radiotherapy. An international code of practice for dosimetry based on standards of absorbed dose to water. IAEA TRS-398*. Vienna: IAEA; 2000.
20. Lourenco A, Subiel A, Lee N, et al. Absolute dosimetry for FLASH proton pencil beam scanning radiotherapy. *Sci Rep13*; 2023:2054. https://doi.org/10.1038/s41598-023-28192-0.
21. Farmer FT. A substandard x-ray dose-meter. *Br J Radiol*. 1955;28:304.
22. Shonka RF, Rose JE, Failla G. Conducting plastic equivalent to tissue, air and polystyrene. *2nd United Nations Conference on Peaceful Uses of Atomic Energy*. New York: United Nations; 1958:160.
23. IPEM. The IPEMB code of practice for the determination of absorbed dose for x-rays below 300 kV generating potential (0.035 mm Al–4 mm Cu HVL; 10–300 kV generating potential). *Phys Med Biol*. 1996;41:2605–2625.
24. IPEM. Addendum to the IPEMB code of practice for the determination of absorbed dose for x-rays below 300 kV generating potential (0.035 mm Al–4 mm Cu HVL; 10–300 kV generating potential). *Phys Med Biol*. 2005;50:2739–2748.
25. IPSM. Code of practice for high-energy photon therapy dosimetry based on the NPL absorbed dose calibration service. *Phys Med Biol*. 1990;35:1355–1360.
26. IPEM. The IPEM code of practice for electron dosimetry for radiotherapy beams of initial energy from 4 to 25 MeV based on an absorbed dose to water calibration. *Phys Med Biol*. 2003; 48:2929–2970.
27. Barish RJ, Lerch IA. Long-term use of an isotope check source for verification of ion chamber calibration. *Med Phys*. 1992;17:203–206.
28. Burns JE, Rosser KE. Saturation corrections for the NPL 2560/1 dosemeter in photon dosimetry. *Phys Med Biol*. 1991;35:687–693.
29. Havercroft JM, Klevenhagen SC. Ion chamber corrections for parallel-plate and thimble chambers in electron and photon radiation. *Phys Med Biol*. 1993;38:25–38.
30. Wickman G. A liquid ionization chamber with high spatial resolution. *Phys Med Biol*. 1974;19:37–48.
31. Gonzalez-Castano DM, Gomez F, Brualla L, et al. A liquid filled ionization chamber for high precision relative dosimetry. *Phys Med*. 2011;27:89–96.
32. Lewis DF. A processless electronic recording medium. *Electronic Imaging Proceedings of SPSE's Symposium*. Arlington, VA: Society for Imaging Science and Technology; 1986:76–79.
33. Grusell E, Rikner G. Evaluation of temperature effects in p-type silicon detectors. *Phys Med Biol*. 1986;31:527–534.
34. Rikner G. *Silicon diodes as detectors in radiation dosimetry of photon, electron and proton radiation fields*. Thesis. Sweden: Uppsala; 1983.
35. Shi J, Simon WE, Ding L, Saini D. Important issues regarding diode performance in radiation therapy applications. *Proceedings of the 22nd Annual Engineering in Medicine and Biology Society (EMBC)*. IEEE, Chicago; 2000.
36. Rikner G, Grusell E. Effects of radiation damage on p-type silicon diodes. *Phys Med Biol*. 1983;28:1261–1267.
37. Khrunov VS, Martynov SS, Vatnitsky SM, et al. Diamond detectors in relative dosimetry of photon, electron and proton radiation fields. *Radiat Prot Dosimetry*. 1990;33:155–157.
38. Kron T. Thermoluminescence dosimetry and its applications in medicine: part 1. Physics, materials and equipment. *Australas Phys Eng Sci Med*. 1994;17:175–199.
39. Jafari SM, Bradley DA, Goldstone CA, et al. Low cost commercial glass beads as dosimeters in radiotherapy. *Radiat Phys Chem*. 2014;97:95–101.
40. Jafari SM, Jordan TJ, Hussein M, et al. Energy response of glass bead TLDs irradiated with radiation therapy beams. *Phys Med Biol*. 2014;59:6875–6889.
41. Fricke H, Morse S. The chemical action of roentgen rays on dilute ferrous sulphate solutions as a measure of radiation dose. *Am J Roentgenol Radium Ther Nucl Med*. 1927;18:430–432.
42. Gore JC, Kang YS, Schulz RJ. Measurement of radiation dose distributions by nuclear magnetic resonance (NMR) imaging. *Phys Med Biol*. 1984;29:1189–1197.
43. Baldock C, Harris PJ, Piercy AR, Healy B. Experimental determination of the diffusion coefficient in two dimensions in ferrous sulphate gels using the finite element method. *Australas Phys Eng Sci Med*. 2001;24:19–30.
44. Appleby A, Leghrouz A. Imaging of radiation dose by visible colour development in ferrous-agarose-xylenol orange gels. *Med Phys*. 1991;18:309–312.
45. Maryanski MJ, Gore JC, Kennan RP, Schulz RJ. NMR relaxation enhancement in gels polymerized and cross-linked by ionizing radiations: a new approach to 3D dosimetry by MRI. *Magn Reson Imaging*. 1993;11:253–258.
46. Maryanski MJ, Schuklz RJ, Ibbott GS, et al. Magnetic resonance imaging of radiation dose distributions using polymer gel dosimeter. *Phys Med Biol*. 1994;39:1437–1455.
47. Fong PM, Keil DC, Does MD, Gore JC. Polymer gels for magnetic resonance imaging of radiation dose distributions at normal room atmosphere. *Phys Med Biol*. 2001;46:3105–3113.
48. Bradshaw WW, Cadena DG, Crawford GW, Spelzler HAW. The use of alanine as solid dosimeter. *Radiat Res*. 1962;17:11.
49. Regulla DF, Deffner U. Dosimetry by ESR spectroscopy of alanine. *Appl Radiat Isot*. 1982;33:1101.
50. Olsson S, Sagstuen E, Bonora M, Lund A. EPR dosimetric properties of 2-methylalanine: EPR, ENDOR and FT-EPR investigations. *Radiat Res*. 2002;V157:113–121.
51. Mascarenhas S, Hasegawa A, Takeshita K. EPR dosimetry of bones from the Hiroshima A-bomb site. *Bull Am Phys Soc*. 1973;18:579.
52. Guskova AK, Barabanova AV, Baranov AY. Acute radiation effects in victims of the Chernobyl nuclear power plant accident. In: Guskova AK, ed. *Unscear report on sources and effects of ionizing radiation, appendix 613-631*. New York: United Nations; 1988.
53. Feinendegen LE, Muhlensiepen H, Porchen W, Booz J. Acute non-stochastic effect of very low dose whole body exposure, a thymidine equivalent serum factor. *Int J Radiat Biol*. 1982;41: 139–150.
54. Bender MA, Awa AA, Brooks AL, et al. Current status of cytogenetic procedures to detect and quantify previous exposures to radiation. *Mutat Res*. 1988;196:103–159.
55. Prosser JS, Lloyd DC, Edwards AA. A comparison of chromosomal and micronuclear methods for radiation accident dosimetry. In: Goldfinch EP, ed. *Radiation Protection: Theory and Practice*. United Kingdom: Institute of Physics, 1989: 133–136.

4

Radiation Protection

Elizabeth Davies and Richard Raynor

CHAPTER OUTLINE

INTRODUCTION

Soon after the discovery of ionising radiation, early radiation workers started to notice its effect on the body. The biological effects of ionising radiation are described in detail in Chapter 5 and are summarised in the following section. While knowledge and understanding of the effects of radiation on the body is an area of constant research, the main sources of data are from radiation accidents, research following the Hiroshima and Nagasaki atomic bombs, follow-up of radiotherapy treatments and the results from animal experiments. International expert groups, principally the International Commission on Radiological Protection (ICRP), have specified levels of radiation which are deemed 'acceptable' when compared with other, non-radiation risks. To allow this level of risk comparison, a quantity that can be measured and associated dosimetric units have been established. This chapter details this system.

To control these risks, most countries have ragulatory requirements that must be met to limit the exposure to individuals arising from the use of radiation. This chapter describes the UK legislative requirements and some of the methods used to ensure compliance with these requirements.

BACKGROUND RADIATION

It is important to remember that, regardless of our occupation, we are all exposed to radiation from natural radiation sources in the environment and from non-natural sources. We often have little control over our level of exposure to these sources of natural radiation, as they arise from everyday lifestyle factors. For example, part of our exposure to background radiation comes from cosmic rays from outer space. These rays are attenuated by the Earth's atmosphere—the more atmosphere there is, the more the attenuation. This means that people who live at high altitudes or travel in high-flying planes will get a greater radiation dose from cosmic rays. Other sources of natural radiation and the proportions they contribute to the overall dose are shown in Fig. 4.1.

The main source of natural radiation are the radioactive gases radon and thoron, which are generated in granite rock and therefore vary around the world based on the amount of granite rock in the area. For example, in Cornwall, England, the level of radon gas is up to three times the national average. The high contribution from radon gas in some areas means that there are specific requirements for the development of homes and work environments to ensure that people do not

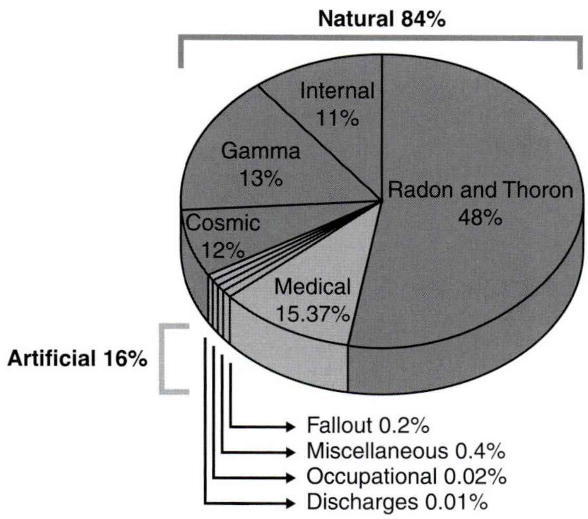

Fig. 4.1 The average background radiation level in the United Kingdon is 2.7 mSv per year from the sources detailed in this pie chart. (Numbers courtesy National Radiation Protection Board, now the UK Health Security Agency.)

have unnecessarily high radon exposure. All the natural sources of radiation we are exposed to lead to an average dose of about 2.3 mSv per annum to a member of the UK population.[1]

Another 0.4 mSv per annum is contributed to by nonnatural sources, making the average total dose 2.7 mSv.[1] While there are contributions to this dose from various sources, the biggest contributor to nonnatural exposures is medical use of radiation. Because this is a controllable exposure, a great deal of effort has been put into reducing both the individual dose per patient and the number of examinations conducted.

BIOLOGICAL EFFECTS OF RADIATION

There are several types of biological effects resulting from exposure to ionising radiation which are caused by the human body absorbing the energy associated with the radiation. *Somatic effects* refer to those affecting the physical human body (Fig. 4.2). Energy absorption can be measured in joules/kg, which is given the special unit of gray (Gy), which is commonly used in radiotherapy (see Chapter 2) . Such energy absorption can cause direct damage by ionisation forming charged particles and indirect damage by the formation of free radicals. Different areas of the body have different degrees of radiation sensitivity, that is

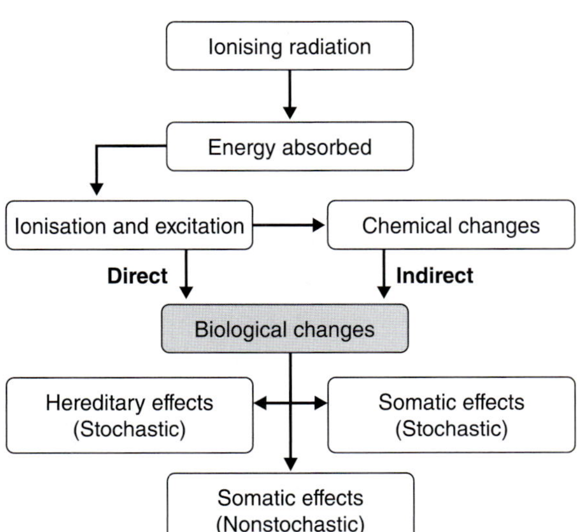

Fig. 4.2 Effects of radiation on the body.

the likelihood of causing damage, which is reflected in the fact that there are different dose limits for specific areas of the body, as will be discussed later. While knowledge of the biological effects of radiation is continually evolving, there are currently thought to be two main types of reactions in the body: stochastic or random effects, and tissue effects (previously termed 'deterministic effects').

Stochastic Effects

Stochastic effects are thought to be effects resulting from damage in a single cell and which are random in nature. In this case, the risk of the effect, rather than the severity of the effect, is dependent on the dose. Examples of stochastic effects are cancer induction or potential hereditary defects in the offspring of exposed individuals. An assumption is made currently that there is a *linear no threshold (LNT)* relationship between dose and risk. That is, there is no threshold at which the effects do not occur, and there is a linear increase in the occurrence as the exposure increases. This relationship is based on scientific observations from high dose exposures. There are competing theories on the relationship at low-doses, such as those seen through occupational exposures, but research has not yet been able to firmly prove any of these. Thus, a pragmatic approach has been to assume that the relationship at high doses can be extrapolated to lower doses.

Cancer Induction

Cancer has several causes, radiation being only one. About 1 in 2 individuals is likely to have a cancer in their lifetime.[2] The current risk estimated by ICRP 103[3] of cancer induction from ionising radiation is 1 in 18,000 for a radiation dose of 1 mSv (see the 'Dose Descriptors' section). The extra cancer risk from very low doses is extremely small and, in practice, undetectable in the population due to the high underlying lifetime risk of cancer incidence. Even after high-dose exposure, it is not possible to be certain that radiation was solely responsible for a cancer arising in an individual.

Hereditary Effects

Hereditary effects are expressed in exposed individuals' offspring, or future generations, rather than the exposed individuals themselves. Examples of natural hereditary defects are having one eye a different colour from the other, or one limb shorter or even missing. Genetic defects appear in the population due to many causes at an underlying rate of about 1 in 200 live births, and there is no way to differentiate natural defects from radiation-induced defects. As such, the possibility of radiation being the cause of any defect can only be shown statistically; the probability is assumed to be dose dependent and rising with increases in dose. The current risk estimated by ICRP 103[3] of severe hereditary effects from radiation is 1 in 500,000 for a radiation dose of 1 mSv (see the 'Dose Descriptors' section). The ICRP note that there is no direct evidence of heritable effects from radiation exposures in human epidemiological studies, and that instead, mutational effects have only been observed in experimental animals. Nevertheless, they justify the inclusion of a component of heritable risk in detriment estimates.

Tissue Reactions

Tissue reactions are caused by cell death. They only occur once the level of dose received exceeds a threshold dose to cause that effect. These effects may occur soon after irradiation (early) or after some time (late). Early (acute) effects may include radiation burns, hair loss, sterility, vomiting and diarrhoea. Neurological effects and cardiovascular disease[4] are thought to be late tissue reactions. The threshold for each type of tissue reaction varies between individuals but is currently defined as the point at which the effect would be produced in 1% of individuals.[5] The severity of the tissue reactions increases with the dose beyond the threshold. While there is some debate regarding whether cataracts are a stochastic

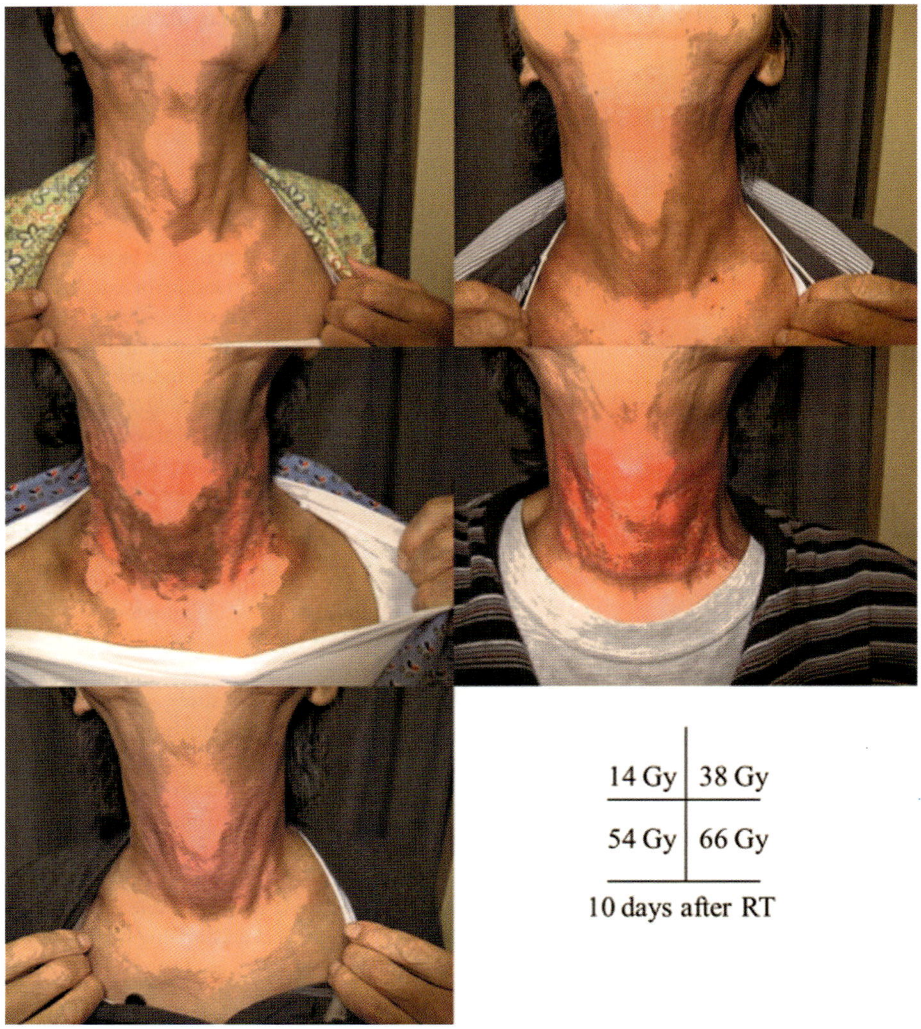

Fig. 4.3 Clinical symptoms of acute radiation erythema. (From Zenda S, Ota Y, Tachibana H, et al. A prospective picture collection study for a grading atlas of radiation dermatitis for clinical trials in head-and-neck cancer patients. *J Radiat Res.* 2016;57(3):301–306. doi: 10.1093/jrr/rrv092.)

effect[6] with no threshold dose or a tissue reaction with a threshold dose, they are generally classified as a late tissue reaction at present.

Dependent on the area irradiated and the level of dose received, tissue reactions can be seen in some patients undergoing radiotherapy exposures (an example is shown in Fig. 4.3). Details of dose thresholds that need to be exceeded for different effects are given in Table 4.1. These thresholds should be considered as minimum dose thresholds and may vary upwards due to variance in the individual and the way in which the dose is delivered (e.g. vascularity of the tissue) or the period over which the dose is delivered.

DOSE DESCRIPTORS

There are two main dose units in use: gray (Gy) and sievert (Sv). ***Absorbed dose*** is a measure of energy absorbed in units of gray (joules/kg). Two other quantities are relevant when discussing radiation protection matters: ***equivalent dose*** and ***effective dose***, which have the unit of sievert.

Equivalent Dose

The total energy deposited is not the only factor which determines the extent of damage. The same absorbed dose delivered by different types of radiation may result in varying degrees of biological damage to body tissues. Equivalent dose was introduced to incorporate the effect of the type of radiation being absorbed on harmful biological effects. Equivalent dose is therefore a measure of the risk associated with an exposure to ionising radiation. Risks caused by exposures to different radiation types can be directly compared when expressed in terms of equivalent dose.

TABLE 4.1 Dose Thresholds for Biological Effects

Acute Exposure Threshold (Gy)	Area Erradiated	Effect
~0.1	Testes	Temporary sterility
~6	Testes	Permanent sterility
~3	Ovaries	Permanent sterility
~4	Skin	Temporary hair loss
5–10	Skin (large area)	Skin burns
~0.5	Eye	Cataracts
10	Skin (large area)	Late atrophy

From Table 4.4 ICRP. ICRP statement on tissue reactions/early and late effects of radiation in normal tissues and organs – threshold doses for tissue reactions in a radiation protection context. ICRP Publication 118. *Ann ICRP.* 2012;41(1/2). https://www.icrp.org/publication.asp?id=ICRP%20Publication%20118

TABLE 4.2 Weighting Factors for Different Types of Radiation

Radiation Type and Energy Range	Radiation Weighting Factor (W_R)
Photons—all energies	1
Electrons—all energies	1
Protons	2
Alpha particles	20

Used with permission from The 2007 recommendations of the International Commission on Radiological Protection. ICRP publication 103. *Ann ICRP.* 2007;37(2–4):1–332. Elsevier.

TABLE 4.3 W_T Values: Tissue Weighting Factors According to ICRP 103 (ICRP 2007)

Tissue	Tissue Weighting Factor W_T	ΣW_T
Bone marrow (red), colon, lung, stomach, breast, remaining tissue[a]	0.12	0.72
Gonads	0.08	0.08
Bladder, liver, oesophagus, thyroid	0.04	0.16
Bone surface, brain, salivary glands, skin	0.01	0.04
	Total	1.00

[a]Remaining tissues: adrenals, extra thoracic region, gall bladder, heart, kidneys, lymphatic nodes, muscle, oral mucosa, pancreas, prostate, small intestine, spleen, thymus, uterus/cervix

Used with permission from The 2007 recommendations of the International Commission on Radiological Protection. ICRP publication 103. *Ann ICRP.* 2007;37(2–4):1–332. Elsevier.

Equivalent dose (Sv) is defined for a given type of radiation by the relationship:

$$\text{Equivalent dose (Sv), H} = \text{Absorbed dose (Gy)} \times \text{Radiation weighting factor, } W_R \quad \textbf{(4.1)}$$

The radiation weighting factor is a dimensionless number which depends on the way in which the energy of the radiation is distributed along its path through the tissue. The rate of deposition of energy along the track is known as the *linear energy transfer (LET)* of the radiation and has units of keV μm^{-1} measured in water, which is considered equivalent to tissue. Types of radiation with a high LET, such as protons and alpha particles, are more likely to damage the small structures in tissue, such as DNA molecules, in a way that leads to biological changes than types of radiation with a low LET, such as x-rays or beta particles. This is because the energy from high-LET radiation is absorbed in a small volume surrounding the trail of dense ionisation produced by this radiation. The radiation weighting factor is related to the LET of the radiation. The radiation weighting factors given in ICRP 103[3] are used to correct for differences in the biological damage to tissue caused by chronic exposure to different radiations (Table 4.2).

Effective Dose

Just as the same absorbed dose delivered by different types of radiation results in different levels of biological harm, the same absorbed dose delivered to different tissues results in different levels of biological harm. If the entire body were irradiated with a uniform beam of a single type of radiation, some parts of the body would react more than others. Equivalent dose accounts for this varying biological effect based on particular tissue types or organs. To take this effect into account, the ICRP have developed a list of tissue weighting factors, denoted W_T, for several organs and tissues that most significantly contribute to an overall effective level of biological damage to the body. Areas of the body with high cell turnover are more vulnerable to stochastic effects than areas with slower cell turnover and thus have a larger weighting factor.

Effective dose (Sv) is defined by the relationship:

$$E = \sum_{\text{All tissues}} \text{Equivalent dose, H(Sv)} \times \text{Tissue weighting factor, } W_T \quad \textbf{(4.2)}$$

Table 4.3 presents values of the tissue weighting factor W_T taken from ICRP 103 based upon age- and sex-averaged population. To arrive at an effective dose for a particular examination, it is necessary to determine the equivalent dose for the different listed tissues or body parts, multiply these doses by the relevant tissue weighting factor and then sum the constituent parts. The unit of effective dose is the sievert, and a worked example is given in Table 4.4. Effective dose was not developed for use in routine medical settings but for radiological protection situations where it was anticipated that the exposure

TABLE 4.4 Effective Dose From a Chest X-ray With a Skin Entrance Dose of 500 μGy

Organ	% Entrance Dose	Absorbed Dose (μGy)	Equivalent Dose (μSv)	Weighting Factor	Tissued Weighted Dose (μSv)
Gonads	0.2	1	1	0.08	0.08
Breast	2	10	10	0.12	1.2
Bone marrow (red)	1	5	5	0.12	0.6
Lung	30	150	150	0.12	18
Thyroid	1	5	5	0.04	0.2
Bone marrow (red)	1	5	5	0.01	0.05
Stomach	5	25	25	0.12	3
Liver	10	50	50	0.04	2
Remainder organs (including heart)	2.1	10.5	10.5	0.12	1.26
				Effective dose (μSv)	25.13

Based on the ICRP figure of 1 in 18,000 cancer incidences per mSv, this implies an additional risk of 1 in 682,335.

would be more uniform across the body. Effective dose requires many assumptions to be made, resulting in potentially high errors.[7] In many applications, such as in radiotherapy, it is more appropriate to provide equivalent or absorbed doses to organs.

LEGISLATIVE REQUIREMENTS

There are two main pieces of legislation associated with the safe use of ionising radiation within healthcare. They are the Ionising Radiations Regulations 2017 (IRR17),[8] which covers the protection of workers and the public from risks associated with ionising radiation; and the Ionising Radiation (Medical Exposure) Regulations 2017 (IRMER17) and amendments 2018, 2024,[9–11] which covers the safe use of ionising radiation for medical and non-medical imaging of the individual. There are other pieces of legislation which also have implications within the healthcare setting, and these are also summarised within this section. In addition to these two major regulations, environmental aspects, transport of radioactive sources and high-activity radiation sources are subject to legislation.

THE IONISING RADIATIONS REGULATIONS 2017

The Ionising Radiations Regulations 2017 (IRR17)[8] cover the protection of staff and the public from practices involving radiation, and breaches of their requirements could lead to prosecution by the regulators, normally the Health and Safety Executive (HSE). To aid implementation of the legislation, the HSE publish the 'Work with ionising radiation' Approved Code of Practice (ACOP) and guidance.[12] Good practice guidance is produced by the Institute of Physics and Engineering in Medicine (IPEM)[13] to support implementation in the medical sector. The Ionising Radiations Regulations require three basic requirements to be met:

- No practice involving radiation will be adopted unless it can be justified that there is a positive net benefit, either to the exposed individuals or to society.
- All exposures must be as low as reasonably achievable (ALARA) or practicable (ALARP). This principle requires that for any source, the number of people being exposed and the likelihood of incurring exposures (where exposures are not certain) be optimised, taking into account social and economic factors. In practice, this assessment must be documented within a risk assessment.
- Doses to individuals must not exceed certain dose limits. The exposure of individuals resulting from the combination of all relevant practices is subject to dose limits. These are aimed at ensuring that no individual is exposed to radiation risks that are judged to be unacceptable from these practices in any normal circumstances.

The original regulations were enacted in 1985 and were revised first in 1999 and again in 2017. Both revisions were triggered by changes in scientific literature leading to the implementation of lower dose limits. The 2017 revision[8] occurred in part because of a reassessment of the risk of radiation to the lens of the eye. This led to a requirement to reduce the previous dose limit to the lens from 150 mSv to 20 mSv per year.

Another change introduced by the 2017 regulations[8] was the introduction of a three-tier system for gaining the approval of the HSE to use ionising radiation. This is known as the *graded approach*, because higher-risk practices require greater oversight and input from both the employer and the regulators. Depending on the level of risk of the ionising radiation work that is undertaken in a hospital, an application will need to be made to either notify the HSE (lowest risk), register with the HSE or get consent from the HSE (highest risk).

Due to the potentially higher risk associated with radiotherapy, consent from the HSE is required. This involves the submission of an application for consent including a safety assessment, payment of a fee and inspections from the HSE.

Risk Assessments

Prior to starting any work with radiation, a risk assessment must be completed to ensure that all doses are kept as low as reasonably practicable. This is similar to the requirement under the Management of Health and Safety at Work Regulations[14] to carry out risk assessments for work involving hazards, but it has more specific requirements. The assessment must be suitable and sufficient to demonstrate that all hazards with the potential to cause a radiation exposure or accident have been identified and that the nature and magnitude of the risks arising from those hazards have been evaluated and reduced where practicable. Where the risk assessment identifies the risk of a radiation accident, the employer must take all reasonable steps to prevent any such accident, limit the consequences of any accident that does occur and provide employees with the information, instruction and training to restrict their exposure. Throughout health and safety, the HSE define the hierarchy of control measures[15] which should be implemented during the risk assessment process. These are illustrated in Fig. 4.4, which provides the preferred order of application of controls.

These risk assessments should be recorded and reviewed regularly to ensure their continued relevance. The factors that should be considered in performing a radiation risk assessment are given in the ACOP[12] and include such things as the nature of the sources and the estimated radiation dose rates to which anyone can be exposed.

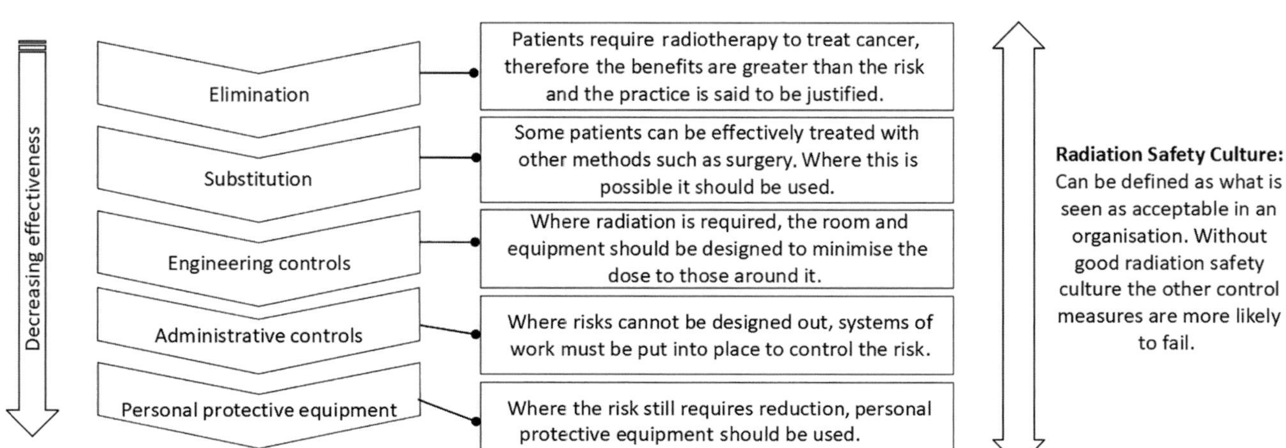

Fig. 4.4 Illustration of the hierarchy of control set down by the Health and Safety Executive and applied to radiotherapy.

Controlled and Supervised Radiation Areas

It is often necessary to impose strict controls on how and where radiation-generating equipment and radioactive materials are used to ensure that doses can be kept as low as reasonably practicable and below dose limits. Radiation-generating equipment and materials should be housed in sufficiently shielded areas so that individuals in adjacent areas will not be subjected to a significant exposure. These are referred to as *engineering controls*. If people are required to enter radiation areas or adjacent locales, engineering controls and design considerations must be used to protect them. A radiation area can be designated as either a controlled or a supervised radiation area under the legislation on the basis of the risk assessment.

Controlled Area

A controlled area is any area where persons entering are required to follow special procedures contained within local rules to limit the risk of a significant exposure (see the 'Dose Limits' section), or where they are likely to receive an effective dose of more than 6 mSv per year or an equivalent dose greater than three-tenths of any other applicable dose limit. Within the ACOP,[12] in Paragraph 297, there is an additional statement which says that an area should be controlled if:

> *'The dose rate (averaged over a minute) exceeds 7.5 μSv/h and employees untrained in radiation protection are likely to enter the area'.*

The guidance further states that when the instantaneous dose rate (IDR) exceeds 100 μSv/h, control of the area is likely to be required regardless of the time-averaged dose. This can cause issues around linear accelerators which utilise very high dose rates but are only irradiating for small portions of the day. This must be considered in the design process and can result in additional shielding requirements to limit the IDR, even when the dose over the entire year would be within acceptable limits. For example, a bunker designed for conventional radiotherapy may be converted for flattening filter free (FFF) treatment, thus increasing the dose rate to the isocentre by a factor of four in some cases. This increases the dose rate from scatter by a similar factor, although the unit is on for less time. To ensure that the 7.5-μSv/h dose rate is met may require additional shielding, although the annual dose and therefore risk may not have significantly changed.

A controlled area must, wherever possible, be defined with reference to physical boundaries; for example, the entirety of a bunker may be defined as a controlled area. Once a controlled area has been defined, access into it must be controlled. Wherever practicable, radiation warning signs and notices are required to be placed on entrances to the area that explain the nature of the radiation and the control measures to help avoid risk. An example of such signage is given in Fig. 4.5, and similar signs are often used in combination with two-stage warning lights which indicate when a controlled area exists and when an exposure is underway. There are some situations in which reliance on physical boundaries is not practicable and alternative approaches have to be taken. This is not generally an issue for radiotherapy.

In a medical situation, access to a controlled area is limited to three main groups:

- The patient undergoing the exposure, for whom there are stringent controls both on the equipment that is used and on the process. These are governed by the Ionising Radiation (Medical Exposure) Regulations 2017.[9]
- Classified workers who are subjected to individual monitoring (see the 'Classified Workers' section).
- Unclassified radiation workers (see the 'Unclassified Workers' section) and others who have been issued written schemes of work which, if followed, ensure that they do not receive a dose greater than any applicable dose limit. Written schemes of work should consider the existing knowledge and training of those entering the area and may be set differently for different subgroups. For example, a radiographer may have to have undergone local training ensuring that they are familiar with safety controls in the area, while an inspector may be expected to be under direct supervision of a radiographer with the necessary knowledge.

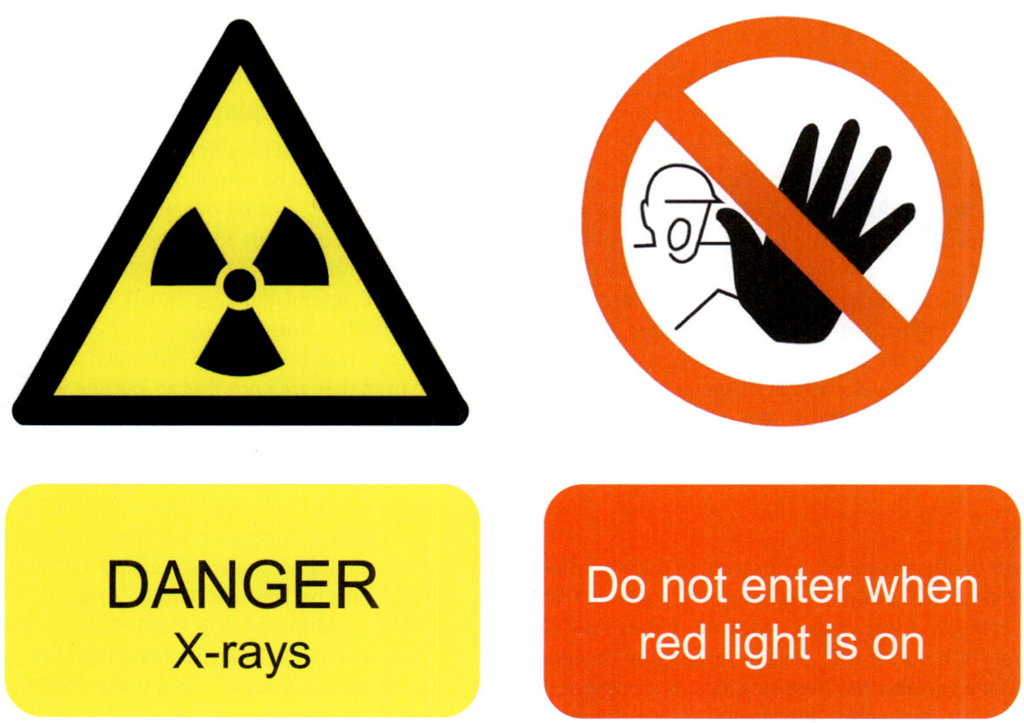
DANGER
X-rays
Do not enter when red light is on

Fig. 4.5 Radiation warning signs.

In some cases, these individuals may be employed by another employer (outside workers) and the regulations require that employers co-operate to ensure the safety of workers.

Supervised Area

A supervised area is any area where the doses must be kept under review to ensure that the area does not require designation as a controlled area. Typically, this means an area which would only require controlling if equipment usage increases above a current limit. Alternatively, supervised areas are required where a person is likely to receive an effective dose of greater than 1 mSv per year, which is the public dose limit, or an equivalent dose greater than one-tenth of any relevant dose limit. Supervised areas should have suitable signage indicating the nature of the radiation source and warning that a supervised area exists and the risks arising therein.

Dose Limits

The whole-body annual dose limit is 20 mSv and has remained unchanged for the past 40 years. Under exceptional circumstances, a limit of 50 mSv within a year can be allowed, but this requires prior approval from the HSE and the dose averaged over a 5-year period must still not exceed 20 mSv per year. For those employees under 18 years of age, a different whole-body dose limit of 6 mSv per year applies. This is also the point at which an individual would need to be classified as a radiation worker, as discussed previously. The current dose limits are summarised in Table 4.5.

TABLE 4.5 Current Dose Limits

	Classified Workers	Unclassified Workers and Trainees Under 18 Years	Members of the Public
Whole body	20	6	1
Individual organ (e.g. skin)	500	150	50
Lens of eye	20	15	15
Foetus of pregnant worker	1	1	

Dose limits per year in mSv.

There are two things to note in Table 4.5. First, there are groups of people with different dose limits: classified workers, trainees under the age of 18 and members of the public. Second, there are different dose limits for different areas of the body, because different organs within the body have different radiosensitivities and because radiation exposures can be nonuniform. An area of the body that has rapid cell division, and is therefore the most radiosensitive, is the foetus. The foetus, in regulatory terms, is a member of the public. The dose limit to the foetus over the declared term of a pregnancy is 1 mSv. Conversely, the skin is not as radiosensitive, and higher levels are permissible.

Classified Workers

Classified workers are those workers who, by virtue of the work they undertake, are likely to exceed the doses set down in regulation 21(1) of IRR17[8] (Table 4.5). Before a worker can be classified, they must be deemed fit for this role by a doctor who meets a recognition criterion issued by the HSE. Once a worker has been classified, the employer is legally obliged to issue the worker an individual radiation dosimeter from an HSE Approved Dosimetry Service (ADS). Continual dosimetry must be used to establish a record of occupational doses received by that person until that person has or would have attained the age of 75 years at least 30 years from when the record was made, whichever is longer. An annual report of the doses received by all classified staff is sent to a body known as the Central Index for Dose Information (CIDI). The aim of CIDI is to allow epidemiological studies to be undertaken in subsequent years and allow national perspectives for the regulator. Reports of any investigation into a real or suspected overexposure of staff, patients or visitors must be retained for the same duration as the dose records. It is rare that workers within a hospital setting receive doses that would require classification under routine work, but there is a requirement to classify an individual if it is reasonably foreseeable that limits would be exceeded in accident situations. Therefore, individuals working in radiotherapy, particularly with high dose rate brachytherapy sources, may be classified despite incredibly low doses in their routine work. The requirement to classify is dependent on the findings of the risk assessment, supported with the outcomes of contingency plan rehearsals. Some centres find themselves able to justify that they do not believe classification is required while other centres choose to classify their staff.

Unclassified Workers

Radiation monitoring has shown that most hospital staff receive very low doses from the work they undertake. Nevertheless, employers are legally obliged to demonstrate that staff working with radiation do not need to become classified, and the best way to do this is to provide them with a radiation monitor.

Members of the Public

Members of the public often do not directly benefit from work undertaken with radiation and often are unaware of the existence of the radiation source. Therefore the risk assessment must ensure that the dose to members of the public is kept both as low as reasonably practicable and within dose limits. This is done by making reasonable worst-case assumptions about the behaviour of individuals and assessing the potential dose associated with this behaviour. Where possible, controls are introduced to reduce this dose (e.g. shielding), and any residual risk once these control measures have been implemented is documented in the risk assessment.

Co-operation of Employers

There is a requirement for employers to co-operate when the work with ionising radiation of one employer presents a risk to the employees of another employer. This co-operation must allow both employers to make informed decisions about the risk to their employees and allow compliance with the regulations.

There are several different situations in which an employer will need to consider co-operation:

- Where a worker enters a controlled area belonging to another employer, they are known as an 'outside worker'. There is a requirement for both employers to co-operate in this situation so that the employer of the outside worker is informed of the risks and potential doses. The nature of this co-operation will depend on the level of the risks involved and how unusual this environment is for the outside worker. For example, a therapy radiographer completing a site visit would require less detailed arrangements than an individual without a background in radiotherapy.
    - If the outside worker is classified, there are additional requirements, and a 'radiation passbook' must be completed which allows the potential doses to be communicated between employers. This allows the employer of the classified worker to estimate the individual's cumulative dose until monitoring results are available.

- If an individual works for multiple employers, the employers must establish an agreement for sharing dose information to track the cumulative dose of that worker over a year.
- Where multiple employers work within an area, an agreement must be in place to ensure that all the requirements of the legislation are met. For example, where an external company employs staff that clean the area, there must be agreements about access restriction, training and monitoring.
- Where an outside engineer comes to work on equipment, it is a common practice for the controlled area to be formally handed over to the engineer to work under their risk assessment and systems of work. Obviously, consideration must then be given to employees who normally work in this area who would then be outside workers if they enter the controlled area.

Local Rules, Radiation Protection Advisers and Supervisors

Once a controlled or supervised area has been defined, it is necessary to have written safety rules, referred to as 'local rules'. These should be drawn up considering the findings of the prior risk assessment. Workers entering the controlled area under these local rules should read and sign the rules to say that they have understood them.

Local Rules

Local rules must contain the following, at a minimum:

- Identification and a description of controlled and supervised areas.
- Names of radiation protection supervisors, discussed below.
- Arrangements for restricting access to radiation areas.
- Dose investigation levels. These are levels of doses which, if received, will trigger an investigation into the circumstances. Because procedures should ensure that doses are ALARP, they must be lower than the applicable dose limit.
- Summary of work instructions, including written arrangements, which are sometimes called *systems of work*, for nonclassified persons to safely enter the controlled area.
- Contingency arrangements for any foreseeable accident or incident (e.g. loss of a source).

The ACOP[12] details a number of additional items which may be 'beneficial in the local rules'. One of these is the name of the radiation protection adviser, discussed next.

Radiation Protection Adviser

Any employer who has set up a controlled area is required to appoint a radiation protection adviser (RPA) whose duty is to advise the employer on compliance with the regulatory requirements, including assistance in undertaking a prior risk assessment of areas where ionising radiation is to be used; the correct identification of controlled and supervised areas; the prior examination of plans for radiation installations; and the acceptance into service of new or modified sources of ionising radiation. An RPA is required to have a certificate of competence to act as an RPA; this certificate is issued by an HSE-approved certification body to candidates who can provide evidence of their suitability to act as an RPA. If there are any questions regarding how IRR17[8] should be implemented in an area, the advice of the RPA should be sought.

Radiation Protection Supervisor

The radiation protection supervisor (RPS) is responsible for ensuring that the work with radiation that is being undertaken on a day-to-day basis follows the local rules. They should also be involved in the preparation of the local rules for the area they supervise to ensure that they are both practical and not prohibitive. To act as an RPS, the person must have received training in a core of knowledge that has been specified by the HSE.[16] In addition, they should be in a position of authority and familiar with the work of the area they are supervising. There must be sufficient RPSs to cover the work carried out in an area, and they should be given sufficient resources by their employer to carry out the work. It can be beneficial to provide a written letter appointing the RPS and detailing their responsibilities to justify the provision of these resources.

Contingency Plans

Contingency plans are required where a radiation accident is reasonably foreseeable. The risk assessment should determine what situations require a contingency plan and whether additional training, including rehearsals to enact the contingency plan, is required. An example of a situation in which regular rehearsals are required is the failure of a high dose rate brachytherapy unit such that the source is retained in the patient. Due to the highly unusual nature of the incident, combined with the potential doses of the individuals involved, full and documented practical training is required for this contingency plan. Where contingency plans involve pressing the emergency stop button, rehearsals may not be appropriate, but the location of the emergency stops should form part of the equipment competency assessment and potentially be reevaluated at a frequency determined by the risk assessment.

The enactment of a contingency plan requires a detailed analysis of the causes, the effectiveness of the plan and the lessons learned from the incident. This analysis must be retained for 2 years. It should be clear if there is a difference between contingency plans and other foreseeable incidents; for example, incorrectly following the procedure for exiting a bunker may be an incident, but with sufficient safety controls in play, it may not result in a contingency plan enactment and use of emergency isolation switches.

Personal Protective Equipment

If risk elimination, substitution, engineering controls and administrative controls fail to reduce risk to acceptable levels, personal protective equipment (PPE) may be required. PPE is rarely appropriate for external beam radiotherapy but may be utilised via lead aprons in planning computed tomography (CT), or gloves, aprons, and tongs used in molecular radiotherapy or brachytherapy. Where PPE is in use, it must be stored appropriately to avoid damaging its protective properties and reusable PPE should be examined at frequent intervals to ensure it is fit for use. For some PPE a visual inspection will be sufficient but lead aprons need to be screened to ensure that no cracks in the protective material have developed. The results of the inspection should be recorded, and the protective devices themselves should be individually identifiable, for example, by a serial number.

THE IONISING RADIATION (MEDICAL EXPOSURE) REGULATIONS 2017

The Ionising Radiation (Medical Exposure) Regulations (IRMER) 2017[9]: Ionising Radiation (Medical Exposure) (Amendment) Regulations 2018,[10] Ionising Radiation (Medical Exposure) (Amendment) Regulations 2024[11] and the Ionising Radiation (Medical Exposure) Regulations (Northern Ireland) 2018[17] are designed to protect a patient undergoing treatment or diagnosis with ionising radiation; they also cover persons exposed to radiation as part of research and non-medical imaging procedures, such as pre-immigration chest x-rays. A set of amendment regulations were published shortly after the publication of the 2017 regulations in relation to safety measures regarding the administration of radioactive substances to patients and again in 2024.[10,11] These regulations are enforced by the Care Quality Commission (CQC).

The key difference to IRR17,[8] which requires limitation of doses of radiation to staff and the public, is that IRMER17[9] requires justification of exposure to individuals with no imposed limits. The Radiotherapy Board, which was established by the Royal College of Radiologists (RCR) in 2013 and is made up of representatives from professional bodies throughout the United Kingdom, has issued guidance on the implementation of IRMER17[9] within radiotherapy.[18] IRMER17 defines set roles, responsibilities and training requirements for individuals involved in exposing patients to radiation. It also requires a standard set of procedures to be implemented to ensure there is a framework of radiation safety around the exposure of patients.

Employer

The employer (e.g. the chief executive of a trust) is responsible for:

- Ensuring that there are specific written procedures in place and that the staff involved adhere to these procedures
- Ensuring that radioactive substances are only administered to humans within their facilities if they hold an employer's licence from the appropriate licensing authority
- Ensuring that training records of those identified as undertaking practitioner or operator roles are maintained
- Holding an up-to-date inventory of the radiation equipment and associated software at each radiological installation they control
- Establishing referral criteria for medical exposures, making these available to the referrers, and ensuring that there are written exposure protocols in place

The employer will not usually carry out these tasks directly but ensures that there is a governance framework in place so that they are completed.

Referrer

The referrer (e.g. a general practitioner or oncologist) must be a registered medical or dental practitioner or other registered health professional who is entitled to act as a referrer under the employer's procedures, usually with additional training requirements. APs are now registered and this does not allow referrals from staff groups such as associate practitioners, as they are not currently registered. The referrer is legally responsible for providing sufficient detail on the referral request to allow for the correct identification of the patient and, where relevant, their menstrual status so that pregnancy can either be ruled out or considered as part of the justification process. They are also required to provide sufficient details of the clinical problem to allow justification and authorisation of the radiation exposure.

Practitioner

The practitioner (e.g. an oncologist) is a registered medical or dental practitioner or other registered health professional who is entitled by the employer's procedures to undertake this role. Their legal duty is to justify a medical exposure based on the information provided to them by the referrer, considering the specific objectives of the exposure, the total potential benefits and risks to the individual undergoing the exposure, and the possibility of using alternative techniques which do not use ionising radiation but which would attain the same objective. An individual can only act as a practitioner for the administration of radioactive substances to humans if they hold a licence from the appropriate licensing authority (discussed later in this chapter). A requirement of the legislation is that practitioners are adequately trained and that they undertake continuing education in radiation protection of the patient. Medical and dental practitioners who act as referrers do not require any additional training, although other health professionals performing this role should be trained in the clinical aspects of a patient's presentation that would warrant an exposure.

Operator

The operator (e.g. a radiographer or a treatment planning dosimetrist) is any person recognised by the employer's procedures who carries out any practical aspect of the medical exposure. This covers a range of functions, each of which will have a direct influence on the medical exposure. Some of these will be undertaken in the presence of the patient (e.g. making the exposure or identifying the patient). Other aspects are performed without the patient being present (e.g. machine calibration and radiotherapy planning). Anyone who evaluates a medical image and records the result of this evaluation is also considered to be an operator. As with practitioners, operators are required to complete continuous professional development.

Medical Physics Expert

A medical physics expert (MPE) is defined as an individual certified to act or give advice on matters relating to radiation physics in a medical setting. An MPE must be closely involved in every radiotherapeutic practice. Their roles in radiotherapy are, among other things, to provide consultation on the suitability of treatment techniques, responsibility for the dosimetry and accuracy of treatment, optimisation of treatments by ensuring that equipment meets adequate standards of accuracy, and the definitive calibration of radiotherapy equipment and dosimeters. MPEs are also required to provide advice to the employer on compliance with IRMER17 (and Amendments).[9]

Carers and Comforters

Carers and comforters are people who knowingly and willingly incur an exposure to ionising radiation by helping an individual undergoing an exposure. Prior to 2017, this requirement was dealt with under the statutory ionisation radiation regulations current at that time; today it is managed by the IRMER17[9] regulations. As such, all exposures must be justified by a practitioner, either directly or via authorisation under a protocol. Justification should consider the benefits and risks to both the patient and the carer and comforter. They must be informed of the risk they are accepting by looking after a patient, and must not be undertaking this exposure as part of their employment, which would fall under IRR17.[8] For example, a care home worker attending with an elderly patient would be an outside worker under IRR17,[2] but a member of the family attending with that patient could be a carer and comforter under IRMER17.[9] A procedure should state the circumstances in which a carer and comforter can be used (see the 'Employer's Procedures' section).

Justification

In radiotherapy applications, there will normally be only one IRMER practitioner for both the treatment exposures and any concomitant exposures that are part of the planning and treatment process, such as simulation, CT scans and verification images. In recent years the number of concomitant exposures has increased, as image-guided radiotherapy makes target- and critical-organ definition an increasingly important aspect of treatment. Estimation of doses and risks to critical organs in the body from all sources is thus necessary to provide the basis for adequate justification of the exposures as required by IRMER17.[9] Although negligible in comparison with the target dose, realistic numbers of concomitant exposures give a small but significant contribution to the total dose to most organs and tissues outside the target volume. In general, this is in the range of 5% to 10% of the total organ dose, but it can be as high as 20% for bone surfaces.[19] These exposures will be justified by the practitioner, and an operator such as a therapy radiographer will check that they are authorised to proceed under this justification at the time of exposure. The number of verification images that are justified must be specified, and any additional imaging must be subject to justification prior to proceeding.

Employer's Procedures

The employer's procedures should be local to radiotherapy, written by those carrying out the work and ratified by the employer to ensure that they are applicable, workable and comprehensive. It is typically recommended that when a procedure does not apply to an area, there should still be a procedure to make this explicit and to avoid any uncertainty.

The regulations require procedures for:

- Correct identification of the person and the area to be exposed.
- Identification of individuals who are entitled to act as referrers, practitioners and operators. It is the responsibility of the employer to decide whom they are willing to let fulfil these roles and to ensure that those undertaking the roles are adequately and appropriately trained, as defined in Schedule 3 of IRMER17.[9]
- Exposures for Non-medical imaging purposes. Although non-medical imaging does not take place within radiotherapy, this must be stated.
- Enquiries of individuals of childbearing age to establish whether they may be pregnant or breastfeeding. Irradiation of the foetus can be detrimental and must be avoided without justification. In addition, radioactive material administered to a breastfeeding patient may be expressed in the breast milk, which could then give a large radiation dose to a breastfed baby. Recent recommendations state that these procedures should be inclusive,[20] and the RCR have issued national guidance on consent forms which take these requirements into account.[21]
- Ensuring that quality assurance programs are carried out. These relate to ensuring that these procedures are adhered to and are still relevant, including schedules for audit of compliance with the procedures, update of procedures, and quality control programs performed on radiation equipment.
- The assessment of patient dose and administered activities. In radiotherapy, this is likely to involve the use of a record and verify system.
- The use of diagnostic or dose reference levels (DRLs). Diagnostic reference levels apply to radiodiagnostic and interventional exposures or radio-pharmaceutical administration while Dose reference levels apply to radiotherapeutic exposures including localisation or verification exposures. Despite the different terms they share the same intent to act as indicative dose levels that are set locally with due regard to any national or international data that are available. Such levels have been set by the UK Health Security Agency (UK HSA)[22] based upon surveys of current national practice. They should be set in units which are related to the patient dose and are easily monitored, for example mGycm rather than effective dose for CT. National DRLs were historically set at the 75th percentile of the room mean distribution, but more recently, there has been a move towards using the median of the room data. Local DRLs should then be set with the aim of ensuring that they are below the national DRL, unless a reasonable explanation can be given. In this way, DRLs alongside changes in technology have had the effect of reducing the doses for medical examinations.
- The conduct of medical research involving exposure to ionising radiation of the participating individuals where no direct medical benefit is expected from the exposure. This should include the use and setting of dose constraints that are levels of dose associated with the research, which are not allowed to be exceeded.
- Giving written information and instruction to patients undergoing treatment or diagnosis with radioactive materials. This information will detail how the exposure from the patient can be restricted to protect other persons in contact with the patient following discharge from the hospital. This only applies to procedures that result in retained activity within the patient.
- Carrying out and recording an evaluation of each medical exposure including factors relating to patient dose. This ensures that, where there is an exposure to ionising radiation there is a medical benefit to the patient. This is usually straightforward and apparent in exposures undertaken in radiotherapy. The dose factors must also be recorded to allow dose estimation and optimisation.
- Ensuring that the probability and magnitude of accidental or unintended doses are reduced as far as reasonably practicable. This should include things such as routine servicing and post servicing quality assurance checks on the equipment.
- Providing an individual or their representative with adequate information on the risks and benefits of the exposure. Wherever practicable, this should be prior to the exposure taking place. This requirement can also be covered by using RCR consent forms.[21]
- Informing the referrer, practitioner and individual of any clinically significant accidental or unintended exposures and the outcome of any analysis. While guidance from the CQC defines Significant Accidental and Unintended Exposures (SAUE),[23] the definitions of Clinically Significant Accidental and Unintended Exposures (CSAUE) are left to the professional bodies. Therefore, depending on the type of exposure, radiotherapy guidance[18] or diagnostic radiology guidance[24] may be applicable.
- The justification and setting of dose constraints for exposures of carers and comforters. This procedure should state the circumstances in which a carer and comforter can be used. For example, it may be acceptable to have a carer and comforter in the room for plain film x-rays, but it would be unacceptable for them to be in the room during a radiotherapy treatment.
- A procedure for carrying out clinical audit and ensuring that appropriate actions are undertaken. This is to ensure that clinical practice is continually monitored against standards and improvements are made where required.
- A procedure for making, amending and cancelling any referrals for exposure. This is to ensure that only appropriate individuals are exposed to radiation and where cancellations occur unnecessary exposures are avoided.

Administration of Radioactive Substances to Humans

IRMER17[9] requires employers to be licenced to administer radioactive materials to humans. A licence is required for each site at which substances are to be administered and for each practitioner undertaking the justification of the administration. The licencing authority depends on the country within the United Kingdom, and advice is provided regarding suitability by the Administration of Radioactive Substances Advisory Committee (ARSAC). The licence will be specific to the radionuclide and the use of the radionuclide: research, diagnosis or treatment. Further details can be found in Notes for Guidance on the Clinical Administration of Radiopharmaceuticals and Use of Sealed Radioactive Sources.[25]

ENVIRONMENTAL PERMITTING (ENGLAND AND WALES) REGULATIONS 2016 WITH EU EXIT AMENDMENT (2018)

The Environmental Permitting (England and Wales) Regulations 2016[26] require that the premises that store, use and dispose of radioactive materials above certain quantities possess permits. The quantities used in a hospital that performs radiotherapy and diagnostic applications of radionuclides generally exceed these limits, and a permit will be required which specifies how storage, use and disposal must be carried out. The inspectors of these regulations differ by country: in England it is the Environment Agency (EA), in Wales it is Natural Resources Wales (NRW), in Scotland it is the Scottish Environment Protection Agency (SEPA) and in Northern Ireland it is the Northern Ireland Environment Agency (NIEA).

There are permits for common activities that are of low hazard and bespoke permits which contain conditions specific to the site. The main permit used in hospital settings is a category 5 sealed radioactive sources permit. However, for larger sources, a bespoke permit will need to be issued considering additional security requirements. Work with unsealed sources will require a bespoke permit. Breaches of the permit conditions are treated as a breach of the legislation. Before a permit is issued for disposal of radioactive materials, an environmental impact assessment must be performed to assess the radiation dose that will arise in the local population, wildlife and environment. The employer must also demonstrate that they are following best practicable means in the storage, use and disposal of radioactive material prior to a permit being issued.

Some substances are defined as 'out of scope' and are not considered radioactive from the point of view of the legislation. However, in some circumstances, practices will be above the 'out of scope' definition but of sufficiently low risk to not require a permit. In these cases the responsible body may provide an 'exemption'. There are several requirements which must be met even when exemptions are applied, such as ensuring that sources are appropriately stored and identified. If the practice would be unable to follow these requirements, full permitting from the regulator would be required. Examples of this include sites which have low-activity sources for educational or training purposes.

HIGH ACTIVITY SEALED RADIOACTIVE SOURCES (HASS)

A sealed source is classified as HASS if the activity exceeds a level corresponding to the level of danger associated with that radioisotope. Where there are multiple sources in an area they are defined as HASS if the ratio of the activity of the source to the specified danger level for that radionuclide is greater than 1 when all sources are added together. The RPA will be able to provide advise on how to determine whether any source that you have is a HASS source.

If a source falls into a HASS category, additional security arrangements are required to be put in place, and the source owner must demonstrate that they have adequate financial provisions in place for its subsequent future disposal. Without this, a permit will not be granted by the relevant environmental agency.

TRANSPORT OF RADIOACTIVE MATERIALS

Anyone transporting radioactive materials should appoint and consult a dangerous goods safety adviser (DGSA) to ensure that they are doing so in compliance with the Carriage of Dangerous Goods and Use of Transportable Pressure Equipment Regulations 2009 and Carriage of Dangerous Goods (CDG) (Amendment) Regulations 2019.[27] These regulations are based on the implementation of the agreement concerning the International Carriage of Dangerous Goods by Road (ADR)[28] which is usually updated every 2 years. During transport, there is also a requirement to ensure compliance with IRR17.[8] As most radiotherapy centres have limited involvement in the transport of radioactive materials, the details of the legislation will not be presented here, but there is detailed guidance presented by the Office for Nuclear Regulation.[29]

PRACTICAL IMPLEMENTATION OF THE LEGISLATION

The legislation sets down the foundation on which radiation safety is built and the limits within which we work. However, often the most challenging part of radiation safety is how to practically implement this legislation.

Protective Measures

The types of protective measures used will depend on the unique situation. However, for radiation, there are a set of core principles that may be used: time, distance and shielding. Minimising the radiation dose people receive will minimise the risk of stochastic effects occurring and will eliminate the risk of tissue effects. Most routine protective measures used in external beam radiotherapy are focused on engineering controls in the form of shielding, with time and distance becoming more pertinent in accident situations.

Time. Minimising exposure time minimises dose. For example, high dose rate procedures or contingency plan enactment can be rehearsed with nonactive material to minimise exposure during work with radiation. Emergency stops should be placed at strategic points to ensure that radiation generation can be stopped rapidly in the event of an emergency. All emergency stops, laser curtains and last man out engineering controls must be fail-to-safe and tested in operating conditions.

Distance. Radiation arising from a point source reduces in intensity in proportion to the square of the distance from the source. Larger bunkers and longer mazes can reduce the doses from linear accelerators outside the bunkers. Using forceps to handle sources can significantly reduce the dose to operators hands. For example, an increase in distance from 0.1 cm to 5 cm will reduce the dose rate by a factor of 2500.

Shielding. The most appropriate shielding material depends on the type and energy of radiation. Several factors need to be considered in designing a radiation room: its walls and barriers must be such that the levels of radiation received by staff, waiting patients and members of the public are kept to a minimum. This can be achieved by the correct use of shielding material. A certified and appropriately experienced RPA should always be consulted in any design process involving radiation. Due to the complexity of the task, detailed reports have been produced to guide RPAs in these calculations.[30]

There are some basic principles that all scientists should be aware of:

- Beta particles should be initially shielded by low-density material, such as Perspex (to prevent production of photons by bremsstrahlung), followed by a denser outer shield such as lead.
- At diagnostic radiology energies, lead is the most used shielding material as its high atomic number is effective for shielding at energies where photoelectric effect dominates.
- With radiation above about 1 MeV (megaelectron volt) in energy, where the Compton process predominates, there is no real advantage in using lead, because all materials show similar attenuation properties depending solely on their density. Therefore concrete may be a more cost-effective solution.
- For high-energy linear accelerator installations, generally taken as a minimum of 10 MV (megavolts), the possibility of neutron generation and activation must be considered and appropriate protective material employed.

Time, distance and shielding may be used at various levels within the hierarchy of control. For example, engineering controls may include shielding of the head of a LINAC device to prevent unnecessary leakage, and shielding of the room and emergency stops to minimise the time to shut down the machine in an accident situation. Administrative controls may include the use of shielding by standing in a CT control room when possible, increasing distance by taking a step back from iodine seed implantation, or using forceps where possible when handling sources. The protective measures appropriate to the task should be considered in the risk assessment and transferred into the local rules.

Contamination

Personnel contamination, either by ingestion, absorption or inhalation, means that exposure time is maximised, distance is minimised and shielding is not possible. Therefore the possibility of contamination of surfaces where unsealed or leaking sealed sources are used needs to be risk assessed. Many controls can be put in place to reduce the likelihood or severity of contamination. These include confining the source; using trays, fume cupboards and glove boxes; and ensuring that the environment in which the sources are being used is well ventilated and easily decontaminated. In addition, good basic hygiene standards, such as wearing gloves and protective clothing and washing hands after dealing with such sources, is essential. These simple precautions will help to reduce the risk of internal exposure rather than eliminate it altogether. Task- and area-based contamination monitoring with a suitable radiation detector should also be undertaken and recorded and may be subject to inspection by the HSE or Environment Agency (EA).

Critical Examinations, Commissioning and Quality Control

Before new equipment is used, the installer has a legal responsibility to carry out a critical examination of the installation to ensure that all safety-critical parts of the equipment are operating correctly. As the critical exam requires an RPA, some installers choose to engage the local RPA to undertake the critical exam on their behalf. A report of the examination should be made to the customer, who should keep it for reference throughout the life of the equipment. The critical examination should be repeated after any major upgrade or repair which may affect the radiation output or other safety-critical factors (e.g. a change of radioactive source or x-ray tube).

Once the installer has performed a critical examination, the user should carry out an adequate number of tests and measurements to set up a quality control baseline and ensure that the equipment is working within the purchasing specification. All safety-related features of the equipment should be checked, including those associated with the room containing the equipment. An MPE should be responsible for acceptance testing of the equipment. For radiotherapy equipment, compliance with sections of British Standard BS EN 60601 relevant to equipment safety[31] should be checked. Further guidance on the acceptance testing, commissioning and quality control of radiotherapy equipment can be found in IPEM publications 81 and 94.[32,33]

Environmental Monitoring

The purpose of monitoring radiation levels is to ensure that all the controls that have been put in place are working as intended. There are essentially two levels of radiation monitoring: environmental monitoring and personal monitoring.

Careful choice of the instrument used is needed to ensure that the combination of low doses outside of shielding with high dose rates can be measured. For more information on radiation detectors and the theory behind them, see Chapter 3.

Initial Monitoring. Initial monitoring of IDRs provides valuable information for the risk assessment and demonstrates that shielding has been installed correctly. At the critical exam, measurements of IDR averaged over 1 minute should be made, and such measurements are required in the safety assessment needed to gain consent from the HSE.

Continuous Monitoring. In some cases, such as high dose rate brachytherapy installations, a radiation detector may be placed within the room or at exits to indicate when a source is present and unshielded. When handling sealed sources (e.g. to carry out leakage tests), it is important to have access to both a dose rate monitor to give an indication of the level of risk (particularly for risk assessment purposes) and a contamination monitor to ensure that contamination is not spread. The RPA will be able to give advice regarding the appropriate monitor to use, and this should be considered in the risk assessment.

Long-Term Monitoring. Longer-duration environmental monitoring should be carried out to ensure that the time-averaged dose rate is acceptable. This is usually carried out using environmental monitoring versions of personal dosimeters. These measurements should be completed following installation and repeated regularly to ensure that workload or other changes have not affected doses in the surrounding environment.

Personal Monitoring

IRR17[8] only requires employers to provide personal radiation dosimeters to their classified radiation workers and to demonstrate that nonclassified workers do not need to become classified. However, in an area where there are potentially high doses of radiation in a brief period, a thorough risk assessment would be needed to justify removal of dosimeters from individuals where they can provide valuable information following an incident.

There are several distinct types of personal radiation dosimeters which can be used to assess the dose individual staff members receive as part of their work activity. Most passive dosimeters use thermoluminescent dosimeters (TLDs) or optically stimulated luminescent (OSL) dosimeters (see Chapter 3 for technical details). Recent developments in semipassive monitors allow for time-stamped dose data to be transmitted through Bluetooth to a central database. To carry out definitive measurements of dose for classified workers which will be accepted by the regulators, the dosimeters used must be of an HSE-approved type. To meet this type of approval, the dosimeters must meet certain minimum performance and measurement specifications.

Personal dosimeters must be worn when at work and must not be exposed to radiation when the person is not at work. Individuals must not wear personal dosimeters during any medical exposure to radiation as part of their care pathway. It is also important that individuals are instructed on how to care for their dosimetry, as failure to do so can lead to significant doses being recorded (e.g. allowing a dosimeter to pass through a baggage scanner at an airport). While the type and location of dosimeter will be decided through a local risk assessment, there is detailed guidance on the considerations available.[34] Some common monitoring decisions are included in Table 4.6, but local risk assessment should consider all parts of the body and document the decision-making process for monitoring various locations. This should include reasons for not monitoring areas (e.g. the eye in routine planning CT).

Equipment Checks and Calibration

On a regular basis, contamination monitors, dosimeters and dose rate meters require calibration, and the results of this calibration should be logged. The calibration of such equipment needs to be traceable back to a national calibration standard for consistency in adherence among centres. This is often arranged by sending one instrument away for calibration by a national calibration service such as the National Physical Laboratory (NPL), and then cross-calibrating other equipment held with the one that was calibrated. The calibrated measurement equipment can then be used with a degree of confidence for carrying out dose measurements on radiotherapy

TABLE 4.6 Summary of Common Dosimetry Practice in Radiotherapy Areas

Area	Considerations for Dosimetry
Planning computed tomography	The routine doses are likely to be low, but due to the potential for doses through unsafe practice, routine whole-body dosimeters are usually used.
Radiotherapy	The routine doses are likely to be low, but there is the potential for high doses in an accident situation. Therefore the usual form of personal dosimetry in this area is a whole-body dosimeter.
High dose rate/pulsed dose rate brachytherapy	Staff are likely to be classified workers due to the potential dose in an accident situation. Therefore it is essential that an approved dosimetry service is used.
	Usual dosimetry will include at least a whole-body dosimeter and ring thermoluminescent dosimeters. It is also advisable to have an electronic personal dosimeter (Fig. 4.6) available to give instantaneous dose feedback in case of an incident. These devices are relatively expensive, may have some energy dependence and are susceptible to damage. However, they supply instant feedback on dose and so are useful in situations where doses may be rapidly accumulated or highly susceptible to work practices. Careful risk assessment is needed to decide the applicable dosimetry.
Manual brachytherapy Iodine seed implants	Risk assessment will depend on the technique used, but it would be expected that whole-body dosimeters are used and that finger dosimetry is used for individuals handling sources. The proper position of the finger dosimetry will depend on the risk assessment.

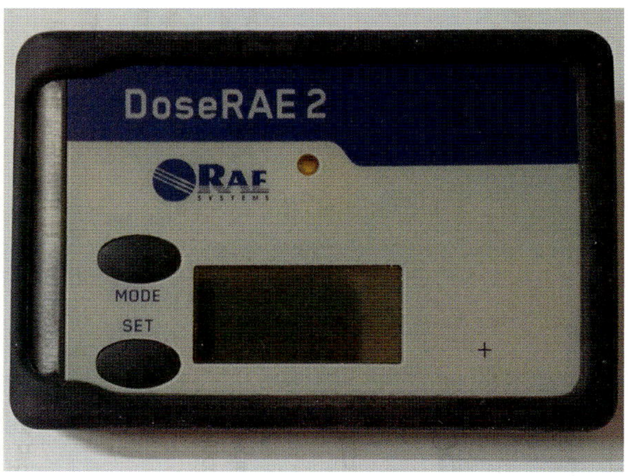

Fig. 4.6 Electronic personal dosimeter.

treatment machines and diagnostic x-ray equipment and for contamination and dose rate measurements. Such measurements in radiotherapy form part of a comprehensive quality assurance program that needs to be in place in every radiotherapy department to help ensure that the risk of incorrect or inaccurate treatments being given is minimised.

RADIATION SAFETY CULTURE

It should be noted that in parallel with the hierarchy of controls in Fig. 4.4, there is an often forgotten but crucial factor that changes the capability of an organisation to effectively implement prescribed controls: radiation safety culture. There are many different definitions of radiation safety culture, but generally it is the result of shared beliefs and values which define the awareness of and level of tolerance for risk around radiation safety. Some sources describe safety culture as 'The way we do things around here'.[35]

Human Factors

Healthcare is a complex, highly variable, uncertain and dynamic system. Often it is not possible to prescribe every step in the care of the patient. Healthcare systems can be modelled by looking at the interactions between various components of the system using methods such as those defined in the System Engineering Initiative for Patient Safety (SEIPS) framework[36] (Fig. 4.7). A slight change in any one component may lead to a favourable or unfavourable outcome from the system. Because there are so many inputs to the system, individuals must work flexibly for the system to work and be efficient. However, too much flexibility in working practices can lead to unintended effects, such as degradation of safety controls.

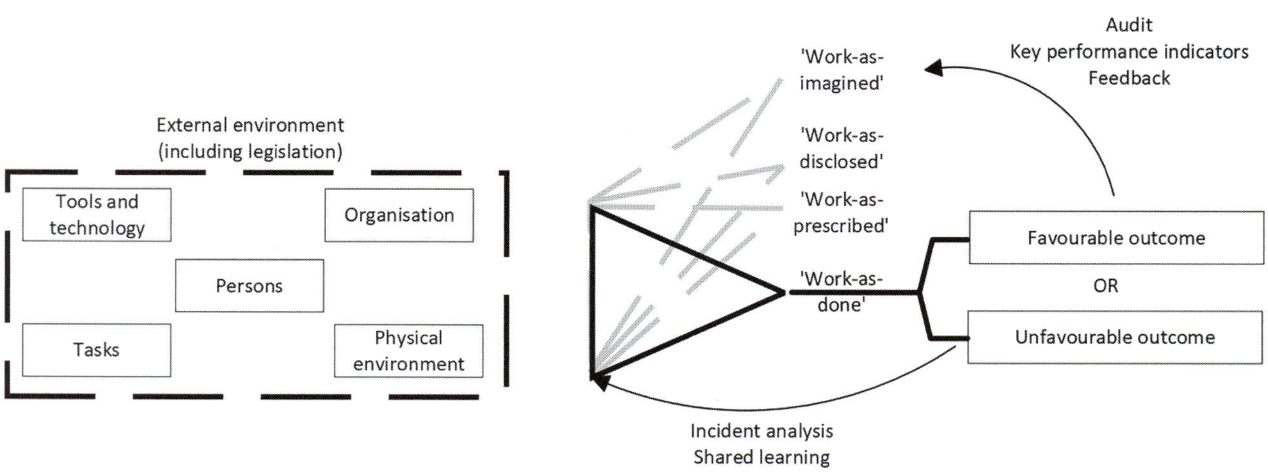

Fig. 4.7 SIEPS model as defined by NHS England combined with representation of the varieties of work. (Adapted from Shorrock S. The varieties of human work. Humanistic systems blog. 2016. https://humanistic-systems.com/2016/12/05/the-varieties-of-human-work/.)

A good safety culture can be defined as a culture in which all types of work defined below, match:

- Work-as-done: How the task is completed
- Work-as-imagined: How managers and other members of staff believe the work is being carried out
- Work-as-disclosed: How the individual carrying out the work describes or records the work that they have done
- Work-as-prescribed: How work instructions state that the task should be carried out

Work-as-Imagined Versus Work-as-Done Mismatch

At an individual level, a person may perceive that they are busier than they are, or they may forget that they do certain tasks. This may cause issues when writing protocols if an individual forgets to mention key steps that are innate to them, and less experienced individuals miss these steps. To overcome this, ensure that draft protocols are checked against actual work-as-done prior to implementation.

If an individual imagines that a task is the responsibility of another individual and therefore assumes it has been done, key stages may be missed. Mapping the work of individuals, their interactions and their responsibilities is key to ensuring that this does not lead to unfavourable outcomes in the system.

Work-as-Done Versus Work-as-Disclosed Mismatch

Work-as-disclosed may not match work-as-done in situations where an individual fears that they will be blamed for an unfavourable outcome. Developing a culture of psychological safety where a just culture is assured is key to ensuring that mismatches do not affect the outcome of the system. A way to seek out these differences is to ensure regular audit and safety walkabouts.

Work-as-Done Versus Work-as-Prescribed Mismatch

This is commonly an issue when managers, who have less day-to-day knowledge of the job, write the protocols or the protocols are known to be impractical and so individuals work around the protocols. Those who carry out the role should be involved in the writing of protocols, and any new protocols should be audited to ensure that they are embedded into local practice. The importance of raising any issues with the practicality of the procedure should be part of staff training.

Failure Mode and Effects Analysis

Because of the complexity of work carried out in radiotherapy and the potential implications of any unintended outcomes, it is important that all potential failure modes are identified and assessed. This requirement is formalised in Regulation 8 (2) of the IRMER17[9] which states:

> *'The employer's quality assurance programme must, in respect of radiotherapeutic practices, include a study of the risk of accidental and unintended exposures'.*

Failure Mode and Effects Analysis (FMEA)[37–39] provides a systematic method of assessing failure modes and the potential effects of those failure modes and has become more popular within radiotherapy. Carrying out FMEA during the process design enables the design of systems that are resilient to errors.

Incident Analysis

It is important to quickly identify near misses and incidents through an incident reporting system and review those incidents for common themes and causes. There is extensive guidance on how this can be done within *Towards Safer Radiotherapy*.[40] There is also a requirement in IRMER17[9] to identify and report trends in incidents regardless of the potential dose associated with these incidents. The aim is to ensure that remedial actions are taken and that learning from incidents is implemented and shared both locally and nationally. It is important that a 'just culture' is shown in the investigation of incidents to ensure that staff feel able to escalate incidents where they occur.

Levels of Safety Culture

While safety culture is difficult to measure, most workers have a general feel for where their organisation lies on the Hudson ladder[41] of safety culture (Fig. 4.8). This tool is useful, as it allows the next step on the ladder to be identified and enables work to be planned to progress.

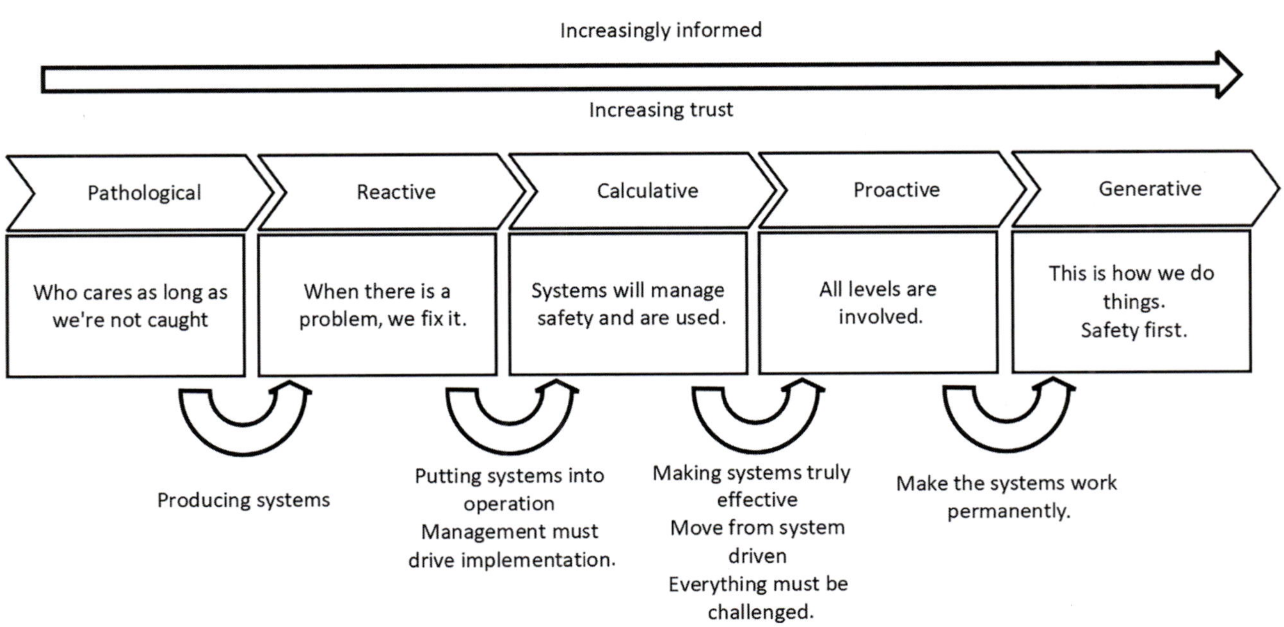

Fig. 4.8 Summary of Professor Patrick Hudson's Ladder of Safety Culture. (From Professor Patrick Hudson. Moving up the culture ladder. Delft university of technology. 2014. https://www.youtube.com/watch?v=XtK6v1pe04Q.)

Changing a safety culture is a long-term process, and taking it stage by stage is the best way to ensure success.

Governance Framework

One of the key elements to ensure a successful safety culture is to ensure that there are strong governance frameworks in place. All trusts should have a radiation safety policy which defines how the governance of radiation safety is set out within the organisation. Individuals need to be empowered to highlight safety issues locally, perhaps to the RPS or manager, and have confidence that these issues will be resolved. However, issues that cannot be resolved locally must be escalated through the management structure. It is common that trusts have Radiation Safety Committees (although the name may vary) which provide assurance to senior colleagues and act as a forum for constructive challenge. These committees might take reports on incident trends, new activities and audits and act as a mechanism for monitoring and ratifying key procedures. It is also common to have one or more local Radiation Safety Groups which monitor, at a more operational level, compliance within a department or area and report up to the Radiation Safety Committee. In addition to these committees, following the publication of the Committee on Medical Aspects of Radiation in the Environment (COMARE)[42] a lot of organisations have implemented Medical Exposure Committees or Image Optimisation Teams. These groups are tasked with continuously working on optimisation of the use of radiation within their areas and should be asked to escalate the results of their work to the local Radiation Safety Committee.

MECHANICAL, ELECTRICAL AND FIRE HAZARDS

While this chapter concentrates on radiation safety, it is important not to ignore the other risks that may be present:

- Mechanical risks are posed by equipment. For example, the rapid acceleration and deceleration of treatment machine movement to direct a radiation beam can cause significant hazards to patients. Collision sensors and regular quality control checks of them minimise this risk.
- Linear accelerators use extremely high voltages. However, even low-voltage electrical equipment has the potential to kill if used unsafely. Therefore all medical equipment must be electrical safety tested and maintained to ensure that this risk is reduced.
- Because of the high voltages employed by radiotherapy, x-ray and other medical equipment, there is an increased risk of fire. If radioactive sources are used in an area, the risk associated with a fire may be compounded by the radiation risk. Therefore detailed fire risk assessments should be carried out in radiotherapy departments and control measures put in place. There should also be a contingency plan for a fire in the local rules.

These are only some of the other risks which will need to be considered in addition to and in conjunction with radiation risks within a radiotherapy department.

CONCLUSION

All employees expect to work in a safe environment. The regulations exist to enable and enforce this. By following these regulatory requirements and guidance, it should be possible to remove the risk of tissue effects and limit the probability of stochastic effects occurring in workers and the public.

While it may not always be possible to remove the risk of side effects in patients undergoing radiotherapy, justification and optimisation should mean that the risks to patients from radiation are kept as low as reasonably practicable and that patients should be consented regarding the residual risks.

The legislation provides the framework to enable these two aims to be met. However, the challenging part of radiation safety is often ensuring and demonstrating that the core governance structures are being followed consistently.

REFERENCES

1. UK Health Security Agency. Ionising radiation and you. UKHSA Radiation protection services. https://www.ukhsa-protectionservices.org.uk/radiationandyou/
2. Cancer Research UK. Cancer statistics for the UK. Accessed 14 April 2023. https://www.cancerresearchuk.org/health-professional/cancer-statistics-for-the-uk#heading-Three
3. ICRP. The 2007 recommendations of the international commission on radiological protection. ICRP publication 103. *Ann ICRP*. 2007;37(2–4):1–332. https://doi.org/10.1016/j.icrp.2007.10.003.
4. Whitlow PL, Muhammad KI. Chronic total coronary occlusion percutaneous intervention: the case for randomized trials. *JACC Cardiovasc Interv*. 2011;4(9):962–964. https://doi.org/10.1016/j.jcin.2011.05.023.
5. Authors on behalf of ICRP : Stewart FA, Akleyev AV, et al. ICRP publication 118: ICRP statement on tissue reactions and early and late effects of radiation in normal tissues and organs: threshold doses for tissue reactions in a radiation protection context. *Ann ICRP*. 2012;41(1–2):1–322.
6. Hamada N, Azizova TV, Little MP. An update on effects of ionizing radiation exposure on the eye. *Br J Radiol*. 2020;93(1115):20190829. https://doi.org/10.1259/bjr.20190829.
7. Martin CJ. Effective dose: how should it be applied to medical exposures? *Br J Radiol*. 2007;80(956):639–647.
8. UK Statutory Instruments. The Ionising radiation regulations 2017. 2017. No. 1075. https://www.legislation.gov.uk/uksi/2017/1075/contents/made
9. UK Statutory Instruments. The Ionising radiation (Medical Exposure) regulations 2017. 2017. No. 1322. https://www.legislation.gov.uk/uksi/2017/1322/contents
10. UK Statutory Instruments. Ionising Radiation (Medical Exposure) (Amendment) Regulations 2018. 2018. No: 121. https://www.legislation.gov.uk/uksi/2018/121/regulation/1/made
11. UK Statutory Instruments. Ionising Radiation (Medical Exposure) (Amendment) Regulations 2024. 2024. No. 896. https://www.legislation.gov.uk/uksi/2024/896/made
12. Health and Safety Executive. *Work with ionising radiation: Ionising radiations regulations 2017 approved code of practice and guidance*. TSO; 2018. http://www.hse.gov.uk/pubns/priced/l121.pdf.
13. Medical and Dental Guidance Notes (Second Edition): A good practice guide on all aspects of ionising radiation protection in the clinical environment: IPEM Report 113. https://doi.org/10.1088/978-0-7503-2332-1
14. UK Statutory Instruments. The management of health and safety at work regulations 1999. SI 1999 No. 3242. https://www.legislation.gov.uk/uksi/1999/3242/contents
15. Health and Safety Executive. Using personal protective equipment (PPE) to control risks at work. Accessed 20 April 2023. https://www.hse.gov.uk/ppe/managing-risk-using-ppe.htm
16. Health and Safety Executive. Radiation protection supervisors. Ionising radiation protection series 6. https://www.hse.gov.uk/pubns/irp6.pdf
17. Regulation NIS. Ionising radiation (Medical Exposure) regulations (Northern Ireland) 2018. Statutory rules of Northern

Ireland 2018 No. 17. https://www.health-ni.gov.uk/sites/default/files/publications/health/doh-ionising-radiation-regulations-2018.pdf

18. The Radiotherapy Board. Ionising radiation (Medical Exposure) regulations: implications for clinical practice in radiotherapy. Guidance from the radiotherapy board. 2020, p. 1-153. https://www.rcr.ac.uk/sites/default/files/guidance-on-irmer-implications-for-clinical-practice-in-radiotherapy.pdf
19. Harrison RM, Wilkinson M, Shemilt A, Rawlings DJ, Moore MLA. Organ doses from prostate radiotherapy and associated concomitant exposures. *Br J Radiol.* 2006;79:487–496.
20. Society of Radiographers. Inclusive pregnancy status guidelines for ionising radiation: diagnostic and therapeutic exposures. 2021, p. 10–11. https://www.sor.org/
21. Royal College of Radiologists. National radiotherapy consent forms. Accessed 14 April 2023. https://www.rcr.ac.uk/clinical-oncology/service-delivery/national-radiotherapy-consent-forms
22. UK Health Security Agency. National Diagnostic Reference Levels (NDRLs). Accessed 14 April 2022. https://www.gov.uk/government/publications/diagnostic-radiology-national-diagnostic-reference-levels-ndrls/ndrl
23. Care Quality Commission. Significant accidental and unintended exposures under IR(ME)R. Guidance for employers and duty-holders. 2020, p. 1-13. https://www.cqc.org.uk/sites/default/files/20200826_saue_guidance_updated_aug20.pdf
24. Royal College of Radiologists. IRMER implications for clinical practice in diagnostic imaging, interventional radiology and diagnostic nuclear medicine. 2020. https://www.rcr.ac.uk/system/filessss/publication/field_publication_files/irmer-implications-for-clinical-practice-in-diagnostic-imaging-interventional-radiology-and-nuclear-medicine.pdf
25. Administration of Radioactive Substances Advisory Committee. *Notes for guidance on the clinical administration of radiopharmaceuticals and use of sealed radioactive sources.* UK Health Security Agency; 2023. https://www.gov.uk/government/publications/arsac-notes-for-guidance.
26. UK Statutory Instruments. The environmental permitting (England and Wales) regulations 2016 No. 1154. https://www.legislation.gov.uk/uksi/2016/1154/contents
27. UK Statutory Instruments. The carriage of dangerous goods (Amendment) regulations 2019. 2019 No. 598. https://www.legislation.gov.uk/uksi/2019/598/contents/made; https://www.legislation.gov.uk/ukdsi/2019/9780111176658
28. UNECE. *ADR 2023—agreement concerning the international carriage of dangerous goods by road.* United Nations; 2022. https://unece.org/transport/standards/transport/dangerous-goods/adr-2023-agreement-concerning-international-carriage.
29. Office for Nuclear Regulation. Guidance and resources. 2023. Accessed 19 April 2023. https://www.onr.org.uk/transport/resources.htm
30. Horton P, Eaton D. *Design and Shielding of Radiotherapy Treatment Facilities.* UK: IOP Publishing; 2017:2053–2563. https://doi.org/10.1088/978-0-7503-1440-4.
31. British Standards. BS EN 60601. Medical electrical equipment. General requirements for basic safety and essential performance (+A2:2021) (Incorporating corrigenda December 2006, December 2007, March 2010, July 2014 and June 2018). 2006. https://www.bsigroup.com/
32. IPEM (Institute of Physics and Engineering in Medicine). *Physics Aspects of Quality Control in Radiotherapy.* 2nd ed. York, UK: IPEM; 2018 IPEM Report 81.
33. IPEM (Institute of Physics and Engineering in Medicine). *External Beam Radiotherapy Treatment Equipment: Acceptance and Commissionssing.* 2nd ed. York, UK: IPEM; 2024 IPEM Report 94.
34. Martin CJ, Temperton DH, Hughes T, Jupp T. *Guidance on the Personal Monitoring Requirements for Personnel Working in Healthcare.* UK: IOP Publishing; 2018.
35. Kennedy A, Deal T. *Corporate Cultures: The Rites and Rituals of Corporate Life.* rev. ed. UK: Basic Books; 2000.
36. NHS England. SEIPS quick reference guide and work system explorer. 2022. https://www.england.nhs.uk/wp-content/uploads/2022/08/B1465-SEIPS-quick-reference-and-work-system-explorer-v1-FINAL.pdf
37. Shorrock S. The varieties of human work. Humanistic systems blog. 2016. Accessed 20 April 2023. https://humanisticsystems.com/2016/12/05/the-varieties-of-human-work/
38. Rassiah P, Su F-CF, Huang YJ, et al. Using failure mode and effects analysis (FMEA) to generate an initial plan check checklist for improved safety in radiation treatment. *J Appl Clin Med Phys.* 2020;21(8):83–91.
39. Cantone MC, Ciocca M, Dionisi F, et al. Application of failure mode and effects analysis to treatment planning in scanned proton beam radiotherapy. *Radiat Oncol.* 2013;8(127):1–9.
40. Briggs G. *Towards safer radiotherapy.* UK: National Patient Safety Agency; 2008:85.
41. Professor Patrick Hudson. Moving up the culture ladder. Delft university of technology. 2014. Accessed 24 April 2023. https://www.youtube.com/watch?v=XtK6v1pe04Q
42. Committee on Medical Aspects of Radiation in the Environment. COMARE 16th report: patient radiation dose issues resulting from the use of CT in the UK. 2014. https://www.gov.uk/government/uploads/system/uploads/attachment_data/file/343836/COMARE_16th_Report.pdf

5

The Radiobiology of Radiotherapy

Alan E. Nahum

CHAPTER OUTLINE

INTRODUCTION

Ionising radiation—photons (gamma rays, x-rays), electrons and protons—kills tumour cells. If the dose of radiation to all actively dividing cells is high enough to halt further cell division, the tumour is said to be *locally controlled*. Unavoidably, however, external beam radiotherapy (EBRT) irradiates tumour-free or healthy parts of a patient's body—that is, *normal tissues*. The aim of radiotherapy treatment planning (RTP) aka dose planning is to deliver the prescribed dose (e.g. 70.0 Gy in 35 fractions) to the *target volume* (the volume encompassing all the cells in the tumour plus a margin for tumour movement and microscopic tumour-cell extension) while keeping doses in the surrounding normal tissues within safe limits (i.e. at **low** risk of any complications).

Fig. 5.1 shows how the probability of local tumour control (or TCP) and the **probability of normal-tissue complications** (or NTCP) vary with the absorbed dose D to the tumour. Here, the prescription dose D_{pr} is ≈73 Gy. The separation of the two curves is known as the *therapeutic ratio*: the greater the separation, the more favourable the outcome. It should be noted, however, that the position and slope of the TCP and NTCP curves vary not only with total dose but also with fraction size.

It is assumed in Figure 5.1 that the dose across the target volume is uniform. For a given total dose and a given fraction size, the position and shape of the TCP curve will be determined by the number and radiosensitivity of the cells in the tumour, and the position and shape of the NTCP curve will depend on the characteristics of the organ(s) at risk (OAR) as well as the **dose distribution** in the OAR *and* the **number of fractions**. For the same total dose, increasing the fraction size will increase the steepness of both curves and will, in general, decrease the *therapeutic ratio*.

TUMOUR GROWTH

The relationship between the mass of a tumour and the number of cell doublings, and therefore the total number of cells, is shown in Fig. 5.2; (there are approximately 10^9 cells per gram of tissue).

The increase in the size and mass of a tumour as a function of time is illustrated schematically in Fig. 5.3. In general, a tumour can only be detected when its mass is at least 1 g. The lower graph in Fig. 5.3 shows the tumour mass on a logarithmic scale in powers of 10.

In a fully grown tumour between approximately 1 in every 100 cells and 1 in every 1000 cells is a *clonogen*. A clonogen is an actively dividing cell, and the number of such cells per unit volume, known as the *clonogen density* (ρ_{clon}), will be between ~5×10^5 and ~5×10^6 cells per cm^3.

CELL KILLING BY RADIATION

Let us assume that a tumour receives a radiation dose of approximately 2 Gy. The effect of this dose on the dividing cells is illustrated schematically in Fig. 5.4.

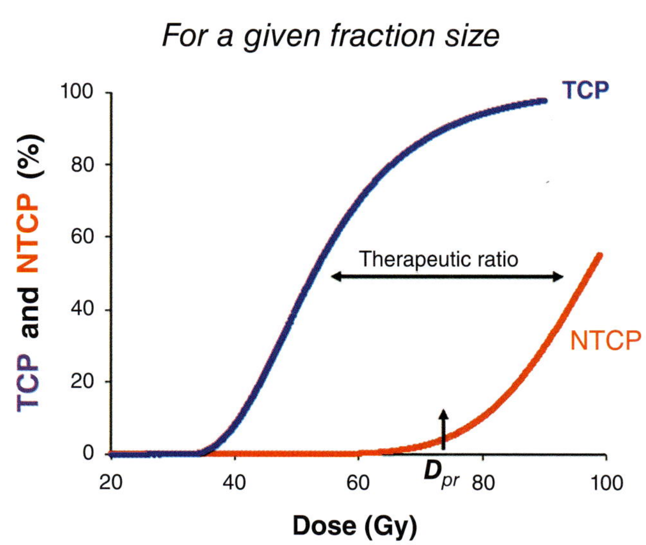

Fig. 5.1 The relationship between the probability of local tumour control (TCP) and of normal-tissue complication (NTCP) on the absorbed dose D to the tumour; the prescription dose D_{pr} is ≈ 73 Gy in this example. It is emphasised that the position and slope of both the TCP and NTCP curves varies with total dose and fraction size. The separation of the two curves is sometimes known as the *therapeutic ratio*.

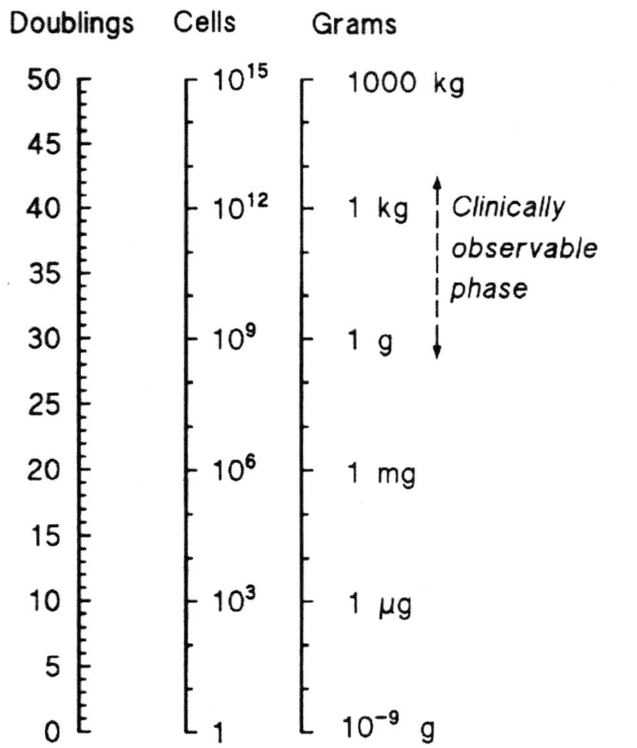

Fig. 5.2 The relationship between the mass of a tumour, the number of cell-number doublings and the total number of cells it contains (assuming 1 g contains 10^9 cells). (From Steel GG [Editor.]. *Basic clinical radiobiology*, 3rd ed. Hodder-Arnold; 2002.)

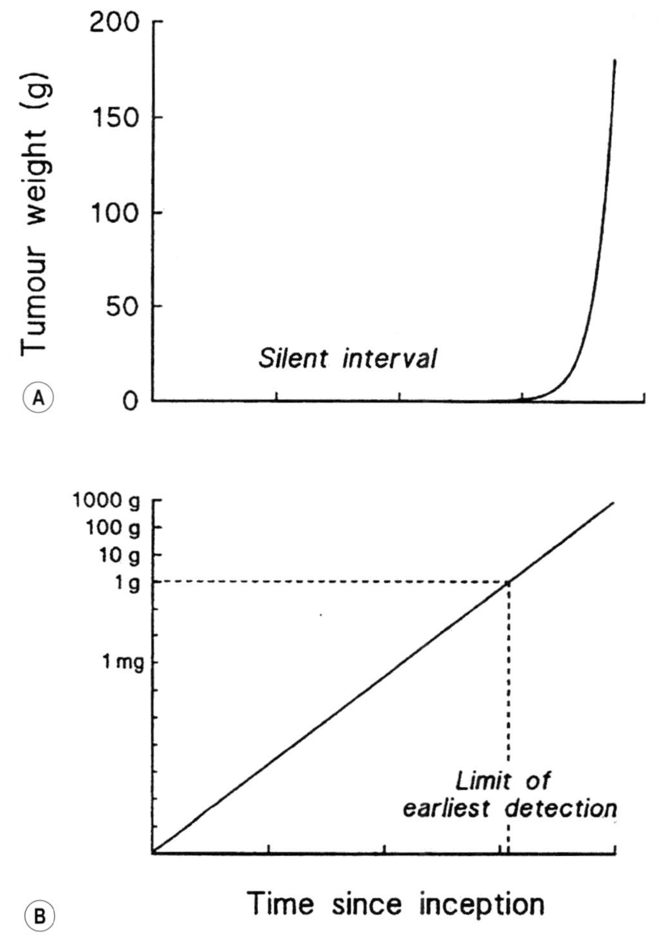

Fig. 5.3 An exponential growth curve plotted on a linear scale *(top)* and on a logarithmic scale *(bottom)*. The clinical growth phase is a minor part of the life history of a tumour. (From Steel GG [Editor.]. *Basic clinical radiobiology*, 3rd ed. Hodder-Arnold; 2002.)

Referring to Fig. 5.4, after two cell divisions, the four cells receive a dose of 2 Gy, which halts further cell division for *two* of the *four* cells. The surviving fraction (*SF*) is therefore 2/4, or 0.5. Radiobiologists have measured SFs for various types of human tumour cells. The cells are irradiated in *Petri* dishes at a series of different dose levels to yield curves of *SF* versus radiation dose in Gy. The SF is the number of *surviving* cells after each dose, divided by the number at the start of the irradiation. Fig. 5.5 shows how SF decreases with dose for four different human tumour cell lines. For HX142, neuroblastoma, a dose of 4 Gy reduces the SF to about 0.001, or 1 in 1000, whereas for RT112, a bladder carcinoma, approximately 14 Gy is required to achieve an SF of 0.001. This emphasises the wide variation in tumour cell killing achieved by a given radiation dose.

LINEAR QUADRATIC MODEL OF CELL KILLING

The continuously downwards-bending form of cell-survival curves, as illustrated in Fig. 5.5, can be described or "fitted" by the following equation:

$$SF = \frac{N_S}{N_0} = \exp\{-\alpha D - \beta D^2\} \quad \textbf{(5.1)}$$

Equation (5.1) applies to a single dose D delivered in less than about 10 minutes. N_S is the surviving number of cells and N_0 is the

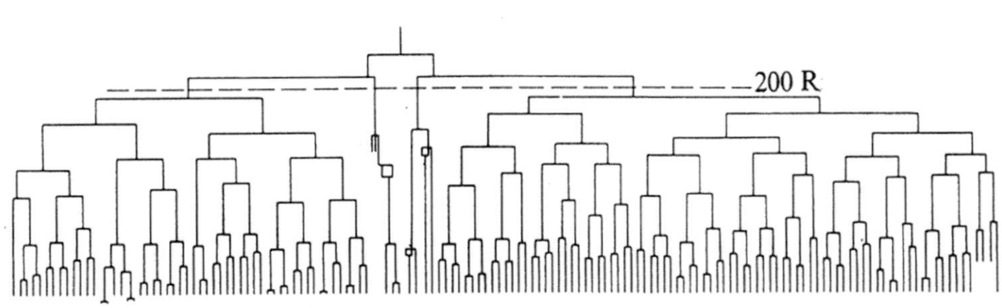

Fig. 5.4 Pedigree of a clone of mouse L-cells irradiated with an exposure of 200 roentgens at the 4-cell stage, illustrating the concept of surviving and nonsurviving clonogenic cells (200 roentgens ≈ 200 rads or 2.0 Gy). (From Trott KR. Relation between division delay and damage expressed in later generations. *Current Top Radiat Res*. 1972;7:336–337.)

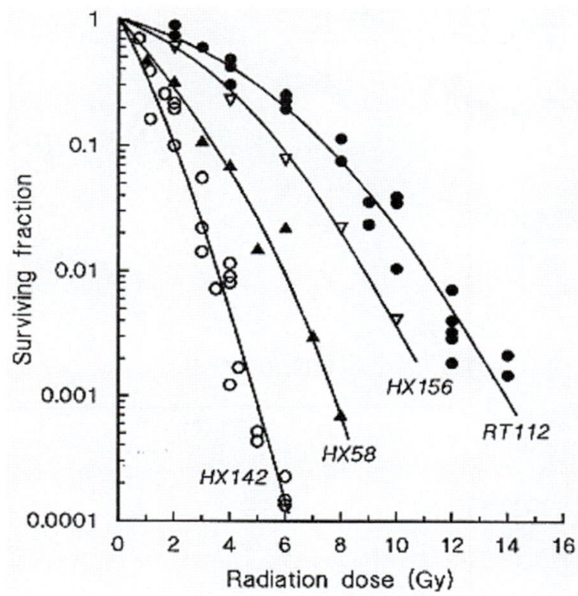

Fig. 5.5 The surviving fraction of irradiated tumour cells as a function of the radiation dose (at high doserate) for four representative human tumour cell lines: HX142, neuroblastoma; HX58, pancreatic; HX156, cervix; and RT112, bladder carcinoma. (Reproduced from Steel 1991.)

number of cells at the start of irradiation. Equation (5.1) is known as the *linear-quadratic (LQ) model.* On a log(*SF*) versus *D* plot the LQ survival curves are continuously bending, with no straight portion either at low or high dose.

In Eq. (5.1), for the two parameters α and β (described below), the smaller the α-to-β ratio the more 'bendy' the curve. The LQ model describes, to a good approximation, both *in vitro* and *in vivo* responses to radiation. The mechanistic interpretation is that the linear component $-\alpha D$ is due to a **single** event, referred to as a *one-hit lethal event*, that halts further cell division. The quadratic component $-\beta D^2$ arises from two *independent sublethal events*. This is consistent with log cell-survival curves becoming straight lines at **low** doserate because those sublethal events occurring in close proximity will be sufficiently far apart in time that at least one of the sublethal lesions will have been repaired.

Fig. 5.6A illustrates the two types of cell-killing events, and Fig. 5.6B illustrates what happens several hours later. The cells subjected to single-hit (or Type A) events remain "killed", whereas only a fraction of the sublethally damaged cells (Type B) result in cell death, the remainder being repaired.

A number of human tumour-cell survival curves are shown in Fig. 5.7A. These range from MO59, the most radiosensitive, to HT29, the most radioresistant. The fits of the data points to Eq. (5.1) in Fig. 5.7A have been transformed, using Eq. (5.2), into straight lines in Fig. 5.7B:

$$-\ln(SF)/D = \alpha + \beta D \quad \textbf{(5.2)}$$

The intercept of each straight line on the y-axis yields an estimate of α, and the slope (or gradient) of each line yields an estimate of β. It can be seen that there is a wide variation in α but a much smaller one in β; it follows that there is a wide range in the values of α/β for tumour cells.

FRACTIONATION AND REPAIR

External-Beam Radiotherapy (EBRT) is generally delivered in a large number of fractions, usually one each weekday. Fig. 5.8 explains why multiple fractions generally yield a *therapeutic advantage.*

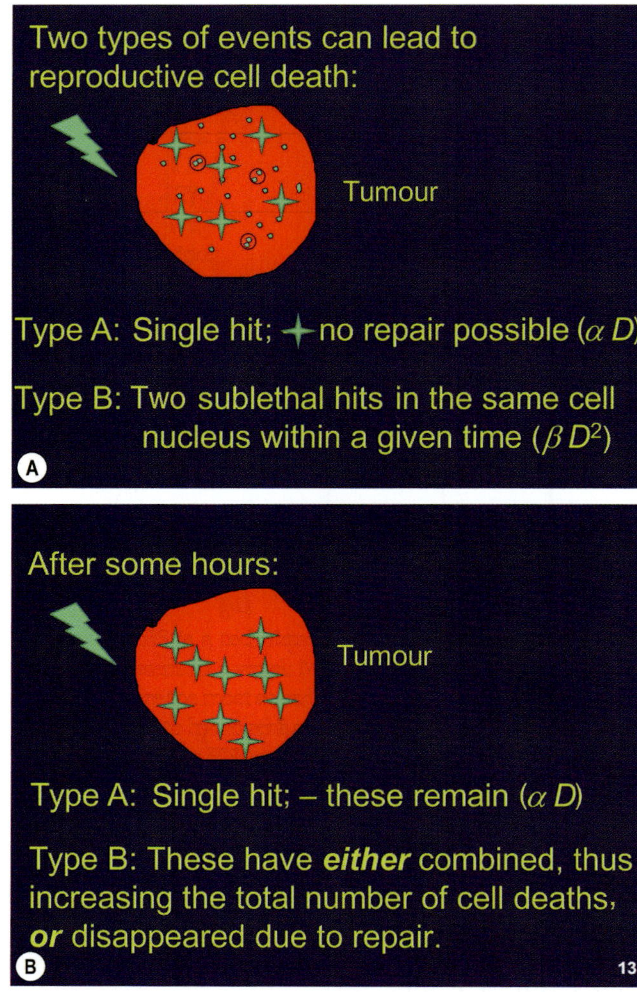

Fig. 5.6 (A) The two mechanisms of cell killing: Type A, single hit; and Type B, two sublethal hits combining within a given time. (B) Several hours later: For Type A (single hit), cell death is **permanent**; Type B: the *sublethal* hits have either combined, resulting in **cell death**, or disappeared due to **repair**.

In Figure 5.8 it is assumed that α/β = 10 Gy for the *tumour cells* and α/β = 3 Gy for the relevant *normal-tissue* (NT) *complication.* The figure demonstrates that delivering the tumour dose in **five 2-Gy fractions** yields a *far smaller difference in SF* between the tumour and normal tissue (N-T) curves compared to the *SF* difference for **a single fraction of 10 Gy.**

Note, however, that if the α/β values for the tumour and NT are *similar in magnitude*, the optimal fraction size can be much larger than 2 Gy. This is referred to as *hypofractionation.*

OVERALL TREATMENT TIME AND TUMOUR REPOPULATION

The number of tumour clonogens increases with time due to cell doubling. However, when a tumour has reached a size or volume such that its presence gives rise to patient symptoms, its overall rate of growth will have usually slowed down considerably. Many of the cells will have died (*necrosed*) because of inadequate blood supply and therefore been starved of oxygen, referred to as *extreme hypoxia.* As the radiation preferentially kills the well-oxygenated cells, the oxygen supply to the surviving, less well-oxygenated or *hypoxic* cells will increase. These cells will start to increase in number, referred to as *repopulation.*

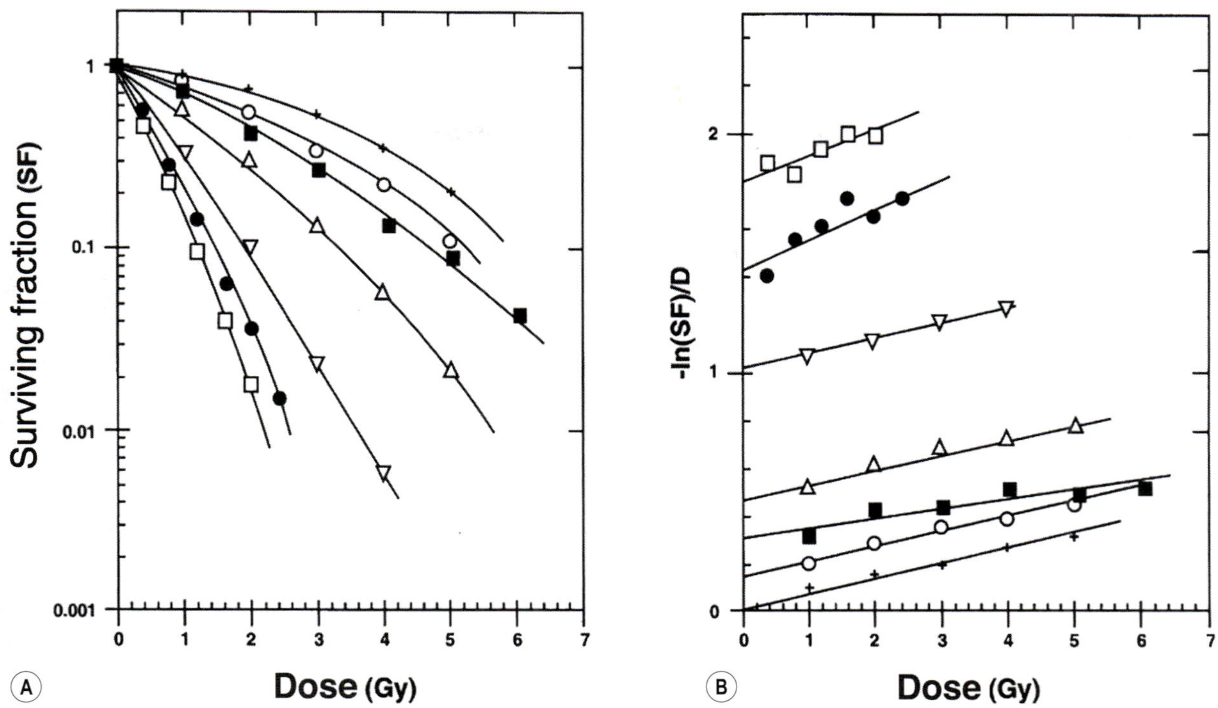

Fig. 5.7 (A) Radiation cell survival curves for asynchronous populations of several human tumour cell lines, ranging from highly radiosensitive (M059J, *open squares*) to relatively insensitive (HT29, *crosses*). (B) Curves in (A) replotted with -ln(*SF*)/*D* on the y-axis against dose *D* (Gy) on the x-axis. The y-axis intercept yields the parameter α; the slope (or gradient) of the lines yields the parameter β.

Fig. 5.9 shows that the total dose required to achieve a given level of local control for tumours in the head and neck region must be increased if the total treatment duration exceeds approximately 3 weeks. The *total* dose shown has been adjusted to be radiobiologically equivalent to 2-Gy fractions. The increase is due to *tumour-cell repopulation* kicking off after approximately 3 weeks. The figure implies that the total number of actively dividing tumour cells starts to increase after the first 3 weeks of radiotherapy. Thus, for radiotherapy schedules of increasing total time, more and more tumour cells must be killed to achieve a given level of local tumour control (e.g. 50%), requiring an increasing number of 2-Gy-equivalent total doses.

In Fig. 5.10, tumour cell repopulation is represented by the short vertical sections of the **SF** versus **Total Dose** curve from the third fraction onwards. Thus a greater total dose, through an increase in the number of fractions, would be required to reduce the SF to the same level as that achieved in the absence of repopulation.

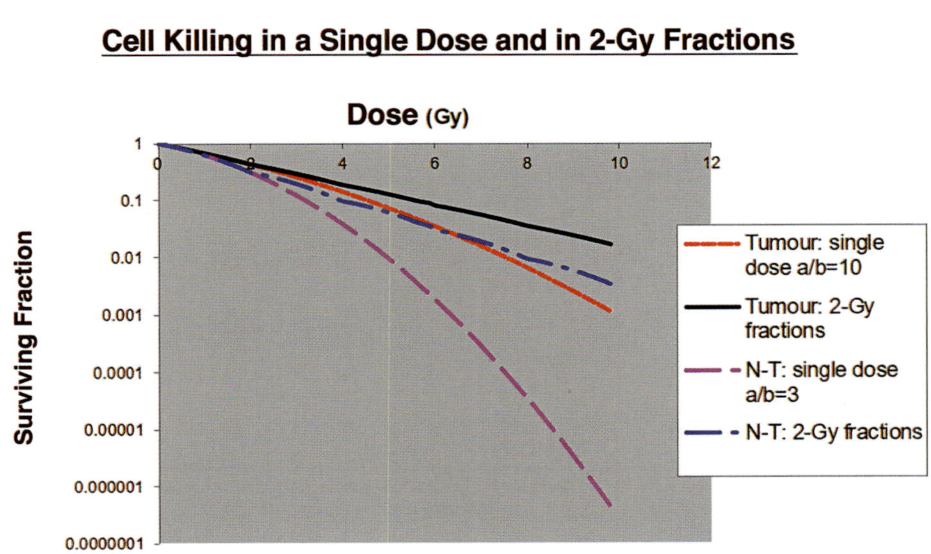

Fig. 5.8 Variation in **surviving fraction (SF)** with dose per fraction, number of fractions and α/β ratios of 3 Gy and 10 Gy.

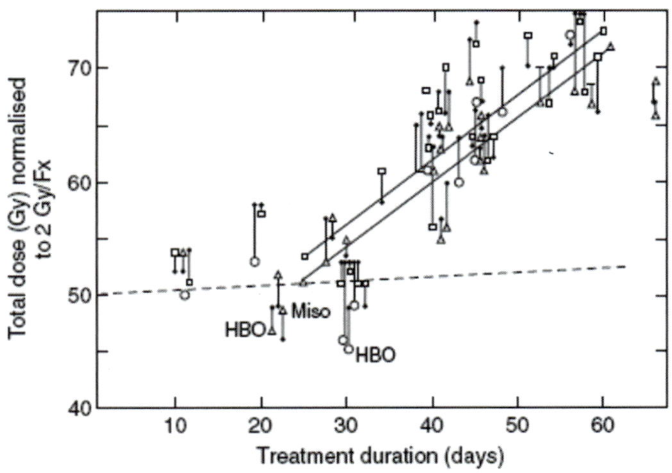

Fig. 5.9 Total dose required to achieve a given level of local control for tumours in the head and neck region.

SIGNIFICANCE OF OXYGEN, HYPOXIA AND REOXYGENATION

The radiosensitivity of tumour cells is strongly influenced by their oxygen supply. The SF versus dose curves in Fig. 5.11 demonstrate clear differences in cell survival between *oxic* cells, which are well oxygenated, and *hypoxic* or oxygen-starved cells. If a significant fraction of the cells in a tumour are hypoxic a dose two to three times greater is required to reduce the SF to the level achieved for well-oxygenated or oxic cells.

The mass of cells on the left-hand side of Fig. 5.12 explain how hypoxia can occur in cells lying greater than a certain distance from a blood vessel, known as *diffusion-limited chronic hypoxia*. Alternatively, a completely blocked or *transiently occluded* blood vessel causes *perfusion-limited hypoxia*, shown on the right-hand side of the figure.

The delivery of a radiation dose fraction will preferentially kill the well-oxygenated cells in the tumour, and hence the proportion of tumour cells that are hypoxic will immediately increase, as shown in Fig. 5.13. If the hypoxic fraction were to further increase with each radiation fraction, the tumour would become increasingly hypoxic after each fraction, and radiotherapy would fail to control most tumours.

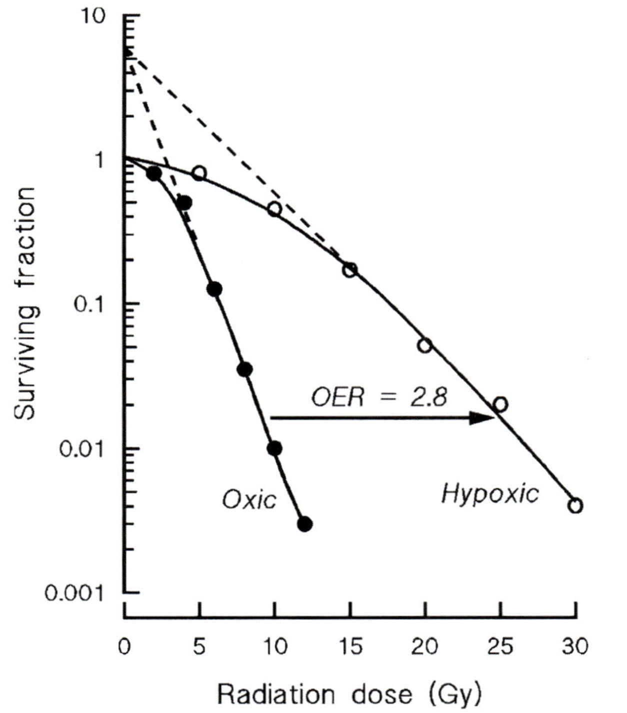

Fig. 5.11 Survival curves for cultured mammalian cells exposed to x-rays under oxic or hypoxic conditions (diagrammatic), illustrating the radiation dose-modifying effect of oxygen. (From Steel GG [Editor.]. *Basic Clinical Radiobiology*, 3rd ed. Hodder-Arnold; 2002.)

Fortunately, this progressive increase in tumour hypoxia as more fractions are delivered *does not happen*, due to the phenomenon of *reoxygenation*. The killing of well-oxygenated cells results in an increase in the supply of oxygen to the remaining viable tumour cells, enabling more and more of these to be killed with each radiation fraction.

EFFECT OF RADIATION DOSE RATE

External-Beam radiotherapy is almost always delivered at a *high dose rate*; a dose fraction of 2 Gy or greater requires a few minutes, at most.

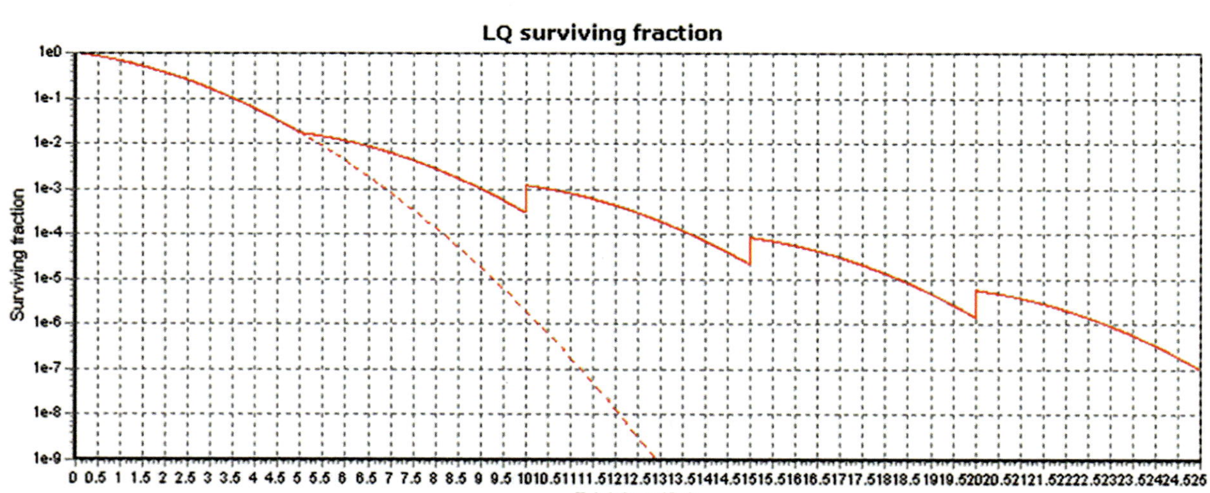

Fig. 5.10 Tumour cell repopulation causes an increase in surviving fraction (SF), from the third fraction onwards. A greater number of fractions would be required to achieve the same final SF as that achieved in the absence of repopulation.

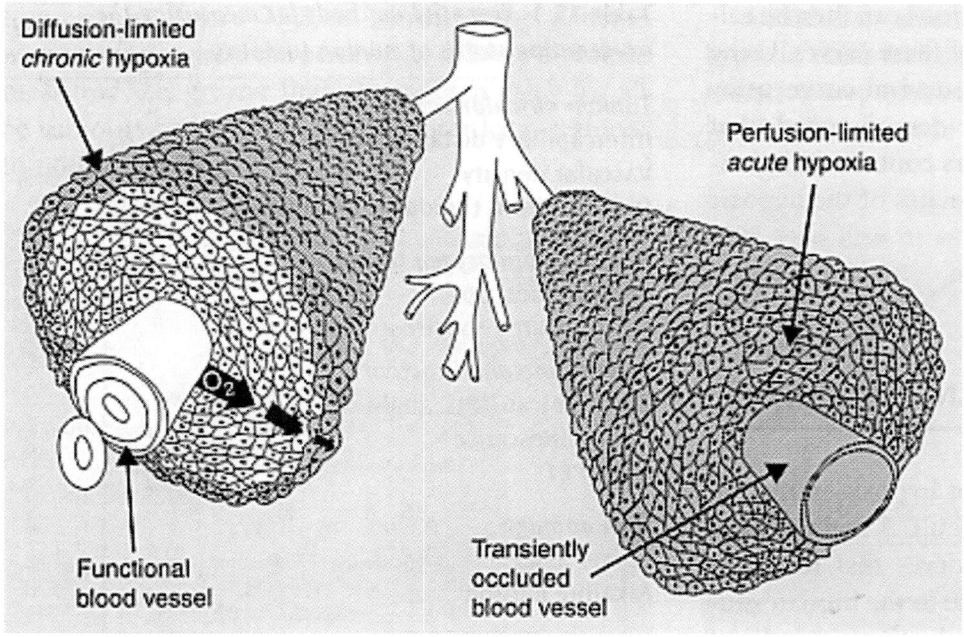

Fig. 5.12 Schematic representiation of diffusion-limited chronic hypoxia and perfusion-limited acute hypoxia within cellular masses clustered around blood vessels. (From Horsman MR. Measurement of tumour oxygenation. *Int J Radiat Oncol Biol Phys*. 1998;42[4]:701–704.)

This ensures maximum cell killing. However, for certain techniques, in particular *brachytherapy*, the dose is delivered over a significantly greater time, and the dose rate is therefore relatively *low*. Fig. 5.14 shows how the cell survival curve becomes progressively less steep as the dose rate is decreased. At the lowest dose rate of 1.6 cGy per minute the curve indicated by open squares lies close to the line labelled B, which corresponds to zero cell killing by the β mechanism of *two independent sublethal events*, as described earlier.

RADIOSENSITIVITY AND TUMOUR TYPE

It used to be assumed that tumour cells were of approximately similar radiosensitivity irrespective of the type of tumour. However, radiobiologists gradually discovered that this was not so: neuroblastoma cells are significantly more *radiosensitive*: i.e. they have a lower Surviving Fraction after 2 Gy than, for example, the relatively *insensitive* tumour cells of melanoma and glioblastoma (see Fig. 5.15).

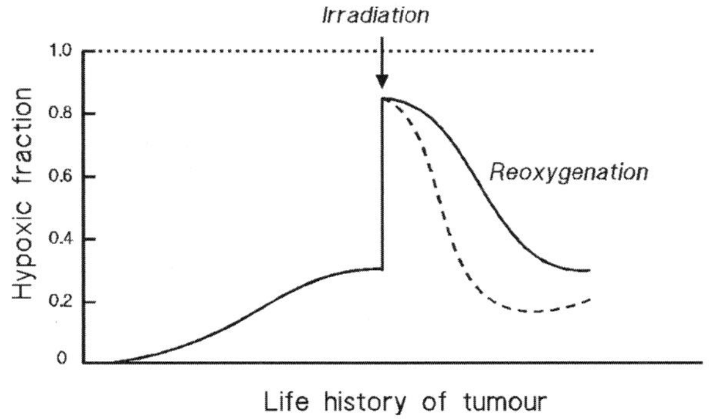

Fig. 5.13 The time course of changes in the hypoxic fraction during the life history of a tumour. A single radiation dose kills the oxic cells, thereby increasing the hypoxic fraction. Subsequently, the hypoxic fraction falls due to reoxygenation. (From Steel GG [Editor.]. *Basic Clinical Radiobiology*, 3rd ed. Hodder-Arnold; 2002.)

CONCLUDING REMARKS

Radiobiology has contributed significantly to the understanding, development and improvements in treatment regimens (e.g. *hypofractionation*). Historically, the radiobiology of tumour-cell killing was summarised with the four Rs: *Repair*, *Reassortment*, *Repopulation*

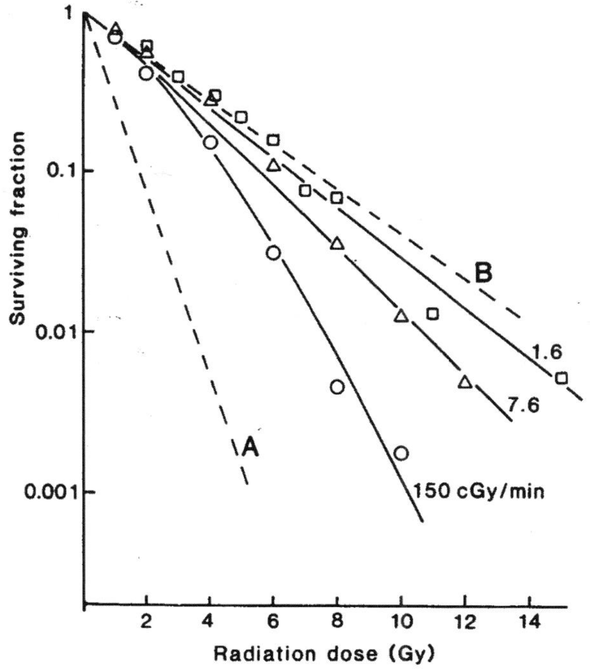

Fig. 5.14 Cell survival curves for a human melanoma cell line irradiated at dose rates of 150, 7.6 or 1.6 cGy min^{-1}. *Line A* represents the high doserate limit and *line B* represents the low doserate limit (*b* cell killing eliminated). (From Steel GG, Deacon JM, Duchesne GM, Horwich A, Kelland LR, Peacock JH. The dose-rate effect in human tumour cells. *Radiother Oncol*. 1987;9[4]:299–310.)

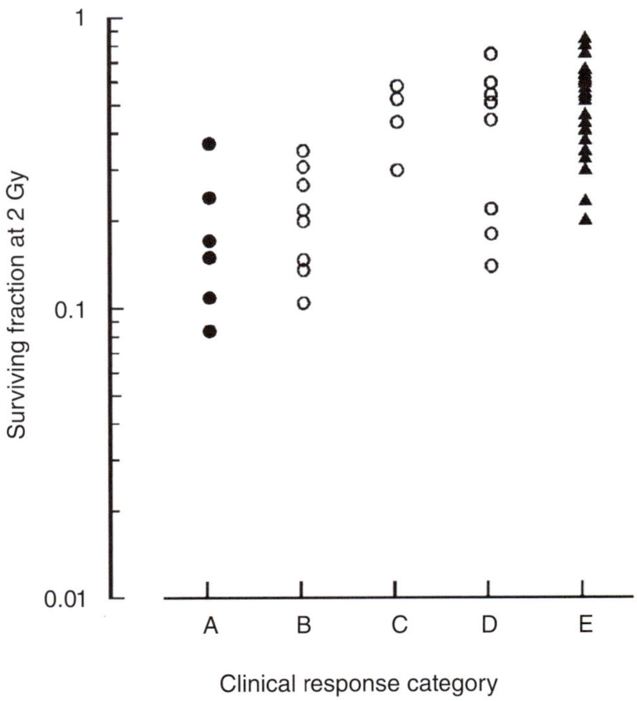

Fig. 5.15 Surviving fraction at 2 Gy for 51 human tumour cell lines, arranged in five categories of clinical radioresponsiveness. *A*, Lymphoma, myeloma, neuroblastoma; *B*, medulloblastoma, small-cell lung cancer; *C*, breast, bladder, cervix carcinoma; *D*, pancreatic, colorectal, squamous-cell lung cancer; *E*, melanoma, osteosarcoma, glioblastoma, renal carcinoma. (From Deacon JM, Peckham MJ, Steel GG. The radioresponsiveness of human tumours and the initial slope of the cell-survival curve. *Radiother Oncol.* 1984;2[4]:317–323.)

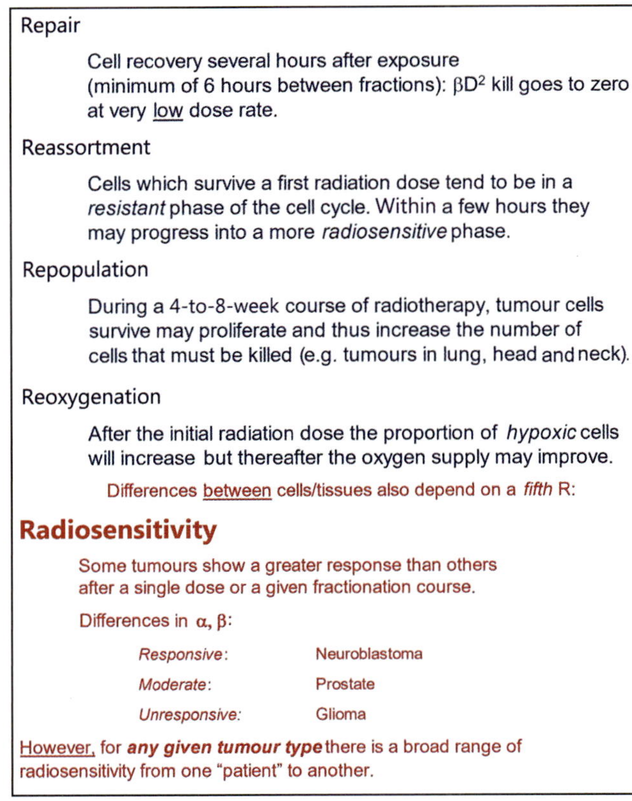

Fig. 5.16 Summary of the factors which modify the response of a given tissue/tumour to repeated doses of radiation.

and *Reoxygenation*. A fifth R has subsequently been added: **Radiosensitivity**; (see Fig. 5.16). The average intrinsic radiosensitivity of tumour cells varies significantly *between* tumours originating in different organs, and *patient-to-patient* radiosensitivity varies between *tumours of the same type*.

ACKNOWLEDGMENTS

I am indebted to Professor Gordon Steel of the Institute of Cancer Research (Sutton, UK) for introducing me to radiobiology in the late 1980s; and to Professor Don Chapman of the Fox Chase Cancer Center (Philadelphia, PA) for deepening my radiobiological knowledge some 15 years later.

FURTHER READING

Chapman JD, Nahum AE. *Radiotherapy Treatment Planning: Linear-Quadratic Radiobiology*. Boca Raton, CRC Press; 2015.

Deacon JM, Peckham MJ, Steel GG. The radioresponsiveness of human tumours and the initial slope of the cell-survival curve. *Radiother Oncol.* 1984;2(4):317–323.

Fowler JF. The linear-quadratic formula and progress in fractionated radiotherapy. *Br J Radiol.* 1989;62(740):679–694. https://doi.org/10.1259/0007-1285-62-740-679

Horsman MR. Measurement of tumour oxygenation. *Int J Radiat Oncol Biol Phys.* 1998;42(4):701–704.

Joiner MC, van der Kogel AJ. *Basic Clinical Radiobiology*. 5th ed. CRC Press, Boca Raton; 2019.

Steel GG. Cellular sensitivity to low dose-rate irradiation focuses the problem of tumour radioresistance. *Radiother Oncol.* 1991;20: 71–83.

Steel GG, ed. *Basic Clinical Radiobiology*. 3rd ed. Hodder-Arnold; 2002.

Steel GG, Deacon JM, Duchesne GM, Horwich A, Kelland LR, Peacock JH. The dose-rate effect in human tumour cells. *Radiother Oncol.* 1987;9(4):299–310.

Trott KR. Relation between division delay and damage expressed in later generations. *Current Top Radiat Res.* 1972;7: 336–337.

West C, Nahum AE. Tumour and normal-tissue radiobiology. *Handbook of Radiotherapy Physics—Theory and Practice*. 2nd ed. CRC Press, Taylor&Francis Group, Boca Raton, London, New York. 2021.

6

Imaging With X-ray, Magnetic Resonance and Ultrasound

Tim Wood, Sarah Bacon and Carl Tiivas

CHAPTER OUTLINE

INTRODUCTION

X-rays, magnetic resonance imaging (MRI) and ultrasonic images play a key role in the diagnosis, staging, planning and delivery of treatment and follow-up of patients with cancer.

In everyday language, an image is a picture and, more generally, a representation of the distribution of some property of an object. It is formed by transferring information from the object to an image domain. In practice, this requires the ordered transfer of energy from some source via the object of interest to a detector system. The detected signal may be processed in some way before being displayed and stored by suitable devices.

Medical imaging modalities covered in this chapter are classified according to the type of energy used to carry information: x-rays, radiofrequency (RF) waves and high-frequency sound waves.

X-ray imaging enables tumours to be localised with respect to normal anatomic structures and external markers. Because x-rays travel in straight lines until they are absorbed or scattered, they can produce images which faithfully represent spatial relationships within the body. It is principally for this reason that x-ray images of various kinds are essential to the planning and delivery of radiotherapy. A further reason is that interactions of ionising radiation with matter are an essential feature of both imaging and therapy so that information on properties of tissues relevant to treatment planning, such as electron density, may be obtained from suitable images.

MRI is an excellent technique for imaging soft tissue and is often used to diagnose and stage cancer in the head, neck and body. It can also be used to monitor the response to treatment. The extent of the cancer can be seen on anatomic images. Other specialised MRI techniques, such as diffusion weighted imaging and dynamic imaging with a contrast agent, can also be used to refine the diagnosis and cancer staging. Magnetic resonance spectroscopy (MRS) provides information regarding the metabolism of the tumours and can also be used to monitor treatment response.

Diagnostic ultrasound imaging has several advantages over other imaging modalities.[1] It is relatively cheap, is safe, gives real-time images and has good soft tissue contrast. As well as anatomic detail, ultrasound can exploit the Doppler effect to give information about blood flow and the vascularity in tissues. The distortion of tissue under pressure in ultrasound images can give images related to the elasticity of the tissue.

Radionuclide imaging, including positron emission tomography–computed tomography (PET/CT), which is primarily concerned with the function of organs and tissues, is dealt with in Chapter 7.

X-RAY IMAGING

Overview of the X-ray Imaging Process

The energy source in medical x-ray imaging is usually an x-ray tube and electrical generator, though in the case of radiotherapy portal imaging, it may be a linear accelerator. As the x-ray beam passes through the patient, some radiation is absorbed or scattered. The intensity of the emerging primary beam varies with position and carries information about the interactions that have occurred in the body. The emerging beam can be detected by a variety of devices, such as a screen-film cassette, image intensifier or flat-panel digital radiography detector. These are typically large-area devices, and the image is a two-dimensional projection of the intervening anatomy. Radiographic film is unique in combining all three roles of image detection, recording and display, but it is rarely used in modern radiotherapy departments. Image intensifiers are usually joined to a charge-coupled device (CCD) camera that allows the capture, digitisation and storage of both static and dynamic images (with the potential of advanced image processing) prior to display on appropriate monitors. In CT, the x-ray beam is collimated in the longitudinal direction to a narrow slit, and this is aligned with an arc of solid-state detectors. The tube and detectors are mounted on a gantry that rotates about the patient. While the x-ray tube/detector assembly is rotating, the patient is fed through the aperture on a moving couch, creating a helix of irradiation on the patient and detector. These projections are processed in a computer to form image slices through the patient which can potentially be in different orientations depending on the clinical application (with the most common being transaxial slices).

Production of X-rays for Imaging

The general topic of x-ray production is covered in Chapter 2. This section highlights some aspects of specific relevance to imaging.

X-rays are generated by the collisions of electrons which have been accelerated to high energies in a vacuum tube with a metal target. The electrical supply is normally from a generator, which takes power from the mains three-phase alternating current (AC) supply and converts it, using a transformer and associated circuits, to an approximately constant kilovoltage (kV) direct current (DC) output. Older models used rectification and smoothing circuits, which resulted in appreciable ripple on the kV waveform such that the output voltage varied by several percent over a mains cycle. For this reason, the kilovoltage is specified as the *peak value*, denoted by the abbreviation kV_p. Modern generators use converters operating at a frequency of several kHz, which produce voltage waveforms with very little ripple. Diagnostic imaging work mostly uses accelerating potentials in the range of 50 to 150 kV_p, though lower values are used in mammography.

At megavoltage energies, as in linear accelerators used for radiotherapy, the x-rays are produced mainly in the forwards direction of the electron beam and hence a transmission target is used. At kilovoltage energies, as used in diagnostic x-ray equipment, radiotherapy simulators and CT scanners, x-rays are produced more isotropically and a reflection target is used. This allows the tube to be constructed with a rotating anode (Fig. 6.1) that permits the heat generated to be dissipated over a much larger area than with a stationary anode. This is important because at kilovoltage energies, only 1% of the electron beam energy appears as x-rays, with the remaining 99% generating heat that must be removed from the x-ray tube. Moreover, to produce images with good spatial resolution, small focal spots are used to minimise geometric unsharpness and short exposure times are used to reduce blurring caused by patient movement. With a stationary anode, this would cause a large quantity of heat to be deposited in a short time over a very small area, which can potentially cause serious damage to the target. For this reason, most x-ray tubes offer two sizes of focal spot; the larger being used for higher exposure rates when there is a higher filament current and the smaller for applications where the best spatial resolution is required.

Bremsstrahlung, as described in Chapter 2, is responsible for the major part of the spectrum, with characteristic radiation peaks defined by the target material being used (see Fig. 6.2). The area under the spectrum represents the total quantity of radiation produced, and the shape of the spectrum determines the quality of the radiation which indicates its penetrating properties. Increasing the tube current (mA) or the exposure time(s) increases the quantity of radiation produced but does not affect its quality. Increasing the applied voltage (kV_p) increases both the quality and quantity of radiation produced. The output is approximately proportional to the square of the applied voltage $(kV_p)^2$ in a conventional diagnostic x-ray tube, although the high filtration seen in some systems, such as CT or cone beam CT, may cause some deviations from this relationship. Other factors, such as anode material and filtration of the beam, further affect the quality and quantity of radiation produced. For imaging, the lower-energy components are usually selectively reduced by suitable filtration, as they only contribute to patient radiation dose and not to the final image.

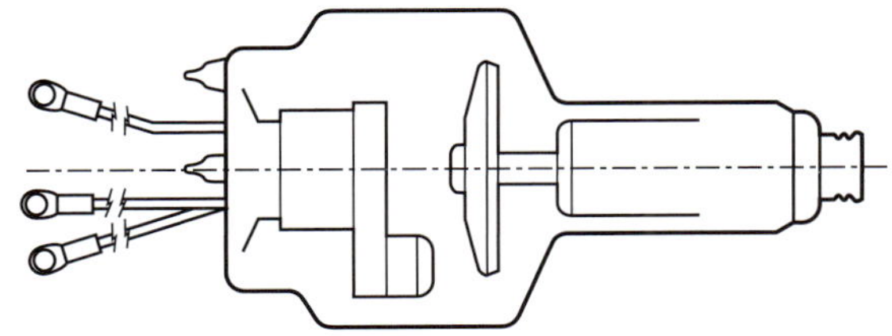

Fig. 6.1 X-ray construction and rotating anode tube. (Courtesy Elekta Ltd.)

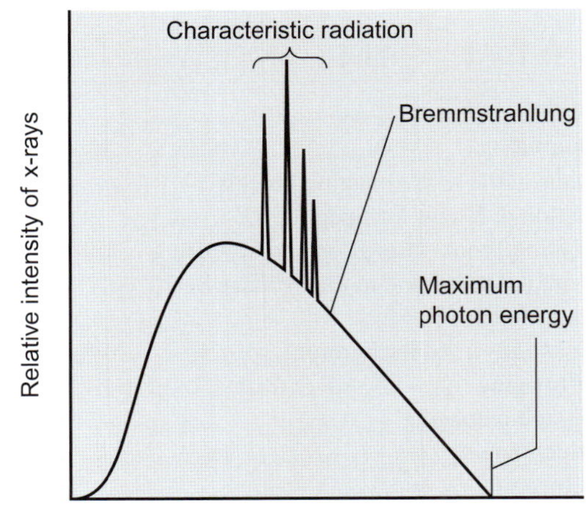

Fig. 6.2 X-ray spectrum produced from a tube.

Information From Absorption and Scattering

When x-rays generated from a suitable source are incident upon an object such as the human body, some pass straight through while others interact with the material in the object by processes of absorption and scattering. In biological tissues at kilovoltage energies, the interactions of importance are photoelectric absorption and Compton scattering. The photoelectric effect depends strongly on the atomic number Z and the energy E of the x-rays. Calcium, found in bone, has a relatively high atomic number and hence strongly absorbs kV x-rays, while soft tissues with their relatively low atomic numbers do not. However, as the beam energy increases, photoelectric absorption falls off rapidly such that at megavoltage energies, it is the Compton effect that dominates and which is primarily dependent on electron density ρ_e.

Hence the beam emerging from the object contains both primary and scattered radiation, and it is the varying intensity of the transmitted primary beam that carries useful information to produce an image. Scattered radiation does not carry useful imaging information and is usually detrimental to final image quality.

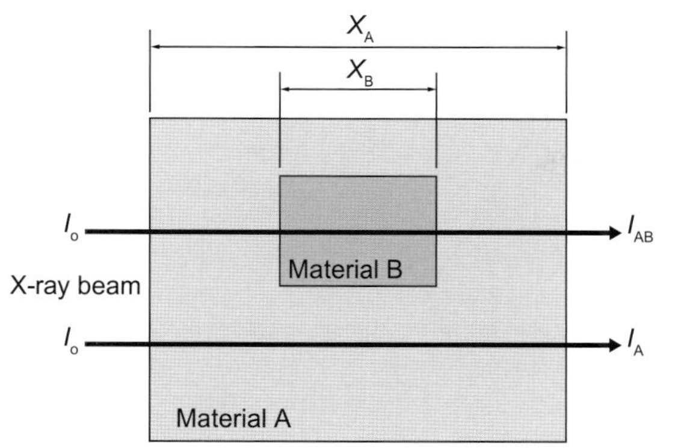

Fig. 6.3 Simple inhomogeneous situation to illustrate contrast.

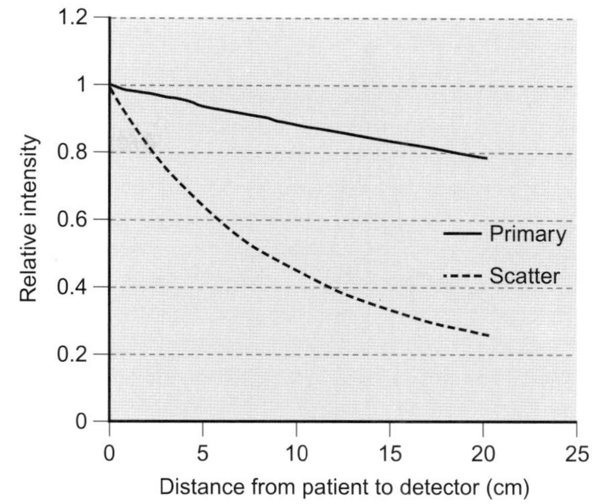

Fig. 6.4 Diagram showing falloff in scatter reaching a detector with distance.

Differential Attenuation in the Primary Beam

Consider the simple situation in Fig. 6.3, which shows a slab of some homogeneous material A of thickness X_A and linear attenuation coefficient μ_A and which contains a region of some other material B of thickness X_B and linear attenuation coefficient μ_B. Suppose a parallel x-ray beam of intensity I_O is incident on this slab. Then, the intensity of the primary beam transmitted through A is:

$$I_A = I_O \cdot \exp(-\mu_A X_A) \tag{6.1}$$

and that transmitted through both A and B is:

$$\begin{aligned} I_{AB} &= I_O \cdot \exp(-\mu_A (X_A - X_B)) \cdot \exp(-\mu_B X_B) \\ &= I_O \cdot \exp(-\mu_A X_A) \cdot \exp((\mu_A - \mu_B) X_B) \\ &= I_A \cdot \exp((\mu_A - \mu_B) X_B) \end{aligned} \tag{6.2}$$

Hence the ratio of the transmitted intensities is:

$$I_{AB}/I_A = \exp((\mu_A - \mu_B) X_B) \tag{6.3}$$

Taking the (natural) logarithm of both sides, this may also be expressed as:

$$\begin{aligned} \ln(I_{AB}/I_A) &= \ln(I_{AB}) - \ln(I_A) \\ &= (\mu_A - \mu_B) X_B \end{aligned} \tag{6.4}$$

This ratio, which determines the contrast visible in the image, increases with the thickness of B (X_B) and with the difference between the linear attenuation coefficients of A and B ($\mu_A - \mu_B$).

The linear attenuation coefficients for air and bone are very different from those of soft tissue at kV energies, so even quite thin structures containing these materials can be visualised on the x-ray image. The differences between the linear attenuation coefficients for different soft tissues are, however, much smaller, and special techniques such as CT are needed to reveal them.

Contrast Media

Some structures may be made visible by deliberately introducing contrast agents, such as air or liquids containing iodine or barium, which have a very different value of μ from the surrounding tissues. This can be particularly useful in cancer and vascular applications where the accumulation or absence of a contrast agent can indicate the presence of pathology.

Scatter as Unwanted Background

Scattered radiation generally contributes a more or less uniform background signal to the image, which does not convey useful information as it is not known where the scattered photons originated. The overall effect is to reduce contrast in the final image. The amount of scattered radiation emerging from the patient can be several times greater than the transmitted primary beam. It increases with the energy of the x-ray beam, the size of the area irradiated and the thickness of the body part being imaged. For this reason, scatter is of greater concern in thicker regions of the patient with inherently poor contrast, such as the abdomen, than it is in less dense regions such as the chest. It is possible to reduce the amount of scatter reaching the detector by using antiscatter grids, an air gap technique or a combination of the two in some cases, such as with cone beam CT. The latter relies on an appreciable separation between the patient and the image detector which reduces the amount of scatter that falls on the detector surface relative to the primary beam, as shown in Fig. 6.4. It should be noted that the air gap technique may require higher radiation doses to the patient to achieve adequate image quality, as both the scattered and primary radiation reaching the detector will be reduced.

The antiscatter grid consists of an array of long, thin, very high atomic number strips and is typically lead, separated by a low atomic number spacer material such as carbon fibre (Fig. 6.5). Only radiation travelling perpendicular to the grid can pass through to the detector, which is most likely to be primary beam photons. Most of the scattered radiation will strike the grid at angles other than perpendicular and is most likely to be absorbed by the lead strips. While some primary beam photons will also be absorbed, the net effect is to greatly increase the ratio of primary-to-scattered radiation reaching the detector, thus improving image contrast.

To ensure that the detector receives the requisite number of photons to guarantee adequate image quality, the use of antiscatter grids may require an increased dose to the patient. However, this is very much dependent on clinical application as the increased contrast may allow the acceptance of higher noise levels in the final image due to an overall improvement in the contrast-to-noise ratio. This should be considered as part of the optimisation process when configuring clinical protocols.

If the angle between the primary beam and the area perpendicular to the grid becomes too great, for example, towards the edge of large fields, a significant fraction of primary radiation will be absorbed. This can be overcome by using a focused grid, as shown in Fig. 6.6. It is of critical importance to ensure that focused grids are used in the correct orientation and at the correct distance to avoid cutoff of the primary x-ray beam. The correct distance should be within a range stated for each specific grid.

To avoid shadows from the lead strips producing distracting lines on the image, there are a range of methods used. One common solution

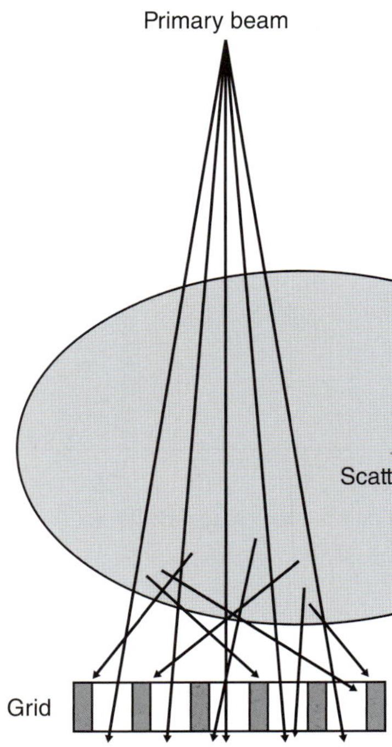

Fig. 6.5 Antiscatter grid principles.

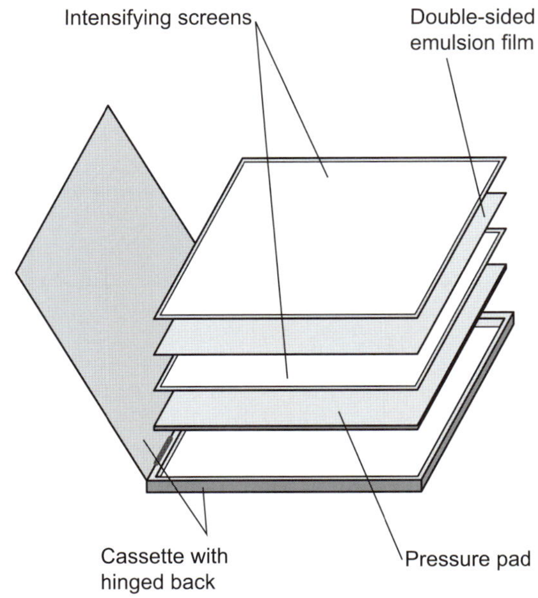

Fig. 6.7 Radiographic film cassette.

is to move the grid to and fro laterally during the exposure to blur out any grid lines in the image, that is, to actively exploit motion unsharpness. However, this is not always possible, such as in LINAC-based cone beam CT. Therefore high line density grids, where the frequency of the grid lines is much higher than the underlying detector sampling, are used to render the lines unresolved in the final image. Also, computer-based postacquisition image processing corrections can actively recognise and remove grid lines, and these are increasingly used on modern systems to remove any grid-induced artefacts.

Planar Imaging

Screen-Film Radiography

For many years, screen-film radiography has been used as a combined detector, storage and display device for x-ray images (Fig. 6.7). However, with the implementation of digital techniques, it is no longer in widespread use in x-ray imaging departments. The intensifying screen (Fig. 6.8) uses a fluorescent material that emits visible light when irradiated with x-rays, and it is this visible light that is then detected by the film. The screens have a higher x-ray absorption efficiency than film and emit many visible light photons for each x-ray photon absorbed. Hence they enable acceptable blackening of the film at much reduced patient doses when compared with film alone. With modern rare earth screens, this reduction may be by a factor of about 100. A cassette is used that contains a separate screen for each side of the film and is constructed so as to ensure close contact between screen and film over the whole area. This reduces blurring.

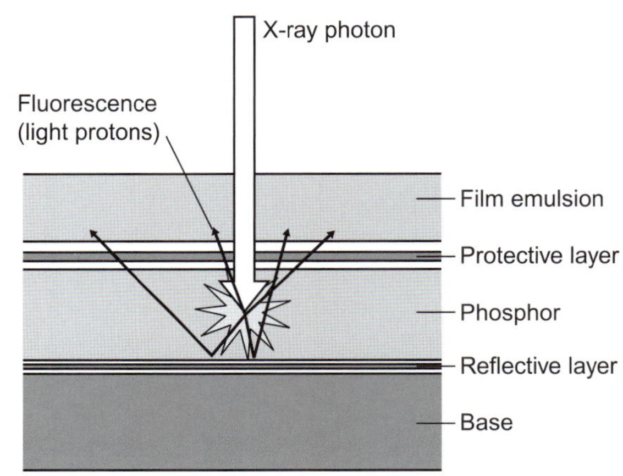

Fig. 6.8 Intensifier screen principles.

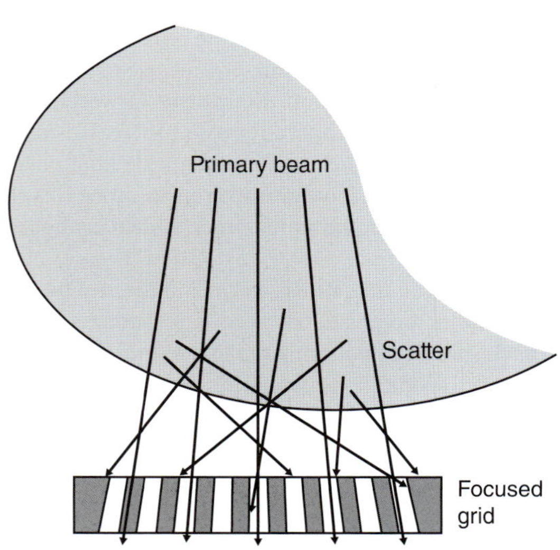

Fig. 6.6 Focused antiscatter grid.

Radiographic film consists of a transparent polyester base, approximately 0.2 mm thick, that usually coated on both sides with an emulsion containing crystals of silver bromide, and this, in turn, is coated with a protective layer. When the emulsion is exposed to light or x-rays, some electrons are transferred from bromide ions to silver ions, which are reduced to silver atoms. These form a latent image which is not visible until it is chemically developed, a process in which the remaining silver ions in the affected crystals are also reduced to silver atoms, which cause blackening of the film. The more silver atoms that are present per unit area in the developed image, the darker the film appears.

Exposed films are normally processed automatically, in several stages:

1. The latent image is developed using an organic reducing agent.
2. The developed image is fixed by dissolving away undeveloped silver bromide from the emulsion.
3. The emulsion is hardened to protect it from damage.
4. The film is washed and dried.

The degree of blackness of the film is measured in terms of optical density (*D*). If a beam of light of intensity I_0 is incident on a piece of film, and intensity I_t is transmitted, then:

$$D = \log_{10}(I_0/I_t) \quad \textbf{(6.5)}$$

Hence a region of film that transmits one-tenth of the incident light intensity has optical density 1.0, whereas a region which transmits one one-hundredth of the incident light intensity has optical density 2.0. A perfectly transparent region would have $D = 0$.

A plot of *D* against $\log_{10}$ (exposure) is called the *characteristic curve* (Fig. 6.9). If an unexposed film is developed, its optical density is a little greater than zero because the film base is not perfectly transparent and some of the silver bromide crystals are reduced to metallic silver (film fog). At very high exposures, all the silver bromide crystals are reduced on development and no increase in *D* occurs for higher exposures; in this case the screen-film response is said to be *saturated*. In between these extremes, and over a *limited* range of exposures, the characteristic curve is approximately linear, and the gradient (slope) in this region is known as *gamma* for that screen-film combination. Note that different screen-film combinations may have different gamma. It is this region which gives rise to contrast in the image as different exposure levels give different optical densities. Under favourable conditions, the human eye can detect density differences as small as 0.02. For high gamma (steep slope) screen-film combinations, the density increases rapidly over a relatively narrow range of exposure values, so the image has high contrast. However, this is at the cost of only allowing a narrow range of exposures to be represented before the image saturates, resulting in an exposure with *low latitude*. Careful radiographic technique is needed to ensure that all features of interest are properly imaged. With a lower gamma screen-film combination, lower-contrast images are produced, but a wider range of exposure levels can be accommodated, resulting in an exposure with *high latitude*.

If only a relatively small exposure is required to produce a given density, the screen-film combination is said to be *fast*, while films requiring high exposure levels are said to be *slow*. Fast films have the benefit of potentially reducing patient doses, but they may suffer from a grainy appearance due to the larger crystals of silver bromide and from increased noise due to fewer photons creating the image, also referred to as *quantum mottle*.

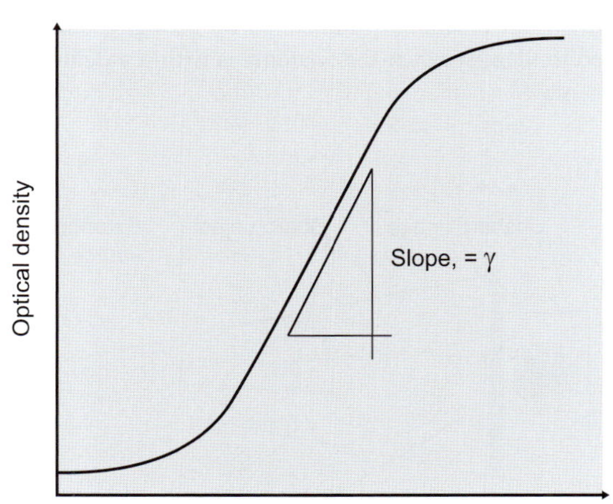

Fig. 6.9 Graphical plot of optical density against exposure.

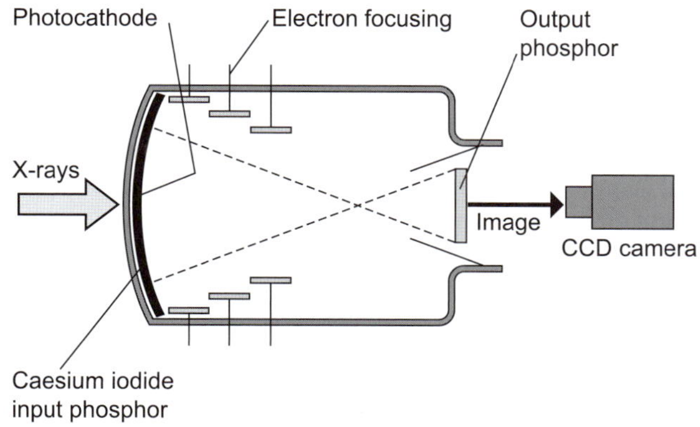

Fig. 6.10 Charge-coupled device camera viewing of the intensifier image (II).

Fluoroscopic Imaging

It is possible to view a *time-varying image*, or *dynamic image*, by using a fluoroscopic system. In older image intensifier–based systems, x-rays are absorbed by a fluorescent material that emits visible light similar to a screen-film cassette. However, the brightness of the resultant image is very low, so the image intensifier is used to increase the brightness, and this secondary image is viewed by a CCD camera via close-coupled optics to minimise any distortions and scatter (Fig. 6.10). The CCD camera signal is recorded in digital format and is usually subject to computer-based image processing prior to display.

The image intensifier tube is an evacuated glass envelope with an input phosphor which is typically in the form of a layer of caesium iodide (CsI) crystals. In contact with this is a photocathode which absorbs the visible light photons and emits photoelectrons. These are accelerated through a large potential difference of approximately 25 kV and focused onto a much smaller output phosphor window which produces visible light when it absorbs these electrons. As a consequence of the energy gained by the electrons and the fact that they are concentrated onto a smaller area, the brightness of the image at the output phosphor is much higher than at the input.

Image intensifiers can be subject to some loss of fidelity, and this can be serious if the electron optics are poorly adjusted or if there is significant interference from external magnetic fields. This can lead to a range of artefacts including veiling glare, pincushion distortion and S distortion, with the latter being due to Earth's magnetic field.

Digital Image Acquisition

Digital imaging technologies have largely replaced these older screen-film and image intensifier–based techniques in modern departments. Digital capture, processing and storage of the image data offers many advantages. There is much improved efficiency and exposure latitude that enables reduced image doses and repeat imaging. Enhanced storage and archiving of images on a digital network enables viewing in many locations at once, and the application of new and advanced image processing algorithms prior to display is possible.

Computed Radiography

An alternative to imaging on radiographic film is computed radiography (CR), which uses photostimulable phosphor (image) plates as the x-ray detector. These are similar to intensifying screens used with film, but instead of emitting visible light immediately on absorbing x-rays, they store a fraction of the absorbed energy by exciting electrons to occupy energy level traps where they remain until stimulated by a suitable light source. The spatial density and distribution of trapped electrons forms the latent image that is subsequently read out by scanning the plate with a red laser beam in a light-tight enclosure. As the trapped electrons return to their ground state, blue light photons are emitted from the image plate, which is then detected by a sensitive photomultiplier tube that produces an electrical signal proportional to the intensity of the light released from the specific point that the laser irradiated. The electrical signal is digitised and stored in a computer as an image matrix, which might typically contain 2000 × 2000 pixels (picture elements).

Digital Radiography and Fluoroscopy

Large-area solid-state detectors based on amorphous silicon (a-Si) technology are now widely available and are commonly referred to as *digital radiography (DR) panels*. These comprise an array of semiconductor elements, each of which acts as a capacitor storing electric charge. Overlying this a-Si matrix of pixels is normally a phosphor layer, such as CsI, as used in the input screen of the image intensifier. This turns the incident x-rays into light photons that are detected by the a-Si photodiodes, which turns the incident light photons into electric charge. The charge pattern is read out electronically by control electronics that open transistor 'gates' in each pixel to allow the charge trapped to flow, thus creating a voltage across readout resistors. This voltage is then turned into a digital signal via an analogue-to-digital converter. This all happens quickly enough to allow up to approximately 4-million-pixel signals to be read out virtually in real time, unlike CR systems, which require the image plate to be transferred to a reader. The digital signal is stored as a digital image matrix in a computer. Because of the imaging speed, dynamic imaging can also be performed with these systems, and pulse mode acquisition is also able to produce higher-quality fluoroscopic and radiographic images. The DR panel is also a fundamental component of the imaging chain of cone beam CT imaging systems on linear accelerators.

Magnification Distortion

Image magnification is always present in any x-ray image as the photons diverge from a small focal spot and travel in straight lines through the patient before reaching the image detector (see Fig. 6.11). Object features which lie in a given plane, parallel to the image detector, are magnified by the same factor. Planes closer to the x-ray source have a higher magnification factor, whilst planes nearer to the image detector have a lower magnification factor. It is often said that a particular image is taken at a certain magnification, though strictly this only applies to one specific plane, usually that passing through the position about which the axes of source and image detectors rotate. Any anatomic feature which does not lie in a single plane parallel to the detector will appear distorted in the image since different parts of it will be magnified to different degrees. In practice, with careful radiographic technique the impact of this can be minimised to the extent that it does not impact on the utility of clinical images.

Resolution, Geometric Unsharpness and Movement

The resolution of an imaging system is a measure of its ability to represent separate features in the object as separate features in the image. Because no imaging system is perfect, the image of a point in the object is blurred to some degree, and sharp edges are rendered unsharp. There are several sources which contribute to the unsharpness of an x-ray image: the finite size of the x-ray focal spot, patient movement and the resolution of the detector system.

X-ray Focal Point Size

Diagnostic x-ray tubes usually offer a choice of two focal spot sizes: *fine*, with a typical diameter of 0.4 to 0.8 mm; or *broad*, with a typical diameter of 0.8 to 1.5 mm. Fig. 6.12 shows how such a source gives rise to a penumbra (blurring) when imaging a sharp edge, with the penumbra wider for a larger focal spot. This is known as *geometric unsharpness*. Because of the bevelled angle of the rotating anode, the apparent size of the focal spot and hence the degree of blurring varies across the image in the direction of the anode's axis of rotation. The blurring is also increased for detail lying in planes with greater magnification. This is especially important for the image of field-defining wires in a physical simulator, as these are located relatively close to the x-ray source and are thus greatly magnified (Fig. 6.13).

Patient Movement

If the patient moves during the exposure, features will be blurred in the image. This can be minimised by using short exposure times, by asking the patient to keep still and to hold their breath and, if necessary, by using patient immobilisation devices. In radiotherapy, when treatments may be long and the patient is breathing normally and spontaneously, motion during imaging may be a desirable property to ensure appropriate representation of the tumour's movement. In contrast, for treatments controlled by gating, gated imaging is required to identify when the anatomy is within a defined range of movement.

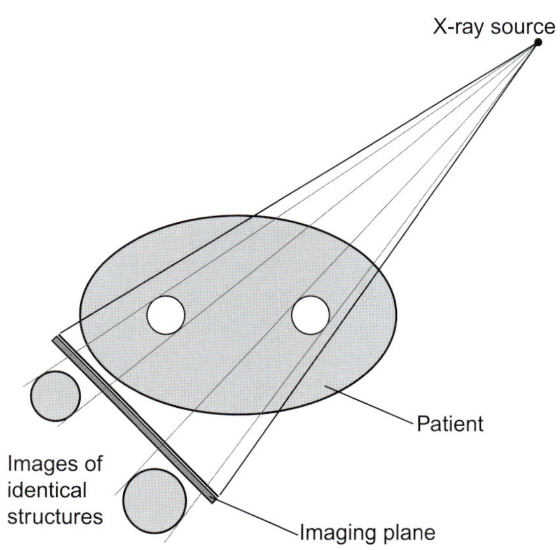

Fig. 6.11 Magnification of objects lying in different planes.

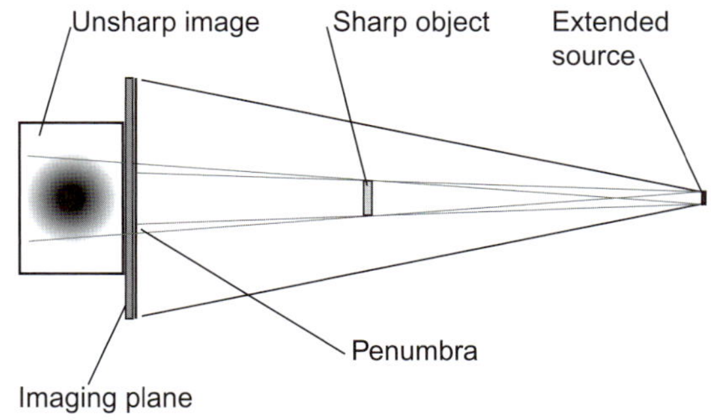

Fig. 6.12 How a source gives rise to a penumbra.

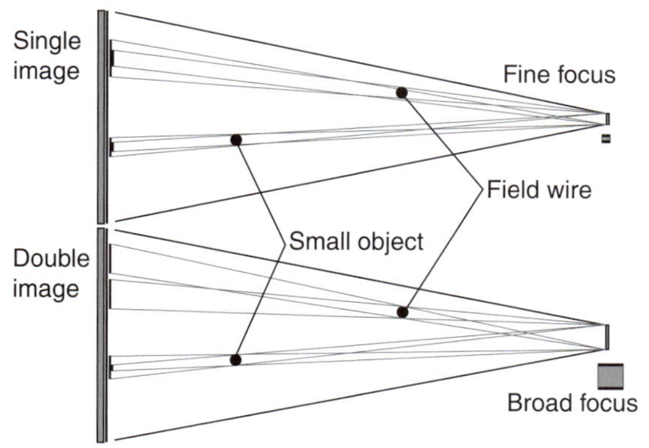

Fig. 6.13 Magnification of the field wires in the physical simulator.

Resolution of the Detector

The detector resolution is inherently related to the number of distinct and independent samples which are detected within the image. This can be thought of as the spatial sampling rate of the detector. For film, the sampling rate is directly related to the grain size, so for example, if the grain size were 1.0 μm × 1.0 μm, a 1-mm^2 area of film would contain 1 million samples. Hence the sampling rate can be expressed as 1 million samples per mm^2. With digital systems, the sampling rate is dependent upon the density of sensitive electronic devices that can be manufactured per square mm. This depends upon the pixel size, which is effectively the size of the a-Si sensitive element in flat-panel detectors. The resolution required is determined by clinical need, and detector design has had to evolve to meet various clinical requirements. Modern flat-panel detectors are typically manufactured with a pixel pitch of between 100 μm and 150 μm. Hence the inherent limiting spatial resolution of digital detectors is much poorer than was possible with film due to the lower sampling rate.

Image Signal and Noise

An ideal x-ray image would represent the distribution of attenuation coefficients in an object with perfect fidelity. In practice, even the image of a homogeneous object of uniform thickness is not perfectly uniform. The signal exhibits variations about its mean level, and these are called *noise*. Noise can make it difficult to distinguish signal levels which only differ by a small amount, that is, areas of low contrast in the image.

There are various sources of noise, but one that is always present to some degree is quantum noise, or mottle. This results from the fact that any image is made using a finite number of x-ray photons (quanta), and the processes of interaction in the patient and of absorption in the detector are random. This means that there is a statistical variation in the number of photons detected even over an area of uniform attenuation. If the average number of photons per unit area is N, the statistical uncertainty in the number detected in any particular unit area is $\sqrt{N}$. Expressed as a percentage of the average number, this is $100 \times (\sqrt{N}/N)\%$ or $100/(\sqrt{N})\%$. So, relative to the detected signal, the noise decreases as the number of x-ray photons increases, but it is never quite equal to zero.

Other sources of image noise can be the finite size of the fluorescent crystals in intensifying screens, the finite size of silver grains in radiographic film, and electrical noise in various components of an imaging chain or digital detector system.

With the development of ever more advanced image processing algorithms, it is becoming possible to minimise the impact of image noise in the final image. This includes methods that employ artificial intelligence (AI) techniques to suppress noise. Care must be taken with the implementation of such technology to ensure that it does not compromise image quality in undesirable ways (e.g. remove clinical features that appear to be noise, introduce artefacts). It should also be remembered that the application of image processing also breaks the statistical link between signal levels and 'noise' presented in the final image.

Dose

All x-ray imaging procedures give some ionising radiation dose to the patient. This is believed to usually entail a small risk of harmful effects, such as future cancer induction. In some diagnostic techniques, deterministic skin injury is also widely reported. It is normally a requirement of national regulations, such as the Ionising Radiation (Medical Exposure) Regulations[2] in the United Kingdom, that the doses from medical imaging exposures should be kept as low as reasonably practicable, consistent with the intended purpose. Doses from different procedures can be measured or calculated in various ways. For a given patient, it is often convenient to combine these into an estimate of the total effective dose received, which may be regarded as an index of the total radiation risk from the combined imaging procedures. However, it should be noted that dose limits for patient exposure do not exist, and each and every medical radiation procedure should be justified on its own merits as contributing to the medical management of the patient.[2]

Tomographic Imaging

Planar x-ray imaging is limited in its ability to show low-contrast features, especially in soft tissues, and to allow accurate localisation of features in all three spatial dimensions. This results from the fact that it projects a three-dimensional object onto a two-dimensional image domain, coupled with a limited ability to reject scattered radiation. Tomographic imaging addresses these limitations by imaging selected planes of the patient separately.

Historically, conventional tomography used linked movements of the x-ray tube with planar detectors to image selected longitudinal planes of the patient in focus, with more distant planes increasingly blurred out into a more or less uniform background. Methods were devised to optimise the use of these systems, and there is continuing interest in digital processing of the component images, for example, in the technique called *tomosynthesis*, which is now widespread in mammography applications. Although these techniques can improve localisation and contrast, they do not reduce the effect of scattered radiation, and they never give a 'true' three-dimensional representation of the patient as there is always a contribution from blurred, out-of-plane structures in the image set.

Computed Tomography

CT uses the principle of mathematically reconstructing the internal structure of an object from a set of images of the object taken from different projection angles. To acquire data from which to reconstruct a single slice, the x-ray beam is collimated and aligned with an arc of narrow solid-state detectors. The tube and detectors are mounted on a gantry that rotates about the patient (Fig. 6.14). With this imaging arrangement, it is possible to reject a large proportion of the scatter while detecting the transmitted primary beam with high efficiency. Essentially, one-dimensional projection images are acquired from many angles, and the data are processed in a computer to form images of transverse slices through the patient. There are several mathematical techniques which can be used to do this, including filtered back projection (Fig. 6.15) and iterative methods. Iterative reconstruction is now the most common method available on modern CT scanners, but it exists with a wide range of implementations between manufacturers. This can lead to different image presentations that can be advantageous in the suppression of image noise, but it can also reduce detectability of low-contrast structures due to the change

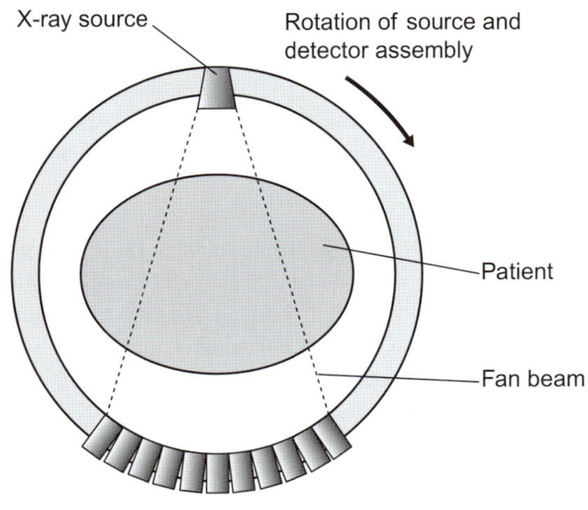

Fig. 6.14 Diagram of a third-generation computed tomography scanner.

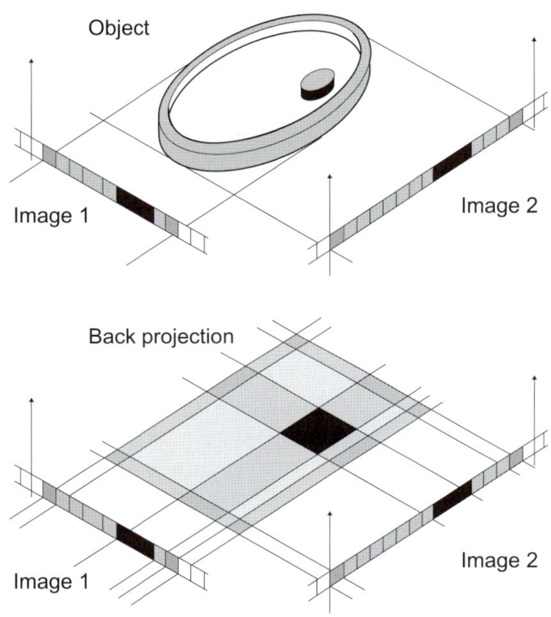

Fig. 6.15 The principle of filtered back projection.

in noise texture. As with DR imaging, AI-based reconstruction technology is finding increased application in CT and may in the future replace iterative as the default method on CT scanners.

Practical Configurations

Almost all modern CT scanners are of the so-called third-generation design shown in Fig. 6.14. Electrical connections with the rotating gantry are made using slip rings and sliding contactors operating at low voltage, with the high-voltage generator being mounted on the rotating gantry itself. This allows the gantry to rotate continuously in the same direction, which is necessary for helical (spiral) acquisitions in which the patient on the table top is slowly advanced through the gantry aperture and data are acquired continuously during several rotations.

Multislice Computed Tomography

Since the early 1990s, multislice CT scanners have been available in which several arcs of detectors are stacked together longitudinally and the divergence of the x-ray beam can be adjusted so as to irradiate them simultaneously. This permits more rapid collection of projection data from a given length of the patient and makes for efficient use of the x-rays generated by the tube, thus easing the heat loading.

Cone Beam Computed Tomography

It is possible to acquire projection data using devices other than a dedicated CT scanner. Using a solid-state DR panel and rotating this about the patient during data acquisition, a set of cone beam projections is obtained from which a set of transverse slices can be reconstructed through advanced reconstruction techniques.

Dynamic Imaging

Many structures in the body move. Some motion is more or less regularly repetitive or periodic, as in the beating heart or respiratory movement. Some may be quasiregular, such as peristalsis, and others more intermittent, such as swallowing or coughing. A single image will only represent the situation within the time frame over which it is acquired. If that is short compared with the time over which the movement occurs, it will be a 'snapshot' of a particular phase of the movement; otherwise, it will be a blurred image, averaged over some range of movement.

By taking a time sequence of images, a so-called *dynamic series* can be acquired which represents the anatomy of interest at its various positions. This can be useful for diagnosis and staging. For example, a barium swallow can demonstrate oesophageal or gastric abnormalities. Also, a dynamic fluoroscopic image or a dynamic CT image can be set to demonstrate the movement of a lung tumour.

Gated Imaging

Where periodic motion is present, gated imaging may be a useful option. This represents data over a typical cycle of the motion as a series of images at different times or phases of the cycle. The image acquisition is linked to some suitable physiological gating signal, such as an electrocardiograph (ECG) signal or a respiratory monitoring device. For treatment planning, a CT image set gated to the respiration cycle may be used in a study of the chest to demonstrate and accommodate the movement of a lung tumour. The latter is known as a *four-dimensional CT (4DCT)* and is increasingly used.

Dedicated Radiotherapy Systems

The basic principles of x-ray imaging have been described earlier. However, there are some x-ray imaging devices which are exclusive to radiotherapy with either x-ray imaging embedded into the device or by using image data obtained with x-rays.

Simulator

The radiotherapy simulator is a machine which replicates the movements and geometry of a megavoltage LINAC or cobalt treatment machine but uses a diagnostic x-ray tube to produce kV images. It includes beam-limiting diaphragms and field-defining wires to allow accurate simulation of the treatment beam and patient geometry. The gantry and couch of the simulator should reproduce all the movements of the treatment machine, to the same accuracy or better (see Chapter 10).

Computed Tomography Virtual Simulator

By acquiring a series of CT slices over a suitable longitudinal range, it is possible to generate a digital representation of the body in all three spatial dimensions. This can be used as the basis of virtual simulation, in which digitally reconstructed radiographs can be generated to provide beam's-eye views of the patient from arbitrary directions for various shapes and sizes of field.

Treatment Verification Systems

A check on the accuracy of positioning of treatment fields can be made by acquiring *portal images*. These are images of the transmitted treatment beam emerging from the patient and may be acquired directly onto film or by an electronic portal imaging device (EPID). Because photoelectric absorption is relatively unimportant with megavoltage (MV) x-rays, contrast between bone and soft tissue is much poorer with MV images than with kV images, so identification of anatomic features depends more on contrast with air.

Manufacturers now offer a range of kV imaging devices integrated with linear accelerators for image-guided radiotherapy. These include kV tubes and amorphous silicon imagers mounted on the same gantry at 90 degrees to the megavoltage beam (Fig. 11.12). Such systems can acquire data during a rotation about the patient to produce cone beam CT images. CT 'on rails' has also been offered on linear accelerator systems to produce three-dimensional data sets of the patient, though this is not common in modern radiotherapy centres now.

Another system uses two fixed x-ray tubes mounted in the floor of the treatment room, in conjunction with ceiling-mounted detectors, to acquire oblique views of the patient. The images can be analysed by computer software to compare with reference images to indicate required setup corrections. It can, however, be difficult for operators to interpret images taken from these angles.

MAGNETIC RESONANCE IMAGING

Overview of the Magnetic Resonance Imaging Process

MRI uses a strong magnetic field, typically between 0.3 and 3.0 T (tesla), and radiofrequency (RF) pulses to manipulate the magnetic properties of hydrogen nuclei in water and fat within the body. Nuclei with odd numbers of protons and neutrons act like tiny magnets, and in the presence of a strong magnetic field, they have a net alignment with the magnetic field. After a pulse of RF energy is applied, some of the nuclei will flip and align themselves against the field. Following the pulse, the nuclei will return to the original alignment, producing an RF signal at the same frequency as the one applied. Images are generated that reflect the distribution of tissue magnetisation within the body. By altering the interval between the RF pulses and the time at which the signals are detected, images with different tissue contrast are produced.

Producing a Signal

Magnetic resonance occurs when a magnetic field is applied to systems that possess both a magnetic moment and angular momentum. The nucleus of a hydrogen atom is a single proton which has both a magnetic moment and angular momentum and can be referred to as a *proton* or a *spin*. When the protons in the human body are placed in a strong magnetic field (B_0), they will experience a 'twisting force' which will cause them to precess around the direction of the magnetic field at a frequency (f_0) given by the Larmor equation:

$$f_0 = \frac{\gamma}{2\pi} \cdot B_0 \quad \textbf{(6.6)}$$

where γ is a constant called the *gyromagnetic ratio*. The $\gamma/2\pi$ is approximately 42.6 MHz T^{-1} for hydrogen protons. When a magnetic field is applied, there is a tendency for the individual proton magnetic moments to align with the field. This creates a net magnetisation vector (M_0)

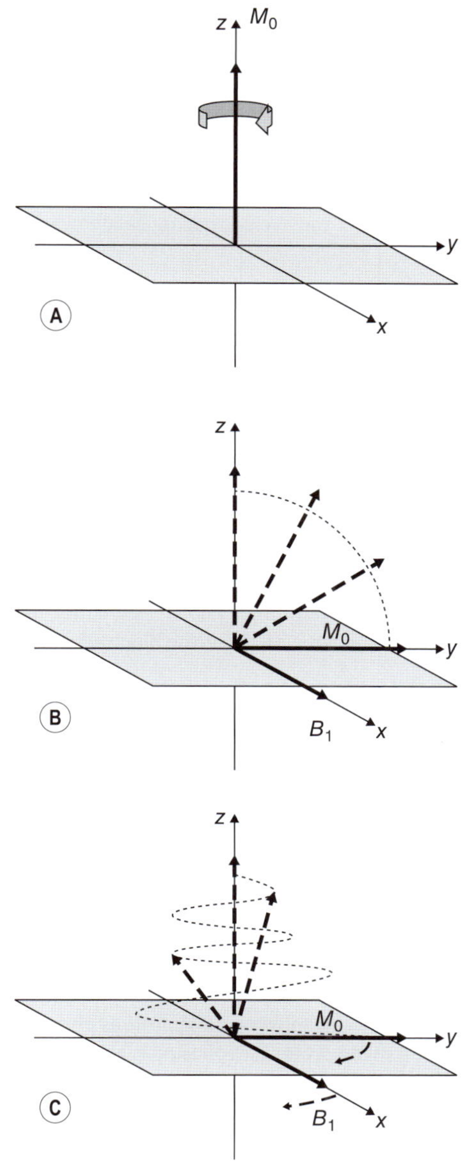

Fig. 6.16 (A) Net magnetisation vector *(Mo)* rotating about the z-axis at the Larmor frequency. (B) Motion of Mo in the rotating frame during the application of a 90-degree RF pulse *(B1)*. (C) Motion of Mo in the lab frame during the application of a 90-degree RF pulse *(B1)*.

parallel to the magnetic field B_0 (Fig. 6.16A) in which B_0 is parallel to the z-axis.

In all MRI sequences, an RF excitation pulse (B_1) is applied perpendicular to B_0 to tip the net magnetisation, (M_0), away from its initial alignment with B_0 so that the magnetisation can be detected. To be effective, the applied RF pulse needs to be at the Larmor frequency. The RF pulse brings all the spins into phase, so the net magnetisation vector rotates about the z-axis at the Larmor frequency, as shown in Fig. 6.16B. The motion of the net magnetisation vector in the rotating frame and the laboratory frame as the RF pulse continues to be applied is shown in Figs. 6.16B and C. The angle through which M_0 is rotated depends on the amplitude and duration of the RF pulse. A 90-degree pulse will rotate M_0 into the *x-y* or transverse plane.

The precessing net magnetisation vector induces a voltage in a receiver coil. The detected signal oscillates at the Larmor frequency and decays exponentially as the individual spin components of M_0 rapidly dephase.

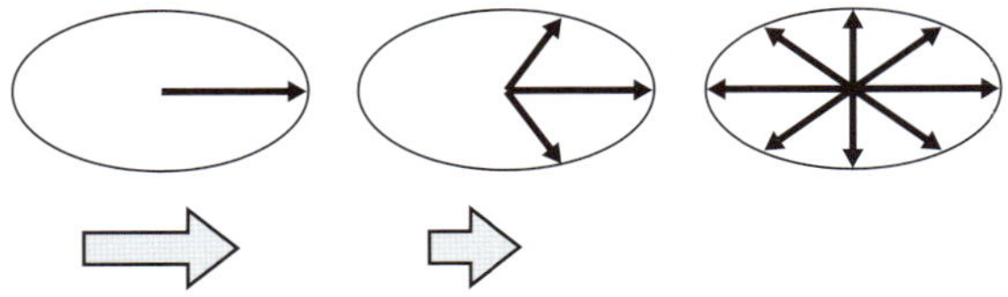

Fig. 6.17 Dephasing of transverse magnetisation over time shown in the rotating frame.

Returning to Thermal Equilibrium

Once the RF pulse B_1 is switched off, the net magnetisation vector will return to its thermal equilibrium state parallel to the magnetic field. Bloch[3] described this process, called *relaxation*, using two different time constants, T_1 and T_2. Different tissues exhibit different T_1 and T_2 values.

T_1 relaxation is also called *longitudinal relaxation*, as it governs the rate at which the z-component of M_0 recovers. The recovery process occurs when spins which have been excited by the RF pulse give up their energy to their surroundings, known as a lattice in early experiments. Following a 90-degree RF pulse, the Bloch equation simplifies to:

$$M_Z(t) = M_0 \cdot [1 - \exp(-t / T_1)] \quad \textbf{(6.7)}$$

The T_2 relaxation occurs because each proton experiences a slightly different magnetic field strength, as the surrounding protons and molecules move around it on a microscopic scale. As a result of these spin–spin interactions, each proton experiences slightly different magnetic fields over time, causing them to rotate at different frequencies, leading to a dephasing of the signal in the transverse plane. This dephasing, viewed in the rotating frame, is shown in Fig. 6.17. Following a 90-degree RF pulse, the Bloch equation simplifies to:

$$M_{xy}(t) = M_{xy}(t=0) \cdot \exp(-t/T_2) \quad \textbf{(6.8)}$$

As well as the random movement of protons and molecules causing the dephasing of the protons, dephasing is also caused by magnetic field inhomogeneities and the change in magnetic field at some tissue boundaries. The combined relaxation caused by random spin–spin interactions and both the magnetic field inhomogeneity and changes at some tissue boundaries is called *T_2* relaxation*.

Imaging Sequences

To determine the location of an emitted signal in the body, the signal must be *spatially encoded*. The spatially encoded signal then needs to be recalled as an 'echo' either by using extra RF pulses, called the *spin echo*, or by using gradients, called the *gradient echo*. The intrinsic tissue properties, such as the T1 and T2 values, and the instrumental variables, such as the timing of RF pulses, affect the relative signals from different tissues and hence the contrast in the image. Image contrast will be discussed; first using the Bloch equations and then using two-dimensional spatial encoding.

How Contrast Is Altered in a Magnetic Resonance Image

To produce an MRI image, a series of RF pulses must be applied. The reason for this will become clear when spatial encoding of the signal is discussed. The time between the 90-degree RF pulses is called the *repetition time (TR)*. The *echo time (TE)* is the time between the 90-degree RF pulse and the central point of the signal detection, or the 'echo'.

If no transverse magnetisation remains when each 90-degree RF pulse is applied, the signal (S) produced at time TE is:

$$S(TE) \sim M_0 \cdot \left[1 - \exp(-TR/T_1)\right] \cdot \exp(-TE/T_2) \quad \textbf{(6.9)}$$

TABLE 6.1 T_1 and T_2 Relaxation Times of Common Tissues at 1.5 T

Tissue	T_1 (ms)	T_2 (ms)
White matter	560	82
Grey matter	1100	92
Cerebrospinal fluid	2060	1000–2000
Fat	200	≈110

An image with the contrast dependent on the T_1 times of the tissues is called a *T_1 weighted image*. From Eq. (6.9), to remove any T_2 weighting requires $e(-TE/T_2) \approx 1$, which is achieved by keeping TE ≪ T_2. To make the signal dependent on T_1 requires a TR around the minimum T_1 time. Typically, brain imaging at 1.5 T would use a TR of approximately 500 ms and a TE of less than 20 ms. Table 6.1 shows the T_1 and T_2 times of white matter, grey matter, cerebral spinal fluid (CSF) and fat. Eq. (6.9), with a TR around the minimum T_1 time and a TE ≪ T_2, also indicates that tissues with shorter T_1 values will produce a higher signal than tissues with long T_1 values. So, on a T_1 weighted image, white matter is brighter than grey matter and CSF is dark. Fat will also be bright because of its short T_1 time and long T_2 time.

To produce a *T_2 weighted image* with contrast dependent upon T_2 times requires T_1 weighting to be minimised. Again, looking at Eq. (6.9), this is achieved when $e(-TR/T_1) \approx 0$, which occurs when TR ≈ three to five times T_1. To make the signal dependent on T_2 values requires a TE around the T_2 time of tissue. For brain imaging at 1.5 T, a TR of at least 3000 ms and a TE of 80 to 120 ms would be typical. Eq. (6.9), with a TR of 3000 ms or higher and a TE equalling 80 to 120 ms, shows that tissues with long T_2 values will produce more signal than those with short T_2 values. So, from Table 6.1, in a T_2 weighted image, CSF is very bright and grey matter is brighter than white matter.

A third type of image, called a *proton density weighted image*, aims to produce weighting dependent only on the density of protons within a given region and is independent of the T_1 and T_2 relaxation times. So, again looking at Eq. (6.9), T_1 weighting is eliminated by using a TR of three to five times the T_1 value. T_2 weighting is minimised by keeping TE≪T_2. The parameters for a brain image at 1.5 T would typically be a TR of at least 3000 ms and a TE of less than 20 ms.

The three image contrasts, using different parameters, are shown in Fig. 6.18.

How Positional Information Is Encoded in the Signal

Positional information is encoded into the MRI signal through a technique called *spatial encoding*. This involves applying magnetic field gradients in orthogonal directions to create variations in the magnetic field along those directions. The strength and timing of these gradients vary throughout the imaging sequence. To generate a single two-dimensional image, a slice select gradient is applied during RF excitation to only excite protons in a slice with a given position and thickness dependent on the frequency and bandwidth of the RF pulse and the strength of the slice select gradient. The plane of the slice can also be altered by changing the direction of the applied gradient or gradients. A phase encoding gradient is then applied, causing the protons to experience a phase shift which is directly related to their position along the axis. Finally, a frequency encoding gradient is applied as the RF signal is read out, which causes the precessing protons to experience a slight variation in the magnetic field strength and results in a corresponding variation in their Larmor frequencies. The resultant spatially encoded signal is digitised and stored as one row in a raw data space, referred to as a *k-space*. To collect the entire data set required for a two-dimensional image, it is necessary to repeat this signal acquisition

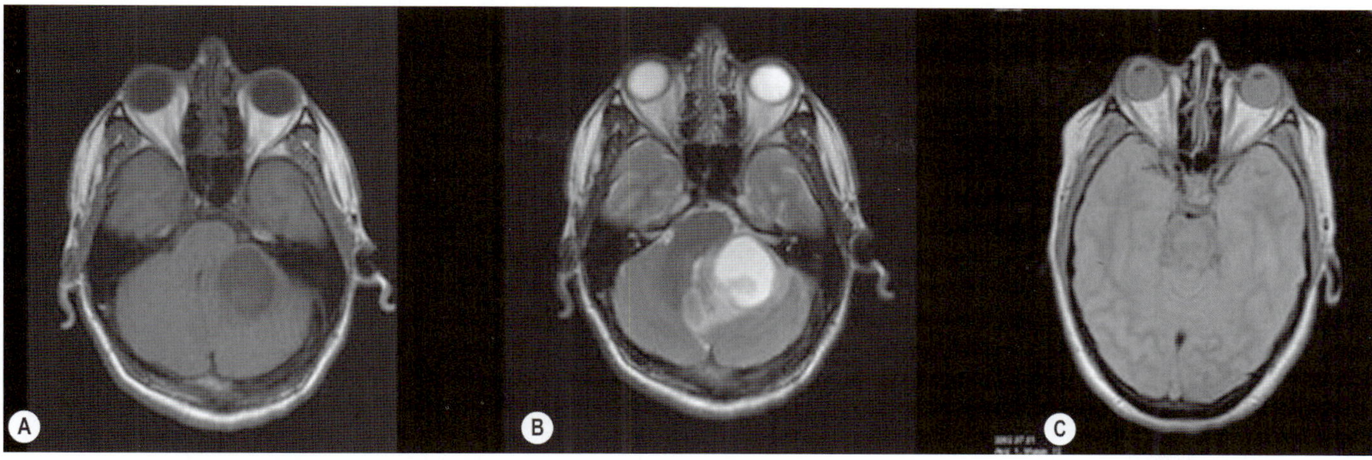

Fig. 6.18 (A) T_1 weighted image (TR = 554 ms, TE = 13 ms). (B) T_2 weighted image (TR = 5070 ms, TE = 98 ms). (C) Proton density (TR = 370 ms, TE = 15 ms).

multiple times, each with different phase encoding gradient amplitudes applied. Each resultant signal is stored in a different row of *k*-space. The number of phase encoding steps required for a fully sampled image is equal to the number of pixels there will be in the phase encoding direction in the final image. The final two-dimensional image is generated by applying a mathematical operation known as a *Fourier transform* to the raw data in *k*-space (Fig. 6.19). Multiple two-dimensional slices in different positions can be acquired separately by repeating this method. Alternatively, three-dimensional images can be generated by initially exciting a thick slice or 'slab' and then performing phase encoding in two orthogonal directions.

For readers who want a much more comprehensive understanding than has been attempted here, a good MRI text reference is *MRI: From Picture to Proton*[4] or online resources such as Mriquestions.com[5] or research by Edelstein et al.[6]

Magnetic Resonance Imaging Scanners

The main components of an MRI scanner are the main magnet; the *x*, *y* and *z* gradient coils; an RF transmitter coil; and a receiver coil. A computer controls the timings of the RF pulses and currents through the gradient coils. Image reconstruction may be performed by the main computer or an additional specialised computer.

The majority of clinical MRI scanners use superconducting magnets in which there is no electrical resistance. These currently have field strengths between 0.5 and 3.0 T, but there are 7- and 8-T research systems. Higher-strength magnets have the advantage of greater signal-to-noise ratios and can be used to improve image quality, imaging speed or both. However, the disadvantage is increased costs, increased artefacts and safety concerns. The superconductivity is achieved by cooling the wire coils, which produce the magnetic field, to around −269°C using liquid helium. These magnets have a cylindrical design, with the patient lying inside the bore or tunnel, and the magnetic field direction is aligned with the bore. A commercial MRI scanner with a superconducting magnet is shown in Fig. 6.20.

Other types of magnet are available in commercial MRI systems, although these are less common. For example, Fig. 6.21 shows an open 0.35-T permanent magnet. Although the magnet is heavy at around 10 tonnes, running costs are low.

The remainder of this section concentrates on the cylindrical superconducting magnet system because it is by far the most common. The

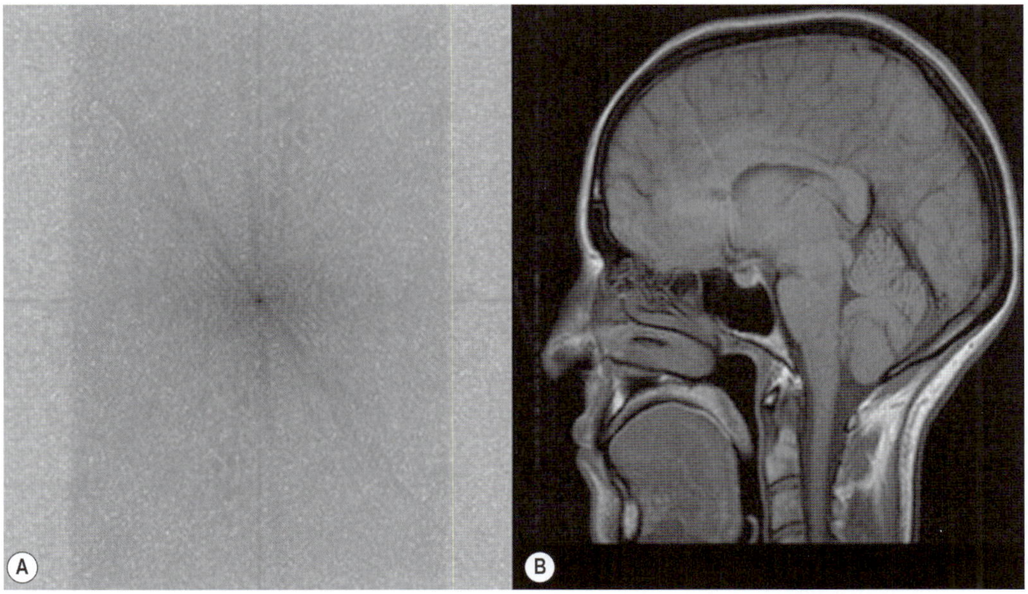

Fig. 6.19 (A) The *k*-space data stored. (B) Two-dimensional Fourier transform of the *k*-space data.

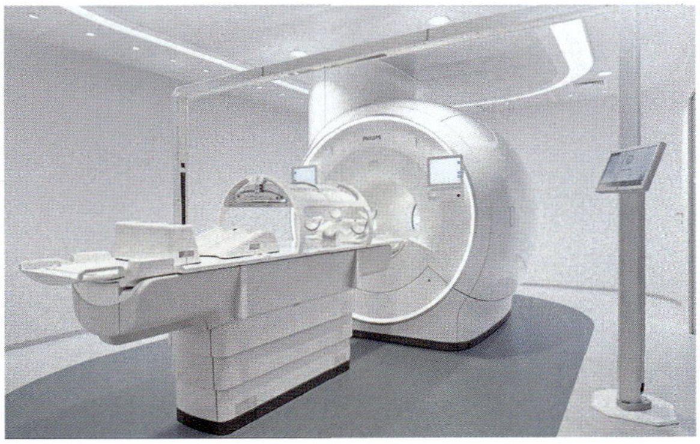

Fig. 6.20 Magnetic resonance imaging system with a cylindrical superconducting magnet.

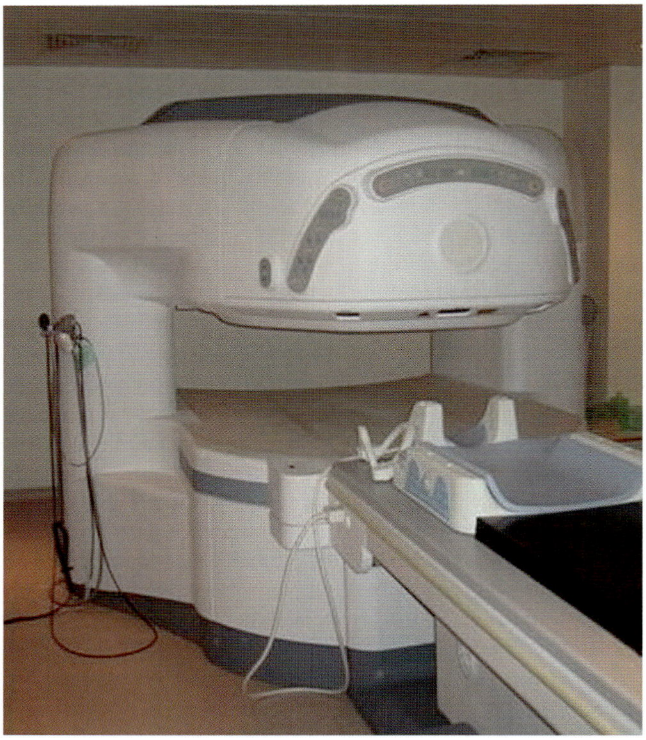

Fig. 6.21 Open magnetic resonance imaging system with a permanent magnet.

field produced by the magnet is not completely uniform and homogeneous, and therefore it must be shimmed. A fixed shim is achieved passively using small pieces of steel positioned around the magnet. However, this may be supplemented or replaced by the use of computer-determined currents inside special superconducting coils called *shim coils*. Because the patient affects the magnetic field homogeneity, additional shimming is also performed each time a patient is imaged. This dynamic shimming uses the gradient coils and sometimes uses extra (resistive) shim coils. The RF pulses are transmitted through a birdcage design, known as the *integrated body coil* (Fig. 6.22), which is inside the bore of the magnet, and the signal is normally received by a dedicated receive coil. At its simplest, this receive coil is a loop of wire, orientated perpendicular to the main magnetic field. Phased array receive coils consisting of multiple small coil elements are designed to sit close to the patient and hence the signal. These may be *surface coils* used, for example, to image the body, spine, breast and extremities; or *volume coils* used, for example, to image the head, knees and feet. Some

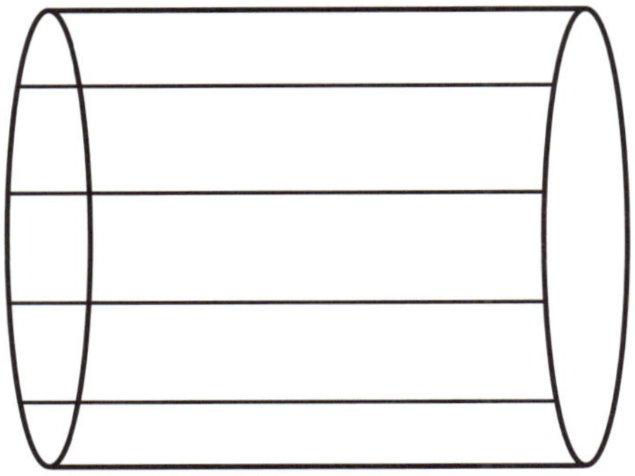

Fig. 6.22 Schematic diagram of a birdcage coil.

of the RF coils can be used to both transmit the RF pulses and detect the signal produced. The most common design of coil which both transmits and receives RF pulses is the birdcage coil (Fig. 6.22). This coil design produces a uniform RF field with good penetration and is often used in knee coils and some head coils.

Spectroscopy

Single-voxel MRS is a technique which produces a spectrum of the metabolites present in a voxel. Most MRS is performed on hydrogen nuclei, as they are the most abundant nuclei and MRI systems and coils are already tuned to hydrogen's resonant frequency. However, MRS can also be performed on ^{23}Na and ^{31}P. In the limited space available here, only hydrogen MRS will be discussed.

The voxel which produces the MRS spectrum is normally selected using RF pulses and gradients. For single-voxel spectroscopy, two techniques are commonly used: *point-resolved spectroscopy (PRESS)*[7] and *stimulated echo acquisition mode (STEAM)*.[7] A Fourier transform of the signal detected from the voxel gives the spectrum (Fig. 6.23). A spectrum is produced because each metabolite has a slightly different local magnetic field strength due to its chemical environment. Therefore each metabolite resonates at a slightly different frequency. The area under each peak is proportional to the amount of metabolite present. The water peak has to be suppressed or this would dominate the spectrum.

Chemical shift imaging is another spectroscopic technique which produces a matrix of spectra from a matrix of voxels encoded with a phase encoding gradient.

Clinical Applications of Magnetic Resonance Imaging in Oncology

Anatomic MRI is often used in the head, neck, abdomen and pelvis for the detection of cancer and for staging the disease. Contrast agents, which are gadolinium based and injected intravenously, shorten the T_1 of tissue. Areas of tumour with high vasculature are therefore highlighted on T_1 weighted images obtained after the administration of contrast agent.

Complete textbooks have been written on the use of MRI in cancer diagnosis, staging, treatment planning and treatment monitoring. In this section the application of MRI in brain tumour imaging is briefly outlined. MRI can be used to diagnose and stage cancer in most organs of the body, including the bladder, pancreas, bowel, cervix, ovaries and prostate. The use of MRI in bowel cancer is concentrated on as an example of this vast area.

Brain Tumours

MRI scanning is unsurpassed as the ideal imaging medium for the diagnosis of brain tumours. Brain tumours make up around 9% of all adult cancers. Approximately one-half are primary tumours and

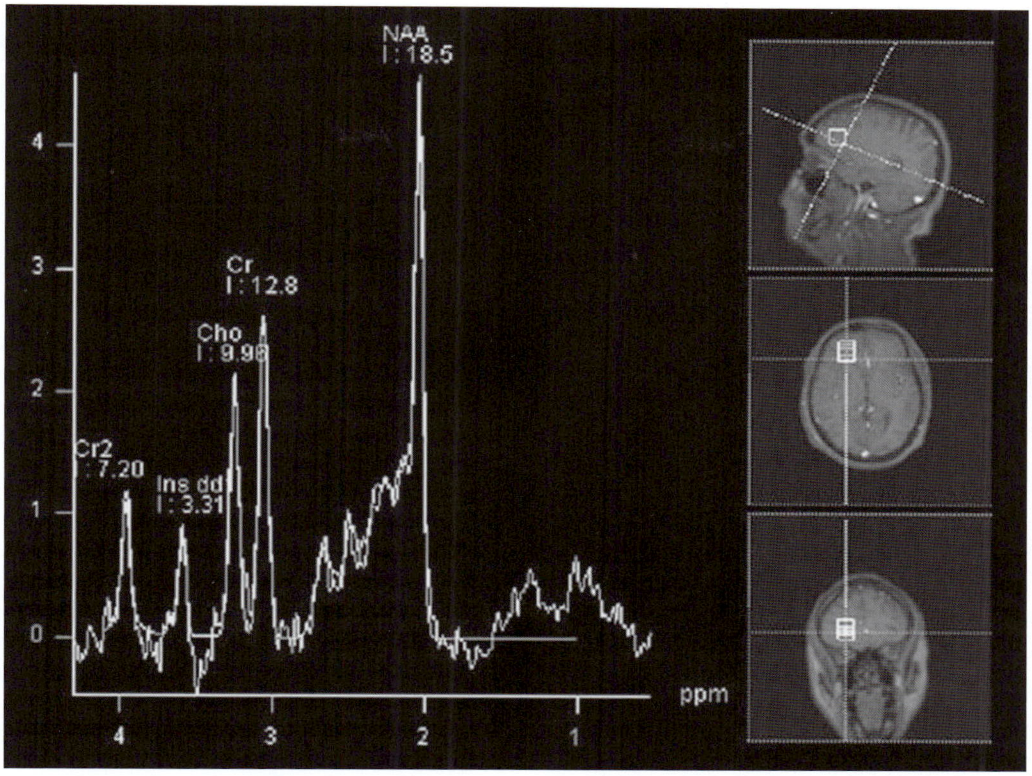

Fig. 6.23 Spectrum from a voxel normal brain tissue showing a high N-acetyl aspartate *(NAA)* peak, and choline *(Cho)* levels below those of creatine *(Cr)*. Obtained using stimulated echo acquisition mode sequence with TE = 30 ms.

the other half secondary. Gliomas are the most common type (45%–50%) of primary brain tumour. Fig. 6.24 of a patient with a large left occipital lobe glioma shows the extent of the tumour, which appears as a bright area of hyperintense signal on the T_2 weighted image. Pathological processes, such as a tumour or infarction, increase the amount of extracellular water, which can lead to cerebral oedema. T_2 weighted images, as in Fig. 6.25A, are best at showing an increase in the amount of extracellular water, which also appears as bright, hyperintense areas. On T_1 weighted images, oedema appears as a dark, hypointense area.

Discrimination between the tumour and surrounding oedema can be helped by the use of a gadolinium-based contrast agent, which can enhance the tumour in the image. Gadolinium is a rare earth metal with seven unpaired electrons. These unpaired electrons enable nearby protons to align more quickly with the magnetic field and therefore shorten the T_1 and T_2 relaxation times. Usually, low-grade gliomas do not enhance on T_1 weighted images with gadolinium-based contrast agents; however, high-grade gliomas enhance avidly, often with a heterogeneous appearance because of haemorrhage or necrosis. Figs. 6.24B and C show areas of strong contrast enhancement where the glioma has broken down the blood–brain barrier. However, isolated tumour cells can penetrate beyond the tumour margins visualised using MRI. This is significant with regard to the margins used in radiotherapy treatment planning (see Chapter 11).

The type of brain tumour can usually be determined by its location and appearance. However, from its visual appearance and location, the tumour shown in Fig. 6.25 could have been a glioma or metastasis.

The single-voxel spectrum from the lesion is shown in Fig. 6.26. For comparison, Fig. 6.23 shows a spectrum obtained from normal brain tissue. The very high level of lactate and only slightly increased choline level in Fig. 6.26 show that this lesion is likely to be a metastasis.

Body Tumours

The role of MRI in body cancer diagnosis and staging is vast. As a purely illustrative example, we will look at the role of MRI in staging rectal cancer and the difference that it makes to treatment.

The very close proximity of the rectum to other organs makes the very exact staging of rectal cancer critical. Figs. 6.27A and B show an early stage of rectal cancer, with the cancer confined within the rectum muscle wall. This patient was managed by surgical resection. Figs. 6.27C, D, and E show a patient with a later stage of rectal cancer; the cancer has extended outside the rectal muscle wall, along the veins and into the surrounding fatty tissue, referred to as *extra mural venous invasion*. This patient required combined radiotherapy and chemotherapy, followed by surgery. MRI was used at the end of the combined radiotherapy and chemotherapy to monitor the response of the tumour. All patients with rectal cancer will have continued monitoring with CT at 6-to-12-month intervals to check for liver and other metastases.

MRI of tumours in the abdomen and pelvis can be fused with CT images for use during treatment planning. However, the nonrigid nature of the anatomy makes fusion more difficult than in the brain.

Clinical Applications of Magnetic Resonance Imaging in Radiotherapy

MRI has a wide range of clinical applications in radiotherapy, including facilitating accurate treatment planning, improving adaptive radiotherapy, enabling real-time image guidance and helping to evaluate tumour response. Unlike other imaging modalities such as CT or PET, MRI does not involve ionising radiation. This is particularly advantageous for paediatric patients and individuals who require repeated imaging over the course of their treatment, reducing the radiation dose to tissues surrounding the tumour that are included in imaging fields of view.

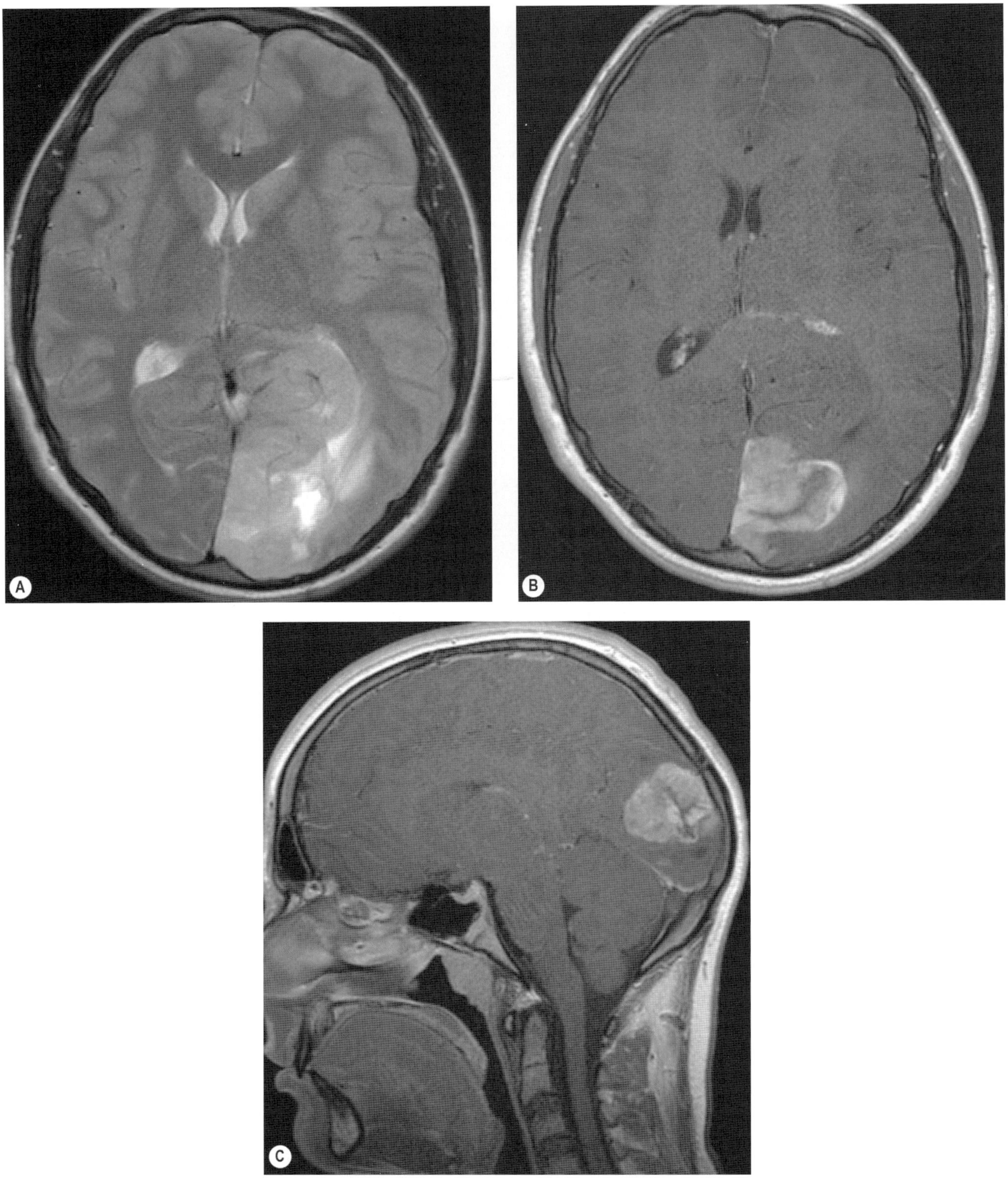

Fig. 6.24 (A) T_2 weighted precontrast axial image showing a large left frontal lobe malignant glioma. (B) Precontrast T_1 weighted axial image. The same slice position is shown as in (A). (C) Postcontrast axial T_1 weighted image. The contrast agent clearly defines the area of the glioma where the blood–brain barrier has broken down.

As discussed earlier, MRI is widely used in the diagnosis and staging of various types of cancer. It offers multiplanar, high-resolution anatomical imaging with excellent soft-tissue contrast combined with functional or physiological information allowing for the visualisation and characterisation of tumours. MRI can accurately determine the location and extent of tumours and identify nearby critical structures that may be exposed to the radiation. Incorporating MRI data into the treatment planning process can improve the precision of the contouring of target volumes and of some organs at risk, enabling optimisation of treatment plans.

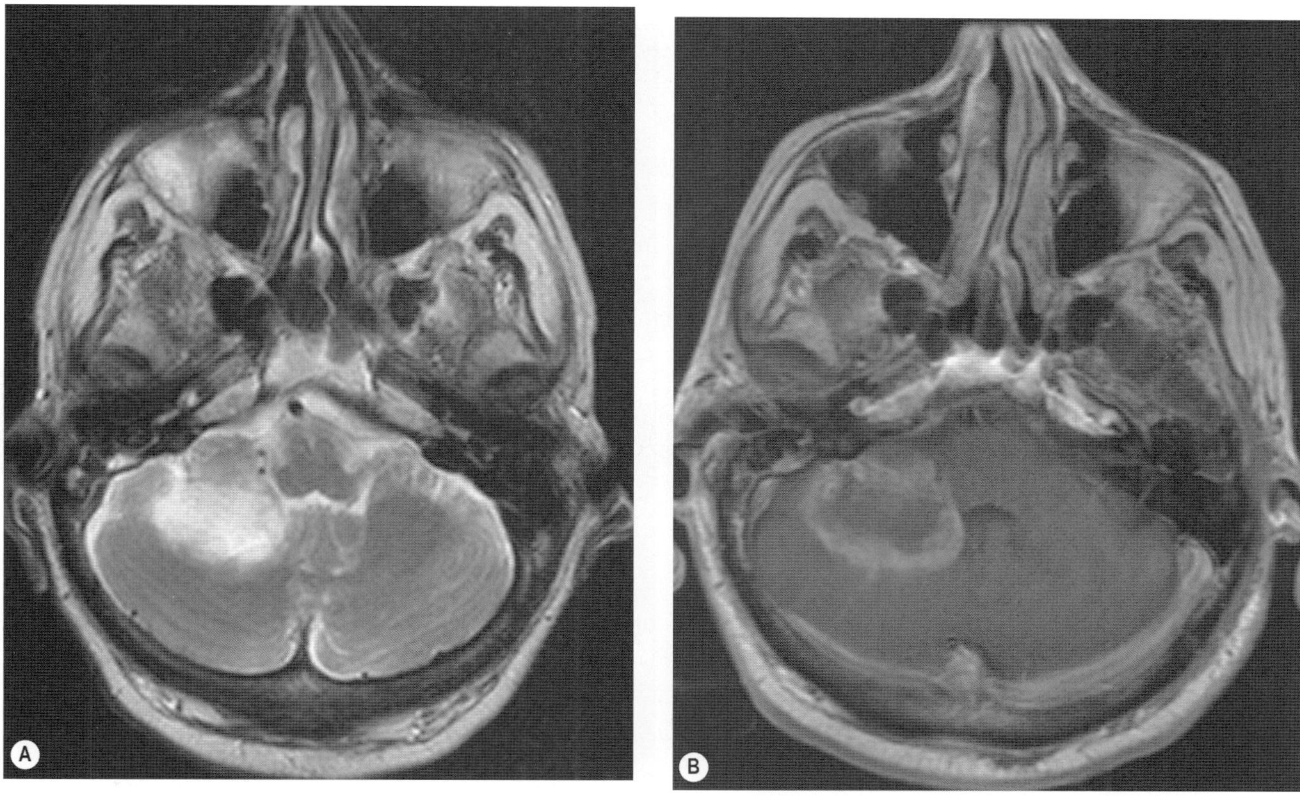

Fig. 6.25 (A) Axial T_2 weighted image of a glioma or brain metastases. (B) Axial T_1 weighted image post contrast.

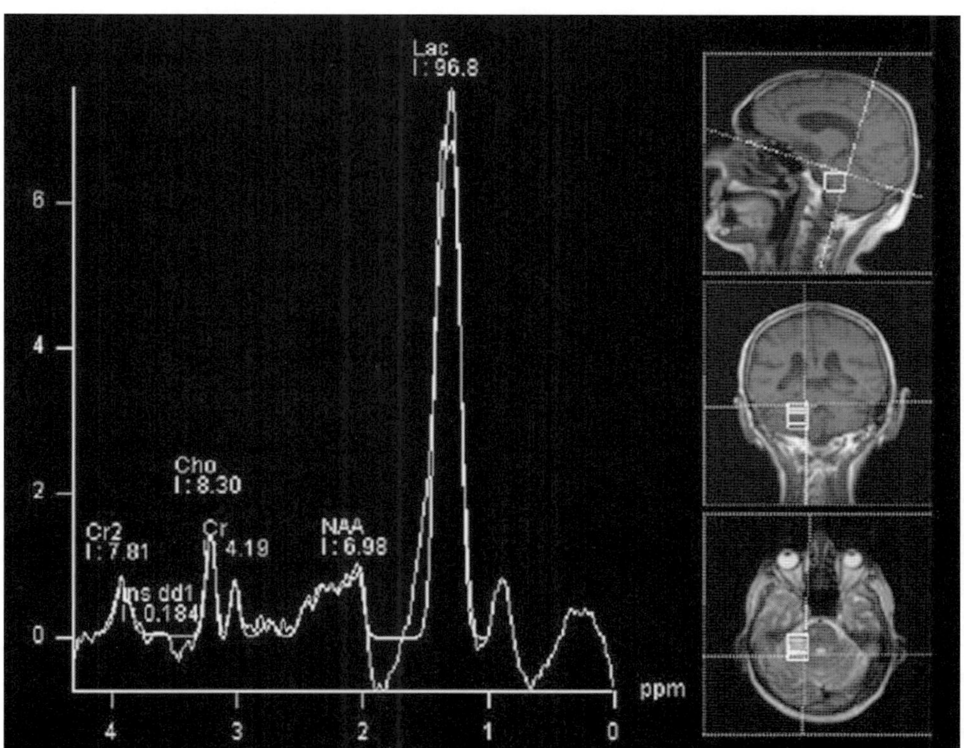

Fig. 6.26 Spectrum from the metastasis showing an extremely elevated lactate peak and slightly elevated choline levels. The spectrum was obtained using stimulated echo acquisition mode with TE = 30 ms.

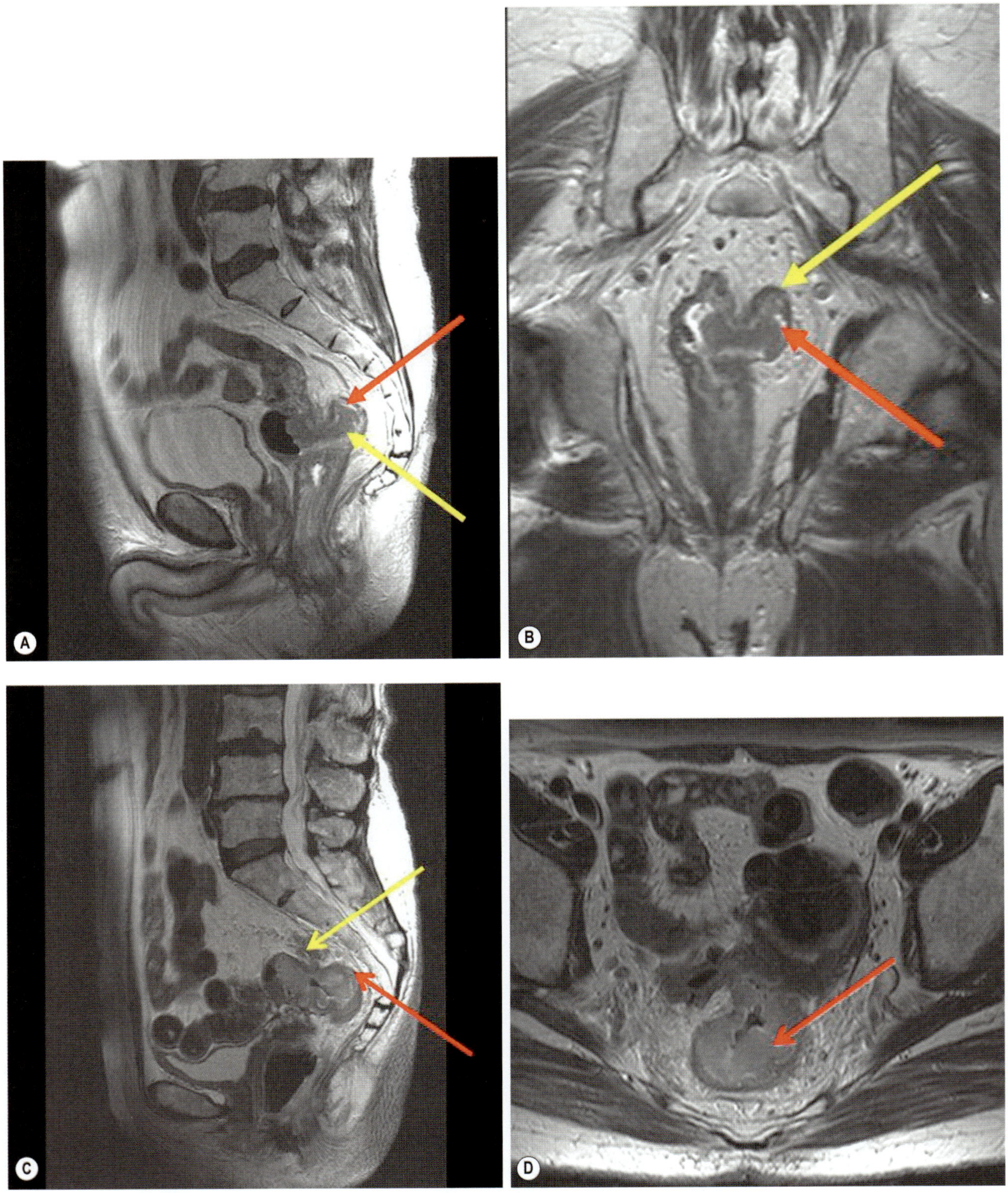

Fig. 6.27 (A) Sagittal image of early stage rectal carcinoma *(red arrow)* still contained within the rectal muscle wall *(yellow arrow)*. (B) Coronal image of early stage rectal carcinoma *(red arrow)* still contained within the rectal muscle wall *(yellow arrow)*. (C), (D) and (E) Sagital, axial and coronal images of a stage 3 rectal cancer, which has extramural venous invasion. The *red arrows* point to the tumour and the *yellow arrows* to areas of extramural venous invasion.

(*continued*)

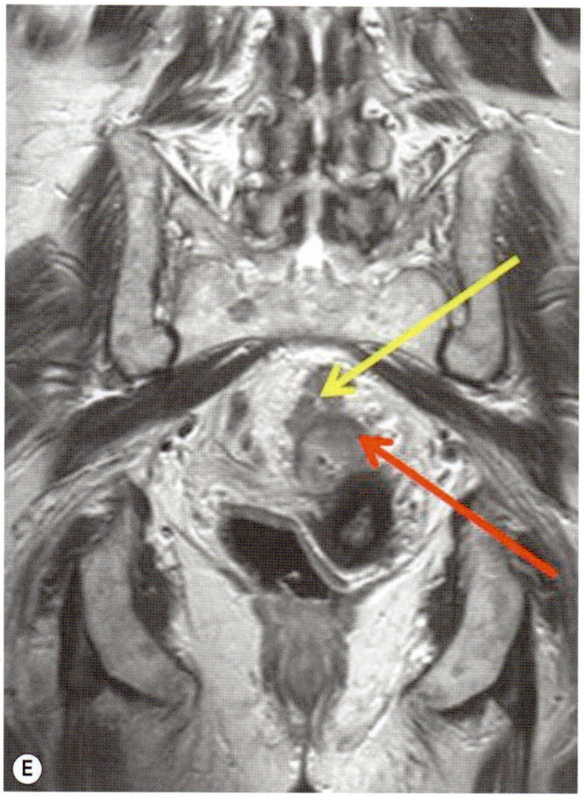

Fig. 6.27—cont'd

MR imaging during the treatment course, with the patient in the treatment position, can allow replanning of later fractions to accommodate changes that would alter treatment, such as changes in tumour size, and functional or physiological changes which may not be apparent on CT. MRI guidance such as on the MRI LINAC treatment machine allows for real-time imaging during treatment delivery. This capability enables real-time adaptive treatment planning, leading to more precise and personalised treatment. MRI can also track respiratory or organ motion with high temporal resolution, allowing for accurate tracking of tumour motion during treatment.

MRI plays a vital role in assessing the response of tumours to radiotherapy. By conducting follow-up MRI scans after treatment, it is possible to evaluate changes in tumour characteristics. This information helps determine the effectiveness of the treatment and guides further decision-making, such as the need for additional treatment. Additionally, advanced MRI techniques, such as diffusion-weighted imaging, dynamic contrast-enhanced imaging and spectroscopy, can provide functional or physiological information about tumour response by assessing changes in tissue characteristics such as cellularity, perfusion, hypoxia and metabolic status.

While MRI has several advantages in radiotherapy, it is important to consider certain limitations and the potential solutions to these issues. MRI scanners are not as widely available in radiotherapy departments compared to other imaging modalities such as CT, and the equipment and maintenance costs are higher. Additionally, MRI-guided LINACs can be prohibitively expensive. There are also staff cost implications related to MRI being a complex modality that requires adequately trained staff of all disciplines, and currently there is a skills shortage. To add to these costs, a range of specialised equipment is required to image radiotherapy patients, including an accurate laser system, a flat couch, immobilisation equipment that is safe to use in the scanner and does not affect image quality, and 'bridges' to suspend surface coils so that they do not distort the patient outline. Efforts are being made to increase the availability of MRI scanners in radiotherapy departments. This includes expanding infrastructure, acquiring dedicated MRI systems for radiotherapy and optimising scheduling to accommodate patient needs. Continued research and advancements in MRI technology aim to reduce the cost of MRI systems, improve the efficiency of MRI workflows and make the workflows more cost-effective for radiotherapy applications.

MRI scans generally take longer to acquire than CT scans, mainly due to complex image acquisition protocols and the need for patients to remain motionless in the treatment position during the scan. This can lead to increased discomfort for patients and potential challenges in imaging patients with limited tolerance for longer scan times. Various techniques are being explored to shorten MR imaging times, including the development of advanced accelerated imaging sequences and the use of AI-based reconstruction algorithms.

MR images are susceptible to various types of distortions and artefacts, including geometric distortion, susceptibility artefacts which are apparent at tissue-to-air or tissue-to-metal interfaces and motion artefacts. These can affect the accuracy of target delineation, potentially impacting treatment planning and delivery. For this reason, geometric accuracy is generally more important in MRI for radiotherapy than diagnostic applications, and consequently there is a focus on quality control and verification of this aspect of image quality. Techniques such as distortion correction algorithms, improved gradient designs and advanced shimming methods are being developed to minimise distortion and associated artefacts in MR images.

Integrating MR imaging with other imaging modalities, such as CT or PET, for accurate registration and treatment planning can be challenging due to differences in image contrast, resolution and geometric distortions. Additionally, replicating organ positions between modalities can be a challenge due to differences in rectal and bladder filling in the pelvis and breath-hold positions in the abdomen. Robust registration algorithms and software tools are necessary to facilitate accurate fusion and integration of MR imaging into the treatment planning process.

Unlike CT, which provides Hounsfield unit (HU) values that correlate with tissue electron density, MRI does not provide direct calibration for dose calculations in radiotherapy. This limits the use of MRI for treatment planning based on tissue electron density information, which is important for accurate dose calculations and treatment verification. Currently, MRI images are generally registered to CT data to enable MRI-based contouring with CT-based dose calculation. However, this requires additional appointments for the patient which can be inconvenient, and it carries additional cost implications for the NHS. It also requires extra data processing steps and introduces scope for errors in the registration stage. Various methods are being investigated and developed to allow MR-only planning pathways, where electron density information is estimated directly from MR images, including machine learning or AI-based commercial solutions.

ULTRASOUND IMAGING

In this section the emphasis is on the use of ultrasound in imaging. However, at higher power levels than those used for diagnosis, ultrasound can be used in various ways in the treatment of cancer and other conditions. These include lithotripsy to smash kidney stones, hyperthermia to enhance radiotherapy and high-intensity focused ultrasound to ablate soft tissue.

Overview of the Ultrasound Imaging Process

Ultrasound is defined as a vibration with a frequency, above the upper limit of human hearing, at 20 kilohertz (20 kHz). One hertz (1 Hz) equals one vibration cycle per second. In fact, medical ultrasound most often uses much higher frequencies, usually between 1 and

20 MHz, and higher frequencies than these can be used for acoustic microscopy. The passage and interactions of the ultrasound wave as it penetrates through tissue, interacts with it and is scattered, reflected and attenuated enables information about tissue to be derived from the wave.[1]

Physical Characteristics of Ultrasound Waves

Ultrasound usually travels as a longitudinal pressure wave moving through the soft tissue and producing areas of compression and rarefaction (low pressure). Consider a small area of tissue. For a longitudinal wave, this will vibrate to and fro along the direction of travel of the ultrasound wave as the pressure wave passes. Transverse or shear waves, where the tissue vibrates at right angles to the direction of wave travel, are possible but are only used for specialised techniques.

The amplitude of the ultrasound wave can be defined in various ways, such as the peak pressure, or if for a small area of tissue, the peak distance displaced or peak velocity of this area. A way of characterising the energy carried in an ultrasound wave is to measure the intensity, which equals the power transmitted per cross-sectional area of the beam in watts per square centimetre.

The speed of sound in tissue, C in metres per second (m/s), is related to the frequency, f, in Hz and wavelength, w, in metres (m) in the usual way:

$$C = f \cdot w \quad \textbf{(6.10)}$$

For soft tissues, the average speed of sound is 1540 m/s. So, for medical ultrasound, the wavelength is from about 0.075 mm at 20.5 MHz to 1.5 mm at 1 MHz. The resolution of ultrasound is related to the wavelength, so higher-frequency ultrasound, which has a smaller wavelength, gives better resolution.

The speed of ultrasound in tissue is related to the bulk modulus and the density of the tissue through which the ultrasound travels. The bulk modulus is defined as the change in pressure divided by the fractional change in volume for a material. So, for harder materials, where a given change in pressure will result in a small change in volume, the bulk modulus and sound velocity are larger than for softer materials. Higher density results in a lower velocity:

$$C = \sqrt{(B/\rho)} \quad \textbf{(6.11)}$$

where C = speed of sound (m/s), B = bulk modulus (N/m^2) and ρ = Density (kg/m^3):

The bulk modulus is expressed by

$$B = dP/(dV/V) = V \times dP/dV \quad \textbf{(6.12)}$$

where P = pressure (N/m^2) and V = volume (m^3).

The speed of ultrasound in different soft tissues is generally within about +/−6% of 1540 m/s. The speed of ultrasound in harder tissues, such as bone, is much higher, at about 3200 m/s. Air, which has a low density and low bulk modulus, has a much lower speed of ultrasound, at 330 m/s. For diagnostic purposes, ultrasound gives us information related to the mechanical properties of tissue. Ultrasound is reflected from interfaces between tissues with different mechanical properties. The amount of ultrasound reflected depends on the acoustic impedance of the material.

Considering a small area of tissue, the acoustic impedance is defined as the ratio of the pressure amplitude divided by the velocity amplitude of the area of tissue as the ultrasound wave passes through it. The acoustic impedance can also be defined relative to the speed of sound and tissue density:

$$Z = \rho \cdot C \quad \textbf{(6.13)}$$

where Z = acoustic impedance, ρ = density and C = speed of sound in tissue.

The fraction of ultrasound reflected from an interface between tissues of different acoustic impedances can be calculated as follows:

$$R = (Z_1 - Z_2)^2/(Z_1 + Z_2)^2 \quad \textbf{(6.14)}$$

where R = the fractional intensity of ultrasound reflected and Z_1 and Z_2 are the impedances on either side of the interface.

Interactions at Interfaces

For interfaces between different soft tissues, the amount reflected is usually between 0.01% and 1%. For a soft-tissue-to-air interface, 99.9% of the ultrasound is reflected. The practical consequence of this is that ultrasound cannot image beyond gas; therefore lung tissue cannot be imaged and bowel gas can be a problem in the abdomen. Also, the air gap between the ultrasound transducer and the skin must be eliminated using ultrasound gel when scanning. Imaging into and beyond bone is usually impractical, as bone both reflects a lot of the ultrasound and highly attenuates the ultrasound beam.

For smooth interfaces between different tissues, the reflection will be mirror like so that the angle of reflection equals the angle of incidence. Also, the transmitted part of the wave may be bent slightly or refracted because of the difference in sound velocity between the materials. Usually, for soft tissues the angle of refraction is small and is neglected.

For rough interfaces the ultrasound will be reflected at a variety of different angles. For small scatterers, which are much smaller than the wavelength, the ultrasound is scattered in all directions. This is called *Rayleigh scattering* and occurs, for instance, with red blood cells.

As it travels through tissue, energy will be lost from the ultrasound beam by scattering of ultrasound away from the beam direction and by energy absorption in the tissue. Energy absorption occurs when the coherent vibration of the ultrasound wave is degraded into random motion of the tissue, resulting in tissue heating. For diagnostic imaging, the amount of heating is very small, but at higher intensities, the heating effect can be used deliberately for therapy.

Attenuation and Interference

Attenuation of the ultrasound beam is usually proportional to the frequency of the ultrasound, so higher-frequency ultrasound is more highly attenuated. This results in a compromise between attenuation and image resolution. For the imaging of superficial structures, a higher frequency is usually used to give better resolution. For deeper structures, a lower frequency with poorer resolution may be needed to allow sufficient ultrasound to penetrate the tissues.

In addition to the aforementioned interactions, because ultrasound is a wave phenomenon, we must consider interference effects. If two waves arrive at a point and the peaks of the waves are aligned, the peaks add up, resulting in constructive interference. If, however, the peak of one wave arrives at the same time as a trough from the other wave, the waves will cancel each other out, resulting in destructive interference.

When considering the intensity of the echo from a small area of tissue, this is the sum of the echoes from a group of microscopic scatterers within this area. The overall intensity of the echo will be a weighted sum of all the echoes from all the microscopic scatterers in this area, which will depend randomly on the degree of constructive or destructive interference. These random interference effects produce variations in echo intensity called *speckle*, which is considered a type of structured noise in the image.

When looking at the texture of echoes in the image of an organ, these will be partly related to the physical variations in underlying mechanical properties of the tissue and partly related to random interference. Luckily, in diagnostic images, speckle is a minor problem and it is possible to minimise its effects.

Ultrasound Scanners

Production of Ultrasound for Imaging

Ultrasound machines use piezoelectric materials to generate and detect ultrasound. The piezoelectric effect was discovered by Pierre and Jacques Curie in 1880 and occurs in some materials where there is a polarised crystal structure. When a piezoelectric material is compressed, it generates a voltage across the crystal structure and an opposite voltage if the crystal is subjected to the low pressure of rarefraction. A piezoelectric crystal will generate an alternating voltage across it as an ultrasound wave passes through, and thus it can be used as a detector. Conversely, if an alternating voltage is applied across a piezoelectric crystal, it will vibrate and hence can be used to generate ultrasound.

The most commonly used piezoelectric material is a ceramic material known as *lead zirconate titanate (PZT)*. Originally, a narrow focused beam of ultrasound was produced by using a flat disk piezoelectric element with an acoustic lens attached to the front. Modern ultrasound transducers use an array of many small piezoelectric elements, often in a row called a *linear array* (Fig. 6.28). A small group of elements are switched on at any one time to produce a narrow beam. The position of the beam can be altered by selecting which elements along the length of the array are switched on.

The depth of focus within the image plane can be controlled electronically using the timing of the pulses applied to each element and altering the relative amount of delay between the voltage pulses. Likewise, continuously incremented electronic delay across the elements can be used to steer the ultrasound beam. Two-dimensional arrays of piezoelectric elements can also be used and allow electronic steering and focusing both within the image plane and across the thickness of the slice being imaged.

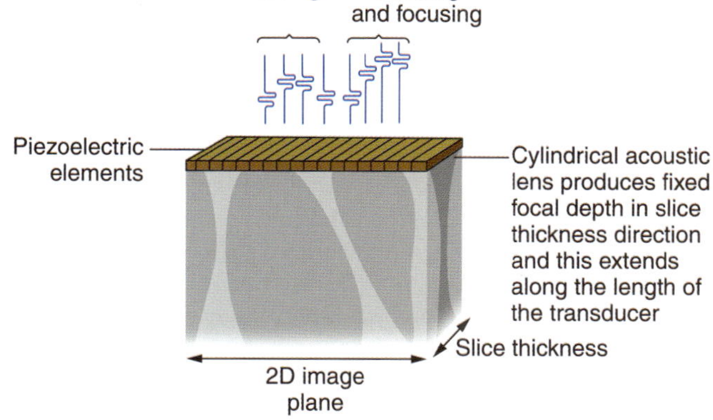

Fig. 6.28 Beam steering and focusing with a linear array.

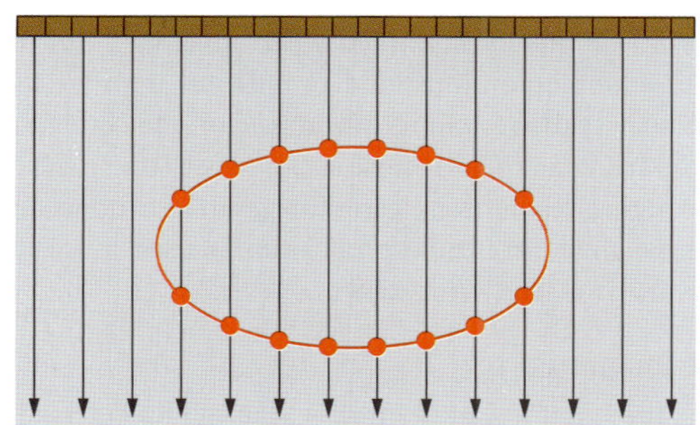

Fig. 6.29 Image production by a linear array.

Derivation of an Ultrasound Image

To produce an ultrasound image, the sound navigation and ranging principle of sonar is used. This was originally used to detect submarines. A short pulse was directed along a narrow beam, and the depth from which the echoes were generated within the tissue was calculated from the time delay from the transmitted pulse to the echoes' return, knowing the speed of ultrasound in the tissue. For each pulse transmitted, the intensity of the echoes can be used to modulate the brightness of the image on a screen along a line in the image. This is referred to as *brightness mode (B-mode) ultrasound imaging.*

In B-mode ultrasound image production using a linear array (Fig. 6.29), a pulse is sent out along a narrow beam and the echoes are allowed to return to the transducer. The strength of the echoes is used to modulate the brightness of the image along a line in the image. More pulses are sent out across the transducer to build up a two-dimensional image. An example of a B-mode image across the neck is shown in Fig. 6.30.

As ultrasound travels very quickly in soft tissue (1540 m/s), each ultrasound image can be acquired very quickly and frame rates of between 5 and 40 images per second can be achieved, allowing real-time imaging. This makes it possible to follow the movements of the heart, guide biopsy needles to sample tissue from lesions in real time and facilitate live image guidance during various invasive ablation techniques.

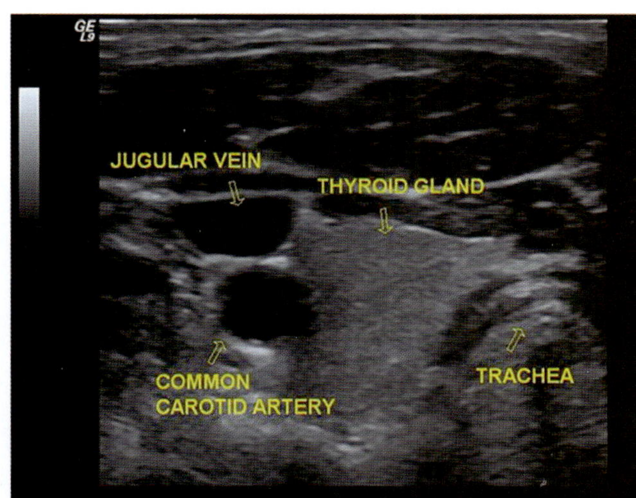

Fig. 6.30 B-mode transverse image of the neck showing a map of the brightness of reflection of ultrasound from different tissues. Blood vessels are dark on B-mode images as blood reflects relatively little ultrasound.

Brightness Mode Ultrasound Imaging Artefacts

When B-mode ultrasound images are produced, simplifying assumptions are made about how the ultrasound beam travels and interacts. The main assumptions are that the ultrasound travels along a straight, narrow path at constant velocity, with similar attenuation across the image. Also, it is assumed that the pulse only bounces once on its path before travelling back to the transducer. Deviations from these assumptions result in various artefacts in the images. For example, in reality the beam is not quite straight because of refraction, and the velocity of ultrasound changes slightly when passing through different tissues. This results in slight horizontal and vertical distortions in the images. Multiple reflections can result in some echoes being misplaced. Ultrasound operators become skilled in recognising these artefacts and minimising their effects. Some artefacts can be useful. For instance, the image beyond a highly attenuating structure will be darker as less ultrasound penetrates beyond the object. Thus a gallstone usually shows a characteristic shadow beyond it. Conversely, a low attenuating structure, such as a clear fluid-filled simple cyst, will show a bright enhancement streak beyond it as more ultrasound penetrates to the tissue below. This can be used as a diagnostic feature suggesting a simple cyst.

Three-Dimensional Ultrasound Imaging

Linear array transducers produce a two-dimensional image. It is possible, by moving the transducer perpendicular to this two-dimensional image plane, to produce a three-dimensional stack of images. The spatial orientation of these images can be determined by using a detector that clips to the ultrasound probe to detect the spatial position of the probe and hence the image plane in space. Alternatively, specialised two-dimensional arrays of piezoelectric elements can be used to produce three-dimensional images by electronically steering the beams across a three-dimensional block of tissue.

Intracavity and Endoscopic Probes

Sometimes image quality is limited when imaging from outside the body. Small endoscopic ultrasound probes can improve local image quality. Intracavity probes can be introduced into the body to allow the ultrasound transducer to be as close as possible to the tissue of interest. This allows higher-resolution, clearer images to be produced. Transrectal and transvaginal ultrasound probes can be used in imaging of the prostate, ovary or uterus, for instance.

Harmonic Imaging

Most of the time in ultrasound imaging, the echoes detected are at the same frequency as the transmitted pulse. However, gas bubbles and soft tissues produce echoes at multiples of the transmitted frequency. Most commonly, these harmonic echoes are detected at twice the transmitted frequency. This technique was originally used in conjunction with ultrasound contrast agents, which consist of suspensions of encapsulated microscopic gas bubbles that are injected into the circulation. The gas bubbles produce strong harmonic echoes, so it is possible to produce an image that largely reflects the distribution of the contrast agent.

Later, it was discovered that soft tissue generates enough harmonic echoes to produce images. These harmonic images of soft tissue tend to have better contrast and fewer artefacts at depth than conventional images.

Dynamic Imaging

The movement of blood and tissues can be measured using the Doppler effect. The Doppler effect occurs when a wave is reflected from a moving structure. If the structure is moving towards the sound source, the wavefronts are compressed and this increases the frequency of the ultrasound. Likewise, the frequency is decreased when the structure is moving away from the source. The most familiar everyday example of this is a car horn, which sounds higher pitched when the car approaches and lower pitched as the car passes by and moves away.

Pulsed mode Doppler ultrasound uses repeated sampling of the ultrasound from a sample volume in a blood vessel and gives a detailed real-time blood flow spectrum, allowing changes in the flow during the heart cycle to be studied and the blood flow velocity calculated. Fig. 6.31 shows a pulsed Doppler mode blood flow velocity spectrum in the lower half of the image. It shows the blood flow velocity spectrum (vertical axis) in a small sample volume as it changes with time (horizontal axis). Each peak represents high systolic flow at the start of the heart cycle. The small upper image shows where the sample volume was located.

Colour Doppler ultrasound measures the shift in frequency from moving blood and overlays this on the B-mode greyscale image. The colour of the image is coded according to the direction of the flow relative to the beam and the size of the frequency shift, which is related to the blood flow velocity. Colour Doppler images can give an idea of the vascularity of tissue. Fig. 6.32 shows a colour Doppler image of blood flow in the common carotid artery.

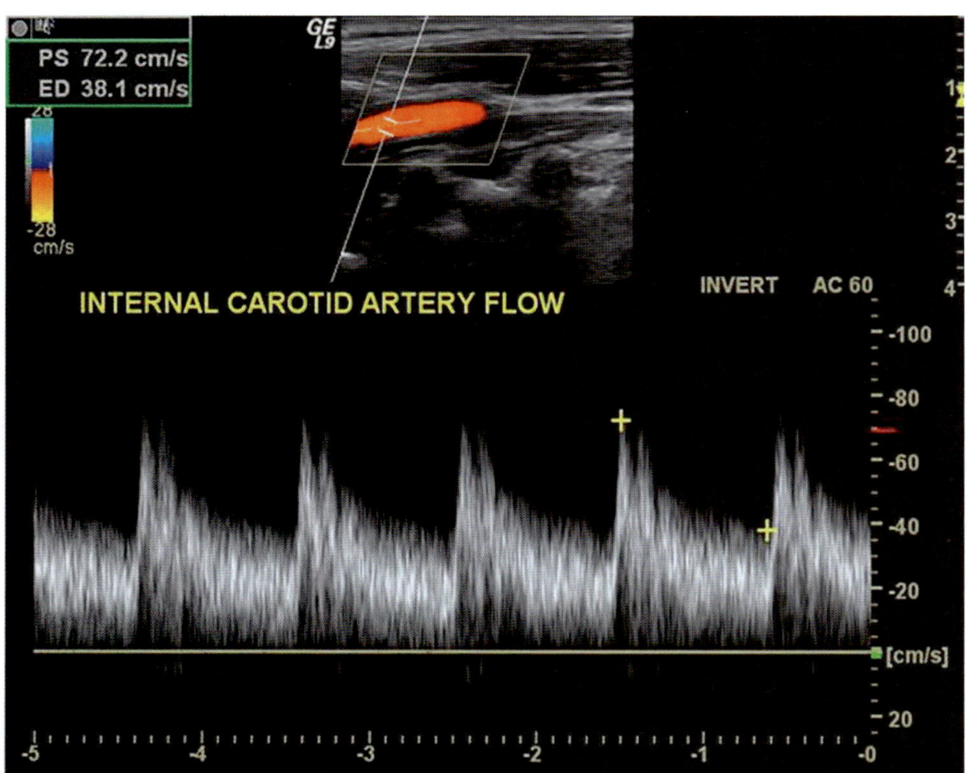

Fig. 6.31 Pulsed mode Doppler sonogram of flow in the internal carotid artery.

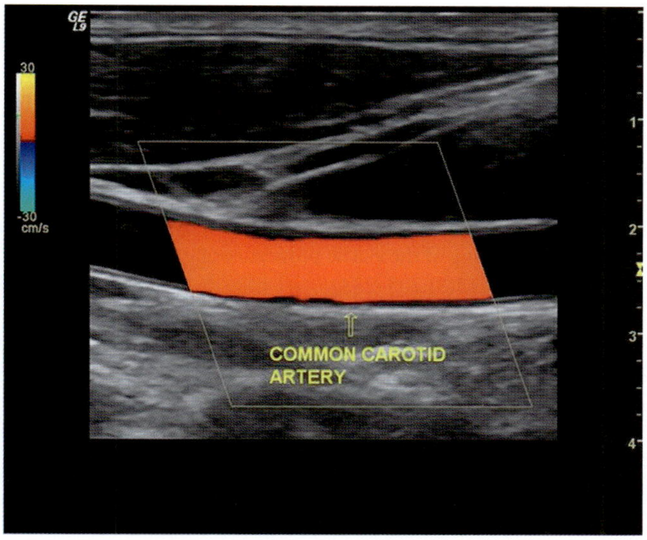

Fig. 6.32 Colour Doppler image of flow in the common carotid artery. The background B-mode information shows the echoes of stationary tissue. Within the colour box, flowing blood is colour coded according to the direction of flow and size of frequency shift, which is related to the blood flow velocity and the angle of the flow relative to the beam direction.

Contrast and Tissue Characteristic Imaging

Encapsulated microbubbles can be injected into the blood stream as a contrast agent to increase the reflection from blood vessels and vascular tissue.[1]

A newer technique, called *elastography*, can give images related to how hard tissues are.[8,9] It achieves this by measuring the distortion of the tissues on ultrasound images with and without applying pressure to the tissue. Other techniques involve generating transverse (shear) waves in tissue. Sometimes elastography can demonstrate changes in the hardness of tissue surrounding a mass demonstrated on the B-mode image. This suggests that infiltration into the surrounding tissue has occurred and that the B-mode image alone may underestimate the extent of the tumour's local involvement in some cases.

Ultrasound has some heating effects, and other biological effects related to the activity of the gas bubbles in the acoustic field (cavitation) are possible. However, if used prudently at diagnostic power levels, it is considered safe.

Clinical Applications of Ultrasound Imaging

General Imaging

Probably the best-known application of ultrasound is its use in obstetrics to image the foetus. The age of the pregnancy, foetal growth and foetal abnormalities can be monitored and detected. It can also be used to guide the sampling of amniotic fluid (amniocentesis) to analyse the genetic makeup of the foetus.

Ultrasound is used widely in cardiology to analyse the size and shape of heart chambers, the pumping action of the heart and the flow of blood through stenosed or faulty heart valves.

In the venous system, ultrasound can be used to detect deep vein thrombosis and analyse the function of venous valves. In the arterial system, ultrasound can detect stenosis, occlusion or aneurysmal disease in the main arteries.

Advantages and Disadvantages

Ultrasound gives good soft-tissue contrast and can identify abnormal structure, size or texture of many different organs of the body. It is one of the cheapest imaging modalities, and small, portable ultrasound machines can be used in clinics, in accident and emergency, by paramedics in the field or in operating theatres.

However, as previously mentioned, the dependence of ultrasound imaging on the transmission and reflection at tissue interfaces and the poor transmission through an air-to-tissue interface limits the application of ultrasound imaging. It is of no value in imaging the lungs. Bowel gas can sometimes limit the quality of images in the abdomen. Ultrasound cannot usually be used for imaging beyond bone, although some useful Doppler flow information can be obtained transcranially by using low-frequency ultrasound directed through the thinnest parts of the skull. Calcified tissue can also cause imaging problems, notably in renal and diabetic patients.

Also, the ultrasound appearance of a solid mass may not be specific enough to diagnose whether a lesion is cancerous, and a biopsy may still be required to establish its histology.

Imaging for Cancer

Ultrasound imaging is used widely in the diagnosis of cancer, assessment of its local extent and staging.[10] Masses can be identified and characterised, helping to differentiate solid masses from benign fluid-filled cysts.[11]

Good images are produced if there is a tissue-to-fluid interface, and therefore ultrasound is particularly effective at showing whether lumps are cystic or solid. For this reason, ultrasound is frequently used to examine the breast. Ultrasound can distinguish solid (sometimes malignant) and cystic (usually benign) lumps within the breast.

Small endoscopic ultrasound probes can be used to assess the invasion of a tumour into the bowel wall and surrounding tissue, for instance.

Colour Doppler can detect the distribution of small vessels within a mass and can help characterise how vascular it is. Vascular lesions are more likely to be malignant.

Ultrasound is a sensitive technique for detecting metastases within the liver, as metastases often reflect the sound waves poorly and produce hypoechogenic areas. The use of gas bubbles as an ultrasound contrast agent can help characterise the blood supply in liver tumours. Liver tumours often derive their blood supply from the hepatic artery, which makes them enhance early in contrast studies. Liver tissue that has a blood supply from the portal vein will enhance later in the study.

Usually, ultrasound contrast agents are eventually incorporated into the liver parenchyma by phagocytosis. Harmonic images taken a few minutes after injection can be used to selectively image the distribution of gas bubbles in the liver tissue. Areas where no gas bubbles are shown often correspond to liver metastases, which sometimes cannot be detected on conventional ultrasound images.

Transvaginal ultrasound can be used to measure the thickness of the endometrial lining of the uterus and is a sensitive measure for screening for endometrial cancer in patients with postmenopausal bleeding. It also produces good images of ovarian cysts, and solid areas within these cysts can be demonstrated, which helps diagnose whether the lesion is benign or malignant.

When the ultrasound appearance of a solid mass is not specific enough to diagnose whether a lesion is cancerous and a needle biopsy is required, this can be done under ultrasound guidance.

Ultrasound imaging can be used to guide various invasive therapies. Ablation devices can be inserted percutaneously or endoscopically into tumours under ultrasound guidance, and the local tumour tissue can be ablated using heat, cold or chemical means.

Clinical Therapeutic Ultrasound

For completeness, it is worth considering the use of ultrasound in direct cancer therapy[12] High-intensity focused ultrasound (HIFU) can be used to ablate areas of soft tissue. A large, focused ultrasound transducer can produce a high temperature increase at the focus and spare surrounding tissue. HIFU machines often combine ultrasound and MRI. MRI is used to image the area to be ablated, and temperature-sensitive MRI sequences can be used to optimise and measure the treatment. This technique has been used in various soft-tissue and bony lesions. It can be used in areas of previous radiotherapy and can be repeated, but it tends to be slow to treat a large tumour area.

REFERENCES

1. Hoskins P, Martin K, Thrush A. *Diagnostic ultrasound: physics and equipment*. 3rd ed. Boca Raton: CRC Press; 2019.
2. UK Statutory Instruments 2017 No. 1322. The Ionising radiation (Medical Exposures) regulations 2017. UK; https://www.legislation.gov.uk/uksi/2017/1322/contents
3. Bloch F. Nuclear induction. New York, USA: *Phys Rev*. 1946; 70:460–474.
4. McRobbie DW, Moore EA, Graves MJ, Prince MR. *MRI: from picture to proton*. Cambridge, UK: Cambridge University Press; 2003.
5. Elster AD. Questions and answers in MRI. ELSTER LLC 2018. https://www.mriquestions.com/index.html
6. Edelstein WA, Hutchison JMS, Johnson G, Redpath TW. Spin warp NMR imaging and application to the human whole-body imaging. *Phys Med Biol*. 1980;25:751–756.
7. Keevil SF. Spatial localization in nuclear magnetic resonance spectroscopy. *Phys Med Biol*. 2006;51:R579–R636.
8. Ophir J, Alam SK, Garra B, et al. Elastography: ultrasonic estimation and imaging of the elastic properties of tissues. *Proc Inst Mech Eng H*. 1999;213(3):203–233.
9. Zaleska-Dorobisz U, Kaczorowski K, Paulus A, Puchalska A, Inglot M. Ultrasound elastography—review of techniques and its clinical applications. *Adv Clin Exp Med*. 2014;23(4):645–655.
10. Diaz-Alejo JF, Gomez IG, Earl J. Ultrasound in cancer therapy: a summary of their use and unexplored potential. *Oncol Rev*. 2022;16(1):531.
11. Rumack CM, Levine D. *Diagnostic ultrasound*. Philadelphia, USA: 2018.
12. Dubinsky TJ, Cuevas C, Dighe MK, Kolokythas O, Hwang JH. High-intensity focused ultrasound: current potential and oncologic applications. *Am J Roentgenol*. 2008;190(1):191–199.

7

Imaging With Radionuclides

Paul Hinton

CHAPTER OUTLINE

INTRODUCTION

Radionuclide imaging plays a key role at all stages in the management of cancer patients, including diagnosis, staging, planning the delivery of treatment (for both radionuclide and external beam radiotherapy), monitoring of treatment response and follow-up for detection of recurrent disease.

An ever-increasing range of radiotracers are available, and the challenge is to localise their distribution as accurately as possible within the patient by the external detection of radiation emitted from the patient (gamma ray photons from single photon-emitting radionuclides, annihilation photons from positron emitters and bremsstrahlung radiation generated by beta particle absorption).

The main advantage of radionuclide imaging is its incredible sensitivity to detect very small amounts of tracer and demonstrate the function of cells, tissues and organs. Other imaging modalities, using x-rays, magnetic resonance imaging (MRI) or ultrasound, primarily provide structural or anatomical information, although the distinction between structural and functional imaging is not absolute.

As new radiotracers become more specific to particular cancer cells, multimodality combinations of imaging systems (hybrid imaging), as in positron emission tomography (PET) combined with x-ray computed tomography (PET/CT) or PET combined with MRI (PET/MR), can provide powerful tools for discriminating between normal and malignant tissues.[1]

A radiotracer is produced when a suitable radionuclide is combined with a pharmaceutical or a molecule which targets a particular biological function or process. The behaviour of this radiolabelled compound is monitored by radiation detectors external to the body, allowing in vivo biochemical function, aspects of tissue function and dynamic biological processes to be investigated noninvasively.

As new targeting molecules are discovered and radiochemistry becomes more advanced, a new branch of nuclear medicine has become established, known as theranostics, where the same targeting molecule can be used with different radionuclides to diagnose and treat several cancers. Firstly, the tracer is labelled to single photon or positron emitters to optimise accuracy of localisation for diagnostic imaging and dose planning studies. This is followed by administering the same tracer labelled with beta- or alpha-emitting radionuclides for delivery of specific therapeutic doses. Radionuclide imaging is now essential for many cancer diagnoses and treatments.

OVERVIEW OF THE RADIONUCLIDE IMAGING PROCESS

A full-range nuclear medicine service includes diagnostic studies using imaging and nonimaging techniques and radionuclide therapy treatments. This chapter covers radionuclide imaging, with radionuclide therapeutic applications being covered in Chapter 8.

A radionuclide is an unstable isotope of an element that will spontaneously 'decay' by the emission of particles and/or electromagnetic radiation. The three most common emissions from radionuclides are alpha and beta particles and gamma rays. There are two types of beta particle: beta minus (β^-) and beta plus (β^+). Both are electrons with negative and positive charges, respectively, with a β^+ particle being referred to as a *positron*. Of the different types of radioactive emissions, gamma rays are the only ones with sufficiently penetrating characteristics to enable them to be detected externally to the patient, although an estimation of the distribution of a beta-emitting radionuclide may be made using a technique called bremsstrahlung imaging.

Radionuclide imaging is generally split into two branches. One uses a relatively limited number of radionuclides that emit gamma rays and is referred to as *single photon imaging*; the other uses radionuclides that decay by emitting positrons and is referred to as *positron emission tomographic imaging* or *PET*. A positron is not a penetrating particle,

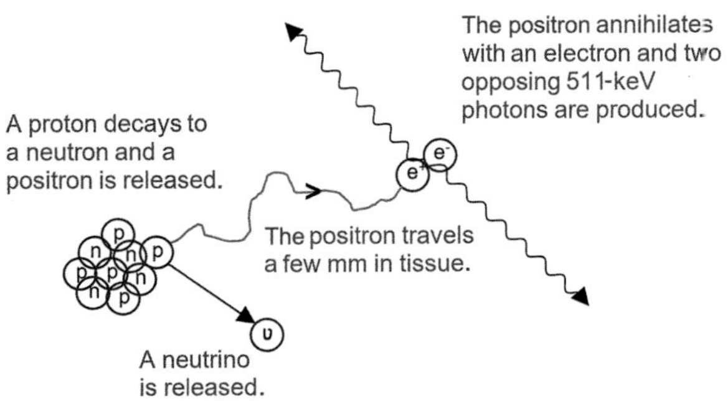

Fig. 7.1 Positron annihilation.

travelling on average a few mm in tissue, but it does then interact locally with an electron, where both annihilate to form two photons travelling in opposite directions (Fig. 7.1). These photons are penetrating and can be detected as they leave the body.

A radiopharmaceutical is formed by attaching a radionuclide to a molecule, a process known as *radiolabelling*. These are introduced into the body by some means, usually by intravenous injection, but can also be administered by oral ingestion, intradermally, intrarterially or by inhalation. Each radiotracer has a known biodistribution within the body which is related to the physiology or function of an organ, tissue or tissue type. This is in contrast to x-ray, MR or ultrasound imaging, which to a large extent provide information on anatomical structure.

Gamma rays are imaged using a device known as a *gamma camera*, and the device used to detect annihilation photons resulting from the decay of positron-emitting radionuclides is referred to as a *PET camera* or *PET scanner*. Gamma cameras are large-area detection devices capable of forming an image of the distribution of a radiopharmaceutical within the body. The majority of devices in current use have two large detector heads, and imaging with a gamma camera can take place in one of three ways: (1) with the detector heads and patient in a stationary position, called *planar mode*; (2) with the detector heads stationary and the patient moving through the heads on the couch, termed *whole-body mode*; or (3) with the detector heads rotating around the body through, typically, 180 or 360 degrees, a mode of acquisition known as *single photon emission computerised tomography (SPECT)*. PET cameras work on the basis of a series of rings of stationary detectors to identify the origin of a nucleus decaying via positron emission, by coincident detection of both annihilation photons within a predefined time window (of pico- to nanosecond length). This is sometimes referred to as *coincidence imaging*.

Most gamma and PET cameras currently being installed are hybrid systems with an x-ray CT scanner incorporated into the gantry. In both types of system, the primary purpose is to allow hybrid three-dimensional imaging that is intrinsically coregistered. Structural (transmission) CT images offer an additional benefit in that they can be used to improve the quality of the radionuclide images by allowing them to be corrected for attenuation of the gamma rays within the patient, which is done by converting the CT scan into an attenuation map.[2] This map is used to correct the functional nuclear medicine (emission) images for attenuation of the gamma rays due to variations of density of body tissue and significantly improves the image quality (Fig. 7.2). Having the CT imaging incorporated into the cameras allows the emission and transmission images to be acquired sequentially in the same patient imaging session. Assuming there is no patient movement between the two scans, the data derived from the transmission CT image can be accurately applied to the emission images. This process is applicable to tomographic images acquired on gamma cameras (SPECT) and all images acquired on PET/CT cameras. Consequently, imaging techniques associated with these devices are known as *SPECT/CT* and *PET/CT*. Historically, the CT scanners used in hybrid systems were not of a comparable standard to the most up-to-date diagnostic CT devices. However, this has changed. Gamma cameras and PET scanners now have high-specification CT units attached, and the registration or fusion of high spatial resolution structural images with the sensitive but poorer resolution functional images results in an imaging device that is extremely effective at identifying and localising pathology.

A commercially available alternative to the PET/CT hybrid scanner replaces the CT scanner with an MRI scanner to take advantage

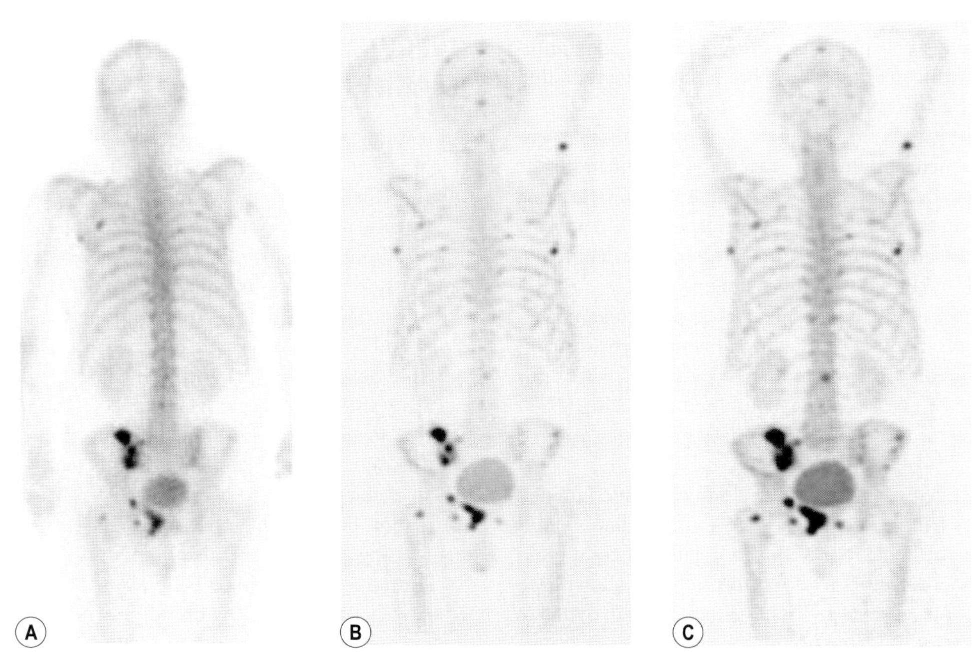

Fig. 7.2 Attenuation correction in single photon emission computerised tomography (SPECT). (A) Planar whole body. (B) Non-attenuation corrected SPECT. (C) Attenuation corrected SPECT.

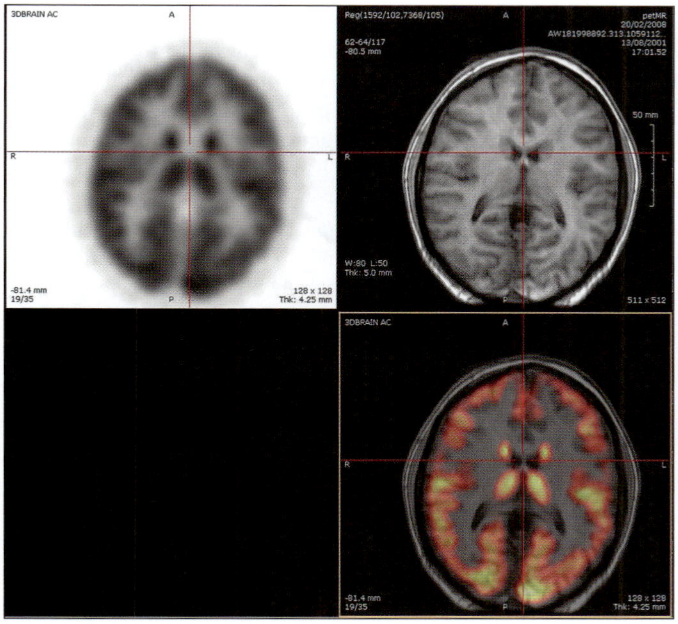

Fig. 7.3 Positron emission tomography (PET)-magnetc resonance imaging (MRI) scan. Clockwise from top left hand corner: PET image, MRI image and PET-MRI image.

of the MRI scanner's superior soft-tissue imaging capability (Fig. 7.3). As MRI scans do not directly represent tissue density, the use of the scans for attenuation correction of radionuclide images has proven to be a difficult challenge to overcome, but this is now an established technique.[3]

GAMMA CAMERAS

Gamma cameras are imaging devices used to detect and record the distribution of a radiopharmaceutical within the body. Historically, these devices have involved the use of large-area scintillation crystal detectors to physically convert the gamma rays into flashes of light, but they are starting to be replaced by large field of view or multihead solid-state detectors (Figs. 7.4 and 7.5).

Scintillation Gamma Cameras

Gamma rays are detected by using large-area crystals, typically 50 cm × 40 cm and around 1 cm thick, of sodium iodide doped with trace quantities of thallium (NaI(Tl)). The crystal structure

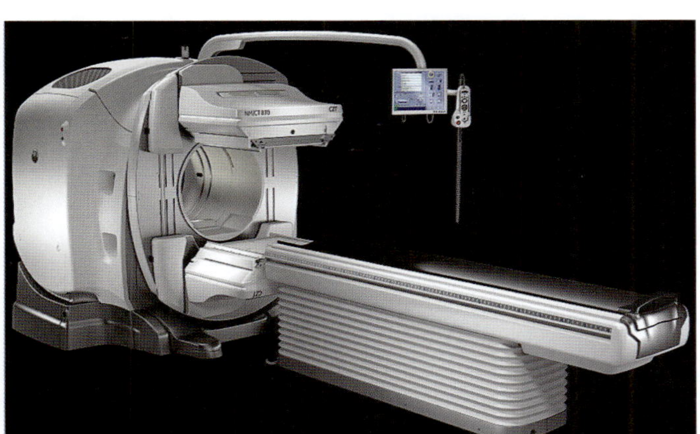

Fig. 7.4 Large field of view cadmium zinc telluride gamma camera.

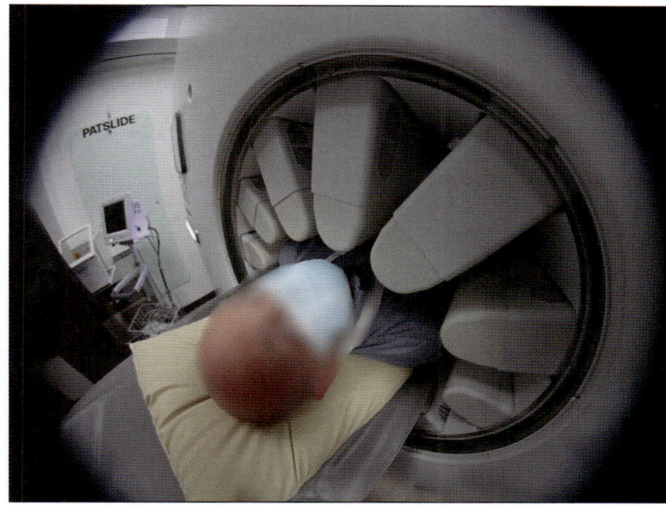

Fig. 7.5 Multiheaded cadmium zinc telluride camera.

has the property of absorbing gamma radiation and reemitting photons of visible light and is referred to as a *scintillator*. Smaller detector systems are available for specialised purposes, such as cardiac or brain imaging. A schematic of a scintillation gamma camera detector head is shown in Fig. 7.6. The crystal, collimator and photomultiplier array are mounted inside a lead shield. Further information regarding the design of gamma cameras may be found in Cherry et al.[4]

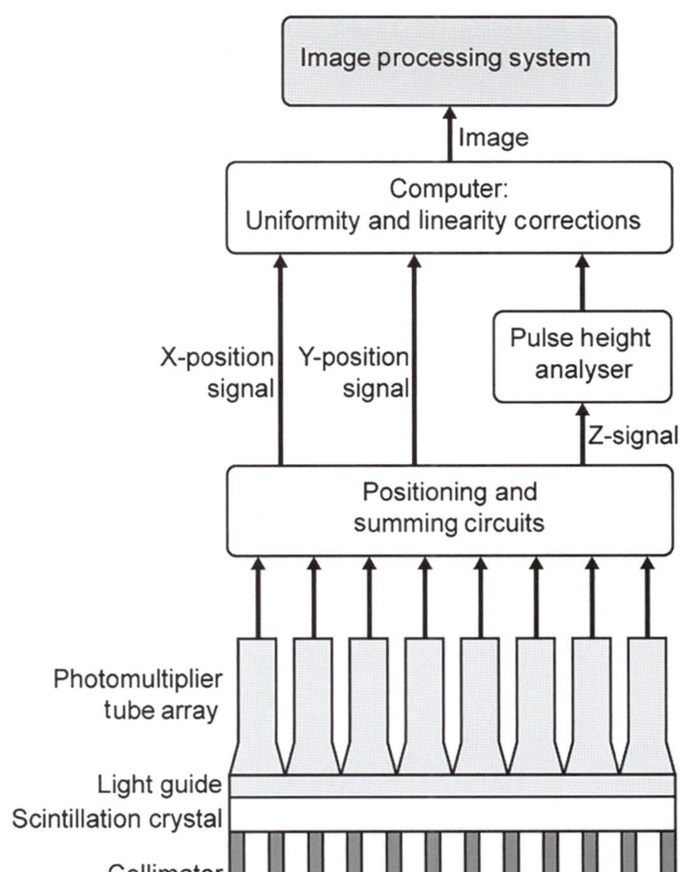

Fig. 7.6 Schematic of gamma camera head.

The process of recording a single gamma ray event by the camera is as follows (Fig. 7.7A):

1. A γ-ray emitted from the body and travelling towards the detector, in a direction approximately parallel to collimator holes (parallel hole collimator), passes through and interacts with the NaI(Tl) scintillator crystal.
2. The γ-ray is absorbed by the crystal and the energy is reemitted as a plume of photons with a wavelength associated with visible light.
3. The light photons travel through a waveguide to the front face of the photomultiplier tube (PMT) array where they are converted into photoelectrons.
4. The photoelectrons are multiplied between the increasing voltage dynodes of the PMT, amplifying the signal.
5. Comparison circuitry between the signal produced by each PMT localises the likely position of the detected event.
6. The total output from the PMT array also gives information about the energy of the detected event. Energy discriminators (windows) allow photons of a specific energy, usually only unscattered photons, to contribute to the image.

Solid-State Gamma Cameras

The scintillation gamma camera has retained the same basic design since its development in the late 1950s. Many attempts have been made to replace the various performance-limiting components, such as photomultipliers, with solid-state devices to improve the gamma camera's capabilities, but only now are fully solid-state gamma camera systems becoming commercially available for routine use in nuclear medicine imaging. The new systems generally use cadmium zinc telluride (CZT) modules sitting behind a collimator. One of the first clinical systems was the Spectrum Dynamics D-SPECT cardiac camera.[5] Today, GE Healthcare are producing large field of view CZT and multihead CZT systems capable of a full range of nuclear medicine imaging studies.[6] In solid-state systems, the gamma rays are directly converted to electron-hole pairs in the CZT crystal (Fig. 7.7B). With the dedicated counting electronics attached to the CZT, several gains in performance are achieved in terms of sensitivity, spatial resolution and energy discrimination.

Image Construction

Images of the distribution of radiopharmaceuticals within the body are made up of hundreds of thousands to millions of detected events, with each event individually detected. Most gamma cameras have two detector heads, and the orientation of these heads is variable. The structure of the collimator directly affects two important performance characteristics of the gamma camera: spatial resolution and sensitivity.

The function of a gamma camera collimator is to permit gamma rays travelling in a predefined direction to reach the detector. This is achieved by absorbing all other gamma rays in the septa between the holes of the collimator. A number of different types of collimators are available, but by far the most widely used are parallel-hole collimators.

Parallel-hole collimators consist of a thick lead plate with several thousand small parallel holes perpendicular to the plane of the plate. For this type of collimator, there is a 1:1 relationship between the size of the distribution of imaged activity and its projection onto the detector. Thus the size of the image is independent of the distance from the subject to the detector face. The characteristics of a parallel-hole collimator depend on the hole diameter, hole length and septal thickness (amount of lead between the holes). Sensitivity and spatial resolution are inversely related; the higher the sensitivity, the poorer the spatial resolution, and vice versa. Parallel-hole collimators are purposely designed to image gamma rays of a specific energy range, usually denoted as low, medium or high energy. Imaging Tc-99m requires

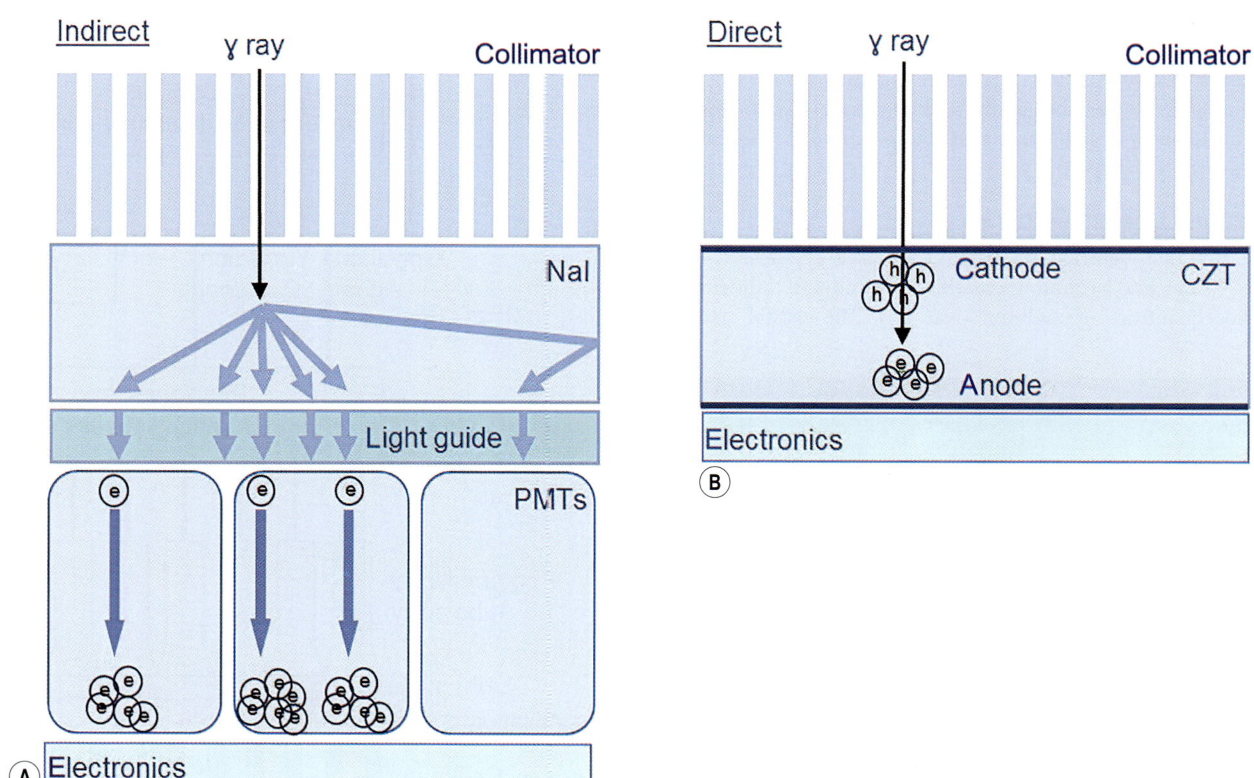

Fig. 7.7 Conversion of gamma rays by (A) Indirect and (B) Direct methods. CZT, Cadmium zinc telluride; PMTs, Photomultiplier tubes.

a low-energy collimator, with medium- and high-energy collimators used for higher-energy photons from different radionuclides. The size of hole, length of septa and number of holes influence the characteristics of a collimator designed for a specific energy. Low-energy collimators are available with slightly different designs to improve one area, such as high sensitivity, high resolution or very high resolution. The exact characteristics of each collimator can vary immensely between manufacturers.

Imaging Techniques

Planar Imaging

Reference has been made to planar and tomographic imaging. Planar imaging can take a number of forms. The simplest is with the camera directed at the part of the body containing the organ or organs of interest and acquiring a predefined number of events or for a predefined period of time. These are sometimes referred to as *spot views*. Keeping two camera heads in a fixed position in front of and behind the patient and moving the patient slowly between the detectors is commonly referred to as *whole-body imaging*. The bone scans shown in Figs. 7.8 and 7.9 use this form of imaging. A dynamic acquisition is when a series of images, often sequential and of the same duration, is obtained. With these data, temporal changes in distribution guide the diagnostic results. An example of dynamic imaging is discussed in the 'Kidney Imaging' section. A final form of planar imaging is when the acquisition is synchronised to a physiological signal obtained from the patient, known as *gating*. Gated blood pool imaging, discussed in the 'Cardiac Imaging' section, is the most widely used form of this mode of imaging for estimating the left ventricular ejection fraction (LVEF). The cardiac cycle is divided into a fixed number of frames (the example shown in Fig. 7.10 includes 24 frames of 41 ms each). The dynamic acquisition is triggered by the R-wave on the patient's electrocardiograph (ECG). Images from multiple heart beats are obtained, and corresponding frames (first, second etc.) are summed together to produce a dynamic series representing a composite beat. Without this technique, the quantity of data in each frame would be insufficient to achieve the accuracy of the ejection fraction calculation required.

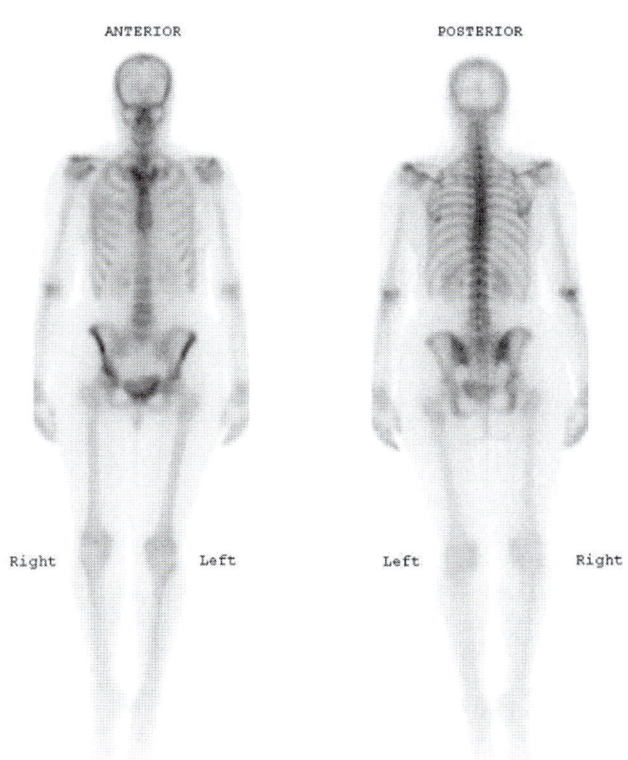

Fig. 7.8 Normal bone scan.

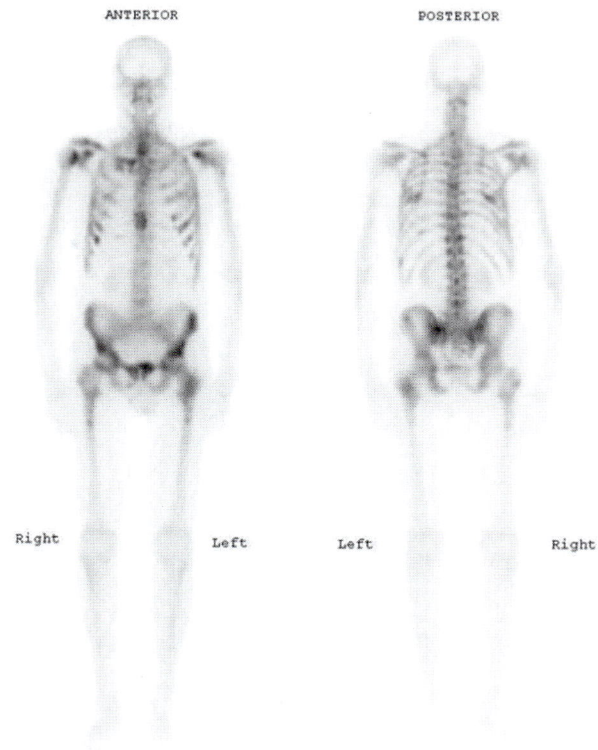

Fig. 7.9 Bone scan with secondary deposits.

Tomographic Imaging

Tomographic imaging is performed with a gamma camera by rotating the detector systems around the patient while acquiring images. The image data may be obtained with the camera heads stationary at a number of fixed positions around the body, known as *step and shoot mode*, or acquired continuously as the camera rotates. Two-dimensional cross-sectional images are reconstructed using mathematical algorithms, in a similar way to x-ray CT. The two-dimensional cross-sectional images can be stacked to form a volume of data which gives the appearance of having acquired a three-dimensional data set.

Knowledge of the three-dimensional distribution of the radiopharmaceutical within the body allows correction for the attenuation of the emitting gamma radiation within the patient if the size and density of surrounding structures can be determined, which is readily achieved using a CT attenuation map. A CT acquisition represents the variation of x-ray absorption throughout the image volume, and a direct relationship can be made between this and the attenuation of the emitted gamma radiation. An example of nuclear medicine images that have been attenuation corrected and fused with the CT structural images is shown in Fig. 7.11.

Post Therapy Imaging

With the requirement to perform routine dosimetry for radionuclide therapy treatments, increasing numbers of patients are being scanned post treatment to assess the distribution of the therapeutic dose.

This is straightforward for treatment agents involving beta-emitting radionuclides that also emit gamma rays (principal gamma emission energies shown in brackets), such as I-131 (364 keV), Lu-177 (113, 208 keV),

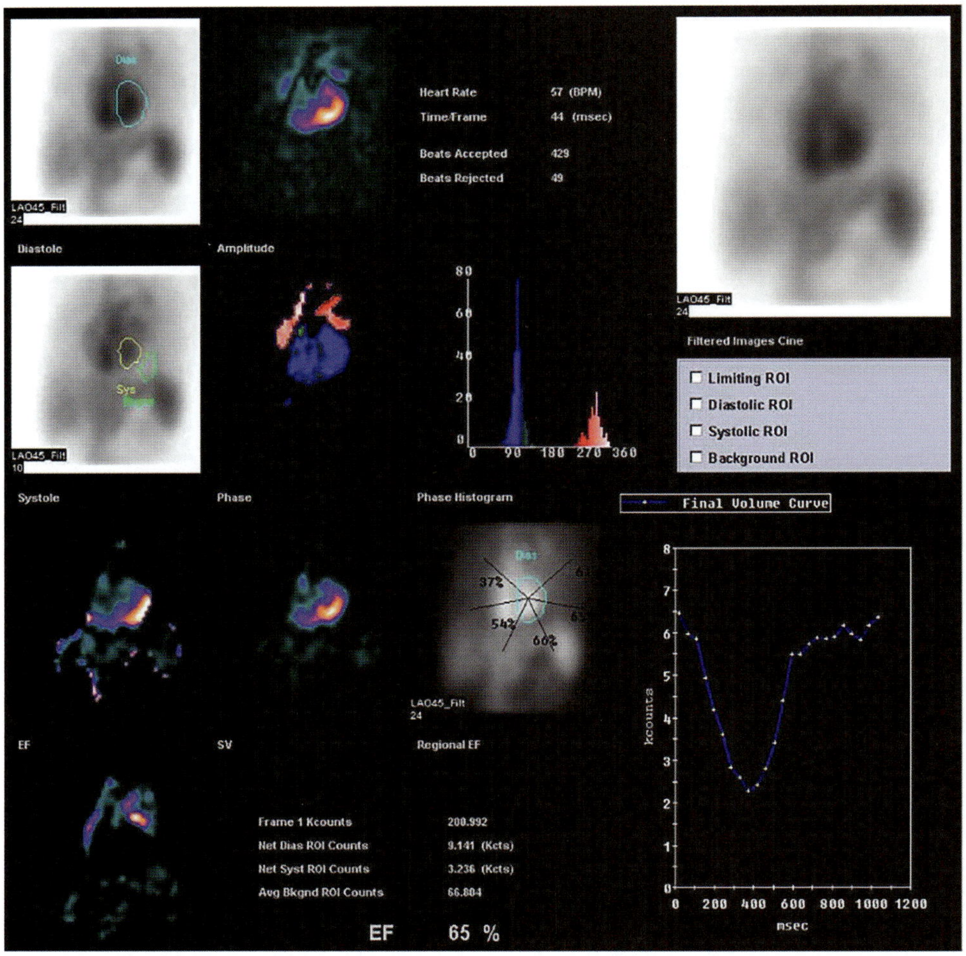

Fig. 7.10 Multiple gated acquisition images from a patient with a normal left ventricular ejection fraction.

Re-188 (155 keV) and Ho-166 (81 keV), which can be imaged on a standard gamma camera, but a commonly used treatment agent, yttrium-90, has no such gammas. These patients can still be imaged due to the high-energy beta particles emitting x-rays as they slow down due to interactions within the patient. This bremsstrahlung or 'braking radiation' is a continuous spectrum of x-rays, but following careful setup of the gamma camera, reasonable images can be obtained which are a useful guide to the therapeutic distribution within the patient and can be used for dosimetric purposes (Fig. 7.12).

Whole-Body Tomographic Imaging

For many reasons, including increased contrast, better localisation and the ability to register with CT images, acquiring three-dimensional radionuclide images of the patient is much more desirable than planar imaging. Tomographic imaging is therefore increasingly replacing planar imaging techniques in nuclear medicine, with some centres now using whole-body SPECT for routine bone imaging. This requires acquiring several (three to five) individual tomographic scans along the patient length and then stitching these together at the image processing stage, as has happened in Fig. 7.2. This technique has been used by PET scanners for decades, but due to the length of time required for each SPECT scan, it can be time-consuming for both patients and staff. Major technological advances will need to occur in single photon imaging to completely replace planar imaging. In PET, this advance has been made by adding sufficient rings of imaging detectors to cover an almost 2-m long field of view incorporating nearly 600,000 individual crystal detectors.[7] Due to the massively improved sensitivity, this scanner has an incredible imaging performance compared to existing PET scanners and offers never-before-seen capabilities to dynamically and quantitatively track tracers as they are administered to patients and distributed throughout the body, which offers enormous potential in the field of drug development.

Gamma Camera Performance Characteristics

It is essential that gamma camera performance is maintained to achieve the highest possible image quality for each investigation undertaken on it. The performance of gamma camera detectors is characterised by a number of parameters:

- Spatial resolution
- Sensitivity
- Uniformity
- Linearity and energy response
- Energy resolution
- Multiple window registration

Detailed descriptions of the precise definitions of these parameters, factors influencing their stability, measurement methodologies and how they may be specified during equipment procurement are covered in two publications: IPEM Report 111 2003[8] and NEMA 2012.[9] Brief outlines are given here.

Spatial resolution. This is the ability to distinguish an object from its surroundings and is a measure of the sharpness of the image. It is defined by a full-width half-maximum distance, which is about 3 mm for the intrinsic (no collimator) resolution of a current gamma camera.

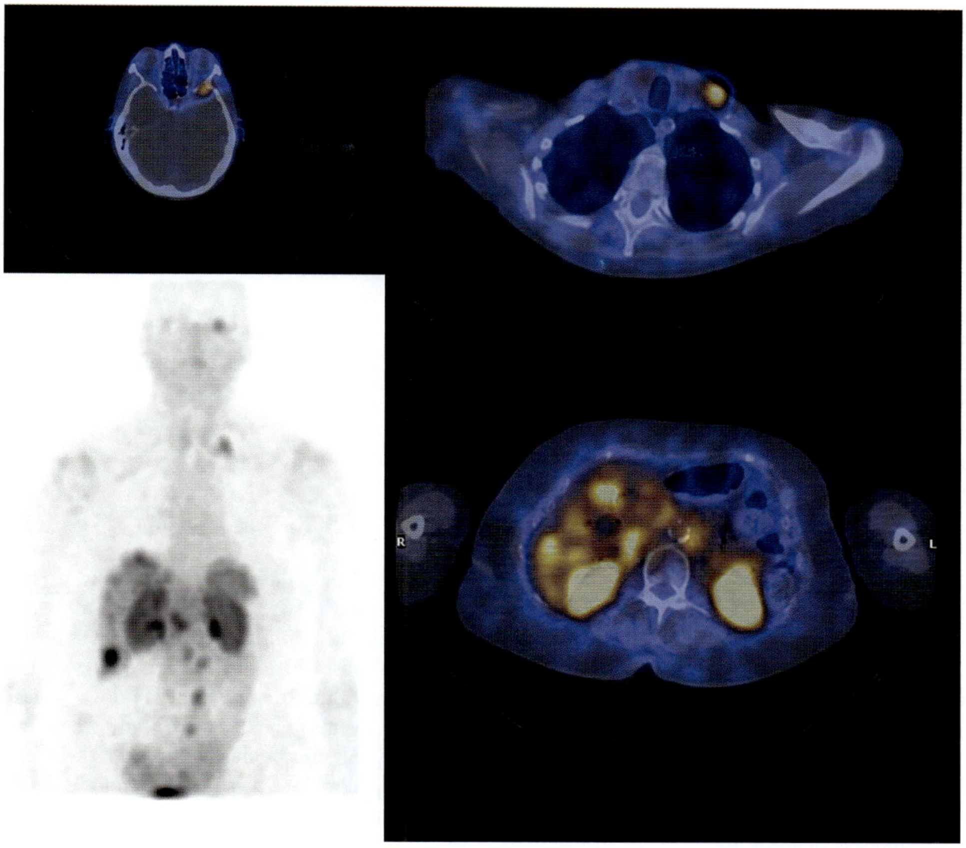

Fig. 7.11 Tc-99m Tektrotyd single photon emission computerised tomography–computed tomography image of a patient with multiple neuroendocrine tumour metastases of the liver.

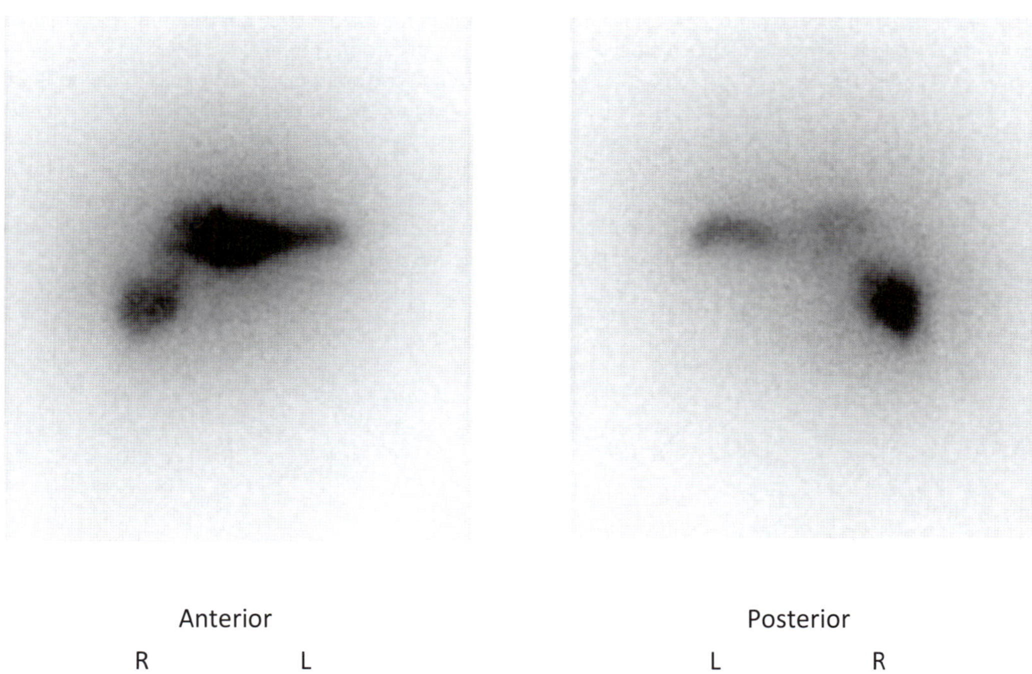

Fig. 7.12 Bremsstrahlung images of yttrium-90 treatment.

Use of collimators degrades this resolution but is essential for creating the images.

Sensitivity. This term relates to the number of gamma events per megabecquerel (MBq) detected by the gamma camera.

Uniformity. This refers to the variations in count rate across the field of view when the detector is exposed to a uniform source of a gamma ray–emitting radionuclide.

Linearity and energy response. These refer to the gamma camera's ability to determine the true location and energy of a gamma ray detected anywhere in the field of view. These are the fundamental parameters that influence detector uniformity.

Energy resolution. Statistical variations in the detection of gamma rays by the crystal and photomultiplier assembly result in a characteristic broadening of the total absorption peak of the energy spectrum. Energy resolution is defined by the full-width half-maximum of the broadened energy peak.

Multiple window registration. This refers to the ability of the gamma camera to determine the location of a detected gamma event as a function of its energy.

Corrections can be made during data acquisition to overcome some of the nonrandom defects in camera performance. These include corrections for nonuniformity of sensitivity, nonuniformity of energy resolution and nonlinearity.

There are additional performance characteristics to take into account when performing SPECT imaging and still further with SPECT/CT. SPECT imaging requires the centre of rotation (COR) of the rotating camera heads to be within predefined limits. Failure to do so will result in artefacts on the reconstructed SPECT images. It is also important that the parameters defining the detector heads' performance remain stable at every angle of rotation. SPECT/CT relies on the accurate registration of the SPECT and CT images, and phantoms should be routinely used to assess the gamma camera SPECT capability and SPECT/CT alignment. The performance of the CT is assessed as for all CT equipment and is covered by IPEM Report 91.[10]

Prior to injecting any patients, quality control should be performed and passed, and a large-area, solid, uniform radioactive (cobalt-57) source can be imaged to check several key performance parameters of gamma camera systems.

POSITRON EMISSION TOMOGRAPHY SCANNERS

PET imaging systems (Fig. 7.13) are designed specifically for imaging the high-energy photons generated following decay by positron-emitting radionuclides. Scintillator crystals with high stopping power are used, such as lutetium oxyorthosilicate (LSO) or lutetium–yttrium oxyorthosilicate (LYSO). These are positioned in rings around a gantry. As coinciding annihilation events need to be detected for PET imaging, incredibly fast electronic timing circuitry registers if two crystals detect a photon within a defined time window (typically picoseconds), allowing 'true' events to be detected. Many 'single' events and 'random' coincidences will also be detected (Fig. 7.14A), but having a small timing window will reduce these. The size of the crystal elements depends on the make and model of the scanner but is generally around 3 to 6 mm^2 by around 25 mm deep—the depth being needed to improve detection of the high-energy (511-keV) photons. The elements are arranged in blocks with, for example, 36 elements per block, and the blocks are arranged into modules with 4 blocks per module (incorporating the photomultipliers) and then into rings with over 30 modules per 360-degree ring. With typically four to five rings per scanner, this gives around 20,000 individual crystal elements per scanner. The crystal size is one of the main factors contributing to the spatial resolution, which is typically around 3 mm (FWHM).

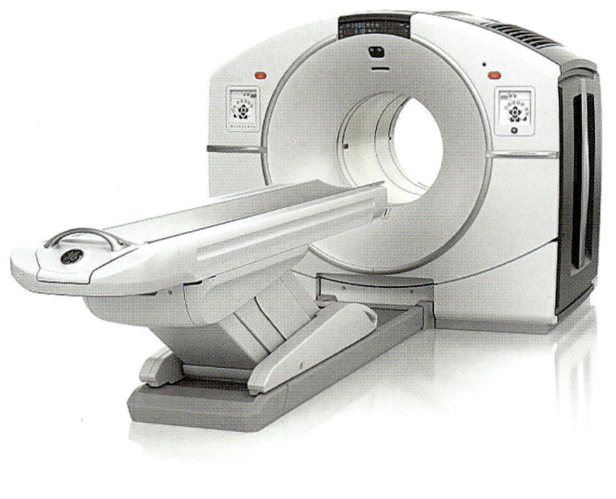

Fig. 7.13 Positron emission tomography camera.

When two events are detected simultaneously within the short timing window, the computer system is able to reconstruct the line connecting these events in opposite crystals as a line of response (LOR). Millions of LORs are acquired over a period of time and reconstructed to form cross-sectional images using appropriate image reconstruction software. Iterative reconstructions are generally used, but other reconstruction techniques are being introduced.[11]

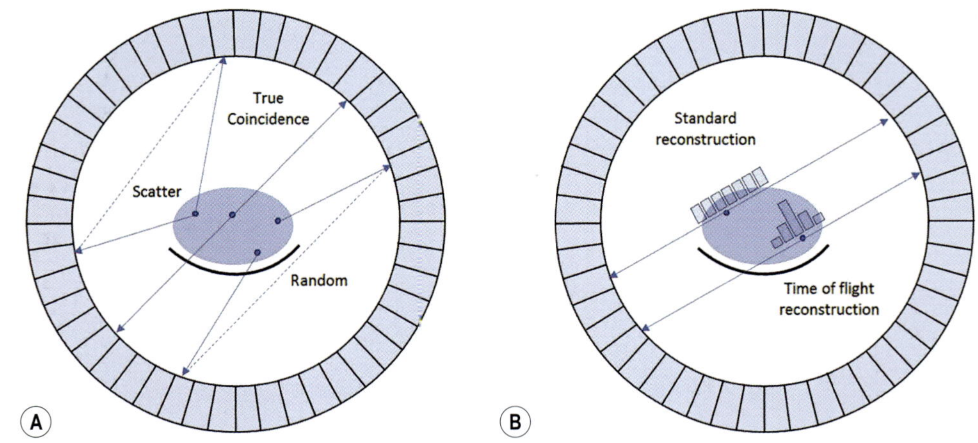

Fig. 7.14 (A) Positron emission tomography (PET) detected events. (B) PET time of flight rebinning.

Attenuation of the annihilation photons within the patient degrades the image quality in a similar manner to SPECT imaging. Ironically, although the 511-keV photon energy is much higher and therefore much more penetrating than the Tc-99m 140-keV emission most widely used in single photon imaging, attenuation effects are more pronounced on the reconstructed PET images. This is because each pair of detected photons will have had to pass through the equivalent of the total body thickness. Correction for the qualitative and quantitative impairment of PET images due to attenuation is achieved by the acquisition of CT attenuation correction maps. Low-quality CT was introduced purely for this purpose in the early 2000s, but the addition of high-quality CT images greatly enhances the diagnostic capability of the modality as functional and structural information is fused in a single set of images.

As with gamma camera systems, there is a move towards solid-state electronics, and although PET still utilises scintillator crystals for the initial detection, these can now be connected to solid-state silicon photomultipliers. This advance allows time of flight (TOF) PET to deliver significantly improved image performance. Being able to measure very small differences in the detection time of the coincident photons means the information can be used to more precisely locate the origin of the annihilation event. In non-TOF image reconstruction, the origin of the annihilation event has equal probability of occurring along the line of response (within the patient outline), but by using exceptionally fast electronics, the slight difference in arrival times at the detectors can be used to weight the rebinning of the events more accurately along the LOR (Fig. 7.14B).

Other reconstruction improvements, such as resolution modelling, have also helped to improve the quality of PET images. Resolution modelling uses known performance characteristics of the imaging system across the field of view and compensates for this in the reconstruction of the images.

PET Scanner Performance Characteristics

As with gamma cameras, it is essential that PET scanner performance is maintained to achieve the highest possible image quality for each scan. The performance of a PET scanner is characterised by a number of parameters:

- Spatial resolution
- Sensitivity
- Count rate performance
- Image quality
- TOF resolution
- Coregistration accuracy

Detailed descriptions of the precise definitions of these parameters, factors influencing their stability and measurement methodologies are covered in two publications: IPEM Report 108 2013[12] and NEMA 2018.[13] Brief outlines are given here.

Spatial resolution. This is the ability to resolve small objects and is measured using very small point sources of radioactivity scanned at specific locations within the field of view (FOV). This can range from around 4 mm centrally to over 6 mm at the edge of the FOV.

Sensitivity. A carefully measured amount of radioactivity is used to calculate the number of counts detected per MBq by the scanner.

Count rate performance. A high activity line source is placed in the field of view inside scatter material, and serial acquisitions are collected as the activity decays. From these scans, data can be generated to demonstrate count rate performance including true events, scatters and randoms plotted against activity concentration with peak values being quoted.

Image quality. A specific test object is used to assess image quality in PET scanners comprising six fillable spheres of size 10 to 37 mm diameter, generally filled with activity concentrations five times that of the background. The contrast of these spheres is assessed to demonstrate the performance of the scanner.

TOF resolution. A line source of radioactivity is used to investigate the timing resolution for each block in the scanner, which is typically hundreds of picoseconds.

Coregistration accuracy. This test uses point sources combining a suitable amount of radioactivity and CT contrast media imaged at various locations within the field of view. Analysis of the PET and CT scans will show the degree of misregistration between the images.

As with gamma cameras, quality control of PET scanners must be performed daily and found satisfactory before patients can be injected. Generally, a uniform test cylinder filled with a solid radioactive (germanium-68) impregnated resin is used for daily quality control tests which can test several of the aforementioned parameters in one short scan.

RADIOPHARMACEUTICALS

A wide range of radiopharmaceuticals are available.[14] Most of these are administered intravenously, but radiopharmaceuticals can be administered by many routes, including orally, by inhalation, intraarterially or subcutaneously. When deciding upon the efficacy of a given radiopharmaceutical, the physical and chemical properties of the radionuclide, together with the biochemical, physiological and pharmacological properties of the pharmaceutical, must be considered.

The Radionuclide

The best possible radionuclide to use for any given procedure will depend upon its properties, which include:

- Type of radiation emitted, its energy and abundance
- Half-life
- Specific activity
- Radionuclidic purity
- Chemical properties of the element

Each of these properties is considered in the following sections.

Type of Radiation

Diagnostic imaging involves external detection of the radiation. Therefore the required physical characteristics include the emission of gamma or x-radiation.

The photon energy should be high enough to avoid serious attenuation in tissue but low enough to allow the photon to be stopped by and interact with the detector. The design characteristics of a scintillation gamma camera favour photons with energies between 75 keV and 300 keV. Selecting radionuclides that have a monoenergetic emission is an advantage as a single energy window will minimise the quantity of scattered radiation incorporated into (and degrading) the final image. Absorbed radiation dose to the patient will be kept as low as reasonably practicable (ALARP) if the radionuclide has no particulate emissions and decays with a high abundance of gamma photons. Technetium-99m does not emit any particles and provides 89 photons of 140 keV for every 100 disintegrations.

Physical Half-life

The half-life of the radionuclide must be sufficiently long to allow for radiolabelling, administration, localisation and imaging of the radiopharmaceutical within the organ of interest. At the same time, it should be remembered that the radiation dose to the patient is proportional to the half-life of the radionuclide, and therefore the half-life should be as short as possible. As a rule of thumb, radionuclides used for imaging ideally have half-lives of similar duration to that of the study.

Specific Activity

Specific activity should not be confused with radioactive concentration, which has units of activity per volume. Specific activity is activity per unit mass, and therefore it has units of becquerel per gram or mole. There is a maximum specific activity for each radionuclide, which depends upon its physical half-life. Specific activity gives an indication of the ratio of radioactive to nonradioactive atoms of the element in the sample.

Generally for radiopharmaceutical production, it is best to use radionuclides with as high a specific activity as possible, as this allows very small quantities to be used which will help to ensure that the radiolabel does not significantly alter the chemical or biological properties of the pharmaceutical to which it is attached. However, carrier-free samples can be difficult to work with because there is so little mass of the element present. For example, 500 MBq of carrier-free technetium-99m has a mass of 2 ng.

Radionuclide Purity

Radionuclide purity is the fraction of the total radioactivity in the sample that is in the form of the desired radionuclide. It is important to have the highest radionuclide purity possible, as any contaminants of other radionuclides will increase the radiation dose to the patient and may degrade the image. Impurities can arise from the manufacturing process, from daughter radionuclides or from parent radionuclides.

Chemical Properties

Even if a radionuclide has ideal physical properties, it is of little value if it has no useful chemical properties that can be used for localisation or if it cannot be efficiently and securely attached to a suitable pharmaceutical. The success of technetium-99m as the radionuclide of choice in diagnostic imaging is due in no small part to the way in which its chemistry has been exploited.

Chemical toxicity is generally not a matter of concern, as radiopharmaceuticals are administered in such extremely small physical quantities, typically of the order of nanograms. This amount is so small that it is uncommon for the administration of radiopharmaceuticals to a patient to cause any interference at all with the physiological effects being investigated.

The Ideal Radionuclide for Imaging

Technetium-99m comes close to meeting the requirements of an ideal radionuclide for imaging. It has a monoenergetic gamma emission of 140 keV, high abundance, no accompanying particulate emissions and a half-life of 6 hours, and it decays to an effectively stable daughter product. It is readily available from a molybdenum-99 generator and in a chemical form that can be simply attached to a range of pharmaceuticals.

Production and Quality Control of Radiopharmaceuticals

Even though radiopharmaceuticals generally have no pharmacological effect on a patient, they are still considered drugs, and the ever-increasing regulatory requirements for drug manufacture compounded by those for using radioactive materials has meant that it is difficult for departments to run a small in-house radiopharmacy. Therefore technetium radiopharmaceuticals are now generally manufactured at large, centralised radiopharmacies. When purchasing technetium-99m radiopharmaceuticals from external suppliers, these providers must be licensed by the Medicines and Healthcare products Regulatory Agency (MHRA) in the United Kingdom. There is an exemption from this in current UK legislation for sites manufacturing radiopharmaceuticals in-house if this is performed under the close supervision of a pharmacist. Nontechnetium radiopharmaceuticals are generally purchased solely from commercial suppliers with a marketing authorisation (product licence) for that particular product.

Technetium Radiopharmaceuticals

These are generally produced using technetium-99m, in the form of liquid sodium pertechnetate, from a generator and 'cold kits' containing the required targeting agent. Production consists of mixing the correct amount and volume of radioactive liquid with the chemicals in the cold kit. The chemicals are supplied freeze dried in vials ready to be reconstituted when needed. These contain the pharmaceutical itself, some form of reducing agent to pull the technetium away from its pertechnetate environment, and additional material required to bulk out the contents so that they freeze dry successfully. There may be additional chemicals to buffer the solution to ensure that it maintains the correct pH and other substances required to ensure optimum chemical binding between the radionuclide and the pharmaceutical. The pertechnetate itself is usually produced by a molybdenum-99 generator, and radiopharmacies will purchase these from a suitable manufacturer once or twice weekly (due to the approximate 3-day half-life of Mo-99) and elute them once or twice daily.

For the majority of diagnostic tests, intravenous injection of the radiopharmaceutical is necessary and so great care must be taken to produce a sterile radiopharmaceutical in a solution that is of the correct pH value and free from foreign proteins arising from previous bacteriological activity (pyrogens). Due to the short half-life of technetium-99m of around 6 hours, these radiopharmaceuticals must be produced on a daily basis. As it is not possible to terminally sterilise the radiopharmaceuticals, a technique known as *aseptic manufacturing* must be used to ensure that the products are sterile, of suitable quality and fit for purpose. The responsibility for the quality control of radiopharmaceuticals lies with the manufacturer.

Manufacture takes place in specialised cabinets (isolators) sited in clean rooms to provide an environment that caters for the conflicting requirements of the radiation safety of the operator and the need for aseptic production. For radiation safety, it is usual to provide an environment in the cabinets at a lower pressure than its surroundings to contain any airborne contaminants. The preparation area must be bathed in a flow of sterile air to minimise risks of microbiological contamination produced by passing the air through a filter which will remove any particulate or bacterial contamination.

Labelling of a patient's own blood cells is possible as a medical procedure and is undertaken in specialised facilities with more stringent requirements for protection of the operator and the product.

Once manufactured and all quality control that can be performed during production has passed, the radiopharmaceuticals can be released for use with a defined 'shelf-life' usually of 2 to 6 hours.

Prior to administration, the label on the vial, syringe or capsule, if for oral administration, is checked against that prescribed for the procedure. The activity given to the patient is checked independently on a radionuclide calibrator which measures the amount of radioactivity (generally in MBq) for the radionuclide specified. The constancy of the radionuclide calibrator is checked daily, and its calibration should be traceable to national standards. The amount of radioactivity administered is noted in the patient record.

If the binding of the radionuclide to the pharmaceutical is poor, the distribution of radioactivity in the patient may appear unusual or abnormal. Poor binding can be due to problems with the radiopharmaceutical or one of its components, or it may be due to a fault in manufacture. Radiopharmacies measure the radiochemical purity, usually by chromatography, to check the binding. Unusual distributions in images should be reported to the radiopharmacy for investigation, although other situations can arise that will modify the distribution. For example, a female who is breastfeeding may exhibit increased uptake of radioactivity in the breast due to uptake into milk. Also, prescribed and over-the-counter drugs taken by the patient may affect the biodistribution of a radiopharmaceutical.

PET Radiopharmaceuticals

Proton-rich radionuclides are generally produced in cyclotrons by irradiating suitable targets with high-energy protons. The most prolific PET imaging radionuclide in use is fluorine-18 (F-18), which is produced by irradiating oxygen-18 as a liquid target in the form of water. Once generated, the F-18 is synthesised into various radiopharmaceuticals using dedicated synthesis units. The most frequently used PET radiopharmaceutical by far is the glucose analogue F-18 fluorodeoxyglucose (FDG), which is a useful generic imaging agent for cancer and infections. Determination by PET scanning of F-18 FDG uptake during and after antineoplastic treatment may be used as an early indicator of response to treatment. The reaction to radiotherapy or chemotherapy treatment may be an initial rise in F-18 FDG uptake, followed by a decrease, the magnitude of which can serve as a marker of treatment response. F-18 FDG is also taken up in inflammatory lesions, giving rise to nonspecificity. This presents interpretational limitations and requires caution in the reporting of PET/CT scans. The optimal timing of posttreatment evaluation by PET/CT is not established, is the subject of current research and will be dependent on tumour type and treatment modality.

A growing body of literature has now led to FDG-PET being used routinely in the clinic for the detection and staging of malignant tumours, determination of the extent of spread of disease (including assessment of the suitability of patients for radical surgery), differentiation of benign from malignant mass lesions, measurement of response to therapy, and long-term follow-up for detection of recurrent disease. Due to the high cost of PET scans, their funding is limited to approved indications, and these are listed in Evidence-Based Indications for the Use of PET-CT in the United Kingdom 2022.[15]

Due to the logistical advantages of F-18, many other compounds have also been labelled with this radionuclide, such as fluorocholine, fluorofatty acids, fluoroamino acids, spiperone derivatives, fluoromisonidazole (FMISO) and fluoroaltanserin. A fluorinated prostate-specific membrane antigen (PSMA) has also been developed and is the most clinically useful fluorinated tracer after F-18 FDG.

Much of PET tracer development uses the germanium-68/gallium-68 positron emitter generator system with the long half-life germanium-68 (half-life 270 days) decaying to the short half-life gallium-68 (half-life 68 minutes). As well as simpler chemistry, the gallium-68 (Ga-68) radiopharmaceuticals tend to have fast blood clearance and rapid target localisation. The use of radiometals for labelling peptide targeting agents also provides an additional value, as the Ga-68 radionuclide can easily be replaced with other beta- or alpha-emitting radionuclides and labelled to the same peptides to allow radionuclide treatment.

Commercial, fully licensed Ga-68 generators are now available, and licensed cold kits analogous to those used for technetium-99m radiopharmaceutical manufacture have also been produced. These are currently available for manufacturing Ga-68 somatostatin analogues for somatostatin receptor imaging in neuroendocrine tumours and Ga-68 PSMA for prostate cancer imaging. The main drawbacks of Ga-68 generators are the limited amount of radioactivity they can produce, which is generally only enough for a small number of patients per day, and the decline in this over time due to the decay of the parent radionuclide, which necessitates replacement on an annual basis. Cyclotron production can yield large amounts of radioactivity, and the almost 2-hour half-life of F-18 makes it more suitable for large-scale production and distribution. Therefore, once Ga-68 radiopharmaceuticals are shown to be useful, F-18 alternatives are sought.

Substantial effort is being invested into developing an agent that targets fibroblast activation proteins, which are overexpressed in many types of tumour. This has resulted in the development of a Ga-68–labelled fibroblast activation protein inhibitor (FAPI), which is showing promising results as an alternative to FDG.[16]

Mechanisms of Localisation

Radiopharmaceuticals can be divided into two major categories depending upon whether or not their localisation within the body involves their participation in a specific chemical reaction. Many traditional radiopharmaceuticals, such as technetium-99m macroaggregated albumin (MAA) for lung perfusion imaging, are not incorporated into specific biochemical pathways but rely for their utility on the correct molecular size and route of administration.

More exciting advances in recent years have involved the development of radiopharmaceuticals whose precise chemical nature has allowed specific biochemical pathways to be investigated. An example is technetium-99m octreotide (Tektrotyd)[17] a somatostatin analogue which is used to localise neuroendocrine tumours that overexpress somatostatin receptors.

A more detailed breakdown of mechanisms that determine the localisation and behaviour of radiopharmaceuticals is given in the following subsections.

Diffusion and Dilution

Tracers may be used that distribute themselves throughout the space in the body into which they were introduced. Imaging of their distribution can identify the extent of these areas or demonstrate where their natural boundaries have broken down. An example is lung ventilation imaging, which depends upon the inhalation of a suitable tracer, such as krypton-81m gas, into the lungs, where it diffuses throughout the functioning air spaces, allowing them to be visualised.

Radiotracer dilution is a quantitative (generally nonimaging) method which depends on complete mixing of a radiopharmaceutical throughout a body space. Knowledge of the administered activity and the radioactive concentration of a sample of the fluid within the space once mixing is complete will allow the volume of the space to be calculated. An example is the determination of red cell mass.

Capillary Blockade and Cell Sequestration

If radioactive particles in the size range 20 to 50 µm are injected into the vascular system, they will partially occlude the first capillary bed they encounter (the size of capillaries is 8–10 µm). An intravenous injection of 200,000 technetium-99m–labelled particles of MAA will block around 0.02% of the capillaries of a normal lung, thus permitting the visualisation of the vascular bed of the lungs. A protein such as albumin is chosen for production of the particles, as it will be broken down naturally and removed from the lungs.

Phagocytosis

The reticuloendothelial cells in the body have the capacity to ingest bacteria and small particles in the range 0.01 to 10 µm. This is known as *phagocytosis*. If a radiolabelled colloid is injected intravenously, the phagocytic action of the reticuloendothelial cells, in particular, the Kupffer cells in the liver and macrophages in the spleen, will remove the colloid from the circulation, enabling the organ to be visualised.

Metabolic Pathway

The metabolic pathway of a huge number of substances can be investigated using radioactive techniques. They may be designed specifically to investigate a particular body function, such as technetium-99m–labelled mercaptoacetyltriglycine (MAG3) for the investigation of kidney function.

Iodine is incorporated into the hormones produced by the thyroid gland, and a study of the metabolic behaviour of iodine in the body gives valuable diagnostic information on thyroid function. Radioactive iodine introduced into the body therefore enables iodine metabolism to be studied easily. Iodine-131 (I-131) and iodine-123 (I-123) are two radionuclides commonly used for imaging thyroid tissue.

Metabolic Trapping

Some radiopharmaceuticals become trapped within the tissue into which they have been transported by metabolic processes. Certain radiopharmaceuticals have been developed specifically to exploit this behaviour. For example, technetium-99m tetrofosmin and methoxy isobutyl isonitrile (MIBI) were developed to mimic the distribution of uptake of thallium-201, the radionuclide originally used for imaging myocardial perfusion. Thallium-201 washes out of the tissues quickly, but the technetium-99m–labelled analogues are trapped, allowing more time for the tracer distribution to be imaged and generating images of much better quality.

F-18 FDG is the most widely used radiopharmaceutical in PET imaging. Fig. 7.15 shows an F-18 FDG PET/CT image of a patient with a lung tumour. It is commonly described as a metabolic marker. Its chemistry is modified by the label so that it becomes trapped within cells, and its method of localisation comes under the heading of metabolic trapping rather than metabolic pathway. Compared to normal cells, tumour cells are highly metabolically active and tend to have higher glucose metabolism. This makes the positron-emitting tracer, FDG, particularly useful in oncology to identify hypermetabolic tissues that may be malignant.

Antibodies and Antibody Fragments

Antibodies are large, *Y*-shaped molecules consisting of proteins. They form part of the body's immune response, and the body manufactures them as needed to neutralise a threat posed to the body by foreign or harmful material. The material that triggers the antibody response is called the *antigen*. Antibodies are produced in the body at the site of need; they are not designed to be carried in the blood, seeking out suitable receptors, but splitting them into fragments can retain their functionality and remove some of the drawbacks of using the whole antibodies, such as nonspecific liver uptake.

Antibodies can also be raised against substances which are not foreign to the body. For example, there are antileukocyte antibodies, and fragments of these can be radiolabelled and used to investigate the distribution of circulating leukocytes and sites of accumulation of them in the body.

Radiolabelling of antibodies has been seen as very promising in nuclear medicine, but nonspecific uptake, particularly in the liver, has

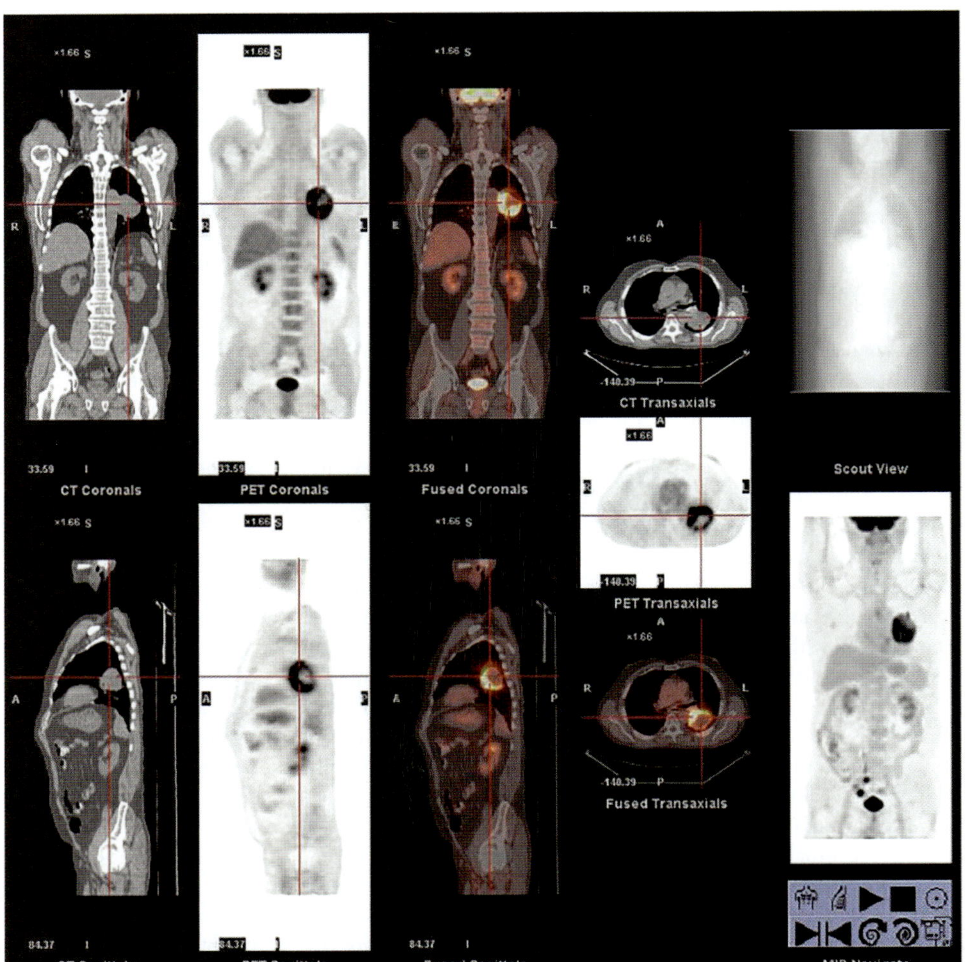

Fig. 7.15 Fluorine-18 fluorodeoxyglucose positron emission tomography–computed tomography image of a patient with a lung tumour.

meant that few radiolabelled antibodies are in routine use for radionuclide imaging.

Receptor Binding

The experience gained in attempting to label antibodies did, however, pay dividends in the area of receptor labelling. Different receptors are found in cells throughout the body, and their specificity has been exploited in various commercially available products. One such example are somatostatin receptors, which can be used to investigate and treat neuroendocrine and other tumours. Other receptor targets which are looking promising for the development of nuclear medicine tracers are PSMA for prostate cancer, human epidermal growth factor (HER) for breast cancer and the previously mentioned FAPI which shows useful uptake in a range of cancers.

CLINICAL APPLICATIONS

Imaging of the distribution of a radiopharmaceutical within tissues, and, in some cases, how it changes with time, enables deductions to be made about the function of that tissue. An abnormal distribution may appear as an increase in radioactive concentration above the surroundings or the expected margins, revealing lesions as 'hot spots' or as reduced activity in the visualised pattern. The appearance of hot spots does not necessarily mean that a lesion is larger than the minimum resolvable power of the gamma camera; if the amount of activity accumulated in the lesion is large enough compared to its surroundings, the lesion will be detected in the image. 'Cold spots' are sometimes referred to as *photopenic areas*, and they are more difficult to detect than hot spots because the margins are blurred with respect to the surroundings.

The purpose of imaging is to investigate tissue function rather than anatomical definition. The following provides a brief description of some of the more important clinical applications of radionuclide imaging that are directly or closely applicable to imaging cancer.

Table 7.1 is a list of commonly used radiopharmaceuticals with notes on their more important uses, details of the diagnostic reference level (DRL), the absorbed dose to the critical organ and the effective dose to the whole body from ICRP 53 and subsequent addenda.[18]

Bone Imaging

Bone imaging is the most widely used investigation in nuclear medicine, and the majority of referrals relate to patients with known primary tumours (breast or prostate cancer) and suspected metastatic spread of the disease to the bones. Bone is made up of collagen and minerals, mainly calcium, phosphates and hydroxides. The minerals form a crystalline lattice known as *hydroxyapatite*. Following intravenous injection, a bone-seeking agent will be transported to the bone and become adsorbed onto the newly forming hydroxyapatite crystals, thus reflecting the bone-forming (or osteoblastic) activity at a given skeletal site. Hence areas where there is an abnormally high increase in bone turnover will show increased uptake and will appear as hot spots on the image. Because localisation on bone depends on transportation in blood, avascular areas will appear 'cold'. Conversely, areas of locally increased blood flow, for example due to infection, may appear as areas of increased uptake on the scan.

All commercially available bone-seeking radiopharmaceuticals today are based on phosphate-containing compounds which can be labelled with technetium-99m. A variety of analogues are available, but the most widely used is methylene diphosphonate (MDP). Typically, 400 to 600 MBq of technetium-99m MDP is administered intravenously, and after a period of 3 to 4 hours (to enable circulating activity to clear), approximately 40% of the injected activity will be localised in the bone, with the majority of the remainder being excreted via the kidneys. Multiple static views or a combination of whole-body imaging and selected static views are acquired. Tomography may also be helpful. A normal bone scan is shown in Fig. 7.8, and a bone scan showing secondary deposits is shown in Fig. 7.9.

The bone scan is a very sensitive technique for demonstrating bone lesions and shows changes earlier than conventional x-rays. For musculoskeletal problems, SPECT/CT scans are particularly useful.

Tumour Imaging

Nuclear medicine can employ many agents to aid in tumour localisation and to follow the progress of the disease and treatment. This section describes nonspecific tumour agents, such as MIBI, as well as several specific tumour agents and studies.

Breast

Technetium-99m MIBI was developed to replace thallium-201 as a cardiac imaging agent, but it was also noted to localise in tumours while it was under clinical evaluation. It has found an application in the localisation of breast tumours.

Neural Crest

Metaiodobenzylguanidine (mIBG) is an analogue of norepinephrine (noradrenaline) and guanethidine. It is available radiolabelled with I-123 for diagnostic imaging and with I-131 for pretreatment dosimetry and therapy. Normal adrenal medulla tissue will concentrate the agent, as will neuroendocrine tumours or tumours of neural crest origin such as phaeochromocytoma, neuroblastoma, carcinoid tumours and medullary carcinoma of the thyroid. Uptake into tumour can be inhibited by many drugs, including tricyclic antidepressants; therefore care must be taken to withdraw any potentially interfering medication well in advance.

Neuroendocrine

Somatostatin is a peptide found in the brain, where it acts as a neurotransmitter, and in the gastrointestinal tract and the pancreas, where it is manufactured. It inhibits the release of neuroendocrine hormones such as growth hormone and insulin. Somatostatin receptors are found in the normal pituitary, pancreas and upper gastrointestinal tract from stomach to jejunum. They are also expressed by a variety of endocrine tumours, such as carcinoids; small-cell lung cancers; tumours of the ovary, cervix, endometrium, breast, kidney, larynx, paranasal sinus and salivary gland; some skin tumours; and tumours arising from glial cells in the central nervous system (CNS). It can be surmised that somatostatin receptor imaging would be clinically useful in a variety of tumours. However, somatostatin has a half-life of only 2 to 3 minutes in the body, so such imaging was not feasible until somatostatin analogues with much longer clearance times were developed.

Initially in single photon imaging, an indium-111–labelled somatostatin (111In-pentetreotide) analogue was used, but now a technetium-labelled somatostatin analogue is available: 99mTc-HYNIC-Tyr3-octreotide (Tektrotyd). Somatostatin analogues can also be labelled with a positron emitter (Ga-68) for PET imaging, which is the diagnostic radionuclide of the theranostics pair used to identify patients suitable for lutetium-177 (Lu-177) SSR radionuclide therapy.

Sufficient uptake for visualisation can occur with many carcinoid tumours, pituitary tumours, gastrointestinal tract endocrine tumours (although disappointing in insulinoma), small-cell lung cancer, medullary carcinoma of the thyroid, neuroblastoma, pheochromocytoma, meningioma and Hodgkin's and non-Hodgkin's lymphoma. Many of these tumours may be better visualised with CT and MRI, but somatostatin receptor imaging may be used to demonstrate small

TABLE 7.1 Examples of Radiopharmaceuticals in Common Diagnostic Use With Critical Organ, Effective Dose and Diagnostic Reference Level Activity

Radionuclide	Chemical Form	Clinical Use	Diagnostic Reference Level (MBq)	Physical Half-life	Route	Critical Organ	Dose to Critical Organ (mSv)	Effective Dose (mSv)
Fluorine-18	Fluorodeoxyglucose	Tumour imaging	400	110 min	IV	Bladder	64	8
Gallium-68	Prostate-specific membrane antigen	Prostate cancer imaging	200	68 min	IV	Kidneys	30	5
Gallium-68	Somatostatin analogue	Neuroendocrine cancer imaging	200	68 min	IV	Kidneys	16	5
Iodine-123	Sodium iodide	Thyroid imaging	20	13.2 h	Oral or IV	Thyroid	90	4 for 35% uptake
Iodine-123	Norepinephrine analogue (mIBG)	Neural crest tumors	400	13.2 h	IV	Liver	27	5 (with thyroid block)
Iodine-131	Sodium iodide	Thyroid metastases imaging	400	8.1 d	Oral or IV	Bladder	244	24 for 0% uptake
Technetium-99m	Sodium pertechnetate	Thyroid imaging	80	6 h	IV	Colon	3	1
Technetium-99m	Phosphonate (MDP)	Bone imaging	600	6 h	IV	Bladder	29	3
Technetium-99m	In vivo labelled red blood cells	Left ventricular ejection fraction measurements	800	6 h	IV	Spleen	22	6
Technetium-99m	Methoxy isobutyl isonitrile or tetrofosmin	Myocardial perfusion at rest or exercise	400	6 h	IV	Colon	7–10	3–4
Technetium-99m	Macroaggregated albumin	Lung perfusion imaging	100	6 h	IV	Lungs	7	1
Technetium-99m	Pentetate (DTPA) as aerosol	Lung ventilation imaging	80	6 h	Inhalation	Lungs	1	0.5
Technetium-99m	Exametazine hexamethylpropyleneamine oxime	Regional cerebral blood flow imaging	500	6 h	IV	Kidney	17	5
Technetium-99m	Hexamethylpropyleneamine oxime attached to leukocytes	Infection imaging	200	6 h	Leukocyte labelling and IV	Spleen	30	2
Technetium-99m	MAG3	Dynamic renal imaging	100	6 h	IV	Bladder	11	0.7
Technetium-99m	Succimer (DMSA)	Kidney imaging	80	6 h	IV	Kidneys	14	0.7
Technetium-99m	Somatostatin analogue	Neuroendocrine cancer imaging	740	6 h	IV	Kidneys	15	3

IV, Intravenous.

symptomatic tumours and metastatic spread, although hepatic metastases are difficult to visualise because of uptake in normal liver. As mentioned earlier, evidence of somatostatin receptor uptake is an essential step when considering radionuclide therapy for these tumours. Fig. 7.11 shows a technetium-99m SPECT/CT image of a patient with multiple neuroendocrine tumour metastases in the liver.

Prostate

PSMA is overexpressed in prostate cancer cells and so labelled radiopharmaceuticals are now key to the management of prostate cancer patients. Again using the diagnostic/therapeutic Ga-68/Lu-177 pair, patients can be assessed for suitability for treatment using a Ga-68 PSMA diagnostic PET scan and then treated using Lu-177 PSMA.

Thyroid

Nuclear medicine imaging of the thyroid plays a minor role in the initial diagnosis of thyroid cancer where ultrasound and fine needle aspiration (FNA) is the first-line imaging technique.[19]

The normal function of the thyroid gland includes the concentration of iodine from the circulation and the synthesis and storage of thyroid hormones. Iodine may also be trapped in the salivary glands and the gastric mucosa. I-131 was once the radionuclide of choice for all thyroid imaging. However, because it delivers a relatively high

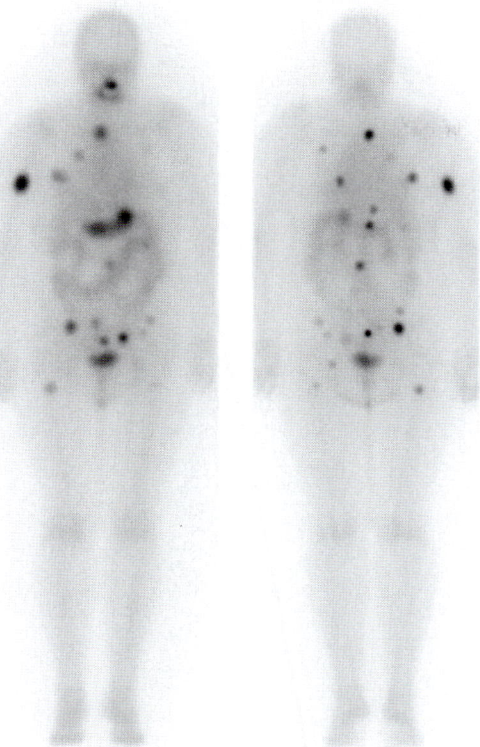

Fig. 7.16 Posttreatment whole-body iodine-131 scan.

radiation dose to the patient and it has poorer imaging properties, it has been almost completely superseded by I-123 and technetium-99m pertechnetate for routine diagnostic thyroid imaging. I-131 continues to be used for therapy (see Chapter 8) and, in some centres, for whole-body imaging in patients who have previously undergone treatment for thyroid cancer and where further disease is suspected.

Fig. 7.16 shows a whole-body I-131 scan on a patient previously treated for thyroid cancer but with widespread metastases. Sometimes suspected thyroid metastases do not appear 'hot' on the I-131 scan. In such circumstances, they may be designated to be 'not iodine avid' and an F-18 FDG study may be considered for further evaluation.

Cardiac Imaging

The most common cardiac investigation performed in the nuclear medicine department on oncology patients is gated blood pool imaging. It is correctly called *equilibrium radionuclide ventriculography* but more often termed a *multiple gated acquisition (MUGA) scan.* It is used to evaluate cardiac function, in terms of LVEF, prior to and in response to the administration of potentially cardiotoxic chemotherapeutic drugs.

The heart is a muscular organ divided internally by a septum into right and left sides, each side having two chambers. The right and left atria receive blood returning from the pulmonary and systemic circulations. The right and left ventricles are pumping chambers and are more muscular, particularly the left ventricle (LV), which pumps the blood to the systemic circulation.

LVEF is one of the major indicators of cardiac function. It can be investigated by means of a MUGA scan, which is performed generally following a two-stage injection procedure. A nonradioactive or 'cold' injection of pyrophosphate is followed 20 minutes later by administration of 400 to 800 MBq of technetium-99m pertechnetate, both administered intravenously. The 'cold' preinjection allows labelling of the patient's red cells to take place in vivo. By using the R-wave of the patient's ECG to gate (i.e. control) image acquisition, a series of 16 to 24 images is recorded during each cardiac cycle and stored in time order on a computer. Data collection continues for 10 to 15 minutes. Images of adequate spatial resolution for the purpose are obtained by summing images of identical time segments from several hundred cardiac cycles. The MUGA images can be processed to produce amplitude and phase images that aid the delineation of the LV and the demonstration of paradoxical motion. *Amplitude* refers to the magnitude of the change of the LV image intensity, while *phase* refers to the timing of the intensity change within the cycle. The LVEF is derived from the maximum counts (C_{max}) and minimum counts (C_{min}) in the LV over the cardiac cycle and is usually expressed as a percentage; see Eq. (7.1). All counts are corrected for background:

$$\mathrm{LVEF} = (C_{max} - C_{min})/C_{max} \qquad \textbf{(7.1)}$$

The technique is still widely used for LVEF estimation, as it does not rely on geometrical approximations to the shape of the heart chamber but derives its values from the entire ventricle, including any effect due to paradoxical motion. It is also less operator dependent than other assessments. Fig. 7.10 shows images from a patient with a normal LVEF.

MUGA scans image radioactive-labelled blood within the heart. Blood flow to the heart muscle itself (myocardial perfusion) can be imaged using technetium-99m MIBI or tetrofosmin. Thallium-201 was once the most common agent, but due to its higher radiation dose, more limited availability and less favourable imaging characteristics, it has been superseded by the tecehnetium-99m agents. This group of radiopharmaceuticals distribute themselves within the heart muscle according to blood flow through the coronary arteries. Tomographic images are taken under stress and at rest, and the results are used in the differential diagnosis of normal myocardial perfusion, ischemia and infarction. These studies have an important role in diagnosis of heart disease in patients with low to medium probability of heart disease and in their prognosis. The LVEF can be derived from gated myocardial perfusion tomography, but the results are not as reliable as those from a MUGA scan, particularly where the position of a substantial part of the myocardial wall must be inferred because there is no blood flow within it.[20] MUGA scanning is used extensively in monitoring cardiac output in patients being treated for breast cancer, particularly those receiving Herceptin and the anthracycline group of cytotoxic agents that can be cardiotoxic.

Kidney Imaging

The kidney produces urine and disposes of metabolic waste products. It is divided into an outer cortical region and an inner medullary region. Urine drains from the medullary region via the renal pelvis into the ureter and into the bladder. Several radiopharmaceuticals are available for imaging the kidney and investigating renal function. The choice of pharmaceutical depends on the specific renal function measurements required and the clinical condition being studied. The most common reason for renal investigation in oncology patients within nuclear medicine is to investigate suspected obstruction to urine drainage through the ureters caused by primary tumours, such as gynecological pelvic malignancy or bladder and prostate carcinomas, or by secondary metastatic disease spread to lymph nodes in the paraaortic or iliac chains, which lie adjacent to the ureters. The nonimaging test, glomerular filtration rate (GFR), is also common in oncology patients as part of the workup for the prescription of nephrotoxic drugs (e.g. carboplatin).

The most widely used radiopharmaceuticals for kidney function imaging are technetium-99m tiatide (MAG3) and pentetate (DTPA). They are suitable for the assessment of individual kidney function and investigation of drainage. With the kidneys and bladder in the field of view of the gamma camera, up to 80 MBq of technetium-99m MAG3 is injected

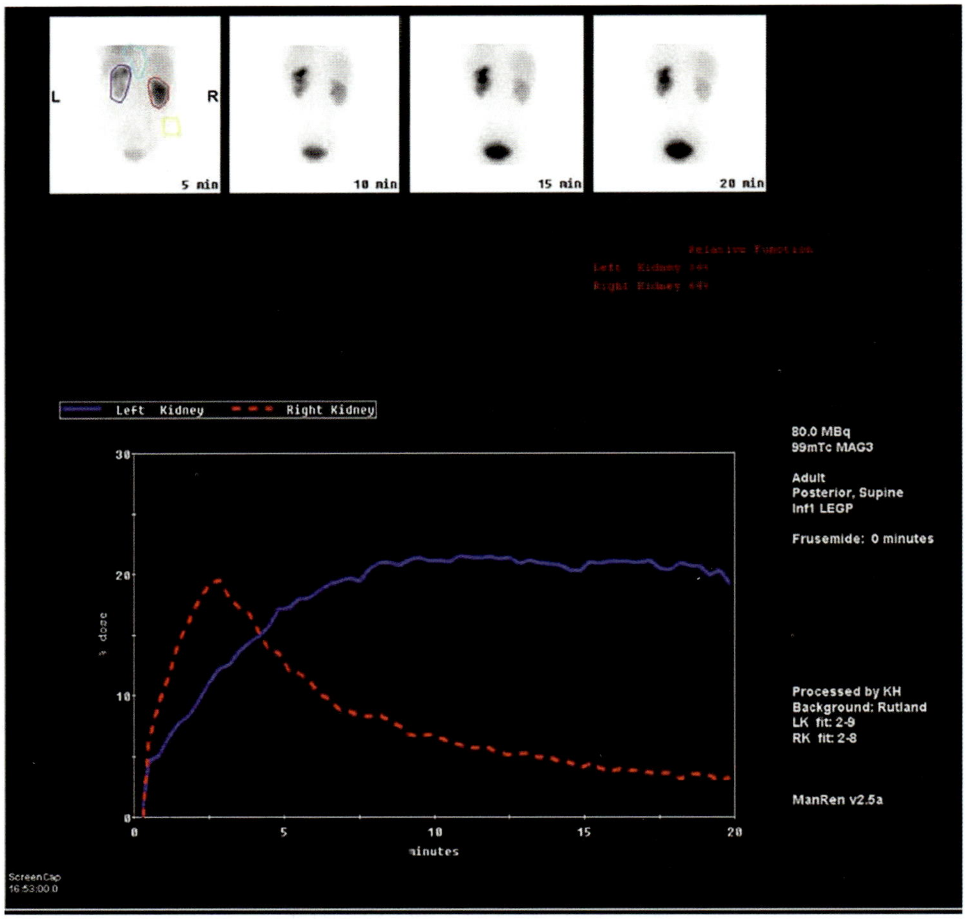

Fig. 7.17 Renogram images and clearance traces.

intravenously. For the following 20 minutes, a series of images (generally 20 seconds per frame) is acquired. Regions of interest are defined around the kidneys and bladder, and after suitable background correction, activity-time curves can be generated for each region. This set of curves is termed a *renogram*. Often, this term is also used to denote the entire investigation.

Fig. 7.17 shows the renogram results from a patient with one normally functioning kidney and one obstructed kidney.

Other renal agents include technetium-99m dimercaptosuccinic acid (DMSA), used primarily in the investigation of renal scarring, often in children.

Infection Imaging

A patient's own leukocytes (white cells) will accumulate at the site of an infection, so one method of localising infection is to label autologous white cells with a suitable radionuclide. Two are available: indium-111 and technetium-99m. Both labelling processes involve taking up to 200 mL of blood from the patient and leaving it to settle under gravity for about 1 hour. This enables reasonable separation of white cells from the rest of the blood. The cells are incubated with either indium-111 as oxine or tropolonate, or technetium-99m as HMPAO, marketed as Ceretec, which was originally developed for cerebral perfusion studies. The labelling technique is not available in many centres, as it is labor intensive, requiring skilled, experienced staff and specialised aseptic facilities. PET imaging using F-18 FDG is a good alternative to white cell labelling.

Sentinel Node Mapping

Lymphatic vessels receive cellular waste and discharge it from the body. The waste is filtered through nodes within the vessels. Metastatic spread from some tumours is carried by the lymphatics, and sites of disease may be found within the lymph nodes. Knowledge of this spread is important when staging a patient's cancer and so sentinel node mapping has become an important technique for many cancers.

Breast cancer is known to spread in this way, and almost all of the associated lymph nodes are located in the axilla. Historically, the usual approach by breast surgeons was to perform a full axillary clearance of lymph nodes along with surgical removal of the breast in patients with breast carcinoma. Should histology have subsequently failed to find any evidence of metastatic spread in the nodes, this signalled a good prognosis for the patient. Unfortunately, some of these patients went on to suffer serious morbidity associated with the removal of the lymph nodes, including severe oedema of the arm.

A technique has been developed, initially for patients being treated for breast cancer[21] to locate the lymph node(s) nearest to the tumour site, referred to as the *sentinel node(s)*. Tc-99m–labelled nanocolloid is injected subdermally or intradermally in the peripheral region of the breast containing the tumour. Gamma camera imaging post injection will identify the location of the sentinel nodes to help guide the surgeon. Fig. 7.18 shows the sentinel lymph node images of a patient immediately prior to surgery. Injection and imaging may take place either on the morning of the surgery or on the previous day. Patients will have the still-radioactive sentinel nodes located in theatre with the aid of an intraoperative probe system (Fig. 7.19). Histological evaluation of the sentinel nodes will influence the patient's subsequent treatment pathway. The technique is now being used for many other tumours and tumour sites including melanoma, vulval, penile and head and neck tumours.

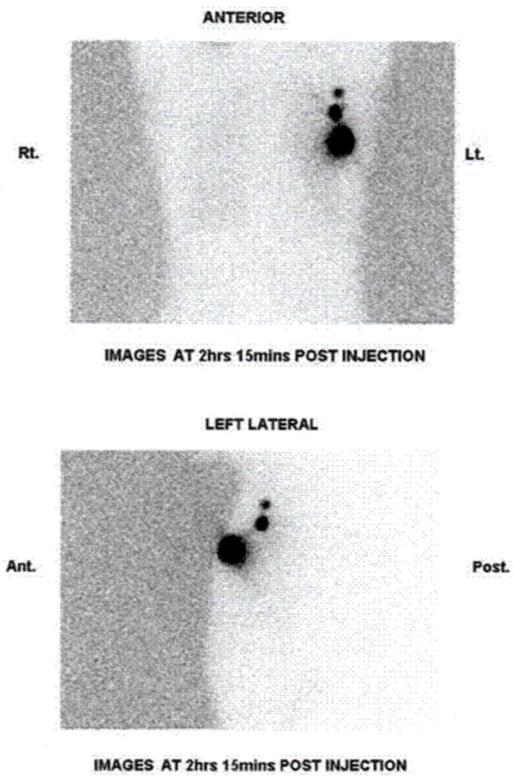

Fig. 7.18 Sentinel lymph node images of a patient immediately prior to surgery.

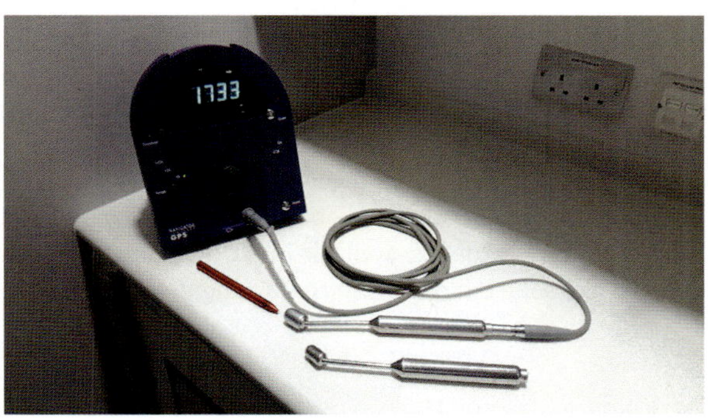

Fig. 7.19 Intraoperative lymph node probe system.

CONCLUSION

Radionuclide imaging is continually developing and plays an invaluable role in the diagnosis, staging and assessment of treatment response in cancer patients.

REFERENCES

1. Mayerhoefer ME, Prosch H, Tamandl D, et al. PET/MRI versus PET/CT in oncology: a prospective single-center study of 330 examinations focusing on implications for patient management and cost considerations. *Eur J Nucl Med Mol Imaging*. 2020;47(1): 51–60.
2. Dendy PP, Heaton B. *Physics for Diagnostic Radiology*. 3rd ed. Boca Raton, FL: CRC Press; 2012.
3. Wagenknecht G, Kaiser HJ, Mottaghy FM, Herzog H. MRI for attenuation correction in PET: methods and challenges. *Magn Reson Mater Phy*. 2013;26:99–113.
4. Cherry SR, Sorenson JA, Phelps ME. *Physics in Nuclear Medicine*. 4th ed. Philadelphia, PA: Saunders; 2012.
5. Patton J, Sandler M, Berman D, et al. D-SPECT: a new solid state camera for high speed molecular imaging. *J Nucl Med*. 2006;47(suppl 1):189P.
6. Keidar Z, Raysberg I, Lugassi R, Frenkel A, Israel O. Novel cadmium zinc telluride based detector general purpose gamma camera: initial evaluation and comparison with a standard camera. *J Nucl Med*. 2016;57(suppl 2):259.
7. Nardo L, Abdelhafez YG, Spencer BA, Badawi RD. Clinical implementation of total-body PET/CT at University of California, Davis. *PET Clin*. 2021;16(1):1–7.
8. IPEM (Institute of Physics and Engineering in Medicine). *Quality control of gamma cameras and nuclear medicine computer systems. IPEM Report 111*. York, UK: IPEM; 2015.
9. NEMA (National Electrical Manufacturers Association). *Performance measurements of gamma cameras*. NEMA NU 1-2012. https://www.nema.org/
10. IPEM (Institute of Physics and Engineering in Medicine). *Recommended standards for the routine performance testing of diagnostic x-ray imaging systems*. York, UK: IPEM; 2010 IPEM Report 91.
11. Aide N, Lasnon C, Desmonts C, Armstrong IS, Walker MD, McGowan DR. Advances in PET/CT technology: an update. *Semin Nucl Med*. 2022;52(3):286–301.
12. IPEM (Institute of Physics and Engineering in Medicine). *Quality assurance of PET and PET/CT systems*. York, UK: IPEM; 2013 IPEM Report 108.
13. NEMA (National Electrical Manufacturers Association). *Performance measurements of positron emission tomographs (PET)*. NEMA NU 2-2018. https://www.nema.org/
14. Kilbourn MR, Scott PJ. *Handbook of Radiopharmaceuticals: Methodology and Applications*. Hoboken, NJ: Wiley; 2021.
15. The Royal College of RadiologistsRoyal College of Physicians-British Nuclear Medicine SocietyAdministration of Radioactive Substances Advisory Committee. *Evidence-based indications for the use of PET-CT in the United Kingdom 2022*. London: The Royal College of Radiologists; 2022. https://www.rcr.ac.uk/our-services/all-our-publications/clinical-radiology-publications/evidence-based-indications-for-the-use-of-pet-ct-in-the-united-kingdom-2022/.
16. Sollini M, Kirienko M, Gelardi F, Fiz F, Gozzi N, Chiti A. State-of-the-art of FAPI-PET imaging: a systematic review and meta-analysis. *Eur J Nucl Med Mol Imaging*. 2021;48(13):4396–4414.
17. Decristoforo C, Mather SJ, Cholewinski W, Donnemiller E, Riccabona G, Moncayo R. 99mTc-EDDA/HYNIC-TOC: a new 99mTc-labelled radiopharmaceutical for imaging somatostatin receptor-positive tumours: first clinical results and intrapatient comparison with 111In-labelled octreotide derivatives. *Eur J Nucl Med*. 2000;27:1318–1325.
18. ICRP Publication 53 and Subsequent Addenda. Radiation dose to patients from radiopharmaceuticals. *Ann ICRP*. 1988;18 1–4.
19. Schoedel KE, Tublin ME, Pealer K, Ohori NP. Ultrasound-guided biopsy of the thyroid: a comparison of technique with respect to diagnostic accuracy. *Diagn Cytopathol*. 2008;36(11):787–789.
20. Bartlett ML, Srinivasan G, Barker WC, Kitsiou AN, Dilsizian V, Bacharach SL. Left ventricular ejection fraction: comparison of results from planar and SPECT gated blood-pool studies. *J Nucl Med*. 1996;37(11):1795–1799.
21. Mansel RE, Fallowfield L, Kissin M, et al. Randomized multicenter trial of sentinel node biopsy versus standard axillary treatment in operable breast cancer: the almanac trial. *J Natl Cancer Inst*. 2006;98(9):599–609.

8

Therapy With Unsealed Radionuclides

Amit Nautiyal, Matthew Aldridge and Sofia Michopoulou

CHAPTER OUTLINE

INTRODUCTION

Radionuclide therapy, *molecular radiotherapy* and *internal radiation therapy* are some of the terms used for treatments involving administration of unsealed or dispersible radioactive sources to patients.

Radionuclide therapy is used for both benign and malignant conditions. Cell targeting can be due to chemical or physical properties of the radiopharmaceutical, such as the mechanical entrapment of microspheres in liver capillaries, or by means of carrier molecules that attach to receptors guiding the radionuclide to the target tissue.

The aim of radionuclide therapy is to deliver a sufficient radiation dose that maximises the cytotoxic effect to the target tissue while sparing normal tissues and thus limiting toxicities to normal organs at risk. This can be achieved by selecting pharmaceuticals that maximise the ratio between the amount deposited in the target tissue and the amount deposited in nontarget tissue. Furthermore, the radionuclide properties are chosen so as to deposit energy locally to the target tissue. Most radionuclide therapies use beta-emitting radionuclides with a soft tissue range of a few millimetres. Recently, alpha-emitting radionuclides were also introduced in clinical practice. Alpha emitters have a range of just a few micrometers in tissue and very high linear energy transfer, resulting in local energy deposition and a highly targeted cytotoxic effect. Some alpha- and beta-emitting radionuclides additionally emit gamma photons which enable imaging the distribution of the radiopharmaceutical in the body using a gamma camera, as described in Chapter 7, and can provide data for dosimetry calculations. The physical properties of radionuclides commonly used in therapeutic applications are outlined in Table 8.1.

Dosimetry for radionuclide therapy is performed using the Medical Internal Radiation Dosimetry (MIRD) scheme.[1] The radiation dose, D, delivered from a source organ, s, to a target organ, t, is given by the accumulated activity, Ã, in the source organ and the S-Factor, S ($t \leftarrow s$), as outlined in Eq. (8.1). The accumulated activity in the source organ is calculated by integrating the radioactivity in this organ over time, as shown in Fig. 8.1C. The details of radiation-absorbed dose-per-unit-administered activity for some radiopharmaceuticals are outlined in Table 8.2. The radioactivity in the source organ clears with an effective half-life (T_{eff}), which depends on the physical half-life of the radionuclide (T_{phys}) and the biological clearance of the pharmaceutical (T_{biol}), as outlined in Eq. (8.2). The S-factor depends on the physical properties of the radiation, that is, the type of radiation and the energy, as well as the size and shape of the target organ and its distance from the source organ. S-factor values are calculated using Monte Carlo simulations based on anthropomorphic models of the body. Tables of these factors are available in the literature for a variety of radionuclides and source-target organ combinations[1,2]:

$$D = \tilde{A} \cdot S \quad \textbf{(8.1)}$$

$$\frac{1}{T_{eff}} = \frac{1}{T_{phys}} + \frac{1}{T_{biol}} \quad \textbf{(8.2)}$$

Radionuclide therapy has been in use since the 1940s, but it has recently experienced rapid growth, with new therapies being introduced into clinical practice[6] such as radium-223 (^{223}Ra) dichloride for bone palliation, lutetium-177 (^{177}Lu)-dotatate for the treatment of neuroendocrine tumours and Yttrium-90 (^{90}Y) for selective internal radiation treatment (SIRT) for liver metastasis, as shown in Fig. 8.2. More recently, lutetium-177 prostate-specific membrane antigen (PSMA) has emerged as a promising treatment for metastatic castration-resistant prostate cancer (mCRPC) and has demonstrated improved progression-free and overall survival compared to standard care regimens.[7]

Many of these new therapies are performed in a theranostic context. The principle of *theranostics* is the utilisation of a diagnostic and therapeutic pair of radionuclides, generally using the same pharmaceutical as a carrier, with pretreatment imaging used to stratify patients for molecular radiotherapy. A good example of a theranostic pair is ^{68}Ga/^{177}Lu, which, when labelled with a somatostatin analogue such as dotatate, can identify appropriate patients using positron emission tomography–computed tomography (PET/CT) imaging, as outlined in Figs. 8.1A and B.

TABLE 8.1 Properties of the Radionuclides Used in Therapy

			ALPHA/BETA EMISSION		GAMMA EMISSION	
Radionuclide	Physical Half-life (days)	Therapeutic Radiation	Mean Energy (MeV)	Mean Range in Soft Tissue (mm)	Energy (MeV)	% Abundance
^{131}I	8.02	Beta	0.182	0.6	0.364	81.7
^{223}Ra	11.4	Alpha	5.78	<0.1	0.154	6.04
					0.269	13.6
^{177}Lu	6.7	Beta	0.13	0.6	0.208	11
					0.117	6.4
^{90}Y	2.7	Beta	0.935	3.6	–	–
^{32}P	14.3	Beta	0.70	3.0	–	–
^{89}Sr	50.5	Beta	0.58	2.4	0.909	0.01
^{153}Sm	1.9	Beta	0.22	0.6	0.103	28
^{169}Er	9.4	Beta	0.099	0.3	–	–
^{186}Re	3.8	Beta	0.33	1.1	0.137	9
^{166}Ho	26.8	Beta	1.79	2.2	0.080	6.7
^{225}Ac	9.92	Alpha	5.8–8.4	0.04–0.08	0.440	26.1
					0.218	11.6

TABLE 8.2 Radiation Absorbed Dose, mGy/MBq, for Some Radiopharmaceuticals[3–5]

Radiopharmaceutical	Target Organs and Average Dose Absorbed per Unit Administred Activity (mGy/MBq)	Typical Administered Activity A (MBq)
^{131}I sodium iodide: carcinoma	Bladder wall: 0.39; marrow: 0.09; kidneys: 0.27; colon: 0.14; salivary:0.19 (considering medium thyroid uptake)	1100–3700
^{131}I sodium iodide: thyrotoxicosis	Kidneys: 0.77; bladder wall: 0.29; marrow: 0.08	400
^{223}Ra dichloride	Kidneys: 3.2; liver: 3; bladder wall: 4	3.85
^{131}I meta-iodobenzylguanidine	Kidneys: 0.12; bladder wall: 0.59; salivary glands: 0.23	11000
^{177}Lu177 dotatate	Kidneys: 0.32–1.67; liver: 0.05–0.21; marrow: 0.02–0.07	7400
^{177}Lu177 prostate-specific membrane antigen	Salivery glands: 0.39; kidneys: 0.50; lacrimal: 2.26	7400
^{90}Y-microspheres	Lungs: 0.01–1.35	2100
^{32}P sodium phosphate	Red marrow: 11	200
^{89}Sr strontium chloride	Red marrow: 19	150
^{166}Holmium microspheres	Lungs: 0.02–1.35	6700
^{225}Actinium prostate-specific membrane antigen	Salivery glands: 2300; kidneys: 700; red marrow: 50	5.55
^{90}Y-zevalin	Red marrow: 0.83; liver: 3; kidneys: 2.3	900

Further theranostic pairs and their properties are outlined in Table 8.3. Furthermore, the diagnostic component of theranostics allows for personalised evaluation of biokinetics and dosimetry, providing a useful tool in predicting which patients will respond optimally to therapy.

In clinical practice, the radionuclide therapy service is delivered by a multidisciplinary team of healthcare professionals. Typically, treatment selection is jointly performed by oncologists and nuclear medicine physicians based on clinical examination, prior imaging and blood indices. Dosimetry calculations are performed by medical physicists. The therapy administration is supported by nuclear medicine physicians, technologists and physicists working together, although this may vary from centre to centre.

IODINE-131 IN THE TREATMENT OF THYROID DISEASE

Iodine-131 (^{131}I) is the radionuclide most widely used therapeutically and has been used in the treatment of thyroid conditions since the 1940s. Iodine accumulates in the thyroid gland, and the use of ^{131}I, with the emission of beta particles with a maximum range of 3 mm in tissue, allows a high-radiation dose to be delivered to the thyroid and a low dose to the rest of the body. It is most commonly used in the form of sodium iodide (^{131}I) for treatment of the benign thyroid diseases thyrotoxicosis and nontoxic goiter and of thyroid carcinoma.

The characteristics of ^{131}I are shown in Table 8.1. As specified by the Society of Nuclear Medicine (SNM)[8] and the European Association of Nuclear Medicine (EANM)[9] it is essential that, before any treatment, all thyroid hormones, iodine-containing preparations and supplements and any other medications that could suppress thyroid uptake are discontinued for a sufficient length of time. Almost all thyroid treatments are given orally, as a capsule or as a liquid.

Thyroid Cancer

Within differentiated thyroid cancer (DTC), the carcinoma retains characteristics of healthy thyroid tissue including expression of the sodium iodide symporter, enabling uptake of radioiodine. The treatment is associated with a 10-year overall cause-specific survival of 85%; see Chapter 24 for more information about thyroid cancer. Radioiodine therapy may be subdivided into *ablation*, a postsurgical procedure used to eliminate

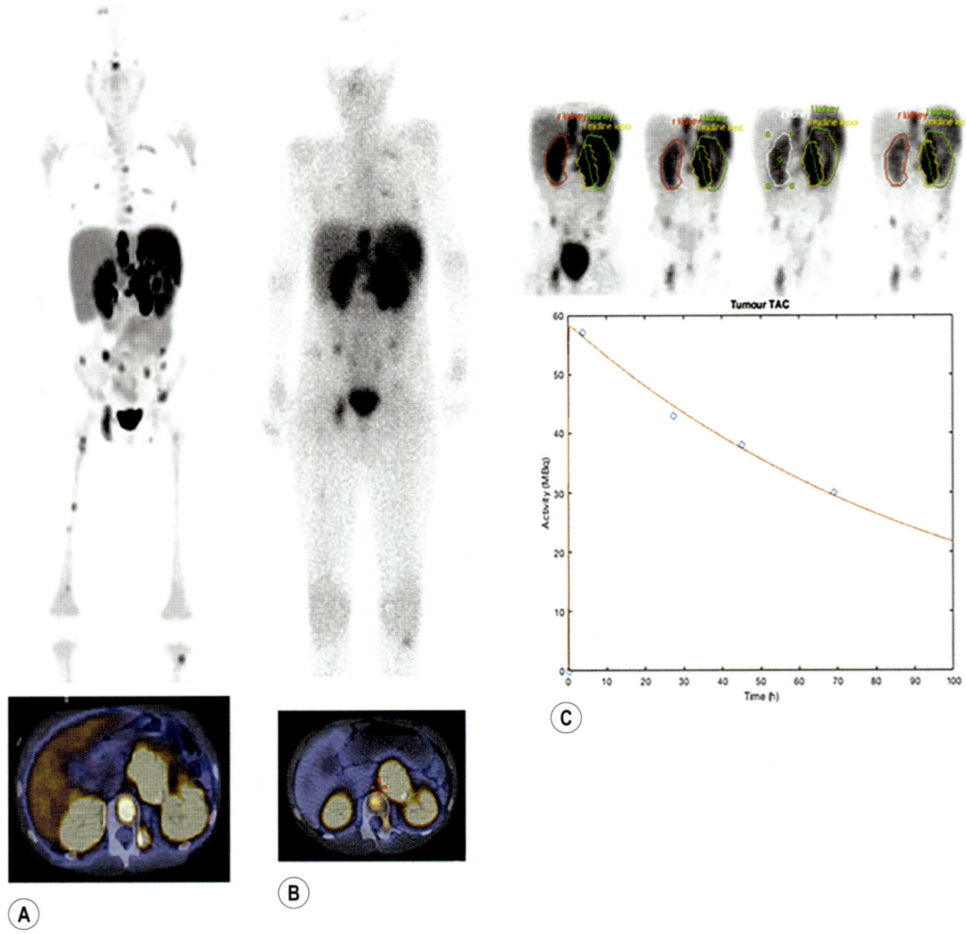

Fig. 8.1 A ^{68}Ga/^{177}Lu-dotatate theranostic example. (A) A diagnostic ^{68}Ga-dotatate positron emission tomography–computed tomography scan showed multiple dotatate avid lesions confirming patient eligibility for treatment. (B) A ^{177}Lu-dotatate posttherapy single photon emission computerised tomography–computed tomography verified distribution of therapeutic activity and facilitated dosimetry. (C) Tumour dosimetry based on planar ^{177}Lu-dotatate therapy scintigraphy. The accumulated activity in the tumour is calculated from the tumour counts obtained at 2, 24, 48 and 70 hours post administration.

thyroid remnants; or as a component of primary curative treatment in the setting of nonresectable or incompletely resectable lesions.

Following total thyroidectomy, the aim of remnant ablation is to destroy any remaining normal thyroid tissue and any microscopic deposits of thyroid carcinoma.[10] The usual activity administered for ablation is 3.7 GBq (gigabecquerels), although in the low-to-intermediate-risk group, lower activity of 1.1 GBq is being used instead.[11] By destroying any remaining thyroid tissue, the theory is that the only remaining source of thyroglobulin production is any remaining malignant cells, thus making the measurement of

TABLE 8.3 Theranostic Pairs Currently Being Used or Evaluated

Diagnostic Component	Therapeutic Component	Target	Disease
^{68}Ga-PSMA, ^{18}F-PSMA, ^{99m}Tc-PSMA, ^{203}Pb-PSMA	^{177}Lu-PSMA, ^{225}Ac-PSMA, ^{212}Pb-PSMA	PSMA	Ca-Prostate
^{99m}Tc-MAA/^{166}Ho-microspheres	^{90}Y-microspheres/^{166}Ho-microspheres	Hepatic microvasculature	Hepatocellular carcinoma/liver metastasis
^{68}Ga-Pentixafor	^{177}Lu-Pentixather	CXCR4	Multiple myeloma
^{99m}Tc-MDP	^{223}Ra	Hydroxyapatite	Ca-Prostate
^{68}Ga-dotanoc, ^{111}In-Octreotate, ^{99m}Tc-Octreotate, ^{64}Cu-dotatate	^{177}Lu-dotatate, ^{90}Y-dotatate, ^{225}Ac-dotatate	SSTR	Neuroendocrine tumors
^{123}I-NaI	^{131}I-NaI	Sodium/iodide symporter	Ca-Thyroid
^{123}I-MIBG	^{131}I-MIBG	Neuroendocrine cells	Neuroblastoma, PCC
^{89}Zr-Trastuzumab	^{177}Lu-Trastuzumab	HER2	Ca-Breast
^{11}C-methylbenzamide	^{211}At-methylene blue	GRM1	Melanomas
^{64}Cu-Tz	^{67}Cu-Tz	Tumour-specific antigens	RIT

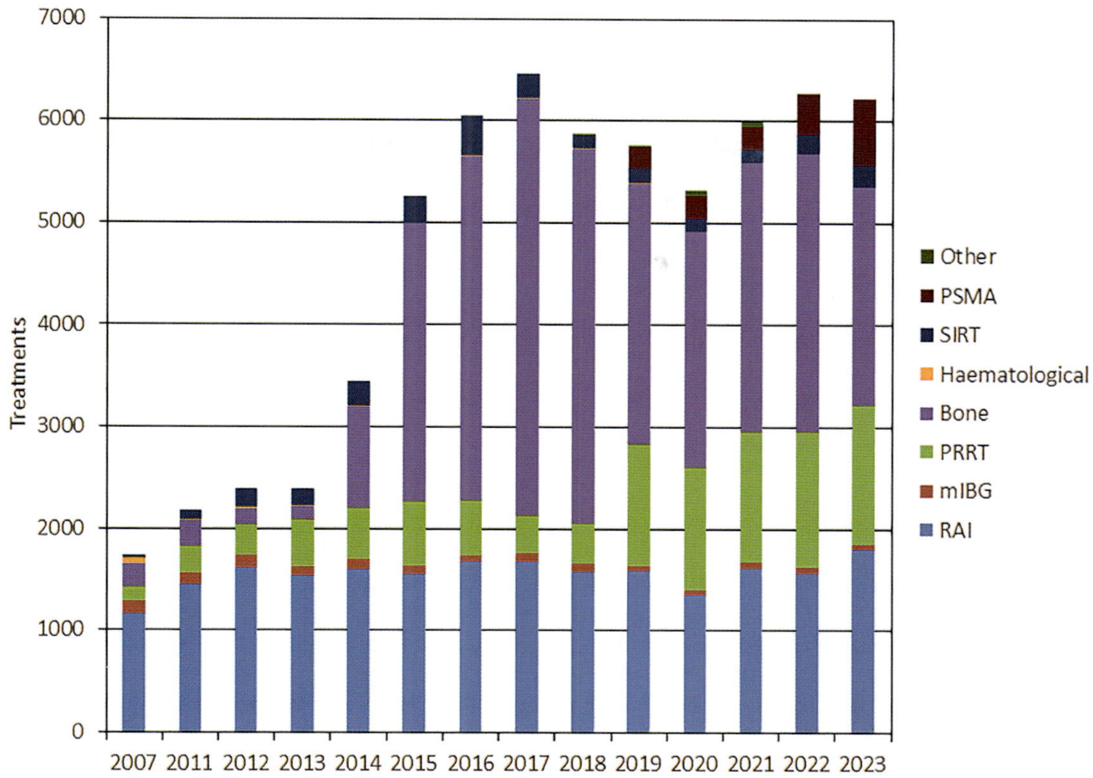

Fig. 8.2 Number of administrations for common types of radionuclide therapy in UK centres participating in the Internal Dosimetry Users Group Survey between 2007 and 2023. (Courtesy Bruno Rojas.)

thyroglobulin level a sensitive test of any local recurrence or metastatic disease.

Metastatic lesions have a lower avidity for iodine than normal thyroid tissue, and it is customary to administer higher activities of 3.7 to 5.5 GBq.[11] Treatments for thyroid cancer require an inpatient stay in a dedicated treatment room with appropriate resources, due to the high external dose rates from these patients contributing to significant dose to the public, their family and any comforter and carer. As such, patients are monitored during their stay until the level of radioactivity has fallen sufficiently for safe discharge, as outlined in the Medical and Dental Guidance Notes (MDGN).[12]

To improve the effectiveness of treatment, the remaining thyroid tissue may be stimulated by elevating the level of thyroid-stimulating hormone (TSH), with the effect of aiding the absorption of radioiodine.[11] One method is to withhold thyroid hormone medication for 2 to 4 weeks and allow TSH to increase. However, this is associated with hypothyroid symptoms in most patients. The alternative is to administer Thyrogen, a protein designed to be identical to TSH, as a prescription medication given in two injections prior to treatment or diagnostic testing.

Gamma camera images, using the 364-keV photons of ^{131}I, may be obtained after treatment to confirm uptake in residual thyroid recurrence or metastases.[11] Scanning protocols may also be used after surgery and before ablation to, for instance, determine the completeness of ablation as part of a patient's treatment. Iodine-123 may provide a suitable alternative for follow-up. Hybrid single photon emission computerised tomography–computed tomography (SPECT/CT) imaging, described in Chapter 7, enables precise anatomical localisation of any residual disease and metastatic spread.

Benign Thyroid Disease

The overproduction of thyroid hormones manifests in patients as hyperthyroidism, arising from benign conditions such as Graves disease, toxic or nontoxic goiter and solitary hyperfunctioning thyroid nodule. As iodine is a component of the thyroid hormones LT4 (tetraiodothyronine, T4) and L-triiodothyronine (T3), it is readily extracted from the blood and incorporated into L3 and L4 when administered as radioiodine. Approaches to radionuclide therapy have included giving sufficient radioiodine to render the patient hypothyroid and giving low activities of ^{131}I in combination with an antithyroid drug.[13] However, the Royal College of Physicians (RCP) recommend that the aim of treatment should be to render the patient euthyroid while accepting that there will be a moderate rate of hypothyroidism.[14]

Assessment of thyroid function and eligibility for treatment may be performed using ^{123}I-labelled sodium iodide or ^{99m}Tc-pertechnetate. Pertechnetate ions are trapped through the active transport mechanism in the same manner as ^{123}I- or ^{131}I-labelled sodium iodide, and thyroid function may be evaluated by measuring the percentage uptake of administered activity.

According to national regulations, the treatment may be given on an outpatient basis, assuming that an appropriate risk assessment has been undertaken, principally with regard to contact patterns with other members of the public.[12] The range of activities currently prescribed varies between 200 and 800 MBq (megabecquerel).[13] If therapy is performed on an inpatient basis, particularly in the case of paediatric patients, this should take place in the appropriate environment with the necessary resources required by national legislation.

PALLIATION OF BONE PAIN

Radionuclide therapy gives an additional possibility for the palliation of bone pain arising from osteoblastic metastases, which are seen in some cancers with a high prevalence, such as prostate and breast carcinoma. This systemic approach may be used for patients with multifocal osteoblastic metastases as an alternative to external beam radiotherapy, or for those whose pain is refractory to conventional analgesia or antitumour therapy.[15] Before administration of the treatment, it is essential to verify that there is evidence of focal increased uptake on bone scintigraphy (Chapter 7). Such increased uptake is due to an osseous reaction to the development of metastases, and if it is not present on a gamma camera bone scan using a ^{99m}Tc imaging agent (e.g. MDP or HDP; see Chapter 7), there will be no selective uptake of the therapeutic radionuclide and therefore no benefit.

A variety of bone-seeking radionuclides are available for bone palliation, including beta emitters such as ^{89}Sr, ^{153}Sm and ^{223}Ra (an alpha emitter). ^{223}Radium-dichloride (Xofigo) is the most widely used radiopharmaceutical and has been shown to not only provide pain relief but also improve overall survival in patients with castration-resistant prostate cancer (CRPC).[16] It is currently undergoing clinical trials to assess its efficacy for breast carcinoma.[17] ^{223}Radium-dichloride selectively accumulates in areas of high bone turnover by forming complexes with hydroxyapatite, the inorganic component of the bone. ^{223}Ra has a half-life of 11.4 days and a mean alpha energy of 5.78 MeV (megaelectron volts). The alpha particles have a high linear energy transfer and can thus deposit their energy over a short range (<100 μm), resulting in double-strand DNA breaks and highly localised cytotoxic effects. Additionally, this short range of ^{223}Ra minimises myelosuppression, a known risk of beta emitters such as ^{89}Sr, with a range of 2.4 mm.[16] ^{223}Ra also emits low-abundance (<2%) gamma photons with energies of 82, 154 and 270 keV. These can be imaged with a gamma camera to confirm uptake on bone metastasis.

A standard treatment course of ^{223}Ra comprises six administrations at 4-week intervals, and the activity delivered is typically adjusted by patient weight, with 55 kBq/kg given to patients with prostate cancer.[18] Posttherapy imaging offers the additional opportunity to perform personalised dosimetry and customise the injected activity of subsequent administration to the individual patient.[19]

^{223}Ra is routinely given as an outpatient treatment and is generally well tolerated, with the most common side effects being diarrhoea or vomiting as the radiopharmaceutical is mostly eliminated through the fecal route. Being an alpha emitter, the posttherapy radiation protection restrictions required are minimal and focus on good hygiene to reduce the risk of radioactive contamination.[18]

MOLECULAR RADIOTHERAPY TREATMENT OF NEUROENDOCRINE TUMOURS

Neuroendocrine tumours are a complex group of tumours derived from the primitive neural crest, which develops to form the sympathetic nervous system (SNS). Malignant neuroendocrine tumours include phaeochromocytoma; neuroblastoma; carcinoid tumours including gastroenteropancreatic tract neuroendocrine tumours; paraganglioma; and medullary thyroid cancer.

Neuroendocrine tumours demonstrate targets for molecular radiotherapy in that they frequently express somatostatin receptors (SSTRs) on their cell surface, enabling them to be imaged with somatostatin analogues such as ^{111}In-pentetreotide (Octreoscan) or ^{99m}Tc-HYNIC-TOC (Tektrotyd) on a gamma camera. More recently, somatostatin imaging has been achieved using PET radiopharmaceuticals such as ^{68}Ga-dotatate and utilising the advantages conferred by PET imaging over planar imaging: improved spatial resolution, contrast and the ability to perform whole-body scanning in a short time.[20]

Peptide receptor radionuclide therapy (PRRT) uses similar somatostatin analogues as in diagnostic imaging but instead is labelled with therapeutic radionuclides, with the most commonly used being yttrium-90 (^{90}Y) and lutetium-177 (^{177}Lu).[21] Both are beta emitters, ^{90}Y having a maximum energy of 2.3 MeV and tissue penetration of 12 mm and ^{177}Lu having a maximum energy of 0.5 MeV and tissue penetration of 2 mm. Both the ^{90}Y and ^{177}Lu peptides demonstrate rapid blood and urinary clearance, with the main dose-limiting organ being the kidneys. For this reason it is common to coadminister the amino acids L-lysine and L-arginine to block the renal tubules and hence afford protection.[21]

^{177}Lu emits gamma radiation of low abundance, making it suitable for gamma camera imaging, and its half-life of 6.7 days enables dosimetric evaluation. Typical administered activities are between 3.5 GBq and 7.4 GBq, although this may be modulated, taking into account renal toxicity and individualised dosimetry. A fractionated approach is optimal, with at least four administrations, each separated by 8 to 12 weeks. Patients may require admission to a dedicated radionuclide therapy room for a period of time determined by national regulations.[21] A phase 3 Neuroendocrine Tumors Therapy (NETTER-1) trial found that ^{177}Lu-dotatate therapy increases progression-free survival in patients with advanced midgut neuroendocrine tumours.[22]

These tumour types offer another target for molecular radiotherapy (MRT) in the form of noradrenaline transporter expression, which can be a predictor of tumoural uptake of meta-iodobenzylguanidine (mIBG). A noradrenaline analogue, mIBG can be labelled with iodine-131 (^{131}I).

Before treatment, any drugs known to interfere with the uptake and/or retention of ^{131}I-mIBG must be withdrawn in accordance with the European Guidelines.[23] A thyroid-blocking agent such as potassium iodide must be prescribed, starting before and continuing for an extended period after treatment, to protect the gland from taking up any free ^{131}I with the subsequent risk of developing hypothyroidism. The dose-limiting toxicity is hematological, and monitoring of blood counts is essential after treatment.

Eligibility for treatment can be assessed by ^{123}I-mIBG imaging on a gamma camera or ^{124}I-mIBG on a PET/CT camera to confirm uptake in tumour sites. Uptake can also be confirmed with a low activity of ^{131}I-mIBG, and all radionuclides exhibit gamma emissions such that dosimetry can be assessed.

In routine practice, the majority of centres administer fixed ^{131}I mIBG activities of 3.7 to 11.1 GBq every 3 to 6 months. Because several therapeutic doses may be required to achieve objective response, these activities are often repeated at varied intervals.[20]

Neuroblastoma is a predominantly childhood cancer that peaks in incidence in young children. Over 50% of patients present with high-risk disease, and ^{131}I-mIBG may also be used in relapsed or refractory neuroblastoma, with 90% of neuroblastoma mIBG avid. Treatment of very young children poses challenges resulting from radiation safety requirements associated with the administration of ^{131}I-mIBG therapy.

Myelosuppresion is the main dose-limiting toxicity, necessitating stem cell reinfusion at higher administered activities.[24]

These treatments are well tolerated by patients, with very few side effects reported.

SELECTIVE INTERNAL RADIATION THERAPY

Selective internal radiation therapy (SIRT) or radioembolisation is a safe and effective treatment for unresectable primary and secondary liver cancer.

SIRT uses yttrium-90 (^{90}Y)-microspheres which are injected through a catheter into the liver vasculature, as shown in Fig. 8.3. The microspheres are mechanically trapped inside the tumour, delivering high-radiation dose to the tumour with a relatively low dose to the normal liver parenchyma.[25] ^{90}Y is a high-energy beta-emitting radionuclide. Its physical properties are provided in Table 8.1. It has an average range of 4 mm in tissue and can travel over 10 metres in air, but it can be easily shielded by 10 mm of acrylic. ^{90}Y does not have any gamma emissions but is accompanied by the emission of secondary bremsstrahlung X photons which can be exploited for imaging.

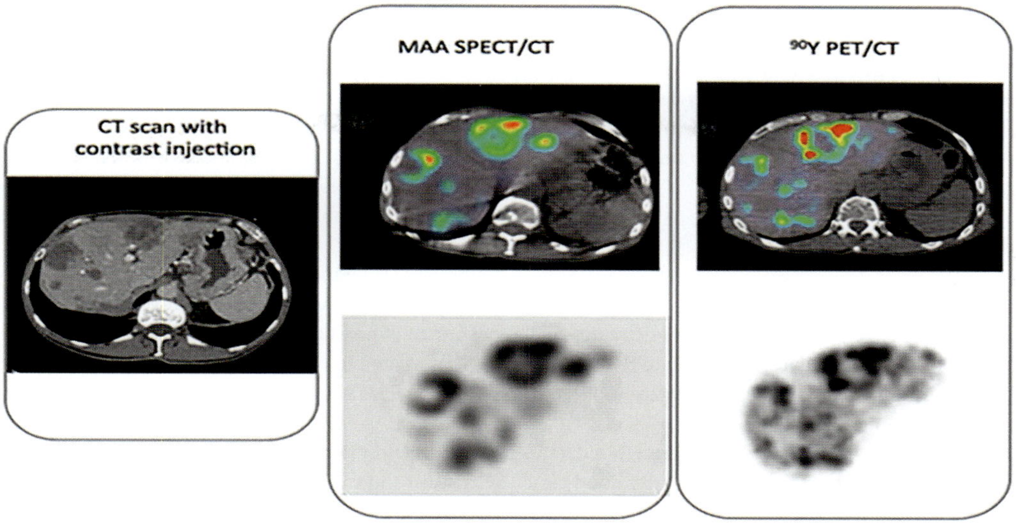

Fig. 8.3 Example of pretherapy imaging and posttherapy imaging in a patient with colorectal metastases. (From d'Abadie P, Walrand S, Lhommel R, Hesse M, Jamar F. A theranostic approach in SIRT: Value of pre-therapy imaging in treatment planning. *J Clin Med.* 2022 Jan;11(23):7245.[49]) *CT*, Computed tomography; *MAA*, macroaggregated albumin; *PET*, positron emission tomography; *SPECT*, single photon emission computerised tomography.

As of 2018, two commercial microsphere products are available worldwide:

- Glass spheres (theraspheres) with a diameter of 20 to 30 µm. These are injected in limited numbers (1 to 4 million particles at 2500 Bq per particle), producing lower embolic effects (blockage of the vessels), which makes them suitable for patients with compromised portal venous flow.[25]
- Resin spheres (SIRTEX) of 20 to 60 µm in diameter which use a large number of spheres for the same desired activity (20 to 60 million particles at 50 Bq per particle), resulting in more uniform distribution of radiation dose and larger embolic effect than theraspheres.[25]

The SIRT patient pathway is complex and requires combined expertise from oncology, interventional radiology and nuclear medicine departments.

In the 2 weeks prior to treatment, a planning angiography is performed to identify the tumour-perfusing vessels and to assess portal vein patency. Once the optimal catheter position has been identified, ^{99m}Tc-labelled macroaggregated albumin (MAA) is administered, acting as a surrogate for the microspheres.

Planar scintigraphy and/or SPECT/CT imaging of the ^{99m}Tc MAA distribution is used to evaluate the tumour perfusion, quantify shunting to the lung which could result in radiation pneumonitis and exclude any reflux to the gastrointestinal tract.[25] Chapter 7 outlines the imaging principles of planar scintigraphy and/or SPECT/CT.

The required therapeutic activity is then determined by dosimetry evaluation of the ^{99m}Tc MAA images using the MIRD methodology, empirical calculations such as the body surface area method, the partition model or Monte Carlo simulation techniques.[26]

Treatment is performed in the angiography suite, with the catheter placed at the same position as for the ^{99m}Tc MAA injection. Following the therapeutic injection, patients are hospitalised for clinical reasons. Radiation protection precautions following therapy relate to external dose rate from bremsstrahlung radiation and a small amount of urinary excretion.[27]

Posttherapy verification of the ^{90}Y distribution can be performed through bremstrahlung imaging using planar or SPECT scintigraphy. Alternatively, posttherapy PET imaging exploiting the low abundance of pair production which occurs in the ^{90}Y decay may be used.

In 2019, holmium-166 (^{166}Ho)-microspheres were approved for liver treatment in the European Union. A beta emitter, ^{166}Ho also has a gamma component which makes it suitable for SPECT imaging, and it's a lanthanide that is detectable using magnetic resonance imaging (MRI). This enables pretherapy dosimetry using the ^{166}Ho-microspheres, which eliminates the need to use ^{99m}Tc MAA as a surrogate for microspheres and has superior predictive value for intrahepatic distribution.[28]

PHOSPHORUS-32 IN THE TREATMENT OF REFRACTORY MYELOPROLIFERATIVE DISEASE

Phosphorus-32 (^{32}P) phosphate is used in the treatment of polycythaemia rubra vera (PRV) and essential thrombocythaemia. Although its use is in decline, it has a role in patients over 70 years of age who are resistant to other treatments such as venesection and conventional chemotherapy.[29]

The ^{32}P radionuclide is a pure beta-emitting radionuclide with a mean particle range in tissue of 3 mm and a maximum of 8 mm. It is typically administered by intravenous injection with an activity of between 150 and 250 MBq, and there is no requirement for an inpatient stay.[30]

INTRAARTICULAR AND INTRACAVITARY TREATMENTS

Radiation synovectomy/radiosynoviorthesis (RS) is a molecular radiotherapy modality used for the treatment of chronic inflammatory joints. It involves the intraarticular injection of radiopharmaceuticals either on an inpatient or outpatient basis, dependent on local regulations.

The beta-emitting radiopharmaceuticals ^{90}Y, ^{186}Re and ^{169}Er (see Table 8.1) can be used to penetrate and ablate the synovial tissue. It is injected as a colloid, with an ideal particle size of 10 nm, which results in a homogeneous distribution within the joint cavity and minimal lymphatic clearance. The affected joint should be immobilised for 48h post injection. Eligibility for treatment can be assessed with ^{99m}Tc MDP/HDP/HEDP, used to detect synovial inflammation.

As a general rule, yttrium-90 (^{90}Y) silicate/citrate is used for large joints such as the knee; rhenium-186 (^{186}Re) sulfide for medium-sized joints such as the hip, shoulder or ankle; and erbium-169 (^{169}Er) citrate for small joints as in the fingers.[31] This is due to the differences in soft-tissue range, with the greater range of ^{90}Y used for larger joints.

Appropriate radiation protection considerations are required to protect both the patient and the medical staff performing the procedure. It is essential to use Perspex syringe shields to reduce radiation exposure to the fingers.

RADIOIMMUNOTHERAPY

Radioimmunotherapy (RIT) uses engineered monoclonal antibodies paired with radionuclides. When injected into the bloodstream, they bind to cancer cells and deliver a high radiation directly to the tumour. In contrast to most treatments already discussed, which are well established, RIT is a relatively new and growing field.

In non-Hodgkin's lymphoma (NHL), ^{90}Y ibritumomab tiuxetan (Zevalin) is an approved treatment targeting the CD 20 antibody, for the treatment of relapsed follicular NHL which is refractory to chemotherapy. It is prescribed as 15 MBq/kg, with a maximum of 1.2 GBq, and the dose-limiting toxicity is haematological.[32]

RADIOLIGAND THERAPY USING PROSTATE-SPECIFIC MEMBRANE ANTIGEN FOR METASTATIC PROSTATE CANCER

Prostate cancer is one of the most common cancers among males. Over the past decades, prostate cancer cases have rapidly increased in populations around the world. Prostate cancer mainly presents with the localised disease inside the prostate gland. However, a significant proportion of patients still show advanced progressive metastatic disease, that is, the metastatic castration-resistant stage of prostate carcinoma (mCRPC), for which no curative treatment is available.[33] There are 48,500 new prostate cancer cases in the United Kingdom every year (2015–2017). Incidence rates are projected to increase by 12% between 2014 and 2035 in the United Kingdom to 233 cases per 100,000 in 2035 (cancer incidence statistics, 2021). Approximately 10% to 20% of patients with prostate cancer will develop castration resistance within 5 years, and 84% of patients have metastatic disease at the time of castration resistance.[34]

In radioligand therapy (RLT), radiation is delivered directly to cancer cells using specific radioligands. In clinical practice, RLT targeting PSMA ligands has recently been introduced for the treatment of mCRPC. PSMA is a transmembrane glycoprotein expressed on the surface of prostate cells.[35] PSMA is also thought to have multiple functions related to nutrient uptake, cell survival and migration.[36] The theranostic PSMA ligand PSMA-617 directed towards the PSMA receptors is an effective treatment option to treat prostate cancers having greater PSMA expression. Patients having advanced prostate cancer or mCRPC disease show greater expression of PSMA compared to the rest of the prostate cancers, as shown in Fig. 8.4. The PSMA receptor has an internalisation process which allows radiolabelled PSMA to enter and bind to the extracellular space of PSMA receptors, resulting in DNA damage to cancer cells, which makes it an ideal target for RLT.[37]

The most commonly used theranostic radiopharmaceutical for RLT is ^{177}Lu-PSMA (β and γ emitter). The indications of this treatment are patients having mCRPC disease who have not benefitted from standard care treatments such as chemotherapy or radiotherapy and who have adequate uptake of PSMA ligands at the time of pretherapy imaging (^{68}Ga-PSMA or ^{18}F-PSMA PET scans).[38] A standard activity of 7.4 GBq ^{177}Lu-PSMA can be administered at 6-week intervals over four to six treatment cycles (depending on response and organ toxicities). Activity is administered by slow intravenous injection. Before administration of activity, the patient should be well hydrated (intravenous or oral hydration). If the patient has a low cardiovascular risk, 1 to 2 L

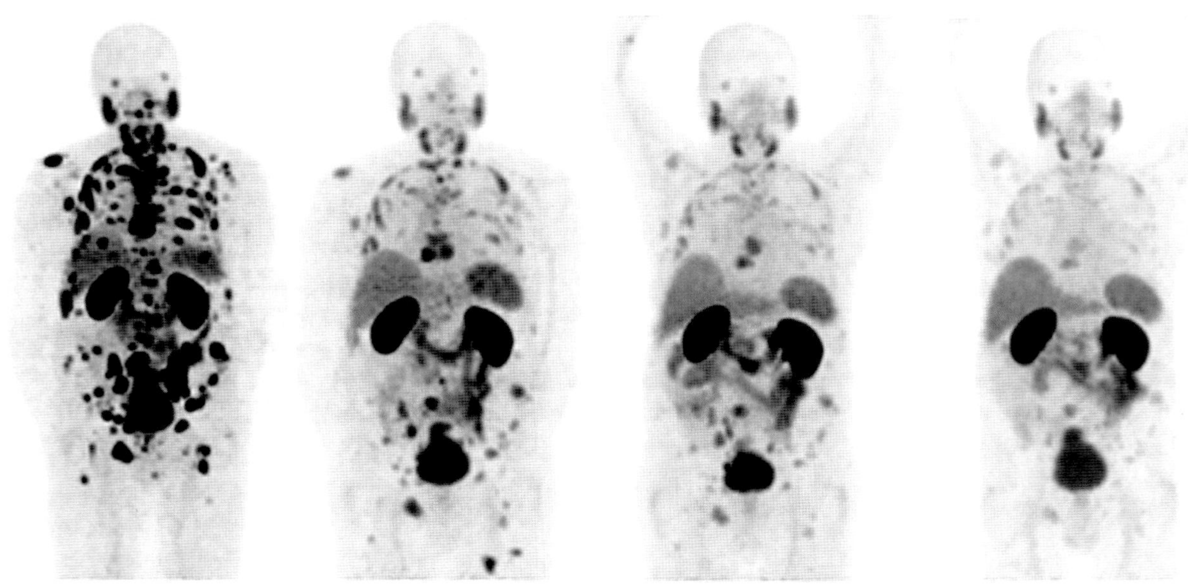

Fig. 8.4 Maximum intensity projection (MIP) of ^{68}Ga-PSMA-11 positron emission tomography images of a patient with disseminated bone metastases and local disease responding to the standard treatment with six cycles and showing further response to the extended radioligand therapy (RLT). Treatment was discontinued due to insufficient prostate-specific membrane antigen (PSMA)–expressing residual disease after 13 cycles of ^{177}Lu-PSMA RLT (progression-free survival [PFS]: 58 months). (From Mader N, Nguyen Ngoc C, Kirkgöze B, et al. Extended therapy with ^{177}Lu-PSMA-617 in responding patients with high-volume metastatic castration-resistant prostate cancer. *Eur J Nucl Med Mol Imaging*. 2023;50:1811–1821. https://doi.org/10.1007/s00259-023-06119-1.[50]) *PSA*, Prostate-specific antigen.)

of normal saline can be given intravenously. Also, concerning patient condition, several recommendations can be considered for the treatment: (1) use of diuretics posttreatment for the clearance of unbound ^{177}Lu-PSMA; (2) use of cold packs to salivary glands to minimise ^{177}Lu-PSMA uptake; and (3) use of antiemetics to alleviate nausea and vomiting. The posttherapeutic emission scans and prostate-specific antigen (PSA) blood results are used to see the treatment response at every cycle. Targeted therapy with the use of actinium-225–labelled PSMA ligands (^{225}Ac-PSMA) has also evolved as a potential treatment option for patients with mCRPC disease. The ^{225}Ac-PSMA is found to be effective in patients having 'superscan' patterns and red marrow infiltration because of higher linear energy transfer and a shorter range of alpha particles. However, this treatment is still a part of clinical trials.

Besides cancer cells, PSMA is also expressed at low levels in normal prostate epithelium and other tissues.[39] Therefore normal physiological expression of ^{177}Lu-PSMA also takes place in the lacrimal glands, kidneys, salivary glands and bone marrow, which are also known as target organs in RLT.[40] Physiological expression of radiolabelled PSMA can result in unintended radiation exposure to healthy tissues and organs. There can be significant adverse effects in lacrimal glands, kidneys and salivary glands, causing lacrimal gland toxicity, renal dysfunction or xerostomia, respectively, which limit the total therapeutic dose delivery and the number of treatment cycles.[41] To ensure maximum dose delivery to the tumour lesions and minimise organ toxicity, individual patient dosimetry plays a significant role in RLT by monitoring treatment cycles, administered activity and organ-absorbed doses in each treatment cycle. Currently, the Medical Internal Radiation Dose Committee (MIRD Committee) formalism is commonly used for measuring patient doses in clinical settings. Imaging methods that can be used for dosimetry in RLT include multiplanar imaging–based dosimetry, multi-SPECT/CT–based dosimetry and hybrid dosimetry combining two-dimensional and three-dimensional data. Techniques that can be adopted for organ-level dosimetry include S-values derived directly from standardised reference models, dose point kernel and voxel S-value.[42,43] Based on the available literature and scientific reports, ^{177}Lu-PSMA treatment can be administered safely for a number of cycles before critical organs including the lacrimal glands, kidneys, salivary glands and bone marrow reach their tolerance limits.[44,45] The maximum tolerance limits are around 40 Gy for lacrimal glands, 23 Gy for kidneys, 20 Gy for salivary glands and 3 Gy for bone marrow.

RADIATION PROTECTION, WASTE AND REGULATIONS

Radiation protection is an important component of molecular radiotherapy for the patient, comforters and carers, and staff involved in both the administration and care of the patient. The type of therapy agent used will affect the protection requirements. Treatments with predominantly beta emitters and low-abundance gamma rays, such as yttrium-90, present a lower external dose rate to others, while radionuclides such as iodine-131, with a long half-life of 8 days and a high abundance of high-energy 364-keV gamma rays, present a more complex problem.

Requirements and guidance are drawn from several sources. In the United Kingdom, the Ionising Radiation (Medical Exposure) Regulations (IRMER17)[46] and the Ionising Radiations Regulations 2017 (IRR17)[47] apply for radionuclide therapies, while the MDGN provides guidance on the implementation of legislation.[12] In particular, an individualised risk assessment is used for each patient to estimate likely contact patterns with other people, their home circumstances and the risk of contamination and ingestion as well as inhalation of radionuclides. Specific requirements can include restricting any contact with young children and pregnant females.

Hospital Requirements

Hospitals delivering radionuclide therapies in the United Kingdom should have the following licenses, certifications and appointed personnel to support compliance with regulations:

- Appointed trust radiation protection advisor (RPA)
- Appointed trust radiation protection supervisor (RPS)
- Medical physics expert (MPE) with expertise in radionuclide therapy
- Appropriate certification for radiopharmaceutical administration from the Administration of Radioactive Substances Advisory Committee (ARSAC)
- Procedures for compliance with IRR2017, such as designation of controlled areas, dose limits, contamination monitoring and risk assessments
- Registration and authorisation for holding and disposing of relevant radioactive materials, referred to as the Environmental Permitting Regulations (EPR2010) License[48]
- Method of checking activity prior to administration
- Facilities for oral and intraveneous administration of radiopharmaceuticals

Facilities

Dependent on national and local regulations, the patient may have to be admitted and cared for in a specialised and dedicated radionuclide therapy facility that includes:

- A room with a sufficient lead lining which is designated as a controlled area.
- Exclusive use of a toilet and shower facility with appropriate disposal route.
- A method for monitoring for room and equipment contamination.
- Facilities for washing and decontamination of bed linen, towels and clothing.
- Appropriate facilities for storage of contaminated items. These facilities should be adequately shielded, labelled and designed with appropriate security measures to prevent risk of escape or theft of material.
- Appropriate personal protective equipment (PPE) such as gloves, gowns and overshoes for staff as well as comforters and carers. They should also have access to appropriate decontamination facilities, including a wash basin and decontamination shower.
- Appropriately trained nursing and care staff who are also trained in radiation protection.

Carers and Comforters

Patients undergoing molecular therapy may require additional support by a family member or friend. For paediatric patients, their parents would typically act as carers and comforters for the duration of their treatment. Carers and comforters are defined in IRMER17 as those individuals who are 'knowingly and willingly helping (other than as part of their occupation) in the support and comfort of patients undergoing medical diagnosis or treatment'. They are not subject to the public dose limit, but their radiation exposure should be justified by the IRMER practitioner. The dose to comforters and carers should be kept as low as reasonably achievable (ALARA), and for this reason, radiation protection measures are put in place and advice is provided to help individuals minimise their personal radiation exposure.[46]

Inpatient and Outpatient Therapies

In radionuclide therapy, radioactivity is administered to patients on an inpatient and outpatient basis for the treatment of various disease and tumours. Prior to both inpatient and outpatient therapies, all patients undertake an individualised radiation risk assessment—dependent on personal circumstances—and advice related to minimise the radiation exposure to others. In inpatient radionuclide therapy, the patient is hospitalised for a few days after administration of radioactivity and is discharged when the level of radioactivity has gone down to a level where exposure to family members and members of the public is below the dose constraints. As per the International Commission on Radiological Protection (ICRP) and IRR17, a member of the public should not receive more than a 1-mSv effective dose per year. The treatment of a patient as an inpatient depends upon the amount of activity administered, type of emission and biodistribution characteristics of radiopharmaceuticals—that is, blood clearance and excretion rates. It is necessary to treat patients as inpatients when they are treated with isotopes having high γ energy and relative abundance (i.e. ^{131}I-NaI therapy for thyroid cancers), because these γ radiations may induce an external radiation hazard to people who directly interact with the patient. The infrastructure of these isolation rooms is usually prepared as per the guidelines prepared by the national authorities. As per the recommendation of the ICRP and MDGN,[12] a patient can be released from the hospital once the ^{131}I-NaI residual activity is less than 800 MBq post treatment, assuming home circumstances are appropriate (e.g. no pregnant females or young children), and alternative arrangements can be made regarding the minimisation of close contact patterns. In many countries a dose rate of 30 to 50 μSv per hour at a 1-m distance from the patient's body is used as the discharge criterion. ^{131}I-NaI can be safely administered for the treatment of hyperthyroidism on an outpatient basis because the amount of administered activity is less and is safer for members of the public in comparison to thyroid cancer treatment. Sometimes biological excretion of radioactivity from the patient is another source of risk, which occurs primarily through the urine and largely occurs within 48 hours of treatment (i.e. ^{177}Lu-dotatate therapy). Therefore many centres recommend inpatient isolation after ^{177}Lu-dotatate administration. However, other centres provide this treatment to outpatients without isolation but require that strict precautions be followed once the patient leaves the hospital. To minimise the dose to family members and small children at home after radionuclide therapy, specific instructions related to radiation safety must be provided. The treatment of patients using pure alpha or beta emitters (high linear energy transfer, i.e. ^{225}Ac, ^{223}Ra, ^{90}Y) is routinely performed as an outpatient procedure.

The MDGN contains a table of restrictions which are suitable when discharging patients who have undergone radioiodine therapy for thyrotoxicosis. This includes restrictions on contact with children and any restrictions on the mode of transport used.[12] Self-discharge must be firmly discouraged on the grounds of the hazards to others.

Where risk assessment has shown it necessary, all patients should be given written instructions on leaving the hospital about precautions to be taken to minimise the dose to others. A card is often given to the patient, outlining restriction durations and contact details of radiation protection advisors in the event of hospitalisation or other concerns. Even many weeks after precautions have elapsed, patients may retain enough radioactivity in their bodies to set off radiation alarms at airports. Travel plans and arrangements should be discussed with patients prior to discharge.

Following discharge from inpatient accommodation, the room may not be reused until it has been monitored and declared free from substantial contamination.

In the case of the death of a patient following the administration of a therapeutic dose of radioactivity, due regard must be given to the safety of the relatives, pathologists and undertakers. The MDGN[12] contains a section giving advice on this, but a local policy should be written for each treatment offered in that centre.

Waste Disposal

The disposal of radioactive waste from a hospital must be organised, carefully controlled and documented in compliance with the UK regulations to avoid hazard to staff, patients and the general public. The Environment Agency will authorise limits of activity for gaseous, aqueous and solid-waste discharge for each site.[48] *Solid waste* refers to items contaminated with radioactivity, such as syringes, swabs and paper tissues. *Aqueous waste* refers to waste discharged to the sewage systems and can include radioactive solutions from radionuclide administration and bodily fluids from patients. The site must show that it disposes of all waste by the best practicable means before authorisation is granted. Detailed records must be kept of all disposals of radioactive materials irrespective of which route has been used. These records should include the type of radionuclide, its activity at disposal, the route of disposal and the date of disposal.

REFERENCES

1. Loevinger R, Budinger TF, Watson EE. *MIRD Primer for Absorbed Dose Calculations*. Society of Nuclear Medicine, New York, USA; 1988.
2. Stabin MG. MIRDOSE: personal computer software for internal dose assessment in nuclear medicine. *J Nucl Med*. 1996;37(3): 538–546.
3. ICRP. Radiation dose to patients from radiopharmaceuticals: a compendium of current information related to frequently used substances. ICRP Publication 128. *Ann ICRP*. 2015;44(2S).
4. Bombardieri E, Giammarile F, Aktolun C, et al. 131I/123I-metaiodobenzylguanidine (mIBG) scintigraphy: procedure guidelines for tumour imaging. *Eur J Nucl Med Mol Imaging*. 2010;37(12):2436–2446.
5. Yonekura Y, Mattsson S, Flux G, et al. ICRP publication 140: radiological protection in therapy with radiopharmaceuticals. *Ann ICRP*. 2019;48(1):5–95. http://doi.org/10.1177/0146645319838665.
6. Rojas B, Hooker C, McGowan DR, Guy MJ, Tipping J. Eight years of growth and change in UK molecular radiotherapy with implications for the future: internal dosimetry users group survey results from 2007 to 2015. *Nucl Med Commun*. 2017;38(3):201–204.
7. Sartor O, de Bono J, Chi KN, et al. Lutetium-177-PSMA-617 for metastatic castration-resistant prostate cancer. *N Engl J Med*. 2021;385(12):1091–1103. http://doi.org/10.1056/NEJMoa2107322.
8. Silberstein EB, Alavi A, Balon HR, et al. The SNMMI practice guideline for therapy of thyroid disease with 131I 3.0. *J Nucl Med*. 2012;53(10):1633–1651.
9. Luster M, Clarke SE, Dietlein M, et al. Guidelines for radioiodine therapy of differentiated thyroid cancer. *Eur J Nucl Med Mol Imaging*. 2008;35(10):1941–1959.
10. Robbins RJ, Schlumberger MJ. The evolving role of 131I for the treatment of differentiated thyroid carcinoma. *J Nucl Med*. 2005;46(1): 28S–37S.
11. Perros P, Boelaert K, Colley S, et al. Guidelines for the management of thyroid cancer. *Clin Endocrinol*. 2014;81(s1):1–22.
12. Medical and Dental Guidance Notes. *A Good Practice Guide on All Aspects of Ionising Radiation Protection in the Clinical Environment*. Institute of Physics and Engineering in Medicine, York, UK; 2002.
13. Stokkel MP, Junak DH, Lassmann M, Dietlein M, Luster M. EANM procedure guidelines for therapy of benign thyroid disease. *Eur J Nucl Med Mol Imaging*. 2010;37(11):2218–2228.
14. Dottorini ME, Mansi L. Radioiodine in the management of benign thyroid disease: clinical guidelines. Report of a Working Party, 2007. Royal College of Physicians (RCP). *Eur J Nucl Med Mol Imaging*. 2007;34(12):2148–2149.
15. Lewington VJ. Bone-seeking radionuclides for therapy. *J Nucl Med*. 2005;46(1 suppl):38S–47S.
16. Parker C, Nilsson S, Heinrich D, et al. Alpha emitter radium-223 and survival in metastatic prostate cancer. *New Engl J Med*. 2013; 369(3):213–223.

17. Coleman R, Aksnes AK, Naume B, et al. A phase IIa, nonrandomized study of radium-223 dichloride in advanced breast cancer patients with bone-dominant disease. *Breast Cancer Res Treat.* 2014;145(2):411–418.
18. Poeppel TD, Handkiewicz-Junak D, Andreeff M, et al. EANM guideline for radionuclide therapy with radium-223 of metastatic castration-resistant prostate cancer. *Eur J Nucl Med Mol Imaging.* 2018;45(5):824–845.
19. Flux GD. Imaging and dosimetry for radium-223: the potential for personalized treatment. *Br J Radiol.* 2017;90:20160748.
20. Gains JE, Bomanji JB, Fersht NL, et al. 177Lu-dotatate molecular radiotherapy for childhood neuroblastoma. *J Nucl Med.* 2011; 52(7):1041–1047.
21. Zaknun JJ, Bodei L, Mueller-Brand J, et al. The joint IAEA, EANM, and SNMMI practical guidance on peptide receptor radionuclide therapy (PRRNT) in neuroendocrine tumours. *Eur J Nucl Med Mol Imaging.* 2013;40(5):800–816.
22. Strosberg J, El-Haddad G, Wolin E, et al. Phase 3 trial of 177Lu-dotatate for midgut neuroendocrine tumors. *New Engl J Med.* 2017;376(2):125–135.
23. Giammarile F, Chiti A, Lassmann M, Brans B, Flux G. EANM procedure guidelines for 131 I-meta-iodobenzylguanidine (131 I-mIBG) therapy. *Eur J Nucl Med Mol Imaging.* 2008;35(5):1039–1047.
24. Gaze MN, Chang YC, Flux GD, Mairs RJ, Saran FH, Meller ST. Feasibility of dosimetry-based high-dose 131I-meta-iodobenzylguanidine with topotecan as a radiosensitizer in children with metastatic neuroblastoma. *Cancer Biother Radiopharm.* 2005;20(2):195–199.
25. Giammarile F, Bodei L, Chiesa C, et al. EANM procedure guideline for the treatment of liver cancer and liver metastases with intra-arterial radioactive compounds. *Eur J Nucl Med Mol Imaging.* 2011;38(7):1393.
26. Garin E, Rolland Y, Laffont S, Edeline J. Clinical impact of 99m Tc-MAA SPECT/CT-based dosimetry in the radioembolization of liver malignancies with 90 Y-loaded microspheres. *Eur J Nucl Med Mol Imaging.* 2016;43(3):559–575.
27. Kennedy A, Nag S, Salem R, et al. Recommendations for radioembolization of hepatic malignancies using yttrium-90 microsphere brachytherapy: a consensus panel report from the Radioembolization Brachytherapy Oncology Consortium. *Int J Radiat Oncol Biol Phys.* 2007;68(1):13–23.
28. Stella M, Braat AJAT, van Rooij R, de Jong HWAM, Lam MGEH. Holmium-166 radioembolization: current status and future prospective. *Cardiovasc Intervent Radiol.* 2022;45(11):1634–1645. http://doi.org/10.1007/s00270-022-03187-y.
29. Parmentier C. Use and risks of phosphorus-32 in the treatment of polycythaemia vera. *Eur J Nucl Med Mol Imaging.* 2003;30(10): 1413–1417.
30. Tennvall J, Brans B. EANM procedure guideline for ^{32}P phosphate treatment of myeloproliferative diseases. *Eur J Nucl Med Mol Imaging.* 2007;34(8):1324–1327.
31. Clunie G, Fischer M. EANM procedure guidelines for radiosynovectomy. *Eur J Nucl Med Mol Imaging.* 2003;30(3):BP12.
32. Wiseman GA, White CA, Stabin M, et al. Phase I/II 90 Y-Zevalin (yttrium-90 ibritumomab tiuxetan, IDEC-Y2B8) radioimmunotherapy dosimetry results in relapsed or refractory non-Hodgkin's lymphoma. *Eur J Nucl Med.* 2000;27(7):766–777.
33. Gosewisch A, Ilhan H, Tattenberg S, et al. 3D Monte Carlo bone marrow dosimetry for Lu-177-PSMA therapy with guidance of non-invasive 3D localization of active bone marrow via Tc-99m-anti-granulocyte antibody SPECT/CT. *EJNMMI Res.* 2019;9(1):76.
34. Labriola MK, Atiq S, Hirshman N, Bitting RL. Management of men with metastatic castration-resistant prostate cancer following potent androgen receptor inhibition: a review of novel investigational therapies. *Prostate Cancer Prostatic Dis.* 2021;24(2):301–309. http://doi.org/10.1038/s41391-020-00299-9.
35. Chang SS, Gaudin PB, Reuter VE, O'Keefe DS, Bacich DJ, Heston WD. Prostate-specific membrane antigen: much more than a prostate cancer marker. *Mol Urol.* 1999;3(3):313–320.
36. Rajasekaran AK, Anilkumar G, Christiansen JJ. Is prostate-specific membrane antigen a multifunctional protein? *Am J Physiol Cell Physiol.* 2005;288:C975–C981.
37. Liu H, Rajasekaran AK, Moy P, et al. Constitutive and antibody-induced internalization of prostate-specific membrane antigen. *Cancer Res.* 1998;58:4055–4060.
38. Kratochwil C, Fendler WP, Eiber M, et al. EANM procedure guidelines for radionuclide therapy with 177Lu-labelled PSMA-ligands (177Lu-PSMA-RLT). *Eur J Nucl Med Mol Imaging.* 2019; 46(12):2536–2544.
39. Chang SS, Reuter VE, Heston WD, Bander NH, Grauer LS, Gaudin PB. Five different anti-prostate-specific membrane antigen (PSMA) antibodies confirm PSMA expression in tumor-associated neovasculature. *Cancer Res.* 1999;59(13):3192–3198.
40. Kabasakal L, AbuQbeitah M, Aygun A, et al. Pre-therapeutic dosimetry of normal organs and tissues of (177)Lu-PSMA-617 prostate-specific membrane antigen (PSMA) inhibitor in patients with castration-resistant prostate cancer. *Eur J Nucl Med Mol Imaging.* 2015;42(13):1976–1983.
41. Privé BM, Peters SMB, Muselaers CHJ, et al. Lutetium-177-PSMA-617 in low-volume hormone-sensitive metastatic prostate cancer: a prospective pilot study. *Clin Cancer Res.* 2021; 27(13):3595–3601.
42. Stabin MG, Siegel JA. RADAR dose estimate report: a compendium of radiopharmaceutical dose estimates based on OLINDA/EXM version 2.0. *J Nucl Med.* 2018;59(1):154–160.
43. Bolch WE, Bouchet LG, Robertson JS, et al. MIRD pamphlet No. 17: the dosimetry of nonuniform activity distributions-radionuclide S values at the voxel level. Medical internal radiation dose committee. *J Nucl Med.* 1999;40:11S–36S.
44. Nautiyal A, Jha AK, Mithun S, Rangarajan V. Dosimetry in Lu-177-PSMA-617 prostate-specific membrane antigen targeted radioligand therapy: a systematic review. *Nucl Med Commun.* 2022;43(4):369–377.
45. Emmett L, Willowson K, Violet J, Shin J, Blanksby A, Lee J. Lutetium 177 PSMA radionuclide therapy for men with prostate cancer: a review of the current literature and discussion of practical aspects of therapy. *J Med Radiat Sci.* 2017;64(1):52–60.
46. UK Statutory Regulations 2017 No. 1322. The ionising radiation (Medical Exposure) regulations 2017. https://www.legislation.gov.uk/uksi/2017/1322/contents
47. UK Statutory Instruments 2017 No. 1075. The ionising radiations regulations 2017. https://www.legislation.gov.uk/uksi/2017/1075/contents
48. UK Draft Statutory Instruments. The environmental permitting (England and Wales) regulations 2010. https://www.legislation.gov.uk/ukdsi/2010/9780111491423/contents
49. d'Abadie P, Walrand S, Lhommel R, Hesse M, Jamar F. A theranostic approach in SIRT: value of pre-therapy imaging in treatment planning. *J Clin Med.* 2022;11(23):7245.
50. Mader N, Nguyen Ngoc C, Kirkgöze B, et al. Extended therapy with [177Lu] Lu-PSMA-617 in responding patients with high-volume metastatic castration-resistant prostate cancer. *Eur J Nucl Med Mol Imaging.* 2023;50(6):1811–1821.

9

Brachytherapy, Low-Voltage X-rays and Gamma Rays

Sarah Aldridge and Charles Deehan

CHAPTER OUTLINE

INTRODUCTION

Radioactive sources and kilovoltage (kV) X-rays have been utilised in radiotherapy for many years. Clinical practice has developed to utilise gamma rays, beta rays and x-rays from accelerating voltages as low as 10 kV.

Kilovoltage x-rays were discovered in 1895 by Roentgen, and at the start of 1896 radioactivity was discovered by Henri Becquerel. In 1898, the naturally occurring radioactive element radium was discovered by Marie Curie, and soon after, the therapeutic potential in treating diseases such as cancer was realised. Radium was still being used for treatments in the 1980s but has now been replaced by artificially produced radionuclides with more favourable characteristics.

For well over 100 years, machines, expertise and techniques have developed which demonstrate clinical response and therapeutic benefit that has become well understood.

Radionuclide Characteristics and Kilovoltage X-rays

Radionuclides provide a range of materials with which to provide ionising radiation. Devices range from teletherapy beams of gamma rays to physical encapsulations of material which enable direct radiotherapy with electrons. X-rays are produced by utilising the process normally referred to as *bremsstrahlung* (Chapter 2).

Gamma Emitters

Radium

Radium-226 was the first radioisotope used in brachytherapy. It has a half-life of 1600 years and a mean photon energy of approximately 800 keV. The major source of gamma rays is the gaseous daughter product, radon. For medical applications, radium was encapsulated in a tube which had to be gas tight and frequently checked for leaks. The gamma rays used are highly penetrating, and very thick lead shields are required to provide adequate radiation protection. Other radioisotopes with more suitable properties are now available, and therefore this material is no longer in use.

Caesium

Caesium-137 is a fission product derived from spent uranium fuel rods used in nuclear reactors. Caesium-137 has no gaseous daughter products and largely replaced radium as the nuclide of choice in the 1960s. It has a half-life of 30 years and a mean photon energy of 662 keV.

Iridium

Iridium-192 has a mean gamma energy of 380 keV and a half-life of 73.83 days. It has been in use since the late 1950s and has a high specific activity. Its physical form for use in radiotherapy is that of a flexible wire, and this has many advantages over traditional radium and caesium needles for implants.

Iodine

Iodine-125 has a half-life of 60 days and has been used clinically since the early 1960s. It is the daughter product of xenon-125, which is produced by a neutron-gamma reaction. The average photon energy of iodine-125 is only 28 KeV.

Cobalt

Cobalt-60 has a half-life of 5.3 years and an average photon energy of 1.253 MeV (megaelectron volts), which makes it a highly penetrating radiotherapy beam. Cobalt-60 is used for teletherapy.

Beta Emitters

Strontium

Strontium-90 has a half-life of 28.8 years. It is only useful when in radioactive equilibrium with its daughter product, yttrium-90, and that equilibrium is achieved with silver encapsulation. Strontium-90 emits electrons of 546 keV and the daughter product, yttrium-90, emits an electron with a maximum energy of 2.27 MeV.

Ruthenium

Ruthenium-106 has a half-life of 369 days. It is a fission product of uranium and decays with a low-energy beta emission to rhodium-106, which has a maximum high-energy beta emission of 3.54 MeV.

Kilovoltage X-ray Production

In x-ray production, accelerated electrons are slowed down in the interaction with a material. In x-ray machines, the interaction takes place in a target, referred to as the *x-ray target*. An energetic beam of electrons is produced by the machine using high-voltage acceleration, and this electron beam is directed at the x-ray target.

It is essential to have a high voltage with which to accelerate an electron beam for x-ray production. On early machines, step-up transformers were used to provide high voltages to excite the x-ray tube. The transformers operated at mains frequency and were very bulky due to the large iron core required.

Modern units employ switched-mode power supply techniques to improve voltage stability and make savings in size and efficiency. The power supply comprises an input rectifier to convert mains AC to a DC voltage. A switching inverter converts the DC to a high-frequency (25-kHz) pulsed waveform that is stepped up to 10 kV via a high-frequency transformer. Finally, the waveform is rectified and passed through a number of cascaded multiplying stages (Cockcroft–Walton) to produce a DC voltage in the 100- to 300-kV range.

The extra high tension (EHT) voltage is monitored and a control signal fed back to alter the pulse width of the waveform leaving the inverter stage. In this way, a stable voltage is maintained across the x-ray tube.

The intensity of the x-ray beam produced at a particular kilovoltage depends upon the number of electrons emitted from the filament. This tube current is a function of the filament temperature and hence the filament current. The filament drive voltage is controlled electronically to respond to changes in the AC supply and stabilise the beam current. A schematic is shown in Fig. 9.1. Typically, for voltages in excess of 200 kV, two high-voltage power supplies are used in series.

The high-tension (HT) generator is controlled externally so that safe operating parameters can be set for the particular tube in use. The generator status can also be fed to the operating system to indicate

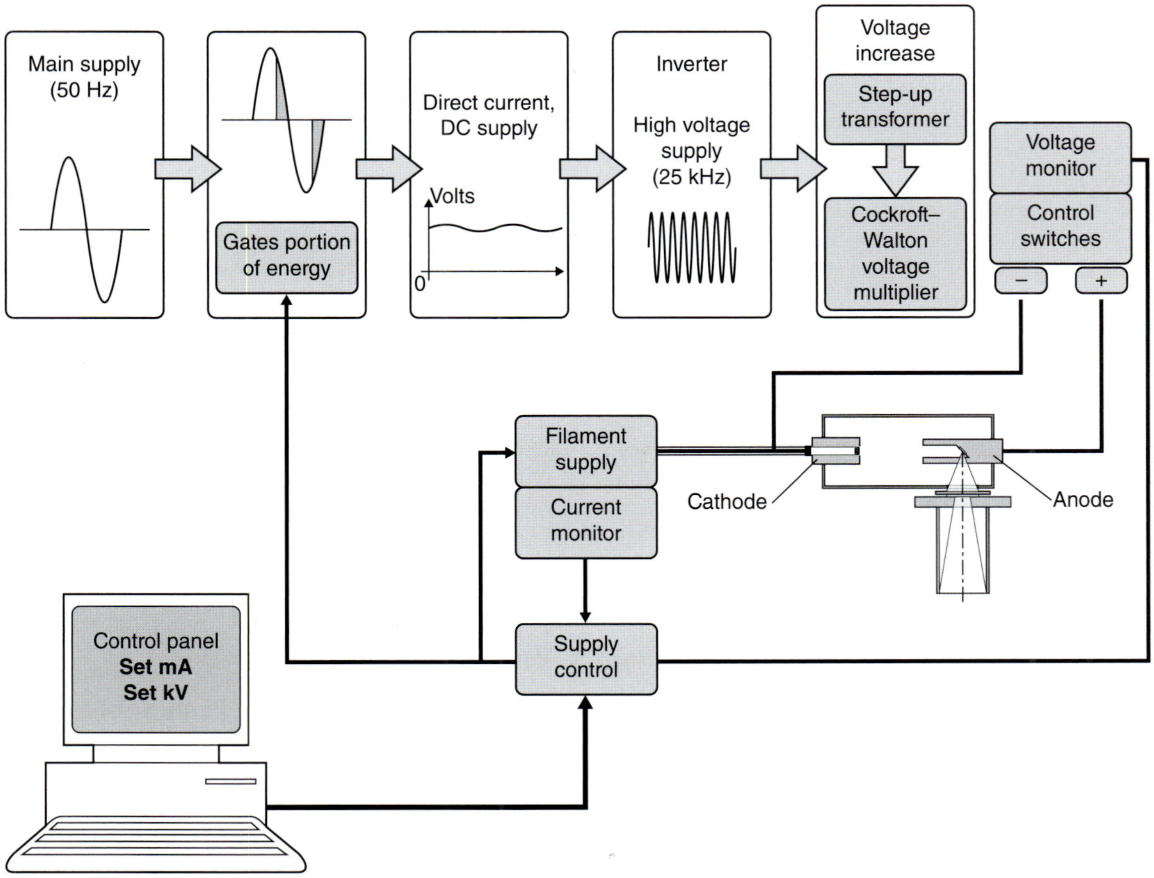

Fig. 9.1 Schematic of high-tension generator with feedback and connection to controller.

faults, to link into the interlock system to ensure safe treatment and to assist in fault diagnosis.

The high voltage and filament power supply is connected to the x-ray tube by means of a high-voltage cable. To prevent voltage flashover in the connectors, care must be taken to keep all parts clean and to use high-voltage insulating grease during assembly and reassembly following maintenance inspection.

Kilovoltage X-ray Characteristics

The x-ray beam from any bremsstrahlung target consists of a range of energies up to the maximum accelerating potential produced by the machine. Hence, for a 120-kV machine, 120 keV will be the accelerated electron energy and, in turn, the maximum x-ray photon energy will be 120 keV. This spectrum of energies is modified using a filter to remove lower-energy x-rays and so reduce the dose to the skin. The beam that emerges from the tube through the x-ray window has undergone what is called *inherent filtration*. However, additional filtration is chosen to provide a beam with the desired depth-dose penetration. The energy characteristics of the beam are often referred to as its *quality* and are dependent upon both the accelerating potential and filtration. The beam quality is normally measured using thicknesses of aluminium or copper and specified in terms of the half-value layer (HVL), which is the thickness of the layer of metal required to reduce the intensity of the beam by one-half. Typically, when this is measured, it is done in a narrow beam which is obtained by additional collimation to a broad clinical beam. The measuring ionisation chamber is also placed at a sufficient distance from the machine, floor and walls to ensure that there is no additional scattered radiation. In practical terms, the penetration of the beam is also due to the source to surface distance (SSD) and the field size. Depth-dose data indicating the penetration of different HVL beams can be compared in the *British Journal of Radiology*, Supplement 25.[1]

BRACHYTHERAPY

Brachytherapy is the delivery of radiation treatment using sealed radioactive sources or miniaturised kilovoltage sources which are positioned within or as close as possible to the site to be treated. The term comes from the Greek word *brachios* meaning 'short' or 'near'. It therefore translates as 'near treatment' or 'near therapy'. It is applicable for a wide variety of tumour sites and can be used as a stand-alone treatment or in combination with surgery or other therapies.

It takes advantage of steep gradients in the dose distribution around the source due to the inverse-square effect. Hence the target receives a sufficiently high dose while the dose to the surrounding healthy tissues is reduced considerably. Another advantage is that the radiation sources are physically connected to the target volume. They move with the target volume, resulting in minimal inpatient variation during treatment and with no need to account for setup error or organ motion. Thus, in brachytherapy, the clinical target volume (CTV) is the planning target volume (PTV). The main disadvantage with brachytherapy is in gaining access to the tumour, which often requires an operative procedure and the skilled personnel to perform it.

Today the manual insertion of radioactive sources has largely been replaced by remote computer-controlled afterloading with the exception of procedures such as low-dose-rate seed brachytherapy.

In the past 25 years, brachytherapy has moved from a two-dimensional dose distribution using conventional x-ray films to full three-dimensional volumetric dose distribution utilising computed tomography (CT), magnetic resonance imaging (MRI), positron emission tomography (PET) and three-dimensional ultrasound imaging. Brachytherapy volumes are no longer defined by the implant itself, and instead the CTV can be defined with the implant in situ. Using the flexibility of stepping the source in an afterloading treatment machine, the dose distribution can be tailored to cover the CTV, enabling conformal dose delivery and better sparing of healthy tissues.

Sealed Sources

Most brachytherapy sources are termed *sealed sources*, that is, radioactive material that is permanently encapsulated in a sealed capsule or closely bound in a solid form. In other words, the activity is fixed to its carrier, and contamination of the environment is not possible as long as the source remains intact. All sealed sources have an activity specified by a calibration certificate. A regular check of source integrity by a wipe test[2] is essential to ensure that the source can still be classified as 'sealed'.

The radioactive isotopes used in brachytherapy sources today are generated in a nuclear reactor as a fission product or as an activation product of a neutron-capture reaction, and in a cyclotron using particle beams for activation of stable nuclides. The process of nuclear fission occurs when large nuclei divide and produce new elements which are radioactive. Often, the desired product has to be separated from other fission products. In neutron activation, a sample of a stable isotope is placed in a neutron field in a nuclear reactor. Some of the nuclei capture a neutron and become a radioactive isotope of the element, with the emission of gamma irradiation. The end product will contain a mixture of the stable and radioactive isotopes.[3]

The Ideal Brachytherapy Sources

As described earlier, radioactive sources have different emission types, radiation energies and half-lives. Different sources have different applications. However, an ideal brachytherapy source would have the following requirements:

1. For temporary implants, the radionuclide should have a long half-life of months to years to enable economical reuse of sources.
2. For permanent implants, a half-life of days to weeks ensures that it is not radioactive for a long period of time in the patient.
3. Charged particle emission should be absent or easily absorbed by the encapsulation, as alpha and beta radiations are so short in range that they can result in very high doses to small volumes around the source.
4. The energy of the emitted radiation should be high enough to treat the target with homogenous dose and low enough to avoid unnecessary exposure to normal tissues and reduce shielding requirements. Ideally, emitted photons should be in the range of 350 keV to 660 keV.
5. The radioactive material should be in a physical form that can be encapsulated to permanently seal the radioactivity, preventing dispersion.
6. No gaseous or liquid products should be produced in the radioactive decay process.
7. The radionuclide material should be available in a high specific activity so that small sources can be produced with an adequate dose rate.
8. The sources should be available at a reasonable cost so that their use is financially viable.

Modern sources come close to this ideal.

The Iodine-125 Low-Energy Photon Source

These low-energy photon seeds encapsulate the gamma emitter iodine-125, as discussed earlier, and are predominately for permanent implants. The low energy has a half-value thickness of 0.025 mm lead (Pb), which makes radiation shielding highly effective.

This source has been available in the form of seeds since the 1960s, and a large number of seed models are now commercially available

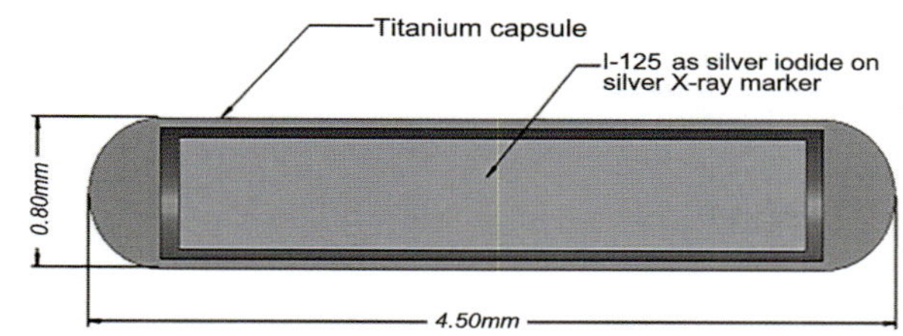

Fig. 9.2 Iodine-125 seed construction. (Courtesy BXTAccelyon Ltd.)

from different manufacturers. They are all based on two basic designs. In one design, the radionuclide is absorbed onto a central silver rod core, and the rod is then encapsulated in 0.5 mm of titanium. In the other design, the radionuclide is absorbed onto an ion exchange resin and then encapsulated in 0.5 mm of titanium. Both seed designs are cylinders measuring 4.5 mm in length and 0.8 mm in diameter (Fig. 9.2).

The Iridium-192 High-Energy Photon Source

Iridium-192 is currently the most widely used radioactive source in the field of brachytherapy (see the 'Radionuclide Characteristics and Kilovoltage X-rays' section for a description of its characteristics). The weighted mean energy spectra of electrons and photons of 176.2 and 346.1 keV, respectively, results in a half-value thickness of 2.5 mm of lead (Pb). Its high specific activity makes it practical to make small radioactive sources which can be used in high dose rate (HDR) afterloading systems. Iridium-192 HDR sources are encapsulated in a thin titanium or stainless-steel capsule or cylinder measuring 0.5 to 1 mm in diameter by 0.5 to 3.5 mm in length (Fig. 9.3), and these sources are laser welded to the end of a flexible cable whose movement can be computer controlled.

The radionuclide is also available as wires composed of an alloy of iridium and platinum with a diameter of 0.5 mm, which is popular in Europe. These wire sources are only suitable for temporary brachytherapy implants, as due to the high average photon energy, this would result in excessive radiation exposure to members of the public if the patient left the hospital with an implant.

Definitions and Doserates

The following terms are frequently used in brachytherapy:

- **Intracavitary:** The insertion of brachytherapy applicators and radioactive sources into an existing body cavity (e.g. the uterine canal or vagina)
- **Interstitial:** The insertion of brachytherapy applicators and radioactive sources directly into tissue (e.g. needles into the breast or prostate)
- **Intraluminal:** The insertion of brachytherapy applicators and radioactive sources into a lumen (e.g. the bronchus or oesophagus)
- **Surface:** The placement of brachytherapy applicators and radioactive sources onto a surface of the patient (i.e. for treating the skin)

Dose rate is an important consideration in the radiobiology of brachytherapy. When changing dose rate, it is important to remember that increasing dose rate increases biological effect and therefore requires dose reduction. There is no universally accepted definition of low, medium and high dose rates, and leading organisations suggest different boundaries.[2,4,5] However, most users accept the following:

- **Low dose rate (LDR)**: Dose rates less than 1 Gy h^{-1}. These are dose rates aimed for in traditional manual brachytherapy applications as the sources are handled directly by personnel.
- **Medium dose rate (MDR):** Dose rates between about 1 Gy h^{-1} and 12 Gy h^{-1}. There is no sharp dividing line between LDR and MDR.
- **High dose rate (HDR):** Dose rates greater than 12 Gy h^{-1}, which is 0.2 Gy min^{-1}. Sources with this dose rate are not directly handled but contained within treatment machines. In practice, most HDR machines operate at dose rates far greater than this boundary; typically about 2 Gy min^{-1}.
- **Pulsed dose rate (PDR):** A technique where HDR 'pulses' of treatment are repeated at short intervals. Each pulse typically lasts around 5 to 10 minutes and is repeated every hour. The intention is to simulate the radiobiological effects of the LDR treatment using an HDR-type treatment machine.

Afterloading

With minor exceptions, up until the late 1960s all brachytherapy sources were inserted directly into the patient manually by the operator. Over the years, concern grew for the possible effects of radiation exposure on the operators. With the aim of reducing the radiation exposure to the operator, the technique of afterloading was developed. Afterloading involves the initial placement of hollow, nonradioactive applicators, templates or needles into or on the patient, followed by the subsequent insertion of the radioactive source or sources.

Manual Afterloading

In manual afterloading, the radioactive source or sources are placed into the applicators, templates or needles using appropriate handling

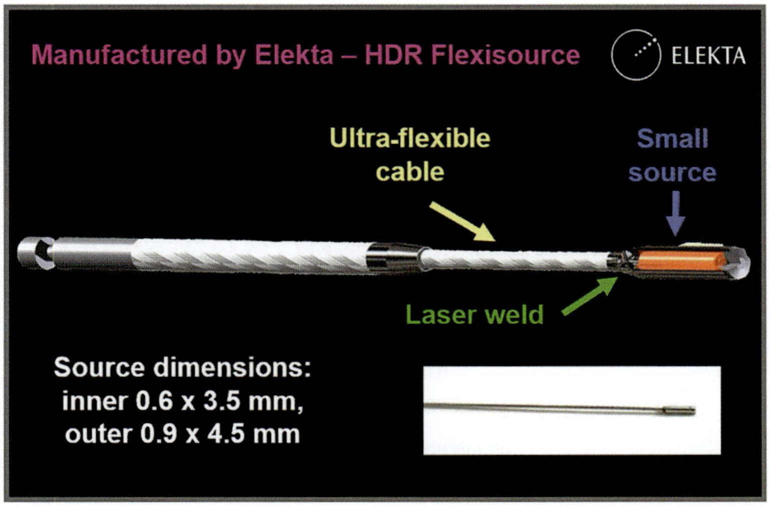

Fig. 9.3 High dose rate iridium-192 source construction. (Courtesy Elekta.)

tools, such as tongs. This is only appropriate for LDR treatments using low-activity sources.

Systems for manual afterloading were developed in the 1960s for gynaecological treatments, and although they are not now used in the United Kingdom, they are still available in many treatment centres around the world. Applicators (hollow tubes) are placed into the uterine canal and vagina in a specific configuration. Their position is then checked using radiographs. The source activities and their arrangement are chosen to match the activities required to deliver the dose according to the Manchester system. Each applicator is then loaded by hand with a source train consisting of low-activity caesium sources and removed again at the end of the patient's treatment. These source trains are stored in a shielded container when not in use. Often, the source trains are mechanically coded to prevent incorrect loading, as in, for example, the source train for the uterine canal being inserted into the vaginal applicator by mistake.

Remote Afterloading

In remote afterloading, a treatment machine using computer control positions the radioactive source or sources within the applicators, templates or needles. With appropriately shielded treatment rooms, this technique facilitates HDR treatments using high-activity sealed sources, although it can also be used for LDR treatments.

Most of the early afterloading machines were designed specifically around the treatment of the cervix. The first HDR afterloading units came into use in the late 1960s. LDR remote afterloading machines were also developed during this time. These used multiple caesium-137 sources with a nominal activity of 740 MBq (20 mCi) and nonradioactive spacers which were loaded as required into source trains in channels connected via transfer tubes to the applicator in the patient in the treatment room. The source trains were pneumatically driven from the safe via the transfer tubes to the patient. As the machine could be controlled outside the patient's room, the treatment could be interrupted and the sources returned to an intermediate safe to minimise the radiation exposure to the staff during nursing procedures.

The High-Doserate Afterloading Machine

The late 1980s saw the introduction of a new generation of afterloading machine, the high doserate afterloading machine, based on a single high-activity iridium-192 source at the tip of a transfer wire (Fig. 9.4). The source can be positioned within applicators or catheters already inserted into the patient and attached to the afterloading machine by a transfer tube. The source activity is typically 370 to 750 GBq (10–20 Ci) and provides an air kerma rate (AKR) of about 50 mGy/h at 1 minute when initially installed. The source resides in a shielded safe when not irradiating a target volume (Fig. 9.5). The single high-specific activity source (see the section titled 'The Iridium-192 High-Energy Photon Source'), with a diameter of only 0.5 mm, allowed the development of new, thinner, flexible applicators and its use for previously inaccessible treatment sites.

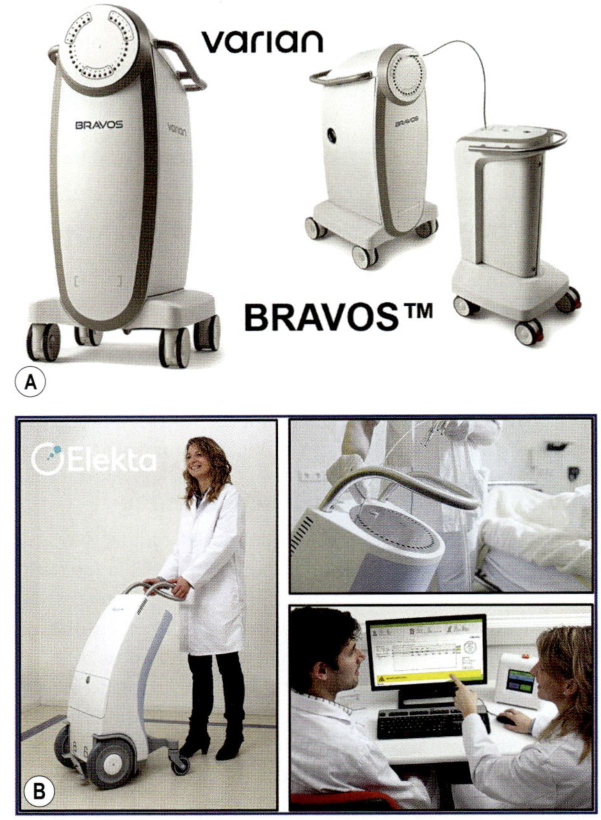

Fig. 9.4 (A) Varian Bravos high dose rate afterloader. (Image courtesy Varian Medical Systems, Inc. All rights reserved.) and (B) Elekta Flexitron high dose rate afterloader. (Image (B) courtesy Elekta.)

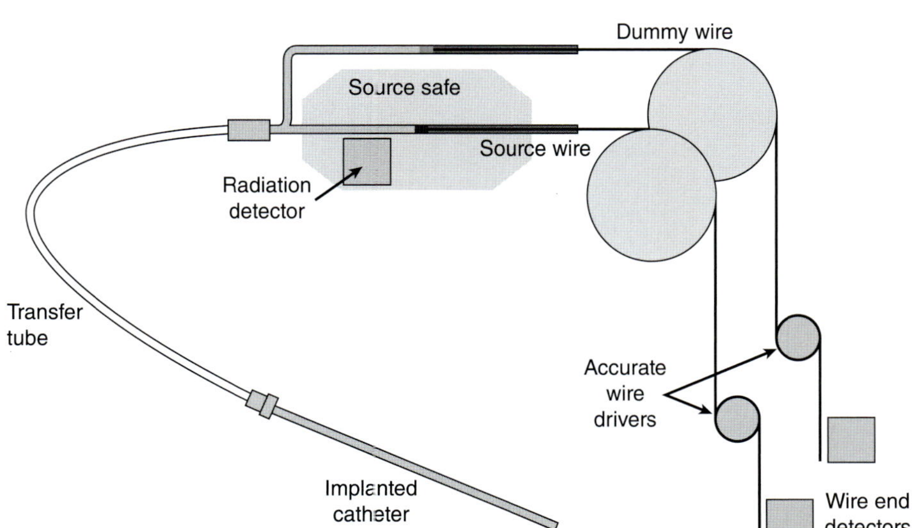

Fig. 9.5 Schematic of the essential features of a high dose rate afterloading machine.

For treatment, the machine is programmed to drive the transfer wire out of the machine along the transfer tube, taking the source out of the safe and into a number of predetermined treating positions for set dwell times. The HDR machine also facilitated complex dose distributions to be produced from the large combination of dwell positions and times available. These treating positions lie within an applicator or catheter located adjacent to or inside the target and previously inserted into the patient. The source can be fed into different types of applicators and catheters for different types of treatment. The HDR treatment units also contain a dummy source wire or check wire (Fig. 9.5) which is used to check connectivity and ensure that the route of the source is clear of any obstructions before the real radioactive source is deployed.

A treatment planning system (TPS) is needed to plan these complex dose distributions. The HDR machine is connected to a treatment control system (TCS), and the dwell positions and times from the treatment plans are transferred directly from the TPS to the TCS, which reduces the risk of transcription errors. In this way, the high-activity source can be positioned as required by the TPS to deliver the chosen isodose distribution. During treatment planning, the dose distribution is manipulated by changing the source dwell time and position before the final approved plan is transferred to the TCS.

Principles of Brachytherapy Dosimetry

Within a brachytherapy implant, the dose distributions are nonhomogeneous. Steep dose gradients occur, and there will be a high-dose region surrounding each source. Between sources, there will be areas of minimum or low dose. A brachytherapy dosimetric system consists of a set of rules for the arrangement of a specific set of radioactive sources to deliver a prescribed dose to a designated point or volume of interest. Over the years, several systems have been developed to calculate the dose distributions of implants resulting from the spacing and geometry of the sources and specifying how dose calculations should be made. For a dosimetry system to be used accurately, the sources must be distributed according to rules of that system and the method of dose specification and prescription maintained. The two systems that modern brachytherapy treatments are based on are the Manchester system[6] and the Paris system.[7] These systems have been adapted as calculations are no longer performed manually, and the rigid division between the Manchester and Paris systems has been eroded as computer algorithms have been developed.

Manchester System

The Manchester system[6] was the most common system used for intracavitary brachytherapy for cervical carcinoma. It was developed in the 1930s using radium tubes and adapted in the 1970s for use with caesium-137. It describes standards, defines reference points to which the dose is specified and defines source strengths to give a predictable and almost constant dose rate to a reference point (Fig. 9.6).

It was originally described in 1938 and later updated in 1953. Although some variations exist, it typically defines a point A dose as the dose at 2 cm above the external cervical os (flange) and 2 cm lateral to midline (tandem) along the plane of the tandem. The point A dose rate was approximately 0.53 Gy/h for all allowed applicator loading patterns. Approximately two-thirds of the point A dose/dose rate contributed from the tandem and one-third from the ovoids. Point B dose/dose rate is typically one-third or approximately 33% of the point A dose/dose rate. The Manchester system specifies a maximum bladder and rectum point dose to be 80% or less than that of the dose to point A. If in any situation, the doses to the bladder and rectum are higher, the source loading should be altered in tandem and ovoids to achieve the goal.

To compare patients' treatment between centres around the world, ICRU Report 38[8] was followed which detailed the reporting information to be recorded.

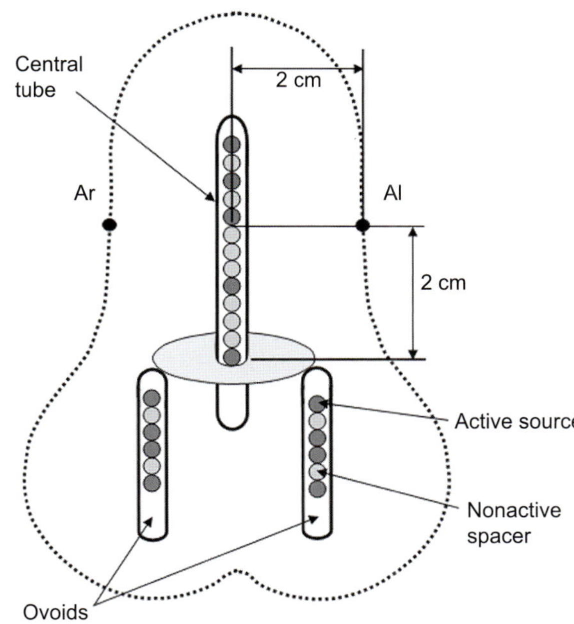

Fig. 9.6 Medium doserate source positions and the Manchester A points.

Paris System

The Paris system[7] was developed for use in determining the dose distributions around iridium-192 wire implants. It is based on a set of implant rules and specifies how dose calculations are to be made. The active sources should be straight and parallel, with no crossing of wires, and ideally should be of equal length and linear activity. They should be evenly spaced between 5 and 20 mm in a geometric pattern. Coils of thin, 0.3-mm diameter wire were cut to convenient lengths and inserted into flexible nylon tubes or rigid hollow afterloading needles similar to hypodermic needles previously implanted into tumours. Thicker wires of 0.6 mm in diameter, in the form of hairpins, were inserted directly into tumours through suitable guides (Fig. 9.7). The system was for low dose rate, 0.5 $Gyhr^{-1}$ to a prescribed reference dose. The reference doserate was 85% of the mean doserates between wires (Fig. 9.8). This reference doserate was used for treatment dose prescription. The Paris system was very flexible, which meant it could cope with a poor implant geometry.

Computer Treatment Planning

Treatment planning in brachytherapy has not developed at the same rate as that for external beam radiotherapy (EBRT) (Chapter 12). The same relatively simple algorithms and calculation methods have been in use for many years. An ideal brachytherapy treatment planning system should take into consideration the effect of the applicator, tissue inhomogeneity, and actual size and shape of the patient while computing the dose distribution.

In 1995, the American Association of Physicists in Medicine (AAPM) published the report of Task Group 43 (TG43)[9] and updated it in 2004 (TG43 U1).[10] The TG43 formalism is based upon the dose rate at a reference point in water from the actual source geometry, which is corrected for relative attenuation in water at all other points using factors such as radial dose function and anisotropy function. This formalism is incorporated into many specialist treatment planning software packages for brachytherapy dose calculation. The TG43 formalism permits consistent and widespread brachytherapy dose calculations with reasonable accuracy under most clinical situations and is recognised as the worldwide standard for low-energy photon-emitting brachytherapy dose calculation.

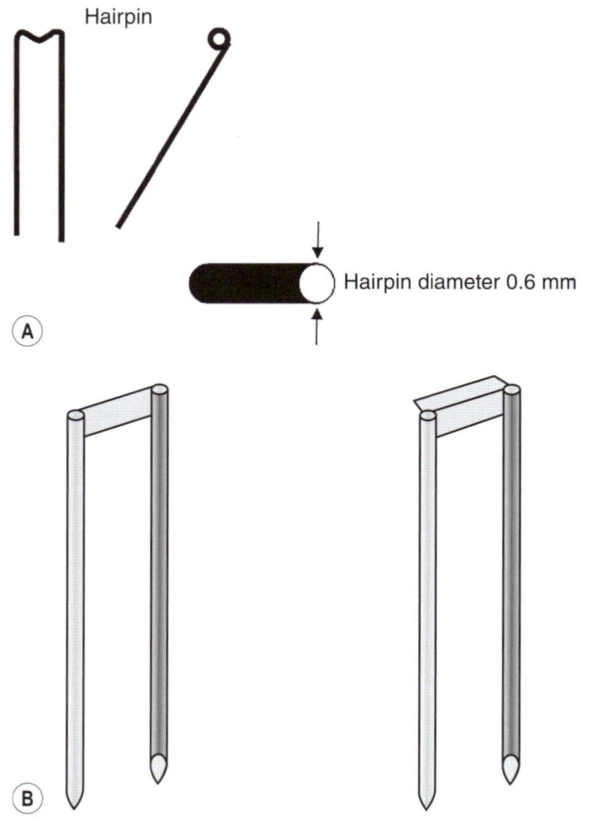

Fig. 9.7 Iridium-192 wire implants: (A) 0.6-mm diameter hairpins and (B) guides for insertion.

In 2012, TG186[11] was published providing recommendations for model-based dose calculation methods in brachytherapy beyond the TG43 formalism. Recent developments have led to improving the accuracy of the dose calculation and dose distributions in a tissue-equivalent medium, and further advances to include the effects of different heterogeneities and intersource and applicator shielding effects providing accuracy comparable to Monte Carlo simulation. There are now several algorithms on the market based on the recommendations published by the AAPM working group in 2012.

Clinical Applications

For a patient to be offered brachytherapy as a treatment option, they should have a localised cancer with a relatively small tumour and have a good performance status, which means they are able to tolerate an operation with general anaesthetic.

A typical patient pathway for an HDR brachytherapy treatment would be as follows:

1. In the operating theatre, the applicator is inserted with the patient under anaesthetic.
2. With the applicator/needle in situ, imaging is conducted, often multimodality (e.g. ultrasound, MR, CT).
3. The required image sets are imported into the TPS and fused.
4. The implant geometry of the applicators or needles is constructed from fused images.
5. The oncologist draws contours (targets and organs at risk (OARs)).
6. The standard plan is viewed.
7. Dose statistics are reviewed and the plan is optimised accordingly.
8. The oncologist reviews and approves the plan.
9. Independent checks are completed and treatment is delivered.
10. Steps 1 through 9 are repeated for all fractions; the patient stays overnight and has multiple treatments using the same applicator/needle insertion.

Prostate

A very popular interstitial treatment is for the radical treatment of localised prostate cancer. Prostate cancer is classified into low-, intermediate- or high-risk disease based on the presenting prostate-specific antigen (PSA), Gleason score and stage. LDR brachytherapy is an excellent option for monotherapy (one single treatment) for low-risk disease using a permanent implant of iodine-125 seeds. HDR brachytherapy with iridium-192 is the preferred option for combination therapy, with EBRT for intermediate- and high-risk disease. HDR brachytherapy capitalises on both the radiobiology of prostate cancer and its high conformal dosimetry by delivering a high dose to the prostate and sparing surrounding normal tissue.

LDR seed brachytherapy is normally performed as a single-stage technique including definition of the target volume and interactive planning during the seed implantation using ultrasound imaging. Most centres use low-activity seeds of 15 MBq per seed, with the final implant having a seed density of approximately 2.5 seeds per cubic centimetre. The target volume is the whole of the prostate, as defined by the capsule with a 2- to 3-mm margin. The advantage of a single-stage technique is that it can be adapted to the patient conditions presented on the day of the implant and is only one session for the multidisciplinary team to attend.

The implant is performed with the patient under a general anaesthetic and in the lithotomy position. A transrectal ultrasound (TRUS) probe is inserted into the rectum attached to a stepping unit that can incrementally advance and retract the probe within the rectum (Fig. 9.9). Attached to the stepper is a template. The coordinates of the template are automatically transposed over the ultrasound images of the prostate (Fig. 9.10). Empty needles are distributed around the periphery of the prostate, with

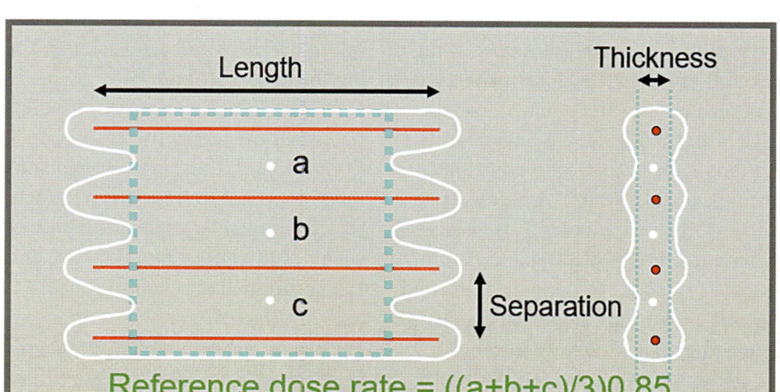

Fig. 9.8 Paris system.

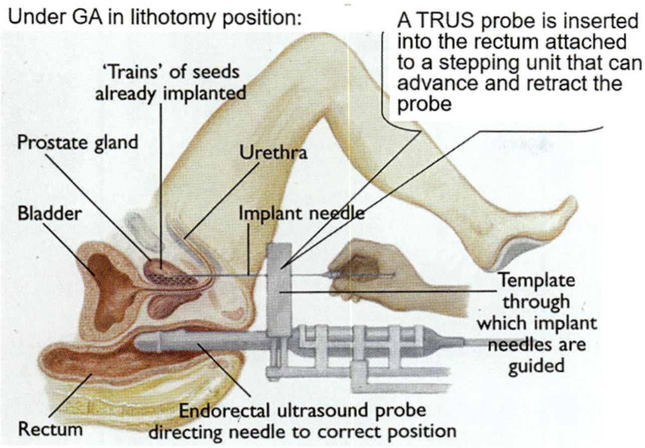

Fig. 9.9 Transrectal ultrasound imaging.

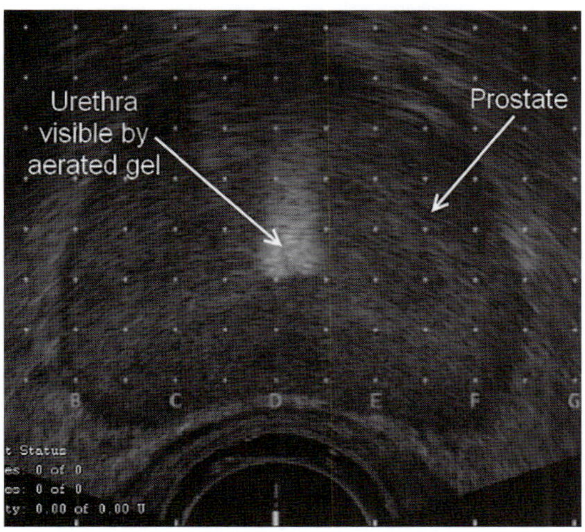

Fig. 9.10 Ultrasound image with superimposed template coordinates. (Image courtesy Varian Medical Systems, Inc. All rights reserved.)

a few additional central needles, avoiding the urethra. Serial images are then acquired from the base to the apex of the prostate in 5-mm intervals. On each image within the TPS, the prostate and OARs are delineated by the clinical oncologist. In Fig. 9.11, the prostate is shown as a red contour, the urethra in pink and the rectum in a blue contour. A 2-to-3-mm margin is added to the prostate, indicated by the orange contour.

A treatment plan is then created using preloaded optimisation rules to speed plan creation and is adjusted to meet the GEC-ESTRO planning recommendations.[12] The seeds are then implanted into the needles, registering the actual positions of the implanted seeds during the procedure on the TPS. The plan is not set in stone and the operator can still adapt it.[13]

HDR brachytherapy for prostate cancer follows a very similar technique. However, instead of inserting iodine seeds into the needles to deposit in the prostate, the needles are connected to the afterloading machine and the seed positions are HDR source dwell positions instead. A different TPS is used to model the iridium-192 source. In general, larger prostate volumes can be treated with an HDR technique, as the needles can be placed outside the prostate to deliver the radiation dose.

If the HDR afterloader is not located in an operating treatment room, the needles would be inserted under ultrasonic guidance in the operating theatre. When the patient has recovered from the general anaesthetic, they would be imaged using CT and/or MR with the needles in situ. These images would be transferred to the TPS and the treatment volume and OARs contoured. The plan would be created following the GEC-ESTRO recommendations[14,15] and sent to the treatment unit. The patient would then be moved to the brachytherapy suite and connected to the HDR machine for treatment to commence.

Gynaecological

From when brachytherapy was first introduced up until the mid-1970s, brachytherapy sources were used in an intracavity technique for treatment of the uterus and the vagina. Radioactive sources were loaded

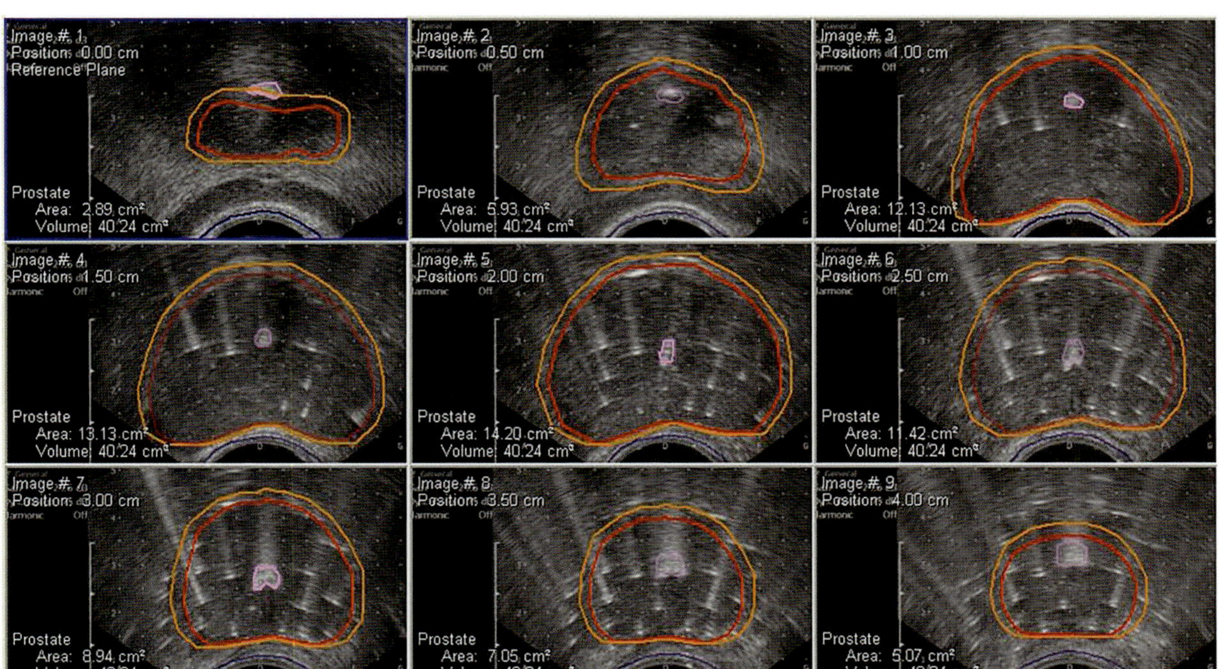

Fig. 9.11 Prostate ultrasound images with contours. (Image courtesy Varian Medical Systems, Inc. All rights reserved.)

into applicators which were positioned by hand. Sources remained in place during the treatment and then were manually retrieved. This, of course, had the consequence that staff involved in the process from beginning to end were exposed to ionising radiation. Manually inserted LDR caesium with or without supplementary EBRT treatment produced excellent tumour control rates unsurpassed by more modern methods of brachytherapy. The serious complication rate was also low, at 5% or less. Such results remain the gold standard against which modern techniques must be judged. The most widely used technique was the Manchester system[6] in which preloaded sources were placed in the uterus and against the cervix, producing a pear-shaped dose distribution around the cervix (Fig. 9.6).

The dose rate at point A was approximately 0.5 Gy/h, which proved to be biologically very advantageous. A typical regimen used to treat an early-stage 1b carcinoma of the cervix was two insertions of approximately 72 hours given 1 week apart, to give a total dose of 75 Gy to point A.

Once the modern HDR afterloader and associated applicators became available, HDR brachytherapy became an essential component of the definitive treatment for locally advanced cervical cancer and is currently the most widely used brachytherapy treatment delivery in the United Kingdom. With higher dose rates, the treatment time is considerably shorter. Increased dose rate has a greater biological effect which needs to be accounted for, and this is done by reducing the overall dose and delivering the treatment in a number of separate fractions. Treatment is completed in a matter of minutes, and rather like EBRT, HDR treatments are fractionated.

Two-dimensional imaging was the standard approach. However, in the past 20 years, image-guided adaptive brachytherapy (IGABT) has resulted in major changes in practice. The GEC-ESTRO gynaecology working group was established in 2000 to support and shape the emerging field of gynaecological IGABT. Their collaboration resulted in the publication of two GEC-ESTRO recommendations for concepts and terms in image-based three-dimensional treatment planning in cervix cancer brachytherapy.[16,17] IGABT, with repetitive MRI, is regarded as the gold standard and is increasingly replacing two-dimensional brachytherapy throughout the world. The GEC-ESTRO recommendations have been used as the conceptual framework for the implementation of IGABT worldwide and have further been included in ICRU Report 89.[18]

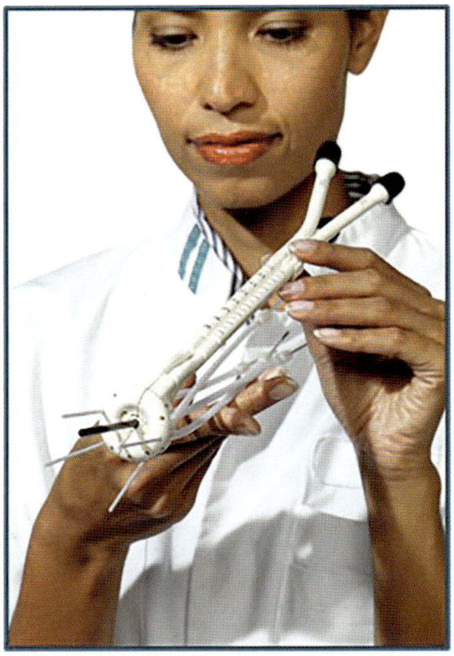

Fig. 9.12 Standard gynaecological applicators. (Courtesy Elekta.)

Today's modern brachytherapy cervix treatments involve insertion of the applicator under spinal or general anaesthetic (Fig. 9.12). During applicator insertions, the cervical os is dilated sufficiently to allow a rigid central tube to be placed in the uterus. Ovoids or a ring applicator is then placed against the cervix in line with the flange on the central tube, and sometimes needles are added through these (Fig. 9.13). These needles provide interstitial brachytherapy in combination with the main intracavitary treatment (Figs. 9.14 and 9.15). To reduce the dose to the rectum, gauze packing was traditionally used to move the rectal wall away from the sources; a rectal retractor can be used instead. The patient undergoes MRI, often in combination with CT. Marker wires inserted into the applicator to aid with applicator reconstruction in the TPS are different for each imaging modality. Target and OAR delineation occurs and an optimised treatment plan is produced following the GEC-ESTRO recommendations.[16,17] Once the final plan has been

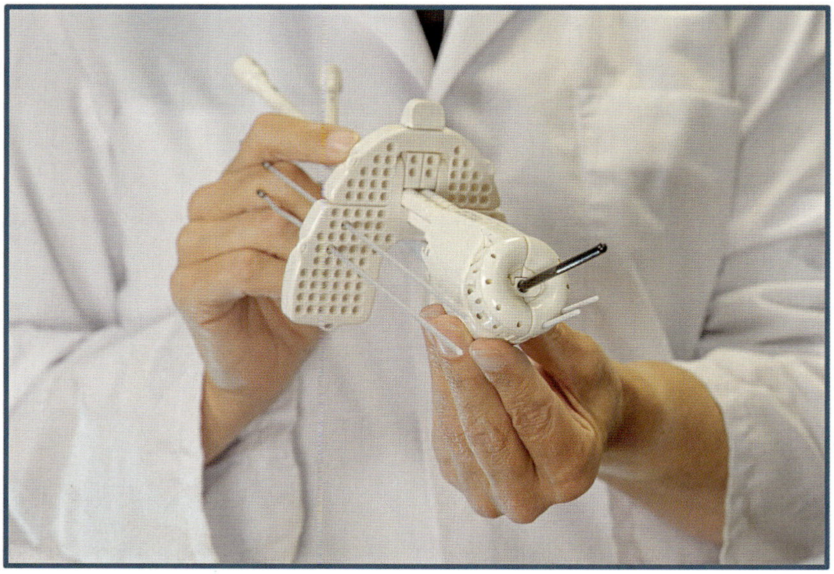

Fig. 9.13 State-of-the-art cervical brachytherapy applicator. (Courtesy Elekta.)

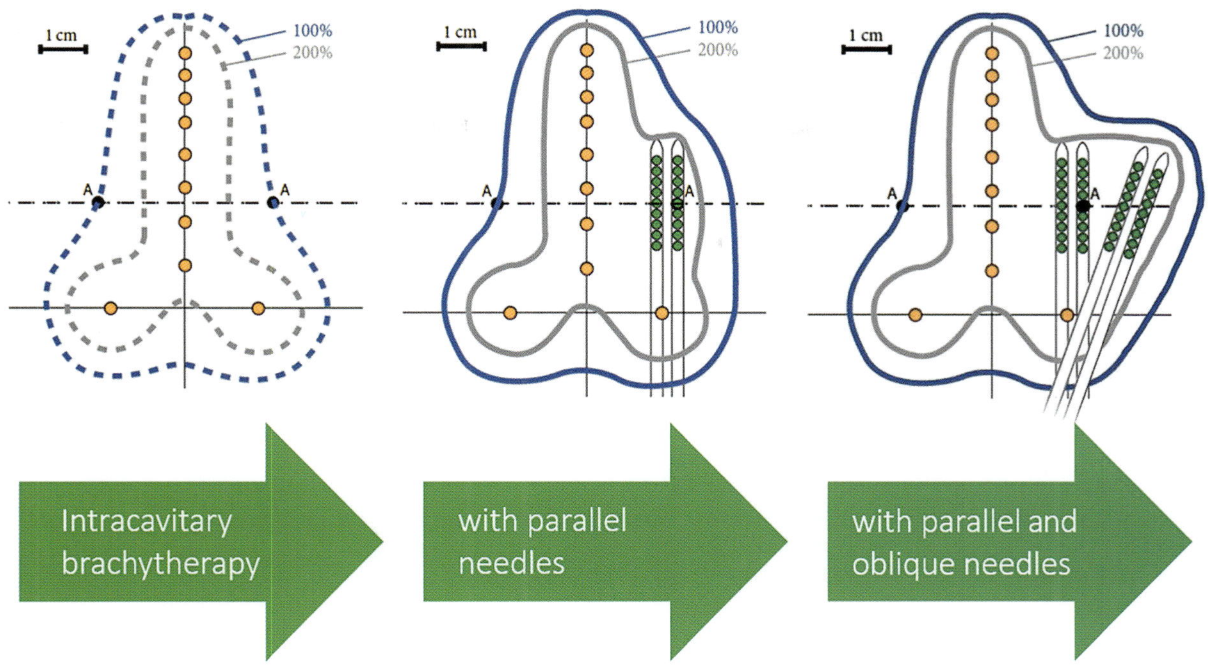

Fig. 9.14 Optimising dose distribution comparison with interstitial needles. (Courtesy Elekta.)

reviewed and approved by the clinical oncologist, various checks are carried out before the patient proceeds to the brachytherapy suite to have treatment.

The publication of the GEC-ESTRO recommendations[16,17] in 2005–2006 was a significant step forwards to reaching international consensus on adaptive target definition and dose reporting in image-guided brachytherapy in locally advanced cervical cancer. However, a unified approach to volume contouring and reporting does not imply unified treatment. Hence the international EMBRACE multistudy[19] was developed to benchmark a high level of local, nodal and systemic control while limiting morbidity, using state-of-the-art treatment.[20]

Brachytherapy for cervical cancer is a continually developing field with extensive research. The EMBRACE study[19] is internationally recognised as the most ambitious study worldwide to evaluate and benchmark image-guided brachytherapy in a prospective multicentre study.

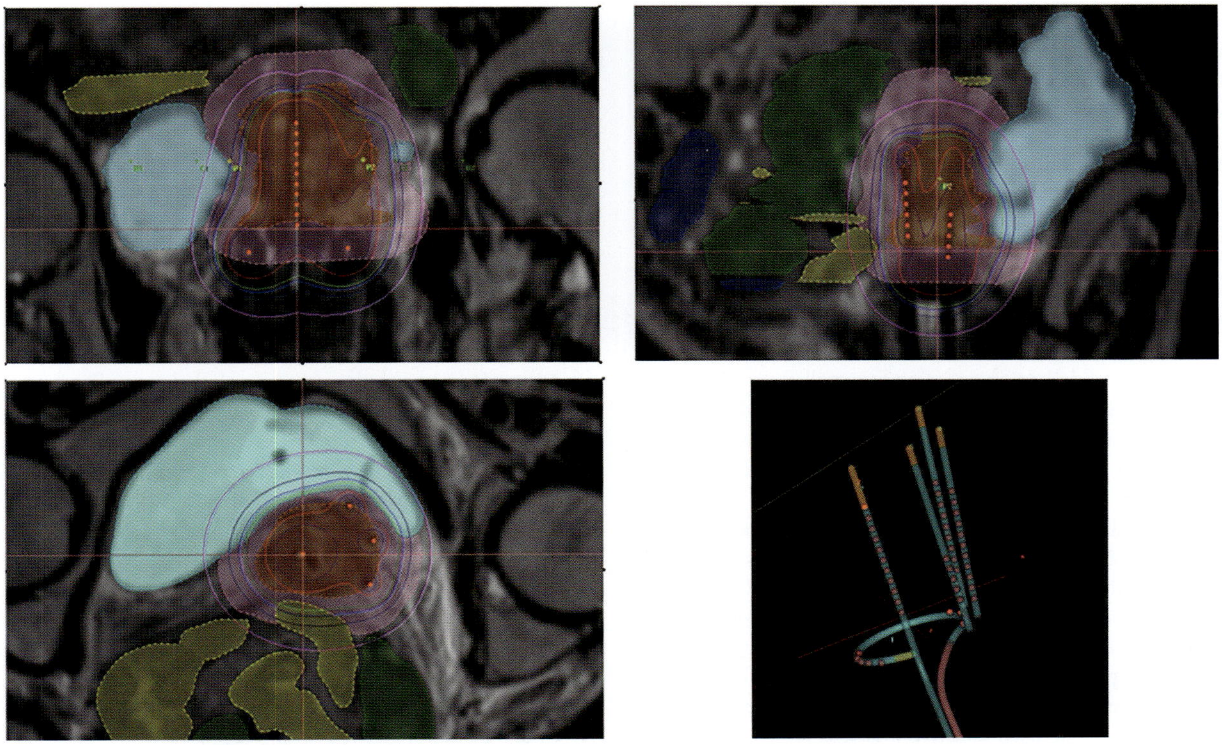

Fig. 9.15 Cervix applicator combining intracavity and interstitial treatment. (Courtesy Elekta.)

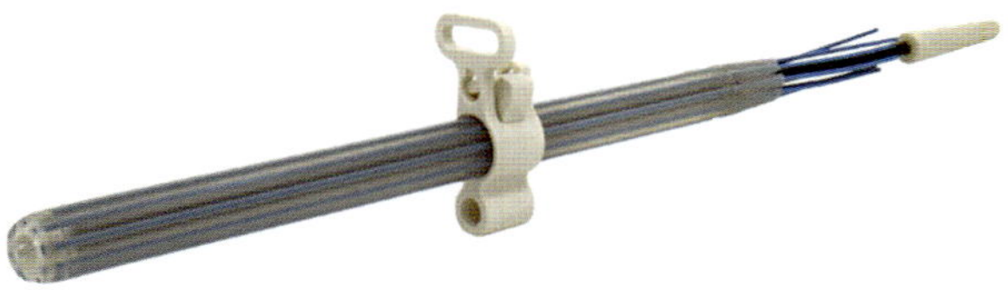

Fig. 9.16 Rectal applicator. (Courtesy Elekta.)

Rectal

Rectal cancer is among the common malignancies throughout the world, frequently affecting patients older than 50 years of age. Colorectal cancer is the third most common cancer and the second leading cause of cancer death globally. Rectal cancer accounts for one-third of these cases.[21,22]

Rectal brachytherapy is an intracavity technique which has increased in popularity in the United Kingdom in recent years. HDR brachytherapy can be used before surgery in patients with cancer in the middle or lower third of the rectum. The aim is to shrink the tumour and 'downstage' it, which may make anal-preservation surgery feasible for more patients.[23]

HDR brachytherapy can also be used as a palliative treatment for advanced inoperable rectal cancer.[24] Local recurrence after curative surgery for rectal cancer occurs in 5% to 30% of patients, depending on the surgical technique, the stage of the tumour and adjuvant treatments.[25] Often, the treatment options for this group of patients are limited due to previous surgery, chemotherapy or radiotherapy. Palliative radiotherapy is considered the standard treatment for these patients, but reirradiation of this previously treated area is made difficult by the tolerance of the surrounding tissues.

For brachytherapy treatment, a single-use flexible endorectal applicator (Fig. 9.16) with eight catheters arranged around its circumference is inserted, with the patient under mild sedation in the brachytherapy suite. The patient then has a CT scan to plan the treatment, and additional images from other imaging modalities are reviewed to inform the target definition. The prescription dose is defined at 1 cm from the surface of the applicator. The applicator is then connected to the HDR treatment machine, and the radiation is delivered to the tumour within the rectum according to the patient-specific treatment plan. The applicator is then removed and the patient goes home the same day.

Lung, Bronchus and Oesophagus

Once HDR afterloading units were using fine catheters of 2 mm in diameter, it was possible to pass these into the bronchus or the oesophagus. This permitted delivery of a high localised dose of radiation to a defined area with relative ease and only requiring moderate sedation. Known as *intraluminal brachytherapy treatment* (Fig. 9.17), it can be given in combination with EBRT as a radical course of radiotherapy or as the sole means of delivering radiation for a palliative treatment.

Oesophageal cancer often presents as advanced-stage disease with a dismal prognosis, with only 10% to 15% of patients surviving 5 years following treatment. Therefore, in a large proportion of patients, palliative treatment is the only option available.

Lung cancer is an area where HDR brachytherapy has been used effectively in the United Kingdom and in many institutions worldwide. It is used largely in the palliative setting when tumours occlude a major airway. It can be used to prevent massive haemorrhage and collapse of the lung as well as providing immediate symptom control for the patient. The technique can be used both for primary lung cancers and endobronchial metastases from cancers originating at other sites. Lung brachytherapy can also be used effectively as retreatment in patients who have received EBRT in the past.

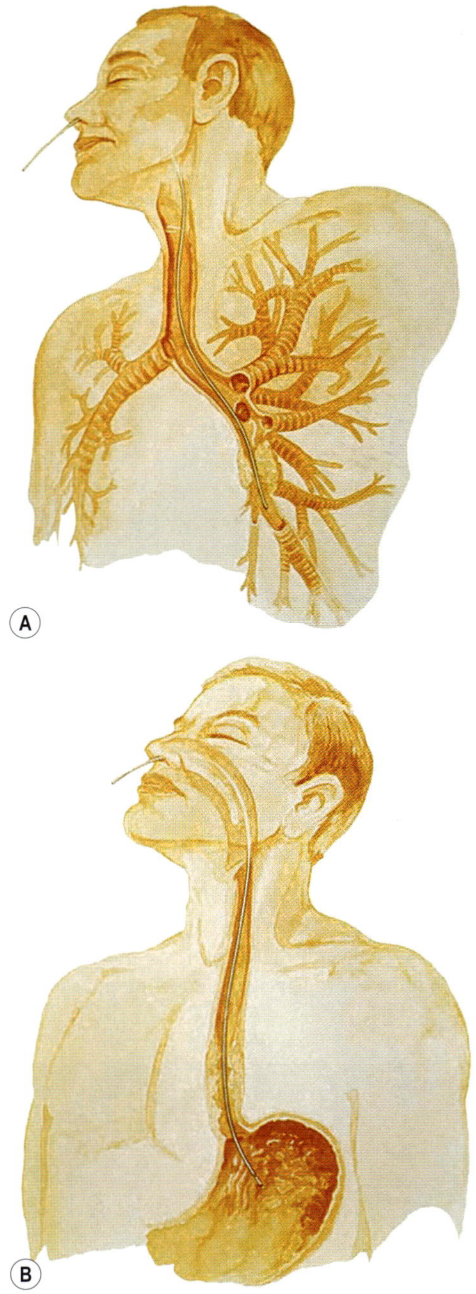

Fig. 9.17 Intraluminal brachytherapy: (A) bronchus and (B) oesophagus. (Courtesy Elekta.)

Most treatments for the oesophagus are delivered in a single dose and is performed as a day case by a skilled team. For bronchus, a full course of brachytherapy is usually between 3 and 5 treatments, depending on the size and location of the tumour. Dose penetration for both sites, however, is limited, with the typical prescription point being 1 cm from the source surface and dwell positions defined along the identified treatment length.[26,27]

Surface and Skin

Radiotherapy has been used to treat skin cancers for over 100 years. Radiotherapy for skin cancer can be delivered by using EBRT, superficial or electron beam therapy, or brachytherapy with radiation sources placed directly onto or into the skin. For the majority of skin cancers which are basal cell carcinomas (BCCs) and squamous cell carcinomas (SCCs), EBRT is the preferred treatment. But in some cases, brachytherapy offers

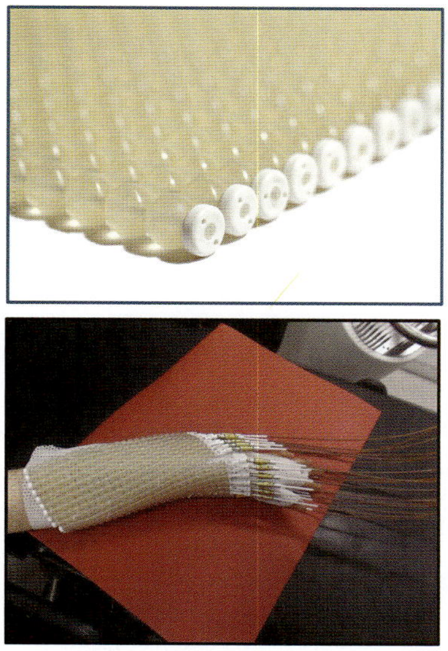

Fig. 9.18 Freiburg flap sewn onto thermoplastic shell using dental floss for a wrist skin treatment. (Courtesy Elekta.)

better coverage of the treatment area, for example in cases of skin malignancies that wrap around skin surfaces such as on the lower limbs, hands and complex curved surfaces on the face, scalp or head and neck. In these situations, moulds of the body part conforming to skin surfaces can be made to hold plastic tubes that allow delivery of HDR brachytherapy. In the past, mould therapy has been used extensively with iridium-192 sources placed across tumours or within wax moulds. Flexible mesh-style surface moulds have now been designed for surface treatments with HDR (Fig. 9.18). The mesh can be easily shaped to fit curved surfaces quickly, rather than needing to make complex wax or thermoplastic moulds.[28]

Custom-made surface moulds, however, can be difficult to manufacture, particularly if there is a lack of experience in superficial HDR brachytherapy techniques or with limited resources. Three-dimensional printing technology has been applied to produce customised skin applicators in HDR brachytherapy. These can improve dose distribution and spare healthy tissue. Jones et al.[29] describe a novel method for manufacturing superficial brachytherapy applicators utilising three-dimensional printing techniques. With the introduction of a preplan, the treatment planning process (Fig. 9.19) allows for an 'ideal' catheter arrangement within an applicator to be determined, exploiting varying catheter orientations, heights and curvatures if required. The preplan arrangement is then three-dimensionally printed to the exact specifications of the preplan applicator design. This results in improved target volume coverage and better sparing of OARs, resulting in a more efficient and improved patient pathway and patient experience.[29]

Plaques for Eye Treatment

The major use of plaques emitting beta radiation is in the treatment of eye tumours.

Strontium-90 compound is incorporated in a rolled silver foil bonded into a silver applicator and formed so that it presents an active concave surface of 15 mm in radius to the cornea. With a surface filtration of 0.1 mm silver, strontium-90 is only useful when in radioactive equilibrium with its daughter product, yttrium-90. The silver filter is designed to absorb low-energy beta particles from the strontium decay (0.546 MeV max) while transmitting the higher-energy beta particles from the yttrium-90 (2.27 MeV max). The back of the applicator is finished with a much thicker (0.9 mm) layer of silver to reduce the transmitted dose rate to a relatively safe level. The plaques are designed to give a useful dose rate of approximately 1 Gy per minute at the surface, reducing to 50% at approximately 2 mm.

The ruthenium-106 applicator is made of silver, with a window thickness of 0.1 mm of silver and a thicker protective layer of 0.9 mm of silver on the back. The applicator is designed for suturing to the sclera for 7 to 10 days. The useful dose rate is typically 0.1 Gy per minute at the surface, reducing to 50% at approximately 2.7 mm. A 15-mm acrylic visor is recommended to protect the eyes of the operator when using the ruthenium applicators.

Treatment of retinoblastoma has been effected using cobalt-60 ophthalmic applicators of similar construction to the ruthenium

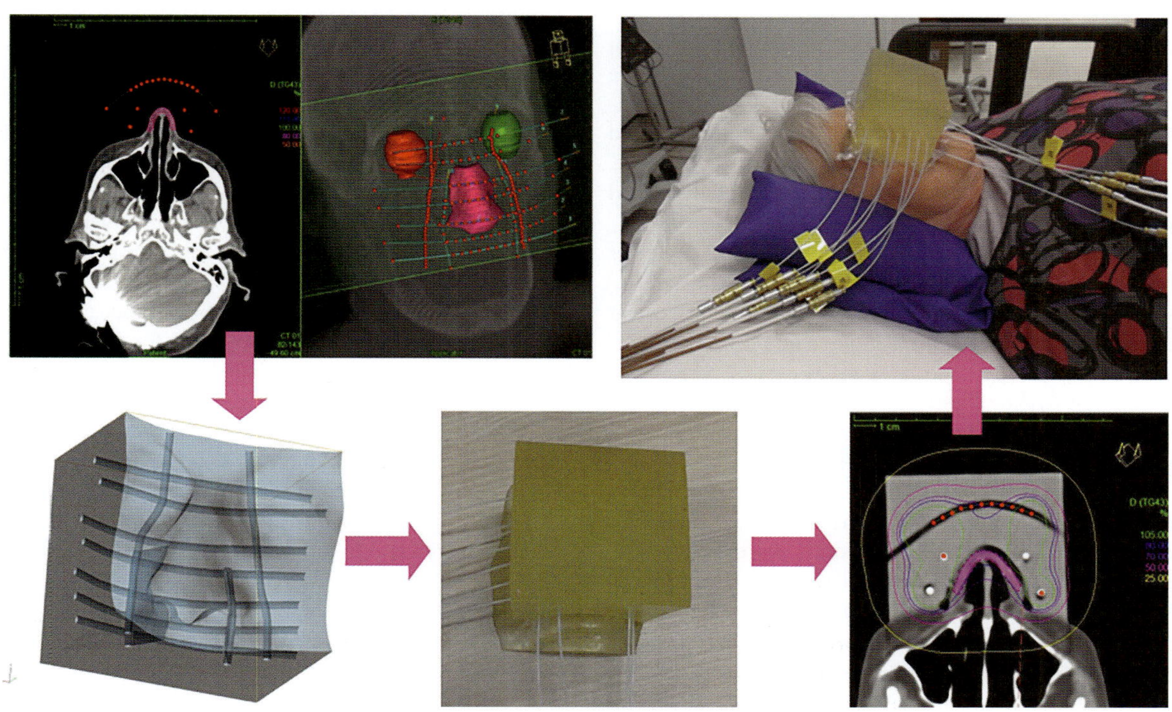

Fig. 9.19 Three-dimensional printed skin applicator. (Image courtesy Varian Medical Systems, Inc. All rights reserved.)

applicator. The longer half-life was an advantage, but the high-energy gamma radiation gave high doses to other vital structures, such as the lens, macula and optic nerve, than with the ruthenium-106 beta particle radiations.

Quality Assurance

The main objective of any brachytherapy treatment is to deliver an optimised dose distribution to the patient so that the prescribed dose is given to the target volume while limiting the dose to OARs and other normal tissues nearby. This is in accordance with the 'as low as reasonably practical' (ALARP) principle. A quality assurance (QA) program ensures that the patient's treatment is delivered correctly and safely by confirming that the equipment continues to perform within an acceptable tolerance. A medical physics expert (MPE) is responsible for management of the QA program and for the acceptance testing, commissioning and definitive calibration of new equipment before its clinical use. Quality control, described comprehensively in Chapter 14, forms part of a QA program which should address every step of the treatment process, from diagnosis through treatment planning to treatment delivery. It should check that all radioactive sources are accounted for, and documentation should be kept for future reference. QA recommendations are provided by IPEM Report 81, ESTRO Booklet No. 8 and AAPM TG41, TG56 and TG53.[30–34]

Source Storage, Security and Records

Radioactive sources must be under the control of an appropriate person at all times. This includes ordering, receiving, storage, handling, use and disposal. The best practice is to utilise electronic records for source stock control. Paper records can be used in addition to these for source movement. Records would be expected to contain the isotope, source serial number, number of sources, reference activity with date/time, date of receipt and date of disposal.

The Statutory Regulations[35] in the United Kingdom ensure a strict regulatory framework for High Activity Sealed Radioactive Sources (HASS). These regulations are defined in terms of activity and nuclide, and in radiotherapy departments these normally only apply to HDR sources.

Permission to hold the sources must be obtained by the Environment Agency, and this will only be granted once the Counter Terrorism Security Advisor (CTSA) has inspected the proposed location of the sources, assessed the level of security measures and deemed them sufficient for the category of radioactive source. Security measures required are expected to include source storage within a locked cage or safe, which is then located in a secure room with an alarm that only limited staff have access to.

The HASS regulations also specify that the source licence holder must have financial provisions in place for the disposal of the radioactive sources. This is often covered by a source takeback or replacement agreement in the service contract with the source supplier.

Source Strength Confirmation and Calibration

Source strength measurements are performed using a reentrant well-type ionisation chamber connected to an electrometer, with different holders used for different sources (Fig. 9.20). The well chamber is unsealed; hence temperature and pressure corrections are required for any measurements. The source holder provides a reproducible position and orientation for every measurement. The electrometer and well chamber should have a calibration traceable to a national standards laboratory such as the National Physical Laboratory (NPL) in the United Kingdom and the National Institute of Standards and Technology (NIST) in the United States. A long-lived calibrated source such as Cs-137 can be used as a reference source to check that the chamber is functioning correctly, which is normally within ±2% of a reference value. The result of the source strength measurement should be within ±5% of the manufacturer's source certificate.

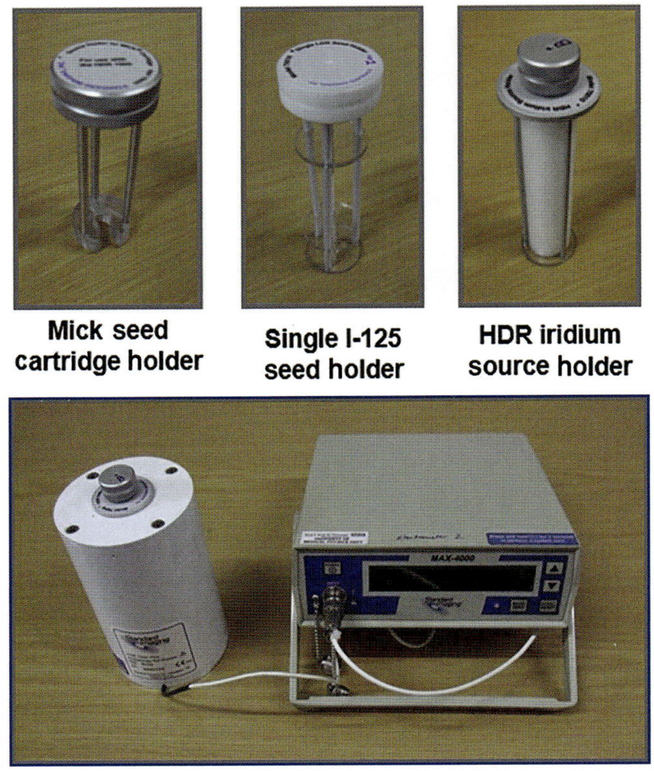

Fig. 9.20 Well chamber and electrometer with source holder.

HDR source calibrations should follow the UK IPEM Code of Practice.[36]

Iodine seed calibrations should follow the AAPM Low Energy Brachytherapy Source Calibration Working Group.[37]

Machine Function Tests

Routine checks on the functionality of the treatment machine should be conducted before every treatment session. These checks should confirm correct functioning of the safety interlocks: that is, the door interlock, interrupt button and emergency stop button. Also, the radiation warning lights should be checked to ensure that they provide an audible warning when exposed to a source. Emergency equipment such as a portable radiation detector, mobile shielded storage safe and long-handed tongs should be in place, and the patient intercom should be functioning along with the CCTV system.

Routine quality control checks should also include visual inspection of the transfer tubes and applicators for damage or constrictions, applicator and transfer tube interlocks, positional accuracy of the source and functionality of the treatment console.

More detailed tests should be performed quarterly in addition to the routine checks. Post source exchange, the source calibration should consist of two independent checks in addition to source position and drive position verification using both CCTV and film. It should be completed with end-to-end testing with a treatment plan.

Treatment Planning System

Treatment planning complexity has increased in recent years due to technological advances in imaging and computational power. Comprehensive commissioning of the TPS should include all aspects of the treatment planning process (image registration, applicator reconstruction, dose distribution optimisation and calculation, data transfer etc.). Once in clinical use, regular QA should then check the integrity of the system. Initial commission testing can be used to form the baseline record against which routine QA measurements can be compared.

In addition, if any software upgrades are implemented or if there are any changes to the data within the TPS, recommissioning should take place.

An individual patient plan will still require an independent check, and this is done by calculating and verifying the dose at one or more points using the source location data from the treatment planning system.

Electronic Brachytherapy

Historically, intraoperative radiotherapy (IORT) has been an important element in radiation oncology. Its use has mainly been to deliver large single doses directly to the tumour bed in the form of a treatment boost, often following surgery. In the past, the use of electrons was preferred because of decreased treatment time, better dose homogeneity and less absorption of radiation by strong absorbers such as bone.

The miniaturisation of x-ray sources has led to the opportunity to implant a nonradioactive source to deliver treatment to a target volume. This is referred to as *electronic brachytherapy (EBT)*. Essentially, these miniature devices generate electrons with 50-keV energy in a very short distance and bombard a transmission target such as tungsten or gold to produce an almost omnidirectional point source distribution of x-rays. As with contact therapy, the source is in direct contact with tissue and has a rapid falloff in depth dose. The aspects of such a device are shown in Fig. 9.21.

More recently, EBT devices able to deliver low orthovoltage radiation during IORT have offered advantages in some cases and have proven to be cost-effective.[38,39] In appropriate cases, EBT provides a novel alternative to conventional brachytherapy techniques. Treatments include partial breast irradiation, rectal cancer and small skin cancers. Because of their low energy, these devices can be used in operating theatres with minimal shielding and radiation safety requirements. In addition, they do not involve the use of a radioactive source and so avoid the need for elaborate source security precautions. Procedures can also be performed with reduced numbers of radiotherapy experts present.

EBT techniques produce steep dose gradients, and as with iodine-125 treatments, care is necessary when treatment delivery is close to structures such as bone, where absorption at low kilovoltage energy is enhanced due to the photoelectric effect.

SUPERFICIAL AND DEEP KILOVOLTAGE MACHINES

Deep x-ray (DXR) and superficial x-ray (SXR) units provide x-ray beams in the keV energy range. The term *orthovoltage* is also used, and this term reflects the arrangement whereby the x-rays are produced in a direction at right angles to that of the accelerating voltage. The units typically take the form of a tube assembly which can be manually manipulated to direct the beam onto the patient. The SSD is typically in the range of 20 to 50 cm, and the field is defined at the surface by a mechanical applicator. An example of such a machine is shown in Fig. 9.22.

Tube Stand

The tube is mounted on a mechanism commonly referred to as the *tube stand* (Fig. 9.23). The design of the tube stand enables manipulation of the beam direction by the machine operator so that it is directed at the patient's lesion. There are both floor-mounted and ceiling-mounted

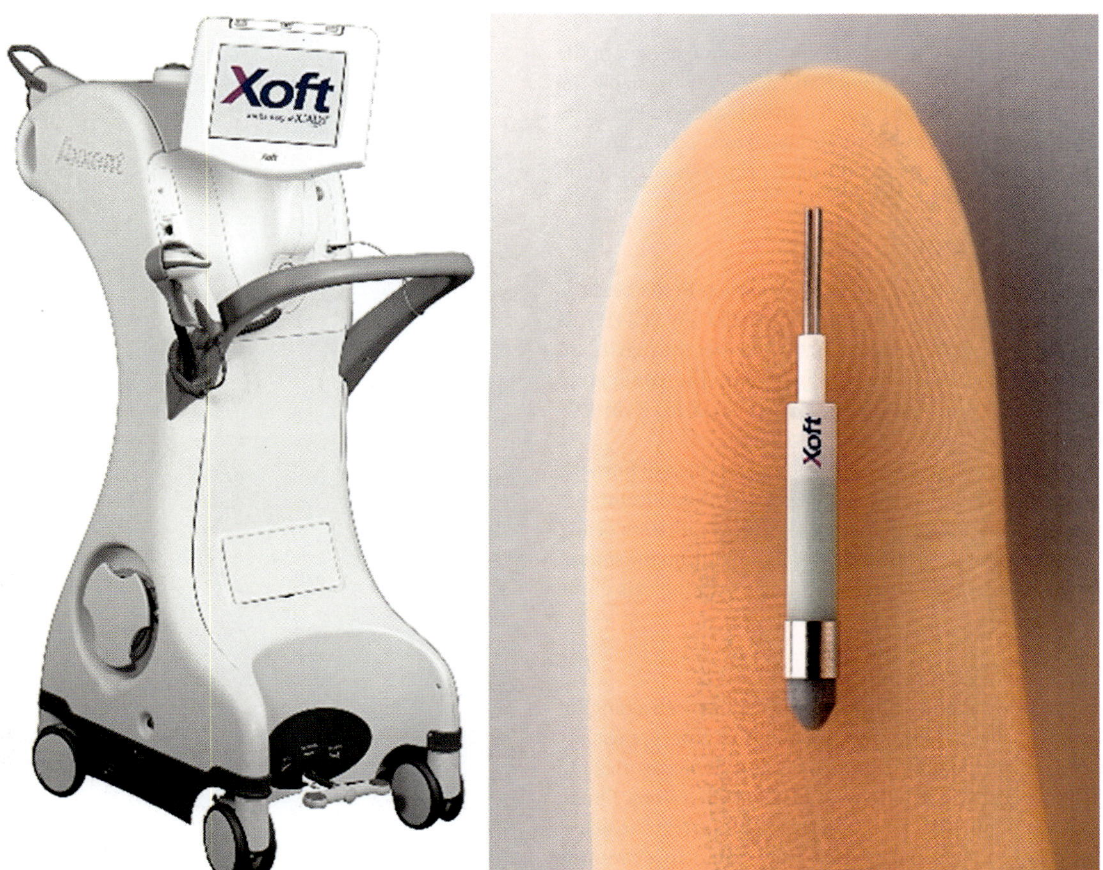

Fig. 9.21 Miniaturised 50-kV x-ray source system for x-ray brachytherapy. (Courtesy Xoft.)

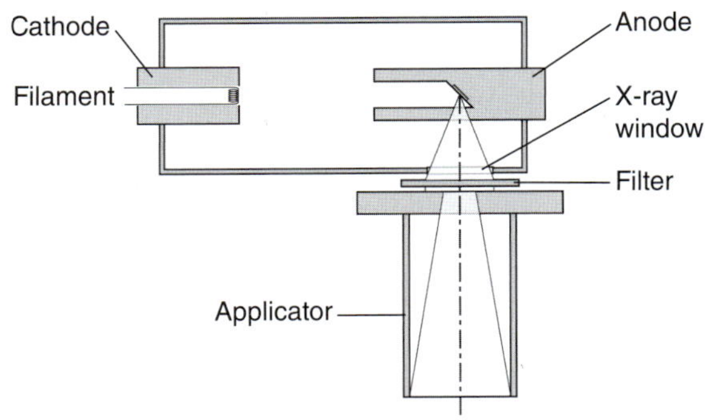

Fig. 9.22 Schematic of an orthovoltage machine.

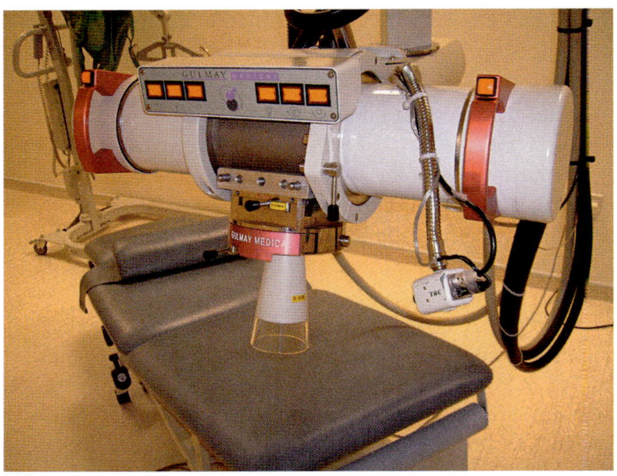

Fig. 9.23 Orthovoltage machine on a stand.

stands. The design allows translational and rotational movement of the beam, and there may be scales of distance and angle which enable the setup position or changes to it to be recorded and monitored. Electrical or mechanical brakes are fitted to the rotational axes and translational runners so that the position can be reliably fixed prior to treatment and monitored during treatment.

Collimation

The anode construction provides the initial collimation of the beam as the x-rays come off the target almost omnidirectionally (Fig. 9.24). This is referred to as a *hooded anode*, and the aperture defines the maximum size of conical x-ray beam that could be provided. The collimation is completed through the use of an applicator which is fixed directly below the tube aperture and provides the following:

- The base of the applicator consists of a collimator which defines the shape and size of the radiation field at the end of the applicator.
- The end of the applicator is the shape and size of the radiation beam.
- The end of the applicator determines a fixed distance from the source.
- The axis of the applicator is mechanically aligned to the axis of the radiation beam.

Skin and Eye Shielding

Beam collimation is provided on orthovoltage machines with a range of applicators which have regular field sizes. These applicators are usually chosen by the user when the unit is purchased. The choice is made to provide a nominal range of sizes for coverage of typical lesions. Often, it is necessary to treat lesions of nonstandard size and irregular shape. It is a common practice to manufacture a lead cutout to define the treatment field exactly to the area specified by the radiotherapist. The cutout is used in conjunction with one of the regular-sized applicators

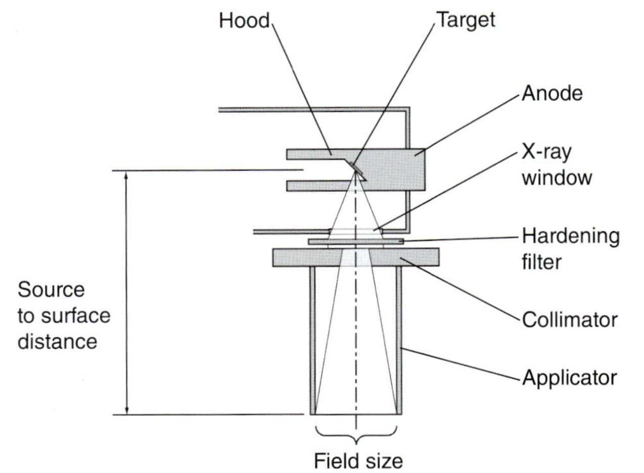

Fig. 9.24 Anode construction, hood and omnidirectional emission with applicator to collimate the beam, set the source to surface distance and define the field size.

to irradiate the treatment area and shield the surrounding normal skin from the rest of the beam. For lesions on the face and in close proximity to the eyes, a lead mask is manufactured based upon a plaster cast of the patient. As well as defining the treatment field and shielding the normal skin and the eyes, the lead mask can also be used to provide direction and localisation of the beam (Fig. 9.25).

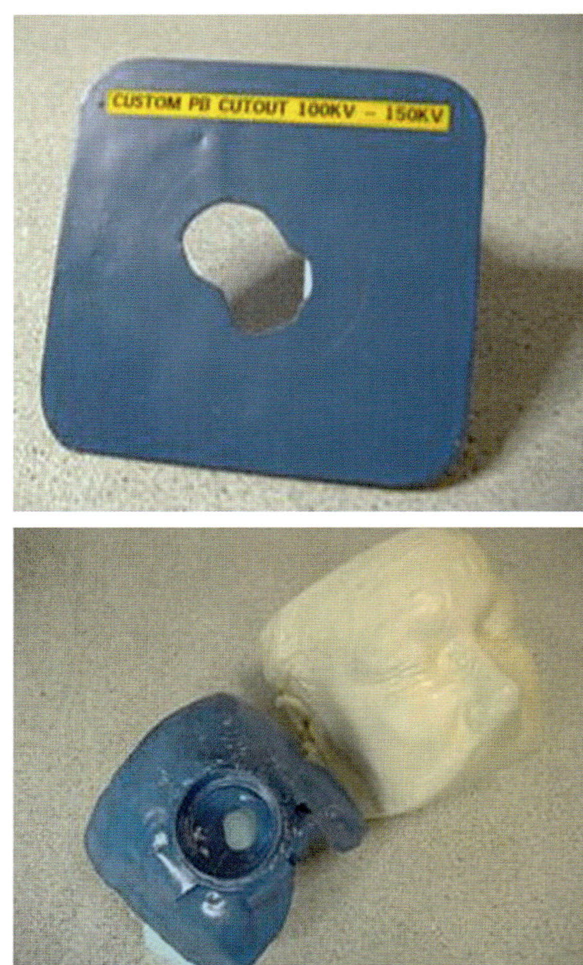

Fig. 9.25 Irregular lead cutout and mask.

To provide effective shielding, the thickness of the lead for the cutout has to be chosen considering the energy of the beam. This can be done from tabulated data of attenuation in lead against field size and beam energy as expressed by HVL (see Chapter 2, Beam Hardening). It is always prudent, however, for radiotherapy physicists to undertake measurements and verify the shielding that is being obtained with the chosen thickness of lead.

When the treatment area impinges onto the eye, it is possible to insert eye shields to provide some protection to the lens. There are commercial lead and tungsten shields available. The problem encountered with eye shields is the contribution from scatter which reaches into the region under the shield from the surrounding field.

Control of Output

The stability of the output from the unit is directly related to the electrical stability of the tube voltage and current. Stabilised electrical supplies, as described earlier, ensure that this is achieved consistently. Typically, a timer is used to control the amount of dose that is delivered. The timer is normally a countdown device and starts to operate when the treatment is initiated and the voltage and current are supplied to the tube. After the set time has elapsed, the voltage and current are switched off and treatment terminates. A timed exposure requires that the output dose rate is stable, which is dependent upon the electrical control stability mentioned earlier. There is always an inherent increase in the dose rate as the voltage and the current ramp up to their operating values, and this effect is normally taken into account using a transit time to accommodate the underdose which this would otherwise lead to. The transit time is added to the calculated time based upon a nominal dose rate to produce a total set time.

Most modern DXR and SXR units utilise a full-field ionisation monitor chamber through which the beam passes. By measuring the charge released against the absolute dose under particular setup conditions, it is possible to control the output from the machine by a system which terminates the beam when the accumulated charge equals the required dose. The units of charge from the ionisation chamber are referred to as *monitor units*, and the specific dose delivered to any individual patient is achieved by calculating the required number of monitor units to be set.

Calibration of Dose Output

As described earlier, there are two types of exposure control utilised on orthovoltage equipment. For a great many years, it has been done utilising a timer. However, in more recent years, exposure is controlled by a full-field ionisation monitor chamber mounted in the radiation beam.

For timer control, the machine operator must know the dose rate of the machine, and for ionisation chamber control, the response of the chamber must be directly related to an absolute dose. The ionisation chamber response is normally quantified in monitor units and calibrated to be dose per monitor unit. Hence, for both systems of control, it is necessary to measure the absolute dose delivered by the beam under a very specific setup, often referred to as *calibration conditions*. The time to be set or the monitor units to be set are then determined using relative factors from the calibration setup. For example, the specific dose rate may be measured for a 5-cm diameter applicator at a 30-cm SSD. To calculate a time to set, relative factors for other applicators, difference in SSD and changes in the irradiated area are used.

The absolute dose is measured in accordance with a protocol or code of practice. This ensures uniformity of practice between institutions. It will utilise the absolute dose calibration of the ionisation chamber being used for the measurement, and this will be traceable to a standards laboratory. The calibration can be done in air with the use of mass absorption coefficient ratios to determine the dose to water or tissue. Alternatively, the measurement can be done directly at depth in water. For superficial kV units with HVL values up to 8 mm Al, it is typical to determine the surface dose rate, as this is where the dose is to be applied. However, for deep x-ray units with HVL values higher than 8 mm Al, it can be preferable to quote the dose deeper than the surface and closer to the target. In the latter case, it is preferable to calibrate at depth in water.

CONTACT KILOVOLTAGE MACHINE

Contact radiotherapy began in the 1940s with very short SSD x-ray treatments. The characteristic of these beams is a rapid falloff in depth dose from the surface due to the short SSD. So, in contrast to moving from SXR to DXR to gain penetration, these beams can provide a very high dose to 1 to 2 mm of the incident tissue while considerably limiting the dose given deeper. This does mean that the depth-dose variation and the incident dose are very sensitive to displacement. For example, a 1-mm standoff at a 20-cm SSD changes the incident dose by 1% whereas at a 4-cm SSD it changes by 5%. Similarly, the change in dose depth at a 1-cm depth is 2% at a 4-cm SSD compared with 0.1% at a 20-cm SSD.

The HT generator is of a standard design, as already described in Radionuclide Characteristics and Kilovoltage X-rays, and typically, a 50-kV accelerating potential is used, with filtration occurring intrinsically in the construction materials as well as the X-ray target, which may well be a transmission design. The design of the target and its cooling system as well as monitoring of the output is challenging. A contact beam will have an HVL of about 0.35 mm Al.[1] These machines have a gantry stand to enable direct treatment onto a surface lesion which may be inside the rectum or intraoperatively aligned to an applicator inserted into the surgical cavity. Such a machine is shown in Fig. 9.26.

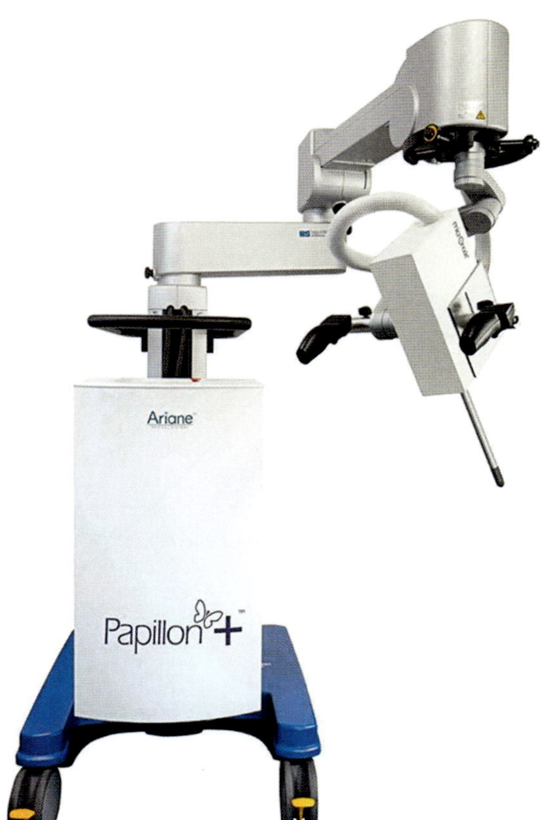

Fig. 9.26 Contact radiotherapy machine. (Courtesy Ariane Medical Systems.)

GRENZ KILOVOLTAGE MACHINE

Very low kV x-ray generation was explored from the 1920s, and the term *Grenz*, which means 'border' in German, was used for beams with HVL of less than 0.04 mm Al, as their biological effect was observed to lie between x-rays and ultraviolet rays for skin conditions. In some designs the x-ray target was the window of the tube. However, in all designs the hardening effect of the tube limited the softness of the x-rays produced. Typical beam characteristics are presented in the *British Journal of Radiolology*.[1] HT generation, cooling and gantry systems remain the same as for superficial and deep x-ray machines.

BETA RAY MACHINE

As mentioned earlier with regard to brachytherapy, beta particle emitters have found applications in superficial treatment utilising the superficial penetration of the beta particles and delivery of a dose to a small thickness of tissue.

A beta ray device has also been developed to deliver a radiotherapy dose from a small strontium-90 source directly to the central area of the retina using an intraocular probe during eye surgery.

Most early teletherapy machines which were developed for both medical and industrial applications utilised gamma-emitting radionuclides such as caesium-137, iridium-192 and cobalt-60. However, one notable attempt was made to deliver a teletherapy beam of electrons for total skin irradiation with strontium-90. It used a 900-MBq source which was 53 cm long by 2 cm wide. The machine traversed along the patient for 40 cm to deliver a skin dose. The treatment times were in excess of 15 minutes to deliver a therapeutic 2-Gy dose fraction, and the penetration of the dose was limited to about 2 mm by the maximum energy of the daughter yttrium-90 emission of 2.27 MeV. The limited penetration and doserate illustrates why there was no widespread use of such a teletherapy machine, and megavoltage (MV) accelerators went on to provide much more effective electron beams for total skin electron treatment (Chapter 10).

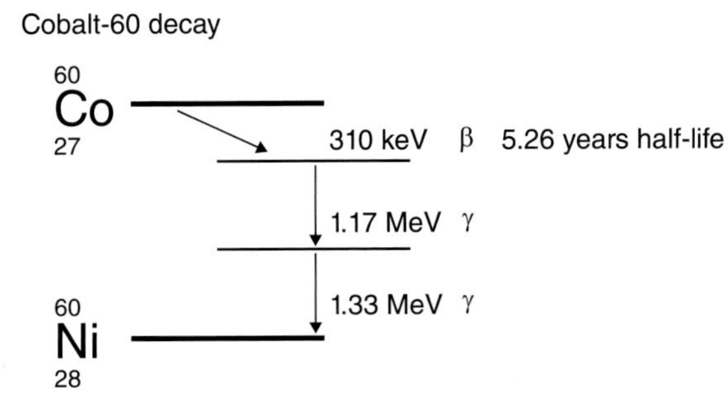

Fig. 9.27 Cobalt gamma ray decay process.

GAMMA RAY MACHINE

The penetrative limitations and high skin dose of even 300-kV x-rays drove the desire for higher-energy x-rays. The radioisotope cobalt-60 (^{60}Co) was discovered at the University of California by Seaborg and Livingwood[42] in the 1930s, and in Canada in 1951 it was used for teletherapy. The isotope is produced by neutron bombardment through the following process:

$$^{59}\text{Co} + n \rightarrow {}^{60}\text{Co} + \gamma \quad \textbf{(9.1)}$$

Nuclear reactors provided an ideal production platform for the substance. The attraction of cobalt-60 was the high-energy gamma emission produced in the radioactive decay process (Fig. 9.27) and the relatively long half-life of the isotope of just over 5 years. The energy of the gamma rays is almost four times that of the highest deep x-ray unit.

The depth-dose characteristics of a nominal 10 × 10 cm cobalt-60 beam at 80 SSD is compared in Fig. 9.28 to that for a 10-cm diameter 0.4-Cu HVL kilovoltage beam. The latter would typically be produced from acceleration with about 300 kV and appropriate filtration. The depth-dose characteristics for a 10 × 10 cm field size 6-MV and 25-MV beam at 100 SSD from a linear accelerator are also shown for comparison.

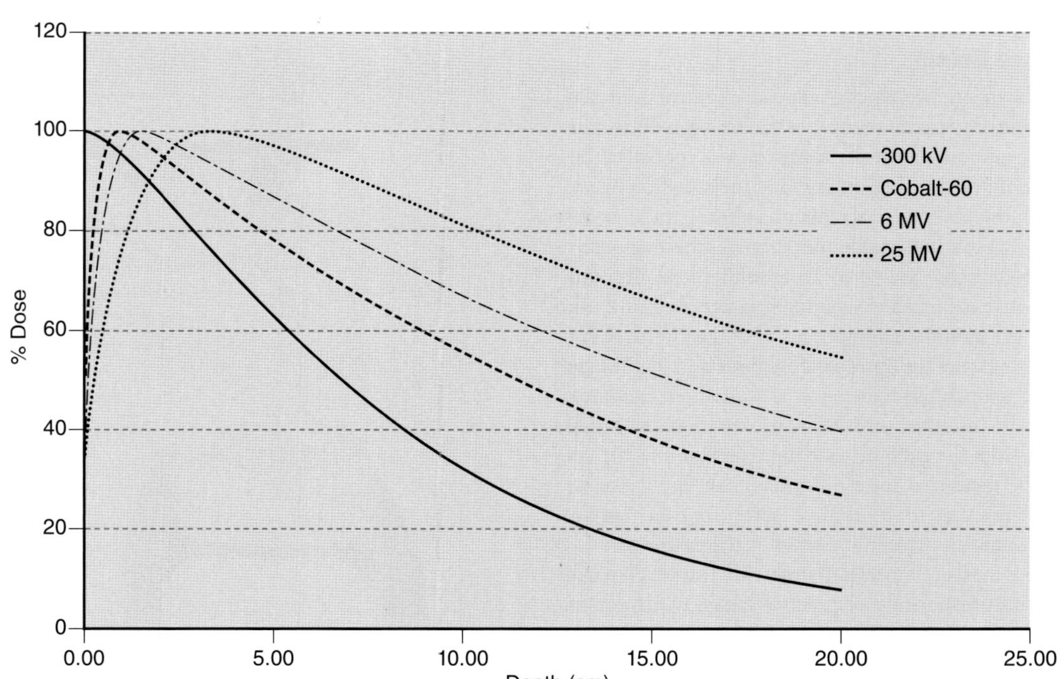

Fig. 9.28 Set of 300-kV, cobalt, 6-MV and 25-MV depth dose curves.

The advantages are immediately obvious. First, for example, the dose at depth 7 cm is increased by almost a factor of 1.5. Second, however, the forwards scattering of the electrons produced from the photon interactions results in the skin sparing effect, with a maximum dose at 0.5 cm depth rather than the surface. Cobalt units provided the clinician with an enormous technical advantage for teletherapy.

The cobalt unit represents an extremely simple method to generate an MV treatment beam. There is no requirement for the highly skilled maintenance and costs associated with linear accelerators, and this enables teletherapy to be provided at low cost in situations where technical support is not readily available. Their simplicity and economy represent an enormous potential for these machines.

Radioisotope Source

The radioactive cobalt-60 source consists of a small container which encapsulates pellets or disks of cobalt with an activity of typically 200 TBq. The typical dimensions of such a container are 2 cm in diameter by 2 cm in length. Herein lies one of the deficiencies of the cobalt treatment unit, as this large source in turn produces a large penumbra in its radiation fields. The source is housed within a large shielded safe which has a shutter mechanism to transport the source into an exposed position. Typical mechanisms are spring-loaded wheels, jaws and a sliding mechanism, and there were electrical, mechanical, hydraulic and pneumatically driven systems developed. Periodic testing is required to ensure that there is no leakage of radioactive material from the source encapsulation. Swabs are taken of the aperture to the safe to detect contamination. Emergency personnel procedures are also required to be in place to ensure that, in the event of a failure of the transport mechanism, the patient can be safely removed from the room and the source returned to the safe by manual means. One noticeable feature of a cobalt head is that it is continually warm, which is testament to the reality of the energy release from the cobalt source. This arises from the radioactive decay and absorption in the shielded housing and, in particular, all the β decay indicated in Fig. 9.27.

Beam Collimation

The collimation of the beam is achieved using a system of primary collimator, secondary collimator and penumbra trimmers, as shown in Fig. 9.29. The primary collimator is adjacent to the source and can form part of the drum assembly within which the source is stored. It forms the initial beam which will set the maximum size possible for the final treatment field. The penumbra of a radiation field is dependent upon three aspects: the size of the source, the distance of the secondary collimator jaw from the source and electron scatter at the edge of the beam (Fig. 9.30). Scatter really only becomes a problem at very high energies above 15-MV photon beams. However, the radiation source at 2 cm is very large. So, if the secondary collimator jaws were placed one above the other, the penumbra across the inner jaws would be larger than across the outer jaws. Therefore, to provide a more equitable size in both directions, the jaws are interlaced, as shown in Fig. 9.29. The distance from the source is extended even further by the use of penumbra trimmers which can be fitted to the ends of the main secondary collimators. Although this technique is effective, it is not always practical because of patient positioning.

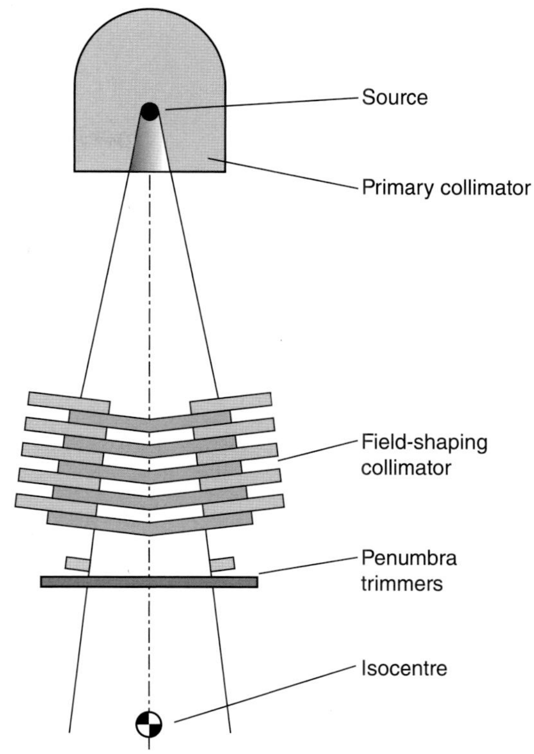

Fig. 9.29 Collimation system for cobalt machine.

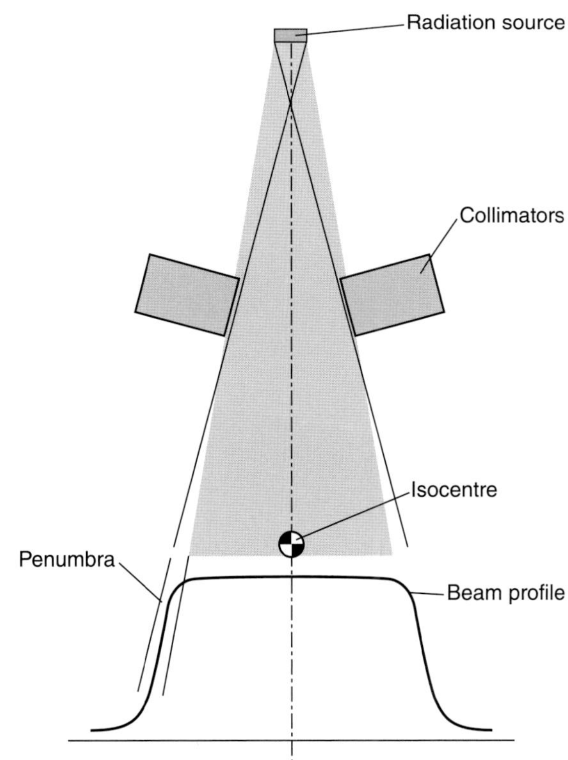

Fig. 9.30 Penumbra diagram.

Design of Gamma Ray Teletherapy Machines

Initially, there were fixed-head cobalt treatment machines followed by rotating gantry–mounted machines (Fig. 9.31). The rotating gantry machines were arranged so that the axes of the radiation head rotation and the gantry rotation intersected. This enabled isocentric treatment, as described for linear accelerators in Chapter 10, with multiple beams intersecting within the target and enhancing the dose there simply by rotation of the gantry. The massive shielding for the radioactive source presented a considerably heavy load and challenge for the gantry assembly. An additional set of movements available on some machines was pitch and roll (Fig. 9.31), which was advantageous for some poorly ambulatory or nonambulatory patients as the beam could be directed for treatment with them upright in a chair or even remaining in their

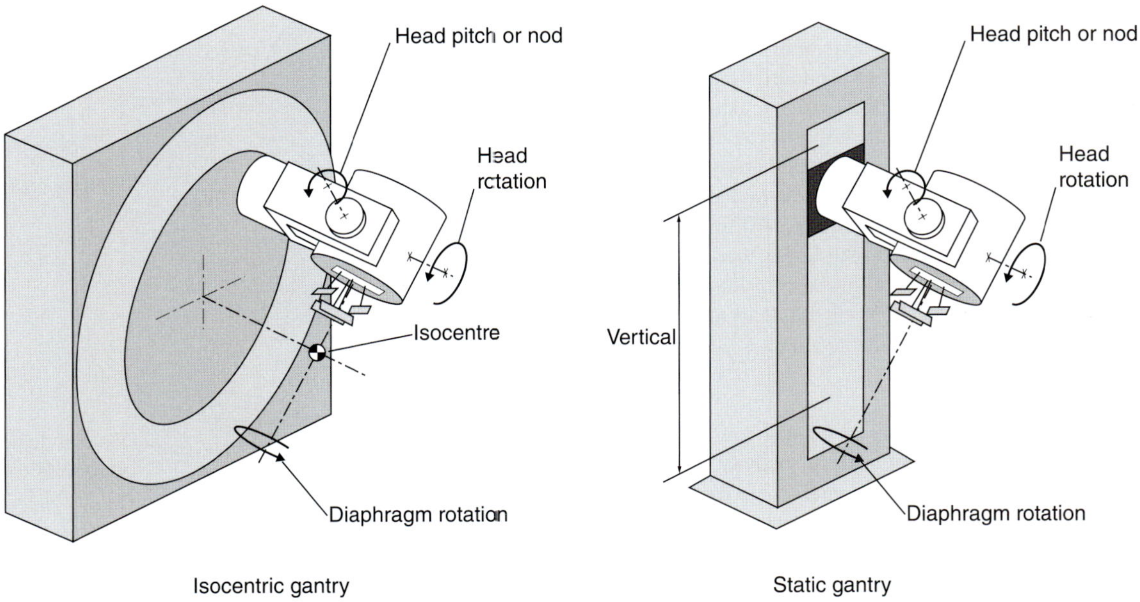

Fig. 9.31 Rotational and static gantry cobalt machines.

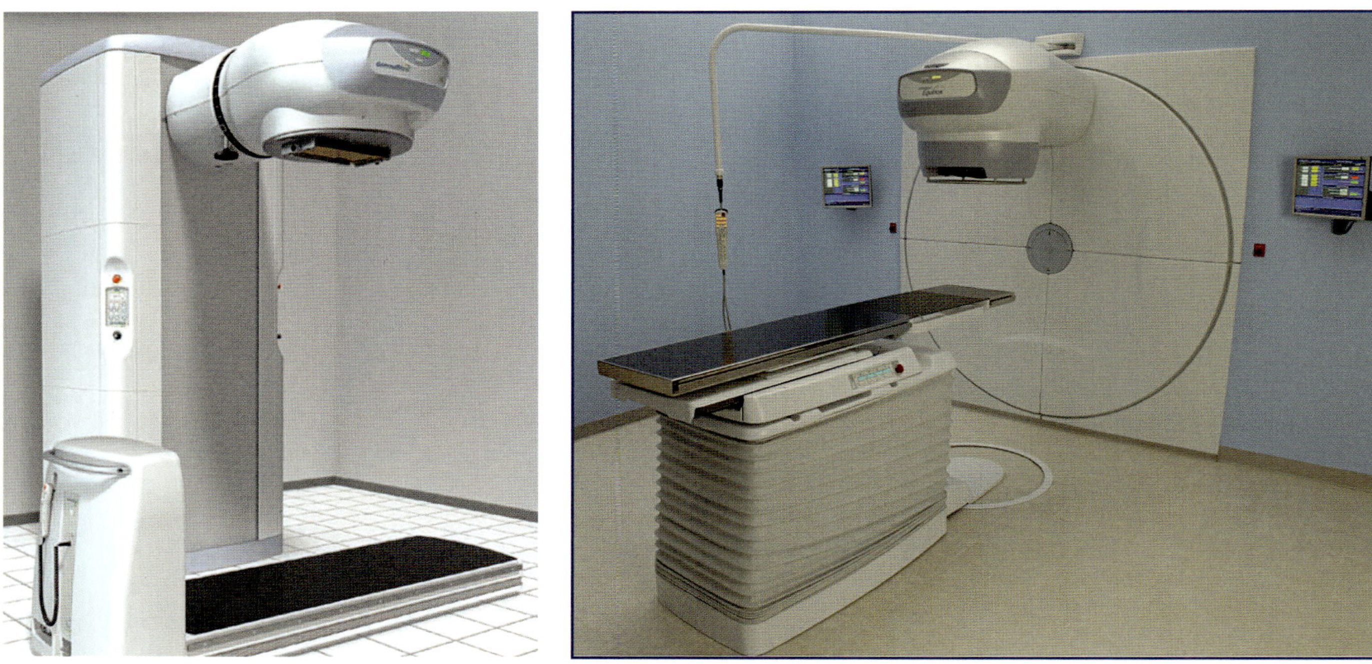

Fig. 9.32 Examples of modern cobalt units on static and rotational gantries. (Courtesy Best Theratronics Ltd.)

bed. Such single-field and often single-shot treatments for palliation provided a valuable treatment technique.

In compact rooms, the radiation head was balanced on the gantry by a shield to reduce the radiation protection requirements in the room. A timer controlled the period the radioactive source was moved out of its safe and the patient irradiated. Because there was a finite time during which the source would be transported to the fully exposed position, this was accommodated by modifying the exposure time with a transit time. The dose rate of the source was checked periodically by absolute measurement under reference calibration conditions. This would typically be monthly and, in addition, a comparison would be made against the known physical decay prediction to ensure the purity of the isotope.

Modern cobalt machines (Fig. 9.32) continue to provide simple treatment delivery as well as field shaping with multileaf collimators (MLCs), MV portal imaging and kV imaging, including cone beam CT, in a manner identical to that described for MV machines in Chapter 10.

RADIOSURGERY

The Gamma Knife or Leksell Gamma Knife is a trademark for a specific commercial device. It is a dedicated cranial radiosurgical machine which uses a large number of collimated cobalt-60 sources to provide an ablative dose to a small treatment volume. The target volume may be on the order of 5 to 40 mm in diameter, and multiple spherical volumes can be used in combination. This machine was pioneered by Lars

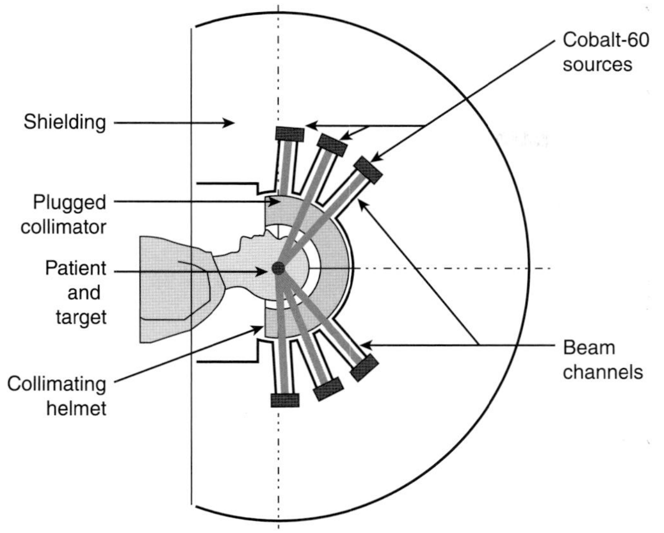

Fig. 9.33 Schematic of collimation system used in radiosurgery with cobalt sources.

Leksell in Sweden in the 1960s to 1980s. The device now has widespread use, and the main principle behind the design of the source collimation is shown in Fig. 9.33. There were up to 200 cobalt sources in the early machines, and all the beams intersect at a point, giving a high dose volume within the patient who was positioned so that the intersection volume is located at the target. In the early machines, there were several helmet collimators with different collimator diameters. Using tungsten plugs, the source and therefore beam array were configured for the particular treatment by helmet selection and arrangement of plugs. In modern machines, there is a single moveable helmet with multiple collimator holes of between 4 mm and 16 mm in diameter, and the combination of beams is automated.

RADIATION SAFETY

Radiation safety, a statutory requirement well set out in Chapter 4, is an intrinsic design feature of radiotherapy devices and facilities. Protection needs to be afforded to the patient, the operating staff and members of the public. Devices are designed to ensure that to the maximum extent possible, the patient is exposed to only the clinically required radiation field and dose. The former aspect relates to the beam shaping and the shielding built into the device to minimise any peripheral radiation present outside the useful beam. Ensuring that an accurate dose is delivered to the patient is dependent upon the operation of machine control systems such as dose monitors, timers and safety interlocks and upon working practices to ensure, for example, the presence of the correct applicator, the correct energy of a beam and the mechanical operation of shutters and drive mechanisms. The design of the machine and the room also includes radiation shielding and design features to provide protection during clinical treatment, equipment testing and maintenance to operational, scientific and technical staff. Lastly, protection of the public is ensured by adequate interlocks and room shielding design.

The types of radiation, range of energies, activity of sources and treatment dose rates make for a varied range of design of the treatment room. For example, in the case of iodine-125 radioactive sources, self-shielding of the body reduces the hazard substantially. In contrast, a high-doserate afterloader poses a substantial requirement on the room design with regard to wall thickness and entrance, possibly requiring a maze. Consideration also has to be given to the direction of therapy beams and where in the room or adjacent rooms or corridors a hazard could occur and can be reduced by design. Room design for cobalt-60 teletherapy machines is comparable to that for high-energy linear accelerators, as described in Chapter 10. Design guidance and principles[40] are readily available.

One final and recent issue with regard to radiation safety has been the possibility of radioactive materials being used for terrorist purposes. While the threat of terrorism has led to heightened security throughout many facets of life, it has also impacted the security provision for radioactive sources, their storage and their transport.

COMMISSIONING AND QUALITY CONTROL

The role of commissioning and quality control to ensure the protection of individuals against the dangers of ionising radiation in relation to medical exposure is set out in Article 8 of the European Commission (EC) Directive 93/47/Euratom.[41] Chapter 14 deals in detail with the principles of quality control. Although quality control applies to all radiotherapy devices, Chapter 14 focuses primarily on examples for MV equipment.

The directive specifies the three aspects with regard to maintaining safe and effective equipment which protects individuals, and these are to:

Commission the equipment by conducting measurements to ensure that it operates within a required specification for clinical use.

Undertake routine quality control checks to ensure its ongoing performance.

Undertake quality control checks following repair and modification to ensure its ongoing performance.

These three principles should be applied to all radiotherapy devices, including those in this chapter. There is considerable guidance available for quality control of all types of equipment, and these are referenced in Chapter 14. However, a readily available and comprehensive guide is from the Institute of Physics and Engineering in Medicine (IPEM).[30]

CONCLUSION

The diversity of radiotherapy machines and devices can be seen to have developed as the need for clinical treatment was explored and scientific, engineering and technical knowledge and expertise grew. This exploration has led to many devices, machines and treatment techniques.

Brachytherapy remains an important component of radical radiation therapy in the modern management of cancer and is a field where physicists, radiographers and clinicians work closely together. For this multidisciplinary team, good communication is highly important. Technical advances in imaging and computing have improved the precision of implantation and accuracy of dose calculation. HDR brachytherapy is the most common delivery mode today. Innovation, including with three-dimensional printing, novel optimisation algorithms and deep learning technologies, is ongoing. It is essential that expertise is maintained and developed, as this provides the optimal means of delivering high-dose radiation therapy to many patients.

In recent years, renewed interest in many devices, particularly intraoperative kV machines, has led to novel equipment developments. At the same time, concerns for radiation safety and security have often discouraged the use of radioactive sources. Overall, however, in the absence of alternative methods along with the continued efficacy of radiotherapy, many useful advances continue to emerge in this area.

REFERENCES

1. British Institute of Radiology and Institution of Physics and Engineering in Medicine and Biology. *Central axis depth dose data for use in radiotherapy. A survey of depth doses and related*

data measured in water or equivalent media. British Institute of Radiology, UK; 1996.
2. Saunderson J, Metwaly M. *Medical and Dental Guidance Notes*. 2nd ed. York, UK; 2024 IPEM Report 113.
3. Aird E. Sources in brachytherapy. In: Joslin C, Flynn A, Hall E, eds. *Principles and Practice of Brachytherapy: Using Afterloading Systems*. Arnold, London, UK; 2001.
4. ICRU (International Commission on Radiation Units and Measurements). *International Commission on Radiation Units and Measurements, Dose and Volume Specification for Reporting Intracavitary Therapy in Gynaecology*. Bethesda, MD; 1985 ICRU Report 38.
5. American Institute of Physics. *Remote Afterloading Technology*. New York; 1993 AAPM Report 41.
6. Meredith WJ. *Radium Dosage: The Manchester System*. Livingstone, UK; 1967.
7. Perquin B, Dutriex A, Paine CH, Chassagne D, Marinello G, Ash D. The Paris system in interstitial radiation therapy. *Acta Radiol Oncol Radiat Phys Biol*. 1978;17(1):33–48.
8. ICRU (International Commission on Radiation Units and Measurements). *International commission on radiation units and measurements, dose and volume specification for reporting intracavitary therapy in gynaecology*. Bethesda, MD; 1985 ICRU Report 38.
9. Nath R, Anderson LL, Luxton G, Weaver KA, Williamson JF, Meigooni AS. Dosimetry of interstitial brachytherapy sources: recommendations of the AAPM Radiation Therapy Committee Task Group No. 43. *Med Phys*. 1995;22(2):209–234.
10. Rivard MJ, Coursey BM, DeWerd LA, et al. Update of the AAPM Task Group No. 43: a revised AAPM protocol for brachytherapy dose calculations. *Med Phys*. 2004;31(3):633–674.
11. Luc Bealieu Tedgren AC, Carrier JF, Davis SD, et al. Report of the Task Group 186 on the model-based dose calculation methods in brachytherapy beyond the TG-43 formalism: current status and recommendations for clinical implementation. *Med Phys*. 2012;39(10):6208–6236.
12. Salembier C, Lavagnini P, Nickers P, et al. Tumour and target volumes in permanent prostate brachytherapy: a supplement to the ESTRO/EAU/EORTC recommendations on prostate brachytherapy. *Radiother Oncol*. 2007;83(1):3–10.
13. Royal College of Radiologists. *Quality Assurance Practice Guidelines for Transperineal LDR Permanent Seed Brachytherapy*. London: Royal College of Radiologists; 2012.
14. Hoskin PJ, Colombo A, Henry A, et al. GEC/ESTRO recommendations on high dose rate afterloading brachytherapy for localised prostate cancer: an update. *Radiother Oncol*. 2013; 107(3):325–332.
15. Henry A, Pieters BR, Siebert FA, Hoskin P. UROGEC Group of GEC ESTRO with Endorsement by the European Association of Urology. GEC-ESTRO ACROP prostate brachytherapy guidelines. *Radiother Oncol*. 2022;167:244–251.
16. Haie-Meder C, Pötter R, Van Limbergen E, et al. Recommendations from gynaecological (GYN) GEC-ESTRO Working Group (I): concepts and terms in 3D image-based 3D treatment planning in cervix cancer brachytherapy with emphasis on MRI assessment of GTV and CTV. *Radiother Oncol*. 2005; 74(3):235–245.
17. Pötter R, Haie-Meder C, Van Limbergen E, et al. Recommendations from gynaecological (GYN) GEC ESTRO working group (II): concepts and terms in 3D image-based treatment planning in cervix cancer brachytherapy: 3D dose volume parameters and aspects of 3D image-based anatomy, radiation physics, radiobiology. *Radiother Oncol*. 2006;78(1):67–77.
18. ICRU (International Commission on Radiation Units & Measurements). ICRU report 89, prescribing, recording, and reporting brachytherapy for cancer of the cervix; 2016. https://www.icru.org/report/icru-report-89-prescribing-recording-and-reporting-brachytherapy-for-cancer-of-the-cervix/
19. Tanderup K, Pötter R, Lindegaard J, et al. Embrace II study protocol v1.0; 2015. https://www.embracestudy.dk/UserUpload/PublicDocuments/Docs/EMBRACE_II_title_page_and_total_protocol_v15_151015.pdf
20. Pötter R, Tanderup K, Kirisits C, et al. The EMBRACE II study: the outcome and prospect of two decades of evolution within the GEC ESTRO GYN working group and the EMBRACE studies. *Clin Transl Radiat Oncol*. 2018;9:48–60.
21. American Cancer Society. *Cancer facts & figures 2017*. Atlanta, GA: American Cancer Society; 2017. https://www.cancer.org/research/cancer-facts-statistics/all-cancer-facts-figures/cancer-facts-figures-2017.html
22. Siegel RL, Miller KD, Fuchs HE, Jemal A. Cancer statistics, 2021. *CA Cancer J Clin*. 2021;71:7–33. http://doi.org/10.3322/caac.21654.
23. NICE Interventional Procedure Guidance 2015. *Preoperative high dose rate brachytherapy for rectal cancer*. https://www.nice.org.uk/guidance/ipg531/documents/preoperative-high-dose-rate-brachytherapy-for-rectal-cancers-consultation-document2
24. Corner C, Bryant L, Chapman C, Glynne-Jones R, Hoskin PJ. High dose afterloading intraluminal brachytherapy for advanced inoperable rectal cancer. *Brachytherapy*. 2010;9(1):66–70.
25. Kolotas C, Röddiger S, Strassmann G, et al. Palliative interstitial HDR brachytherapy for recurrent rectal cancer. Implantation techniques and results. *Strahlenther Onkol*. 2003;179(7):458–463.
26. Potter R, Van Limbergen E. Oesophaeal cancer. In: Gerbaulet A, Potter R, Mazeron JJ, Meertens H, Van Limbergen E, eds. *The GEC ESTRO Handbook of Brachytherapy*. ESTRO, Brussels, Belgium; 2002:505–514.
27. Van Limbergen E, Potter R. Bronchus cancer. In: Gerbaulet A, Potter R, Mazeron JJ, Meertens H, Van Limbergen E, eds. *The GEC ESTRO Handbook of Brachytherapy*. ESTRO, Brussels, Belgium; 2002:545–560.
28. Vijande J, Ballester F, Ouhib Z, Granero D, Pujades-Claumarchirant MC, Perez-Calatayud J. Dosimetry comparison between TG-43 and Monte Carlo calculations using the Freiburg flap for skin high-dose-rate brachytherapy. *Brachytherapy*. 2012;11(6):528–535.
29. Jones EL, Baldion AT, Thomas C, et al. Introduction of novel 3D-printed superficial applicators for high-dose-rate skin brachytherapy. *Brachytherapy*. 2017;16(2):409–414.
30. Institute of Physics and Engineering in Medicine. *Physics aspects of quality control in radiotherapy*. 2nd ed. York, UK; 2018 IPEM Report 81.
31. ESTRO. In: Venselaar J, Perez-Calatayud J, eds. *A Practical Guide to Quality Control of Brachytherapy Equipment. European Guidelines for Quality Assurance in Radiotherapy Booklet*. Brussels: ESTRO; 2004 No. 8.
32. Glasgow GP (Chairman), Bourland JD, Grogsby PW, Meli JA, Weaver KA. Remote afterloading technology. *AAPM 41. A report of the AAPM Radiation Therapy Committee Task Group*: AAPM; 1993. American Institute of Physics https://www.aapm.org/pubs/reports/rpt_41.pdf
33. Nath R, Anderson LL, Meli JA, Olch AJ, Stitt JA, Williamson JF. Code of practice for brachytherapy physics: report of the AAPM Radiation Therapy committee Task Group, No. 56. *Med Phys*. 1997; 24(10):1557–1598.
34. Fraass B, Doppke K, Hunt M, et al. Quality assurance for clinical radiotherapy treatment planning: report of the AAPM

Radiation Therapy Committee Task Group, No. 53. *Med Phys.* 1998;25(10):1773–1829.
35. UK Statutory Instruments. High Activity Sealed Sources (HASS) and orphan source regulations 2005. 2005 No. 2686. London, UK: HMSO. https://www.legislation.gov.uk/uksi/2005/2686/contents
36. Bidmead AM, Sander T, Locks S, et al. The IPEM code of practice for the determination of the reference air kerma rate HDR Ir-192 brachytherapy sources based on the NPL air kerma standard. *Phys Med Biol.* 2010;55(11):3145–3159.
37. Butler WM, Bice WS, De Werd LA, et al. Third party brachytherapy source calibrations and physicist responsibilities: report of the AAPM low energy brachytherapy source calibration working group. *Med Phys.* 2008;35(9):3860–3865.
38. Park C, Yom SS, Podgorsak MB, et al. American Society for Therapeutic Radiology and Oncology (ASTRO), emerging technology committee report on electronic brachytherapy, electronic brachytherapy working group. *Int J Radiat Oncol Biol Phys.* 2010;76(4):963–972.
39. Eaton DJ. Electronic brachytherapy: current status and future directions. *Br J Radiol.* 2015;88:20150002.
40. IAEA. *Radiation protection in the design of radiotherapy facilities.* Vienna, Austria: IAEA; 2006 IAEA Safety Report Series No. 47.
41. Council directive 93/47/Euratom. *Off J Eur Commun.* 1997;180: 22–27. https://eur-lex.europa.eu/eli/dir/1997/43/oj/eng
42. Glen Seaborg. Remarks by Dr. Glenn T. Seaborg, Chairman U.S. Atomic Energy Commission at the 17th Annual Meeting of the Society of Nuclear Medicine Washington, D.C. July 10, 1970. "Reminiscences on the Development of Some Medically Useful Radionuclides."

10

Megavoltage Beams: Acceleration, Modulation and Image Guidance

Steve Hunt, Andrzej Kacperek and John A. Mills

CHAPTER OUTLINE

INTRODUCTION

Megavoltage radiation beams of x-rays, electrons and protons are now the most widely used in radiotherapy. Although the physical form of the accelerator and beam delivery system varies, implementation of the isocentric gantry has proven to be the most practical for all beam types and has been widely applied for treatment delivery. Clinical practice and technology development are synergistic in that, until beams were readily available, the clinical application could not be extensively trialed to further inform the development of the engineering and technology. In that respect, we await the development of very high-doserate beams to explore FLASH radiotherapy. There is also the prospect of very high-energy electron beams.

With regard to current machines, for x-ray and proton beams, patient imaging for target localisation has become a major aspect of the treatment machine and is integral to it. Further, beam delivery technology has been extensively developed to modulate the beam to shape the dose distribution to the target, both to avoid and minimise the detrimental effect on normal and critical tissue as well as provide the possibility to vary the dose within the target and tailor it to the disease. This has resulted in new radiotherapy treatments such as lung ablative treatment.

Thus, when we consider modern megavoltage beams, there are three major components to the machines. First, there is the basic acceleration of particles to provide the radiation beams. Second, the beams are modulated to shape and vary the intensity of the beam. And third,

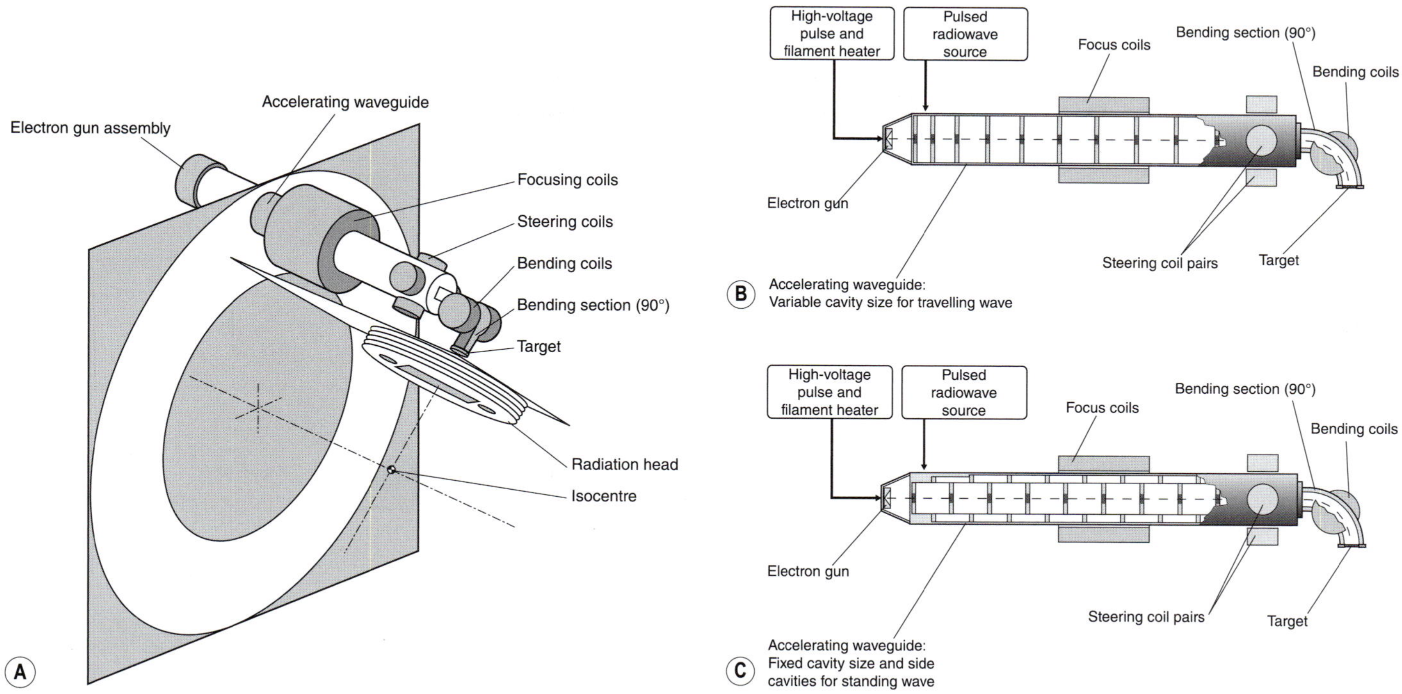

Fig. 10.1 Typical layout of the major components of a medical linear accelerator. (A) General waveguide. (B) Travelling waveguide. (C) Standing waveguide.

imaging systems are critical to providing ongoing tracking of the target and directing beam delivery.

In this chapter, x-ray, electron and proton machines are described to provide an insight to the complexity, engineering and technology which make image-guided, modulated megavoltage treatment beams possible.

X-RAY AND ELECTRON BEAMS

The medical linear accelerator (LINAC) produces x-ray and electron beams. The x-ray beam energy typically ranges from 6 to 15 MV, although higher-energy beams have been produced and used. A range of electron beam energies are typically produced by a single machine to exploit the variation of electron depth-dose range with energy. The electron beam energy usually ranges from 6 MeV to 18 MeV. It is an accepted convention to describe x-ray beams or photon beams in terms of megavoltage (MV) and electron beams in terms of megaelectron voltage (MeV). The actual energy of the beam depends, for example, on whether it is considered at the end of the acceleration, at the surface of the patient or at some depth within the patient.

Electron Acceleration and X-ray Production

The basis of beam acceleration within the modern medical LINAC was born out of the development of megavoltage treatment machines since the 1950s. Betatrons, resonant transformers and Van de Graaff generator designs were used to accelerate electron beams to high energy. However, the elegance of acceleration based upon radiofrequency (RF) electromagnetic waves became universally adopted to provide high dose rate (HDR) megavoltage treatment beams.[1,2] This produces a high-energy electron beam which can be used directly for treatment. An x-ray beam is produced through bremsstrahlung, or braking radiation, by bombardment of a tungsten transmission target by the electron beam.

Electron Acceleration

There are three major parts to an electron linear accelerator: an electron source, a source of RF electromagnetic waves and an accelerating waveguide. These core sections can be found in isocentric medical treatment machines as well as custom machines such as the TomoTherapy.

In addition to the major core components, a modern medical LINAC consists of a gantry assembly to direct the beam into the patient and a radiation head which enables beam shaping. The x-ray beam target, which is bombarded by the electron beam to produce the x-rays, is contained in the radiation head. Steering and stability of the electron beam require magnetic fields generated electrically with inductive coils. These coils focus, bend and steer the electron beam. Also essential are high-voltage and current sources as well as vacuum and cooling systems to create a stable machine environment for beam production.

Fig. 10.1A illustrates the typical layout of the major components of a LINAC. The gun filament assembly produces electrons by raising tungsten to a sufficiently high temperature through electrical heating. There are two types of waveguide: standing waves (Fig. 10.1C) and travelling waves (Fig. 10.1B). Although this affects the waveguide structure, both types use electromagnetic waves at an RF of approximately 3 GHz. In the travelling type, the electrons are carried along on an accelerating wave, whereas the standing type uses the electric component of the wave to exert an accelerating force on the electrons.

The source of the RF is either a klystron or a magnetron. The klystron uses a low-power RF source—essentially a small-cavity oscillator. The low-power RF is applied to a high-power electron stream in the klystron, causing the high-power stream to oscillate and emit a high-power RF wave. In contrast, the magnetron is a multiple-cavity device which produces a high-power RF wave directly. Waveguide sections transport RF from the magnetron or klystron to the accelerating waveguide section.

The other essential ancillary aspect of the LINAC is the need for the accelerating waveguide to be under high vacuum. For machine designs in which higher vacuums are required, the waveguide is factory sealed. This limits the possibility of maintenance to ancillary waveguide components in the field, such as with RF interfacing and electron gun assemblies. In other designs, trained personnel can replace vacuum system components on-site where external high-vacuum pump-down equipment is available. However, both designs still require onboard high-vacuum pumps that work continuously to maintain the high vacuum required to cater for outgassing from surface gas desorption and from gas permeation in the physical waveguide walls and other components exposed to the high vacuum.

Because electrons are charged particles, there is a tendency for an electron beam to disperse as it travels along the accelerating waveguide. Fortunately, this can be countered by using the interactive force which is experienced by a charged particle as it passes through a magnetic field. The magnetic fields that are used to counter this dispersion are produced by focusing coils which are wound around the accelerating waveguide and produce a magnetic field flux parallel to the direction of the electron beam.

This interactive force between a magnetic field and a moving electron is used in two other systems, both with the magnetic field at right angles to the direction of the electron beam. One system, referred to as the *bending magnet*, steers the electron beam into a trajectory appropriate for the radiation head. This magnet also plays a crucial role in the selection of beam energy. The strength of the magnetic field, controlled by the electrical current flowing in the bending magnet coil, selects the appropriate beam energy.

The other system steers the beam into and out of the accelerating waveguide. To maximise the number of electrons that are accelerated and minimise beam losses, these steering coils adjust the trajectory correcting the beam alignment by controlling the electric current in the coils.

X-ray Production

Bombardment of a tungsten transmission target by the electron beam produces an x-ray beam through the bremsstrahlung process. The tungsten target is placed directly in the path of the accelerated electron beam, immediately after it exits the bending coil section, as shown in Fig. 10.2. This raw x-ray beam is collimated into the useful beam by the primary collimator. The raw beam has a peak intensity in the forwards direction (Fig. 10.3).

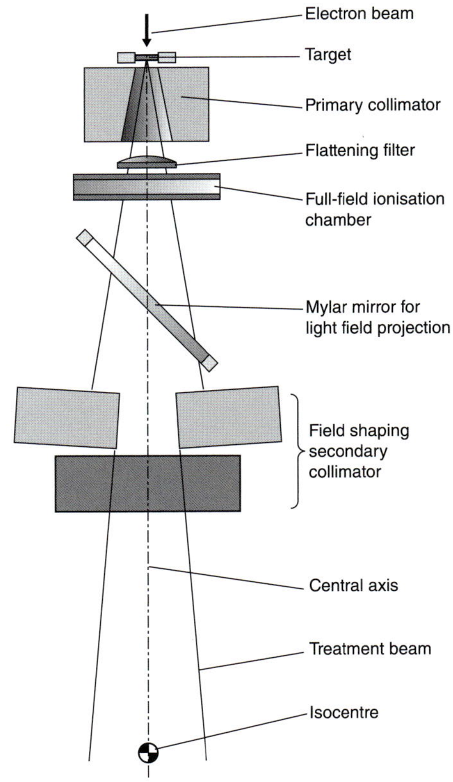

Fig. 10.2 Linear accelerator radiation head.

Gantry Assembly and Beam Stability

The modern medical LINAC consists of a gantry assembly to direct the beam into the patient through the radiation head, which enables beam shaping. The gantry construction of the standard medical LINAC is referred to as being *isocentric*. In effect, this means that all the main axes of rotation concerning the gantry, radiation head and patient couch intersect within a sphere 2 mm in diameter, referred to as the *isocentre*. This is illustrated in Fig. 10.4. The benefit of this isocentric system is that placement of the patient such that the tumour is centred on the machine's isocentre simplifies treatment with the superposition of multiple beams.

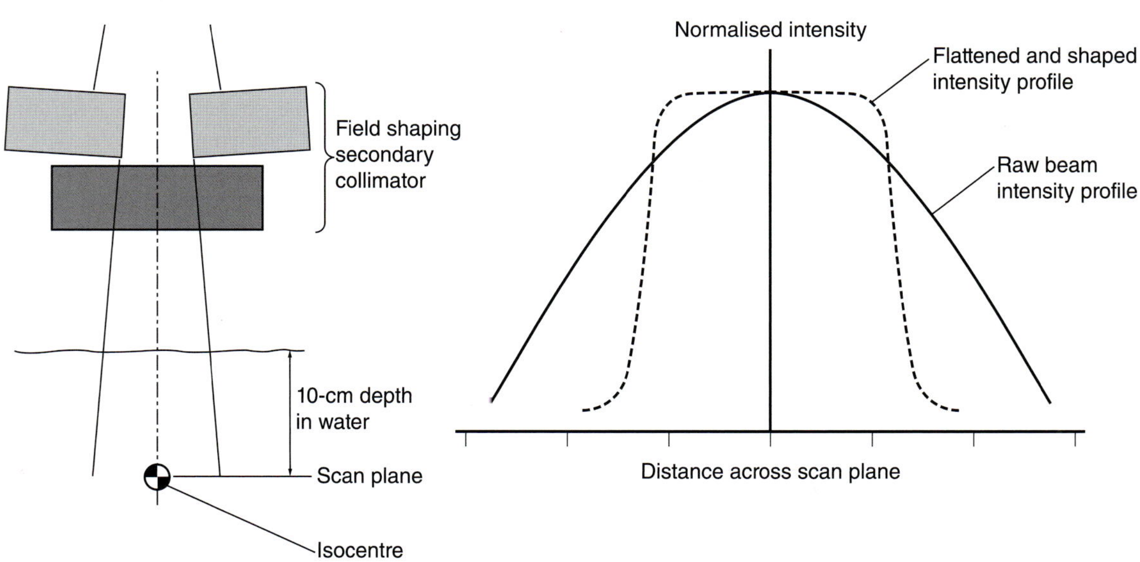

Fig. 10.3 Raw beam profile after target and flattened uniform beam under International Electrotechnical Commission (IEC) conditions.

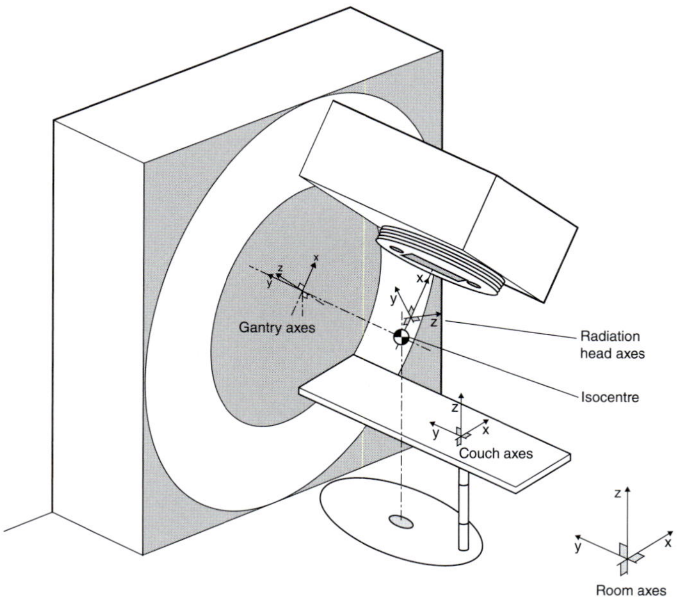

Fig. 10.4 Linear accelerator axes: gantry, collimator and couch conventions.

The imaging devices as well as the beam shaping and modulating radiation head are mounted on the gantry assembly and rely upon its mechanical stability for accurate beam delivery and verification.

Beam production is not an energy-efficient process, and a lot of energy is dissipated within the machine as heat. The stability of beam production relies on the stability of component dimensions. For example, the RF cavities in the waveguide can be subject to expansion and contraction with heating. Hence there is a need for a great deal of water cooling on the machine for the target, all the magnetic coils, the accelerating waveguide, the RF source and large electrical devices such as transformers. Adequate and stable cooling is essential for effective beam production.

FORMING THE CLINICAL BEAMS

Two types of clinical beams are produced following acceleration. These are often referred to as *x-ray mode* and *electron mode*. The processes for forming these beams are quite different, and forming the x-ray beam has become very complex compared with the simplicity of the electron beam.

X-ray Beam Shaping

Following x-ray production in the target and primary collimator, final beam shaping is done using a substantial secondary collimation system. In early machines, these consisted of simply two orthogonal sets of collimators which could set rectangular field shapes by movement in their orthogonal directions (Fig. 10.2).

The two sets of orthogonal jaws of early machines have either been replaced entirely, replaced in part or supplemented by systems referred to as *multileaf collimators (MLCs)*, with leaf widths at the isocentre ranging from 4 mm to 10 mm. This has provided the opportunity for simplified conformal shaping of the beam to the target volume. The MLC is now established in modern machines and in clinical practice. Current designs typically employ up to 160 leaf pairs in two parallel banks, fabricated in a high-density material such as tungsten, where opposing leaf pairs can interdigitate to allow complex field shapes and structures.

Mechanically, each leaf requires high accuracy and constancy of position during patient treatment. To achieve this, each leaf is moved by a motor-driven leadscrew and drive nut assembly commanded by a motor control system. Furthermore, a method to measure the physical position of each leaf is incorporated, and it is here where MLC designs vary, with some optical monitoring systems based on mirrors and cameras and others employing motor encoders and potentiometers.

The overall hardware is generally split into two physical locations. First, the physical MLC, the motors and associated drive electronics as well as the leaf position monitoring are all contained within the radiation head of the LINAC. Due to limited space, a high level of system integration is required. Subsequently, motor drive commands, leaf position feedbacks and interlocks are networked to an MLC control system computer at a second location that is generally close to the primary LINAC computer. A high level of confidence is required in the control system to supervise leaf movement during gantry and collimator rotations, where the influence of gravity is dynamic on the leaf banks during patient setup and is critical in advanced therapies such as volumetric modulated arc therapy. A control algorithm running on the MLC control system computer continually computes the required MLC motor drive commands to resolve the difference between the current and prescribed leaf positions. Any deviation outside set limits will result in an interlock fault and subsequent termination of the treatment beam.

The Uniform X-ray Beam

Conventionally, the aim in RT has been to deliver as uniform a dose as possible to the tumour. To achieve this simply from a direct beam, the raw beam is made uniform or flattened using a flattening filter made from steel (Figs. 10.2 and 10.3). The profile of the flattening filter provides the maximum attenuation in the centre, and the detailed shape of the filter is specific to the profile of the raw beam, which is energy dependent. Following flattening of the beam, the x-rays pass through an ionisation chamber before going on to field shaping with the secondary collimation system (Fig. 10.2).

Uniformity and symmetry of the radiation beam as well as beam width and penumbra are well-established critical performance parameters by which a beam is monitored to ensure satisfactory beam production and control (Fig. 10.5).

The Intensity Modulated X-ray Beam

The standard conventional method of varying the intensity of the beam has been the use of metal wedges placed manually across the beam to modify the uniformity of the beam profile in a controlled manner (Fig. 10.6). Known as *fixed wedges*, the variation of beam intensity was extremely useful in obtaining a uniform dose distribution within the treatment volume by, for example, compensating for oblique incidence. In the past, metal wedges were fitted manually by the operator. Then, by having a metallic wedge mounted on a motorised platform in the radiation head, a variable tilt in uniformity across the beam could be produced by automatically moving the wedge into the radiation beam for a portion of the irradiation. These were referred to as *motorised wedges*.

The same variation in uniformity was also achieved by moving one of the orthogonal secondary collimator jaws (Fig. 10.2), which could form rectangular fields across the field during radiation. For example, at the start of the radiation, the jaws would be entirely closed, with both jaws on the same side of the central axis. As beam delivery was underway, one jaw would open and traverse across to the opposite side of the central axis. This method is referred to as *dynamic wedges*.

A greater complexity of varying beam intensity can be achieved using two approaches with an MLC. The first approach is to deliver a sequence of static beams through a series of fixed MLC shapes; this is known as *step-and-shoot intensity modulated radiotherapy (IMRT)*. Each of these beams is known as a *segment*, and the LINAC is paused

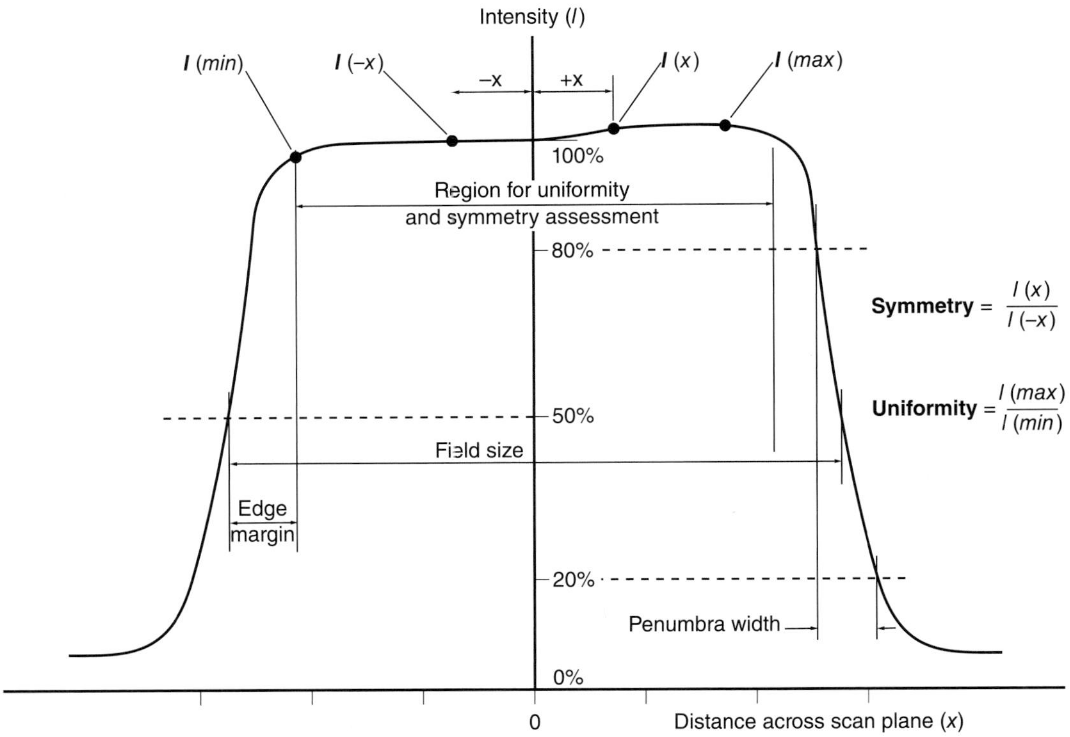

Fig. 10.5 Uniformity and symmetry profiles.

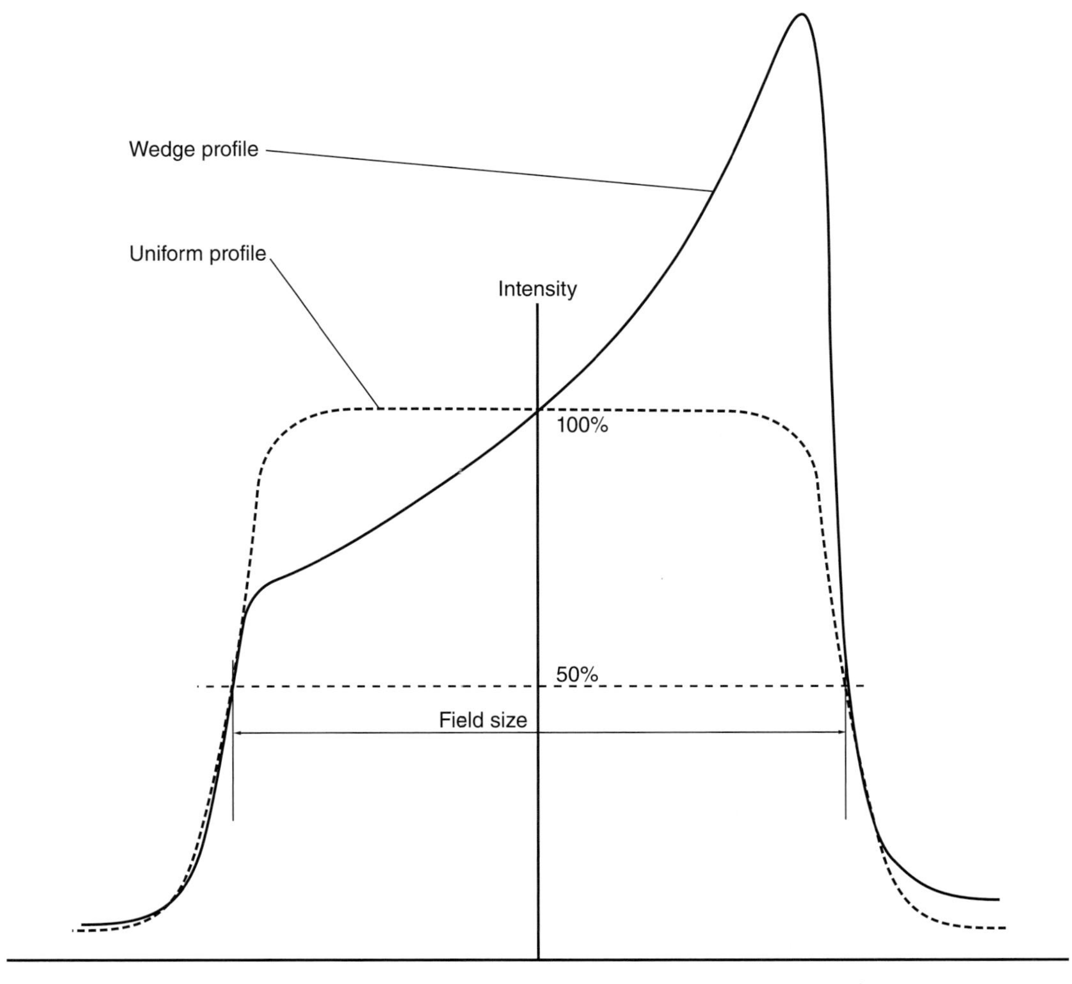

Fig. 10.6 A uniform and wedge beam profile.

in between the delivery of each segment to allow the MLC to drive to the next shape in the sequence. These segments are stacked together to produce the prescribed dose distribution. The second method is to use opposing leaf banks to produce a dynamically shaped, moving beam aperture across the treatment field. Each opposing leaf pair moves at a different speed as a function of time, and this aperture opening creates a window of variable intensity fluence across the treatment field. This is called *dynamic multileaf collimation (DMLC)*.

Volumetric Modulated X-ray Radiotherapy

While modulation of the intensity of the beam within its boundary provides great flexibility to irradiating the target, it is the combination of multiple modulated beams which enables the target volume to be encompassed by a dose distribution tailored to a specific shape for the geometry of the target, sparing of the adjacent critical tissue and even tailored to the distribution of the disease within the target. Hence the beam needs to be formed in a volumetric manner, modulating the beam intensity for multiple beams coincident at the isocentre of the machine. This is referred to as *volumetric modulated arc therapy (VMAT)*.

VMAT delivers a radiation dose as the linear accelerator gantry rotates through arcs around the patient, resulting in a highly conformal treatment. This is achieved by a coordinated modulation of dose rate, gantry speed and MLC aperture. An adequate level of synchronisation and accommodation of the limitations of machine control parameters for these elements is essential for effective VMAT delivery. To achieve this, current machines designed to deliver complex therapies encompass internal control data networks to realise low latency and high data throughput between control system components. One example is the controller area network (CAN) bus that is specifically designed for communications in critical systems. This results in a high level of integration between dose rate, gantry speed and MLC aperture control.

However, a number of constraints need to be imposed on these due to the mechanical limitations of the machine hardware. For gantry rotation, the mass of the gantry structures, including the beam arm containing the accelerating waveguide and associated counterbalance weights, limits the available acceleration and deceleration rates due to mechanical stresses and gantry motor drive capacity. Likewise, the MLC requires time to advance the moving beam aperture across the treatment field. Control system parameters that influence satisfactory treatment delivery are continuously monitored, and those found to be outside set criteria will result in a fault interlock and subsequent termination of the treatment beam.

The Flattening Filter Free X-ray Beam

With the development of intensity modulated beams, the need for a uniform intensity beam was removed and a flattening filter could be considered unnecessary. In fact, the field area over which effective modulation can be done is dependent upon the intensity variation across the raw beam. For example, to produce a uniform field of a specific size would require use of a small field which would be moved systematically across the specific field area, allowing irradiation for varying times. This may well extend treatment time in spite of the high doserate which can be achieved with the flattening filter removed. Indeed, it is this high doserate that has proved to be an advantage in the irradiation of small fields for stereotactic lung treatments where a modest amount of intensity modulation is required.

The Electron Beam

In the electron mode of operation, the transmission target is automatically moved out of the beam so that x-rays are no longer deliberately produced. As mentioned earlier, x-ray production is not efficient, and with the target removed, an electron beam dose rate comparable to that of an x-ray beam can be obtained with approximately 5% to 10% of the electron beam required from the accelerating waveguide for x-ray production. With this significant reduction in beam current, the problem of radiation leakage from the accelerating waveguide is significantly reduced. The accelerating waveguide can be set to produce a spectrum of energies, with the magnetic field produced by the bending section used to select the required energy. The bending section thus acts as a spectrometer, only allowing passage of electrons with the required energy into the primary collimator for production of the treatment beam.

The electron beam as it emerges from the window after acceleration and bending has a very narrow width compared with typically required field sizes for treatment, and scanning and scattering systems have been developed to provide adequate field coverage. Scanning systems employ electromagnets to steer the electron beam across the treatment field. However, by far the most predominant technique employs a dual scattering system along with an applicator attachment to the radiation head (Fig. 10.7). In a dual scattering system, a primary scatterer is introduced to the electron beam before the primary collimator. A secondary scatterer is substituted for the flattening filter, and this may be profiled for the specific electron beam energy which has been selected. These scatterers, along with the x-ray flattening filters, are mounted on a carousel which moves them automatically into the beam with the energy and mode selection. Typically, a treatment machine would have two photon beams and five or six electron beams, each with a

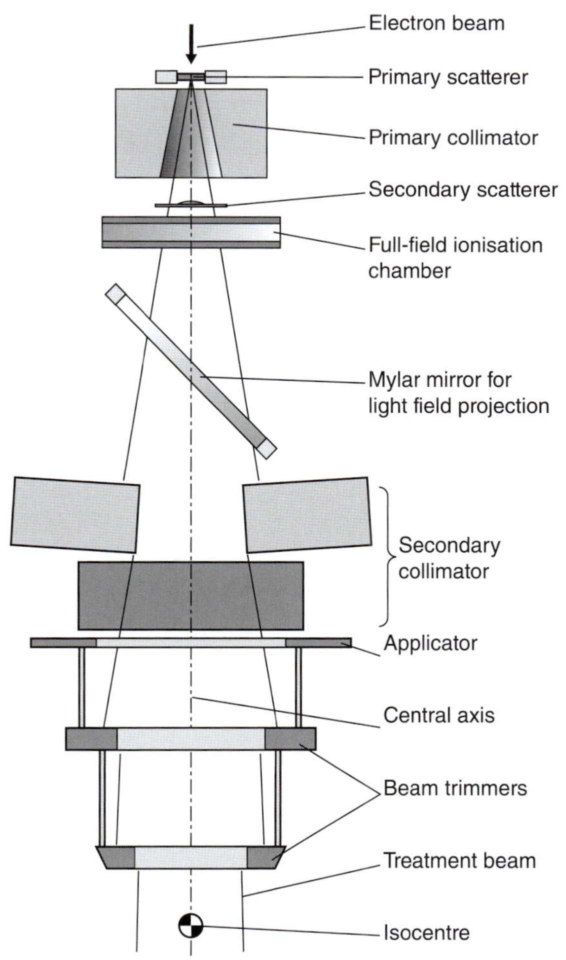

Fig. 10.7 Double-scattering foil system with applicator for electron beam production.

different energy. Both primary and secondary scatterers are specific to the energy selected. The secondary collimator system used for shaping the photon fields is used to set an initial field size for the electron beam as it leaves the radiation head. The electrons are scattered by air and so an applicator is used to produce a sharp edge to the treatment field at the patient. The applicators have open sides and consist of a set of field trimmers which reduce the field down to the required size. The treatment is either with the applicator in contact with the patient or with a small standoff of typically 5 cm. Surface masks in lead (Pb) and alloy are also used to provide a sharper beam edge, particularly close to critical organs such as the eye. The practice at any centre depends upon local preference.

Controlling and Steering the Beams

The ionisation chamber through which the beam passes consists of three sections, with each section covering the full area of the useful beam (Fig. 10.8). The first two sections are dosimetry channels one and two (Ch1 and Ch2). Ch1 is the primary channel, which provides a signal to terminate the beam after a required dose has been delivered. Ch2 is identical to Ch1 and acts as a safety backup to guard against excessive overexposure should a fault occur with Ch1. The third section is a segmented chamber, and the signals from the segments are used to monitor characteristics of the beam such as uniformity and symmetry. The *uniformity* (Fig. 10.5) refers to the variation of dose across the beam and will be characteristic of the beam energy. The *symmetry* refers to a tilt in the beam between positions equidistant from the central axis of the beam and is dependent upon alignment of the electron beam onto the target. The uniformity will vary with beam energy and can be used to control gun filament electron emission, and the symmetry can be used to control the beam steering coil currents in the accelerating waveguide (Fig. 10.8).

The electron beam passes through the same ionisation chamber with multiple sections and segments as the x-ray beam. The signals from these are used to monitor and control the performance of the beam and ensure delivery of the correct dose.

IMAGE GUIDANCE ON MEGAVOLTAGE LINEAR ACCELERATORS

Image guidance has long been used in megavoltage treatment. Slow film was used to obtain a portal image of the beam exiting from the patient. However, megavoltage x-rays have low contrast between bone and soft tissue, and even with copper screens in the film cassette, their value could be very limited. Nevertheless they provided considerable reassurance regarding field coverage and alignment of the beam where there were some identifiable bony landmarks. To provide greater accuracy of treatment delivery, imaging flat panels were developed, followed by cone beam computed tomography (CT), and now magnetic resonance imaging (MRI) has been built into machines.

Flat-Panel Portal Imaging

These panel imagers, known as *electronic portal imaging devices (EPIDs)*, are a standard fixture to modern machines and are retractable

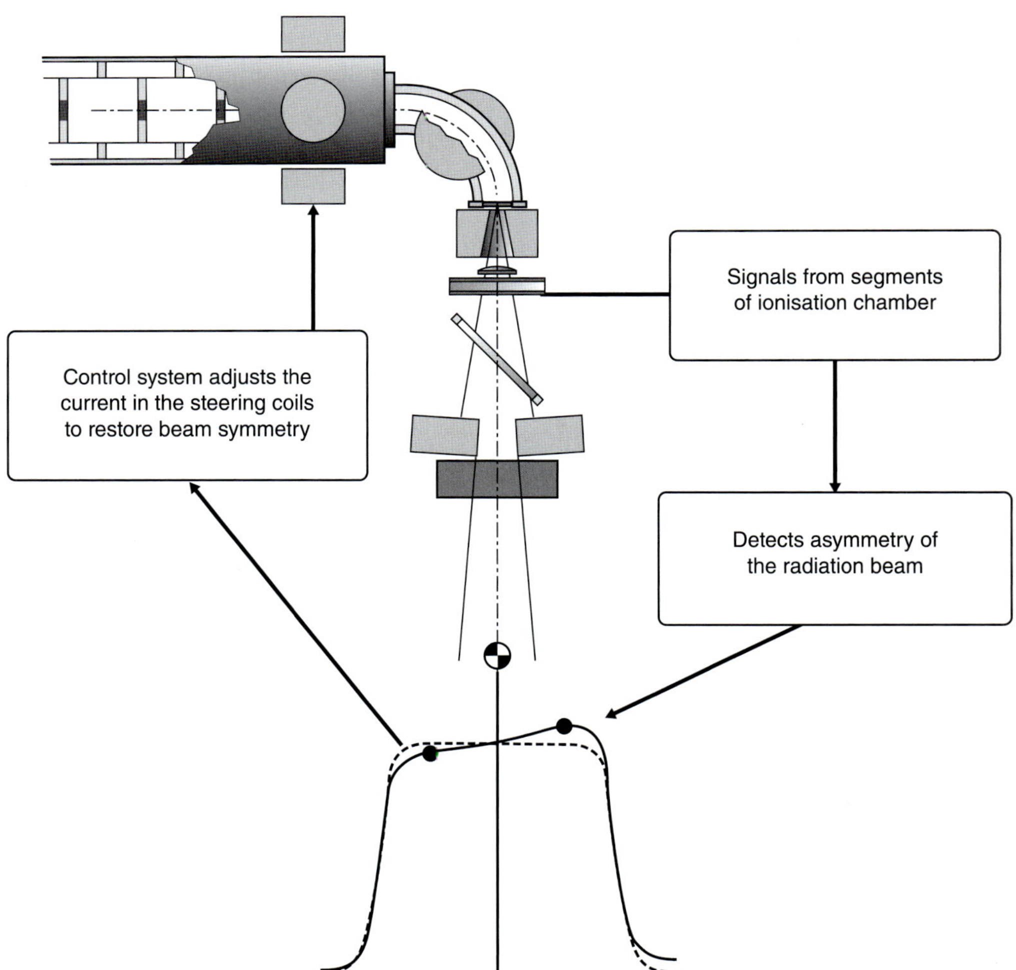

Fig. 10.8 Control system to maintain a symmetric field.

when not required. An image is formed onto a light-sensitive amorphous silicon flat panel by first converting the x-ray image to visible light. A metal plate, for example, copper, and a gadolinium scintillator are used for this purpose. The flat panel is arranged as an array of pixels, each containing a photo-sensitive element that stores an electrical charge relative to the light level produced by the gadolinium scintillator at that position. The array of pixels is read from the array by addressing the row and column of each element in turn using an electronic switch and transferring the signal onto a common bus line. This signal is digitised and stored in an image array for imaging processing.

Cone Beam Systems

Accurate patient positioning and conformation to target volume are essential steps in the pathway to desired treatment outcomes. However, errors and deviations in setup can occur. A kilovoltage (kV) x-ray source of 30 to 140 kV and flat-panel imager pair are mounted on the linear accelerator gantry assembly with the ability to acquire static and, more recently, CT image data. These are located on an axis orthogonal to the accelerator beam arm and share a common isocentre to the treatment beam (Fig. 11.12).

To acquire a volumetric data set in traditional CT requires a fan-shaped beam and a moving patient couch. However, to exploit the technology already available for static imaging on a therapy machine, a cone-shaped beam is employed to acquire a volumetric data set during rotation of the linear accelerator gantry. Thus a cone beam reconstruction algorithm is used to produce a volumetric image set.

MRI Systems

The MR LINAC is a new radiotherapy technology that integrates MRI into a treatment delivery system sharing a common isocentre. Although, Co^{60} has been employed as the radiation source, the LINAC is now the accepted method and is of a flattening filter free (FFF) design. This MRI-guided radiotherapy (MRgRT) uses an MRI scanner combined with the treatment machine, allowing unprecedented motion tracking and visualisation of the target in real time to be achieved. However, integrating these technologies is technically complex, because both utilise highly sensitive detectors in conjunction with high-level magnetic and electrical power systems. Sensitive detectors, such as the receiving coils for the MRI and ion chamber dosimetry components for the LINAC, are susceptible to collective interference from power supply and magnetic systems on both the MRI and LINAC platforms, and suitable electrical isolation and magnetic shielding between these is a critical requirement. Furthermore, there are two orientations of magnetic field lines where the LINAC is parallel or perpendicular to the MR magnet. Current designs favour the perpendicular implementation. An example of just one of many possible interactions is the interaction between the MR magnetic field and the LINAC beam transport system, where a resultant deflection of the electron beam in the LINAC accelerating waveguide and its final position on the x-ray target will influence x-ray symmetry and output. These points considered, successful integration has been achieved, resulting in clinical machines and ongoing development.

DIGITAL CONTROL AND ADVANCED ENGINEERING

The Analogue Nature of LINAC Control

The physical world in which we live is analogue, and this is also the case for LINAC systems. The machine control system needs to be able to set the physical positions of the gantry, collimator and treatment table, and it needs to set the configuration values for the beam accelerator, such as the current flowing in the bending magnet, steering and focusing coils. Conversely, the control system requires input of the sensory data, such as radiation field geometry and the actual and user-required positions of the gantry, collimator and treatment table. Other instrumentation examples are temperatures, pressures and flow rates of cooling water. This analogue world of machine control is therefore two way. The parameters to be set are sent from the control system to electromagnets, motors, power supplies and so on, while signals are read back as analogue voltages and currents from transducers such as ionisation chambers, potentiometers, current shunts, voltage dividers and pressure sensors.

The generation of high-energy electron beams requires precise control of the accelerator and its associated systems, where the optimal electron trajectories are accomplished by means of electric and magnetic fields. As mentioned previously, beam transport requires both focusing and steering to achieve the desired path. It also requires focus of the beamline to the target for successful x-ray delivery or to the electron window for electron beam delivery. Furthermore, the correct operating parameters for the klystron or magnetron components in the RF generation process are generally established by the setting of electric and magnetic fields. The same is true for the electron gun. Overall, this requires high-voltage power supplies for thermionic devices and high-current power supplies for electromagnets. To configure the machine for x-ray and electron operating modes as well as FFF beams over a range of different energies, these power supplies are programmable over a continuous range of voltages and current values. It is an accepted good engineering practice in critical systems to 'read back' and confirm important values once set, and not just to accept that the setting process has worked correctly. An example of this is to read back the value of current in the beam-bending magnet and ensure that it is within acceptable limits of the required setting value. If it is not, an error condition is flagged.

Early Analogue Machines

There is a requirement for adjustment and setting of machine configuration and calibration to be located outside the treatment room so that running parameters can be adjusted to provide the required beam performance. In early analogue machines, this meant cabling signals between the LINAC machine in the treatment room and the cabinet of analogue control electronics in the control area outside the treatment room. Each division of the control system would consist of a circuit board with a multitude of setting potentiometers for the adjustment of calibration and configuration. Furthermore, for a multienergy dual-mode (x-rays and electrons) machine, there would be one potentiometer on each circuit board for each of the beam energies and modalities. This limited the number of presettable parameters available at the design stage. There was also a possibility of confusion to which potentiometer has been adjusted during service and beam setup activities, leading to a potential hazard to loss of calibration of other energies and modalities. Furthermore, because a LINAC platform consists of systems that are sensitive to electrical noise and systems that generate considerable amounts of it, long, complex cabling runs are undesirable. This is due to inductance, intercable capacitance and triboelectric noise generated by cable movement in these cabling schemes. Additionally, the sheer volume of cabling looms required, considering these need to be 'reeled' onto a rotatable gantry assembly, limited the number of signals that could be successfully managed. Downtime on these machines due to cabling problems was not uncommon.

The Digital Machine

Digital communication between the machine and the control area outside the room offered many advantages over the analogue system. It also provided the communication capacity to develop the complexity of the LINAC to deliver advanced radiotherapy treatments as we now see in VMAT and image guidance. Digitisation of control elements and communications was the way many industrial control systems have developed, and LINAC manufacturers followed suit with varying levels of digital instrumentation and control in their emerging digital machine platforms.

As described in the 'Early Analogue Machines' section, configuration, calibration and control are located outside the treatment room. This is still the case for digital machines, where the majority of the control system data are communicated via a digital control data network to and from the accelerator by a dedicated LINAC control computer located in the treatment control area. This negates many of the restrictions imposed by machine cabling described previously, drastically lowering the amount of cabling required, improving electrical noise performance and expanding the possible number of system elements that can be processed.

Within the accelerator electronics located in the treatment room, the digital control data network interacts with the physical machine. This is achieved using digital to analogue convertors (DACs) and analogue to digital convertors (ADCs) as well as using encoders that directly produce digital signals. The digital signals from the machine convey digitised analogue signal levels as well as logic-level signals and status data to the control computer. Likewise, digital control signals are sent from the dedicated LINAC control computer to the DAC systems on the machine. Software on this computer utilises control algorithms for the many systems required to realise a working machine. Configuration data sets are applied to these control algorithms to facilitate initial machine setup and necessary adjustments after major service work. Furthermore, calibration data sets are also applied, allowing for software calibration of parameter readouts and values to set radiation beam geometry. Both data sets are stored on the LINAC control computer.

The benefits of the digital machine are many and include:

- Service diagnostic tools, such as parameter plotting, data logging and analysis
- Superior fault reporting, enabling rapid fault analysis, repair and restoration of treatment
- System calibration, including the use of software wizards
- Software lookup tables to remove static components of error signals in servo control systems
- Improved dual-channel instrumentation for confirmation of critical parameters, with redundancy
- Local and off-site remote diagnostic connectivity

The use of digital technology has realised high reproducibility in machine manufacture. Use of sophisticated controls, multiple parameters and error analysis has allowed for implementation of new advanced technologies such as the fast tuning magnetron and the use of higher-precision waveguides, leading to more stable beam startup and delivery at a higher dose rate. This is reflected in the application of present and developing treatment regimens such as FFF x-ray beams, HDR electron therapy and the development of FLASH radiotherapy delivery systems, ultimately bringing about superior treatment delivery to patients, reduced maintenance and downtime, fewer quality assurance issues and the reduced installation time of beam-matched machines.

However, having said all this, early lessons learnt in the development of the digital machine have resulted in a level of integration of some of the simple interlock techniques found on the early machines. These were based on breaking the circuit of series-connected switches and relays in the accelerator systems to detect fault states. On modern machines, this 'low-level' protection is used to underpin the computerised control and stands alone from the digital hardware and software systems. Generally, if this low-level structure detects an error state not first identified by the digital control, the machine is locked out and requires a reset by a senior operator. The safety of the patient and staff is always of the utmost importance.

PATIENT ALIGNMENT FOR X-RAY AND ELECTRON THERAPY

In both the x-ray and electron modes of operation, the radiation beams are aligned with the mechanical rotation axis of the radiation head (Fig. 10.9). Alignment of the beam to the patient can be considered in three parts. The first consists of mechanical and optical indicators which are aligned with the axis of the radiation head rotation and hence the radiation beam. The second consists of indicators which locate the isocentre of the machine in space. The third is image guidance, the final verification of alignment, which involves registration of patient anatomy with reference images and is described in Chapter 11.

The main indicators of the radiation beam axis are the treatment front pointer, treatment back pointer and light field cross wires. These are illustrated in Fig. 10.10 with the pointers attached to the radiation head, as during patient setup. Light field cross wire projection is achieved through an optical system in the radiation head. A light source is effectively positioned at the x-ray target by using mirrors. Cross wires are introduced into the light field using a thin transparent sheet, and with the light source and the cross wire centre exactly on the radiation head axis of rotation, an optical projection of the axis is produced.

The isocentre is indicated by three systems. The first is the tip of the front pointer, which is set to the isocentre (Fig. 10.10). The second is a distance meter, which effectively this uses the coincidence between the cross wire projection and the distance meter projection to determine distances from the x-ray source to the surface of the patient (Fig. 10.11).

The third indicator, the alignment lasers, are independent of the machine and consist of room-mounted lasers that, through cylindrical

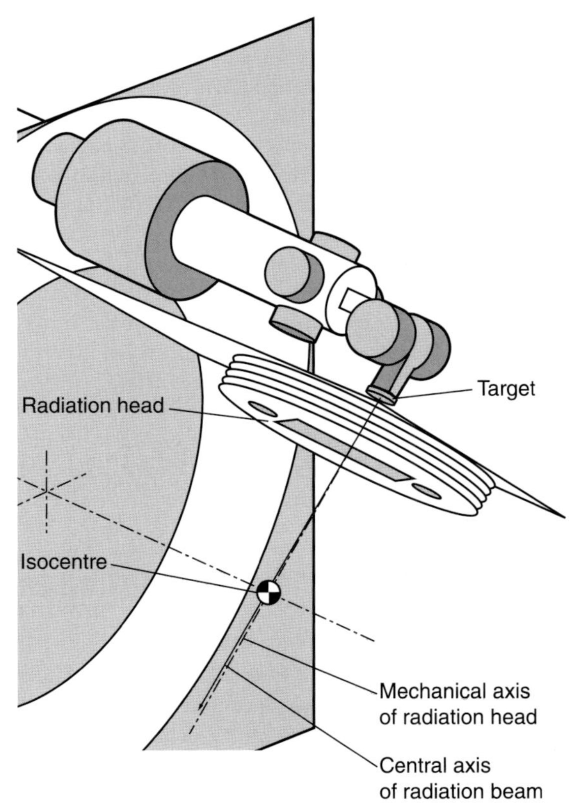

Fig. 10.9 Alignment of mechanical and radiation beam axes.

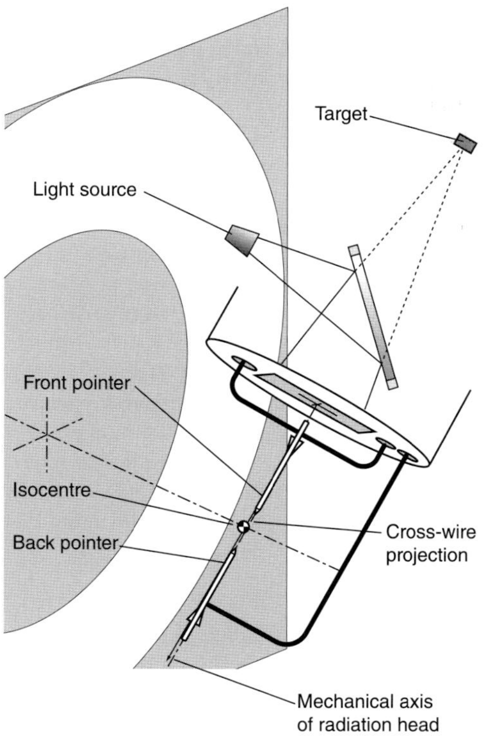

Fig. 10.10 Cross wires and treatment pointers; front and back.

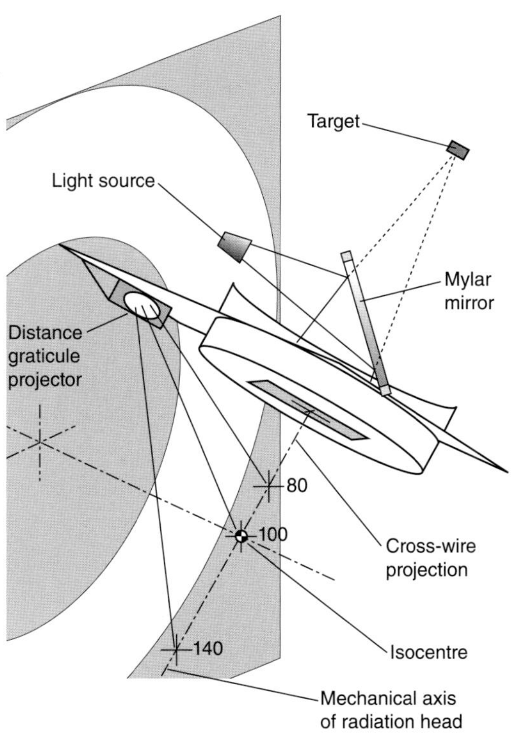

Fig. 10.11 Distance meter for isocentre indication.

lenses, project sheets of light through the isocentre, providing a set of cartesian coordinate planes with the isocentre at the origin. Using surface marks from the patient's treatment planning, the laser sheets enable the patient to be set up with the isocentre at the appropriate place within the patient.

An additional laser, mounted on the treatment machine and projecting a sheet from the base of the gantry through the isocentre and the axis of gantry rotation, provides by intersection with the lateral vertical laser sheets a line coincident with the axis of the diaphragm rotation. This enables visual verification of the exit location of the beam if that was required. For a comprehensive diagram of the laser alignment system, see Fig. 9.14 in Chapter 9 of the Walter and Miller's *Textbook of Radiotherapy: Radiation Physics, Therapy and Oncology*, 8th Edition.

SPECIALISED MEGAVOLTAGE LINEAR ACCELERATORS

The basic waveguide system for the acceleration of electrons has been incorporated into specialised gantry systems for treatment.

CyberKnife

Technological development in industry has led to robots with a very wide-ranging directional and positioning ability. Whereas with a standard treatment machine the beams were almost always delivered in the same plane, the dexterity of a robotic arm meant that the beam could be directed in any direction in space with high accuracy and precision. The CyberKnife is a commercial system which exploits this. The LINAC is mounted at the end of a robotic arm. Small-diameter x-ray beams are produced and directed into the target, shaping the dose distribution around the target in a conformal manner by combining multiple beams. This treatment machine has found applications in the treatment of targets close to critical tissue, such as the spine.

TomoTherapy

The pioneering development of IMRT led to the development of TomoTherapy, a commercial device now widely used. A standard waveguide producing a 6-MV photon beam is mounted on a CT scanner gantry so that an IMRT beam can be delivered around and along the patient. The radiation beam consists of a strip across the axis of the machine gantry rotation. To encompass a target volume, the patient is translated along the axis of the scanner in steps while a fast MLC device modulates the beam. This enables multiple target volumes to be treated in a single irradiation treatment.

Stereotactic Ablative Radiotherapy

Another adaptation of the LINAC has been stereotactic RT and radiosurgery with a standard isocentric LINAC. This is also referred to as *stereotactic ablative radiotherapy (SABR)* and *stereotactic body radiotherapy (SBRT)*. Although dedicated small-field collimators were initially used, micro-MLC and even the higher-resolution standard MLCs are used for the small fields involved. These small fields are delivered statically or, in arc treatment techniques, with very accurate patient positioning. Stereotactic techniques are used for liver, lung and cranial tumours and are also used cranially for arteriovenous (AV) malformation.

Gyroscopic Radiosurgery

Another adaptation for radiosurgery has been the mounting of a 3-MV LINAC on a dual, independent gantry system enabling stereotactic delivery of multiple small fields with a tight penumbra for head and neck treatments. Marketed as Zap-X, the system is comparable to the Gamma Knife (Chapter 9) and benefits from its clinical experience, but with an x-ray source rather than the cobalt-60 radioisotope.

RADIATION SAFETY

Radiation safety is of paramount importance with regard to treatment machine construction and operation. The legislative requirements and practical means to achieve effective radiation protection are described in Chapter 4, and a significant aspect with regard to megavoltage machines is the room design described shortly in the 'Treatment Room Design for X-ray and Electron Protection' section.

There is also a need for protection of the staff and patients by the provision of machine interlocks and shielding. The radiation head itself is constructed with shielding to minimise radiation leakage outside the treatment beam. For electron treatment, this is also addressed within the applicator design and the diaphragm settings.

Room door and maze barrier interlocks are used to minimise the likelihood of accidental irradiation of staff. Besides these, the treatment machines have many interlocked circuits. These interlocks are of two types. The first type is to ensure that the beam is operating within chosen performance limits. An example of such a type would be the monitor for beam uniformity and symmetry discussed earlier in the 'Controlling and Steering the Beams' section. Another example would be the monitoring of the bending current which ensures that the energy of the beam remains stable and detects any fault in the electrical circuit that could affect it and hence the energy of the beam. The second type ensures that fitments on the machine are correctly set; for example, that the flattening filter for photons and the scattering foil for electrons are in position, that the x-ray target is present for photons and that the electron applicator was correctly fitted and agrees with that selected at the treatment console or in the treatment prescription.

The beam control described earlier also provides a safety system, with Ch2 as a backup chamber so that a difference between Ch2 and Ch1 will be detected and the irradiation terminated. Ch2 will terminate the treatment with a very small additional dose than intended if Ch1 has failed. There is also a tertiary timer termination system which should be set so that it terminates the treatment in the event of both Ch1 and Ch2 termination failure, and only a small additional dose will be given to the patient.

ACCEPTANCE, COMMISSIONING AND QUALITY CONTROL

Following supply of a treatment machine, two conditions have to be established. The first is that the equipment supplied meets the specification required by the customer. This involves a formal acceptance of the machine by the customer based upon a demonstration by the supplier that the machine meets the performance and safety specifications upon which the purchase of the machine was agreed.

It is then essential that the characteristics of the machine's beams and performance of the machine are established by measurement. This commissioning period sets out to provide the data upon which all calculations and dose predictions will be made for a patient's treatment. In addition, it provides the baseline set of performance data against which subsequent checks or quality control measurements will be made. Besides measuring standard data such as output factors, depth dose and tissue phantom ratios, specific data for beam-dose algorithms in the computer treatment planning systems along with verification data for dose predictions are gathered and used for validation. In the case of imaging and any other ancillary equipment, relevant commissioning measurements should also be devised.

Quality control (see Chapter 14) of the equipment is required to ensure subsequent satisfactory operation. It is required routinely on a periodic basis to demonstrate the continued satisfactory operation of the machine. It is also required following machine changes, breakdown and repairs to ensure that operation has been returned to a satisfactory level. Lastly, it is required following adjustments to the running of the machine. All these checks ensure that satisfactory operation of the machine has been maintained.

Formal acceptance, the period of commissioning and quality control are an established practice and are recognised in the Euratom 97 and IRMER 2017 statutory legislation.[3,4]

TREATMENT ROOM DESIGN FOR X-RAY AND ELECTRON PROTECTION

The details of treatment room design are very dependent upon the treatment machine, and there are two main aspects to consider. The first concerns radiation safety and protection of personnel[4] whereas the second concerns the ergonomics of the room. The layout of the room is important to ensure efficient treatment, patient access and machine maintenance.

For radiation protection, many of the features employed and materials used can also be related to the actual location of the room, either its adjacencies to public areas or whether it is a new room or a reused and modified room. Although there can be many aspects to detailed room design, there are general features that all room designs use to exploit very fundamental characteristics of radiation.

The purpose of shielding is to protect members of the public and workers associated with the treatment centre, particularly those who will spend a considerable portion of their working day in the vicinity of the room and are involved with patient treatment in the room.

These general features concern first the direction of the primary beam and providing sufficient shielding to attenuate the direct beam. Also with regard to beam direction, the position of room access and the access of penetrations into the room for services such as water and electrical supply, cabling and ventilation should be placed to avoid primary beam irradiation. Away from the primary shielding, the room walls should be adequate to attenuate scattered radiation.

The next feature concerns room access, which may be direct or via use of a maze. Here there are considerations such as staff access and the patient's apprehension of being left alone in a room. Direct access requires a substantial shielding door to be fitted which will be motorised, extend the time for entry and require contingency for access in the event of motor failure. For a maze entrance, three aspects are of significance: the cross-sectional area, distance along the maze and bends in the maze. The cross-sectional area concerns the area of the maze entrance inside the room. In effect, this limits the amount of scattered radiation in the room which enters into the maze. The smaller this can be made consistent with patient access including a bed, the less radiation will enter the maze. Reduction of the cross-sectional area of the maze at the room by use of a lintel can make a substantial contribution to protection. Second, the length of the maze will increase the distance between entrance and exit and provide a dose reduction in line with the inverse-square relationship. Lastly and significantly, the scatter from a right-angled bend within a maze can make a very significant contribution to reducing the dose which can be measured at the end of the maze outside the room.

In Fig. 10.12, a typical megavoltage medical LINAC room layout is shown with the aforementioned features indicated for clarity.

For high-energy photon beams, neutron production because of a photon–neutron interaction in the nucleus needs to be considered. This interaction occurs at megavoltage photon energies but is nominally considered a problem at 10 MV and above. It occurs in, for example, the collimation system on the machine. The aspects described earlier are not readily applicable, and expert advice needs to be sought. Nevertheless, despite the problems which neutrons bring, there are readily available solutions which enable safe room design with direct and maze access, even up to 25 MV. Several aspects concerning neutrons are worth mentioning. First, sharp corners in the room aid in reduction of the neutron flux. Second, care should be taken to avoid

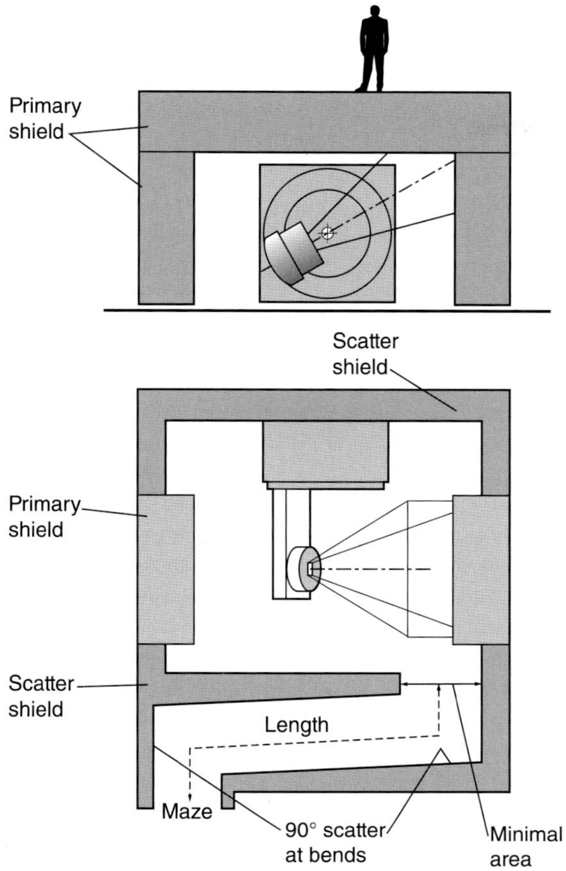

Fig. 10.12 Major features of radiation protection for a linear accelerator treatment room.

metal content in the construction materials, including the concrete aggregate, as gamma activation can occur and result in a neutron problem being traded for a photon problem. This is also the case for wood lining, which was considered appropriate in the past. Lastly, specialised lining, including commercial lining substances for the maze and other penetrations, can be used to significantly reduce the problem to well below radiation protection limits.

For more details on protection requirements and legislation, see Chapter 4, which also includes reference to guidance on room design.[5,6]

Besides safety, the layout within a room for equipment and storage should be given consideration. Adequate storage will ensure that treatment machine accessories such as applicators and specific patient devices such as immobilisation shells can be stored properly. This will help avoid damage which may compromise treatment because of incorrect to operation of the equipment (e.g. electron applicators or treatment pointers). It also avoids treatment delays by having equipment readily available and avoiding repair of damaged devices. Also worth considering at the room design stage are (1) the layout of the room, (2) access to the room and treatment control terminals, (3) visibility of information screens and (4) location of alignment lasers. Furthermore, hand controls for manoeuvering the machine should be accessible and readily available to avoid damage and enhance the ease of treatment. Distance and access from the treatment control area into the room are important to maximise throughput and ease workload. In addition to patient and treatment staff considerations, it is important to facilitate speedy access to the machine for repairs. This will reduce downtime by enabling effective equipment, such as hoists, to be used easily, and ensuring that adequate clearance is available for the removal and fitting of components. Lastly, adequate lighting and dimming controls will ease patient setup and again assist with increasing patient throughput and easing workload. Similarly, clear and controllable CCTV equipment is essential.

SPECIAL TECHNIQUES WITH LINEAR ACCELERATORS

Although LINACs have been designed to deliver beams which will superimpose on each other within the patient in an effective manner, they have also been adapted to fulfil some other treatment requirements.

One of the major adaptations has been to provide total-body irradiation (TBI) treatment with x-rays and total-skin electron (TSE) treatment. For both types of treatment, the limitation of the accelerator is its field size. However, by treating patients at a greatly extended distance of up to 4 m, full-body coverage has been achieved for megavoltage TBI (Fig. 10.13). Likewise, techniques to provide electron fields large enough to entirely cover the patient have been devised for TSE, and Fig. 10.14 shows the well-acknowledged Stanford technique. However, there are other techniques involving gantry rotation and patient movement, and for these extended source-to-patient TSE treatment distances, high dose rates can be specially generated by the LINAC to reduce treatment time.

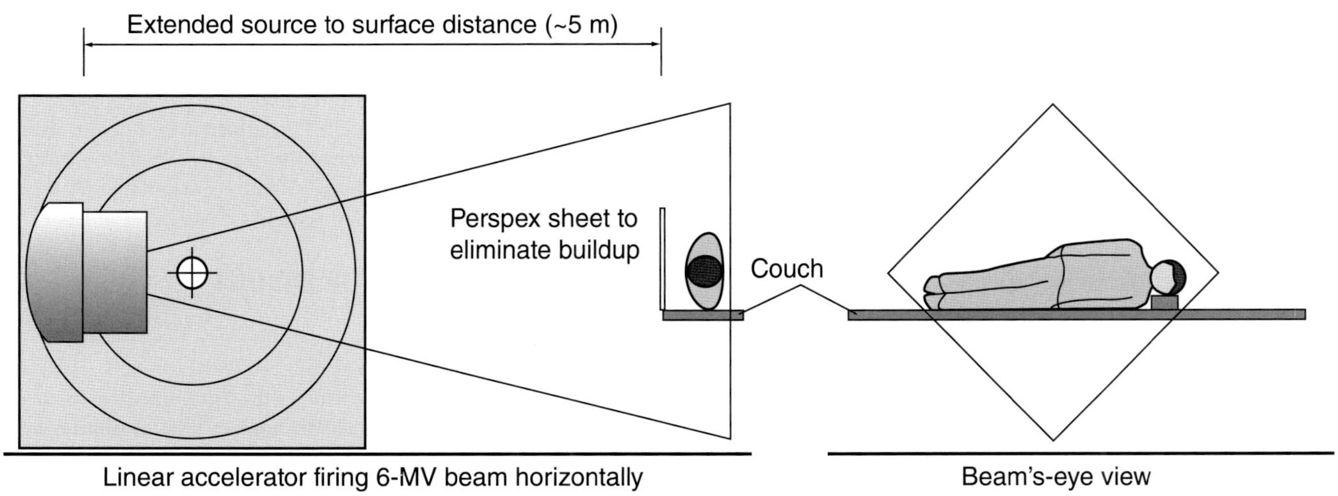

Fig. 10.13 Linear accelerator for total-body irradiation.

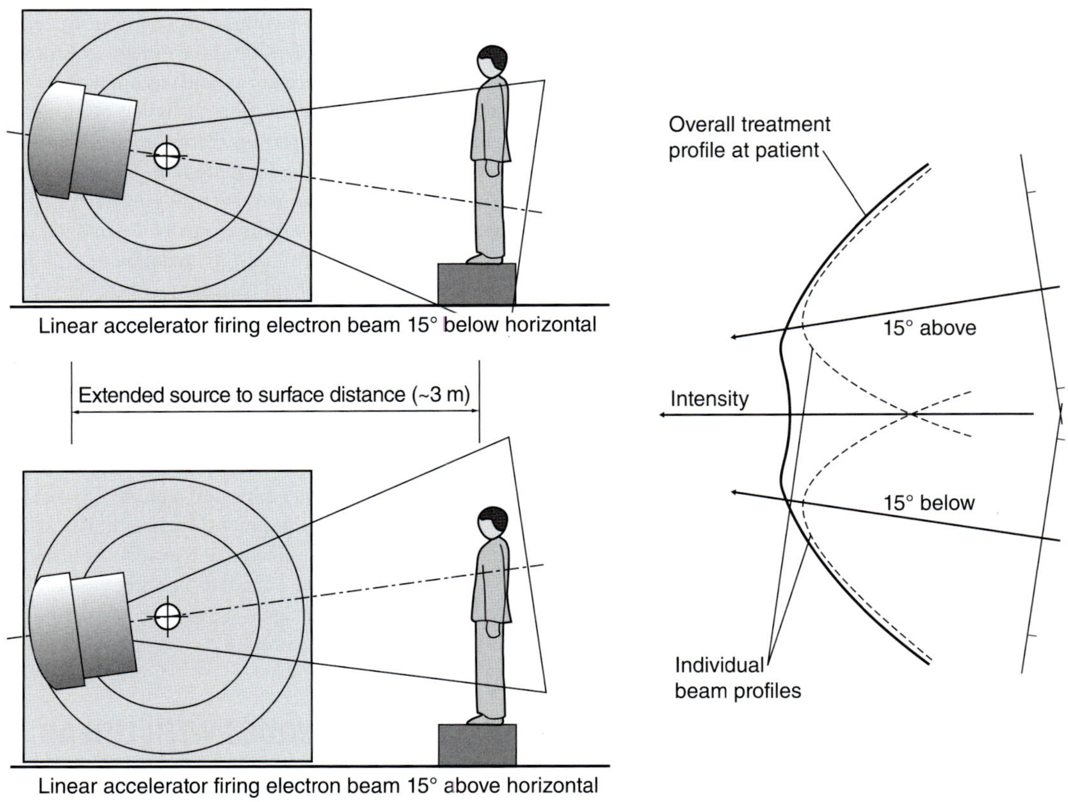

Fig. 10.14 Linear accelerator for total skin electron treatments.

THE DEVELOPMENT OF CLINICAL PROTON AND HEAVIER CHARGED PARTICLE ACCELERATORS

Treatments using heavier charged particle beams, particularly protons, have now moved from decades of development in research centres to being accepted as a formidable tool in mainstream radiotherapy. Despite considerable improvements in x-ray treatments in terms of precision, conformal quality and speed, proton and carbon therapy beams are addressing lesions that are both radiation resistant and positioned adjacent to critical organs. The much-reduced level of secondary integral dose makes this form of therapy of particular interest in paediatric treatments. Commercial and technical developments have helped to produce accelerators that are highly reliable, compact in size and more economically priced. The quality of treatments has been further improved by exploiting the latest developments in image verification and patient positioning. However, the heavier mass and energy of therapy protons requires the use of large, heavy gantries to support powerful bending and focusing magnets and the beam delivery head. Equally demanding is a gantry rigidity that must demonstrate mechanical isocentre reproducibility no different from that found on x-ray linear accelerator machines.

It is estimated that the number of patients who are currently receiving x-ray radiotherapy but could benefit from proton therapy varies from 2% (United Kingdom) to 12% (Sweden). This would represent a substantial patient throughput and has stimulated the current expansion of this radiation modality.

Early proton beam treatment (PBT) facilities were necessarily based in research centres, particularly in the United States (Berkeley, 1954; Harvard, 1961) and Sweden (Uppsala, 1957). This was followed in other countries such as Russia (JINR, 1967; ITEP, 1969) and Japan (National Institute of Radiological Sciences (NIRS), 1979; Tsukuba, 1983).[7–9]

The first hospital-based PBT centre commenced treatment in 1989 at Clatterbridge in the United Kingdom, albeit with an energy only suitable for treating ocular tumours. The first purpose-built high-energy proton centre began patient treatments in 1990, at the Medical Center at Loma Linda in California. This pioneering project used a synchrotron to provide proton beams with selected energies directed to three large gantries, as well as a fixed horizontal beam.[10]

The majority of PBT centres are now based in clinical environments rather than research centres and are considered a part of mainstream radiotherapy. By 2023, there were 130 ion therapy centres in operation worldwide, with 40 in North America alone. Eleven other centres provide carbon beam therapy alone or with PBT. The annual growth of patient treatments and treatment facilities is shown in Fig. 10.15. There were 42 centres in 2012 compared with 120 in 2022, operating with 270 treatment rooms.

An accumulated total of 354,000 patients were treated with PBT by end of 2023, of which 48,000 were ocular treatments. In addition, another 48,800 patients were treated with carbon beams. Ocular treatments with a low-energy proton beam commenced in 1975,[11] and though the basic technique has changed little in over four decades, it has been improved by adoption of digital imaging for diagnosis and treatment verification. This remains the most successful PBT treatment in terms of local tumour control, with 20 centres performing this treatment modality. Treatments consist of 4 or 5 high-dose fractions,[11,12] with the lower-energy cyclotrons providing particularly sharp beam penumbrae and distal falloffs.

PARTICLE ACCELERATOR LAYOUT AND COMPONENTS

The majority of PBT beams are produced with circular particle accelerators. Development of the cyclotron was prompted by the need to produce higher proton energies as a tool in nuclear physics experiments. It was necessary to overcome the limitations of the drift-tube linear accelerator of Wideröe, the Van de Graaff generator and the Cockcroft–Walton accelerator tube. Ernest Lawrence extended the

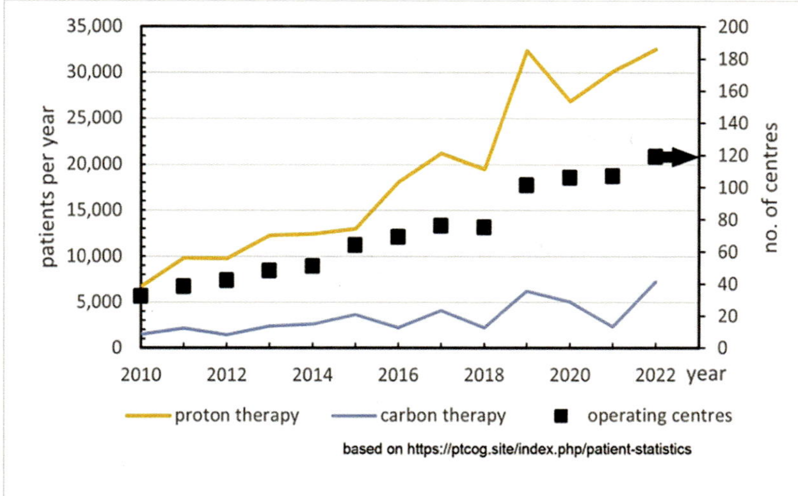

Fig. 10.15 The growth in proton and carbon beam patient treatments and treatment facilities.

Wideröe concept by accelerating particles, in a circular path due to a strong magnetic field, through small 'kicks' in energy which were gained by crossing an electrical potential, with the increase in ion energy leading to an increasing spiral path until the ions exit the magnetic field.

In 1931, after earlier attempts, the group of Ernest Lawrence built an 11-inch (approximately 280 mm) diameter circular accelerator which produced protons of over 1 MeV, albeit at very low currents. Within seven years, a 60-inch (1525 mm) version was being used to produce medical radioisotopes and supply deuterons for neutron therapy. The cyclotron concept was thus established, and the main components of a cyclotron are described in Table 10.1.

Basic Theory of Classical Cyclotron Operation

Positive ions, in this case protons, are accelerated by incremental amounts across an alternating potential between the dees, as shown in Fig. 10.16. The protons travel in a plane which lies at right angles to a uniform magnetic field; this causes the protons to travel in a circular path. The circular path can be described as a balance between the rotational centripetal force and the magnetic Lorentz force which acts normal to the magnetic field and the direction of motion (inset in Fig. 10.17). It can be shown that the radius of the ion orbit will increase with increasing ion momentum (Fig. 10.18). However, the 'period' of the ion orbit is independent of the ion momentum and orbital radius. Thus, although the ion energy and path length increase for each orbit, if the ions arrive in phase with the alternating potential at the accelerating gap at the correct time, they will receive a further increment of energy. This is called *cyclotron resonance*. The beam will have a finite energy spread, so faster charged particles will arrive earlier at the gap and will experience reduced acceleration due to 'phase slip', and slower particles which arrive later at the gap will experience smaller or no acceleration and may be lost to the beam; this is termed *isochronicity*. This type of circular accelerator is termed *isochronous*, as the ions and the RF accelerating potential remain in phase. Thus the repeated traversing of the dee gap by the circulating proton beam incrementally increases the beam energy by the amount of RF potential (V_{dee}) between the dees, which is typically 30 to 100 kV. In this way, high energies are achieved on leaving the magnetic field after multiple passes across the dees. For example, if the dee potential was sufficient to increase the proton energy by 200 keV per orbit, a final beam energy of 240 MeV would be achieved in 1200 proton orbits. An overview of the construction and path of the accelerating protons is shown in Fig. 10.17.

The RF potential across the dees acts as a focusing 'electrostatic' lens[13] which helps to maintain the proton beam in the central plane. However, this effect decreases at increasing proton energies, and the main focusing is provided by the main magnetic field. Thus the design

TABLE 10.1 Main Components of a Cyclotron

Component	Function	Details
Ion source	Provide a source of charged particles by ionising a neutral gas (usually hydrogen)	Types: PIG, ECR, duoplasmatron or microwave
RF power source	Provide an alternating potential to the dee electrodes	30–50 kV; 20–50 MHz
Main magnet	Provide a high magnetic field	Resistive or superconducting
Vacuum tank	Include the dee electrodes, the accelerating beam and deflector assembly	Main accelerating chamber
Dee electrodes	Provide an acceleration gap between the two electrodes	The hollow dee-shaped conductors provide a field-free cavity between accelerations.
Electrostatic deflector	A channel, at negative potential, to provide an exit from the cyclotron tank into a beam pipe	Other types of deflector are used in synchrotrons.
Vacuum pumps	Provide high vacuum required (10^{-5}–10^{-7} mbar) to avoid beam losses	Oil diffusion pumps or ion getter pumps; turbomolecular pumps are not used due to vulnerability of stray magnetic fields.
Cooling system	Provide water cooling to dissipate heating of magnets, RF and all magnet power supplies	Ensure that water is of correct pH to avoid corrosion in copper coils.

ECR, Electron cyclotron resonance; *mbar*, megabar; *PIG*, Penning Ionisation Gauge; *RF*, radiofrequency.

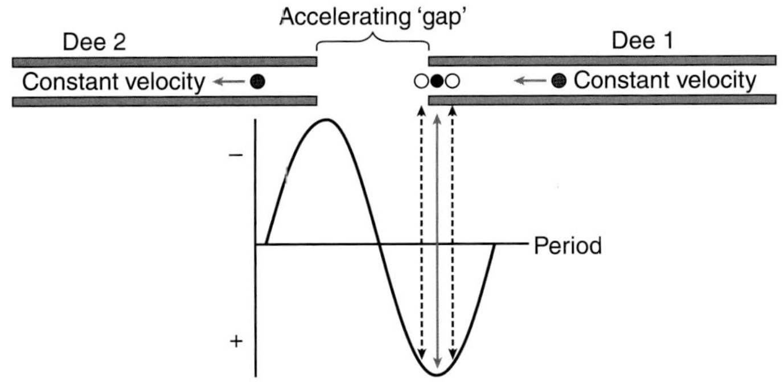

Fig. 10.16 Phase stability of ions in a cyclotron. The dees are viewed edge-on.

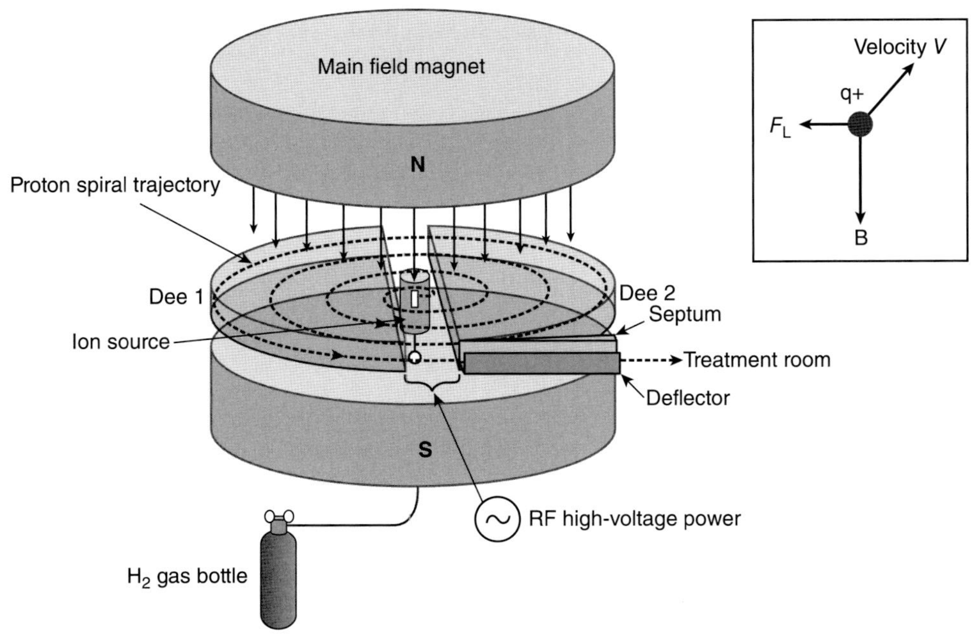

Fig. 10.17 Proton or charged particle path in a constant magnetic field.

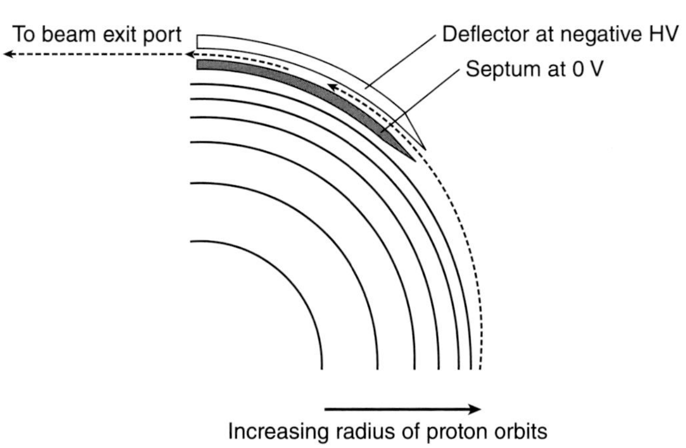

Fig. 10.18 Simplified quarter-plan view of proton orbits and conventional electrostatic deflector.

of cyclotrons requires the frequency and power of the RF to be stable with precise and constant magnetic fields for optimal performance.

The ability of a magnet to bend a charged particle beam is termed *magnetic rigidity* and is expressed analytically in terms of the magnetic field intensity, B, the bending radius, the ion beam momentum and the charge on the ion. This parameter is useful when considering the bending required for ions of different mass, charge and energy in switching magnets, scanning beam magnets and accelerator fields.

The limitations of the classical Lawrence cyclotron became apparent when progressing to higher particle energies and beam currents. Relativistic effects begin to become significant when increasing the proton energies beyond 30 MeV due to the increase in proton mass. The latter will increase by 6% at 60 MeV and by 27% at 250 MeV. The increase in ion mass will reduce the proton velocity and orbit period, thereby causing the particles to become gradually 'out of step' with the RF accelerating potential and thus lose isochronicity. The classical cyclotron uses a uniform magnetic main field, but the weakening of the field at the edge of the magnetic poles creates a vertical focusing component which maintains the beam in the central plane and improves beam output. This is called *weak focusing*. However, the increase in proton energy with the use of wider pole diameters to encompass the increasing orbit radius causes difficulty in radial and axial focusing, which is required to maintain the ion beam in a medial plane, leading to significant loss of beam current. The classical cyclotron design is limited to low energies of <20 MeV and low-current applications. Design improvements have led to higher currents (in the mA range) needed for the production of PET and longer-lived isotopes for medical application.

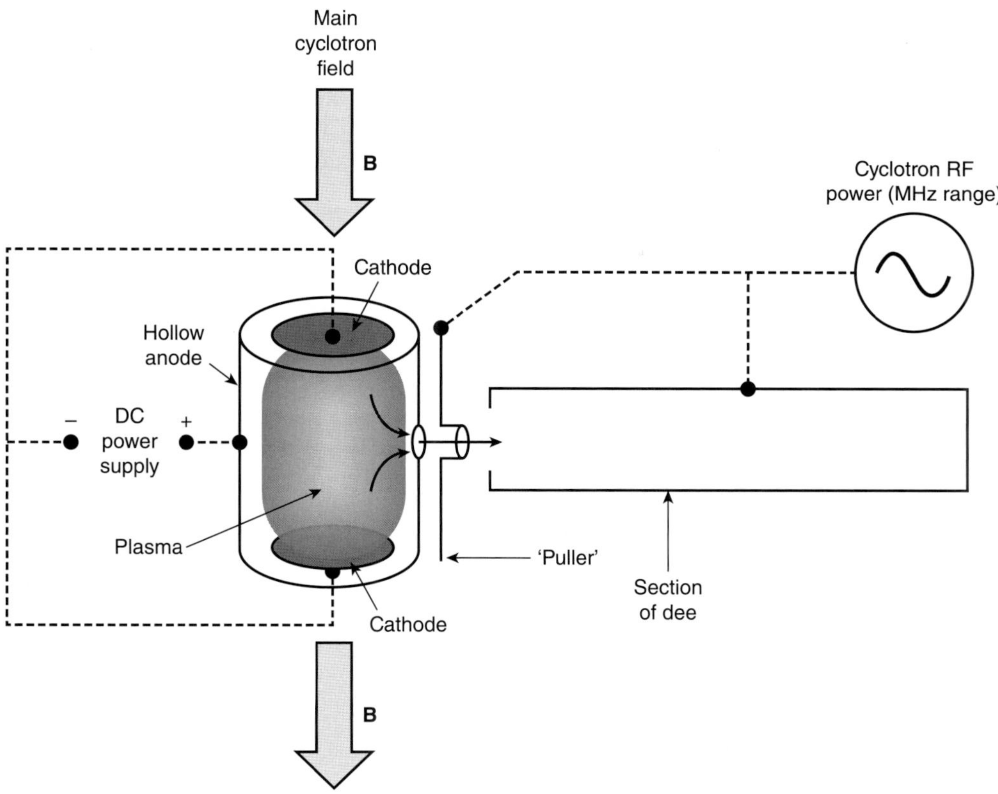

Fig. 10.19 Simplified operation of a Penning Ionisation Gauge (PIG) ion source.

Ion Source Operation

Protons or other light ion charged particles are produced in an ion source, where, for example, for protons, hydrogen gas is ionised by various means to create a localised plasma of protons and electrons. This is illustrated in Fig. 10.19 in the case of a cold-cathode Penning Ion Gauge (PIG) ion source. Electrons are emitted from the two opposing cathode surfaces by a strong electric field, and as they oscillate between the cathodes, they ionise the hydrogen gas. The ionisation is intensified by the main magnetic field of the cyclotron, and with the heating of the electrodes it produces a self-sustaining plasma. The protons are then introduced into the cyclotron tank by diffusion through a 'chimney' slit and by attraction from a 'puller' electrode, which is at the same potential as the dee RF power. At this point the protons come under the influence of the RF accelerating potential of the dees and of the main cyclotron magnetic field. The earliest 'ion source' operated by ionising hydrogen gas using energetic electrons from a hot tungsten filament. Due to the high-availability requirements in modern clinical ion therapy facilities, ion sources are required to provide more intense currents, reliability and ease of maintenance. Types of ion sources which create ion plasmas, such as PIG, duoplasmatron, electron cyclotron resonance (ECR) and microwave plasma, are described in detail elsewhere.[14,15] Ion sources are required to contain intense plasma produced with high-power input (AC, DC, RF or microwave), usually with a strong magnetic field. The gas flow must be sufficient to maintain the plasma but not overload the main tank vacuum system. The ECR and microwave-driven ion sources are considered to deliver high currents reliably with lower maintenance requirements. However, clinical research centres delivering different particle beams require separate ion sources due to quite different operating conditions.

Characteristics and Limitations for Therapy

Clinical therapy requires an accelerator to produce a maximum particle energy to achieve a range of penetration depths required by the prescription. A sufficient beam current should be available to deliver clinical dose fractions in minutes. This requirement refers to accelerators with continuous beams; it is noted that many modern clinical machines are configured to produce narrow pencil beams for spot-scanning or raster beams. These necessitate the production of necessarily short but high dose-rate pulses; thus mean and maximum currents must be specified. The maximum beam current must account for beam losses along beam transport tubes and gantry systems, as well as energy selection systems (ESSs) which function by slit collimation and energy degradation.

Synchrocyclotrons

This type of circular accelerator was developed to increase the beam energy of the proton or heavier ion beams and reduce the size of the diameter of the main magnet. A limitation of the classical cyclotron design was the loss of accelerating phase with increasing proton energy due to a weakening magnetic field with orbit radius and a reduction in proton velocity due to a relativistic increase in proton mass.

The synchrocyclotron incorporated the reduction of the RF to match the reduction in the ion orbit period. Thus the increasingly energetic protons would remain 'in phase' until extraction at the edge of the main field. In earlier designs, this was achieved by a rotating-vane condenser which functions with a duty cycle of several hundred cycles. The frequency variation of the RF power from f_{intial} to f_{final} is approximately 30%. An additional feature which reduces beam losses is where the accelerating phase occurs at a voltage which is offset from the maximum voltage. Thus later-arriving protons will receive an additional 'boost' in acceleration while those more energetic protons arriving at the gap earlier will

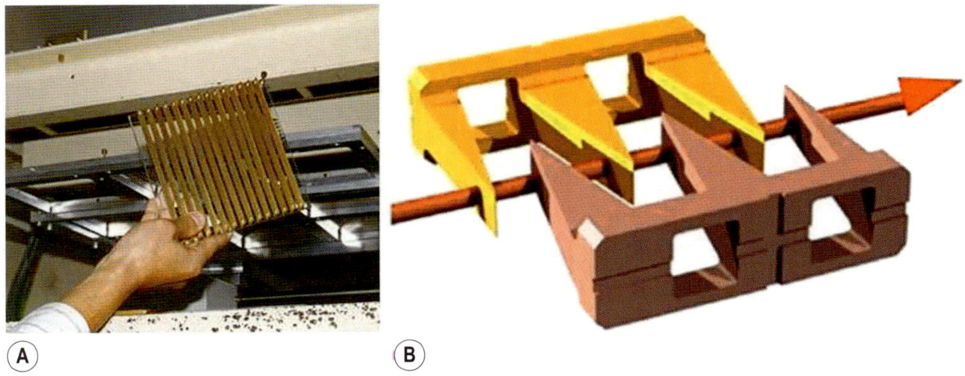

Fig. 10.20 (A) Static ridge energy modulator (NIRS, Japan). (B) Fast-moving carbon multiwedge degrader as part of energy selection system used at PSI. *Red arrow* indicates beam direction. (Courtesy PSI, Villigen, Switzerland.)

receive reduced accelerating potential. This type of synchronisation can be seen as a self-correcting feedback loop and is more tolerant of RF and magnetic field variations. Although beam losses are reduced during orbits, the varying phase synchronisation means that 'bunches' of protons are produced which match the varying RF frequency, and those which are out of phase will be lost to the beam. Overall, synchrocyclotrons will produce a significantly reduced beam current of less than 1% compared to the continuous beam current from a classical cyclotron. This type of circular accelerator has been used in passively scattered beam mode, but it also lends itself for spot scanning. The pulse frequency, with a suitable pulse duration of the order of 1 kHz, can be programmed to complete the required dose spots of individual energy layers, accompanied with 'fast' mechanical energy degraders to decrease the depth of the 'beam scan', as shown in Fig. 10.20. Several commercial PBT synchrocyclotrons, such as the Proteus S2C2 and Mevion Hyperscan 250i, are used in single-room treatment configurations (Table 10.2). These machines benefit from the use of powerful superconducting main field magnets to reduce size and weight; the latter can be related to the magnetic field by $1/B^3$.[16] Thus relatively small increases in magnetic field can improve the compactness of cyclotron accelerators.

Isochronous or Azimuthally Varying Field Cyclotrons

The Azimuthally Varying Field (AVF) was an early concept proposed by Thomas in 1938. The classical cyclotron accelerator used 'weak vertical focusing' due to a reduction of the main field with orbit radius to maintain beam stability. To increase final proton energy or design a smaller cyclotron pole diameter would necessitate an increase in magnetic field, with radius to compensate for the relativistic mass increase of the protons and maintain synchronicity with the dee gap RF. However, this results in vertical defocusing with increasing orbit radius, and thus loss of beam intensity. The solution was to apply strong vertical focusing by means of a stepped variation of the main magnet field intensity along the proton orbit or azimuthal direction. This is produced using alternate stronger and weak fields by wedge-shaped sectors machined within the pole face, as shown in Fig. 10.21. These are known as *hills* and *valleys*, respectively, due to the stepped changes of the pole gap. The sharp change of field at the hill and valley interface causes a deviation in orbit radius from a circular path, depending on whether a hill or valley sector is being traversed. The proton path is no longer perpendicular to the field change, a fact that causes vertical focusing and defocusing. The overall effect, referred to as *isochronicity*, is for strong vertical focusing which is maintained with the increasing main field, B, and proton orbit, resulting in much reduced beam losses. At energies greater than 30 MeV, the wedge-shaped sectors are modified to produce swirl-shaped sectors which greatly enhance strong vertical focusing. Most modern therapy cyclotrons are of this AVF design. For example, the Varian ProBeam and IBA Proteus C230 are of this type. Fig. 10.22 shows the curved dees and pole gap swirls of a high-energy isochronous cyclotron.

TABLE 10.2 Comparison of Compact Accelerators With Single-Room Systems

Vendor	Model	Machine Type	Proton Energy (max)	Weight/ Size	Magnetic Field (tesla)	Dose Rate	Field (cm)	Beam Delivery Options
Mevion	S250 (mounted on gantry; room footprint)	Synchrocyclotron (500 Hz)	250 MeV	22 T; 1.8 m (gantry 80 T)	8–10 T; superconducting (Nb_3Sn)	2–0.4 Gy.min^{-1}	20 × 20	Passive beam; scanning (Hyperscan option)
IBA	S2C2 ProteusOne (centre footprint = 395 m^2)	Synchrocyclotron (1 kHz; 1-μS pulse)	230 MeV	50 T; 2.5 m	5.7–5.0 T; superconducting (NbTi)	2 Gy	24 × 20	Pencil beam scanning
Varian, now Siemens	ProBeam Compact (Superconducting); centre footprint = 260 m^2	Isochronous cyclotron	230 MeV (4–30 cm)	90 T	1.4 T (max); NbTi	>2 Gy.L^{-1}. min^{-1}	30 × 40	ProScan (IMPT)
Hitachi (Hokkaido)	Compact synchrotron (machine footprint = 27 m^2)	Synchrotron (slow extraction)	70–220 MeV	N/A; (mean 5.1-m diameter)	N/A			Spot scanning and passive scattered

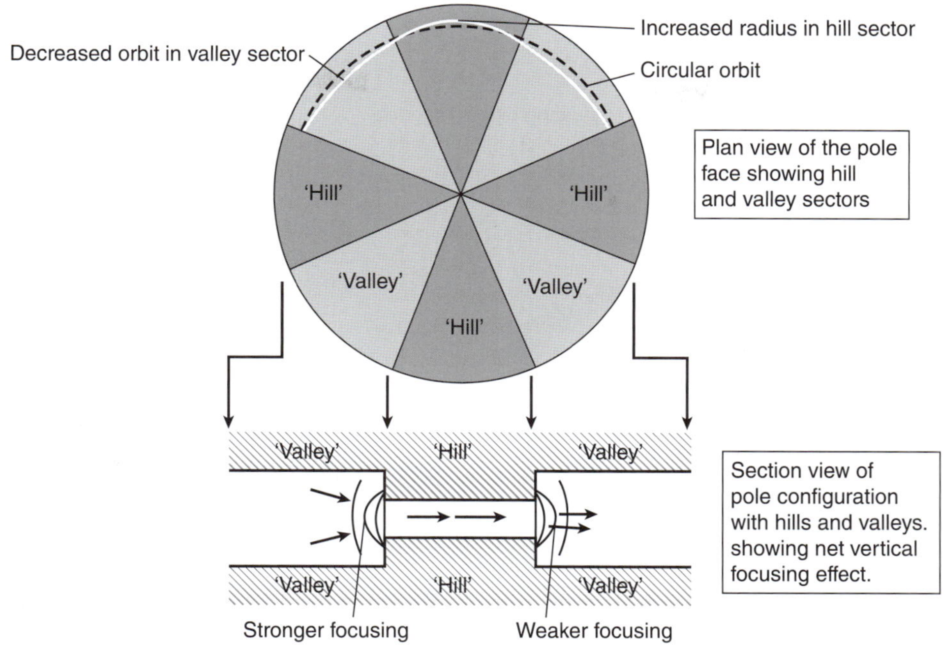

Fig. 10.21 Focusing effect of dees acting as electrostatic lens to maintain beam on central plane.

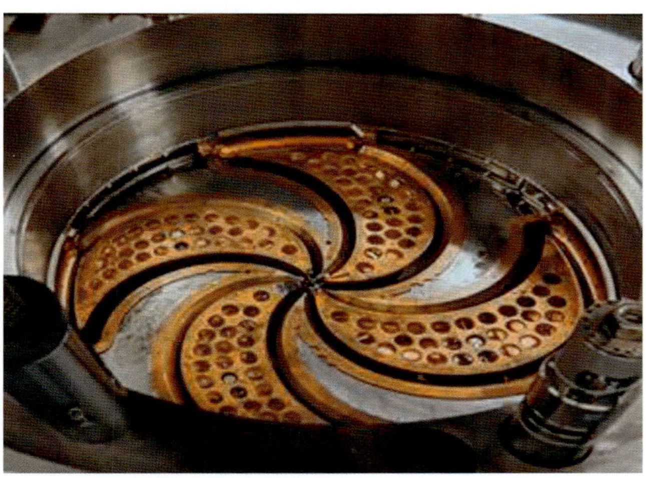

Fig. 10.22 Example of swirl-shaped wedged sectors.

Synchrotrons

This type of circular accelerator was developed at the same time as the synchrocyclotron in the late 1940s to increase the final energy of the accelerated protons and heavier ions. The concept lies in maintaining an ion beam path circumference of fixed radius where individual dipole magnets guide the beam in a circular path. Particles are preaccelerated to low energies of, say, 5 to 8 MeV, by means of a radiofrequency quadrupole (RFQ) and LINAC accelerator before injection into the synchrotron ring. Particle energy increase is provided by an RF accelerator cavity as shown in Fig. 10.23, with an RF deflector or 'kicker' to extract the required amount of beam and at the requested energy. Thus low-energy protons or ions have their energy increased by simultaneous ramping of both the frequency of the RF cavity gap and the magnetic field of the individual dipole magnets. This configuration can be considered figuratively as dividing the single pole face of a cyclotron main magnet into individual magnets, as in equal slices of a cake. As more magnets are employed, each dipole magnet would have a lesser beam-bending or magnetic strength requirement. Thus the final design circumference is dependent on the magnet strength of the bending dipoles, the required final energy and the particle to be accelerated.

As in the case of synchrocyclotrons, the beam is bunched rather than continuous. As the low-energy ions are introduced into the synchrotron ring, an increase in dipole magnet field strength is synchronised with the increasing RF accelerating field. After the required particle energy is attained, the steering and accelerating field strengths are maintained constant for durations of seconds during which time the beam is extracted by means of an electrostatic kicker.[17,18] This beam is of sufficient intensity and duration to complete a layer of spot scanning at a particular proton energy corresponding to the required depth. If all the spots in the required depth slice have been completed, the following proton bunch may be of a reduced energy, E_2, to spot-scan the next shallower depth. The beam is decelerated by a decrease in the accelerating and steering fields.

The average beam intensity is much reduced compared with that from a cyclotron, but the extraction process is highly efficient (typically >90%). In addition, modern clinical synchrotrons are designed with fine energy selection which can control penetration down to 1-mm precision. This avoids the significant beam losses of fixed-energy accelerators which use energy degradation to alter depth penetration. These losses can exceed 95% for both passively scattered and pencil scanning beam modalities. The fast-changing magnetic fields for energetic ions require these magnets to be resistive, with iron cores. The footprint of synchrotrons is necessarily large to accommodate ohmic dipole bending magnets if smaller superconducting magnets are not used. The greater the number of magnets, the smaller the magnetic strength required of each dipole. Synchrotrons can accommodate the acceleration of heavy ions of higher magnetic rigidity, such as helium, carbon and oxygen, as well as protons, with the appropriate ion sources.

A synchrotron footprint is larger than for other circular accelerators, depending on whether it is intended for heavier ion therapy and if it was designed with superconducting dipole magnets. Carbon therapy beamlines are usually fixed and horizontally oriented, as the bending magnet requirements for a carbon beam gantry are challenging. The magnetic rigidity is approximately three times that required for a proton beam of similar penetration of 30 cm. The first carbon

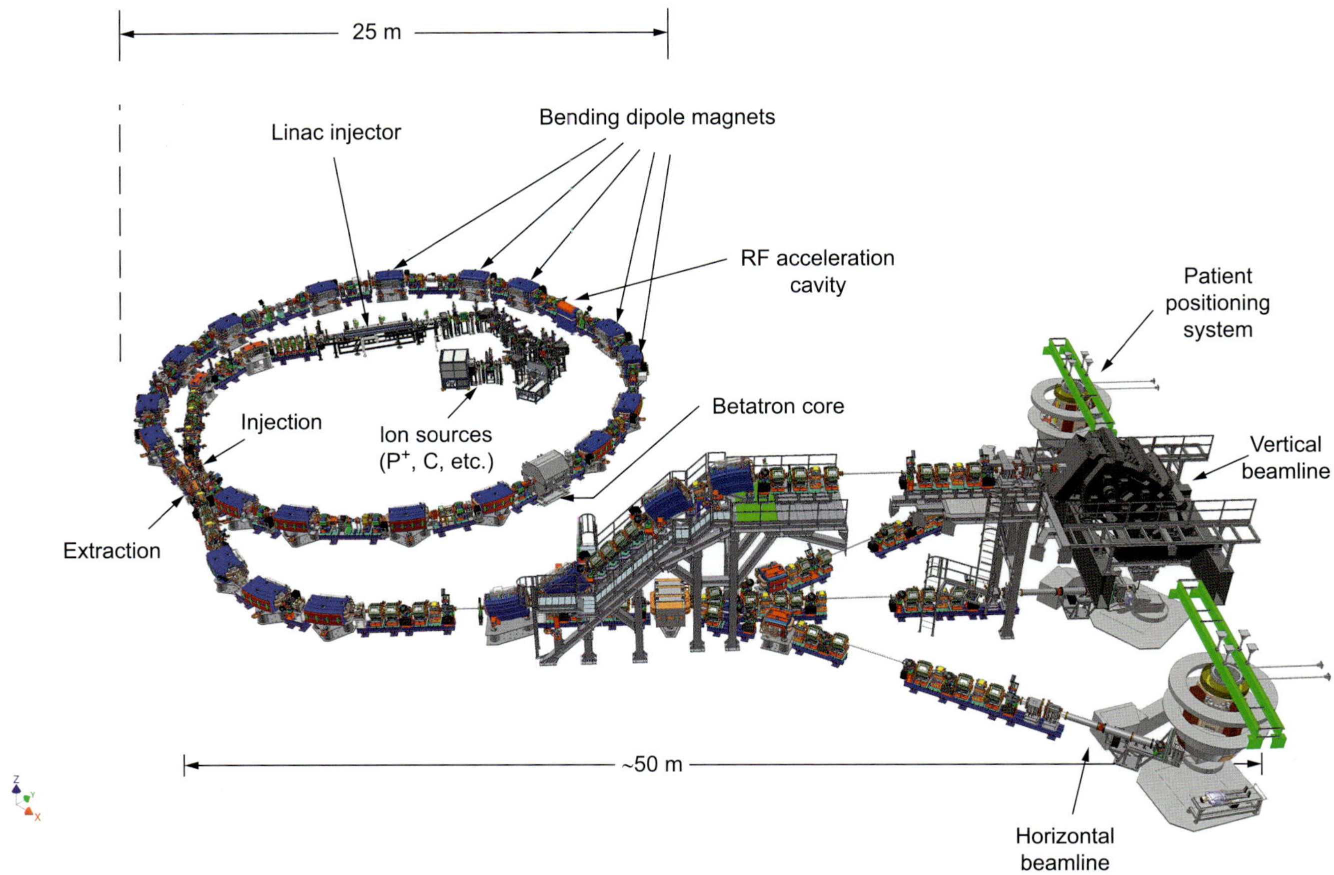

Fig. 10.23 Schematic plan view of clinical synchrotron, based loosely on Hitachi and Siemens configurations (not to scale). The beam transport to treatment rooms is a notional disposition but similar to that used at the Heidelberg Ion Therapy Centre, the National Centre of Oncological Hadrontherapy and MedAustron.

therapy gantry, at the Heidelberg Ion Therapy Centre (HIT), uses resistive magnets and is 22 m long and 13 m high. It weighs approximately 600 tonnes, which is about four times that required of a proton therapy gantry. This is compared with the 1 to 2 tonnes for a rotating x-ray linear accelerator. Recent constructions incorporating superconducting magnets have reduced the weight of carbon beam gantries to 200 to 300 tonnes, such as for the Toshiba machine at the National Institutes for Quantum Science and Technology (QST) Hospital in Japan. A rotational deviation at the isocentre of <1 mm is achieved despite this mass and size. The more compact superconducting designs will significantly reduce the footprint of the gantries and accelerator rings.[19]

PASSIVELY SCATTERED BEAMS AND PENCIL BEAM SCANNING BEAMS

The advantage of proton therapy lies in delivering a three-dimensional dose distribution which is both uniform over the treatment volume and highly conformal to the outlined tumour shape. This exploits sharp proton beam penumbrae, particularly at shallower depths, and rapid distal falloff due to the Bragg peak phenomenon. The incident beam area can be shaped to the tumour outline at a particular depth, and beam penetration can be conformed to the posterior edge of the treatment volume and uniformly spread across the target, as shown in the spread-out Bragg peak (SOPB) in Fig. 10.24. The proton beam delivery techniques to a patient can be simply grouped into two types:

- Passively scattered beams, with energy modulation and collimation
- Pencil beam scanning (PBS), with moving narrow monoenergetic beamlets

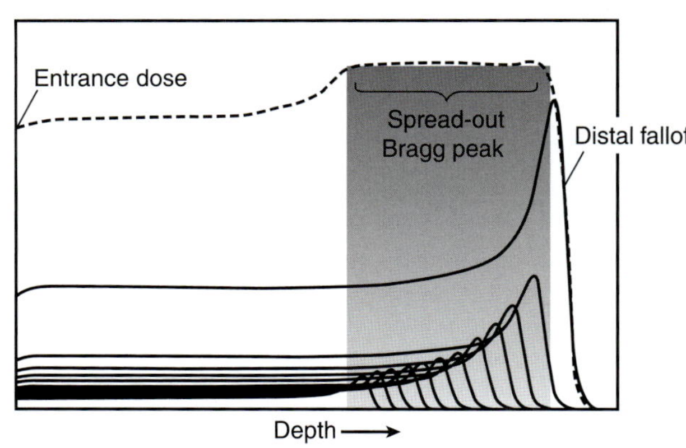

Fig. 10.24 Typical spread-out Bragg peak (SOBP, *dashed line*) depth dose for a high-energy proton beam showing the component Bragg peaks *(solid lines)*. The SOBP region covers the target volume and margins.

The optimisation of both delivery methods requires consideration of the type of accelerator producing the proton beam and, in particular, its pulse structure. Early developments in proton therapy used the passive scattering technique to produce large and uniform treatment fields, particularly with synchrocyclotrons. Although there are several possible configurations of passive scattering, the technique is analogous to those found in linear accelerators producing x-ray and electron beams and consists of one or two high-Z metal foils placed upstream of the patient nozzle, normal to the beam. These serve to scatter the raw

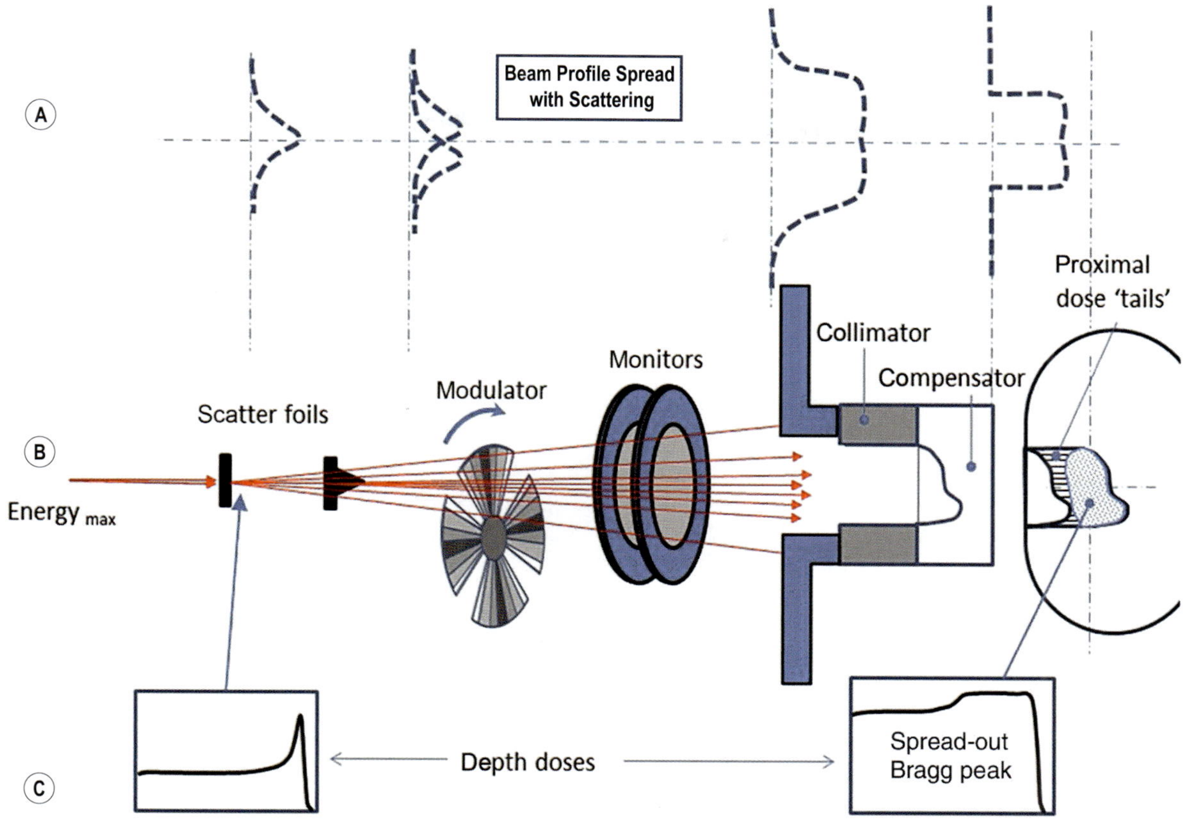

Fig. 10.25 Schematic of proton beam modulation and shaping.

beam into an approximate Gaussian distribution which broadens along the beam direction, as shown in Fig. 10.25. This creates a clinically satisfactory homogeneous central region, which is then collimated at various stages along the beamline by antiscatter diaphragms and the treatment nozzle. The selected scatter-foil configuration depends on the following four criteria:

- The maximum field size required
- The amount of beam energy and beam current losses that can be accepted
- The uniformity of dose and beam energy over the beam aperture
- The activation of beamline components, production of secondary neutrons and appropriate shielding and radiation protection issues

Single- or double-scattering foils, with or without a central stopper, or contoured double scatterers are selected according to the aforementioned criteria and have been used in all types of circular accelerators with fixed horizontal beamlines or rotating gantries.[7,18,20] The thinner double-scattering foil combinations have much greater beam and energy efficiency than single thicker foils.

Passively scattered beams require energy selection to attain the maximum prescribed treatment depth and a method of modulating the pristine Bragg peak in depth to produce a uniform dose over the target volume. The component Bragg peaks are produced by a variable energy absorber, as shown in Figs. 10.25 and 10.26. This is a rotating wheel, often called a *modulator*, with precisely machined thicknesses of plastic or metal, which intercepts the proton beam upstream. Examples are shown in Fig. 10.26, including a static 'pin' modulator.

The time structure of the accelerator beam needs consideration when employing rotating modulators. For example, the short pulses and kHz range of duty cycle of synchrocyclotrons require the rotation speed to be either much faster or slower than the beam pulse frequency to ensure even sampling of beam energies. This poses little problem with the almost direct beam current from cyclotrons due to the high MHz range of RF frequency on the dees and the 'slow' extraction of synchrotron pulses, which are on the order of seconds. In some cases, for example, at the NIRS (Fig. 10.20), a static modulator called a *ridge filter* is used due to its triangular wedge-shaped

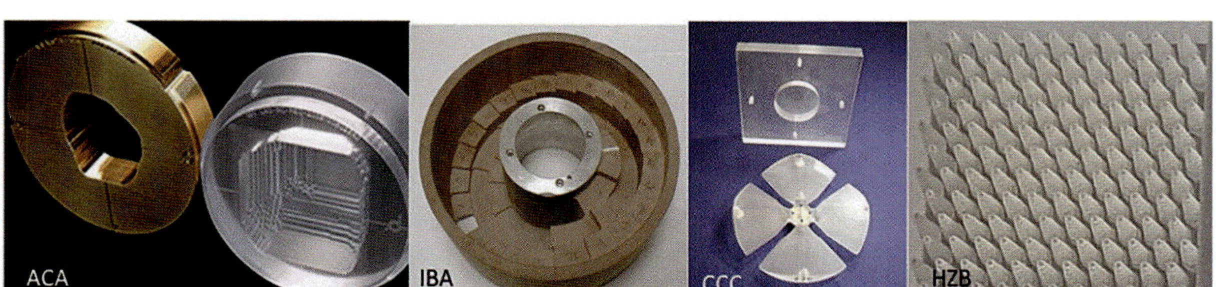

Fig. 10.26 Examples of proton beam shaping and spread-out Bragg peak modulators. (Courtesy ACA, IBA, CCC and HZB.)

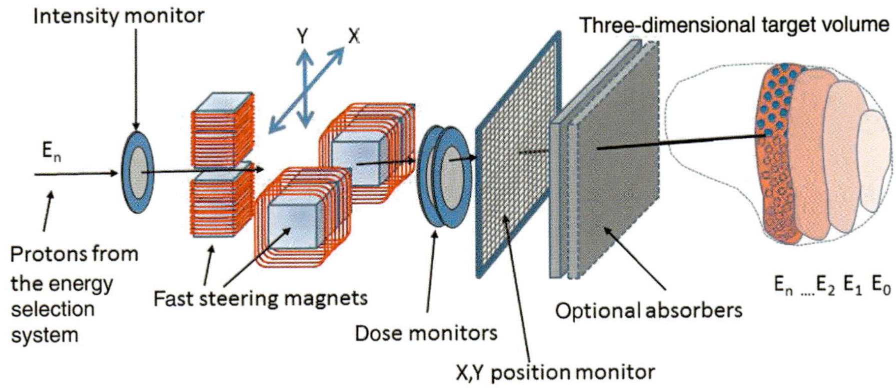

Fig. 10.27 Schematic of proton beam scanning control and Bragg peak depth control using energy change.

absorber strips. The wedge angle and maximum thickness define the extent of the SOBP.

The lateral field is shaped by patient-specific collimators, which are machined by computer controlled (CNC) milling machines using planning data (Fig. 10.26). Collimators for proton therapy were usually manufactured with brass 350. However, the low-melting-point metal compound Cerrobend has been used, which is moulded to the required aperture shape and thickness, allowing economic reuse of the material. Multileaf collimators in passively scattered beamlines were not developed, due to the required weight, control complexity and coarseness of the leaf thicknesses, which would not match the precision of a machined brass aperture. Recently, multileaf collimators are being employed in some PBS systems to improve lateral penumbrae, particularly at lower energies, as in the Mevion S250i.

Patient-specific compensators are used in conjunction with brass apertures for each treatment field. They are designed to contour the dose to the posterior edge of the target volume. These are machined from either polymethacrylate (PMMA) or blue wax. Like the apertures, the process requires the use of CNC milling machines. Several sets of apertures and compensators would be required for each treatment field. A disadvantage is that the compensators cause some full doses proximal to the tumour edges,[7,20] as shown in Fig. 10.25.

Cyclotrons and synchrocyclotrons produce a single maximum energy at extraction. The prescribed treatment energy is thus obtained by reducing the primary energy by an energy degrader, which is simply a graphite absorber of either fixed or adjustable thickness, and an ESS. This can be situated after beam extraction from the accelerator in multigantry facilities or on individual gantries. The ESS beam analysis device consists of adjustable slits which reduce beam emittance and energy spread. However, the degrader and ESS are a source of beam scattering, leading to significant instantaneous neutron and gamma ray dose rates and high induced radioactivity in beamline components. This requires design of neutron and gamma ray shielding appropriate to personnel and public radiation protection limits.

Rapid developments in beam control technology have enabled PBS with proton or ion beams to offer the best dose conformity to a three-dimensional tumour volume, with significantly reduced integral dose. Multiple fields reduce higher dose levels in normal tissue. PBS is achieved by scanning monoenergetic pencil beamlets at programmed intervals in the transverse direction, also referred to as an *energy slice*. This is repeated in the longitudinal depth direction by stepped energy changes. The distribution of beamlets, or spots, in a depth slice is dependent on the spot size and planned transverse area. The beam characteristics (beam position, intensity, energy, magnet settings, etc.) required for a treatment fraction are generated by the proton TPS, in a *log file*, which is then sent to the machine control system. While the beamlets describe the pristine Bragg peak depth doses, the spots refer to the proton dose due to the Bragg peak, and the intensity of the spot delivered takes into account the dose from the Bragg peak tails from higher-energy beamlets. Equally, the beam energy changes corresponding to changes of transverse slice depth are dependent on the resolution of the Bragg peak beamlets and energy change interval of a facility. These may lead to ripple effects that need to be minimised, and the planned spot distributions are calculated to deliver dose homogeneity of <2.5% in the transverse and depth directions. *Intensity modulated proton therapy (IMPT)* is the application of PBS where multiple heterogeneous fields are used to create a uniformly irradiated volume. As with x-ray IMRT, this reduces exposure to organs at risk (OARs), improves sparing of healthy tissue and potentially offers better target dose conformity for complex tumour volumes with much reduced integral dose. This leads to robust proton beam planning techniques where OAR doses are critical.

PBS techniques require fast-acting scanning magnets, rapid changes in beam energy, fast-responding power supplies with range sufficient for required beam rigidities and online, in-beam dose and position monitoring for precise beam spot control. A simplified diagram of the main features of spot scanning beams is shown in Fig. 10.27. The beamlet must be of sufficiently narrow divergence to fulfil the spatial resolution required for a conformal treatment but of sufficient width and spacing to produce the required field uniformity of less than 2.5%. The interval of energy change, hence of scanned depth, is dependent on the ESS and the inherent depth width of the monoenergetic Bragg peak. Many commercial vendors now provide a finely spaced range of available beam energies in approximately 60 to 100 steps in the 70-to-250 MeV range, corresponding to depth slices of only a few mm. The lower-energy limit is mainly due to severely reduced beam intensity and difficulties in beam scattering and focusing. It is noted that the continuous beam from cyclotrons and slow extraction synchrotrons requires beam currents on the order of nAs for PBS, whereas the short pulses with longer-duty-cycle machines require higher instantaneous current availability to complete volume scans in clinically acceptable times. Typical parameters for PBS are summarised in Table 10.3.

At present, there are two basic techniques of moving and delivering pencil beam dose to the required spatial position or volume element (voxel).[9,17,18,21] These can be described as:

- Dose-dependent scanned delivery
- Time-dependent scanned delivery

Dose-dependent scanned delivery requires the beamlet to remain at a fixed voxel coordinate until the planned dose is delivered, and then move to the next adjacent voxel. In time-dependent delivery, the beamlet or spot will remain in the voxel position for a fixed time interval and then move to the adjoining voxel. This necessitates the machine beam current

TABLE 10.3 Basic Parameters Required for Pencil Beam Scanning

Basic Requirements	Lateral: Scan Speed ($cm.mS^{-1}$)	Speed of Energy Change	Range of Field Size (mm × mm)	Spot Diameter (mm)	Dose Delivery ($Gy.Litre^{-1}.min^{-1}$)	Gantry Switching Time (s)
Small beam divergence; spot; spot interval	1–0.2	100 mSec per 5-mm depth	200 × 200–400 × 400	<5 mm @ full width at half maximum	1–2, with dose uniformity of <2.5%	<30

being relatively stable; otherwise, returning to the voxel would be necessary. In both cases, the beam monitoring and intensity control must be rapid to minimise errors in the finite beam switch-off time. A lower beam current reduces this uncertainty at the expense of longer treatment times.

The beam movement options may be briefly summarised as:

- Spot-scanning, where the beam is switched off between voxels, thus creating a dead time between spots.
- Raster scanning, where the beam is on between spots, albeit reduced in intensity. The beam is off only for longer spatial intervals. This is a commonly used option.
- Line scanning of continuous modulated dose in one-dimensional lines. This is in development at Paul Sherrer Institute (PSI) where a second gantry potentially offers fast and flexible scanning, with fast dose redelivery as required.[21,22] The scanned beam, in the one-dimensional direction, is delivered at a constant high velocity, and the planned spot dose is modulated along a horizontal axis.

Although PBS is capable of almost ideal target conformity and dose homogeneity, there are several inherent issues. Patient or organ movement could cause significant dose heterogeneity with hot and cold dose spots. Development of very much faster scanning speeds with advanced beam diagnostics and feedback control offers the possibility of multiple dose redelivery during a single field. Gating of the scanned beams with organ or body respiration and inadvertent movements may increase treatment time but permit tighter conformal margins. Likewise, fast scanning speeds would allow breath-hold gating, which has been practised with cyclotron beams and slow-extraction synchrotrons.[21]

Adaptive pencil scanning is being investigated to address interfractional and intrafractional anatomical changes. It is easier, as imaging and replanning can be performed rapidly and patient-specific beam modifiers are not required with PBS machines. The structure of a PBS system is shown in Fig. 10.28. In some configurations, the long beam traversal in air causes significant beam dispersion which is countered by use of helium- or vacuum-filled chambers. The second scanning magnet is necessarily larger than the first, as the spread of the beam in space and velocity is increased by the first magnet. Note that some more superficial fields may need penetration depths shallower than the 70-MeV low-energy limit. This is addressed by application of calibrated range absorbers at the nozzle to minimise proton scattering and maintain satisfactory field penumbrae. The sharpness of the penumbrae is dependent on the Gaussian width of the beamlets, particularly at the field edge. Several approaches at improving edge penumbrae include the use of multileaf collimators or the use of heavier weighting factors to the edge beamlets.[23]

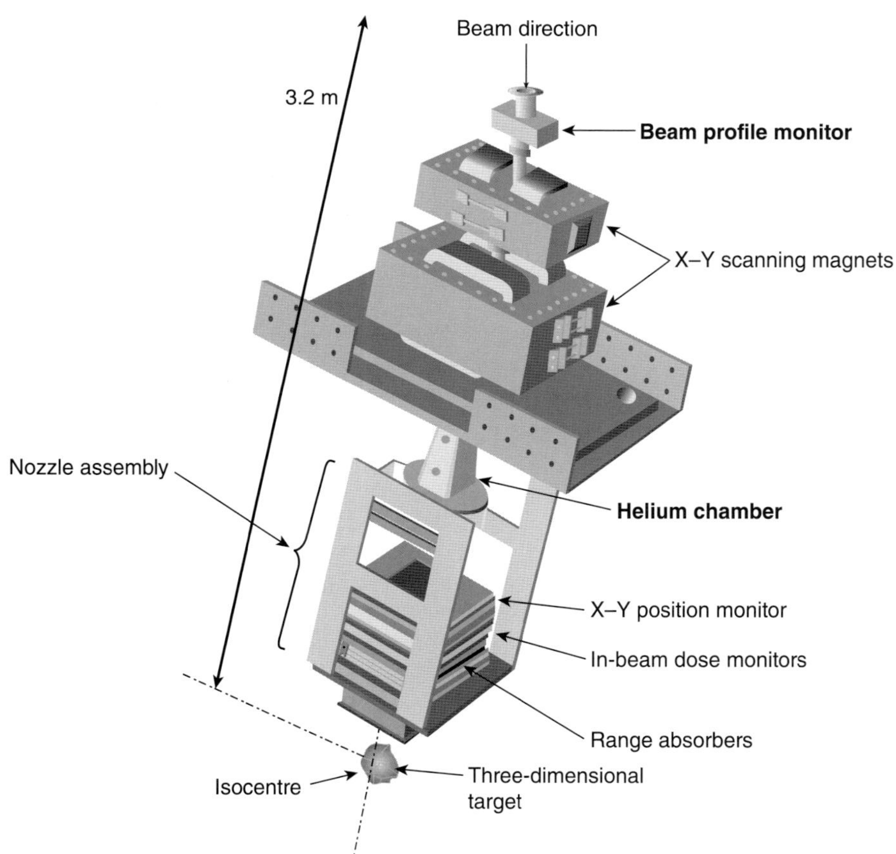

Fig. 10.28 The structure of a pencil beam scanning (PBS) system, similar to Hitachi.

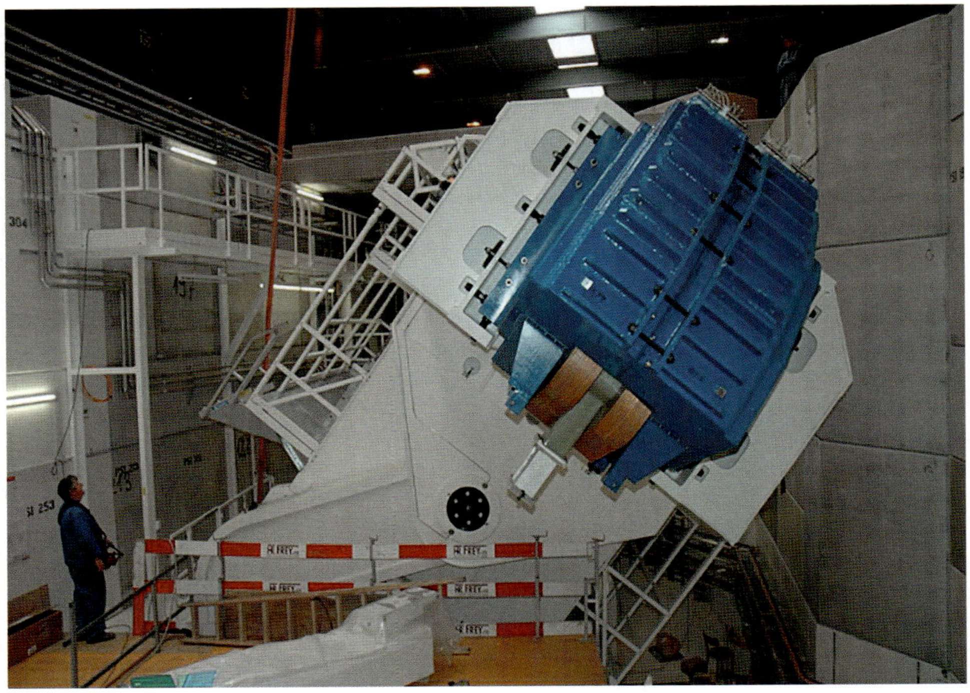

Fig. 10.29 PSI (gantry 2) compact isocentric design at commissioning, showing main bending dipole *(blue)* weighing approximately 40 tonnes. Note the scale; diameter of rotation is 7.5 m and total weight is 220 tonnes. The maximum treatment field at isocentre is approximately 12 × 20 cm. (Courtesy David Meer, PSI, Villigen, Switzerland.)

PROTON AND ION BEAM GANTRIES

The use of fully rotational gantries permits the optimisation of planning and delivery of treatments in conventional x-ray LINAC therapy. To fully exploit the advantage of proton and carbon therapy, most vendor systems provide rotational gantries (Fig. 10.29). However, these gantries require considerable mechanical and beam transport design. The weight of the focusing quadrupoles and bending dipoles and the shielding and beam monitoring devices leads to a total weight of more than 100 to 200 tonnes for a 250-MeV proton beam gantry. The beam rigidity required for a high-energy carbon therapy beam gantry is three times that of proton beams, which leads, for example, to the HIT carbon beam gantry components having a total weight of 600 tonnes.

Where compact PBT facilities are planned at existing hospital sites, the floor footprint is an important consideration for both the accelerator and the gantry system. Many vendor systems now offer reduced gantry rotation such as 270 degrees to 180 degrees for compactness. The MEVION FIT system furthers reduces the space requirement by only using a fixed beam with 6-D patient treatment chair. The rotational axis is necessarily large to obtain as near a parallel beam as possible. This was motivated by near-parallel beams presenting a much reduced surface dose than finite source beams which have their focal point downstream of the beam scanning dipole. Fig. 10.30 illustrates the PSI designed gantry (+180 degrees to −30 degrees), but the scanning X-Y magnets are situated upstream of the main bending dipole which necessarily has to have a large acceptance aperture.

TYPES OF PROTON AND ION ACCELERATORS

A simplified summary of the main features of circular accelerators used clinically and available commercially is given in Table 10.4. This does not include the beam transport or the treatment rooms. It is noted that the footprint is related to magnet size and field strength. A proton LINAC is included for comparison. Energy change and thus the depth of the beam for cyclotron and synchrocyclotrons is by use of hardware absorbers, while for the synchrotron and proton LINAC this is achieved by RF and magnet control.[24]

It has been proposed[25] that a linear accelerator using high-gradient (15–20 MV m^{-1}) 3-GHz LINAC technology is used for producing therapeutic range protons for image-guided hadron therapy (LIGHT). Considerable development has been undertaken by a spinoff company from the European Council for Nuclear Research (CERN). This consists of a low-energy proton source which passes protons into an RFQ device. This is a radial arrangement of four long vane electrodes which provide alternating RF electrostatic fields. The transverse fields provide focusing and the longitudinal fields acceleration. It bunches and accelerates the beam up to 5 MeV, and further acceleration with linear acceleration increases the energy to 38 MeV. Finally, acceleration to the therapeutically useful 180-to-230-MeV range is obtained by the addition of a cell coupled LINAC (CCL) with each cell providing 13 MeV. A maximum energy of 230 MeV would require a length of approximately 25 m. The 200-Hz pulse repetition rate is similar to existing radiotherapy x-ray LINACs and is very suitable for clinical spot scanning. A degree of energy selection is possible by altering the accelerating gradient of the cells. Further developments suggest variable control of beam intensity and proton energy between repetition pulses. The low beam divergence promises minimal beam losses, with shielding needed mainly for the treatment rooms. Testing has demonstrated beam energy of more than 200 MeV, and the Advanced Oncotherapy (AVO) consortium are developing a clinical therapy installation in an existing UK clinic coupled to a reduced-rotation gantry. Further advantages over circular accelerators include reductions in size, weight and space footprint.

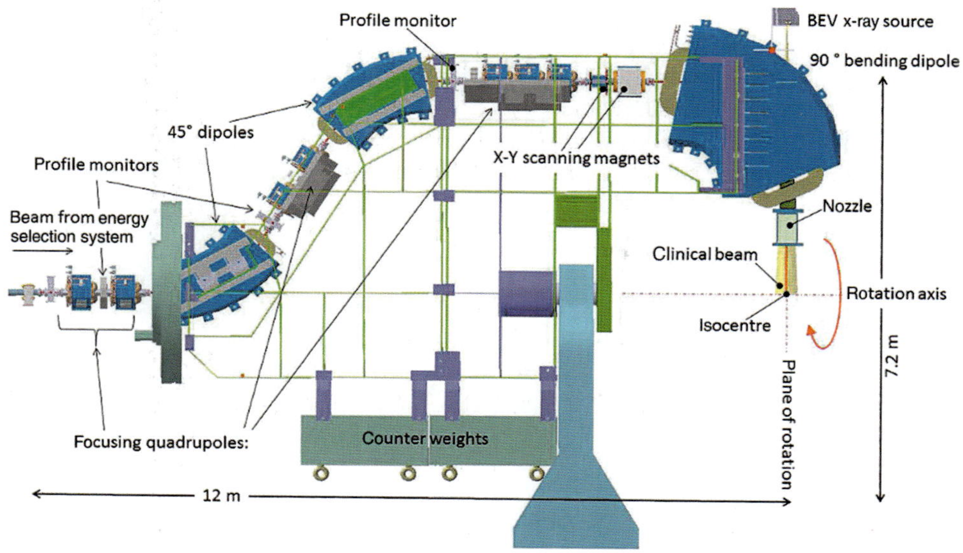

Fig. 10.30 Profile schematic view of the PSI gantry 2 with raster scanning capability. The nozzle can be extended to reduce the air gap from the exit window to the patient. This system features parallel scanning in x- and y-axes, with a fast energy degrader. (Courtesy E. Pedroni, PSI, Villigen, Switzerland.)

TABLE 10.4 Main Features of Circular Accelerators Used Clinically and Available Commercially

	TYPE OF ACCELERATOR			
Feature	**Cyclotron**	**Synchrocyclotron**	**Synchrotron**	**Proton LINAC**
Radiofrequency	Fixed	Variable	Variable	Variable
Magnetic field	Fixed	Fixed	Variable	–
Proton radius	Fixed	Variable	Fixed	–
Particle energy	Fixed	Fixed	Variable	Variable
Energy change	Manual	Manual	Electronic	Electronic
Particle current	High	Low	Low	Low
Beam waveform	Continuous	Pulsed	Pulsed	Pulsed
Footprint	Compact	Compact	Large	Compact

FLASH PROTON THERAPY, PROTON MINIBEAMS, PROTON ARC THERAPY AND MRI-GUIDED PROTON THERAPY

There are several technical developments in PBT being undertaken[26] to enable and explore the clinical benefits which may be attained from their use.

FLASH Proton Therapy

Ultrahigh dose rate (UHDR) therapy, also referred to as FLASH radiotherapy, has shown potential clinical benefit by reducing normal tissue toxicity while maintaining tumour control at curative dose levels. In vivo studies have demonstrated tissue sparing at dose rates of 40 Gy·s^{-1} and above. This modality is being adapted to proton therapy in addition to benefitting from three-dimensional dose conformity. Beam currents of about 500 nA are required to produce treatment doses in less than 1 second.[27] This dose rate is readily attainable with isochronous cyclotrons (see Table 10.4), requiring little hardware modification.[27] At present, pulsed beams from synchrocyclotrons and synchrotrons, with their low duty cycles and space charge limitations, would not achieve the FLASH dose-rate level. However, the Mevion 250i and IBA Proteus One synchrocyclotron dose rates have been increased to FLASH levels by optimising the ion source output and lengthening the pulse width to more than 20 μs, although the duty cycle remains unchanged.

FLASH irradiation with PBS spot scanning is challenging, as individual beamlets in a typical target volume would require beam currents two orders of magnitude greater than available on present systems,[27] particularly at shallower dose layers. Also, the energy changes of a typical ESS may be on the order of 1 second. These factors may make PBS FLASH rates difficult to achieve. Several alternatives have been proposed for clinical FLASH trials. First is the classical 'shoot-through' technique which has fixed high-energy protons with full-dose anterior and posterior to the target volume. Second is a version of the passive-scattering technique using a three-dimensional printed compensator or pin filters (Fig. 10.26) with a range shifter to produce the SOBP encompassing the target. However, the latter method would produce a variation of dose rates in the anterior healthy tissue. The shoot-through or transmission beam would deposit full dose anteriorly and posteriorly to the tumour volume. This technique was used at the Proton Therapy Center at Cincinnati Children's Hospital for the FAST-01 study of clinical palliative irradiations on extremities.[28] This has now progressed to the FAST-02 trial on chest wall metastases.

It remains unclear whether the FLASH sparing effect is sensitive to the irradiation time of the total average dose, dose fractions or individual beamlet dose rates. An alternative to increasing beam current in PBS

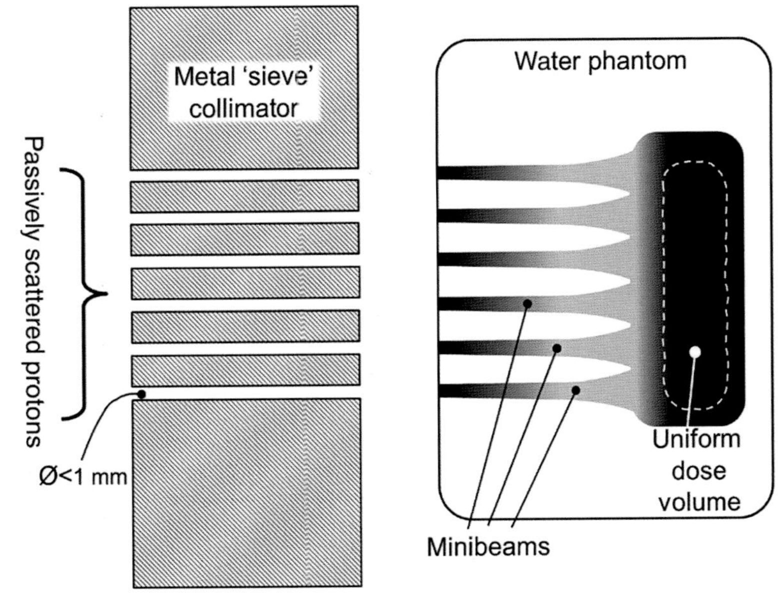

Fig. 10.31 Multihole beam collimation to produce minibeams which produce a uniform dose at depth.

mode is to use FLASH dose rates for small fields or for smaller fields within a larger treatment field in areas where OAR sparing is critical.

Minibeams in Proton Therapy

Minibeam proton therapy (MBPT) involves the use of multihole beam collimation or grid therapy, which may be termed *spatially modulated radiotherapy*. A matrix of submillimetric parallel beams is produced in a collimator, which creates peak-and-valley dose profiles. In vivo studies with electrons and x-rays have shown significantly increased dose tolerance in normal tissue while maintaining tumorcidal dose and increased cell survival. As yet, the biological mechanism is not fully understood, although the sparing effect is related to the size of the peak-to-valley ratio (PVR). In proton beams, the proximal dose profile is also characterised by sharp peaks and valleys. Multiple Coulomb scattering causes the minibeams to merge and provide a uniform dose in the tumour volume (Fig. 10.31), thus the principal advantage lies in proximal tissue sparing but with the possibility of higher treatment dose. Optimising the PVR is dependent on beam energy, hole diameter, spacing and the volume to be irradiated. However, the minibeams require a near parallel beam and sufficient dose rate, hence the technique is limited to smaller fields suitable for research beams.

PBS beams from vendor treatment nozzles offer another approach to MBPT, but this is challenging due to the required longer source to axis distance and beam broadening due to air scattering. However, developments in this approach are in progress and include reducing the beam diameter to the order of 1 mm and optimising the beam spacings.[29]

Proton Arc Therapy

Proton arc therapy (PAT) is analogous to VMAT x-ray treatments on LINAC machines for speed and complex treatment volumes. Some proton gantries (e.g. Varian, Mevion) have been modified to examine the clinical advantages of PAT over IMPT.

Planning studies by Carabe-Fernandez et al.[30] have suggested that there is little difference in terms of dose conformity between PAT and IMPT but that PAT reduces integral dose and improves planning robustness and speed. The greater angular flexibility available with PAT may reduce variations of the RBE of treatment fractions and smooth the effect of range and SOBP uncertainties. Fast energy switching and gantry rotation are a requisite for rapid treatment delivery and the reduction of arcs. PAT offers the interesting possibility of reduced range to place the higher LET portion of the SOBP in the target volume rather than in the distal falloff, thereby increasing the biological effectiveness of the tumour dose.

MRI-Guided Proton Therapy

The advances in image-guided radiotherapy with MRI LINACs have significantly improved radiotherapy treatment quality. This has prompted developments in the utilisation of MRI guidance in proton therapy (MRIgPT) where the capability of monitoring and adapting treatments 'in-beam' is of especial interest when targeting soft tissues of the tumour and OARs.[31] Organs which are subject to interfractional changes and intrafractional movement would reduce the advantage of the sharp conformal dose gradients of proton beams. Studies have focused on the magnetic field interactions between proton beams, particularly with PBS systems, and the MR imaging system. The effects of PBS scanning magnets and MRI fields on image quality and beam distortion, respectively, need detailed examination. As MRI images contain no electron density information for stopping power estimation, this requires conversion to 'pseudo' CT-HU numbers before use in proton treatment planning. A nonclinical prototype MRIgPT system, using a fixed horizontal beamline, at Dresden-Rossendorf (HZDR) in Germany is being used to investigate these challenges and confirm the potential of MRIgPT in improving proton treatment.

CLINICAL PROTON THERAPY CENTRES

The proton therapy systems that are being built by commercial vendors are listed in Table 10.5. These consist of a single accelerator feeding beams into multiple treatment rooms with either gantries, fixed beamlines or a combination of both. The beam control systems are required to switch rapidly from one room to another as soon as patient setup has been achieved. The larger purpose-built proton therapy centres are designed for higher patient throughput and specialist treatments (e.g. paediatric tumours) using multiple treatment rooms with gantries or fixed beams. Although the proton gantries are up to three stories in diameter, the patient treatment room appears quite small. The matching of treatment beam characteristics between rooms is required to achieve optimum treatment flexibility.

TABLE 10.5 **Comparison of Commercial Proton Beam Treatment Centres With Multiroom and Gantry Systems**

Vendor	Machine	Type	Weight	Max Energy Range	Dose Rate or Max Current	Room Switching Time (s)	Field Size (cm)	Beam Delivery Options
IBA	Proteus PLUS, C230	Isochronous cyclotron	220 T; 4.3 m	230 MeV	2 Gy/min	20	30 × 40	Pencil beam, scattered
Varian, now Siemens	ProBeam	Superconducting (NbTi); isochronous cyclotron	90 T; 3.1 m	250 MeV	800 nA	<30	30 × 40	Pencil beam
Hitachi	ProBeat-V (footprint = 42.5 m^2)	Synchrotron (slow extraction)	25-m diameter	70–230 MeV	Approx. 1.5 Gy/L/min	<0.45	30 × 30	Spot scanning
Proton International	Radiance 330	Synchrotron	16 T; 4.8-m diameter	330 MeV imaging; therapy (70–250 MeV)	2 GyL/min	<1.2	30 × 40	Pencil scanning only

Additionally, the majority of new treatment rooms now offer spot or raster scanning for optimal three-dimensional radiation conformity. Fast, in-room CT scan verification and precise positioning by six-dimensional robotic couches further underpin accurate beam volume delivery, with treatment setup and irradiation times similar to conventional x-ray therapy.

With the wider acceptance of PBT, and allied with technical developments particularly in smaller, superconducting magnets, vendors offer more compact accelerators or 'single-room' solutions, as shown in Table 10.2. As can be inferred, these systems have footprints considerably larger than LINAC rooms areas, which are approximately 30 to 50 m^2. However, these are considered sufficiently small to be installed in or adjacent to existing cancer hospitals. In 2022 the Mevion 250-FIT offered a gantry-less configuration with a reduced footprint of 47 m^2, suitable for a single LINAC bunker. This was achieved by a compact synchrocyclotron, with a short beamline to the treatment nozzle. The patients are treated in an upright or inclined chair with six-dimensional movement and dual-energy vertical CT imaging for image guidance. A study at *Massachusetts General Hospital* (MGH) has shown that a significant percentage of patient treatments may not require the flexibility of gantry beams, which implies considerable cost-saving benefits.

There is a continued requirement for proton energies in the 60-to-75-MeV range to treat rare intraocular tumours, with annual treatment numbers increasing from 1650 in 2015 to 2000 in 2022. Ocular treatments constituted 7% of total proton referrals in 2022. The first ocular proton therapy was performed in 1975 at the Harvard Cyclotron Laboratory (HCL) in Cambridge, Massachusetts, followed by European centres. The beam quality produced with accelerators which have little or no energy degradation exhibits highly conformal falloff and penumbrae characteristics.[12] They are well adapted to such small field treatments which require submillimetric precision. In 2025, 22 centres reported ocular treatments, with the majority using chair patient positioning and head restraint and with the patient's gaze angle optimised for a particular treatment. Two eye treatment centres have been adapted from high-energy neutron therapy, such as at Clatterbridge and Nice. Also, there were adaptions from research machines at Berlin, Catania, San Francisco and Krakow. The others have degraded high-energy beamlines, either shared or dedicated. Four centres (3 in the USA and one in Austria) have developed eye treatment attachments onto the nozzles of high-energy gantries with couch patient positioning. The beam characteristics, although adequate, do not achieve those of low-energy beams.

CLINICAL CARBON ION THERAPY CENTRES

Synchrotrons, which are designed specifically for proton beams, have diameters of 6 to 8 m, while synchrotrons for carbon beam therapy are at present 22 to 25 m. This was necessary to achieve what is referred to as the *high magnetic rigidity* of the carbon beams used clinically. Table 10.6 describes the basic information on carbon therapy facilities which are currently treating patients. For the present, their size and cost render them to be clinical research facilities rather than routine radiotherapy centres. They are suitable for clinical trials, studying the effects of highly conformal isodose and elevated RBE on radiation-resistant tumours. Included in Table 10.6 are three of the earlier Japanese facilities which represent the world's largest clinical experience, having treated half of the 57,500 carbon beam patients by end of 2023.[32]

It is to be noted that recent developments in superconducting magnets to counter the high magnetic rigidity of carbon beams have enabled the adoption of compact gantries for carbon beams offering stronger bending fields at three of the European centres. All the European centres have adopted either raster beam or spot scanning to optimise three-dimensional dose conformity and minimise extraneous secondary radiation from the treatment nozzles. It is noted that the Heavy Ion Medical Accelerator Centre (HIMAC) in Japan has added both three-dimensional spot scanning and a compact gantry to their facility. The latter weighs 200 tonnes compared with the 600 tonnes of the HIT gantry mentioned earlier in this chapter. The design of the HIT facility emerged from a collaboration of GSI-Darmstadt and Siemens Medical, while the National Centre of Oncological Hadrontherapy (CNAO) in Italy and MedAustron designs were based on a proton-ion medical machine study (PIMMS) initiated at CERN.[33] This offered the advantage of a smaller surface area with the ion injectors and drift-tube LINAC situated within the synchrotron ring.[34] While present facilities are solely based on synchrotron acceleration, an isochronous superconducting cyclotron–based C-400 design is proposed by IBA and would be capable of accelerating protons to 250 MeV and carbon ions to 400 MeV/u. While heavy at 700 tonnes, it has a diameter of only 6.6 m and a height of 3.4 m. The design incorporates ion injectors beneath the cyclotron.

NEUTRON AND OTHER BEAMS

Fast Neutron Beam Therapy

In the 1970s and 1980s, there was great interest in using collimated neutron beams for treating radiation-resistant solid tumours. Due to the high LET of neutrons and decreased dependence on the oxygen enhancement

TABLE 10.6 Comparison of Carbon Ion Centres

Centre	Country	Type of Accelerator (diameter)	Max Carbon Beam Energy (proton energy)	Particle Types	Field Size (cm^2), Scanning Mode	Treatment Rooms	Year of Clinical Start
HIT, Heidelberg	Germany	Synchrotron (20 m)	88–430/u (221 MeV)	C (p, He, O)	20 × 20, raster scanning	1 gantry; 2 H beams	2009
CNAO, Pavia	Italy	Synchrotron (25 m)	120–400/u (60–220 MeV)	C (p, He)	20 × 20; spot scanning	1 H + V; 2 H beams	2011
MIT, Marburg	Germany	Synchrotron (21 m)	430/u (221 MeV)	C (p)	20 × 20, raster scanning	4 fixed beams (3 × H; 1 × 45)	2015 (recommissioned)
MedAustron	Austria	Synchrotron (25 m)	400 MeV/u (60–250 MeV)	C (p)	Quasidiscrete spot scanning raster	2 fixed beam (1V + 1H); 1 gantry (p)	2017
HIMAC (NIRS), Chiba	Japan	Synchrotron (2 rings) (41 m)	100–800 MeV/u	C (He)	22 × 22; 3D scanning (in 2012); broad beam	1 × h; 1 × V; 1 × V + H beams. Gantry in 2016	1994
HIBMC, Hyogo	Japan	Synchrotron (30 m)	70–320/u (190 MeV)	C (p, He)	15 × 15; wobbler + filter	3 + H; 1 × V and 45 degrees; 2 p gantries	2001
GHMC, Guma	Japan	Synchrotron (22 m)	400 MeV/u	C	15 × 15; wobbler + filter	3 rooms (H, H + V, V)	2010

3D, Three-dimensional.

ratio (OER), these beams were able to deliver highly effective clinical doses with an RBE of approximately 3.0. Neutron beams were shown to be highly penetrating in tissue, depositing dose mainly by collisions with tissue hydrogen which produce low energy but highly ionising 'knock-on' protons. Most clinical neutron beams were produced through proton or deuteron bombardment of beryllium, or sometimes lithium, targets. These accelerators could produce the large proton currents of 30 to 50 μA required for delivering clinical neutron doses of 2 Gy/min. These beams were achieved with cyclotrons, although at the Fermilab in Chicago, a 66-MeV proton LINAC was used. It should be noted that neutron beams required significant developments in collimation which usually consisted of steel, tungsten and high-density polythene and weighed up to 1 tonne. Earlier machines such as deuterium-tritium (D-T) generators had limited neutron penetration in tissue. Later versions were designed with higher acceleration energies to produce fast neutron penetration characteristics similar to 6- and 8-MV x-ray LINACs. In addition, facilities with isocentric gantries, improved collimation, wedges, blocks and couch rotations enabled comparative studies and randomised trials between neutrons and x-rays to be performed. The initial promise was not fulfilled mainly due to increased normal tissue toxicity. This was related to uncertainties in RBE, difficulties in neutron collimation and dilution of the RBE by a significant gamma-ray beam component. Results from parotid and air sinus lesions showed some benefit, but this benefit may now have been eclipsed by highly conformal x-ray therapies. There are now few active centres offering fast neutron therapy. It should be noted that the first gantry-mounted and super-conducting cyclotron was developed by H Blosser for the Wayne State University Medical Center (Detroit, MI) and commenced operation in 1991. This produced neutrons by the d(48.5) + Be reaction; it weighed only 25 tonnes, with a 360-degree gantry, and offered multirod collimation as well as blocks for improved dose conformity. The experience gained with this compact superconducting cyclotron on a gantry mounting eventually led to the development of the Mevion proton therapy configuration and the single-room proton therapy concept.

Helium Beam Radiotherapy

In 1952, alpha particle beams were the first positive ions to be used clinically at the LBL at Berkeley, although they were superseded by the wider availability of proton beams. Helium ions are heavier than protons, thus scatter less and have sharper fall-off. The RBE of helium beams is greater than for protons but less than for carbon beams. However, helium ions have much reduced fragmentation particles beyond the Bragg peak. Some synchrotron-based ion therapy centres are considering using helium beams in addition to carbon and protons, and have been used clinically at HIT (Germany) in 2021.[35]

Boron Neutron Capture Therapy

Boron neutron capture therapy (BNCT) involves the labelling of a tumour-seeking compound with target nuclei followed by slow neutron irradiation. It is a twofold form of radiotherapy based first on the administration of a boron-10 (^{10}B)–labelled compound such as boronophenylalanine (*BPA*) and sodium borocaptate (*BSH*). The compound concentrates on or in tumour cells. This tumour volume is then irradiated with a low-energy neutron beam. The nuclear reaction which occurs for thermal energy neutrons of typically 0.0025 eV has a high probability of 94% and excites ^{10}B to ^{11}B. The excited atom then disintegrates into lithium-7 (^{7}Li), an alpha particle (^{4}He) and a 478-keV gamma ray. As seen in Fig. 10.32, the particles have a high LET compared with gamma rays and so produce highly ionising short-range tracks of 5 to 9 μm, respectively, and would wholly or partially traverse the width of a tumour cell.[36]

Fig. 10.33 shows a schematic view of a clinical irradiation using epithermal neutron beams from a nuclear reactor. The efficacy of BNCT

$$n(\text{thermal}) + {}^{10}B \rightarrow {}^{4}He + {}^{7}Li + \gamma\text{-ray}$$

	Energy	LET	Range
^{7}Li	840 keV;	175 keV/μm	5 μm
^{4}He	1470 keV	150 keV/μm	9 um
γ-ray	478 keV	~1 keV/μm	-----

Fig. 10.32 Nuclear process and physical data of boron neutron capture therapy.

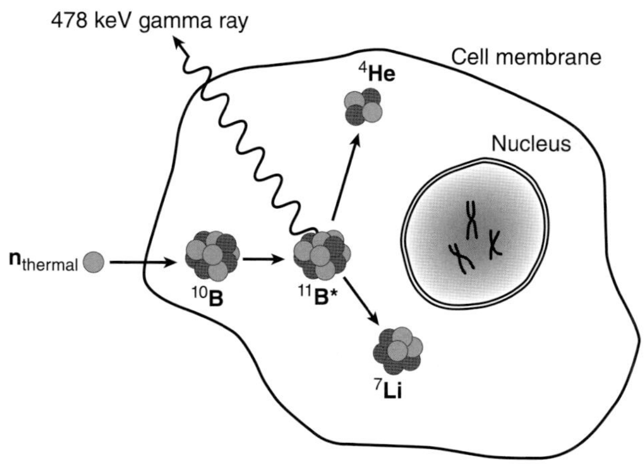

Fig. 10.33 Schematic of boron neutron capture therapy.

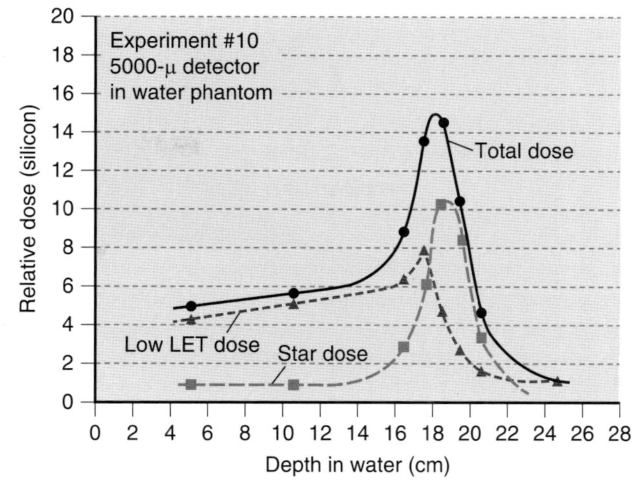

Fig. 10.34 Pion beam starburst phenomenon, enhancing the low linear energy transfer (LET) dose with that of the short-range high-LET particles. (Courtesy A Smith, M Kligerman [LAMPF, NM USA].)

is still being tested by clinical research centres. Due to the decrease in availability of reactor neutron beams, developments of BNCT are directed towards low-energy proton cyclotrons producing mA current proton beams,[37] RFQ LINACs or electrostatic accelerators. The protons bombard Be or Li targets to produce an epithermal neutron beam. All the tissue traversed in the body, including the target volume, acts as a moderator which slows the epithermal neutron beam to the important thermal neutron energies. The thermal neutron uniformity is further optimised by reflecting materials of Al or Bi. In 2023, there were 22 BNCT centres worldwide that were active or being commissioned. Seven were situated in Japan, where this technique was approved for treatments involving unresectable locally advanced tumours.[38]

Proton Boron Capture Therapy

Recent work has suggested that boron capture of low-energy protons[39] may amplify the dose released at the Bragg peak and form a dose enhancement. This proton boron capture therapy (pBCT) is also described as a proton-boron fusion reaction, as it resembles a nuclear fusion reaction with the proton being absorbed. However, as in BNCT, the therapeutic effect is dependent on the boron compound uptake in tumour cells compared with healthy tissue.

The phenomenon is described by the following reaction:

$$\text{proton} + {}^{11}\text{B (80\% abundance)} \rightarrow {}^{12}\text{C} \rightarrow 3 \text{ alphas} ({}^{4}\text{He}) (\sim 4\,\text{MeV})$$

The dose enhancement is achieved at the Bragg peak by the release of three short-range, highly ionising alpha particles and by the greater (80%) abundance of the ^{11}B isotope. The ranges of the 2-to-3 MeV alphas are about 30 μm and with high probability of traversing the cell nucleus.[39] This proposal would combine the physical advantages of low-LET proton therapy with the biological enhancement of localised high-LET particles. Like BNCT, the decay of the immediate carbon nucleus produces a 719 keV gamma ray, which offers the potential of real-time monitoring and range verification with gamma camera imaging. Unlike BNCT, this technique would be a dose enhancement to conventional low-LET proton therapy, without needing a source of thermal neutrons.

Pion Therapy

This accelerator-based therapy involved creating negative pi-meson (pion) beams by bombarding proton beams onto low-Z target nucleons. This produces pions, with mass 278 times that of an electron. These charged particles produce increasing ionisation along their path length, culminating in a 'broad' Bragg peak at the end of their range. At the end of the range, the pion is captured by an oxygen or carbon nucleus, causing disintegration of the nucleus into short-range high-LET particles such as protons, alphas, deuterons, neutrons and electrons. This is the starburst phenomenon which enhances the dose delivered by the pions alone. The combined total dose from a pion beam is shown in Fig. 10.34. In the 1970s pion treatment was considered of interest in treating radiation-resistant tumours. Clinically useful pion beams require the bombardment of beryllium (Be) or carbon targets with high currents (0.1–1 mA) of high-energy protons in the 500-to-800 MeV range. This produces pion beams with penetration from 22 to 31 cm. The short lifetime of pions (2.5×10^{-8} sec) necessitates short beamlines on the order of 10 m, with collimation and focusing magnets. Generally, clinical pion beams used programmable-movement patient couches to enable the fixed beam to cover the required treatment area. The Piotron at PSI used the channelling of 60 radial pion beams into a cross-sectional slice with axial patient couch movement to irradiate a three-dimensional treatment volume.

There have been three clinical pion programs, as shown in Table 10.7. The majority of treated indications were in the brain, mainly

TABLE 10.7 Pion Treatment Centres

Institute (country)	Accelerator Type	Years of Operation	Proton Beam Energy MeV and Beam Current	Clinical Pion Beam Arrangement	No. of Patients Treated
LAMPF (USA)	Linear accelerator	1974–1981	800 (1 mA)	Vertical beam	230
PSI/SIN (Switzerland)	Isochronous ring synchrotron	1980–1993	590 (100 μA)	Horizontal with 3D scanning (Piotron)	503
TRIUMF (Canada)	Large-pole (50′) diameter cyclotron, negative ion	1979–1994	500 (100 μA)	Horizontal beam, scanning couch	367

3D, Three-dimensional.

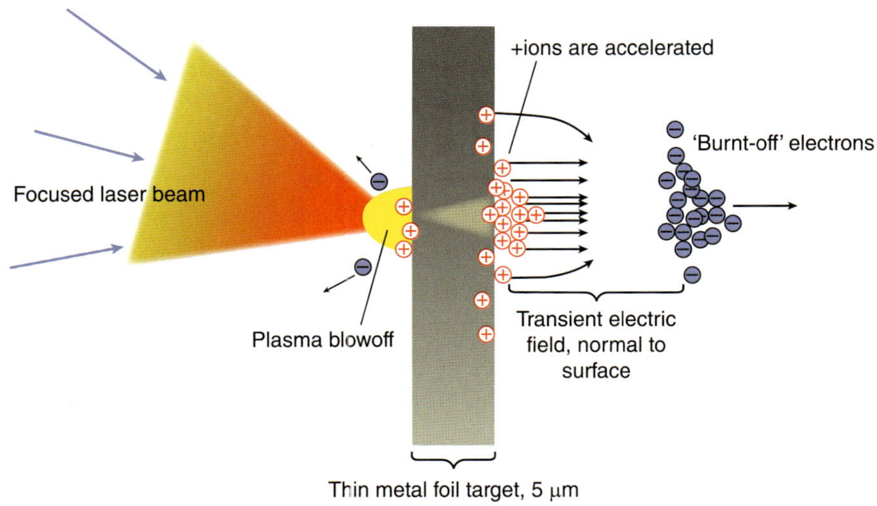

Fig. 10.35 The process to produce particle fluence using very short-pulse, high-intensity laser light.

glioblastomas, and also prostate cancers. Although the high-LET component in the starburst was attractive clinically, spreading this depth dose over larger volumes diluted the biological effectiveness of the starburst. Much of this was due to dispersion of neutron energy from the starburst peak. In addition, the pion beams had significant contamination with muons and electrons. The effective RBE was estimated to be 1.1 to 1.5. Although much was learnt from biological and physical dose treatment planning, normal tissue response and precise beam delivery, the clinical results were considered to show no significant benefit compared with x-ray therapy. The power and size requirements of pion-producing accelerators would have prohibited their development in a hospital environment. For example, the TRIUMF cyclotron required 18 kA (kiloamperes) for supply magnet currents, with a weight of 4000 tonnes.

Antiproton Therapy Beams

The potential use of antiprotons has been studied by the CERN consortium.[40] Antiprotons are known to have slightly greater range than protons with double the dose at the Bragg peak. The latter is caused by the annihilation of the slowing antiproton with a nucleon where a rest mass energy of 1.8 GeV is released by pions and about 20% of these are absorbed by the nucleus. This leads to nuclear fragmentation and the release of short-range and highly ionising particles. This is reflected in an increased relative biological effect (RBE) of up to 2.0. However, as with pion therapy, the biological effectiveness may be diluted by modulating the antiproton energy and by the accompanying whole-body dose from neutrons and pions. The penumbrae have been shown to be poorer than protons at depth, and the mixed-field dosimetry is complex. The requirement of a very high-energy accelerator, as well as sufficient antiproton fluence, limits this technique to a few international research laboratories. The emission of energetic pions during therapy offers real-time monitoring of the annihilation peak position, and hence of the treatment range.

Laser-Driven Proton and Particle Beams

The use of very high-intensity laser beams, in the peta-watt range (10^{15} W), to produce particle fluence has important attractions, and recent progress[41–43] has demonstrated therapy level doses in conventional treatment times. The protons are produced by extremely short, intense pulses of laser light incident on a small area of thin metallic foil. This impact creates a localised plasma where the faster accelerated electrons will almost instantaneously create extremely high electric fields, on the order of 10^{12} V.m^{-1}, when leaving the back of the target material. Protons and other positive ions emerging from the foil will be accelerated by this electric field, normal to the surface of the foil, to energies of tens of MeV. This process is illustrated in Fig. 10.35. Intensities of at least 10^{19} W.cm^{-2} are required in the laser pulse. Measurement results have produced a maximum cutoff energy of up to 80 MeV, albeit with a quasiexponential distribution in the proton spectrum. The inhomogeneous transverse field results in a distribution of proton energies with the maximum proton energy related to the square of the laser beam intensity. Also, significant quantities of other contaminant ion particles are produced. Reduction of the target area and use of cryohydrogen jet targets have been shown to improve beam intensity, increase proton energy and narrow the energy spectrum of the protons with significantly fewer ion and debris contaminants, compared with metal target foil.[44]

The application to proton and ion therapy lies in the possibility of very compact layout and infrastructure. A single power laser would be used to distribute light beams by optics to treatment gantries, where the planned beam intensity and energy would be produced. This would eliminate the beam transport, steering magnets, beam monitoring and vacuum systems, as well as reducing stray neutron production and shielding. This will be dependent on reducing the cost and size of lasers as well as increasing both the laser pulse rate and power intensity to peta-watt levels. Improvements in energy selectivity and spatially narrow beams make laser-driven proton beams well suited for the spot-scanning technique, as well as providing FLASH therapy dose rates.

SHIELDING OF PROTON THERAPY ACCELERATORS AND TREATMENT ROOMS

Many of the design criteria in reducing scattered radiation in high-energy linear accelerators are also applicable to proton therapy accelerators and their treatment rooms. More detailed considerations are given in reference handbooks.[5,44,45]

One significant difference is that, with the exception of the MEVION single-room facility (Table 10.2), all proton therapy centres have separate bunkers for the accelerator with long beamlines and associated diagnostic equipment directing the beam into different treatment rooms when required. The principal radiological concern is secondary neutron dose rates produced by the scattering of the proton beam in the accelerator, beamline diagnostics and treatment head. Higher-energy neutrons are rapidly reduced in energy by high-Z elements such as iron, then further moderated by low-Z elements such as the water content in concrete, and then finally absorbed by doping elements such as B or Li, if required.

As in other radiation treatment facilities, the building shielding design is dominated by staff or public usage of adjacent areas. Space limitations will determine the nature and economic cost of the planned shielding. For example, earth fill would be more economical than doped concrete, while Pb-backed boron-doped polythene composite material would represent significant space savings but at an increased cost.

Activation of air by primary proton beam and secondary neutron fluences produces short-lived positron-emitting isotopes such as ^{11}C, ^{13}N and ^{15}O. Their half-lives are 20.3, 10 and 2 minutes, respectively, and the activity produced will depend largely on field size and whether scanning or passive-scattered mode is employed. However, the short-lived nature of these isotopes and adequate ventilation in the treatment room should minimise any radiological concern, although longer-lived isotopes such as argon (^{41}Ar), with a half-life of 1.8 hours and produced by scattered neutrons, should be considered.

Activation of the concrete shielding by secondary neutrons will demand the most consideration around the accelerator and beamlines, due to longer running times and beamline losses. Most radioisotopes produced in normal high-density concrete will be short-lived. However, other additive or trace elements may produce radioisotopes of, for example, Co, Ba (barytes concrete) and Eu, some of which have much longer-lived isotopes.

NANOPARTICLE-ENHANCED THERAPY

The use of high-Z nanoparticles (NP) as radiosensitisers has been shown to enhance the dose effect in both in vitro and in vivo studies with x-ray therapy. The effectiveness with x-ray beams is due to interaction with the high-Z atom and the subsequent creation of low-energy secondary electrons. The enhancement is highest for x-ray photons in comparative studies using different ionising radiations. The modelling of gold nanoparticles[46] and in vivo studies with protons have shown some degree of radio enhancement in clinical SOBP proton beams, depending on the size and quantity of NP absorbed internally through the cell wall. Although the radiosensitisation mechanism of high-Z NPs is not fully understood, it has been shown that the secondary electron spectrum from protons is of considerably lower energy than that induced by x-rays, meaning that for protons, high-Z NPs need to have penetrated into the cytoplasm to achieve dose enhancement.

RECORD AND VERIFY SYSTEMS

For the machine operators who deliver the treatment, setting up the patient and the machine for the treatment has involved checks being made as independently as possible before treatment is delivered. The increasing complexity of machines and treatments and the introduction of quality systems which require the process to be traceable have made automatic verification of the treatment setup essential. With the availability of fast computing systems, record and verify systems (RVSs) have been developed to fulfil this role automatically. Essentially, the RVS consists of three distinct components: storage, check and record. The patient prescription is stored, a check is made that the machine parameters at treatment match the prescription and a record is built up of the treatment delivered. The structure of such a system is illustrated in Fig. 10.36.

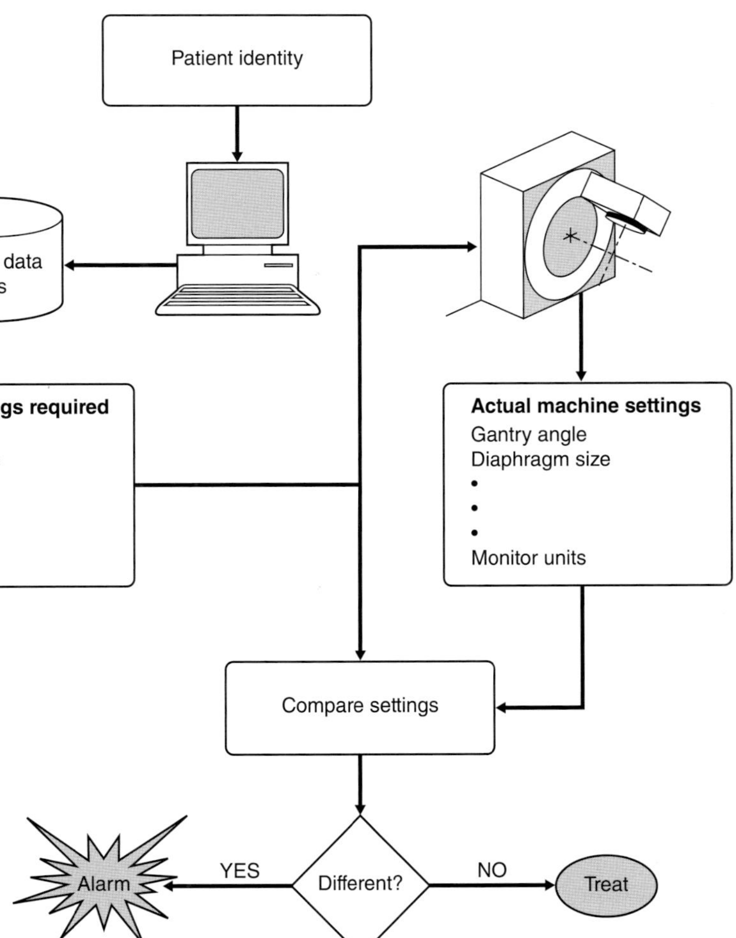

Fig. 10.36 Structure of record and verify system.

For each patient, a treatment parameters file is held and the parameters are downloaded from the RVS to the treatment machine at each occasion of treatment. The machine is then set up for treatment of the patient by the operators, and the RVS compares the settings on the machine with the values stored in the system file. Any differences must be resolved by the operators before treatment can commence. This will normally be done by adjustment of the patient and machine setup to bring it in line with the treatment parameters. However, in exceptional circumstances, parameters can be overridden subject to appropriate checking and supervision. The patient's file is also used to record the dose delivered to the patient on each treatment to maintain an accumulated record of the treatment dose to the patient.

Although these systems provide an invaluable aid to treatment delivery, it should be kept in mind that such systems can fail. As with any computerised data transfer process, acceptance checks and routine checks are required to verify that systems assign the data correctly to a patient's treatment.

FUTURE DESIGN OF PROTON AND ION BEAM MACHINES

It has been shown that much expertise from nuclear physics and engineering has been directed to the commercial provision of particle accelerators, particularly for proton beams. Clinical proton accelerators are required to have reliability or uptime at least equal to that of modern x-ray LINACs. This is due in part to the extended treatment hours necessitated by the capital outlay and expected patient throughput, and as accelerators are unique at a clinical facility, they represent a single point of failure as patients cannot be easily transferred to another proton facility. Any gantry or nozzle downtime at multigantry facilities can be mitigated by redirecting patients to neighbouring gantries. Single-room proton facilities are intended to operate within radiotherapy departments, or in some cases may be planned to operate as a suite of single-room treatment rooms as proposed by the Mevion configuration. Equally, the siting of proton beam therapy in larger radiotherapy centres has the advantage of transferring treatments to x-ray LINACs if required.

The ability of ion accelerators to deliver prescribed dose and conformal fields reliably and in conventional treatment times has been described. Future developments in proton or heavier charged particle accelerators and their advance into tertiary radiotherapy centres will depend on several factors:

- The accumulation of long-term follow-up patient data.
- The increase of treatment sites, following patient trials in which clinical indications show advantage compared with advanced x-ray treatments.
- Reduced fractionation.
- Reduction in the capital costs and footprint sizes of accelerators and single-room facilities, lower-beam energies and adoption of gantry-less treatments.
- Optimising the advantages of proton and ion dose conformality by improved precision of beam delivery, including proton end of range.
- Improved precision regarding the end of range. This needs improved accuracy of proton treatment planning by precise determination of proton stopping powers when converting from x-ray CT-HU data or from direct patient-specific CT obtained from proton tomography using high-energy (>300 MeV) protons. It also requires in vivo monitoring of proton end of range by measurement in two or three dimensions of gamma rays induced by protons, either high-energy inelastic scattered photons or positron emissions.
- Beam gating and dose repainting to reduce effects of patient, organ and target movement.

CONCLUSION

The x-ray and electron beam medical LINAC has become very well established and reached a very consistent level of performance. Although 20 years ago individual machines could vary, even from the same manufacturer, they can now have identical beam characteristics and are interchangeable as machines. The availability of these machines is high and widespread, with satellite treatment centres made easier because of the high reliability of the equipment. Beam shaping with high-resolution MLC, VMAT, FFF beams and SABR has taken megavoltage x-ray machine treatment delivery to a very sophisticated level. The inclusion of onboard imaging with MV treatment beam imaging, kV cone beam and MRI has meant that treatment accuracy and reproducibility have been enhanced. These MV imaging systems have also enabled the development of onboard MLC calibration systems, routine quality control systems and transit dosimetry. This has improved the efficacy of machine maintenance and monitoring of machine performance. Transit dosimetry has provided the means for rapid treatment verification of dose delivered.

The worldwide advent of heavy charged particle therapy in hospital or clinical research facilities in the past two decades has confirmed its place in mainstream radiotherapy for certain clinical indications. The commercially available facilities have achieved:

- Automated and stable operation
- High availability of at least 98%
- Low-maintenance designs, with long-term service contracts
- Lower power requirements
- Smaller-sized accelerators with smaller treatment room 'footprints' becoming available

Modern proton beam therapy facilities are now expected to have the same reliability as modern radiotherapy x-ray linear accelerators. This is a necessity to service the expected large patient throughputs for PBT. The latter will be driven by the experience of the growing number of proton and carbon therapy centres. The larger PBT centres in particular will rapidly accumulate clinical evidence from trials and follow-up data. The commercially available smaller, one-room PBT facilities are to be considered an addition to existing large radiotherapy departments, while developments in circular accelerator-based machines are directed at smaller weight, size and reliability, particularly with the adoption of superconducting main coils. The main developments in alternative accelerator technology in the next decade are LINAC-based proton beams and possibly laser-driven proton sources. Progress in further PBT machine development remains predicated on increasing patient throughput and proven clinical indications.

REFERENCES

1. Thwaites DI, Tuohy JB. Back to the future: the history and development of the clinical linear accelerator. *Phys Med Biol.* 2006;51:R343–R362.
2. Karzmark CJ, Morton RJ. *A primer on theory and operation of linear accelerators in radiation therapy*. 2nd ed. Madison, WI: Medical Physics Publishing; 1998.
3. Council of the European Union. Council Directive 97/43/Euratom of 30 June 1997 on health protection of individuals against the dangers of ionizing radiation in relation to medical exposure, and repealing Directive 84/466/Euratom. *OJ L.* 1997;180:22. http://data.europa.eu/eli/dir/1997/43/oj.
4. UK Statutory Instruments. The Ionising radiations regulations 2017. Statutory instrument 1999 No. 3232. UK: HMSO: 2017.

5. Stedeford B, Morgan HM, Mayles WPM. The design of radiotherapy treatment room facilities. York: IPEM; 1997.
6. Horton P, Eaton D. *Design and shielding of radiotherapy treatment facilities*. Bristol: IOP Publishing Limited, 2017:2053–2563. https://doi.org/10.1088/978-0-7503-1440-4
7. Paganetti H, ed. *Proton Therapy Physics*, 2nd ed. Boca Raton FL, USA: CRC Press; 2018. https://doi.org/10.1201/b22053
8. Smith A. Proton therapy. *Phys Med Biol*. 2006;51:R491–R504.
9. Flanz J, Smith A. Technology for proton therapy. *Cancer J*. 2009; 15(4):292–297.
10. Coutrakon G. Accelerators for heavy-charged-particle radiation therapy. *Technol Cancer Res Treat*. 2007;6(4 suppl):49–54.
11. Gragoudas ES. Proton beam irradiation of uveal melanomas: the first 30 years. The Weisenfeld Lecture. *Invest Ophthalmol Vis Sci*. 2006;47(11):4666–4673. https://doi.org/10.1167/iovs.06-0659.
12. Kacperek A. Ocular proton therapy centers. editor. In: Linz U, ed. Berlin, Heidelberg: Springer; 2012. *Ion Beam Therapy. Biological and Medical Physics, Biomedical Engineering*. 320. https://doi.org/10.1007/ 978-3-642-21414-1_10.
13. Baird D, Faust T. Scientific instruments, scientific progress and the cyclotron. *Brit J Philos Sci*. 1990;41(2):147–175.
14. Muramatsu M, Kitagawa A. A review of ion sources for medical accelerators (invited). *Rev Sci Instrum*. 2012;83(2):02B909. https://doi.org/10.1063/1.3671744.
15. Kleeven W. *Injection and extraction for cyclotrons. CERN Accelerator School (CAS) – small accelerators, zeegse, The Netherlands, 24 May–2 June 2005; proceedings CERN-2006-012.* Zeegse, NL: CAS - CERN Accelerator School; 2006:271–296. http://doi.org/10.5170/CERN-2006-012.271.
16. Owen H, Lomax A, Jolly S. Current and future accelerator technologies for charged particle therapy. *Nucl Instrum Methods Phys Res A*. 2016;809:96–104.
17. Owen H, Holder D, Alonso J, MacKay R. Technologies for delivery of proton and ion beams for radiotherapy. *Int J Modern Physics*. 2014;A29:1441002.
18. Schippers M. Proceedings of the CERN accelerator school 'accelerators for medical applications', CERN-2017-004-SP, 2015, 165–176. arXiv:1804.08551.
19. Mizushima K, Yang Y, Fujimoto T, Iwata Y. Concept design of a superconducting magnet for a compact heavy-ion synchrotron. *IEEE Trans Appl Supercond*. 2022;32(6):1–5.
20. Goitein M. *Radiation Oncology: A Physicist's-Eye View*. Springer Verlag, New York, NY; 2008. http://doi.org/10.1007/978-0-387-72645-8.
21. Yap J, De Franco A, Sheehy S. Future developments in charged particle therapy: improving beam delivery for efficiency and efficacy. *Front Oncol*. 2021;11:780025. http://doi.org/10.3389/fonc.2021.780025.
22. Pedroni E, Scheib S, Böhringer T, et al. Experimental characterization and physical modelling of the dose distribution of scanned proton pencil beams. *Phys Med Biol*. 2005;50(3):541. http://doi.org/10.1088/0031-9155/50/3/011.
23. Safai S, Bortfeld T, Engelsman M. Comparison between the lateral penumbra of a collimated double-scattered beam and uncollimated scanning beam in proton radiotherapy. *Phys Med Biol*. 2008;53:1729–1750.
24. Graeff C, Volz L, Durante M. Emerging technologies for cancer therapy using accelerated particles. *Prog Part Nucl Phys*. 2023;131:104046.
25. Ronsivalle C, Picardi L, Ampollini A, Bazzano G. First acceleration of a proton beam in a side coupled drift tube linac. *Europhys Lett*. 2015;111(1):14002.
26. Mazal A, Prezado Y, Ares C, et al. FLASH and minibeams in radiation therapy: the effect of microstructures on time and space and their potential application to protontherapy. *Br J Radiol*. 2020;93(1107):20190807. http://doi.org/10.1259/bjr.20190807.
27. Jolly S, Owen H, Schippers M, Welsch C. Technical challenges for FLASH proton therapy. *Phys Med*. 2020;78:71–82. http://doi.org/10.1016/j.ejmp.2020.08.005.
28. Mascia AE, Daugherty EC, Zhang Y, et al. Proton FLASH radiotherapy for the treatment of symptomatic bone metastases: the FAST-01 nonrandomized trial. *JAMA Oncol*. 2023;9(1): 62–69.
29. Meyer J, Eley J, Schmid TE, et al. Spatially fractionated proton minibeams. *Br J Radiol*. 2019;92:20180466.
30. Carabe-Fernandez A, Bertolet-Reina A, Karagounis I, Huynh K, Dale RG. Is there a role for arcing techniques in proton therapy? *Br J Radiol*. 2020;93:20190469.
31. Hoffmann A, Oborn B, Moteabbed M, et al. MR-guided proton therapy: a review and a preview. *Radiat Oncol*. 2020;15(1):129. http://doi.org/10.1186/s13014-020-01571-x.
32. Jermann M. Particle Therapy Cooperative Group (PTCOG). https://ptcog.site
33. Degiovanni A, Amaldi U. History of hadron therapy accelerators. *Phys Med*. 2015;31(4):322–332. http://doi.org/10.1016/j.ejmp.2015.03.002.
34. Amaldi U, Bonomi R, Braccini S, et al. Accelerators for hadrontherapy: from Lawrence cyclotrons to linacs. *Nucl Instrum Methods Phys Res A*. 2010;620(2–3):563–577.
35. Vretenar M, Adliene D, Benedetto E, et al. *Conceptual design of a compact synchrotron-based facility for cancer therapy and biomedical research with helium and proton beams.* In: *14th International Particle Accelerator Conference (IPAC 2023)*. Venice, Italy; May 7–12 2023, THPM058. http://doi.org/10.18429/JACoW-IPAC2023-THPM058.
36. Sauerwein W, Wittig A, Moss R, Nakagawa Y, eds. *Neutron capture therapy: principles and applications*. 1st ed. Springer Heidelberg New York Dordrecht London: Springer Science & Business Media; 2012.
37. Forton E, Stichelbaut F, Cambriani A, Kleeven W, Ahlback J, Jongen Y. Overview of the IBA accelerator-based BNCT system. *Appl Radiat Isotopes*. 2009;67(7–8):S262–S265.
38. Matsumura A, Asano T, Hirose K, Igaki H, Kawabata S, Kumada H. Initiatives toward clinical boron neutron capture therapy in Japan. *Cancer Biother Radiopharm*. 2023;38(3):201–207. http://doi.org/10.1089/cbr.2022.0056 Erratum in: *Cancer Biother Radiopharm*. 2023;38(4):273.
39. Cirrone GAP, Manti L, Margarone D, et al. First experimental proof of proton boron capture therapy (PBCT) to enhance protontherapy effectiveness. *Sci Rep*. 2018;8(1):1141. http://doi.org/10.1038/s41598-018-19258-5.
40. Bassler N, Holzscheiter MH, Jäkel O, Knudsen HV, Kovacevic S. The antiproton depth–dose curve in water. *Phys Med Biol*. 2008; 53(3):793–805.
41. Schwoerer H, Pfotenhauer S, Jäckel O, Amthor K, Liesfeld B, Esirkepov T. Laser–plasma acceleration of quasi-monoenergetic protons from microstructured targets. *Nature*. 2006;439(7075): 445–448.
42. Ledingham K, Bolton P, Shikazono N, Ma C. Towards laser driven hadron cancer radiotherapy: a review of progress. *Appl Sci*. 2014;4(3):402–443. http://doi.org/10.3390/app4030402.
43. Rehwald M, Assenbaum S, Bernert C, et al. Ultra-short pulse laser acceleration of protons to 80 MeV from cryogenic hydrogen jets tailored to near-critical density. *Nat Commun*. 2023;14(1):4009. http://doi.org/10.1038/s41467-023-39739-0.

44. International Atomic Energy Agency; (Consultants Morgan HM, Wu RK, et al.). Radiation Protection in the Design of Radiotherapy Facilities, Safety Reports Series No. 47, Vienna: IAEA; 2006.
45. Sunil C. Analysis of the radiation shielding of the bunker of a 230 MeV proton cyclotron therapy facility; comparison of analytical and Monte Carlo techniques. *Appl Radiat Isot*. 2016;110:205–211. http://doi.org/10.1016/j.apradiso.2016.01.023.
46. Lin Y, McMahon SJ, Paganetti H, Schuemann J. Biological modeling of gold nanoparticle enhanced radiotherapy for proton therapy. *Phys Med Biol*. 2015;60(10):4149.

11

Techniques for Accurate Planning and Delivery of Radiotherapy: Immobilisation, Volume Definition and Verification Techniques

Robin Taylor and Daniel Leach

CHAPTER OUTLINE

INTRODUCTION

This chapter covers some key techniques for minimising and accommodating changes and uncertainties in patient anatomy and positioning to ensure that radiotherapy is delivered accurately and reproducibly.

The fundamental aim of radiotherapy is to deliver the prescribed radiation dose to the treatment target(s) in full while keeping doses to nearby healthy tissues within acceptable limits. A treatment planning scan, usually computed tomography (CT) (Chapter 6), is used to create a bespoke plan for each patient. Ideally, the patient anatomy and position at treatment would be identical to their planning scan. This would allow delivery of the treatment exactly as planned. However, in reality, changes are inevitable. This is partly because it is not unusual for days or weeks to pass between acquisition of the planning scan and delivery of treatment, and the course of radiotherapy is itself usually delivered over numerous daily treatments. Over this time, anatomical changes such as weight variation, movement and changes in internal organs are unavoidable. Additionally, it is very difficult to exactly reproduce patient positioning on a daily basis.

If significant, these variations have the potential to cause the delivered radiation dose distribution to deviate from the treatment plan. As a result, they must be identified, minimised, corrected for and/or accommodated for. Some of the main techniques for doing this are covered in the following sections and include:

- **Immobilisation:** Devices used for patient positioning to aid reproducible setup
- **Volume definition:** The way the treatment target and other internal structures are defined on the treatment planning scan, incorporating the potential for change
- **Verification:** Ways of assessing/ensuring the accuracy of treatment delivery, including using imaging on the treatment unit to guide radiotherapy treatment

This chapter also covers adaptive planning, an approach in which the plan itself is changed or adapted on the basis of these variations.

IMMOBILISATION, TARGET DEFINITION AND VERIFICATION WITHIN THE PATIENT PATHWAY

For the purposes of this chapter, a typical radiotherapy pathway can be broadly split into three stages (Fig. 11.1):

1. A *pretreatment appointment*, which includes the acquisition of a treatment planning scan
2. The *treatment planning process*, where a bespoke treatment plan is created using a computer-based treatment planning system
3. *Treatment delivery*, which typically occurs over several daily fractions

Decisions made at each stage can have significant onward implications. This means that awareness of and consideration for the whole pathway is important for all staff. A review of the patient pathway can also help contextualise the important roles played by immobilisation, volume definition and verification.

Pretreatment Appointment

A typical patient pathway begins with a *pretreatment appointment* where a treatment planning scan is acquired. This scan is used to establish up-to-date information on the size and location of the radiotherapy target and proximal healthy tissues. It is also used during the planning process to calculate radiation doses and design the radiotherapy plan. This scan defines the baseline anatomy and position that should be

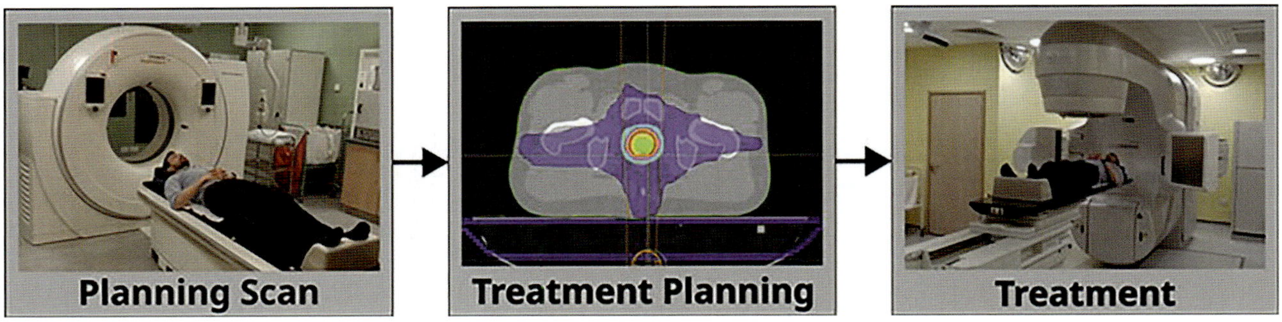

Fig. 11.1 The typical stages in a radiotherapy pathway.

reproduced during treatment. Patient positioning during the scan is therefore crucial.

Immobilisation

Immobilisation refers to the use of specialised devices or equipment to position the patient in a reproducible way and keep them comfortable and still during treatment. Immobilisation depends on the treatment site and intent and may be specifically made or customised for an individual patient's anatomy. Immobilisation is selected at the pretreatment appointment and used during the planning scan, thereby defining the baseline anatomy and positioning. The same devices are then used every day at treatment. It is important to note that no piece of equipment can *truly* immobilise a patient or keep them perfectly still. But appropriate use of immobilisation can help make setup as reproducible and stable as possible.

Treatment Planning

Treatment planning makes use of the planning scan within specialised software known as a *treatment planning system (TPS)*. The TPS allows a user to simulate and model different configurations of radiation beams to achieve the desired dose distribution. This process does not require the patient to be physically present. For most patients, this process will span numerous days/weeks to accommodate the planning process itself as well as meticulous checking and other procedural and confirmatory measures.

Volume Definition

A crucial part of the planning process is *volume definition*. This consists of identifying and outlining treatment targets as well as nearby organs at risk (OARs). In practice, this mostly relies on drawing around structures of interest using contouring tools within the planning system. Sometimes this can be done purely on the basis of the planning scan. However, it can also be aided by reference images of the patient acquired using other modalities such as magnetic resonance imaging (MRI) (see Chapter 6) and positron emission tomography–computed tomography (PET/CT) (see Chapter 7). Volume definition is one of the key stages where accommodation is made for the inevitability of changes in setup and anatomy as well as other sources of uncertainty. For example, for the target, this is done by ensuring that the prescribed radiation dose doesn't just cover the clinical target but also encompasses a larger volume, including a margin around the target.

Treatment Delivery

When the treatment plan is ready, the patient is required to attend *treatment*. The course of radiotherapy is usually split into multiple *fractions*, and the patient is usually required to attend for several days in succession, sometimes spanning several weeks.

At each treatment appointment, every effort is made to reproduce the anatomy and positioning defined at the treatment planning scan. This includes following any protocols for anatomical preparation that were used at the pretreatment appointment. Additionally, the same immobilisation and positioning aids from pretreatment are used to position the patient on the treatment couch. Some form of *verification* will usually also be performed.

Verification is the process of using data, usually images, to assess the accuracy of treatment delivery. Most frequently, some form of image is acquired (e.g. a planar x-ray) on the treatment machine just before treatment and is used to fine-tune the patient setup and ensure accurate delivery. Verification can also extend to monitoring *during* treatment to ensure that the patient remains correctly positioned, as well as detailed review and checking of images between treatments.

Adaptive Radiotherapy

Adaptive radiotherapy offers a different approach to address variations in patient setup and anatomy. Immobilisation, volume definition and verification can reduce the impact of changes but cannot always fully eliminate them or completely mitigate their impact. For example, they cannot always compensate for changes such as weight loss or significant changes in tumour volume. Adaptive radiotherapy is an approach where the anatomy is assessed and the plan itself is altered to compensate for changes. There are different approaches to achieving this. The most advanced techniques, which involve adapting the plan rapidly while the patient lies on the treatment couch, are only beginning to see widespread uptake more recently due to advances in the required hardware and algorithms and their commercial availability.

IMMOBILISATION

Immobilisation can vary in complexity, and some items of equipment can be more restrictive of movement than others. The specific equipment used will depend on the treatment site and what is achievable for any individual patient.

The success of any patient positioning equipment used relies on a number of factors including:

- The available equipment within each radiotherapy centre
- Staff ability to optimise equipment and materials for patient-specific/site requirements, creating sensible, reproducible and stable setups within the scope of limits of the treatment machines and treatment techniques
- Patient comfort, tolerability and compliance

All these points are essential and can make the difference as to whether treatment can be successfully delivered.

Some treatment sites require further consideration of aspects which can impact their setup position, their pretreatment scan and how their treatment is delivered. Therefore patient positioning equipment alone often cannot achieve the desired reproducible treatment position and must be used in tandem with treatment site–specific patient preparation. Common examples are left breast and prostate, explained in more detail later in this chapter.

Another type of treatment that requires special consideration alongside the use of positioning equipment includes treatment of tumours within the lung, where breathing can often cause the target itself to move. In cases such as these, approaches to compensate for motion may include scanning and treating the patient in breath-hold, using compression devices to minimise motion and/or using advanced imaging techniques such as four-dimensional CT (4DCT) to characterise the motion for use in creation and delivery of treatment plans.

The increasing use of the MR LINAC to facilitate real-time imaging and/or adaptive planning during treatment brings its own unique limitations in terms of patient immobilisation. Traditional immobilisation methods, such as rigid masks or vacuum bags, can cause image artefacts and specialised, MRI-compatible equipment should be utilised. These can be expensive and can potentially compromise patient comfort. Another challenge arises from the limited bore size which can significantly reduce positioning and immobilisation options. Patients who are claustrophobic or have specific anatomical requirements may face challenges in finding appropriate solutions that fit within the bore. Finally, the extended times associated with MR LINAC treatments can strain a patient's ability to remain still, particularly for those with discomfort or anxiety.

Common Forms of Immobilisation

Following are descriptions of some of the more common treatment sites and the equipment used to help aid patient positioning.

Head and Neck

The small field sizes used when treating head and neck patients require a high degree of beam positional accuracy because of the proximity of critical organs such as the eye and spinal cord. A similarly high degree of patient positioning reproducibility is therefore required that minimises any variation and movement in patient setup.

Patients receiving radiotherapy to the head and neck region would generally be positioned using commercial systems that employ a combination of a frontal face mask and back neck rest (Fig. 11.2) to achieve a reproducible treatment position. These systems can vary from one another in the detail of how they work, but they tend to have the same fundamental concept of how they are manufactured and used. This tends to involve a perforated thermoplastic material softened in a hot water bath or warm oven and then moulded directly over the patient's face, neck and shoulders. A customised 'back half'/headrest might also be made, or a standard shaped headrest may be used, with a choice of different shapes available and the optimal one chosen for the patient. The thermoplastic masks available from different suppliers can look very similar to one another but can have unique characteristics that set them apart, such as their composition, mouldability, working time and rigidity.

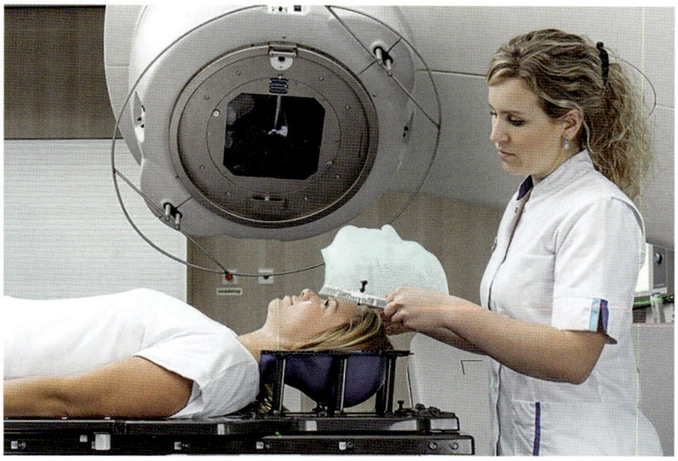

Fig. 11.2 Double Shell Positioning System (DSPS) mask. (Image courtesy MacroMedics.)

The development and increasing use of surface-guided radiotherapy (SGRT) (described further in section titled Verification Using Nonionising Radiation) has allowed thermoplastic masks to evolve into shoulderless and faceless variants whereby the mask is only moulded over the forehead, chin and sides of the face, leaving an open area where the patient's skin surface is visible (Fig. 11.3). The SGRT equipment can then be used to fine-tune and monitor the patient position in detail before and during treatment in absence of where a mask would traditionally be.

Stereotactic Frames

Stereotactic frames were originally designed for stereotactic intracranial surgery, biopsy and electrode placement but have since been extensively adopted for radiosurgery head immobilisation. The high level of precision required for *radiosurgery*, such as with the Gamma Knife and X-knife systems, necessitates a means of relating three-dimensional patient image coordinates to three-dimensional locations in frame coordinates to submillimetre accuracy. The most common system in use is the Leksell Stereotactic System frame, which is rigidly attached to the patient's head using four small screws placed with local anaesthetic. The frame provides the basis for target coordinate determination and is used to immobilise and position the patient's head

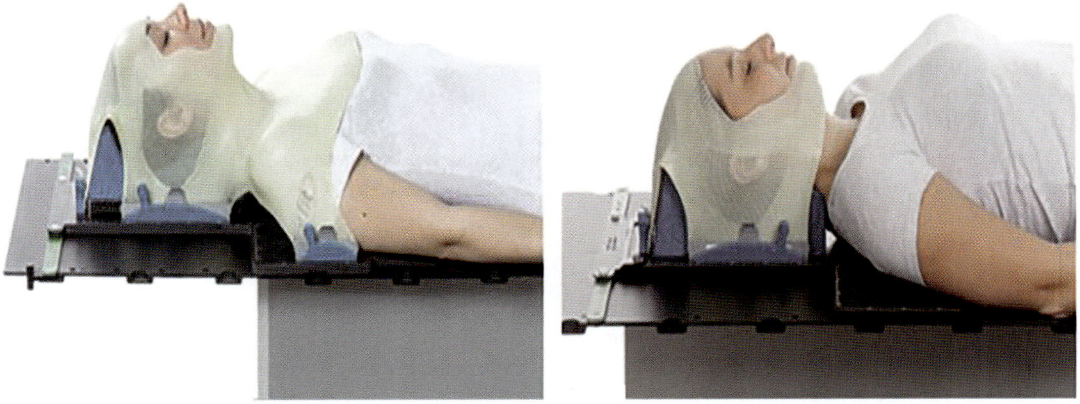

Fig. 11.3 Open face hybrid head, neck and shoulder mask. (Courtesy Orfit industries.)

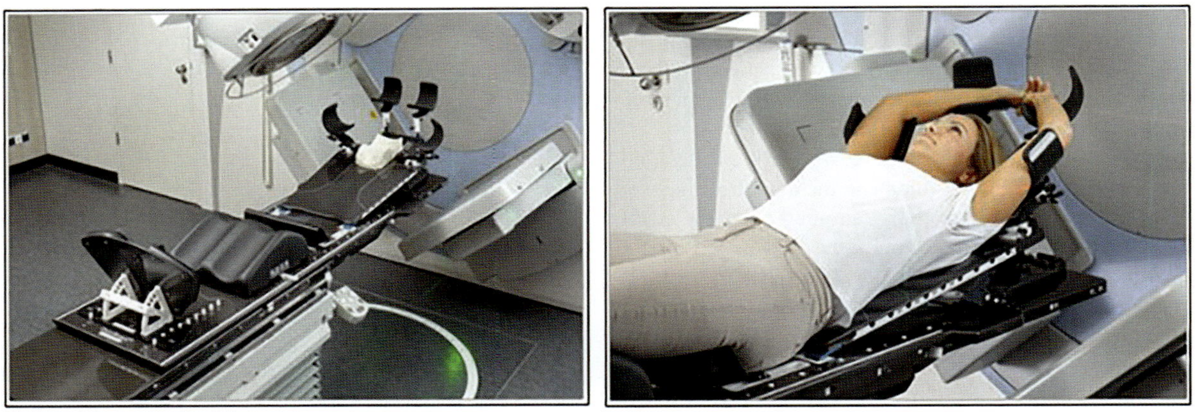

Fig. 11.4 Breastboard LX. (Image courtesy MacroMedics.)

within the radiosurgery collimator helmet. The coordinates of the target volume centre are positioned at the intersection of the beams, such as with the multiple cobalt sources for the Gamma Knife, so that 'target centering' is always achieved within this geometrically rigid system. Relocatable versions of the stereotactic frame are available based upon an accurately fitting mould of the hard palate in the mouth.

Breast

Patient positioning equipment for treatment to the breast or chest wall usually involves the use of a specially designed breast board with many adjustable parts that can be set to suit the individual patient (Fig. 11.4). The settings can then be recorded at the pretreatment stage and replicated at treatment. The board usually inclines the patient's upper body and provides head, elbow and wrist support, all with several setting options to allow the arms to be supported in a raised position superior to the head. Inferiorly, a 'bottom stop' can be adjusted to meet the patient's bottom to help hold their position on the inclined board.

This position allows tangential field access to the required treatment area. If treatment is to be delivered using arcs, as with volumetric modulated arc therapy (VMAT), it may be more suitable to use a similar patient setup but with the patient lying flat to allow the treatment machine gantry to rotate freely around the patient without risk of collision.

There is significant evidence that cardiac doses received by patients undergoing left-breast radiotherapy lead to increased risk of long-term cardiovascular side effects.[1] As such, patient positioning equipment must be used in tandem with specific patient preparation to achieve an optimal reproducible position. *Deep inspiration breath-hold (DIBH)* is a treatment technique in which the patient inhales and holds their breath to a volume that is comfortable and reproducible. This technique utilises the patient's own anatomy to reduce dose to the heart and lung.[2] An inflated lung pushes the breast tissue up and away from the body, isolating it more while simultaneously pushing the heart inferiorly and posteriorly away from the treatment field. This means that in addition to standard patient positioning equipment used for breast patients, pretreatment procedures must ensure that the patient can achieve a reproducible breath-hold position before they are scanned and planned to ensure that the same breath-hold position can be achieved and maintained at treatment. Treatment will be delivered in the breath-hold positions, and in some cases systems will be employed to monitor the patient and automatically halt delivery of the beam if the patient comes out of their breath-hold position.

For patients with large pendulous breasts, which can become problematic for treatment planning purposes and radiotherapy skin reactions due to self bolusing, there are several immobilisation devices available, such as the Vac-Fix bag, a wireless bra or breast cups which could also be implemented if deemed necessary.

Lung and Thorax

For lung and thorax setup, the patient positioning equipment can be the same as that used for breast VMAT. The patient lies flat with support to their head and with adjustable arm and wrist supports, commonly called *wing boards* or *thorax boards*. Dependent on technique, centres may also use vacuum bags in addition to the wing board to help improve stability and reproducibility. A vacuum bag is a reusable commercial product that is known by various names dependent on supplier. It is essentially a sealed bag loosely filled with beads, and the patient lies on the soft pliable bag. A vacuum pump is attached to draw the air out, allowing it to be shaped and moulded while being vacuumed rigid to support the patient as required and prevent any significant movement (Fig. 11.5).

The bag has a valve on it allowing it to be removed from the vacuum pump. The pressure within the bag is maintained, and the bag keeps its shape and rigidity throughout the course of treatment until the pressure is released. Vacuum bags are available in many shapes and sizes and can be used in many applications for different treatment sites to help aid in patient position setup.

When treating tumours within the lung, respiratory motion must often be mitigated or avoided. If the tumour moves while a patient breathes, this movement must either be characterised and taken into account during planning, or minimised or avoided by control of the patient as in breath-hold. One common way to accommodate motion in the treatment plan is to use a 4DCT planning scan, whereby multiple images are acquired over time. In this approach, a sequence of CT images (which can be played back like a movie) allow visualisation of tumour movement during the breathing cycle. These images can be used to ensure that any treatment plan will cover the tumour throughout its range of motion as the patient breathes during treatment. However, to minimise or avoid the motion, a compression belt/plate may be used to apply pressure to the patient's abdomen and reduce respiratory tumour motion. An alternative approach is to avoid motion altogether by scanning while the patient holds their breath at a particular point in the respiratory cycle. Treatment is then delivered with the patient in the same breath-hold position.

The lung is also one of the most frequent sites to be treated with stereotactic ablative body radiotherapy (SABR), a type of treatment where very high doses are delivered to small targets in a small number of fractions. Patient positioning equipment and setup for these patients is therefore particularly important.

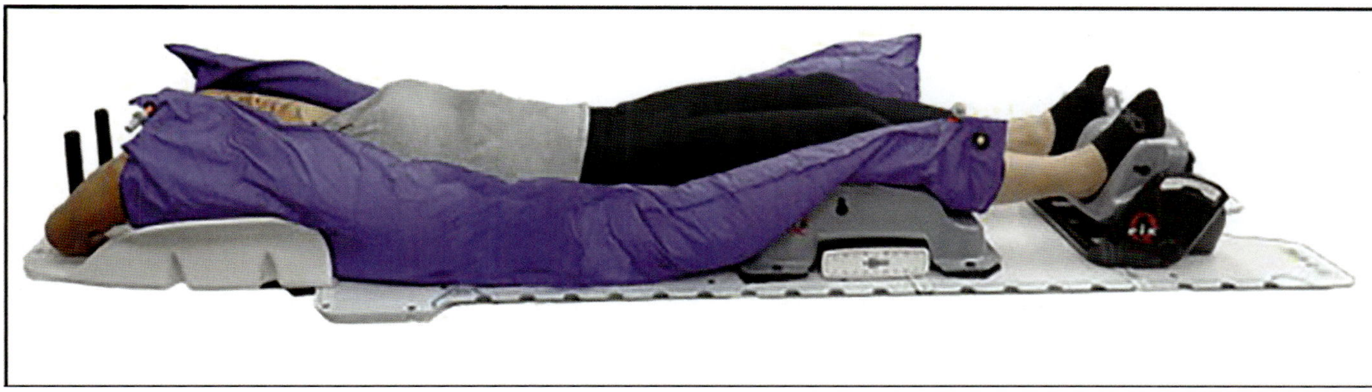

Fig. 11.5 Vacuum bags. (Images courtesy CQ Medical.)

Pelvis

The pelvic region is one of the more difficult areas of the body to provide effective immobilisation and setup reproducibility. Setup equipment can range from simple to complex and will frequently be combined with site-specific patient preparation to achieve a satisfactory reproducible result.

A standard pelvic setup will have the patient lying supine with their head on a combination of standard-shaped foam cushions and wedges. A shaped support is placed under the knees to provide some level of stability and comfort, and a foot rest is placed under the feet; these are fixed to the couch in a position that can be reproduced at treatment. The patient has their hands held together on their chest to ensure that they are out of the way of any treatment beams.

This equipment and setup is of a simplistic nature and is not 'immobilising' the patient in particular, although it can minimise movement of the internal anatomy.

Patient-specific controls for the rectum and bladder are needed for use in conjunction with immobilisation equipment to help create a satisfactorily reproducible setup.

Prescan preparation can consist of bladder filling and rectal emptying. Departments will differ in how they aim to achieve this. Examples could be emptying the bladder, then drinking a measured amount of water and using an enema to aid emptying the rectum prior to the scan.

Prostate radiotherapy, as an example, can have specified maximum tolerances for bladder and rectal size, which can be attained by the pretreatment radiographers at the planning scan appointment. Linear anterior-posterior and lateral measurements can be taken from the CT scout prior to the scan, or total volume can be measured using ultrasound or the planning system, dependent on departmental equipment and workflow. Steps can then be taken to reproduce this at each treatment appointment.

Some centres will take further steps to help aid setup accuracy by using vacuum bags (Fig. 11.5) or pelvic thermoplastics.

DIGITAL MOULD ROOM AND THREE-DIMENSIONAL PRINTING

The development of three-dimensional printing technology has reduced the cost and accessibility to use of this technology in a range of materials. The soft-tissue nature of a patient's surface enables low-cost surface scanners to be used with adequate accuracy. From a surface scan or directly from the CT images in a TPS, printable bolus structures can be generated. This has made it possible to print in flexible, tissue-equivalent bolus for intricate locations on the patient. It is also possible to print a mould to produce bolus in silicone. Fig. 11.6A shows an example of a bolus printed in flexible resin from a TPS-generated file. In Fig. 11.6B a silicone bolus is shown along with the printed mould used to cast it. The mould was derived from a CT scan. Bespoke printed and moulded bolus enables accurate, reproducible and speedy treatment setup.

A digital surface scan can be done in 2 to 4 minutes and is totally noninvasive. The surface scan eliminates the need for an alginate impression and the trauma and discomfort of that to the patient. This increases the accessibility to masks for elderly and apprehensive people. From the surface scan, a number of items can be generated for printing. First is a mould from which a cast can be made in plaster (Fig. 11.7A). While such a cast can be worked on to produce a lead (Pb) shielding mask, a mould for casting the mask in low melting point (LMP) alloy can be printed (Fig. 11.7B). As mentioned earlier, a print file for bolus can be produced from the surface scan; an example for use with an LMP mask is also shown in Fig. 11.7B.

Skin treatment with high dose rate (HDR) brachytherapy (see Chapter 9) has also benefited from having three-dimensional printed moulds with catheter guides embedded. Fig. 11.8 shows three examples: a directly printed mould, a mould cast in silicone and a directly printed shell with embedded guides.

Lastly, a mask to assist in setup and used in conjunction with standard thermoplastic masks, see Fig. 11.3 can be printed such as with an embedded mouth-bite (Fig. 11.9).

A further opportunity with three-dimensional printing is to produce phantom objects for checks, validation and development. Fig. 11.10 shows a soft-tissue and bone insert with air cavities for use in a stereotactic radiosurgery phantom.

VOLUME DEFINITION

Volume definition or delineation is performed within the TPS. Contours are defined on each relevant slice of the planning scan to create three-dimensional representations of structures of interest. The creation of these structures is an essential prerequisite to the planning process to allow prescription, recording and reporting of doses. Accuracy is clearly fundamental, and accommodation must also be made during this stage for the inevitable changes in anatomy and setup that the patient will undergo.

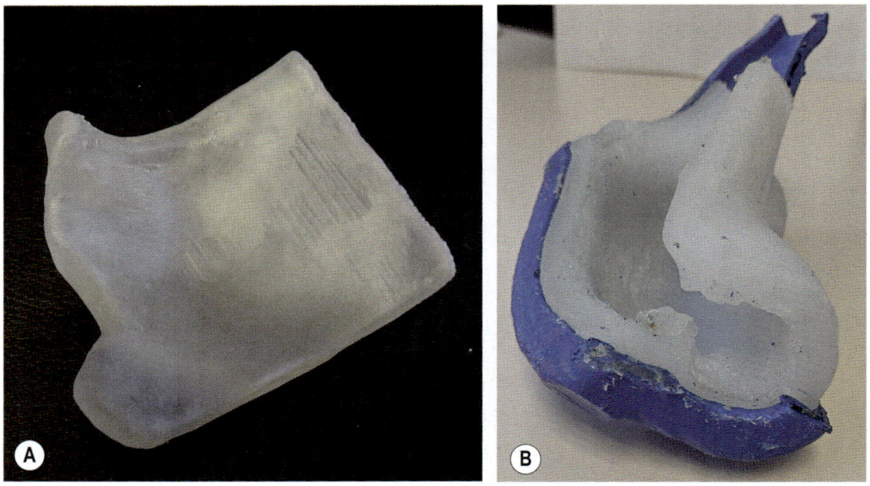

Fig. 11.6 (A) Bolus printed in resin from a treatment planning system file. (B) Silicone bolus cast from a three-dimensional printed mould.

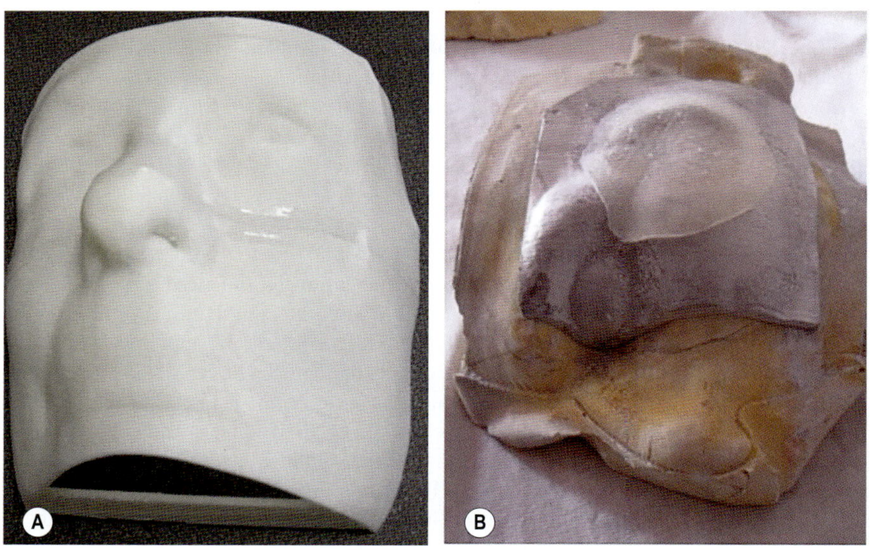

Fig. 11.7 (A) Printed mould from a surface scan. (B) Plaster cast with a low-melting-point shielding mask and printed bolus.

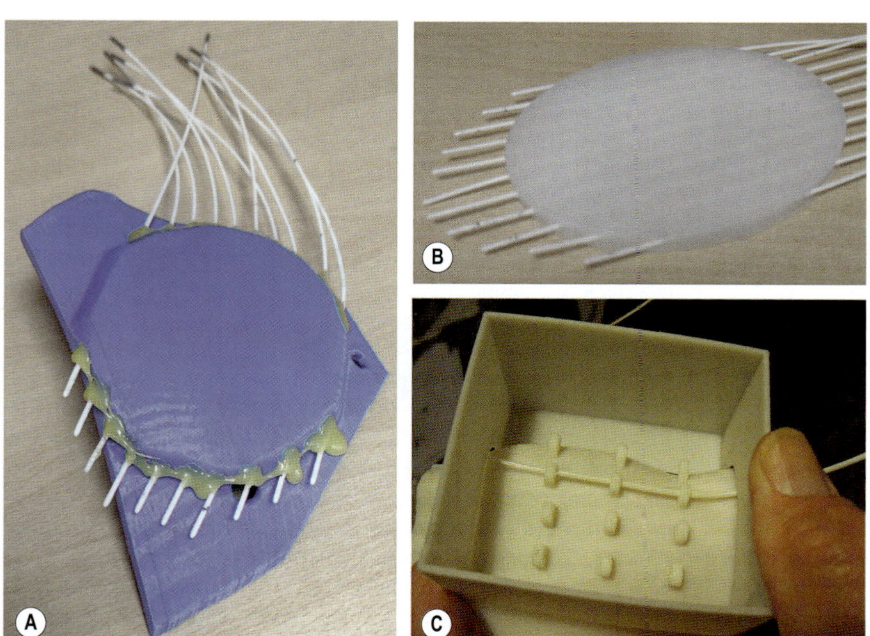

Fig. 11.8 (A) A printed mould with high dose rate (HDR) guides. (B) A silicone cast mould with HDR guides. (C) A printed shell with embedded HDR guides.

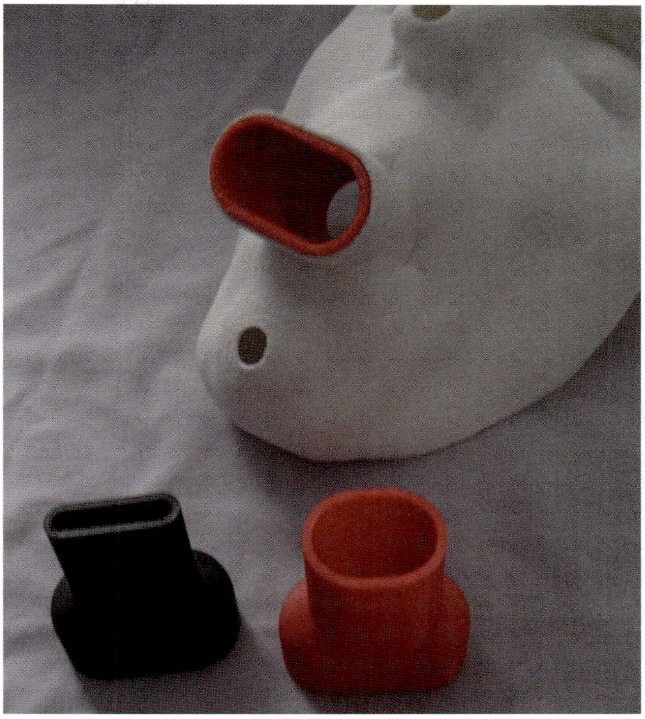

Fig. 11.9 A printed mask with embedded mouth-bite.

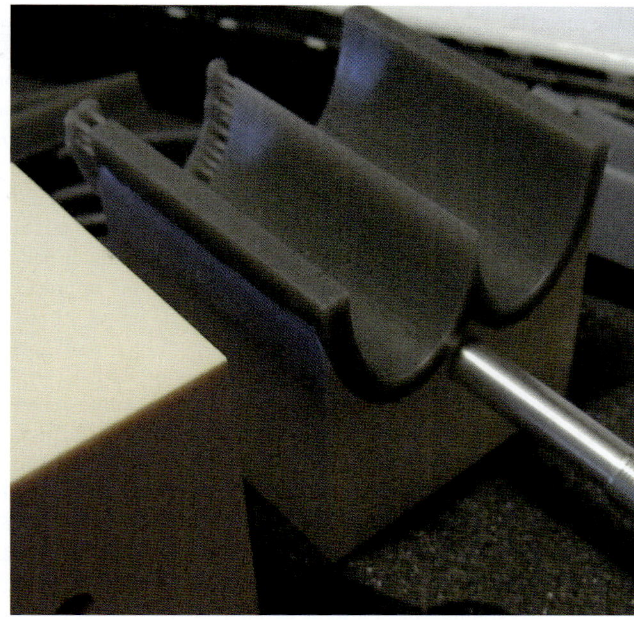

Fig. 11.10 A printed phantom insert with chamber cavity.

Target Volumes

When defining radiotherapy targets, the visible/demonstrable extent of the malignant growth is usually outlined first, creating a volume known as the *gross tumour volume (GTV)*. A series of larger volumes is then created based on the GTV. The purpose of each of these expanded target volumes is standardised, defined and described in depth in a series of reports from the International Commission on Radiation Units and Measurements (ICRU).[3–5] Guidance on volume definition is also issued in the United Kingdom by the Royal College of Radiologists.[6] The most universally applicable target volumes are summarised in Fig. 11.11, together with transcribed ICRU definitions from ICRU Report 50.[3]

Practically, when creating a treatment plan, the GTV is usually outlined by the clinician responsible for the patient's care. The GTV, however, does not take into account the possibility that there may be some microscopic malignant disease which should be treated but which might not be visible on the available imaging. The clinical target volume (CTV) is therefore created, typically by expanding the GTV with a margin based on the likely growth and spread of a particular tumour type.

The radiotherapy plan should ensure that the prescribed dose is delivered to the CTV every day on treatment. As described throughout this chapter, changes in anatomy, movement and variation in setup are inevitable. This means the CTV may move or change over the course of treatment. The planning target volume (PTV) is a geometrical concept created to account for this as well as any other uncertainties by a further expansion applied to the CTV.

In the planning process, the radiation dose is shaped in the planning system with the aim of adequately covering the PTV to ensure

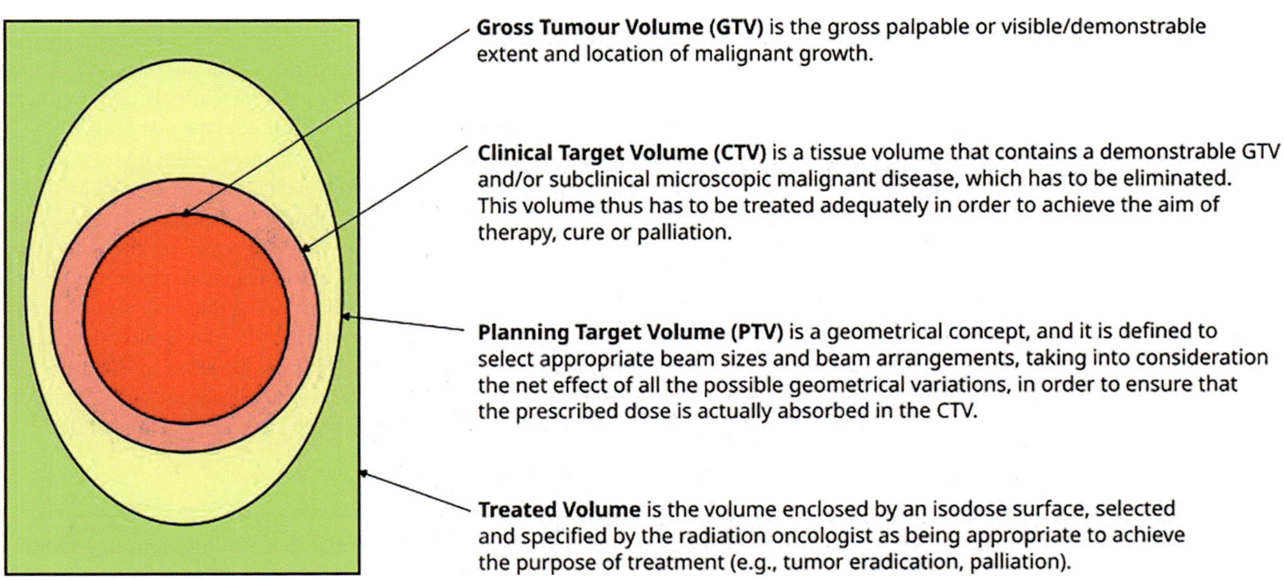

Fig. 11.11 Schematic diagram illustrating target volumes defined by ICRU.[3]

that the prescribed dose is delivered to all parts of the CTV every day on treatment. The CTV-to-PTV margin may depend on the site as well as imaging and treatment techniques. It may also not be uniform: for example, if the target is more likely to move in the superior-inferior axis than it is to move left-right, the PTV expansion may be larger in the superior-inferior axis than left-right to accommodate this.

The *treated volume* is the volume of tissue enclosed within a specific isodose envelope, with the absorbed dose specified by the radiation oncology team as appropriate to achieve tumour eradication or palliation. Ideally, this would perfectly conform to the PTV, but in practice, this might not be the case.

Organs at Risk

In addition to treatment targets, planning will also take into account OARs. OARs are defined as 'tissues that if irradiated could suffer significant morbidity and thus might influence the treatment planning and/or the absorbed-dose prescription'.[5] Tissues considered as OAR will depend on the treatment site: for example, OARs for a prostate radiotherapy treatment could include bladder, rectum and femoral heads, whereas for a left-breast treatment, they might include the lungs and heart. OAR volumes must also be defined by outlining during the treatment planning process so that the dose they will receive can be assessed. The process of creating an optimal plan will consider dose to the target as well as dose to OAR volumes.

Like targets, OARs are subject to potential changes in shape, setup variation and movement. For organs where damage to a small volume of normal tissue may result in very serious side effects (such as the spinal cord), this potential motion can be explicitly taken into account in the planning process. This can be done by adding a margin to the OAR to create a planning risk volume (PRV), a geometrical concept defined by ICRU which is analogous to the PTV. By ensuring that the PRV dose remains within the acceptable tolerance in the plan, the organ itself should be adequately spared, provided movement and changes over the course of treatment are within the PRV margin.

Internal Target Volume and Respiratory Motion

The internal target volume (ITV) is an additional target volume defined by ICRU as the CTV plus an internal margin. It is described in ICRU Report 83 as an optional tool in helping to delineate the PTV and 'might be useful only in clinical situations in which uncertainty concerning the CTV location dominates setup uncertainties and/or when they are independent'.[5]

The ITV concept is based on dividing the CTV-to-PTV margin into two parts. The CTV-to-ITV margin is known as the *internal margin* and is defined to accommodate for the variations in size, shape and position of the CTV as a result of anatomical variations caused by organ movement. The ITV-to-PTV margin is known as the *setup margin* and allows for the uncertainties of patient and beam position. Whereas the internal margin is required to allow for a physiological process, the setup margin is required to allow for the technical factors that cause uncertainties. The setup margin may be reduced by improved immobilisation of the patient and improved setup accuracy. When used, the ITV will therefore be larger than the CTV but smaller than the PTV.

As an example, the Internal Target Volume (ITV) approach might be employed in certain lung or oesophagus radiotherapy cases where targets have the potential to move significantly as the patient breathes. In such cases, instead of a standard planning CT scan, a respiratory-gated 4DCT is usually acquired, during which time the patient is allowed to breathe normally. This allows motion of the tumour to be visualised throughout the breathing cycle. A composite GTV can then be created and expanded to an ITV to account for movement in each plane. The PTV is then created in turn by expanding the ITV by a predefined margin.[6] Having followed this method the patient can breathe normally on treatment and the target should remain covered throughout their breathing cycle.

Automatic Volume Definition

The process of volume definition can be time consuming and delineation can vary, even between experienced radiation oncologists.[7] Automatic OAR contouring aims to improve this and is increasingly available within TPSs. This is one of several areas within radiotherapy where artificial intelligence (AI) and deep learning are being implemented, reportedly leading to improved speed and accuracy.[8] Automatic contouring, including AI-based automatic contouring, is being used clinically in some centres, and increased usage is predicted.[9] AI algorithms/models are adaptive and are trained to undertake a task such as contouring by setting them up using large, high-quality data sets. Validation must be undertaken to confirm that any contours produced by the algorithm are appropriate before going into clinical use.[10]

MULTIMODALITY IMAGES FOR PLANNING

Oncologists increasingly make use of imaging from multiple modalities when localising targets and organs at risk.

Positron Emission Tomography

Positron emission tomography (PET) imaging (see Chapter 7) is a form of functional imaging which can provide information about molecular and metabolic changes associated with a disease.[11] PET makes use of radioactive substances (known as *radiotracers* or *radiopharmaceuticals*) which are introduced into the patient's body. The PET scanner consists of an array of detectors which can detect the distribution of the substance within the patient. The most commonly used tracer for cancer imaging is the 18F-labelled glucose analogue fluorodeoxyglucose (FDG), which accumulates in tissue in proportion to glucose utilisation. Increased glucose consumption is characteristic of most cancers.[12] This means ^{18}F-FDG PET can have multiple uses in oncology. For example, for lung cancer, an FDG PET scan can help with staging, selection for curative radiotherapy, defining and delineating the target volume in the radiotherapy planning phase and detection of residual or recurrent disease.[13] The PET scan is usually accompanied by a CT scan which is 'coregistered', allowing anatomical localisation of the FDG uptake.

Magnetic Resonance Imaging

MRI (see Chapter 6) is an imaging technique which, like CT, can produce three-dimensional images. MRI offers superior soft-tissue contrast compared to CT and so it is increasingly used to improve the accuracy of tumour outlining in radiotherapy planning.[14]

In addition to using MRI to *augment* outlining on a planning CT scan, some treatments are now planned on the basis of MRI scan only. TPSs require electron density information to calculate radiation dose, which CT scans provide directly. MRI scans, on the other hand, provide information relating to certain magnetic properties and physical structures of tissues. MRI-only planning therefore requires conversion of the MRI into a so-called synthetic CT scan to allow dose calculation. This may be done by assigning bulk densities to different structures such as dense bone, spongy bone, muscle, fat and air. Other approaches include using AI and deep learning to create synthetic CTs.[15]

VERIFICATION

Verification is another essential element in minimising the impact of changes in patient anatomy and setup. Two influential reports have been particularly important in guiding the approach to verification used in most UK radiotherapy centres: 'On Target: Ensuring Geometric Accuracy in Radiotherapy'[16] and 'On Target 2: Updated Guidance for Image-Guided Radiotherapy'[17] both jointly published by the Society and College of Radiographers, the Institute of Physics and Engineering in Medicine, and the Royal College of Radiologists. 'On Target 2' defines verification as 'the process by which the accuracy of a fraction of radiotherapy is assessed'. In practice, verification typically consists of a comparison of images of the patient to expected reference images based on the plan.

Verification can occur at various time points throughout the patient pathway, and different methods of verification can be used dependent on the systems available and the clinical needs of the patient.

Online, Offline and Intrafraction Verification

Online treatment verification occurs immediately prior to treatment. At each treatment appointment, every effort is made to replicate the patient's planning scan anatomy and position, including following the same anatomical preparation used at their pretreatment appointment and the same immobilisation devices. The treatment couch is then moved to the expected treatment delivery position, and verification images are acquired. Comparison to reference images allows identification of and correction for residual differences before treatment is delivered. Corrections can be made by manually repositioning the patient on the couch and by moving the treatment couch. Couch corrections can consist of translational movements: moving the patient in the superior-inferior, left-right and anterior-posterior axes. Some couches also allow rotations about these axes, referred to as *yaw*, *pitch* and *roll* corrections.

Offline verification is another approach, in which images taken within the treatment room are compared to reference images *after* the treatment has been given. This is often performed independently, and any identified issues would be acted on during the next treatment fraction. This may include review of images acquired during treatment delivery.

Real-time monitoring and intrafractional verification allow the patient position to be monitored *during* treatment delivery. Various systems are available for this purpose, and some have the ability to control the treatment beam itself. This may involve halting the beam if the patient moves beyond predetermined tolerances or synchronizing beam delivery with a specific anatomical state, such as breath-hold.

Verification Using Two-Dimensional Radiographic Imaging

Most modern linear accelerators are equipped with kilovoltage (kV) and megavoltage (MV) imaging capabilities. The kV images are typically acquired using an x-ray tube and flat-panel detector mounted onto arms that can be extended and retracted (Fig. 11.12A). MV imaging also makes use of an on-board detector which can be extended or retracted but is diametrically opposite the treatment head, with the treatment beam serving as the radiation source (Fig. 11.12B). It should be noted that some stand-alone kV imaging systems are also available for specific purposes and may have kV tubes and detectors mounted in the floor and on the ceiling of the treatment room, but these are usually used for specific purposes such as stereotactic radiotherapy.

Both kV and MV systems can be used to acquire planar images to be used for matching with expected images generated at the treatment planning stage. Each imaging mode has a different dose associated with it and offers a different image quality, making them suitable for different purposes. To assess the patient position, a comparison is made to expected images produced from the TPS and known as digitally reconstructed radiographs (DRRs).

Single planar kV or MV images only allow positional verification in the imaging plane. In other words, an image acquired in the anterior-posterior direction cannot allow accurate verification of the patient's

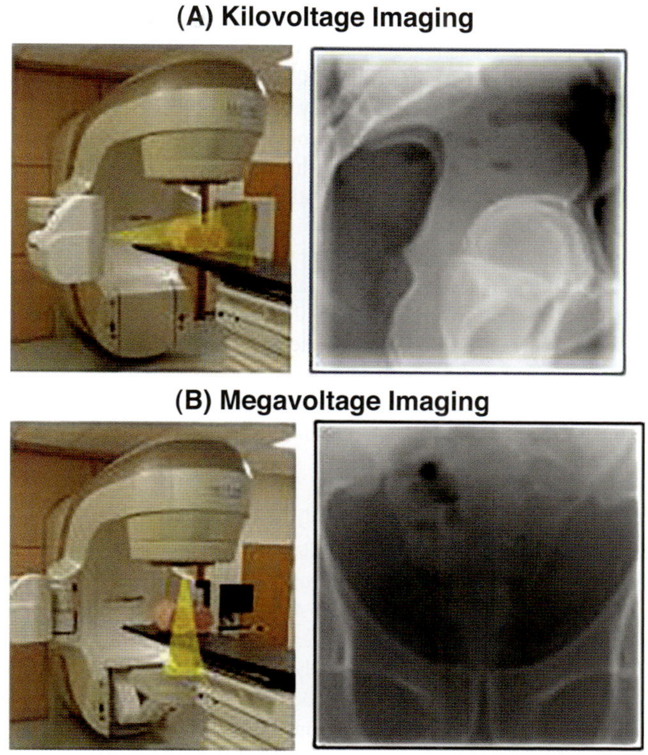

Fig. 11.12 Example images of pelvis phantom using (A) kilovoltage (kV) imaging, and (B) megavoltage (MV) imaging.

vertical height. Acquiring images in pairs, at orthogonal angles, allows verification and position correction in three-dimensional space. The use of two-dimensional imaging can be appropriate to determine setup errors by registration of bony landmarks or implanted fiducial markers, but it may not be sufficient for sites requiring good soft-tissue discrimination.[17]

Verification Using Cone Beam Computed Tomography

Most modern linear accelerators are also capable of acquiring cone beam CT images. In this case the linear accelerator rotates around the patient, with the kV imaging hardware acquiring numerous kV projections which can be reconstructed into a three-dimensional image. The cone beam CT can then be compared on a slice-by-slice basis to the planning CT. This can be particularly useful for matching soft tissues to reference images. As part of this process, structures such as PTVs can be visualised to ensure that the intended anatomy aligns with expected positions, as illustrated in Fig. 11.13.

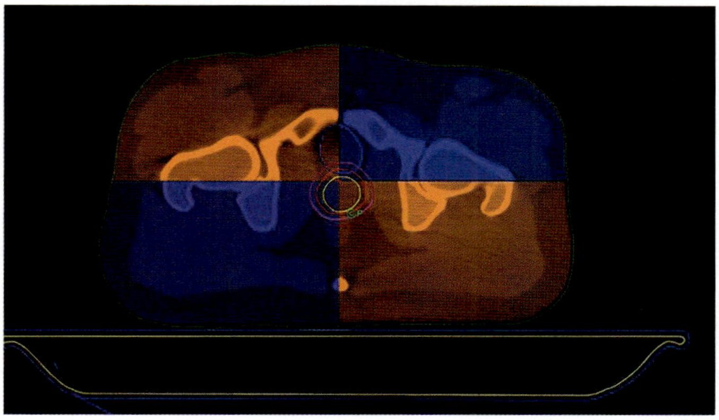

Fig. 11.13 Matching using cone-beam CT: Reference CT in blue, cone-beam CT in red.

It is possible, with appropriate hardware, to acquire four-dimensional cone beam CT images. Like four-dimensional planning CT scans, these are acquired more slowly than standard cone beam CTs and with a higher dose, and they can be used to produce movie-loop style images of respiratory motion.[17] This can be useful to ensure that moving targets will remain within the expected target margins throughout the breathing cycle. Another approach is to only acquire cone beam CT data when the patient is in a specific predefined part of their breathing cycle. This is known as *gated cone beam CT*. In this case the same four-dimensional system can also be used for gate delivery of the beam so that treatment is only delivered when the patient is in a predefined part of their breathing state and is halted at all other times. This aims to deliver treatment more precisely to moving tumours.

Another three-dimensional imaging approach is the use of megavoltage CT, which is available on some treatment systems including TomoTherapy units.

Verification Using Nonionising Radiation

Other methods of verification are available. An example is the use of MR imaging, which is available on some commercial treatment systems such as the MRI LINAC (see Chapter 10). Another implementation has seen an MRI scanner 'on rails' within the treatment room, allowing the patient to have an MRI acquisition immediately before treatment, in the intended treatment position. As with diagnostic MRI, this approach offers very high-quality soft-tissue definition compared to cone beam CT.

SGRT is another method of online verification which aims to augment existing image guidance systems in radiotherapy. These systems can be used to acquire three-dimensional representations of the patient surface which can be compared in real time to the expected contour of the patient from the planning CT scan. Approaches to acquire patient surfaces include the use of structured light, stereovision systems, time-of-flight systems or lasers. The addition of this equipment can help with setup, as it will show setup errors as the patient is being positioned, and can also be used to confirm the patient remains still during treatment. The ability to capture real-time confirmation of patient position can be particularly useful when delivering radiotherapy in breath-hold treatments, and many systems can allow the beam to be stopped if the patient moves from their expected position.

Offline Verification and Verification of Delivered Dose

Offline verification has become less common in recent years, as most linear accelerators have the capacity to quickly perform online verification and allow automatic corrective shifts. However, offline review remains an option, with images acquired in the treatment room being compared to reference images such as DRRs. This can include MV images acquired during treatment. These 'portal images' were of particular importance to verification prior to the widespread uptake of image-guided radiotherapy. Before the development of the MV imager, they were captured using radiographic film.

The use of MV images acquired during treatment can be further extended for dosimetric verification. Some specialised software packages can use these images as an input, together with the planning CT scan, to independently compute the dose that must have been delivered to the patient. This computed dose can be compared to the original treatment plan and give validation that the treatment has been delivered correctly, a process known as *transit dosimetry*. This is covered in more detail in Chapter 14.

Another approach to verifying the delivered dose is to import a cone beam CT acquired on treatment into the TPS, copy the plan onto the cone beam and recalculate the delivered fraction dose. This type of investigation can demonstrate the impact of any anatomical changes on the dose distribution and coverage of targets. When performing this type of analysis, approximations are required and attention must be paid to the resultant limitations. These are largely due to the fact that cone beam CTs are acquired differently from conventional CT scans. For example, cone beam CT is particularly prone to artefacts such as those caused by scatter radiation and generally reduced image quality. Additionally, the density information required for a dose calculation is inherently less reliable on a cone beam CT, often leading to a need to approximate values.

ADAPTIVE RADIOTHERAPY

The methods of immobilisation, volume definition, use of margins and verification are some of the most commonly used approaches to minimise the impact of anatomical changes and day-to-day setup variation on patient treatment. However, they cannot account for every circumstance. Sometimes it can be beneficial to modify the treatment plan itself over the course of treatment to ensure that the clinical intent is met. This concept, known as *adaptive radiotherapy*, can be implemented in different ways and with a range of complexity.

The most prevalent form of adaptive radiotherapy used currently is offline adaptation between treatment fractions in response to an anatomical change observed on treatment.[18] Almost all radiotherapy treatment delivery involves some form of verification imaging. In reviewing these images, an anatomical change might be identified that could impact the treatment plan. For example, it might be noted that a head and neck patient has gradually lost weight. Typically, this will lead to some form of investigation, possibly including recalculation of the treatment dose using the cone beam CT. If adaptation or replanning is required, it will usually require repeating the planning process with a new planning CT. However, the replan must take into account the dose already delivered. The main issues with this type of reactive planning are the resources required in rescanning and producing the replan as well as the inevitable time delay before the replan is ready. Workflows for departments and sites will differ, and it is a common practice to consider the safety of continuing treatment with the original plan until the new plan is ready.[17]

Another common form of adaptive radiotherapy, which can be used when anatomical changes are predicted, is proactive adaptive radiotherapy using a library of plans approach, known as *plan-of-the-day radiotherapy*. The library of plans process involves creating multiple treatment plans which are made available for selection to suit the anatomy of the day. For example, if this approach were used in treatment of the bladder, multiple plans may be created to account for variation in filling. A plan could then be selected that best achieves the clinically required coverage of the target while minimising unnecessary dose to surrounding tissues. The library of plans may be created using a single treatment planning scan, with various sizes of PTV based on expected changes, or alternatively multiple planning scans may be acquired in different anatomical states with plans created on each. A third option is to start with only one plan but acquire and review on-treatment images, creating plans that suit the anatomical variation seen over the course of the first few fractions.[17]

An emerging approach to adaptive radiotherapy is online, real-time adaptive radiotherapy, where a new treatment plan is created while the patient, having been imaged, is on the treatment couch and in the treatment position. In this approach, a baseline or reference treatment plan is prepared as normal. On each treatment, verification imaging is acquired. Before treatment is delivered, the OARs and targets are outlined on the verification images and the plan is calculated on the verification image. This allows prediction and assessment of the dose that would be delivered if treatment were given as per the reference treatment plan. If this were not to be clinically acceptable—for example, if the tumour has grown or moved and is no longer fully covered by the prescription dose—the treatment plan could be adapted at the treatment unit before delivery. This approach requires daily volumetric imaging of sufficient quality and has been closely associated with the development of MRI-guided radiotherapy.[17] However, it is also possible using cone beam CT.[19] Because replanning happens while the patient is positioned and ready for treatment, the process must be orders of magnitude faster than conventional planning. A particular bottleneck is contouring the structures in the on-treatment volumetric imaging. Recent commercial solutions have seen the application of AI and deep learning techniques to speed up automatic contouring (see Chapter 13).

REFERENCES

1. Taylor C. Radiation-related heart disease following treatment of breast cancer (abstract). *Radiother Oncol.* 2011;99(Supp 1):76.
2. Latty D, Stuart KE, Wang W, Ahern V. Review of deep inspiration breath-hold techniques for the treatment of breast cancer. *J Med Radiat Sci.* 2015;62(1):74–81.
3. ICRU (International Commission on Radiation Units and Measurements). *Prescribing, recording and reporting photon beam therapy,* ICRU Report 50, Bethesda, Maryland: International Commission on Radiation Units and Measurements; 1993.
4. ICRU (International Commission on Radiation Units and Measurements). *Prescribing, recording and reporting photon beam therapy (supplement to ICRU Report 50),* ICRU Report 62, Bethesda, Maryland: International Commission on Radiation Units and Measurements; 1999.
5. ICRU (International Commission on Radiation Units and Measurements). *Prescribing, recording, and reporting intensity-modulated photon-beam therapy (IMRT),* ICRU Report 83, Bethesda, Maryland: International Commission on Radiation Units and Measurements; 2010.
6. RCR (Royal College of Radiologists). *Radiotherapy Target Volume Definition and Peer Review.* 2nd ed. London: RCR Guidance; 2022.
7. Brouwer CL, Steenbakkers RJ, van den Heuvel ER, et al. 3D variation in delineation of head and neck organs at risk. *Radiat Oncol.* 2012;7:32.
8. Harrison K, Pullen H, Welsh CR, Oktay O, Alvarez-Valle J, Jena R. Machine learning for auto-segmentation in radiotherapy planning. *Clinl Oncol.* 2022;34(2):74–88.
9. Hindocha S, Zucker KD, Jena R, et al. Artificial intelligence for radiotherapy auto-contouring: current use, perceptions of and barriers to implementation. *Clin Oncol.* 2023;35(4):219–226.
10. Vandewinckele L, Claessens M, Dinkla A, et al. Overview of artificial intelligence-based applications in radiotherapy: recommendations for implementation and quality assurance. *Radiother Oncol.* 2020;153:55–66.
11. Fletcher JW, Djulbegovic B, Soares HP, et al. Recommendations on the use of 18F-FDG PET in oncology. *J Nucl Med.* 2008;49(3):480–508.
12. Boellaard R, Delgado-Bolton R, Oyen WJG, et al. FDG PET/CT: EANM procedure guidelines for tumour imaging: version 2.0. *Eur J Nucl Med Mol Imaging.* 2015;42(2):328–354.
13. Vaz SC, Adam JA, Delgado Bolton RC, et al. Joint EANM/SNMMI/ESTRO practice recommendations for the use of 2-18F] FDG PET/CT external beam radiation treatment planning in lung cancer V1.0. *Eur J Nucl Med Mol Imaging.* 2022;49(4):1386–1406.
14. Speight R, Dubec M, Eccles CL, et al. IPEM topical report: guidance on the use of MRI for external beam radiotherapy treatment planning. *Phys Med Biol.* 2021;66(5):055025.
15. Boulanger M, Nunes JC, Chourak H, et al. Deep learning methods to generate synthetic CT from MRI in radiotherapy: a literature review. *Phys Med.* 2021;89:265–281.
16. Royal College of Radiologists, Society and College of Radiographers, Institute of Physics and Engineering in Medicine. *On target: ensuring geometric accuracy in radiotherapy.* London: The Royal College of Radiologists; 2008.
17. Radiotherapy Board. *On target 2: updated guidance for image-guided radiotherapy.* London: The Royal College of Radiologists; 2021.
18. Bertholet J, Anastasi G, Noble D, et al. Patterns of practice for adaptive and real-time radiation therapy (POP-ART RT) part II: offline and online plan adaption for interfractional changes. *Radiother Oncol.* 2020;153:88–96.
19. Archambault Y, Boylan C, Bullock D, et al. Making on-line adaptive radiotherapy possible using artificial intelligence and machine learning for daily re-planning. *Med Phys Internat.* 2020;8(2):77–86.

12

External Beam Treatment Planning: Dose Calculations, Principles and Practice

Maria Mania Aspradakis

CHAPTER OUTLINE

INTRODUCTION

Radiation therapy is administered using teletherapy, brachytherapy and radioisotope therapy. Teletherapy is externally applied radiation beams of low-energy (kilovoltage, kV) or high-energy (megavoltage, MV) photons, electrons, protons and heavy ions. Brachytherapy is internally or superficially applied radiation sources (Chapter 9) and radioisotope therapy is described in Chapter 8. Whatever type of radiation is used, treatment planning (TP) is the necessary step in the patient pathway (Chapter 11) that enables the treatment of a patient with radiation.

This chapter is specifically concerned with teletherapy, where the goal is to determine a dose distribution within the patient that will destroy the tumour while sparing healthy tissue as much as possible. In palliative radiotherapy (RT), the goal is to provide relief from pain, usually from metastatic disease. In curative or radical RT, the aim is to kill cancer cells while taking into account the radiosensitivity and proximity of healthy organs—organs at risk (OARs). Table 12.1 contains examples of typical dose tolerances for normal tissues.

Appropriate imaging techniques are needed to identify tumour volumes (Chapter 11). Treatment volumes for TP, referred to as the planning target volume (PTV), usually contain those outlined from imaging, as it is important to account for uncertainties in volume definition and motion during treatment. The methodology followed for the prescription and reporting of radiation therapy, which includes the definition of involved volumes, is provided in reports by the International Commission on Radiation Units and Measurements (ICRU).[1–6] Compilations of tolerance doses for conventionally fractionated radiation therapy can be found in the journal article 'Quantitative Analyses of Normal Tissue Effects in the Clinic (QUANTEC)'[7,8]; in sreports on hypofractionated and high-dose-per-fraction regimens by the American Association of Physicists in Medicine (AAPM) Task Group 101[9]; in publications by the Hy Dose per Fraction, Hypo-fractionated Treatment Effects in the Clinic initiative (HyTEC)[10]; and in tables collated by Timmerman.[11]

Serial organs are those that lose functionality when they receive a dose above a certain threshold; an example is the spinal cord. Organs

TABLE 12.1 Typical Normal Tissue Tolerance Doses for Generally Accepted Risks

Organ	Typical Dose Limits		Comments
Spinal cord	45 Gy		Although a serial organ, the length of the cord receiving the dose may be taken into account.
Lung	V20 (e.g. <32%) mean lung dose <18 Gy		Normally consider total volume of both lungs (if the gross tumour volume or planning target volume lies within the lung, its volume should be subtracted from the total lung volume and higher V20 volumes may need to be accepted).
Heart	<40 Gy to entire heart No more than one-third of heart volume to receive 60 Gy		Normally the heart volume outlined will include blood.
Kidney	Whole kidney 12 Gy One-third of the 1/3 kidney 16 Gy		Essential to ensure that the unirradiated kidney is functioning or a nonfunctioning kidney is preferentially sacrificed.
Liver	Whole liver <21 Gy One-third of the liver 30 Gy		
Lens	6 Gy		If cataract formation is the concern, consider the consequence of any treatment compromise against future cataract removal.
Rectum	% of 2-Gy/fraction dose for 74-Gy prescribed dose	(%) Max. vol.	
	68	60	An example of a dose volume histogram–based dose constraint rather than a single volume or dose threshold.
	81	50	
	88	30	
	95	15	
	100	3	

Note: These values may vary for individual situations because of clinical condition and other therapies increasing radiosensitivity. Therefore correction must be made for different fractionation.

classified as parallel continue to provide functionality even if part of them is completely damaged by radiation (e.g. lung), and there are organs that respond as both serial and parallel, such as the heart. In this case it is important to minimise the volume of the organ that receives more than a threshold dose. For example, in the case of the lung, the aim is to minimise the volume of lung receiving more than 20 Gy, because it is known that doses above this threshold lead to radiation pneumonitis.

The first step in TP is volume definition, often referred to as contouring and dose prescription. Target volumes and OAR together with the dose prescription are specified by clinicians. A prerequisite for this step is the information on the anatomy of the patient. Modern radiation therapy in most cases uses three-dimensional patient information from computed tomography (CT) or magnetic resonance imaging (MRI). As described in Chapter 11, the patient is ideally imaged in the treatment position, and planning volumes are identified either exclusively on these images or with the aid of additional imaging modalities such as positron emission tomography (PET), providing further information on the location and extent of the tumour.

The second step in TP involves the generation of a treatment plan. A treatment plan contains all the information needed to realise the dose prescription. A prerequisite for this is an adequate description of the radiation device used for the treatment, the anatomical information of the patient and a method to calculate the dose in the patient. This task is carried out by medical physicists, planning radiographers, dose planners or dosimetrists specifically trained in the generation of treatment plans and almost exclusively using computerised systems. Modern treatment planning systems (TPSs) are software suites comprising different tools for the visualisation of patient anatomy, definition of volumes and simulation of the treatment unit. An essential tool concerns modelling radiation transport and energy deposition in different media, as well as tools for the calculation of dose statistics and the evaluation of metrics on plan quality.

The final step in the TP chain is quality assurance (QA) and verification of the planned treatment. This is typically referred to as plan- or patient-specific verification, where the treatment plan is checked and its parameters are verified through an independent dose calculation method and/or measurement, depending on the complexity of the plan.

In what follows, the key aspects regarding TP are discussed in detail: patient data, beam modelling and dose calculation. Following this, the most common TP techniques implemented in external beam RT are presented together with tools for the evaluation of treatment plans. Basic concepts on QA in TP are discussed in the final section of this chapter.

REPRESENTATION OF THE PATIENT FOR TREATMENT PLANNING

The Planning CT

Approximate representation of the patient anatomy for the purpose of TP is almost completely a practice of the past. Nowadays the planning CT is the minimum requirement for information about the anatomy of the patient needed to generate a treatment plan. The CT scan (Chapter 6) provides a three-dimensional reconstruction of the patient anatomy required for volume definition. Sophisticated software tools on these systems allow clinicians and planners to specify the extent of volumes of interest and design any additional volumes that could aid the production of an optimal treatment plan.

CT images, by definition, are reconstructed from the attenuation of kilovolt x-rays through the imaged body and thus also reflect the attenuation properties of the different materials present in the body at the particular kilovolt energy used for imaging. For megavoltage x-rays the electron density is required for modelling the radiation dose. Through a calibration procedure, using materials of known electron and mass density, a relationship between the type of material and the CT is derived, referred to as the *calibration curve*. It defines the relationship between the relative mass and/or electron density of media and the CT numbers or Hounsfield units (HUs). Thus CT images also provide information in three dimensions on the properties of tissues. This is used to calculate how radiation is attenuated and how particle energy is deposited in the patient. One of the first tasks in setting up a TPS for clinical use is to provide the correct mapping between CT numbers and relative material density and/or additional material properties depending upon the requirements of the dose calculation method.

In three dimensions, and for the purpose of dose calculation, the matrix of CT numbers is divided into voxels. The size of these becomes important when dose is to be calculated in volumes of organs of size comparable with the resolution in the original CT image study. Typical CT image separation and voxel size used for calculations in standard TP calculations is 2.5 mm. The resolution of the CT image data set can affect how faithfully volumes are represented in a treatment plan and subsequently how accurately dose can be calculated for these volumes.

To improve visualisation of certain organs (e.g. nodes in head and neck images) in CT images, contrast materials may be injected into the patient before the acquisition of the CT scan. This aids volume definition, but depending on the contrast agent used, the material composition in the patient, as present in the CT scan, may differ from that during treatment where there is no contrast material present. In most cases, it has been shown that these differences are negligible, but this is something that requires verification for the contrast materials used in a clinic.

Another consideration when using CT images for TP is the presence of high-density materials in the patient, such as dental fillings and metal prostheses. Such materials create artefacts on the images where regions of the anatomy around the metal appear distorted and with incorrect CT numbers assigned to these regions. The use of CT scanners operating in an extended CT range (up to about 30,000 HU) together with the appropriate CT calibration derived for that range can ensure that the correct material density is assigned to very large CT numbers. In addition, some CT scanners provide artefact reduction algorithms to process images and improve image quality. In the absence of both techniques to address the presence of artefacts, and as an approximation for dose calculation, it is a common practice to manually identify regions with artefacts and override the CT numbers in these with those of the neighbouring structures as appropriate. Detailed guidance on the dosimetric considerations with implanted hip prostheses can be found in the report of the AAPM Task Group 63.[12]

The latest generation of dual-energy CT scanners (DECTs) offers the capability to produce image projections from 2-kV beam spectra.[13,14] The resultant composite images from two energies leads to improved image quality with an enhanced contrast-to-noise ratio, because the scans at the lower energy offer information at better contrast, whereas the scans at the higher energy have less noise. In addition to the improvement in image quality, with CT scanning at dual energies it is possible to better discriminate materials from the attenuation coefficients corresponding to the different beam spectra used for scanning. This could lead to more accurate modelling of the dose deposited in the patient in dose calculations during treatment planning. The clinical implementation of DECT necessitates a review of how staff look at images and implement appropriate scanning protocols.[15]

Implanted devices in the patient, such as cardiac pacemakers, also produce artefacts, but with these the primary concern is the influence of radiation and electromagnetic interference from a treatment machine on the operation of the device. Before undertaking the TP, it is advisable to obtain information from the manufacturer of the implanted device and in any case to limit the dose received from scattered radiation to below 2 Gy.[16,17]

Patient Immobilisation for Treatment Planning

Planning CTs are typically acquired using a flat couch top, similar to that used for treatment. However, modern patient immobilisation devices available on treatment machines use couch tops that differ in design and composition than those used during CT. In this case, it is important that the couch top and any immobilisation device used to reproducibly position the patient for treatment are taken into consideration during TP, especially when the irradiation beam traverses through the device. A comprehensive report by the AAPM Task Group 176[18] summarised the dosimetric implications when different couch tops and immobilisation devices are involved in the treatment plan. Careful dosimetry is needed to evaluate skin doses as a result of build-up effects from such devices. It is important that these devices are modelled in TP calculations. This can be achieved by including these as part of the patient anatomy, for which it is essential that they have been present during CT scanning. These include body immobilisation bags or thermoplastic masks/shells (Chapter 11). Another common approach in planning systems is to add these from a library of support models representing each particular device.

Motion Management in Treatment Planning

Respiratory motion of thoracic and abdominal regions not only causes artefacts during image acquisition but also has implications on the delineation of tumour volumes. As described in detail in Chapter 11, following the nomenclature from ICRU 62,[4] margins are added to the gross tumour volume (GTV) to account for suspected microscopic spread, intrafraction and interfraction motion and patient setup errors. An additional margin to account for tumour motion could lead to either an overestimation or an underestimation of the dose delivered to the moving tumour.[15] From the methods to account for respiratory motion reviewed by AAPM Task Group 76[19] the most commonly used are motion-encompassing methods and, in particular, deep inspiration breath-hold (DIBH), four-dimensional CT (4DCT) approaches and respiratory gating methods. In all cases, initially the patient's free-breathing pattern is recorded. In DIBH the planning CT is taken during deep inspiration and the treatment plan is prepared using this, with treatment being delivered in DIBH. In 4DCT approaches, CT scanning is correlated with the breathing pattern, with multiple CT scans taken during at least 10 different breathing phases. Respiratory gating methods include approaches in which treatment is gated based on the patient's breathing pattern as monitored by a motion surrogate device placed on the patient. Gating is also possible using external three-dimensional infrared cameras to monitor the movement of the patient's surface; a technique known as *surface-guided radiotherapy (SGRT)*.[20,21] From all these data sets, typically two single-CT data sets are reconstructed and registered. In the maximum-intensity projection scan, each voxel in the image is assigned the maximum CT number from all phases. In the average scan, each voxel is assigned the average CT number from all phases. The former is used for the delineation of the volume encompassing the tumour in its full range of motion, whereas the latter is used for dose calculation.

The Role of Magnetic Resonance Imaging in Treatment Planning

MRI offers superior soft-tissue contrast in comparison to CT. In addition, MRI allows full flexibility of orientation of the imaging planes, and certain MR sequences can provide information about physiological or chemical properties of the tumour (Chapter 6) which can be used to assess the progression of disease and evaluate and adapt treatment.[22] In a CT-based treatment planning workflow, it is a common practice to register MR images with CT so that tissue delineation is carried out on the MR image with contours transferred to the CT for planning and dose calculation. This practice has generally improved the contouring of structures and volumes for treatment planning. However, MR-to-CT coregistration introduces geometrical uncertainties of the order of 2 to 3 mm, depending on treatment site, which leads to systematic errors throughout treatment and as a result could compromise tumour control.[23] In recent years, considerable efforts are being directed into MRI simulation and MRI-only treatment planning, and this has been demonstrated to be feasible. With such a transition in working practice, improved target definition and use of optimal treatment margins will be followed by reduced geometric uncertainties originating from image registration, possibly leading to efficient and cost-effective treatment strategies involving adaption of treatment during the course of treatment, as well as a marginal reduction in exposure of ionising radiation from CT. The combination of MR and LINAC technology is the next step enabling daily adaptation of treatment.[24,25] Challenges in the design of all technology for MR-only treatment planning include management of artefacts and geometric distortions that MR images are subject to, as well as development of methods to translate MR images to what is known as *synthetic CTs* (also referred to as *pseudo-CT*, *MRCAT* or *MRCT*) for the purpose of dose calculation and the generation of digitally reconstructed radiographs (DRRs), typically used for the verification of patient anatomy in the treatment position. Methods to generate synthetic CTs include voxel-based methods, atlas-based methods and a combination of these two. In the former, there is voxel-by-voxel mapping of MR signals to preclassified tissue signals, which are then assigned to a bulk HU and relative electron density. In atlas-based approaches, atlases of average patient anatomy are registered to the MR images using deformable image registration and this produces an approximate HU.[23]

MRI-based workflows and treatment planning have been shown to work well for certain anatomical sites, such as in the pelvic region, where large changes can be observed during treatment. However, it is expected that other treatment sites, such as in the head and neck, would benefit the most, as it is in these regions where difficulties exist in accurate image registration between CT and MR and in correct localisation of structures.

BEAM MODELLING AND DOSE CALCULATIONS FOR MV PHOTON BEAM TREATMENT PLANNING

Dose calculation algorithms must model all particle transport and energy deposition in arbitrary irradiation geometries and be flexible in their implementation. They should be accurate to better than 3% and fast enough to be practically useful in the clinical environment. Designing models that fulfil these requirements has been challenging, and the introduction of computer technology and its availability in hospitals from the early 1990s led to development of the sophisticated methods currently available on most commercial TPSs. The physical processes that need to be accounted for in megavolt photon beams are shown in Fig. 12.1.

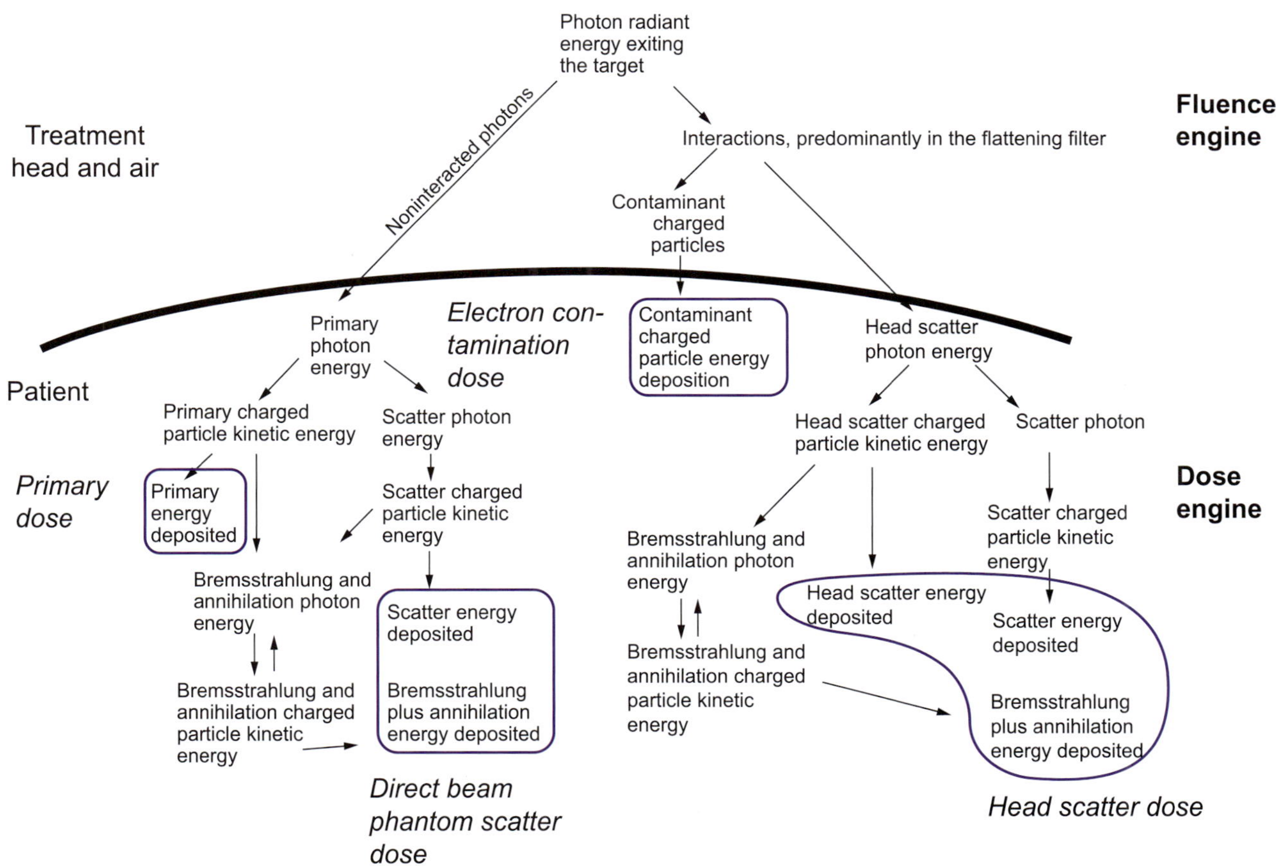

Fig. 12.1 The physical processes to be modelled in megavoltage MV photon beams. From these, the different components of dose are classified: primary dose, phantom scatter dose, head scatter dose and dose from contaminant electrons. The physical processes taking place in the treatment head are modelled by the fluence engine, whereas the physical processes in the patient are modelled by the dose engine. (From Ahnesjö A, Aspradakis MM. Dose calculations for external photon beams in radiotherapy. *Phys Med Biol.* 1999;44[11]:R99–R155. With permission.)

From these processes the different components of dose are classified. These are primary dose, phantom scatter dose, head scatter dose and dose from contaminant electrons. The physical processes taking place in the treatment head are modelled by the fluence engine, whereas the physical processes in the patient are modelled by the dose engine.[26]

Modelling the dose in the patient is a two-step process. In the first step, referred to as *energy fluence modelling*, the energy fluence reaching the patient surface is calculated. This is the distribution of the number of photons with a particular energy leaving the treatment head. In the second step, *dose modelling*, this energy fluence is transported and energy is deposited in the patient. Mathematically the combination of the two steps is described as the multiplication of two factors[27]:

$$\frac{D(x,d;A)}{M(A)} = \frac{D(x,d;A)}{\Psi(x;A)} \cdot \frac{\Psi(x;A)}{M(A)} \quad \textbf{(12.1)}$$

where D is the dose, x is an arbitrary calculation point, d is the treatment depth, A is the beam aperture, M is the monitor signal from the accelerator and Ψ is the energy fluence (Fig. 12.2). The first factor on the right-hand side in Eq. (12.1) is the absorbed dose in the patient per energy fluence from direct photons at the plane of the isocentre in air, and this is the outcome of dose modelling. The second factor in the equation is the calibration of the dose engine. Dose engines refer to the mathematical models that characterise and model particle transport and energy deposition in the irradiated medium. So, the second factor is the relationship between direct energy fluence and the signal from the monitor chamber of the linear accelerator under reference irradiation conditions. The following sections provide some insight into fluence and dose engines as well as the calculation of monitor units (MUs) as implemented in modern TPSs.

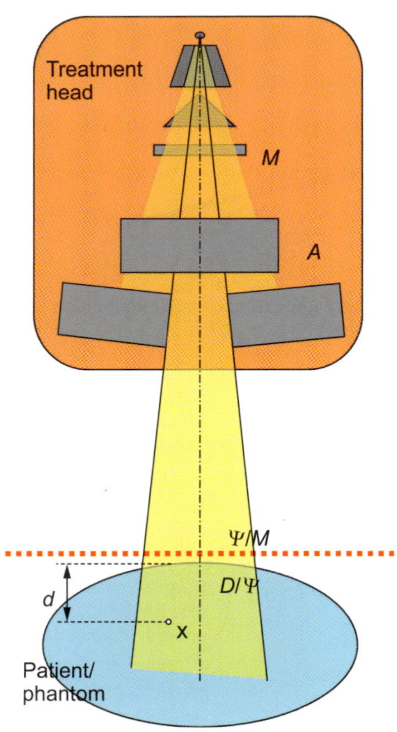

Fig. 12.2 Illustration of the separation of energy fluence modelling and dose modelling. (From Vassiliev ON, Wareing TA, McGhee J, Failla G, Salehpour MR, Mourtada F. Validation of a new grid-based Boltzmann equation solver for dose calculation in radiotherapy with photon beams. *Phys Med Biol.* 2010;55[3]:581–598. With permission.)

Modelling of the Source of Radiation

The radiation reaching the patient surface comprises of primary and extra-focal radiation. Primary radiation originates directly from the primary source, which for linear accelerators operating in photon mode, is the target. Extra-focal radiation, also referred to as head-scattered photon radiation, is the radiation that is scattered from the flattening filter, primary collimator, secondary jaws, physical wedges and multi-leaf collimators (MLCs). Extra-focal radiation can amount to 10% of the total radiation reaching the isocentre at the largest collimator setting, and 12% of this can originate from the flattening filter alone.

An energy fluence engine needs to model the finite size of the radiation source, geometrical penumbra, all sources of head-scattered radiation, the backscatter into the monitor ionisation chamber, leakage radiation from collimating devices, transmission between MLC leaves, transmission through the rounded MLC ends and changes in beam spectrum and electron contamination in the photon beam. The design of such an engine needs to be flexible and tailored to different designs of treatment heads and easily configurable using a small amount of measured data.

Energy fluence engines provide the number, energy and location of particles that reach the patient. With Monte Carlo (MC) methods, the total photon energy fluence and contaminant electron fluence exiting the head of the accelerator can be modelled explicitly. In practice, it has proved efficient and sufficient to implement what are known as *multisource beam models* instead. In these models, different parts of the treatment head are handled as different sources of scattered photons, which can be modelled separately. The algorithms modelling each of these sources implement semianalytical functions to describe the separate physical processes that take place when primary particles interact with different components in the treatment head. The parameters of these functions are typically derived through processes that minimise the differences between measured and calculated data under predefined irradiation conditions. The main source of head-scattered photon radiation is the flattening filter. Charged-particle contamination in high-energy photon beams is usually handled as a separate effect. Modelling the finite size of the direct radiation beam exiting the target, for example, becomes important at narrow collimated fields, where the field size becomes comparable to the size of the source and this influences both beam output and the shape of the penumbra profile.[28,29] Multisource beam models and the consideration of effects such as transmission from the ends and edges of MLC leaves differ among TPSs, and there are only a few scientific publications and TPS manuals that describe these in detail.[26,27,30]

Modelling of Dose in the Irradiated Medium

Dose engines, which mathematically model particle transport and energy deposition in the irradiated medium, are classified into two categories (Table 12.2): factor based and model based. It is the methods in the second category that are of interest nowadays and are discussed in more detail in this chapter.

Explicit Dose Modelling

In explicit dose modelling, the paths, interactions and location of energy deposition from particles traversing the irradiated medium are simulated in detail. These are calculations from first principles and with few approximations to radiation transport physics.

The radiation transport problem is described by the radiation transport equation, also known as the Boltzmann transport equation (BTE). The equation is mathematically established by considering energy conservation when particles traverse a small volume, and it separately addresses the number of particles entering and

TABLE 12.2 **Classification of Dose Engines**

Category	Method	Modelling Approach	Characteristics/Remarks
Factor-based	**Empirical**	Based on broad-beam measured data stored as fan-line matrices divergent from a point source	Implemented together with sector integration methods to model scatter dose in irregular fields together with one-, two-, or three-dimensional heterogeneity corrections
Model based	**Explicit modelling** of secondary particle transport and interaction	Deterministic solvers to the Boltzmann transport equation	Accurate approaches; distributions tend to be influenced from discretisation effects. Only one type of this method is available on a commercial treatment planning system (Eclipse Acuros).
		Stochastic approaches based on the Monte Carlo method	Accurate approaches; distributions tend to be noisy.
	Implicit modelling kernel–based approaches	Pencil beam kernel convolution methods	Not accurate in heterogeneous media. Ideally suited for optimisation calculations and second checks.
		Point kernel methods (superposition/ collapsed cone approaches)	Accurate in heterogeneous media, with limitations at media interfaces and high-density media. These are the current workhorses in treatment planning calculations.
		Hybrid approaches: finite-size pencil beam with lateral scattering	Performance analogous to that of point kernel methods. Only one type of this approach is implemented on a commercial treatment planning system (Eclipse AAA).

leaving this volume and being attenuated or generated in the volume. The equation provides a deterministic solution for the calculation of the total number of particles at a given energy and direction and referred to as differential particle fluence in the irradiated medium. For the radiation transport problem in photon dose modelling, it is assumed that positrons can be treated as electrons, bremsstrahlung radiation is neglected and photons transported in the medium are treated as either primary or scattered photons.

Once the primary energy fluence reaching the patient is computed by the multisource fluence engine, photons are ray-traced in the irradiated medium. The medium is divided into a grid matrix of calculation points, and particle transport equations are solved for this grid so that the electron fluence is calculated. The multiplication of electron fluence with appropriate stopping powers gives the dose deposited at each point on the grid. At the time of this writing, only one commercial TPS offers this approach for external photon beam and brachytherapy planning.[31–33]

An alternative to solving the BTE is the stochastic approach based on the MC method.[34,35] This is a numerical method where pseudo-random numbers are used to sample from probability functions that describe physical processes. Input data to probability distributions are radiation attenuation data and particle interaction cross sections.

A detailed description of the irradiation geometry is required, and sampling of the cross-section data determines the type of interaction that each particle will undergo.

With the MC method, modelling the transport of photons is more straightforward than for electrons. Photons undergo fewer interactions than electrons as they traverse media. Electrons undergo on the order of 10,000 interaction events for an electron with energy of 1 MeV. Modelling electron transport involves the use of special modelling techniques. These consider many electron transport steps or interactions in groups of fewer events and are necessary to achieve realistic computation times. Variance reduction techniques are employed to practically implement techniques based on the MC method for radiation dosimetry and TP applications. These are computational methods to reduce the uncertainty in the results, with the aim to increase efficiency in the simulation while faithfully addressing all involved physical processes. Energy thresholds are set below which particles are halted and the energy is deposited locally. The implementation of appropriate electron transport physics and of variance reduction techniques differs between implementations of MC dose engines for TP.

Keeping track of the location of each particle in relation to the irradiation geometry and its energy in comparison to the energy thresholds defined for the simulation is essential for calculation of a dose distribution. During the simulation, the following properties are assigned to each particle: its type, energy, location and direction of travel. A further assigned property is weight, which relates to the contribution and importance of the particle in the simulation as a result of the different variance reduction techniques employed. In an MC simulation, random numbers are generated and used to transport a particle and determine the position where the next interaction will occur. The next type of interaction is subsequently generated, and for each particle originating from this event, its properties (energy, position, direction and weight) are stored. Particles are placed on a priority list, called the *stack*, and the simulation continues for each particle on the stack until the particle leaves the medium or until the energy of the secondary electrons produced is less than a specific threshold; in this case, further transport of this particle stops and its energy is deposited at that location. As one can imagine, the number of simulated events is enormous, requiring substantial computing power.

Implicit Dose Modelling: Kernel-Based Approaches

Implicit solutions to the radiation transport problem are known as *kernel-based* methods. These use precomputed data, the *energy deposition kernels (EDKs)*, which describe the spatial distribution of the expectation value for the energy deposition caused by an elemental beam in water. EDKs are classified into different types, with the most common being the point kernels and the pencil kernels. Point kernels describe the energy distribution from monoenergetic photons forced to interact at a given location, which is usually at the centre of a homogeneous water medium. Point kernels are calculated from simulations using the MC method.[36] They can be separated into different components depending on the interaction history of particles. The primary dose component results from energy deposited by the first-scattered charged particles, and the scattered dose component originates from first-scattered photons and their descendants.

Pencil kernels describe the distribution of energy in a semiinfinite homogeneous medium from a monodirectional photon beam which is an infinitesimally narrow monoenergetic beam (Fig. 12.3). There are several ways to compute pencil kernels. One way is through simulations

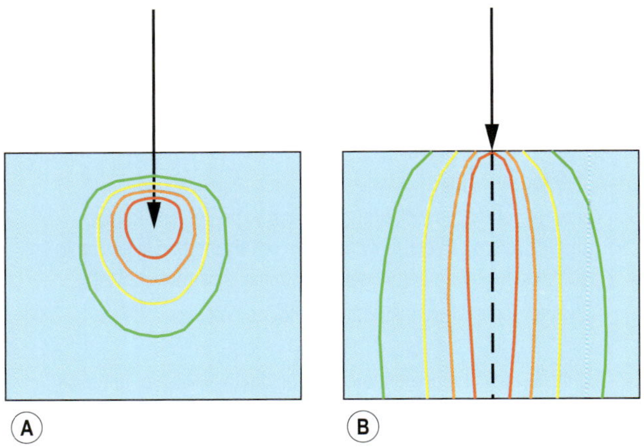

Fig. 12.3 The most common types of energy deposition kernels: (A) point kernel; (B) pencil kernel. (From Ahnesjö A, Aspradakis MM. Dose calculations for external photon beams in radiotherapy. *Phys Med Biol.* 1999;44(11):R99–R155.)

using the MC method or from an integration of point kernels along the direction of the pencil beam. Other methods use radial differentiation of measured scatter functions, or deconvolution of measured dose profiles, or curve fitting to kernels originally generated with the MC method. The latter approach has been recently extended so that the fitting parameters can be obtained as a function of a single beam parameter, the beam quality index, which is the tissue phantom ratio at the depth of 20 cm and 10 cm in water TPR.[10,20,37]

It is important to clarify the difference between two common terms that appear similar but have different meanings: *pencil beams* and *beamlets*. Pencil beams result in dose distributions from a monodirectional, infinitesimally narrow beam. That is a beam of zero area, and this is not the same as a beamlet. A beamlet is a *finite-size pencil beam (FSPB)* that is very small in cross section. By *small beam*, one typically refers to beams with an area greater than that of a beamlet and less than 3 × 3 cm.

Pencil Beam Models. In pencil beam methods, the dose is calculated from the convolution of the two-dimensional energy fluence with the pencil beam kernel over the area of the beam aperture (Fig. 12.4).

This convolution is straightforward for uniform circular beams. In the case of rectangular and irregular field apertures, the field can be divided into sectors of constant energy fluence over the sector area. Pencil beam convolution can be executed using fast convolution algorithms, such as Fast Fourier Transform (FFT). Such an implementation is only appropriate in a homogenous medium, when the pencil kernel is assumed to be laterally invariant and when changes of the energy spectrum off-axis (*off-axis softening*) are ignored. To account for heterogeneities, pencil beam models incorporate scaling of the pencil kernel with changes in the medium density, usually in two dimensions, along the kernel axis and off-axis position at the depth of the calculation point. A correction for off-axis spectral variations is possible in principle, but it differs among implementations of this model. If ignored, it can lead to errors in dose calculations up to 5% at large off-axis distances.[27]

Point Kernel Models. Point kernel models, also known as *convolution/superposition models*, calculate dose from the integration of point kernels with the total energy released through primary photon interactions per unit mass, or Terma (T), in the irradiated medium.[38–40] Terma includes the energy imparted to both charged particles and scattered photons; in other words, it is the energy lost or removed from the primary beam per unit mass. Before performing the integration, these models first calculate Terma. Terma is calculated by tracing and attenuating the incident photon energy fluence along rays of transport in the three-dimensional calculation volume. Once Terma at each voxel is known, point kernels are weighted by their value and the dose distribution is then calculated from an integration over the entire three-dimensional matrix (Fig. 12.5).

The advantage of these approaches is that they enable a complete three-dimensional modelling of the energy deposition process. Important modelling considerations that can introduce approximations include beam divergence, beam hardening, off-axis softening and electron contamination. These approximations differ between commercial TPSs.

To model beam divergence accurately, point kernels need to be tilted to be aligned with the divergent path of primary photons as they are transported in the medium. The polyenergetic nature of the megavoltage photon beam is taken into account from the knowledge of the beam spectrum and from an additional integration over this. Some TPSs use published generic beam spectra as an approximation of the clinical beam, but most derive an estimate of the clinical spectrum through an optimisation procedure, which minimises the difference between measured and calculated depth-dose data for a range of field sizes. The spectrum is used for the calculation of a polyenergetic Terma and kernels. As with pencil beam models, spectral changes laterally can be modelled by taking into consideration the variation off-axis of the mass attenuation coefficient.

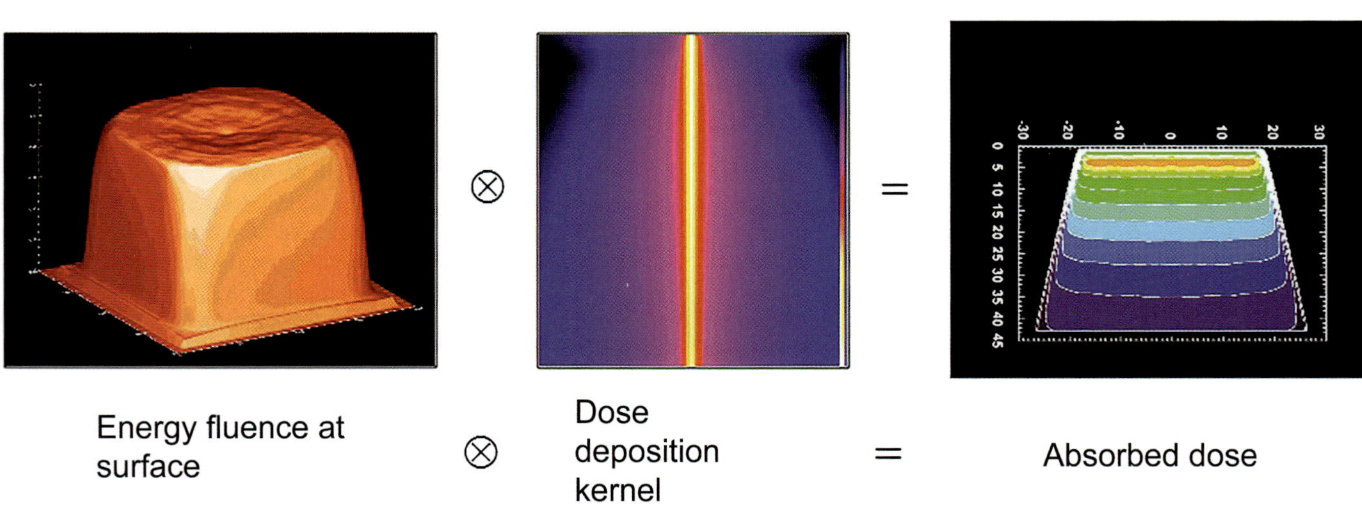

Fig. 12.4 Pencil beam model showing the convolution of energy fluence with a pencil beam kernel.

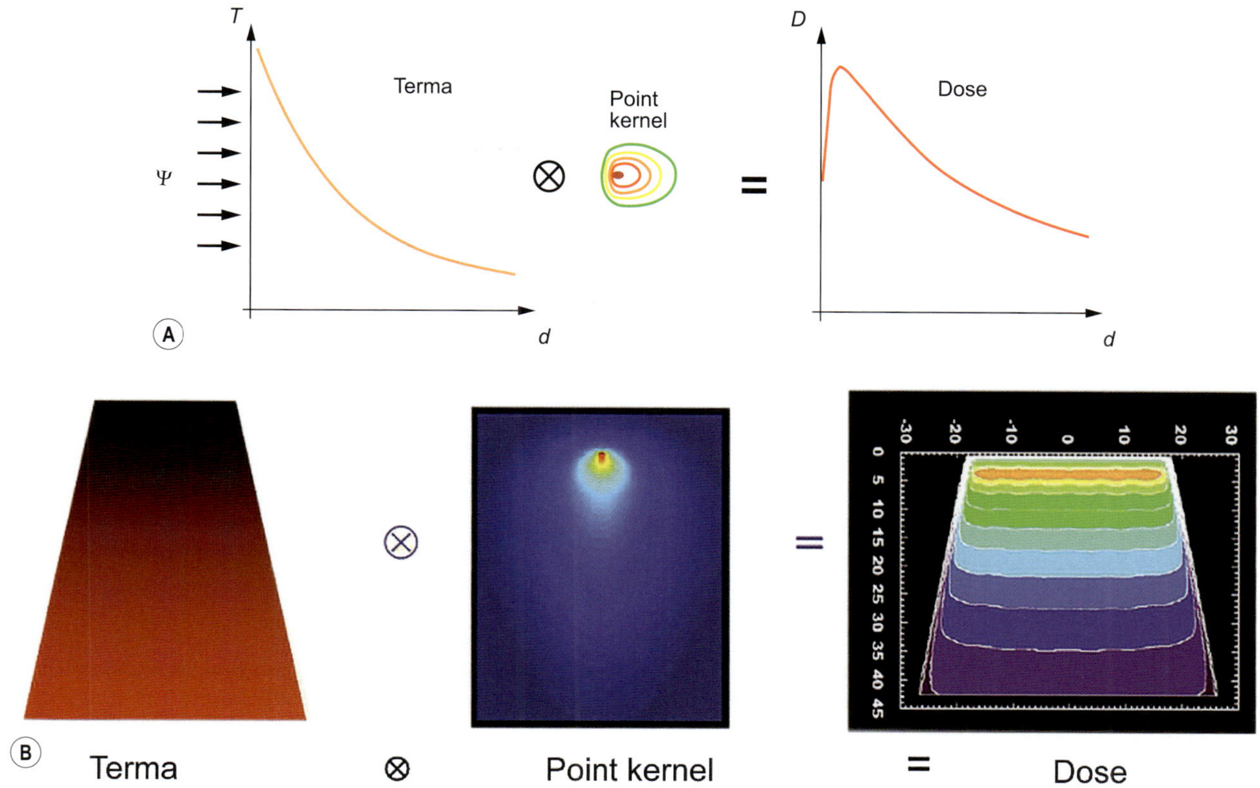

Fig. 12.5 Illustration of the convolution of Terma and a point kernel in one and two dimensions: along the depth (A) and on a plane (B). (From Vassiliev ON, Wareing TA, McGhee J, Failla G, Salehpour MR, Mourtada F. Validation of a new grid-based Boltzmann equation solver for dose calculation in radiotherapy with photon beams. *Phys Med Biol.* 2010;55[3]:581–598. With permission.)

In MV photon beams, there is electron contamination originating from the flattening filter, monitor chamber, collimator and air. For contributions to dose in the build-up region from the contaminant particles, kernel-based approaches incorporate a separate model. Contaminant electrons can be dealt with as an additional source in the multisource model or can be modelled from a separate dose engine using pencil kernels that describe the change of dose from contaminant electrons laterally and with increasing depth.

The heterogeneous and finite nature of the patient is more accurately accounted for in point kernel models than in pencil beam models because scaling of Terma with changes in medium density is possible along the path of transport of primary photons, and rectilinear scaling of point kernels with variations in density between points of interaction and energy deposition can be performed in three dimensions, thus taking full advantage of the available three-dimensional information from CT data sets.

A challenge in the implementation of superposition models in the clinical environment has been the reduction in computation time to perform all numerical operations for the direct summation of the energy deposited in each voxel by each other voxel in three dimensions. Superposition may offer high accuracy in the calculation of dose, but it is time-consuming. FFT techniques can be employed, but these require that point kernels remain spatially invariant and cannot be scaled with density variations. This is not sufficiently accurate for modelling dose in heterogeneous media. As a compromise between accuracy and speed of calculation, approaches have been developed in which the resolution of the dose matrix is varied depending on the gradients present in the Terma matrix. The most common approach, however, has been the collapsed cone approximation.[41] With this, the space around a point kernel is discretised into cones, and energy is transported and deposited only along the axis of these cones. To calculate the dose deposited in the medium, one integrates energy contributions along transport directions that are aligned with the axes of several cones. With the collapsed cone approach, the numerical operations are proportional to the total number of voxels in the dose calculation matrix multiplied by the number of transport directions chosen for the calculations (Fig. 12.6).

Finite-Size Pencil Beam Models. In FSPB models, the beam aperture is divided into small beams of identical, finite cross sections over which energy fluence is considered constant.[42] FSPBs are precomputed, usually from pencil kernels calculated using the MC method. FSPB-based models sum up contributions from individual FSPBs weighted by the incident energy fluence. The best-known implementation of this approach is the analytic anisotropic algorithm (AAA). In the AAA model of Varian's Eclipse TPS, the FSPB kernels are represented by an analytical fit to a weighted sum of four Gaussian distributions, and this implementation reduces computation time.[43,44] Beam divergence, depth hardening, off-axis softening and electron contamination are taken into consideration similar to point kernel models. Because FSPB kernels are scaled with density variations along the axis of the FSPB as well as laterally, the performance in terms of dose accuracy of the AAA in heterogeneous media is better than pencil beam models and comparable to that of superposition/collapsed cone approaches.

Factor-Based Approaches

Traditionally, dose calculations for high-energy photon beams were entirely based on the use of large sets of stored measured data such as percentage depth doses, profiles, tissue-to-air ratios, tissue-to-phantom

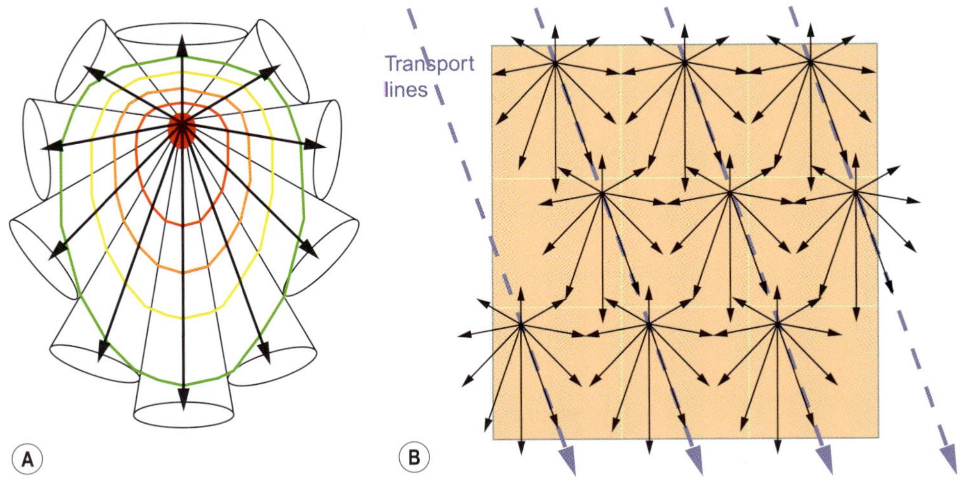

Fig. 12.6 Illustration of the collapsed cone approximation. (A) The point kernel is divided into cones. (B) Superposition is performed along transport lines aligned with the axis of each cone. (From Vassiliev ON, Wareing TA, McGhee J, Failla G, Salehpour MR, Mourtada F. Validation of a new grid-based Boltzmann equation solver for dose calculation in radiotherapy with photon beams. *Phys Med Biol.* 2010;55[3]:581–598. With permission.)

ratios and so on. Dose was calculated from the multiplication of a series of factors, each of which described a change in the dose with a change of a parameter in the irradiation geometry, such as depth or field size, from that under reference conditions.[45–48] These methods are classified as factor-based or broad-beam data–based models where some factors were derived directly by interpolation from the stored data or from simple modelling, if possible. Additional algorithms were needed to provide an estimate of the dose in heterogeneous media. Typically, the stored data corresponded to collimator settings down to 4 × 4 cm. Factor-based approaches have been used extensively in TP for conformal RT where the aim is to encompass the planning target by a homogeneous dose and where the penumbra is not contributing to the dose in the target. They have limited application when it comes to the accurate prediction of dose from complex irradiations, which differ substantially from those during the measurement of the input data. In complex irradiation geometries such as in intensity modulated radiotherapy (IMRT), beam portals comprise many narrow collimated beams, and in these cases it is often desirable to plan an inhomogeneous dose distribution to the target volume. To accurately compute the dose in such cases, it becomes important to model the beam penumbra, the influence of collimating devices such as MLCs and/or the occlusion of the direct beam source.

Factor-based approaches are ideally suited to the calculation of dose at a point on the central axis with an irradiation geometry not substantially different from that in which the measured data were acquired. These methods may still play a role as a secondary independent method for the verification of dose at a point, but they are no longer implemented in modern TPSs.

Conclusion on Model-Based Approaches

Accuracy in the calculation of dose in homogeneous and heterogeneous media has been the subject of many investigations and comparisons. One can conclude that the most accurate approaches are those based on the MC method and the deterministic solution of the BTE. However, the workhorses in TP calculations are (1) point kernel models using superposition and collapsed cone approaches and (2) the AAA method based on an FSPB approach. These are less accurate in computing dose in the build-up region, media interfaces and high-density media in comparison to the solutions based on the MC method and the deterministic solutions, but they are more accurate than pencil beam models in computing dose in heterogeneous media. They are more computationally intensive than pencil beam models but are fast enough to be used in the clinical routine.

Nevertheless pencil beam models have an important role in RT planning. They are used in plan optimisation engines during inverse planning and for independent dose calculations as part of plan-specific quality assurance (PSQA). In addition, they are being implemented in software tools together with complex detector systems designed specifically for the verification of IMRT and volumetric modulated arc therapy (VMAT) treatment plans as part of pretreatment QA.

Dose per Monitor Unit Formalism

The outcome of any explicit or implicit dose calculation model is essentially dose per amount of incident radiation (Fig. 12.1). LINACs are calibrated to a given dose per Monitor Unit (MU) under reference conditions. The MU is the signal derived from the full-field ionisation chamber in the radiation head of a megavoltage treatment machine, referred to as Channel 1 (see Chapter 10). This calibration has traditionally been 1 cGy/MU at the depth of maximum build-up, at a source to surface distance (SSD) of 100 cm and a field size of 10 × 10 cm, but it may be at a 5- or 10-cm depth with SSD of 95 cm and 90 cm, respectively, with a 10 × 10 collimator setting. Thus, for model-based dose engines to calculate MUs, it is necessary to calibrate the dose engine by measurement and determine the relationship between incident radiation under reference conditions and MU.

The approach used to calibrate dose engines varies among TPSs. Strictly, an additional model is needed to account for the effects of backscattered radiation into the monitor chamber at different collimator settings.[3,26,35] Depending on the design of the LINAC head and its monitor chamber, the signal from the chamber can be affected from particles which have backscattered from the upper part of the collimator system into the chamber. For collimator settings narrower than 10 × 10 cm, the amount of backscattered radiation into the monitor chamber increases, influencing the signal of the monitor chamber so that the chamber would reach its preset value more quickly, leading to a decrease in relative output. At collimator settings greater than 10 × 10 cm, the amount of backscattered radiation is less that than at 10 × 10 cm, leading to an increase in relative output. In factor-based approaches, this effect is inherently accounted for in the measured data using measured total output and in air output factors. Most commercial TPSs with model-based dose engines do not explicitly consider this effect. The increase can be on the order of 2%

at a 40 × 40 cm field and is approximately accounted for with a correction factor derived from a limited set of measured output factors.

TREATMENT PLANNING TECHNIQUES IN EXTERNAL MV PHOTON BEAM RADIOTHERAPY

This section concerns treatment planning with megavoltage photon beams generated by linear accelerators. The terminology of forward and inverse planning applies to the planning process of any type of beam arrangement and to treatment planning with photons, electrons or protons. Forward planning has been the tradition for many years and is what RT clinical experience has been built upon. Basically, from a knowledge of the beam characteristics in terms of field size, depth dose and even intensity modulation with wedges (Chapter 10) and compensators, the dose planner would iteratively devise a treatment beam arrangement that can deliver the prescribed dose.

In inverse planning, one starts with the required dose distribution and finds the beam delivery method to achieve this. Inverse planning was introduced together with the concept of IMRT and the use of computer optimisation algorithms to predict an optimal radiation pattern.[49,50] Since the introduction of inverse planning in the early 1980s on a racetrack microtron and of MLCs for beam shaping,[51–53] an enormous technical effort led to the development of software and hardware to enable the MLC to modulate the beam intensity.[54,55] The individual treatment beams for IMRT can be delivered with MLC in either dynamic mode or multiple-segment mode, also called *step and shoot*. There are advantages and disadvantages to each method; however, both methods require the intensity of each beam profile to be determined to deliver the intended dose to the target, normal tissue and critical structures. In Volumetric Modulated Arc Therapy (VMAT), there are more degrees of freedom available to the optimisation software to generate dose distributions, through simultaneous changes in MLC, gantry position and beam dose rate.

The inverse planning process requires sophisticated computational algorithms involving a variety of control theory–type processes. In inverse planning, it is necessary that the planner has the understanding and skill to steer the optimisation software to reach meaningful results for the various clinical sites and individual clinical situations. The number of possible solutions for the delivery is theoretically infinite. However, there are some limiting aspects dictated primarily by the design of the machine and MLC hardware: the width of the leaves, minimum separation between opposing leaves, leaf speed and speed of rotation of the gantry. These can be taken into account in the computation, but the planner brings an overview which is essential to control the inverse planning process and obtain a robust solution.

Forward Planning With Standard Beam Arrangements

An enormous amount of clinical practice, knowledge and treatment grew from the many years of forward, three-dimensional and conformal radiotherapy planning. This clinical experience is still relevant today with regard to the management of patients and practical delivery of treatment. It also provides simple solutions where that may be appropriate. This section does not attempt to provide a comprehensive atlas of treatment plans or an in-depth planning guidance for each site but uses a few clinical examples to demonstrate forward planning techniques.

The first step in preparing a plan is to decide on the position of the isocentre. Although the centre of the PTV might appear to be the best location, in practice it may be preferable to set the isocentre to predefined skin marks which have been set at the time of CT scanning. The skin marks will have been chosen to lie on a stable skin location, perhaps at a standard anatomical point or height above the couch and avoiding steep body contour gradients. This results in a simpler and safer setup and the fields may then be aligned to the PTV by asymmetric collimator settings.

Another strategy is to select the isocentre position based on the internal anatomy of either the PTV or adjacent critical structures. This can minimise the dose to critical structures by eliminating beam divergence without complicating the field arrangement. Examples are breast treatments without the beams diverging into the lung or abutting nodal fields, or brain treatments avoiding beam edges diverging into critical structures such as the lens of the eye. Another aspect regarding choice of internal anatomy relates to the dose computation algorithm and placement of the isocentre in solid material and not in an air cavity so as to improve the dose prediction accuracy at that point for checking.

The beam energy is chosen by considering the depth of maximum build-up, d_{max}, and the penetration properties of the beam. Table 12.3 shows typical values for commonly used energies. Low-energy beams (4–6 MV) are suited to more superficial volumes such as head and neck PTVs, whereas deep pelvic PTVs will require energies between 10 and 20 MV. Beam energies above 15 MV do not give a great benefit to the planner, but their frequent use on a LINAC can introduce radiation protection problems because of neutron production.

The build-up region is a significant feature of the MV beam in that it gives skin sparing, allowing doses that would severely damage the skin to be delivered deep into the patient. However, a PTV which extends from near the surface to a depth treated with MV photons may require bolus to be added to the skin. By placing this tissue-equivalent material on the skin, the build-up region is shifted into the bolus and the maximum dose of the beam is delivered onto or near the skin. Unless the PTV is superficial, the planner should consider the impact of patient immobilisation devices acting as build-up and increasing the surface dose.

Standard field arrangements may be modified for specific patient situations such as metal hip implants. Here, it is preferable to avoid beams entering through the implant, so a three-field arrangement must be modified such as that shown in Fig. 12.7.

ICRU Reports 50 and 62 describe the requirements for dose prescription and reporting in three-dimensional conformal radiotherapy planning. Dose is prescribed at the ICRU reference point located at the centre of the PTV and onto or close to the beam central axis, and a minimum

TABLE 12.3 Typical Depth-Dose Characteristics for 10 × 10 cm² Radiotherapy Beams

X-ray Energy	Source-to-Surface Distance (cm)	D_{max} Depth (cm)	$D_{80\%}$ (cm)	Dose at 10 cm (% of D_{max})
60 kV	30	0	0.5	2
100 kV	30	0	1.0	10
220 kV	50	0	2.5	29
4 MV	100	1.0	5.9	63.0
6 MV	100	1.5	6.7	67.5
10 MV	100	2.3	8.0	73.0
15 MV	100	2.9	9.1	77.0
25 MV	100	3.8	10.9	83.0
Electron Energy (MeV)				
4	95	0.9	1.4	1
6	95	1.3	1.9	1
10	95	2.2	3.2	1
15	95	2.6	4.9	3
20	95	2.6	6.7	10

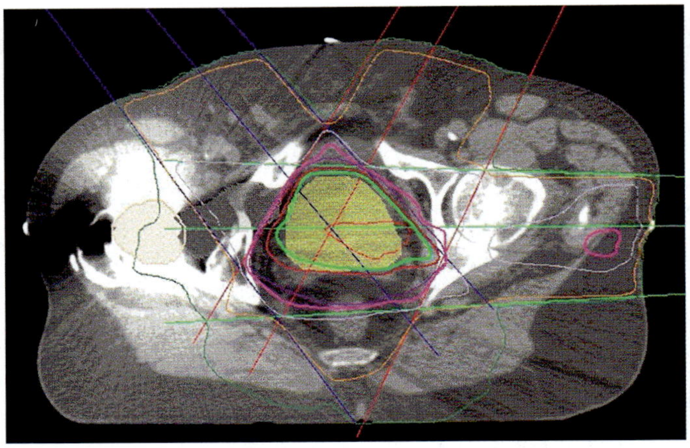

Fig. 12.7 Modified three-field beam arrangement to avoid prosthesis.

requirement is to report the minimum and maximum doses to the PTV as well as the maximum dose to OARs and planning risk volumes (PRVs).

Single Fields

Most plans are based on the intersecting of multiple field paths to create a high-dose region, but single fields may sometimes be the ideal choice, especially for superficial PTVs. The spine can be treated with a single posterior field, although this will usually be done as part of a multifield arrangement to treat the whole central nervous system (CNS), see Fig. 12.18 for example. To cover a PTV length of greater than 40 cm, the field may need to be treated at an extended SSD and with the isocentre positioned off the skin surface as shown in Fig. 12.8. To produce a uniform dose to the cord lying at varying depths, a compensator may be employed, but the most efficient technique is to use top-up fields, all centred on a single isocentre, delivering a few MUs to otherwise underdosed sections of the PTV.

Turned Wedges

Wedges are usually most beneficial with the wedge in the plane of the plan which is usually the transverse patient plane. However, if the patient contour varies out of this plane, a turned or longitudinal wedge may be required to produce an even dose in the superior–inferior direction. This may be accomplished by overlying two fields with identical dimensions but with the collimator rotated 90 degrees. For multibeam plans, it may be possible to achieve uniform dose with a single turned wedge on one field only.

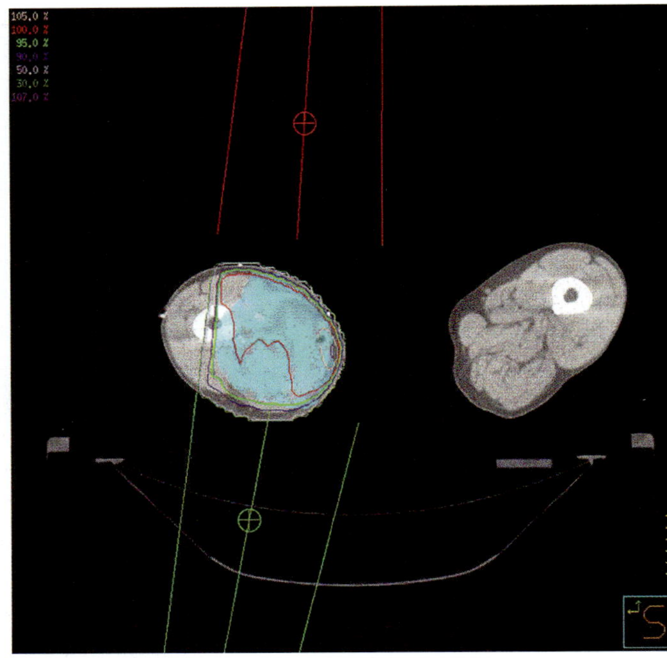

Fig. 12.8 Sarcoma with parallel opposed field and with isocentres outside the target.

Parallel Opposed Fields

The typical isodose distribution arising from a parallel opposed field is shown in Fig. 12.9. If the separation is not too great for the available beam energy, a dose range of +7% to −5% is perhaps just achievable. The high-dose regions may present a problem at wide separations, and the hourglass-shaped contour at about the 90% to 95% level may result in unacceptably low doses at the midplane of the volume. Wedges may be employed where the contour slopes or internal heterogeneities are present, and the use of shielding can produce irregular dose distributions conforming to complex PTV shapes. Clinical applications include large pelvis volumes and whole-brain treatments. For parallel opposed treatments and direct single fields, a treatment plan is unnecessary and the MU required for individual beams is usually obtained by a manual calculation. Manual calculations are undertaken using tabulated beam data such as depth dose, tissue phantom factors (TPRs), output factors, SSDs, tray factors and if necessary wedge factors.

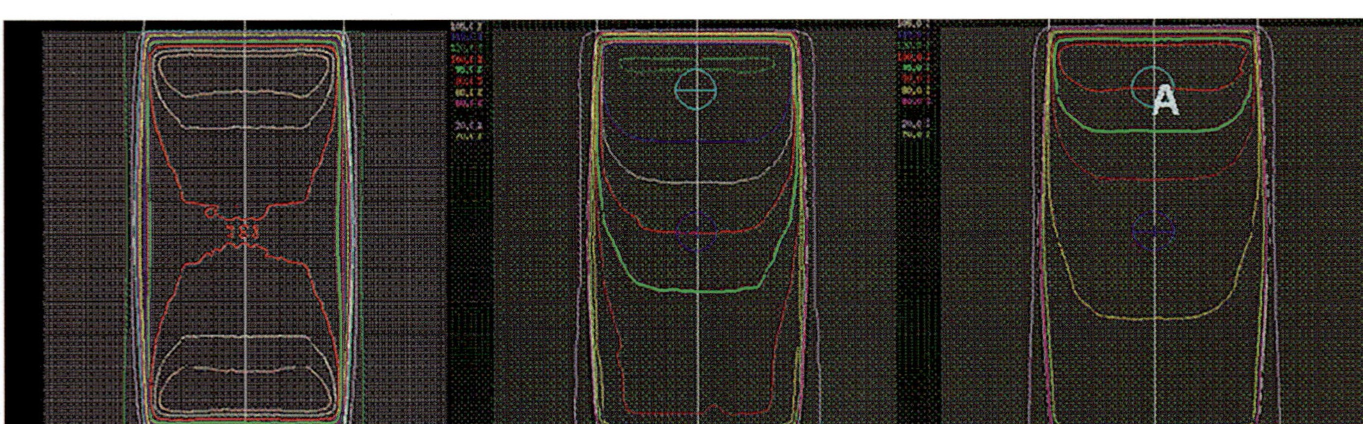

Fig. 12.9 Isodose distributions produced by parallel opposed beams. On the *left*, beams are equally weighted. In the *centre*, weighting is 2:1 at the midplane. On the right, weighting is 2:1 at point A.

Beams Weighted in 2:1 Ratio

The standard parallel opposed distribution can be modified to deliver a higher dose to one side of the PTV without resorting to a more complex plan. It must be clear what the plan request means by 2:1 weighting. For simple, manually calculated plans to deliver a specified dose to the midplane of the patient separation, it would usually mean that the ratio of MU set is 2:1. However, with computerised plans, a dose reference point may be positioned somewhere other than at the midplane depth, so it must be clear to which point the 2:1 ratio applies. The presence of heterogeneities further complicates the issue as the TPS may adjust the set MUs to deliver equal dose from each field to a point by compensating for the different densities each beam has traversed. This demonstrates the potential hazards arising from changing from basic manual calculations to CT-based dosimetry where a seemingly simple request for 2:1 weightings can take on several different interpretations (Fig. 12.9).

Breast Treatments

The breast can be treated with a parallel opposed pair, but the technique is generally refined to minimise lung dose by creating a non-diverging edge, either by fully asymmetric fields with the central axis along the field edge or by slightly angled fields such that the central axes are not parallel to one another but the back edges are (Fig. 12.10).

Wedges will usually be required to produce a uniform dose across the PTV by compensating for the missing tissue and the presence of lung. The PTV is normally defined during simulation or virtual simulation. The gantry angles are determined by the acceptable amount of lung in the field. For postmastectomy chest wall treatments, the contour shape combined with the significant presence of lung may result in open fields or even a wedge orientated with the thin end at the apex of the breast.

A beam of typically 5 or 6 MV is adequate for most breast treatments, but as the separation between the medial and lateral fields increases beyond about 22 cm, a higher-energy beam is required. The higher-energy beam results in reduced breast tissue coverage superficially because of the increased build-up depth, so it should be avoided unless essential.

Segmented fields can produce a more uniform dose, especially in larger or irregular outlines (Figs. 12.10B and C). Usually, a single segment on one field is sufficient to bring the dose range within ICRU 50 and ICRU 62 requirements. For left-sided breast treatments, it may be necessary to shield the heart.

Limb Sarcomas

Limb sarcomas are usually treated with two opposed fields slightly angled to produce a sharper dose gradient to maximise the drainage channel along the limb. The PTV is often greater than 40 cm long, and in that case extended SSD treatments are necessary for a standard LINAC. These require carefully described setup instructions (Fig. 12.8).

Wedged Pairs

For superficial PTVs that extend quite deep in tissue, the wedged pair can produce the optimum dose distribution (Fig. 12.11). Highly wedged beams are required to maintain a uniform dose across the depth of the PTV. A greater angle between the beams, called the *hinge angle*, tends to produce a more uniform dose gradient and may be necessary for deeper PTVs but is likely to increase normal tissue dose adjacent to the PTV. The exit doses from a two-field plan can be significant for critical structures, such as the mouth or spinal cord in parotid treatments, and sometimes a lightly weighted third field can be beneficial if the relative weighting of the two fields cannot be sufficiently adjusted to achieve the required dose distribution.

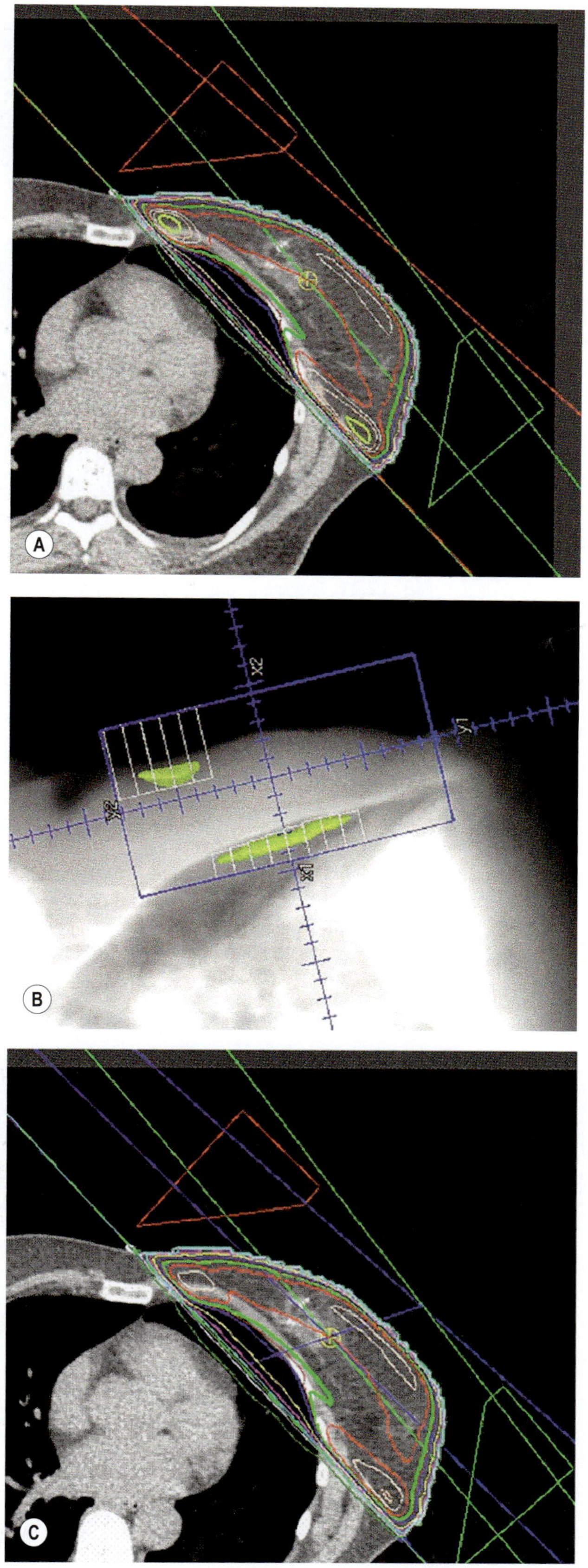

Fig. 12.10 Aspects to consider to produce a satisfactory dose distribution: (A) varying wedge angle and beam weights alone, which may not be satisfactory; (B) adding a segmented field with the high-dose regions shielded and the lower-dose regions thus boosted; and (C) introduction of a segmented field to enhance (A).

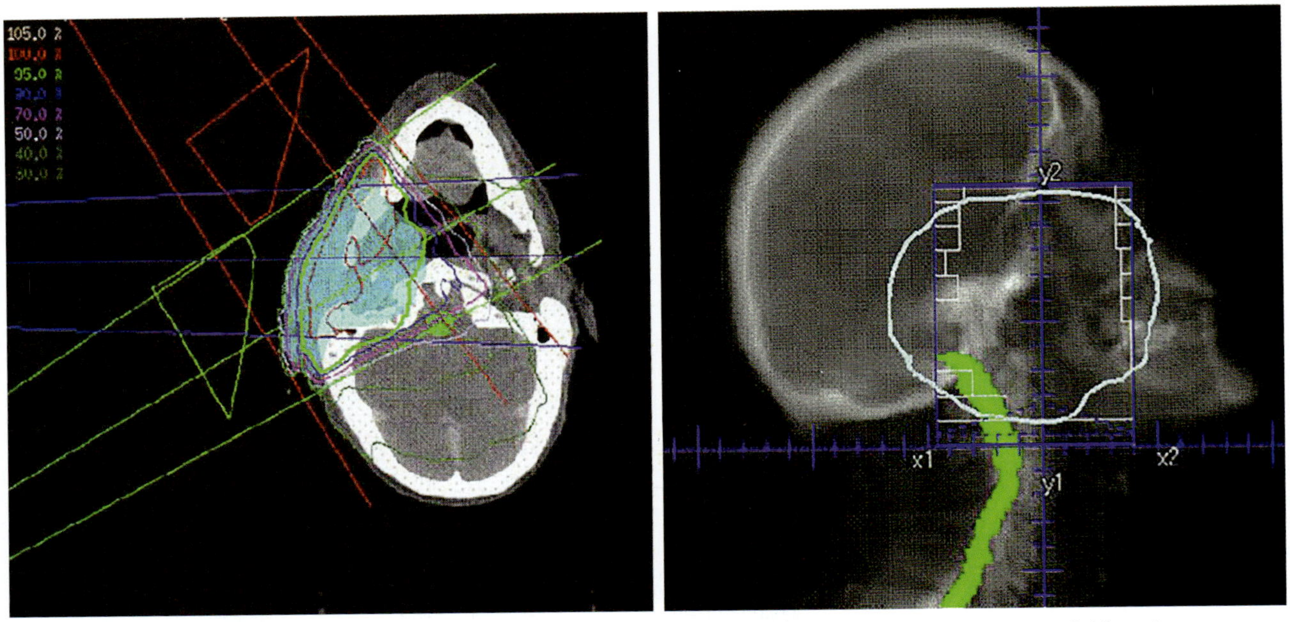

Fig. 12.11 The *left image* shows a transverse view of a wedged pair with a low weighted segment field used to boost the dose to part of the planning target volume *(shown in blue)*. The *right image* shows the beam's-eye view of the boost field showing partial shielding of the cord.

Multiple-Field Plans

For PTVs lying deeper in the patient, three or more fields with paths intersecting at the PTV usually offer the best dose distribution for the PTV while avoiding excessive dose to normal tissue. The clinically useful dose will normally only be delivered where all the beam paths overlap, unless complex inverse planning is employed or an intentional dose gradient is required inside the PTV. The field arrangement is designed to ensure that the treated volume conforms as closely as possible to the PTV as defined in ICRU 50 while complying with critical structure constraints and minimising the volume of normal tissue irradiated.

Pelvis Plans

Three fields will often be sufficient to deliver the required dose to the PTV while maintaining acceptably low normal tissue doses. Unless the PTV extends close to the surface (e.g. some rectum PTVs), a high energy (10 MV or more) is desirable. One posterior and two lateral fields, as shown in Fig. 12.12, represent a good starting point for a plan.

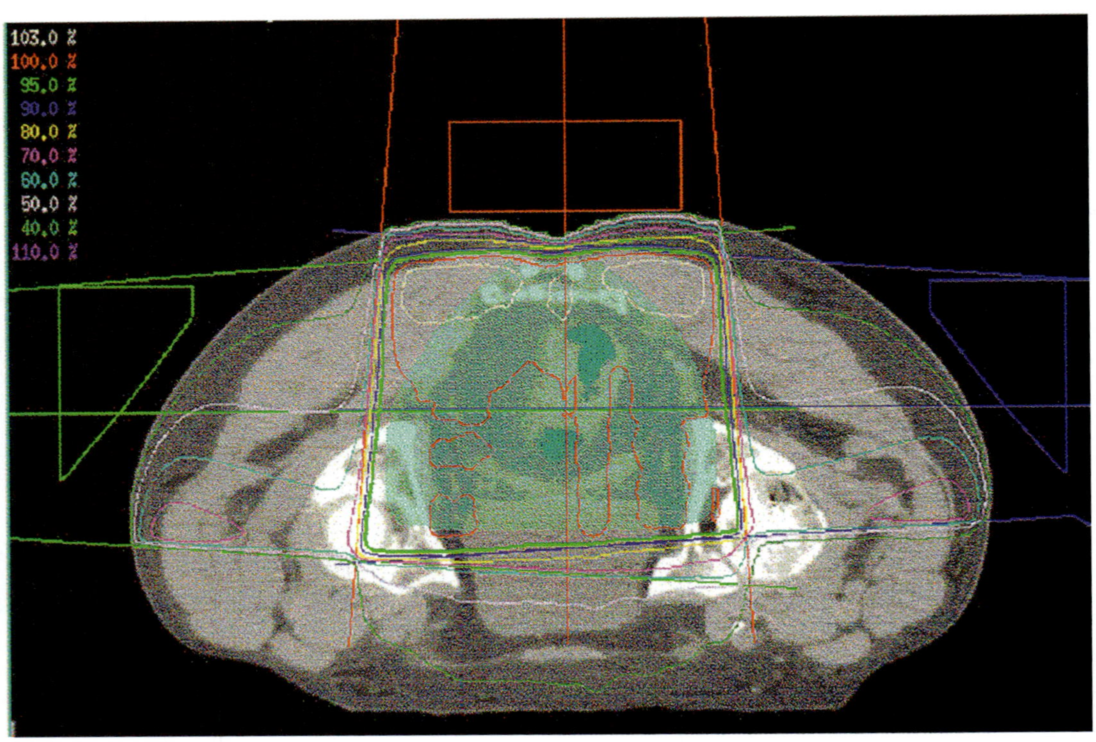

Fig. 12.12 Three-field rectum treatment.

The wedges on the lateral fields compensate for the falloff in dose from the posterior field and also the missing tissue because of the patient contour. The weightings are adjusted to obtain an acceptable PTV dose distribution while also considering the normal tissue doses in the beam entry path and, in this case, the beam exit path from the posterior field. The lateral maximum doses for typical pelvis patients may be around 80% of the PTV dose, or more for patients with a wide separation. The maximum dose that the posterior field contributes to normal tissue will usually be lower—typically 60% of the prescribed dose because of the presence of more radiosensitive structures within its entry and exit paths. Four fields may be required, especially for large volumes in large patients, a four-field box arrangement being the standard technique.

The lateral fields in the three-field plan may be angled posteriorly by up to 20 degrees or more. Angling posteriorly in a supine patient will produce a sharper dose gradient on the posterior PTV edge, which can reduce the dose to the adjacent critical structure, such as the rectum in the case of a prostate PTV. Angling the fields more posteriorly will reduce the normal tissue doses as the exit dose from one lateral dose will not contribute so much to the contralateral entrance dose. For some PTV shapes, a better conformality may be achieved with oblique angles, but in many cases, the rectum dose will be increased by the use of posterior oblique fields.

Thorax Plans

The optimum field arrangement will significantly depend on the location of the PTV in the chest. Three fields are usually required, although occasionally a parallel opposed pair is the best arrangement. Examples of bronchus PTV field arrangements are shown in Fig. 12.13. The cord dose tolerance must not be exceeded and the heart dose minimised where relevant. The total left and right lung volume must be outlined so that the dose distribution and irradiated volume can be correctly evaluated, for example, with a dose volume histogram, discussed later in this chapter. A field arrangement that minimises the lung volume irradiated should then be found usually by inspecting the volume of the lung receiving more than 20 Gy.

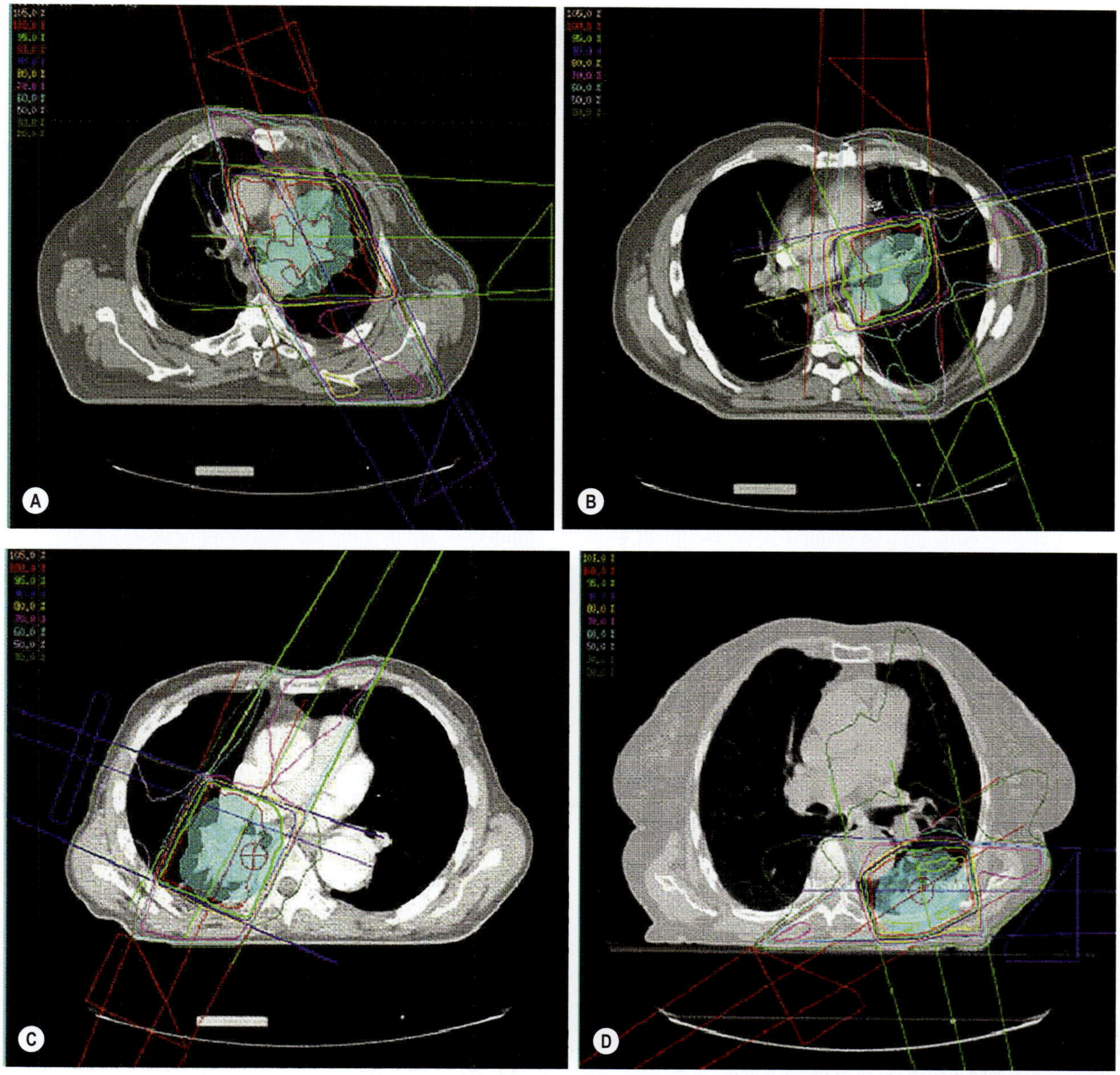

Fig. 12.13 Bronchus treatment ((A) to (D)), with segments used in the left anterior oblique (E) instead of a wedge (C).
(continued)

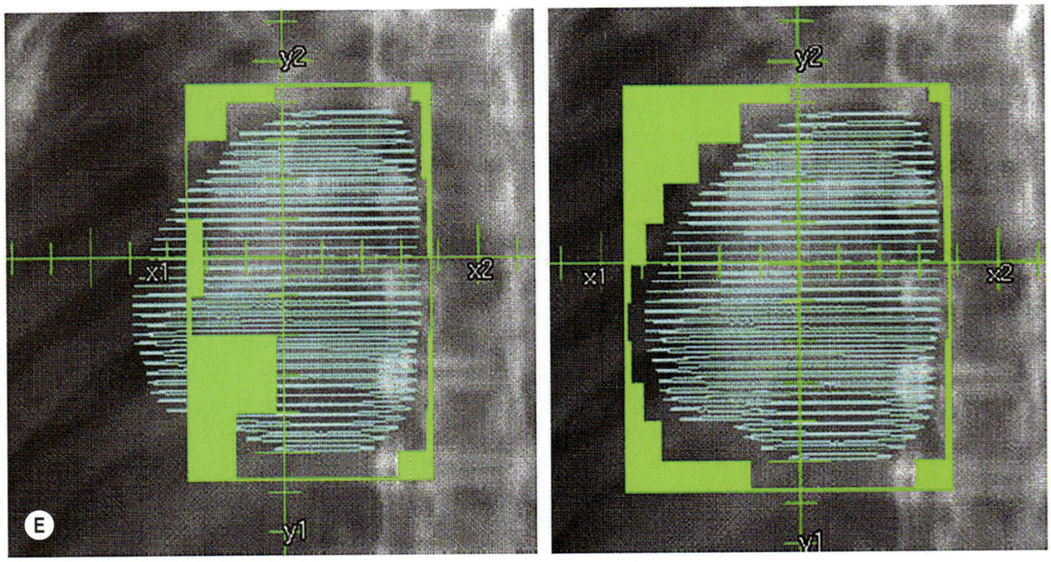

Fig. 12.13—Cont'd

The choice of beam energy needs careful consideration, as at high energy, the increased path length of the electrons released can be detrimental to the target coverage if the target is adjacent to low-density tissue and air. Most dose algorithms do not provide accurate dose predictions at tissue interfaces, and generally the choice of a low-energy beam is considered preferable.

Phased Plans

For many sites the treatment plan will comprise two or occasionally more phases. For example, phase one will deliver dose to a known primary lesion and to surrounding nodal involvement or other disease spread. Phase two will then be a reduced PTV covering the primary lesion only.

Another reason for phased treatment would be to spread the dose to critical structures by employing a different field arrangement in phase two but still targeting the same PTV.

A further form of phased treatments is the use of feathered junctions when treating large PTVs to minimise the risk of overdose or underdose occurring at matched field edges, and typically three phases are employed in this technique. An example is the treatment of the entire CNS with a spine field matched to brain fields, with collimators angled to follow the divergence of the spine field (Fig. 12.14).

There may be radiobiological and/or practical advantages in delivering the phases concurrently in each daily fraction rather than consecutively, when a new plan must be produced and checked for each phase. Simultaneous integrated boosts (SIBs) are nowadays easily feasible using inverse planning techniques.

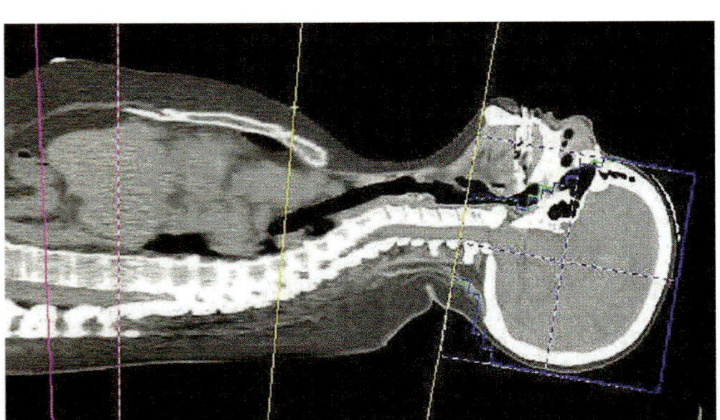

Fig. 12.14 Central nervous system junction.

Oesophagus

Traditionally, the oesophagus has been treated with two phases with the intention of minimising the doses to the cord and lung. Phase one is an anterior–posterior parallel opposed pair, which also irradiates the cord usually to a dose slightly higher than the dose the PTV receives during this phase. As cord dose tolerance is approached, a phase two plan is introduced, usually an anterior and two posterior oblique fields. The oblique fields avoid the cord completely, but it continues to receive an exit dose from the anterior field. Therefore it is essential to plan both phases together to ensure that the total cord dose does not exceed the tolerance over both phases. This arrangement is intended to minimise lung dose by using the phase one and two beam arrangements up to cord tolerance. More recently, cardiac toxicity has become a concern, especially where chemotherapy is also administered, and the heart is outlined as a critical structure. The treatment is delivered using a single four-field plan, and the lateral fields are angled and shaped to conform to and cover the PTV while shielding the heart from as much high dose as possible. Thus the cord maximum dose and the lung and heart volume doses are all optimised in a single plan.

Noncoplanar Planning

The majority of plans have the central axes of all the fields in one plane, which is usually the axial patient plane, although a sagittal, coronal or oblique plane may be preferable in some circumstances, such as a wedged pair to treat the orbit (Fig. 12.15).

Coplanar planning simplifies the planning process, because if all beams project the same out-of-plane dimension, they will each cover the out-of-plane PTV dimension equally. Beam path lengths through normal tissue are minimised and collimator rotations on opposing fields can be easily matched. For most of the body, coplanar fields are preferable, with a few exceptions when small angulations from the treatment plane are used. Examples of such angulations are some breast treatments where floor and collimator rotations are introduced to establish a vertical junction between the breast and nodal fields (Fig. 12.16) and treatments avoiding the shoulders in lateral neck beams.

One disadvantage of coplanar fields is that the exit path of one field will often overlap the entrance path of another, with potentially significant cumulative doses. Noncoplanar plans can be most beneficial in the skull, where the beam paths can avoid each other except

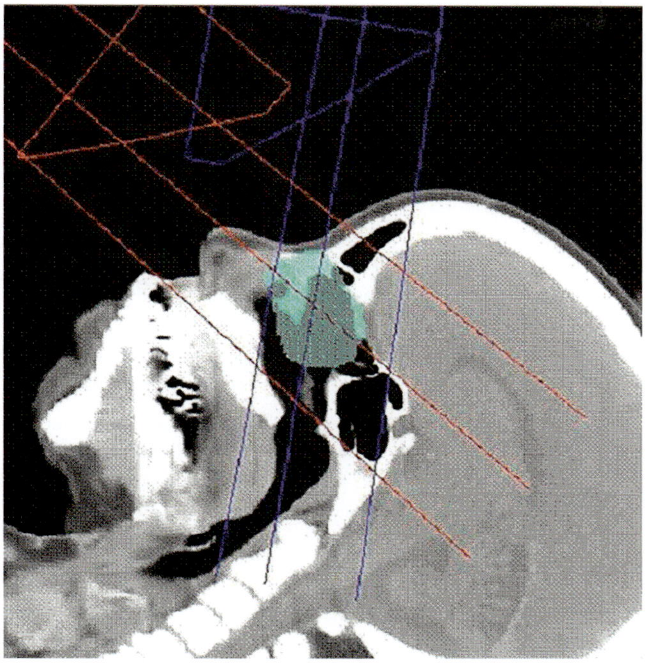

Fig. 12.15 Planning in the sagittal plane to avoid adjacent critical structures, in this case the contralateral eye.

at the PTV, without increased path lengths because of the approximately spherical body contour. However, greater care is needed to avoid critical structures in three dimensions, as beams can deliver significant dose well beyond the PTV area. An example would be the thyroid irradiated by beams in the sagittal plane also irradiating the brain (Fig. 12.17).

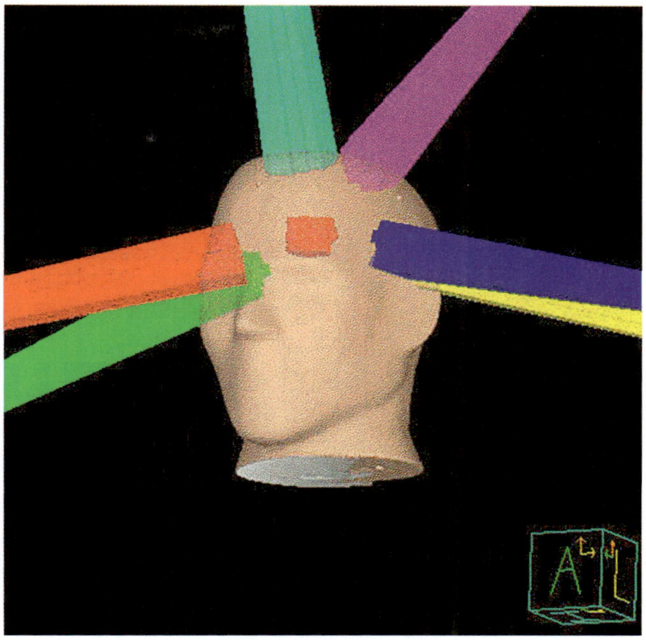

Fig. 12.17 Treatment gemoetry to the skull with non-coplanar beams.

Field Matching

Matching two fields may be essential to treat large volumes, as described in the previous section, with feathering used to spread the uncertainty of the setup, especially when a single isocentre technique cannot be utilised. Figs. 12.18A and B show how asymmetric fields can simplify field matching and are commonly used, especially in head and neck treatments, to match two distinct but abutting PTV shapes into a single treatment.

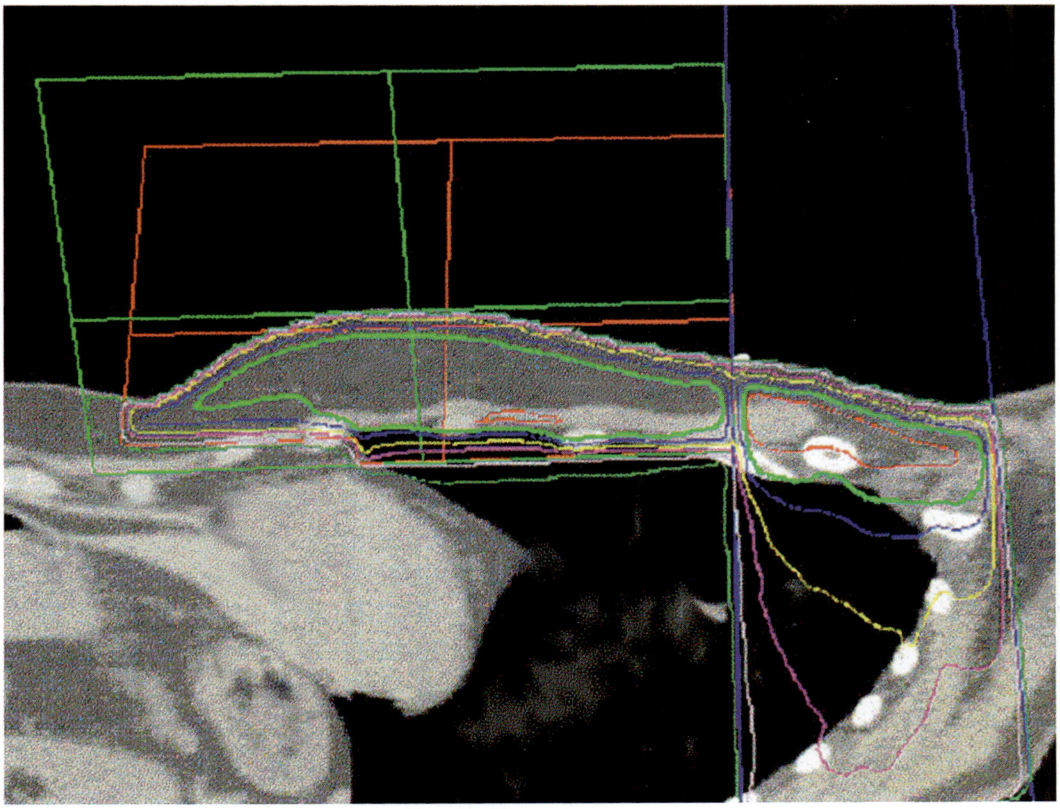

Fig. 12.16 Breast junction.

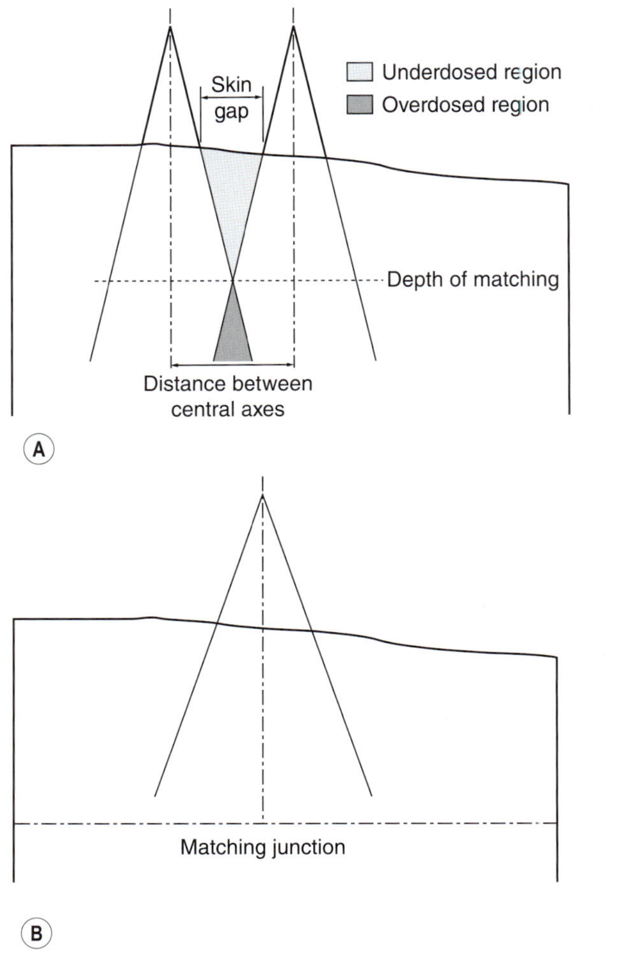

Fig. 12.18 Field matching with (A) divergent beams and (B) asymmetric fields.

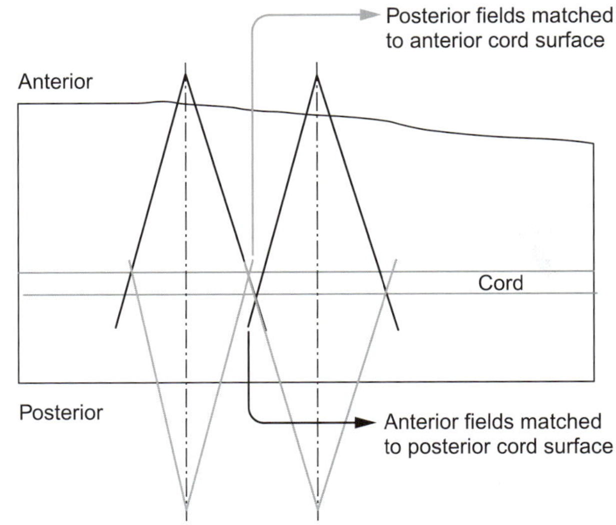

Fig. 12.19 Field matching at different depths.

However, matching may also be necessary when a previous treatment is adjacent to a PTV currently being treated. Matching diverging fields can be complex, and a compromise is usually a pragmatic approach, especially in palliative, low-dose treatments. If the planner has confidence in the location of the previous setup, an attempt to match the beam divergence may be practical. Alternatively, the match may be made at a critical structure, such as the spinal cord, and the overdose and underdose regions adjacent to the cord are accepted (Fig. 12.19).

Forward Planned Intensity Modulated Radiotherapy

In forward planning, additional segments of radiation beams within the overall treatment field can be used to produce improvements in homogeneity and deliver integrated boosts and improved sparing of OARs. The technique is referred to as *field-in-field*, and a simple example is a forward planned breast technique which retains the preferred tangential beam arrangement described earlier but allows shaping of dose to areas within the breast that would be underdosed or overdosed without such customised compensation. This is illustrated in Fig. 12.20B, where the dose uniformity has been improved compared with that in Fig. 12.20A by the addition of four segments within the standard field.

Patients with prostate cancer can also be treated using a forward planned technique. This is done where the aim is simultaneously to boost the dose to the prostate while delivering a lower dose to prostate and seminal vesicle PTVs within the same treatment fraction. This can be achieved using a three-field technique, with two to three segments per beam. Segment shapes can be determined according to rules based on the patient anatomy and the beam weights adjusted to give the required dose distribution.

Forward intensity modulated planning can also be used to generate more complex dose distributions, such as concave dose distributions in the pelvis or head and neck. While the dose distribution of such plans may not be quite as conformal as those produced by inverse planning, they may be an improvement on a standard three-dimensional conformal treatment plan.

Inverse Planned Intensity Modulated Radiotherapy

Inverse planned IMRT involves the use of dose-volume constraints which, once entered into optimisation software called the *optimisation engine*, lead to the generation of an optimal solution to the treatment planning problem. For a given number of beam orientations, the software calculates appropriate beam intensity patterns and the positions of the beam collimating device that would lead to the desired dose distribution in the patient.[56,57] Essential to this is a fully outlined set of three-dimensional volumes of interest as well as the corresponding doses to be delivered to these.

ICRU Report 83[3] provides recommendations on volumetric prescription and reporting of doses in intensity modulated planning. Prescribed doses are given as the dose, D_V, to be received by a fraction, V, of the PTV volume and/or the volume, V_D, to receive at least the absorbed dose, D. Typically, the prescribed absorbed dose is given to 50% of the PTV (D_{median}), with the near minimum dose being the dose received by 98% of the PTV ($D_{near\text{-}min} = D_{98\%}$) and the near maximum absorbed dose being the dose received by 2% of the volume of the PTV ($D_{near\text{-}max} = D_{2\%}$). The prescription also includes dose-volume indices which are upper dose-volume limits for OARs and PRVs. From the treatment planning aims, as dictated by the volumetric prescription, the planner defines for the optimisation software appropriate dose-volume goals and sets priorities for their fulfilment.

Inverse Planned IMRT With Fixed Beam Configurations

There is a lot of published work on appropriate class solutions for IMRT plans, the number of beam angles and the energies of beams. A number of authors have found that for some sites, a small number of appropriately selected beam orientations can provide dose distributions as satisfactory as those produced by a large number of unselected equispaced orientations. The general increase in numbers of incident gantry angles means that lower energies are suitable for deep-seated tumours, although some groups have preferred to continue using higher energies.

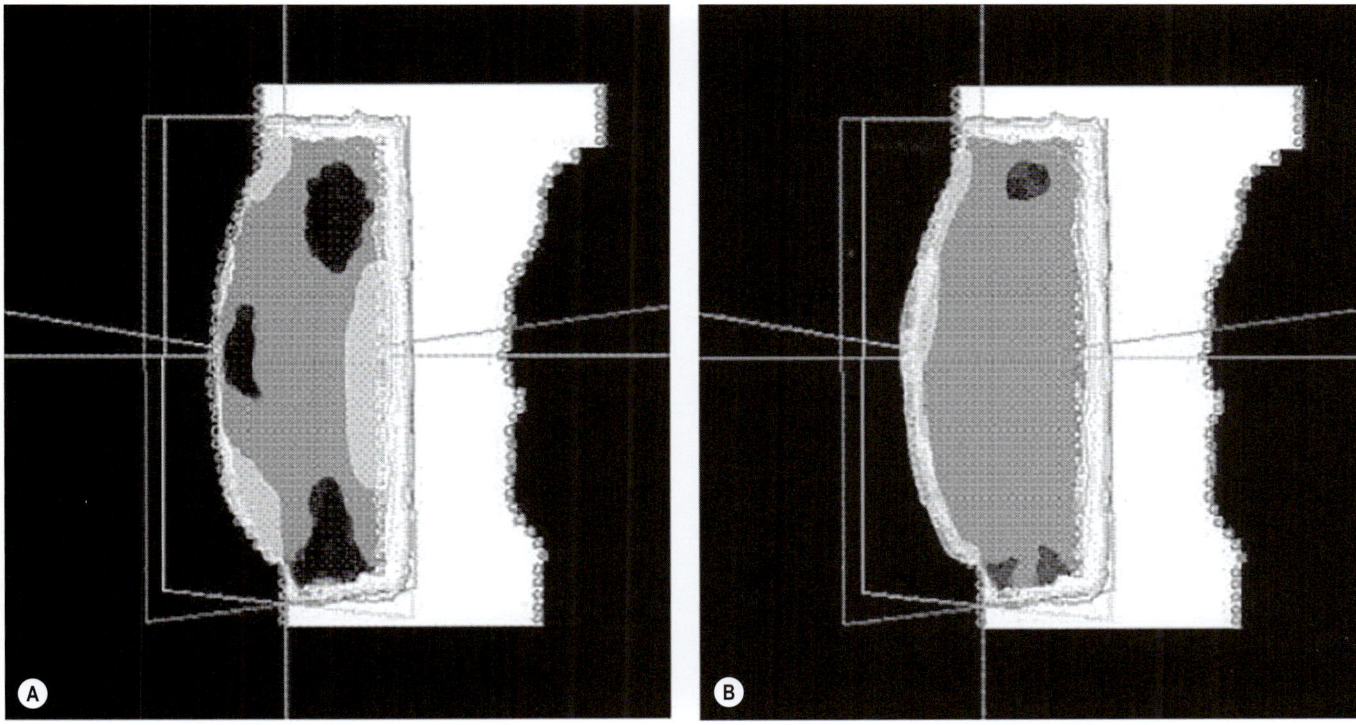

Fig. 12.20 The use of additional segmented fields within the two wedged fields which alone produced the dose distribution on the *left*. Image (A) improves the dose uniformity to that shown in image (B).

During the inverse planning process, the optimisation engine will only attempt to cover or spare those volumes that have been completely outlined. It may therefore be necessary to outline volumes where strict dose sparing is not required but the planner would prefer to avoid hot spots. This enables the dose within these volumes to be reduced and ideally avoid the hot spots. A volume that does not strictly relate to anatomy may be drawn to apply a dose constraint with a relative low priority that will help to avoid dose overspill in this area. Expanded volumes with extra margins can be used to ensure coverage of targets. Depending on the leaf widths and motions, this may require differing margins in different directions.

Optimal ideal beam fluences are converted to deliverable leaf motion sequences which must take into account limitations by the machine hardware. This should be considered when choosing beam orientations and selecting gantry and collimator angles to ensure, for example, that the width of the target volumes in beam's-eye view (BEV) is not larger than the maximum beam width that can be delivered at one time. Deliverable fluences can be realised by using multiple static-field segments (known as *segmental MLC* or *step-and-shoot IMRT delivery*) or by having pairs of leaves dynamically move across the beam portal at varying speeds during beam-on (known as *dynamic MLC* or *sliding window IMRT delivery*).

Each planning system has its own characteristics. Therefore skilled expertise with the system when developing class solutions to achieve local planning techniques is essential.

The calculation process is in two stages. First, the TPS calculates the optimum energy fluence for each beam. Then, this is converted to a set of field segments that the treatment unit can deliver. There may be significant differences between the ideal and achievable fluences, so the planning process will be more efficient if it permits ready access to the predicted dose distribution as it is being calculated. The planner must still ensure that the calculated plan is reasonable and deliverable, and skilled manual intervention to an inverse plan calculation is usually required (e.g. removing very small segments or those with a low number of monitor units (MU)). The planner must also be aware of the limitations of the dose calculation algorithm, as there may be significant errors in calculations of small or elongated fields, or fields with small MLC apertures compared with the secondary collimator settings.

Inverse Planned IMRT With Rotating Arcs

Tomotherapy. The first implementation of a rotating arc approach was based on the serial or sequential tomotherapy concept.[58] This concept used a narrow photon beam collimated with two sets of binary MLCs. The MLCs were binary in the sense that the jaws were either open or closed and were mounted as an add-on on the gantry of a conventional linear accelerator. During a gantry rotation and stationary couch position, two slices were irradiated at once, and following this, the couch was translated along the axis of couch rotation for the irradiation of the next two slices. This was the Peacock system with the pneumatically driven MIMiC binary collimator. The couch motion was controlled by the Crane system, and the patient was immobilised with an invasive head immobilisation device, the Talon system. Treatments were inversely planned using the Corvus optimisation engine. The Peacock was the first commercial solution for the treatment of patients with IMRT. It was marketed by the Nomos Corporation and was primarily available in the United States. It has nowadays been superseded by helical tomotherapy and other rotational therapy solutions.

The concept of helical tomotherapy uses a single bank of binary MLCs with a compact LINAC rotating around the treatment couch, translating in a continuous manner and thereby delivering a fan beam similar to a CT scanner.[59,60] The photon beam is a flattening filter free (FFF) beam. Each leaf delivers a pencil beam, and modulation is achieved by changing the fraction of the time the leaf is open during gantry rotation so that the desired energy fluence can be delivered from each gantry angle. There is a backup collimator that is used to adjust the field width. An integrated planning system is used for optimisation and dose calculation. The original helical tomotherapy system, Hi-Art by TomoTherapy Inc., has been further developed into the Tomotherapy and Radixact systems of Accuray Inc.

Volumetric Modulated Arc Therapy. VMAT is a rotational IMRT delivery technique which is now widely available on a conventional LINAC using a standard MLC. VMAT is possible through continuous gantry rotation, with the MLC leaf, gantry rotation speed and dose rate varying throughout a chosen arc which could be up to the full 360-degree rotation of the gantry.[61] It is a volumetric delivery, with the patient on a static couch and with the patient volumes irradiated during gantry rotation. Optimisation calculations for VMAT delivery are performed in a series of stages, starting initially with an arc that is subdivided into a small number of gantry positions at which the MLC leaf positions are determined. Subsequent stages continue the optimisation using an increasingly larger number of gantry positions with beam segment apertures interpolated from gantry positions used in the previous optimisation stage. The optimisation engine and treatment delivery software are available nowadays on all modern TPSs and LINACs and have become the most commonly used approach for realising IMRT.

Specialised Techniques With MV Photons

Over the years, highly specialist treatment techniques have been developed, often with dedicated treatment machines. Although often some form of the treatment can be delivered on a conventional LINAC with specialised accessories or modification, there are also examples of highly specialised treatment facilities being developed to exploit and explore the potential of specialised treatment techniques.

Total-Body Irradiation

Total-body irradiation (TBI) is employed in the treatment of leukaemia to kill leukaemic cells and to suppress the immune system before a bone marrow transplant. The target site is therefore all malignant stem cells, cells of the immune system (immunocytes) and bone marrow stem cells. The most important critical structure is the lung, as radiation-induced pneumonitis is a common side effect and can limit the total dose administered. TBI is administered in conjunction with chemotherapy before bone marrow transplant, so reliable treatment delivery is essential, as once the chemotherapy commences, the bone marrow transplant cannot be delayed.

The only practical RT technique is to give a uniform dose to the entire body, including the skin. There are wide variations in the delivsery technique, dose administered, dose specification point and dose rate.[62] However, most techniques employ a standard LINAC beam with the patient at an extended SSD of approximately 4 to 5 m treated with lateral fields (Fig. 10.13). A Perspex sheet is placed in the beam to reduce the depth of the build-up region, and bolus may be placed close to the patient to even out the body contour and provide a more uniform dose. The low density of lung means that the thorax will receive a higher dose than the rest of the trunk, so it is important to provide some form of lung compensator. This can range from simply positioning the patient's arms over the chest to the use of the MLC.

The beam characteristics will differ considerably from those at the standard treatment distance, so extensive measurements are required to establish baseline data for planning TBI treatments. The effect of scatter from the wall behind the patient, the floor and the air creates a unique beam condition, and these affect not only the patient dosimetry but also the in vivo measuring devices such as thermoluminescent dosimeter (TLD) and diodes, which must also be calibrated in these conditions.

TP may be based on CT data if the system can accurately account for extended SSD fields. However, all techniques rely on in vivo surface dose measurements to confirm or establish the MU required. These surface dose measurements must be carefully related to the dose at depth—usually the midplane dose at the abdomen or dose to the lung—and may be significantly influenced by electron contamination and the unpredictable scattered radiation in this setup.

Stereotactic Radiotherapy and Radiosurgery

The term *stereotactic radiotherapy (SRT)* refers to the precise irradiation of a tumour with a high radiation dose and in a small number of fractions. The first radiotherapeutic use of stereotactic radiotherapy was in the treatment of brain tumours, following the principles that had evolved with neurosurgery. In early applications of intracranial stereotactic radiosurgery (SRS) with delivery of treatment in a single fraction or intracranial SRT with delivery in multiple fractions, a point in the centre of the tumour was localised in three dimensions by a unique set of coordinates that related to a fixed external reference frame, as seen in Fig. 12.21. In intracranial SRT, well-defined beams of radiation are focused precisely onto a small target, and it is important to minimise the dose to sensitive structures such as brain stem and optic nerves.

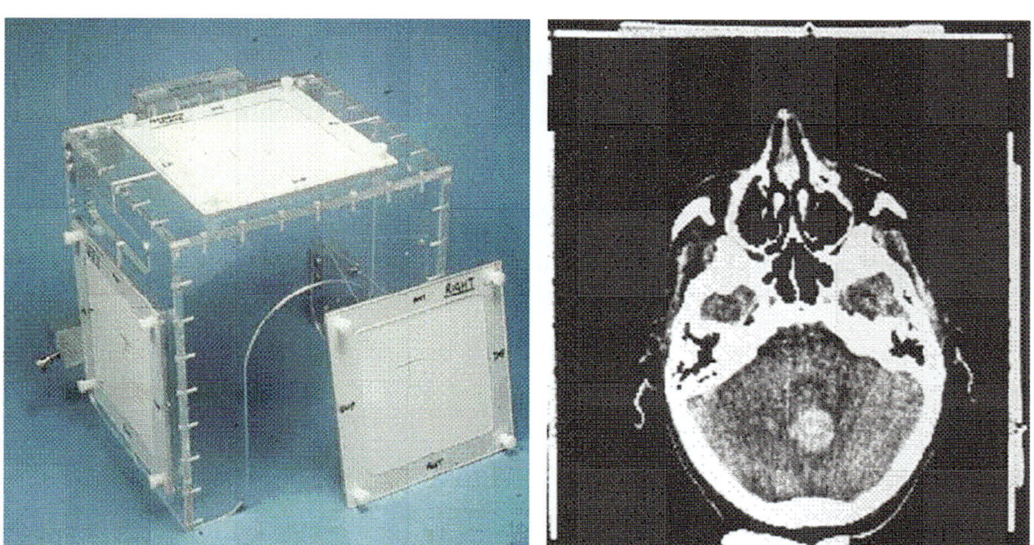

Fig. 12.21 Fiducial marker system with isocentres shown.

In SRS in particular, precise patient fixation, target localisation, treatment delivery and verification allow the PTV margins around the GTV to be generally smaller than for fractionated treatment.

Although initially used in the brain, stereotactic principles have been extended and are now used to treat any tumour site in the body; what is known as *stereotactic ablative body radiotherapy (SABR)* or simply *stereotactic body radiotherapy (SBRT)*. It is essential that patient immobilisation during treatment remains precise and is reproducible, irrespective of the number of treatment fractions. Collectively, SRT/SRS/SBRT treatments are referred to as *stereotaxy* and can be realised on conventional gantry-mounted LINACs as well as on other types of treatment delivery systems.

Stereotaxy on Gantry-Mounted Delivery Systems

Modern gantry-mounted LINACs provide the capability to treat using narrow radiation fields collimated with MLCs or special add-on collimators or cones. It is imperative to maintain the alignment of mechanical, radiation and imaging isocentres to within 1 mm. FFF beams allow deliveries at high dose rates, thus enabling fast deliveries.[63] MLCs with leaf widths between 2 and 5 mm are preferable for use in stereotaxic applications. LINAC-mounted and external imaging systems are available for image-guided radiotherapy (IGRT) and imaging prior to treatment and/or during treatment. Surface guidance systems can also be used to monitor patient position during SGRT.

Stereotaxy on Specialised Delivery Systems

In addition to gantry-mounted LINACs, there are a range of other technologies available for stereotaxy. For intracranial SRT, multisource systems use a large number of Co-60 sources, which are focused onto the volume to be treated. The most commonly used commercial systems in this category are Elekta's Gamma Knife model C and Perfexion systems (Chapter 9). More recently the ZAP-X System by ZAP Surgical Systems Inc. has become available (Chapter 10). This is a self-shielded, self-contained SRS system using a LINAC mounted on coupled gimbals that rotate around a common isocentre. At an accelerating potential of 2.7 MV, isocentric treatments are delivered at dose rates of 500 MU per minute using beams collimated to circular field apertures with diameters between 4 and 25 mm.[64]

A commercial solution for both intracranial and extracranial stereotaxy is the robot-mounted LINAC, the CyberKnife system by Accuray. This is a compact LINAC with a single-energy FFF beam at a dose rate of 1000 MU per minute collimated with either cones of different diameters, an adjustable collimator made of two hexagonal banks of tungsten or an MLC with a leaf width of 2.5 mm. The robot has six movable joints and typically treatments are planned and delivered using predefined irradiation geometry, referred to as *treatment templates* or *paths* and dictated by the body site to be treated.

Image-Guided Stereotaxy

More recently, radiation therapy systems are being developed by research groups or are commercially available that combine MRI together with radiation delivery. These systems offer superior imaging capabilities for volume definition, IGRT and adaptive RT. The challenges still under investigation are the interference of radiation delivery and MR systems, the limited MR field of view, image distortion issues and artefacts, correct assignment of electron and material properties to voxels for dose calculation purposes, and accounting for the deviation of the paths of charged particles in magnetic fields for dosimetry and TP calculations.[25,65,66]

Stereotactic Treatment Planning

The determination of dosimetric parameters needed for factor-based dose calculations often used in TPSs dedicated for intracranial stereotactic TP is challenging because of the perturbations introduced by the size and material composition of detectors used for the measurement of dose in very narrow collimated fields.[67,68] It is recommended to follow careful experimental methodology and use more than one detector with appropriate corrections for the determination of dose. Comprehensive guidance on small MV photon field dosimetry is provided in the dosimetry code of practice of the International Atomic Energy Agency (IAEA)/AAPM.[69] The accuracy in dose calculations for stereotactic planning using model-based approaches relies primarily on the design of the fluence engine. A prerequisite for this is that the finite source size is modelled because of source occlusion effects as well as the influence of the rounded MLC leaf ends on shaping the overlapping beam penumbras.

The TPS needs to have the facility to plan multiple noncoplanar arcs focused to one or more isocentres or to use multiple, fixed, noncoplanar conformal beams using either narrow add-on collimators or MLCs. Planning systems will generally allow planning with dynamic noncoplanar conformal arcs linked to a microleaf delivery system. This directly replaces the original multiple arcs of pencil beams produced with tertiary collimators. VMAT technology with appropriate narrow MLC leaf width is also available. Analysis of brain treatment plans has shown that three to five arcs provide sufficient normal tissue sparing and good dose uniformity to the PTV. However, if stereotactic treatment is being used for young patients or for benign conditions, it is relevant to consider increasing the number of arcs to reduce the exit dose to the whole body from any sagittally orientated arcs. For larger, irregular target volumes (35–70 cc), four to six fixed, noncoplanar fields are probably a better technique, with either conformal blocking or MLC-defined shielding based on the BEV evaluation tool described later in this chapter.

Three different beam configurations which can be used in such a stereotactic plan to treat an elliptically shaped brain lesion can be evaluated using the dose volume histogram, as described later in this chapter. Fig. 12.22 presents the three dose volume histograms to enable comparison. The sparing effect of conformal beam shaping for four and six fixed fields compared with a spherical treatment volume produced by single-isocentre, multiple arcing with a circular collimation is clearly shown. Although MLCs make it very efficient to produce conformality, conventional 1-cm leaf systems are often unacceptably coarse for SRT and SRS. Typically, MLCs with leaf widths of 0.5 cm and 0.25 cm are being used.

In SRT, where the target PTV diameter is equal to or smaller than 3 cm, it is a common practice to prescribe the absorbed dose to the

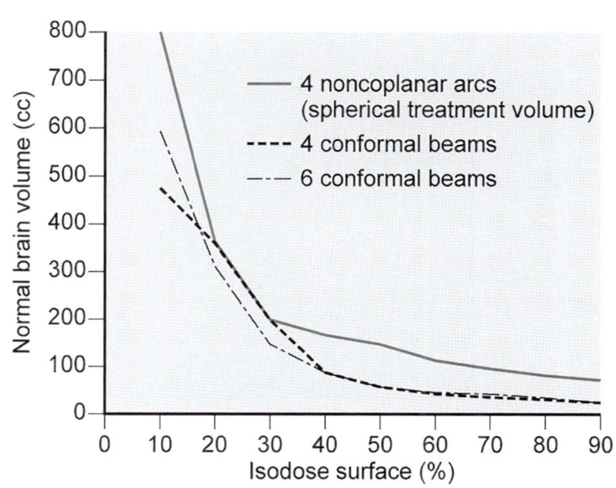

Fig. 12.22 A simple comparison of DVH's for an ellipsoid volume.

outer border of the PTV or to an isodose surface that most optimally conforms to the outer surface of the PTV as a percentage of the maximum dose located near the centre of the PTV. This approach for prescription originated from intracranial SRT delivered with multiple narrow beams and without intensity modulation.

With the introduction of IMRT and the application of this to extracranial SRT, and in line with the recommendations on volumetric prescription in ICRU Report 83,[3] ICRU Report 91[6] recommends that in SRT, the absorbed dose is prescribed to the isodose surface, D_V, that covers an optimal percentage volume, V, of the PTV while optimally restricting dose to OARs and PRV. As an example of this type of dose prescription and treatment plan normalisation, the UK SABR Consortium quotes the dose distribution to be normalised so that 95% of the target volume receives at least 100% of the quoted prescription dose and, in the special case of stereotactic treatment of a lesion in the lung, 99% of the target volume to receive a minimum of 90% of the prescription dose.[70]

Absorbed doses to target volumes are to be reported in terms of median, near-minimum and near-maximum absorbed doses, as defined in ICRU Report 83.[3] For PTVs with volumes smaller than 2 cm^3, however, the near maximum is replaced with the absorbed dose received by an absolute volume of 35 mm^3 ($D_{near\text{-}maximum} = D_{35mm^3}$). The near minimum is subsequently defined as the absorbed dose received by an absolute volume of V − 35 mm^3, where V is the volume of the PTV ($D_{near\text{-}maximum} = D_{V-35mm^3}$).

ELECTRON THERAPY

Electron beams provide an ideal treatment for superficial PTVs extending from the skin surface typically down to a depth of 5 cm. The major advantage over photon beams is the sharp falloff in the dose at depth. The relative biological effectiveness (RBE) is the same as that for x-rays. The field is defined by an applicator and end frame (Chapter 10). Besides the standard fields of circles, squares and rectangles defined by the end frames at the patient end of the applicator, custom cutouts may be constructed for individual PTV shapes.

Electron beams interact with patient contours in unexpected ways, and these interactions vary significantly over the clinical range of electron energies, which are typically 4 to 20 MeV, so computer planning and experimental verification can be essential in some treatments. The computer dose predictions can result in great uncertainty in nonuniform conditions, and they should be used with care and along with dose measurements such as the experimental determination of output factors when appropriate.

Conventionally, electron treatments are not computer planned as the setup is fairly straightforward and the patient can be considered as a uniform water medium. In these cases, standard depth doses and output factor charts may be employed to select beam energy and calculate the MU required. Manual calculations are usually based on the central axis depth dose of the standard applicators as described in the next section, but it is important to understand the limitations of applying these standard data to real clinical conditions.

Energy and Depth-Dose Characteristics

The depth-dose variation of electron beams with energy is shown in Fig. 12.23. Using these data, an electron beam energy is selected for a specific PTV depth. At low energies, the surface dose may be less than 95% of the prescribed PTV dose and bolus may be needed to increase the surface dose. Bolus may also be used to modify the treatment depth if a limited range of electron energies is available. The bolus may be applied to the patient's skin in the form of wax or other flexible tissue-equivalent material, or it may be more convenient and comfortable for the patient if the bolus is attached to the end of the applicator when a solid material such as Perspex may be used. In the latter situation, standoff of up to about 5 cm between the bolus and the patient surface will produce the same penetration of the beam in the patient as if the bolus had been applied directly to the skin surface.

Recommendations on prescription and reporting of doses in electron beam therapy are given in ICRU 71.[5] One approach involves the prescription at the ICRU reference point located close to the centre of the PTV and with an acceptable variation of the dose within the PTV of ±10%. Alternatively, the prescription is at the minimum dose to the PTV; namely, the dose to the isodose level or surface encompassing the PTV. For example, if the 90% isodose is selected to cover the PTV and the dose is prescribed to this isodose, this will result in a 111% maximum dose, and this will always be within the PTV. Usually the latter approach is selected, typically choosing to prescribe at the 90% or 95% isodose level, as this provides a useful dose range to cover the PTV.

Penumbra

The penumbral region of any treatment beam determines the field margin that must be applied around the PTV. Because this is complex

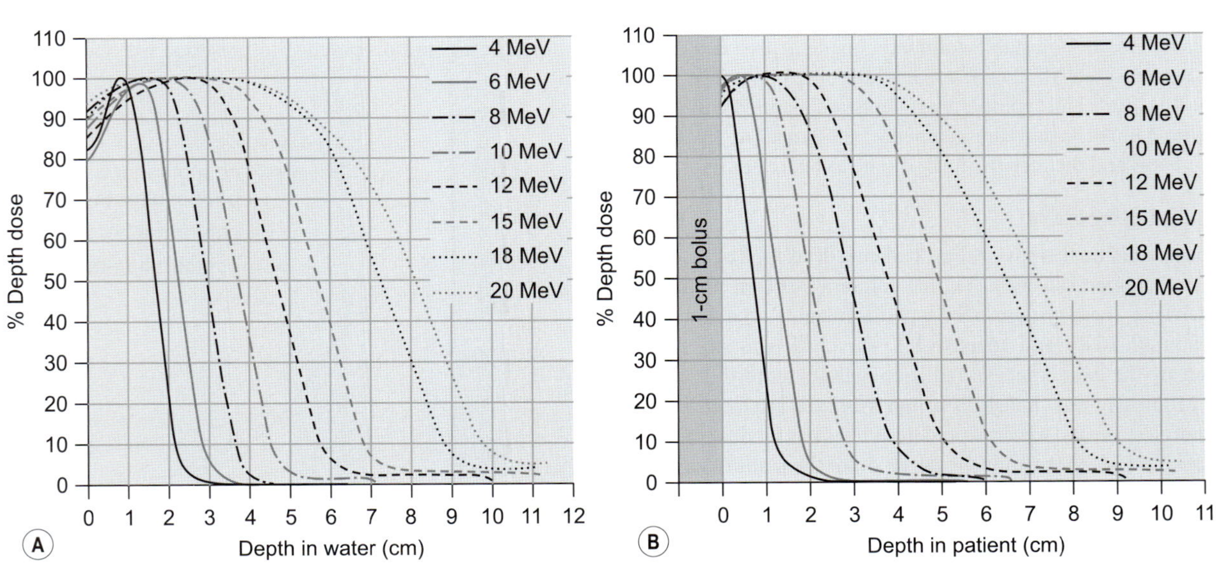

Fig. 12.23 Typical central axis percentage depth doses in water for 10 × 10 cm electron fields. On the *left* there is no build-up, and on the *right* there is a 1-cm build-up.

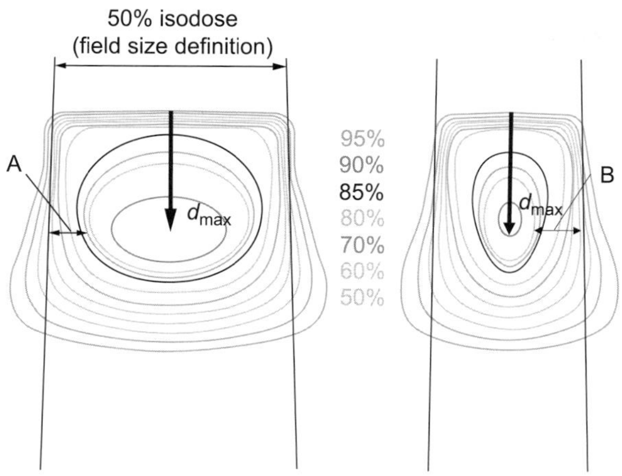

Fig. 12.24 Electron isodose distributions for (A) 8 × 8 cm and (B) 3 × 3 cm fields.

in electron beams, varying with depth and energy, the clinician must appreciate the dose profile and whether adequate coverage at the field edges will be achieved. If coverage of the 95% isodose at d_{max} is the only point of interest, the margin can be taken as A in Fig. 12.24A. However, for small fields in particular, the rounded isodose profile of the 95% contour becomes significant, and the field could be described as being entirely formed of penumbra, as shown in Fig. 12.24B.

Stand-off and Stand-in

It may be impossible to position the applicator at the standard treatment position, which can be at the isocentre or at the end of the applicator. For example, in neck treatments the patient's shoulder may obstruct access to the patient surface, which may result in a variable SSD across the field area. An inverse-square law correction using the nominal SSD cannot usually be applied in the same way as for photon beams. This is because, for each electron energy, the effective source of the beam is not at the exit window of the accelerator but at a position downstream as a result of electrons scattering from the scattering foils through to the photon collimators and the electron applicator. A virtual SSD needs to be employed in inverse-square law corrections instead, or stand-off corrections derived experimentally can be used. Where the patient contour varies within the field, it is a matter of clinical judgment as to where the prescribed dose is delivered and where an overdose or underdose is acceptable.

Patient Contour Effects

If an electron beam is incident on a steep gradient in the patient surface, the uniform scattering that produces the standard isodose and depth-dose characteristics no longer exists, and the light field projected onto the skin gives a misleading indication of good coverage. Electrons are cascaded along the edge of the steep patient surface gradient to greater depths before depositing their dose. For shallow gradients, this effect may only result in a small modification to the depth dose, but for steep gradients, the cascaded electrons deposit a significant dose, often beyond the targeted volume. All these effects are highly energy dependent and therefore require a reliable planning algorithm or careful experiment to confirm the actual dose distribution. Whenever practicable, this situation should be avoided. The beam angle of incidence should be carefully set up by gantry, collimator and couch rotations to minimise nonorthogonal incidence. If the electron beam is incident on a cavity such as the ear, the ear should be filled with a wax plug or wet gauze. Bolus should always extend beyond the field edge so as to avoid a sharp gradient, and variations in bolus thickness should be gradual. It may be necessary to employ bolus to block up some target volumes such as around the ear pinna or the nose to provide lateral scatter into the PTV and to generate the uniform dose distribution predicted by the standard isodose distributions.

Note that field-defining collimation with shaped end frames will not produce a significant scatter contribution, because of self-absorption. However, shielding placed within the field, such as internal nasal and mouth shields, to prevent the beam from penetrating beyond the PTV must be coated with wax or similar materials to prevent backscattered electrons from enhancing the dose to tissue adjacent to the shield tissue.

Heterogeneities

Bone will attenuate an electron beam because of its higher density, and this can be advantageous where the PTV lies above bone, as this reduces the dose to underlying tissue. The lung and other air cavities can be a significant hazard in electron beams, as their absorption is minimal compared with water and the electron beam entering the lung will not be significantly attenuated until it passes through the lung and reaches the lung–tissue interface. Care should be taken when using beams with energy higher than 12 MeV to ensure that the dose limits of critical structures underlying the air cavity are not exceeded. The most common example of this is in electron breast boosts where the heart may receive a significant dose.

The use of CT planning can demonstrate the effects of heterogeneities, but unless the calculation algorithm has been verified under all conditions, the isodose distributions should be considered for indication only. CT planning can be useful for identifying the depth of critical structures such as the spinal cord in neck node treatments, even if the TPS dose calculation is not used.

Dose Calculations for Electron Beams

Dose calculation models for electron beams implemented on TPSs have been based on either pencil beam methods or the MC method. The first commercial pencil beam method was that developed by Hogstrom et al.[71,72] Pencil beam models assume Gaussian characteristics of the incident beam. Hence deviations from these characteristics as a result of collimator scattering, for example, yield errors in the calculation of profiles, leading to an inaccurate prediction of the beam output. To accurately model the penumbra, corrections are required to the incident pencil beam, and these tend to give inaccurate results in the presence of heterogeneities. The width of the incident electron pencil beam is narrow at shallow depths and widens as the depth increases. Dose deposition in small volume elements (voxels) at shallow depths tends to be modelled well in the presence of heterogeneities because the size of the voxel is larger than the width of the pencil beam. Dose calculations at voxels located at greater depths, towards the end of the electron range, where the pencil beam widens, do not account for the influence of heterogeneities localised at those depths. Methods to correct for such effects are usually computationally intensive. Pencil beam models tend to be used for the display of a dose distribution, whereas a factor-based formalism is used for the calculation of the MUs. These models are no longer implemented in modern treatment planning and are replaced with more accurate approaches.

There is increasing use of dose calculation models based on the MC method. One implementation is based on the macro Monte Carlo (MMC) method developed by Neuenschwander et al.[73] The key concept to this approach is use of precomputed energy deposition data stored in macroscopic spheres of various radii and for a variety of media. Using these data, electrons are transported in macroscopic steps through the absorber. The method proves efficient for implementation in a clinical setting. An alternative dose calculation model based on the MC method is the voxel-based Monte Carlo (VMC) approach by Kawrakow et al.[74] Unlike the MMC method, the VMC approach does not use precomputed data but introduces approximations and simplifications in the elementary electron processes without significant losses in accuracy for TP applications and with substantial savings in computation time.

Over the next few years, it is likely that electron beam planning will no longer be carried out manually and most commercial treatment planning systems will offer accurate and robust models based on the MC method.

Field Matching

A perfect match between electron–electron or electron–photon fields is not possible, and a compromise is always needed—either to underdose at the junction and risk recurrence or to overdose and accept potential tissue damage. The underdose or overdose regions are not in the same location and are dependent on the electron beam energy.

Typically, a gap of 2 mm at the skin surface between the 50% isodose edges of an electron and photon beam will give an acceptable compromise. No gap will produce doses of typically 120% or more, whereas a 5-mm gap will result in a significant low-dose region of 70%. Angling the photon beam a few degrees away from the electron beam will give a very small reduction in the overdose region. The use of spoilers, for example, Perspex build-up, in the electron beam can broaden its penumbra and make the setup less critical.[75]

Matching two electron beams is similarly very difficult and will often be complicated by the fact that the beams are not parallel to one another, as the reason for matching is to cover a large or highly curved contour (e.g. the skull). The match border on a curved surface may be created by a lead strip which shields the surface from one field and is then positioned on the other side of the junction to shield the surface from the abutting field. Even with careful immobilisation, such junctions are prone to significant overdosing or underdosing, especially with oblique fields and where the lead cannot be perfectly positioned in direct contact with the skin. Therefore junctions should generally be feathered by moving the junction two or three times during the treatment course to reduce severe overdosing and underdosing. However, many electron treatments are boost fields, so a high-dose region of 120% of the boost dose may only be present for, say, 25% of the overall treatment and thus represents a total high dose of 105%.

Verification measurements should be performed with TLD or film to estimate the dose distribution in unusual electron treatment setups.

Specialised Techniques With Electrons

The majority of electron treatments are undertaken with direct single fields using the standard beams on the LINAC. However, there are two established special techniques which, although not used widely, are worthy of description.

Total Skin Electron Therapy

The treatment of mycosis fungoides and similar malignancies requires irradiation of the entire skin surface and, given the rarity of the disease, this complex treatment delivery is performed at only a few specialised centres. An even dose distribution is required to a depth of only typically 6 mm for the 90% isodose level but often encompassing the entire skin surface of the body. It is extremely difficult to come close to achieving 95% to 107% uniformity however complex the treatment technique may be.

A wide variety of techniques have been developed to attempt to achieve this dose coverage. A small single field at an SSD of 1 to 2 m which scans, or arcs, over the patient is one option, but the most common technique is to use an extended SSD of between 3 and 7 m so that the patient is covered in one or two beams (Fig. 10.14). The dose rate of a standard LINAC is increased to reduce treatment times, and the dose is delivered in daily fractions over several weeks, for example, 36 Gy in 1-Gy daily fractions, as not all treatment positions are delivered in each fraction. The x-ray component of the electron beam is in the range of 1% to 4% of the maximum electron dose for these techniques, so the whole-body dose is not normally of concern.

Beam energies of between 4 and 10 MeV are usually employed, although the energy at the patient is reduced by scattering in air, and energy degraders and scattering screens are placed in the beam to improve dose uniformity and beam penetration.

The standard depth doses will not be applicable under these conditions, and extensive commissioning work is required to determine depth dose and dose rates under these unique treatment conditions. The patient is usually standing and will adopt a different pose at each fraction to be treated effectively at different beam angles to deliver an even dose and to minimise self-shielding. Additional static fields may be required to boost regions that have not received sufficient dose because of self-shielding or extreme obliquity of the incident beam, for example, the soles of the feet and top of the head.

Evaluation of the dose delivered is difficult, as the dose from different beams with a wide range of angle of incidence must be measured at very shallow depths. TLD is ideal in this area. There is limited scope for accurate TP of individual patients before treatment delivery, and in vivo dosimetry is important in verifying the delivered dose to the individual patient and potentially leading to small adjustments in treatment position in subsequent fractions.

Arcing Electron Treatment

Initially, many treatment sites appear to be good candidates for arcing electron therapy, where multiple fixed fields are replaced by a single beam arcing over the patient and thus eliminating problems of matching junctions. However, in practice, arcing therapy is of no practical value in all but a small number of cases. The cross-sectional view of an arc with a narrow slit beam, typically between 2 and 5 cm wide, centred on a deep isocentre and sweeping over the patient is shown in Fig. 12.25. The arc commences and terminates with the slit irradiating shielding so that each part of the patient receives the same exposure to the slit beam. This treatment is rarely applicable to widespread surface lesions, because the dose to each point depends on the dose rate of the treatment machine, the slit width and the time that each point of the patient is in the beam. This in turn depends on the arcing speed

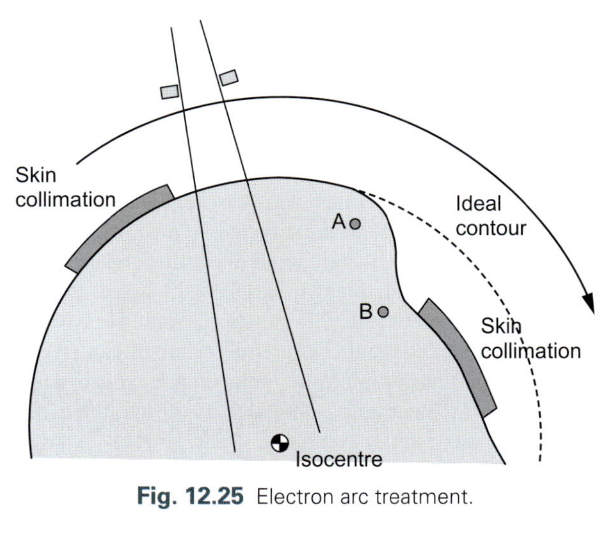

Fig. 12.25 Electron arc treatment.

but, more crucially, it also depends on the distance from the isocentre. If points A and B in Fig. 12.25 are at the same depth and the SSD at point B is 3 cm greater than that at point A, the dose at point B will be approximately 6% less than that at point A because of stand-off variations. However, point B is closer to the isocentre, so the sweeping beam will spend longer irradiating this point than point A, resulting in a higher dose at this point. Therefore contours with any significant variation in curvature can introduce large dose variations across the arc. There are few sites where this can be achieved for more than 30 degrees of arc, and the back is probably the best location for this treatment. The head is unlikely to be a site where arcing therapy offers any advantage over fixed fields, even when the matching of abutting fixed fields is the alternative.

In principle, varying the slit width during the arcing could adjust the output, but this requires specialised technology to perform and is not available as a standard treatment option. A specialised TP computer is also required to design this complex treatment, as the contour will vary along the slit as well as around the arc. As arcing beams have entirely different characteristics to fixed fields of the same energy and the inevitable variation of contour through the arc, many hours of pretreatment phantom measurements and in vivo verification during the treatment are required to design the treatment.

KILOVOLTAGE PHOTON THERAPY

Although opposed fields may be suitable if the separation is small, kilovoltage beams are generally used as a single field to treat very superficial lesions. The field size may be defined by the applicator, but often a lead cutout will be placed on the skin surface to define the field (Fig. 12.26). This needs to be only 2 mm thick for beam energies up to 160 kV. The sharp penumbra of the kV beam means that the high-dose part of the field can be matched to the PTV edge. At depth, however, there is some lateral bowing out of the low-value isodose contours.

Although there is some variation of depth dose with field size, this tends to be pronounced beyond the clinically useful depths so will usually only be relevant if considering the dose to underlying structures.

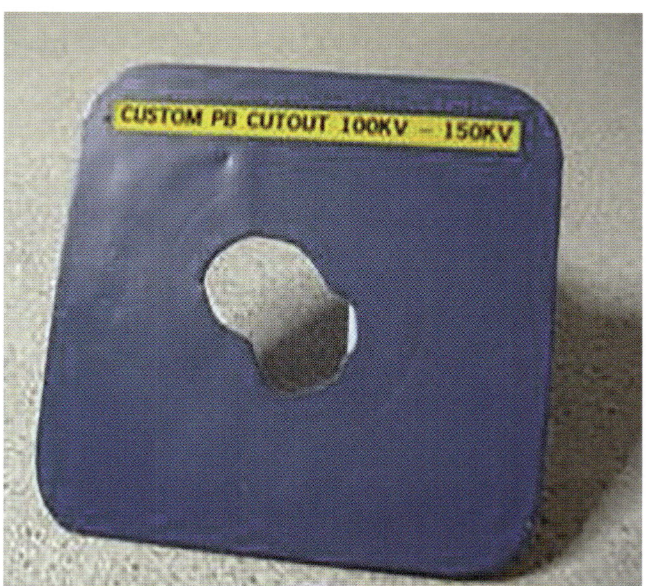

Fig. 12.26 Irregular lead cutout and mask.

If a lead cutout on the skin is used, the calculation of treatment time or number of MUs must be based on the cutout size as well as the applicator output. To calculate the dose in a cutout, the applicator output must be corrected by the ratio of the backscatter factors for the applicator and cutout dimensions. The backscatter factor for the cutout is less than the backscatter factor for the applicator. Hence the treatment time or number of MUs is increased in comparison to treatment with the applicator alone.

The limited applicator size means that fields may have to be abutted to treat long PTVs or for high-curvature surfaces. The sharp penumbra means that fields can be abutted and give a uniform dose. The most practical method of achieving this is to use lead on the skin to define the junction rather than an applicator. Care should be taken to ensure that the beams are as parallel to each other as possible to minimise overdosing at depth.

Differences Between Kilovoltage Beam and Electron Beam Therapy

Although both electron and kilovoltage (kV) photon beams are suited for superficial treatments, the mechanism of dose deposition is different, resulting in clinically significant differences in the features of the dose distribution.

Depth-dose characteristics will usually favour electron beams because of the sharp falloff in dose beyond the PTV, although if the prescribed dose is to be delivered to the patient surface, as mentioned above, bolus material may be required for lower-energy electron beams. This is because of the build-up effect present in electron beams and which is negligible in kV x-ray beams where the maximum dose is at the surface (Fig. 12.27).

The predominant interaction of a low-energy kV photon beam is photoelectric absorption with a probability of interaction in tissue approximately depending on Z^4, where Z is the atomic number. Therefore there is an enhanced dose absorption in bone, which can be significant if high doses are prescribed to superficial regions with underlying bone, such as the scalp. For a 100-kV beam with a half-value layer (HVL) of 3 mm aluminium, the dose absorption in bone will be 4.5 times greater than in water. For a 300-kV beam with an HVL of 3 mm copper, this is reduced to 1.05 times the dose in water, as Compton interactions predominate and the atomic number of the absorbing material is no longer an important factor in energy absorption.

The relatively high energy of electrons in an electron beam compared with those generated in a kV beam results in a large range of lateral scatter, and they can therefore penetrate into tissue well beyond the field edge. The consequence of this is a much broader penumbra region than is present in a kV x-ray beam, and this penumbra varies with depth. Therefore the use of electron beams to treat PTVs very close to critical structures, such as the lens in the eye, should be avoided if possible. The sharp penumbra of a kV beam makes it the ideal modality where critical structures are adjacent.

The SSD of a kV machine will typically be far shorter than a LINAC, ranging from 25 to 50 cm. Therefore the inverse-square law dependence of dose will be far more significant in kilovoltage than electron treatments. For example, a 2-cm air gap results in a dose reduction of approximately 12% at an SSD of 30 cm compared with a reduction of approximately 4% for an electron beam produced by a standard LINAC at 100-cm SSD.

There is usually less demand on a kV treatment machine than on a LINAC, so where the physical differences in the beam are of no clinical significance, the choice of treatment with kV may reduce treatment waiting times in the department and facilitate a treatment starting sooner than on a LINAC. For a few patients, the increased treatment

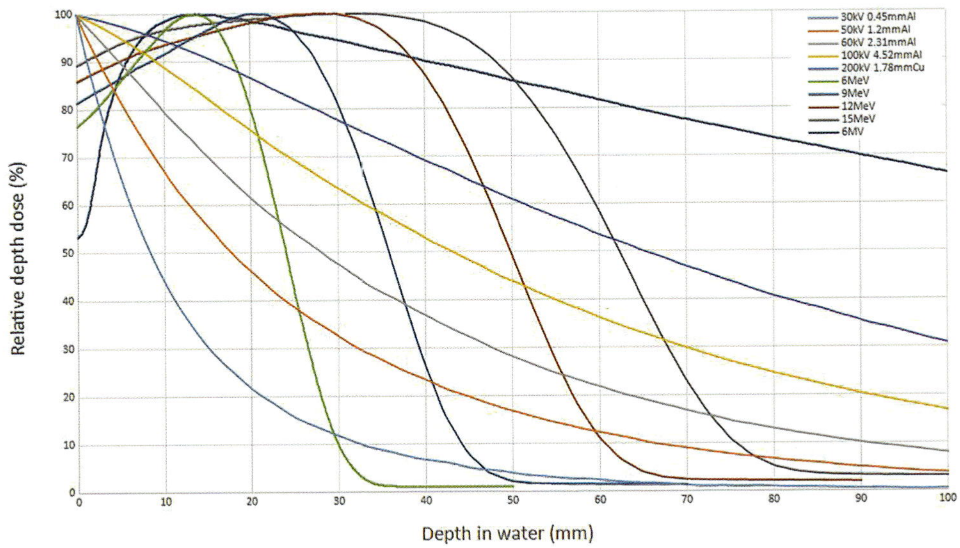

Fig. 12.27 Percentage depth doses (PDDs) for kilovoltage x-ray beams for a field size of 10 × 10 cm at a source to surface distance (SSD) of 40 cm. These are compared to PDDs from electron beams for a field size of 10 × 10 cm at SSD = 100 cm and with the PDD of a 6-MV photon beam at the same field size and SSD.

time arising from the lower dose rates of a kilovoltage unit compared with those from a LINAC may be a disadvantage.

PROTON AND HEAVY-ION BEAM THERAPY

The general formula for a proton pencil beam algorithm for both passively scattered and scanned beams is similar to that of photons. The dose distribution within the pencil beam, $D(x, y, z)$, may be described with a single- or double-Gaussian spread across the transverse beam dimensions in x- and y- axes and the dose distribution along the z-axis for a particular proton range depth. These characteristics alter with different incident proton beam energies.

The principal benefit of clinical proton beam therapy is the adjustable range, with its sharp distal falloff. This, however, is also the cause of its inherent uncertainty in target coverage, as there is no exit dose to be monitored on treatment. There are several important considerations when planning with proton and ion beams which differ from conventional x-ray and electron planning, mainly relating to uncertainties in calculating proton or ion beam range:

- The conversion of Hounsfield CT data to proton stopping power, or range
- The proton beam modality employed, that is, whether it is a scanning pencil beam or a passively scattered beam with collimation and compensators
- The use of planning robustness where uncertainty of complete target volume coverage, particularly at the distal falloff, or avoidance of adjacent OARs necessitates planning of beam directions which rely preferentially on beam penumbrae rather than on proton range to achieve complete target coverage
- Compensation for biological effectiveness for high linear energy transfer (LET) ion beams, as well as the high-LET portions of proton beams

The Hounsfield CT number to proton stopping power conversion has been the subject of much research and development where there was particular concern in regions of bone and air gap interfaces, as well as the proximity of high-Z metal implants.

Robust planning has particular importance in pencil beam scanning (PBS) where nonideal setups and inadvertent intrafraction movement or respiratory motion would cause significant errors in delivered dose volume. These issues are less problematical with passively scattered beams, which are planned with static beams and appropriate range and lateral margins.

Pure Bragg peak beam data at each preferred energy for either passively scattered or pencil beams would be tabulated in the TPS. In addition, PBS requires precise knowledge of the pencil beam dimensions with energy. These may be described by the full-width half-maximum or a Gaussian distribution profile factor, sigma, as well as the position of the delivered beam spots. Recent developments in proton TPSs have included the option of correcting for the increasing biological effects with increasing proton LET or RBE at the distal falloff. Although these effects are not generally considered significant, they are subject to much discussion. The proton range uncertainty when considering all aspects of the planning and measurement processes has been estimated by Paganetti to be between 2.7% and 4.6% + 1.2 mm of the computed range.[76]

Ion beam therapy, for example, with carbon ion beams, is known to produce beams of high RBE, although these are not uniformly distributed. The physical dose distribution of the ion depth-dose distribution has to be modified to produce a uniform biologically effective depth dose (Fig. 10.24). The increasing LET of the ion tracks, with decreasing beam energy towards the Bragg peak, causes the ions to become increasingly ionising. Thus biological survival data, which would be dependent on tumour type to be treated, fractionation and total dose, are folded into the pencil dose algorithm. An additional complexity arises from the effect of carbon beam fragmentation into short-range high-LET particles such as helium and lithium. This dose correction can be shown to amount to 30% to 40% at the carbon beam distal falloff.

In general, single Bragg peak data are tabulated for each energy and then used to form a prescribed spread-out Bragg peak (SOBP) to cover the target. Typically only two to three different fields are employed in modern proton beam therapy plans, whether PBS or passively scattered beams.

The need for an inverse-square correction for variation in SSD depends on the beamline setup and the apparent origin of the proton source. In passively scattered systems, the scatter foils and/or modulators may be only several metres upstream of the isocentre and thus need an inverse-square correction. The same would apply to a pencil beam setup where the scanning magnets would act as the virtual source. Some gantries, for example, the Gantry 2 at Paul Scherrer Institute, have been designed to produce a parallel beam as they arrive at the patient. In effect, the beam has infinite source to axis distance, and this reduces surface dose and simplifies the use of matched fields when large target areas need to be treated.

The need for custom modulation wheels depends on whether the conformity produced by a scanned pencil beam is needed or whether treatment using a passively scattered beam would suffice. The latter would apply to centres with beamlines that offer both proton beam modalities: scanned and passive. Passively scattered techniques require a large set of modulator wheels, whether for a gantry or fixed horizontal beamline, and also require some setups to use these in conjunction with beam timing to produce the required modulation and uniformity. However, most commercial systems offer PBS with a finely spaced range of energies, as explained in Chapter 10. This enables millimetre resolution in depth.

For passively scattered beams, the coverage is according to the prescribed SOBP and range, thus the modulator is custom made. The modulation depends upon energy resolution and affects the quality of the SOBP—that is, the ripple effects.

The aperture is always tailored to the target. Usually, brass apertures and polymethyl methacrylate (PMMA) compensators are used in passively scattered beams; these are created from planning data of the target shape and volume. The manufacture of patient-specific beam modifying equipment is normally not required for PBS, as the intensity and positioning of the beamlets or spots deliver the prescribed three-dimensional dose volume. However, certain improvements have evolved to improve the field edge penumbrae by using collimators. Plastic energy absorbers, which are applied at the beam nozzle and close to the patient, are used to achieve very superficial penetration depths, but in these cases the increased lateral spread of the beamlets would be incorporated at the planning stage.

With passively scattered beams, there are beam output factors to account for the beam aperture area, metal collimators, distance and energy. This does not apply to PBS, where the intensity of each beam spot or beamlet is calculated to deliver the prescribed field, whether in a uniform field mode or in an intensity modulated mode.

TREATMENT PLAN EVALUATION TOOLS

In the ideal radiotherapy treatment plan, the target volume is completely encompassed by the prescribed dose while the surrounding normal tissue is given the lowest possible dose. For the evaluation and comparison of complex three-dimensional plans, a number of tools are available on most modern TPSs. This section reviews several of these tools.

Isodose Distributions

Isodose information is presented as lines or surfaces of equal dose. They show either relative or normalised dose, expressed as a percentage of a reference dose. Or they display the absolute dose in units of gray (Gy) or centigray (cGy). It is a matter of local protocol as to which method is used, although prescriptions specifying different doses to different volumes within the same plan are best displayed in terms of units of dose in Gy or cGy.

To calculate dose to a surface or volume, a matrix of reference points spread over the volume of interest is required. The number of points and their spatial resolution is always a trade-off between speed and accuracy. The finer the grid of calculation points, the greater the calculation accuracy in regions of steep dose gradients, such as close to the beam edge. The disadvantages of a fine grid are the increased computation time and the creation of large data files. In general, two criteria are specified:

- The desired dose accuracy
- The maximum acceptable distance between the estimated and actual isodose contours

For example, 2% dose accuracy or 2-mm isodose positional accuracy will be achieved with a grid spacing of 5 mm. Typically, the *x* and *y* coordinates of these points are in the transverse plane and the *z* coordinate is in the superior–inferior plane. The *z* coordinate is frequently interpolated because the slice thickness of the planning CT scan can vary. The isodose contours are produced by linear interpolation between points; therefore the separation of these points needs to be small enough to allow sufficient dose detail at organ and PTV boundaries.

Conventionally, isodose curves were normalised to give 100% to a reference point, in accordance with the recommendation in ICRU Reports 50, 62, 71 and 78[1,2,4,5] on dose-at-a-point prescription and reporting. In complex intensity modulated radiation therapy, the normalisation of isodose distributions follows the recommendations in ICRU Reports 83 and 91[3,6] on dose–volume prescription and reporting. In the latter case, isodoses are being normalised so that 100% of the prescribed dose is delivered to the median of the target. The aim is typically to cover the target volume with the 95% isodose curve while ensuring that the maximum dose within the volume does not exceed 107%.

The dose distribution can be displayed on a single screen with multiple views of reconstructed sections; with transverse, sagittal and coronal sections; and on a three-dimensional reconstruction of anatomy with isodose surfaces displayed.

Useful features include the following:

- Opaque and translucent colour wash displays. These give a good overall impression of the dose distribution but can obscure target volumes, so they should be interchangeable with conventional isodose lines (Fig. 12.28).
- Zoom and pan facilities.
- Isodose surfaces displayed as wireframes superimposed on rendered surfaces, with real-time manipulation.
- A volume of regret. This is a dose reduction technique applied to the dose distribution. A window of acceptability of dose level is chosen and portions of organs outside this window can be highlighted. For critical organs, this is a one-sided test, in which regions where the dose is above the acceptable level are displayed. For target volumes, regions of either too high or too low dose can be shown. This display feature is particularly useful when checking the coverage of arcing beams such as in stereotactic RT.

Beam's-Eye View

A useful three-dimensional tool for field placement is the BEV, which shows the patient's anatomy from the source position of the therapy machine, looking out along the axis of the radiation beam. The BEV approach is useful for identifying the optimal beam angles at which to irradiate the target and avoid irradiating adjacent normal structures, by interactively moving the patient and the treatment beam. Using BEVs, it is possible to set up noncoplanar radiation beams.

Because there can be a great deal of information displayed via the BEV, it is important to show different structures in colour and be able to highlight, include, exclude and shade them interactively while adjusting beam parameters.

A visual and quantitative representation of machine and treatment couch parameters is also necessary, together with customisable limits and restrictions of beam, collimator and couch angles for specific treatment machines.

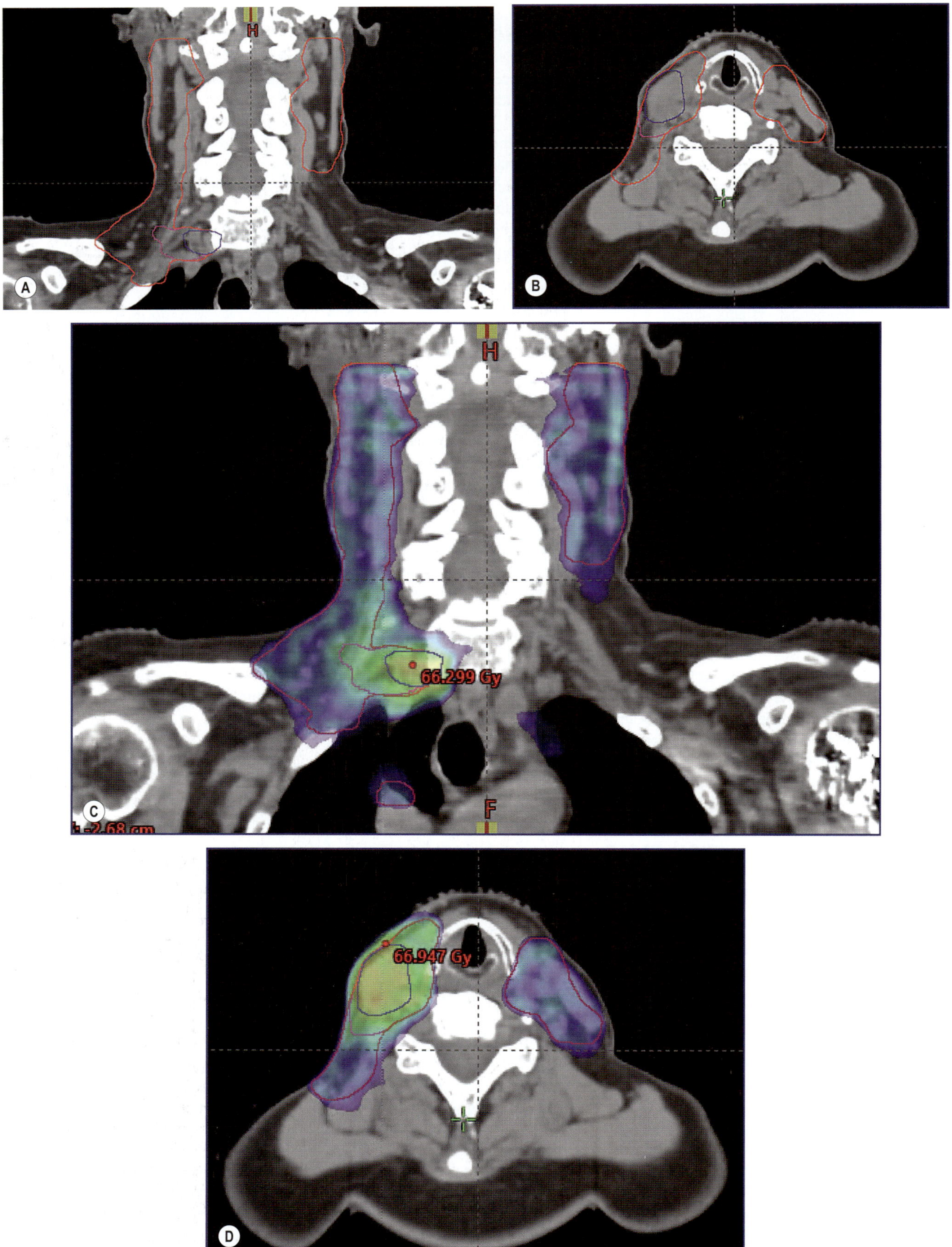

Fig. 12.28 (A) and (B) show sagittal and transversal views of tumour and nodal volumes *(top row)* (C) and (D) show the dose distribution from an intensity modulated plan *(bottom row)* in the corresponding planes. The differences in doses are simultaneously planned to the different volumes using inverse plan optimisation and intensity modulation.

The limitation of BEVs is that it is a one-field presentation, so field overlap is not immediately observed until the dose calculation is done.

Another view available on some planning systems is the physician's-eye view or observer's-eye view, which enables the viewer to look at the patient from all angles to obtain an overview while multiple fields are being displayed.

An extension of the concept of a BEV is to use a DRR. The DRR is reconstructed by various methods from the CT scan data set, which has been used for patient volume definition and planning. The accuracy of the reconstruction of the DRR depends on the slice thickness of CT data and the computing tools available to reconstruct the radiographs. CT information can be enhanced to extract more bony structure from the CT data and suppress the soft tissue to obtain an image with well-differentiated bony landmarks. Using such tools, one can also produce an image that is closer in appearance to either a megavoltage portal image or a diagnostic image.

Dose Volume Histograms

Volume calculations on a three-dimensional TPS provide a large amount of data that can be difficult to interpret and evaluate when displayed as isodose curves on several transverse, sagittal and coronal planes. It is much easier to condense the three-dimensional dose distribution data to a graph which displays the radiation distribution within a specifically defined volume of interest so that summarising and analysing the data are possible. Such a graphical representation is called a *dose volume histogram (DVH)*. The DVH can be expressed as the summed volume of elements receiving dose in a specified dose interval against a set of equally spaced dose intervals. This is a differential DVH and shows the absolute or relative volume in each dose interval directly. The dose interval is referred to as a *bin*. An example for the evaluation of a breast dose distribution is shown in Fig. 12.29 using selected dose bins as the measure of homogeneity over the treatment volume for two differently compensated plans. The standard plan gives a wider spread of dose over the volume of interest compared with the compensated plan, which shows a large volume receiving much less variation in dose.

More often used are cumulative DVH. These are dose volume frequency distributions and plot the volume receiving a dose greater than or equal to a given dose. The volume accumulates starting at the highest dose bin and continuing towards zero dose, eventually reaching 100% of the total volume. In most cases, the volume is specified as the percentage of the total volume of a particular structure receiving dose within each dose interval; however, it may be expressed as absolute volume in some cases.

DVHs can be used during the planning process to check whether the dose is adequate and uniform throughout the target volume. They show that hot and cold spots exist but do not indicate where they occur nor whether there are several of them. However, because they do not display spatial information, they should not be the only method of plan evaluation used.

The main use of DVHs is as a plan evaluation tool. They can be used as a graphical way of comparing different treatment plans on a single graph, for specifically identified OARs and PTVs. Comparisons of PTV coverage by means of DVH should show a uniformly high dose throughout the volume—the shape approximates to a step function and a steep slope shows that a large percentage of the volume has a similar dose (Fig. 12.30A).

For OARs, the shape of the DVH curve should have a concave appearance (Fig. 12.30B), but for different critical organs, it may be acceptable to deliver either a relatively high dose to a small volume or a low dose to a large volume.

An example of plan comparison for three different dose distributions is shown in Figs. 12.31A and B. Fig. 12.31B shows comparative DVHs for a rectal volume where 50% of the volume is receiving 60, 63 or 66.5 Gy depending on the treatment plan. It is also useful to display both absolute dose and absolute volume together with normalised values on the same graph.

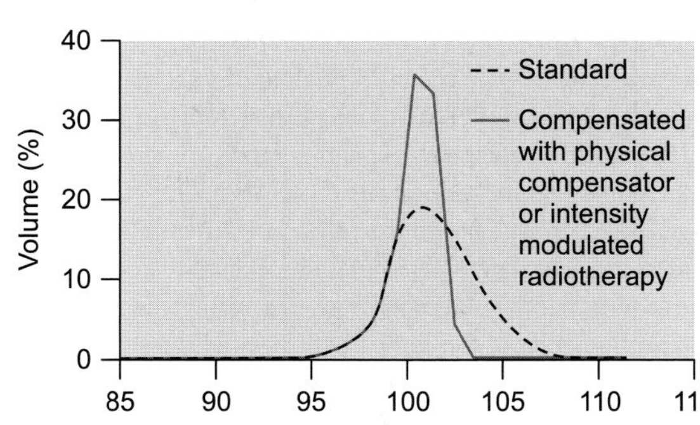

Fig. 12.29 Differential dose volume histogram comparing a standard and a compensated breast plan.

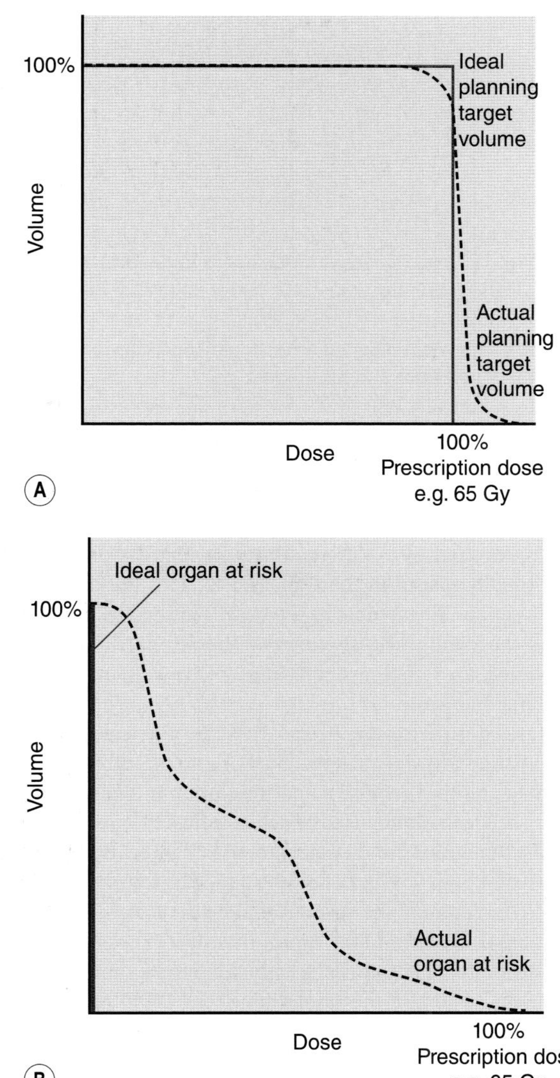

Fig. 12.30 Ideal and typical dose volume histograms: (A) for planning target volume and (B) for an organ at risk.

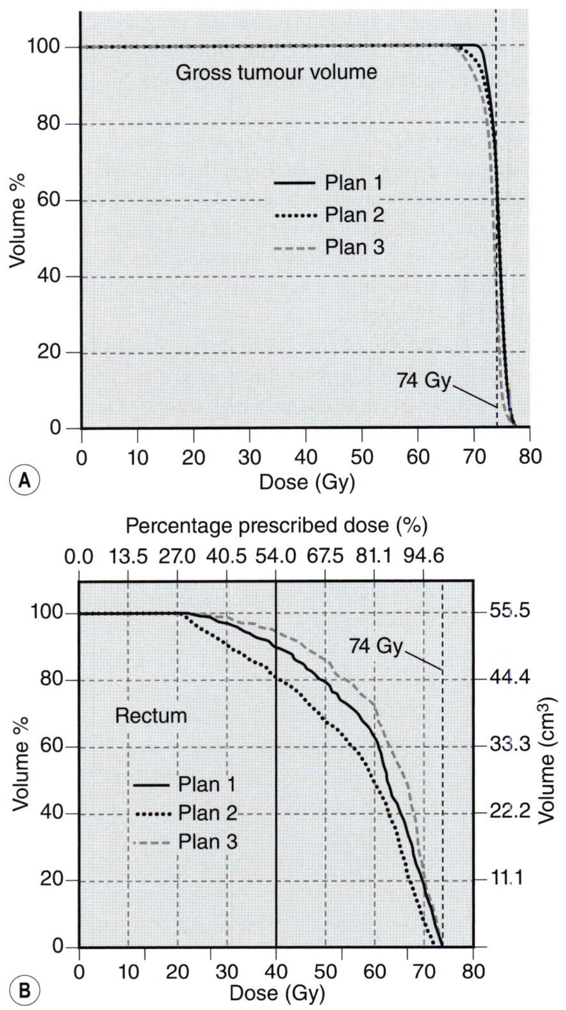

Fig. 12.31 Dose volume histogram comparison of three isodose distributions for (A) the target and (B) the rectum.

Dose Volume Histogram Calculation Requirements and Methods

The three-dimensional DVH is made up of a sequence of CT scans. This can be represented as a three-dimensional grid with cubic volume elements equally spaced in the *x* and *y* directions but not necessarily in the *z* direction. The volume of the voxel can then be defined by the product of the *x* and *y* grid spacing and the slice thickness. A reasonable resolution for sampling the volume of typical anatomical structures is about 2 to 3 mm.

Structures with irregular boundaries can give calculation errors when calculating with a regular rectangular grid. In addition, structures that are long and thin require a finer resolution in one direction than the other. The ideal solution is to be able to adjust the voxel size dynamically to the dimensions of the structure in *x*, *y* and *z* independently.

The dose for each voxel can be determined by linearly interpolating the dose to the centre of the voxel from the dose matrix. All contributing voxels are collected into the appropriate dose bins of the histogram for each structure. The user can specify the number and dose interval of the bins to customise the resolution of the DVH plots. These bin values can then be expressed in graphical form. It is important that the dose and volume calculation windows are large enough to completely include all the voxels in any specific structure.

The range of expected dose values is divided into equal intervals when constructing a histogram. For each interval, the volumes of the voxels receiving dose within that interval are accumulated in the appropriated element of an array, or bin. Cumulative DVHs are obtained by adding volumes accumulated in each bin with the volumes in all bins corresponding to higher dose intervals. For cumulative DVHs, the appropriate dose interval for the bins depends on the dose–response curve for the structure of interest. A dose of 0.5 Gy has been shown to be reasonable, whereas 2 Gy is too wide an interval. Differential DVHs treat the volume in each bin as a separate quantity, and a bin interval between 2 Gy and 5 Gy is reasonable.

Clinical Use and Limitations of Dose Volume Histograms

Interpretation of the DVH plot is fairly subjective, and implications of small differences between DVHs are not well understood. This indicates the usefulness of an objective numeric score such as tumour control probability (TCP) or normal tissue complication probability (NTCP) to provide a ranking when comparing plans. Small changes in DVH often result in significant differences in the computed TCP and NTCP values.

DVHs do not indicate the complexity of the field arrangements and will not show any use of illegal couch, collimator angles and so on.

In summary, the DVH is a very useful tool for three-dimensional plan comparisons and as an input parameter for TCP and NTCP calculations. TCP and NTCP are quantitative methods of predicting the likelihood of local control. DVHs and the predicted behaviour of the cell population in question are used as input data. There is, however, large uncertainty in the clinical data, so absolute probabilities are not attainable, but relative probabilities can be used to assess different treatment plans. DVHs should, however, be used in conjunction with other plan evaluation tools, especially those which will give spatial information. They can also be used to compare different treatment modalities such as protons and photons when performing TP studies, before doing clinical trials.

Dose Surface and Dose Wall Histograms

In some clinical organs, such as the rectum, it can be more relevant to consider the wall of the organ rather than the whole volume. Dose to rectal wall is more likely to represent patterns of morbidity than dose to volume, and rectal dose maps can be extracted from dose surface histograms to give an estimate of areas of high dose that may relate to patterns of morbidity. An example of such a map is shown in Fig. 12.32.

Dose Statistics

Dose statistics as outlined in Table 12.4 give a simplified view of the dose in a specified structure for evaluation purposes. For details and examples of the use of dose statistics from DVHs in treatment planning, the reader is referred to the reports by the ICRU.[1–6]

Other Plan Comparison Tools

Artificial intelligence (Chapter 13) has been shown to provide the potential for treatment plan comparison. Willoughby et al.[77] describe a system of evaluating and scoring RT treatment plans using an artificial neural network. Treatment plans were assigned a figure of merit by a radiation oncologist using a 5-point rating scale. DVH data extracted from a large training set were correlated with the physician-generated figure of merit using an artificial neural network which was then tested on another set of plans. The accuracy of the neural network in scoring plans compared well with the reproducibility of the clinical scoring, and the system is promising for the reliable generation of a clinically relevant figure of merit.

Also useful are:

- Side-by-side transverse/sagittal/coronal plans
- Video loop stepping through two plans displayed side by side, particularly with colour wash displaying isodoses

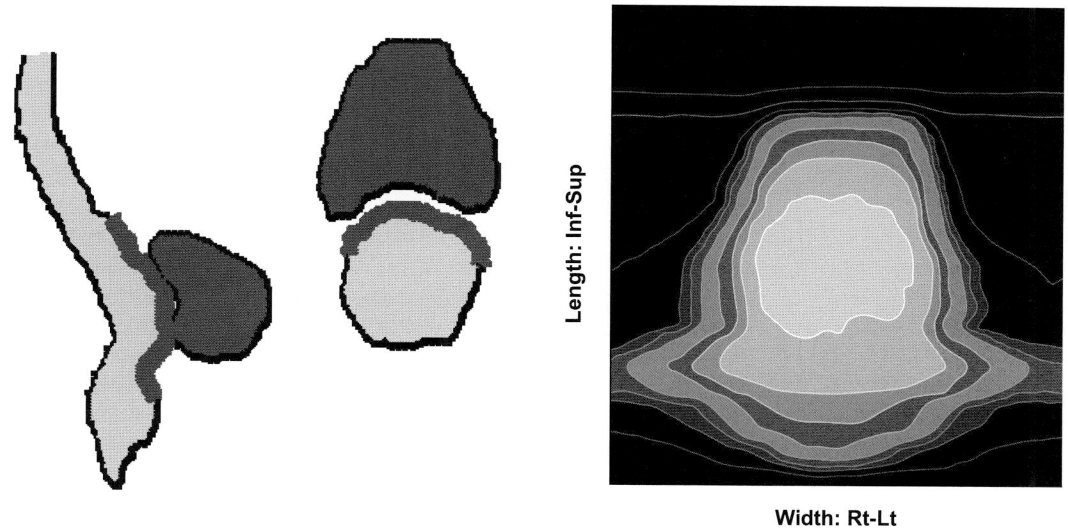

Fig. 12.32 Dose surface map.

- Zoom facility over the relevant area to be compared
- Dose at a point interactively integrated and displayed simultaneously on both plans
- Dose difference displays
- Surface dose display, for example, on the surface of the spinal cord

The other aspect of plan evaluation which has not been addressed here is the accuracy of the actual dose delivery, which is dependent on the size of the margins, complexity of the plan, reproducibility of set up and so on. Some sort of uncertainty analysis should be developed to include these other aspects of treatment plan evaluation.

With IMRT and VMAT technology, it is nowadays possible to generate very complex fluence and dose delivery patterns. This makes it difficult to assess plan quality in terms of complexity, robustness and deliverability. To this effort, metrics derived from treatment plan parameters such as changes in MLC leaf position and aperture, speed, doserate, gantry speed and so on are being proposed to relate complexity to the measured dose from plan-specific quality assurance, as discussed in the following section on quality assurance (QA).[78] If evaluation of such metrics is incorporated in the planning process, this would further assist in comparing treatment plans and choosing the plan which optimally fulfils the prescription and which can be verified with available dosimetry systems with confidence.

TABLE 12.4 Definitions of Absorbed Dose – Structure Volume Indices

Statistic	Definition
Total volume of a structure	The sum of all voxels found within the boundary of the contour defining a given structure
Mean dose	The sum of doses assigned to each voxel within the boundary of a contour defining the structure divided by the total number of voxels within the contour
Median dose	The dose given to half of the total volume of a structure
Minimum dose, D_{min}	The minimum dose in the total volume of a structure
Maximum dose, D_{max}	The maximum dose in the total volume of a structure
D_V: Dose received by fraction V of the total volume	The dose received by the sum of voxels assigned to the structure with volume V, reported as a fraction of the total volume of the structure
V_D: Volume receiving at least dose D	The proportion of the total volume of the structure receiving absorbed dose above a given threshold (given in Gy)

MANAGEMENT OF RE-IRRADIATION

Re-irradiation is increasingly used for the curative and palliative treatment of loco regional recurrences. Type 1 re-irradiation is a new course of radiotherapy to the previously irradiated volume, irrespective of toxicity concerns, while Type 2 is to previously non-overlapping irradiated volume where the cumulative dose raise concern of toxicity. When the new course of radiotherapy is delivered to a target volume within the same organ (e.g. contralateral lung) but without overlap of irradiated volumes and concern for toxicity from cumulative doses, it is considered repeat-organ irradiation. This definition helps distinguish re-irradiation from repeat irradiation.[79] Fig. 12.33A,B summarises the consensus on the definition of re-irradiation by ESTRO. With the increasing availability of high-precision radiotherapy techniques, re-irradiation is being considered as early as 3 to 6 months after the last course of radiotherapy. To minimise radiation side effects, re-irradiation target volumes tend to be smaller, with no CTV margins, treating only residual volume after salvage surgery or chemotherapy.

Planning and QA processes for re-irradiation follow the same principles as any radical radiotherapy course described earlier in this chapter. Re-irradiation in the palliative setting is less complex, as the intent for treatment is short-term palliation rather than long-term disease control with acceptable late toxicities.

To safely account for previous irradiation in the assessment of cumulative doses to organs at risk it is necessary to follow careful methodology on registering anatomical changes between treatment courses in order to transfer (map) doses to organs from previous courses to the current treatment course. At present there is limited guidance and tools for optimal image registration and bioeffect modelling (including calculations of equieffective doses and the application of tissue recovery factors over time).[80,81]

Ideally, the patient should be in the same position with similar localisation settings to achieve a high-quality image registration of previous and current radiotherapy plans. Image registration becomes challenging when there are significant changes in the body anatomy of the patient (e.g. growth and development of children), including missing tissues and differences in co-registration platforms. Current

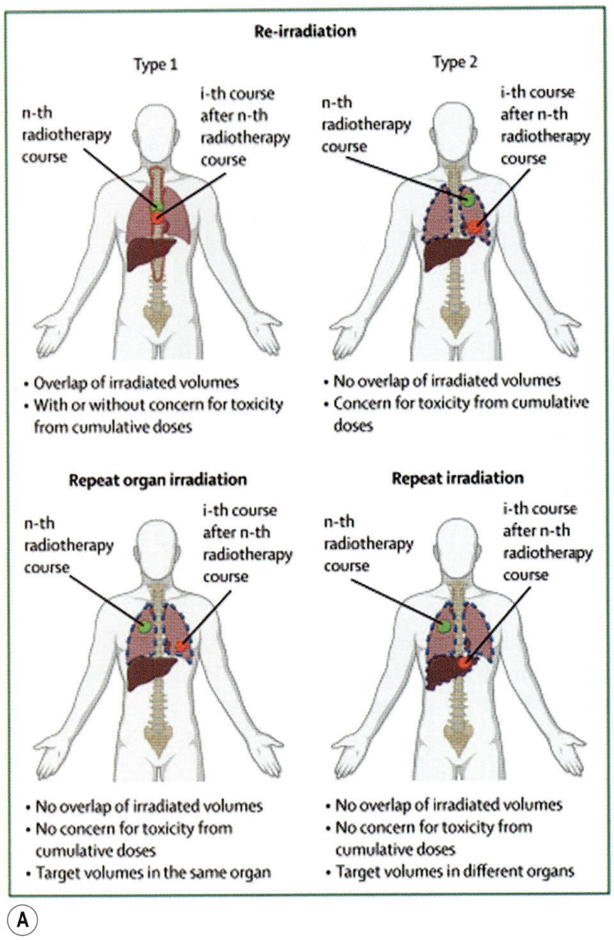

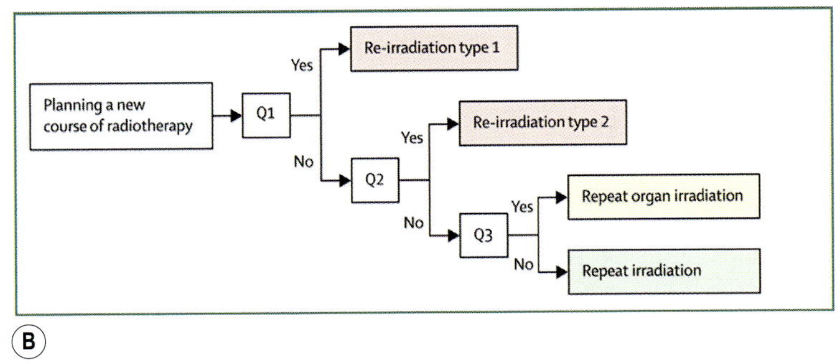

Fig. 12.33 (From Andratschke et al. European Society for Radiotherapy and Oncology and European Organisation for Research and Treatment of Cancer consensus on re-irradiation: definition, reporting, and clinical decision making. *Lancet Oncol.* 2022 Oct;23(10):e469–e478. https://doi:10.1016/S1470-2045(22)00447-8)

practice relies on performing rigid, followed by deformable image registrations between images sets.

Images sets between treatment courses need to be registered in order to be able to transfer doses delivered to organs at risk from the previous courses to the current treatment course. When considering irradiations from treatment plans with different fractionations schemes and dose per fractions other than 2 Gy, physical dose distributions must be converted into equieffective dose maps. Equieffective dose, $EQDX_{\alpha/\beta}$, is defined as the total absorbed dose delivered by the reference treatment plan of fraction size X (typical 2 Gy) that leads to the same biological effect as a test treatment plan that is conducted with absorbed dose per fraction other than X. Currently there is no consensus on the values of α/β to be used in the calculations of $EQDX_{\alpha/\beta}$. Studies comparing spatial differences between rigid and deformable dose registrations showed a highly variable spatial dose difference, and deformable dose registrations may be generally better.[82] The cumulative dose uncertainties are usually low in the shallow dose gradient areas and high in the steep dose gradient areas. This necessitates a clear quality assessment of the dose mapping process.

QUALITY ASSURANCE IN TREATMENT PLANNING

The TPS is an essential component in the RT process, as it is used to define treatment volumes and design and evaluate treatment plans. Its role is illustrated in Fig. 12.34. It is a software suite comprising a range of different software tools, of which the most unique and complex are the fluence and dose calculation engines. QA in TP can be examined in two parts. The first part incorporates all quality control checks on different aspects of functionality of the TPS. The second part is specific to the individual patient's treatment and is referred to as patient- or plan-specific quality assurance (PSQA).

Treatment Planning System Commissioning and Performance Testing

The general performance of a TPS is first checked by its vendor. The vendor and the user are subsequently responsible for the generic performance of the system in the clinical setting. As with other medical equipment, this second step refers to the acceptance testing of the system on site, just after installation. Following this, it is the user's responsibility to check the system's performance under the specific conditions in which it is to be used clinically. The medical physicist is solely responsible for this task. This involves commissioning the system, verifying its performance before clinical use and designing an appropriate program for periodically checking its performance.

Commissioning a TPS incorporates planning and performing all measurements required to configure the fluence and dose engines. The responsible user must carefully select the appropriate detector system for each measurement, perform the measurement with low uncertainty and correctly define and import the data into the system.[83–85] Most systems have a configuration package to process data, calculate the parameters for the fluence and dose engines and review the results. Following commissioning, the user validates its performance for an extended set of irradiation geometries that are encountered in the clinic. Performance testing can be an overwhelming task, considering the large number of different situations that one could check. There is a wealth of guidance and recommendations available on how to design relevant checks to encompass the uses of the system.[84,86–90] There is also guidance

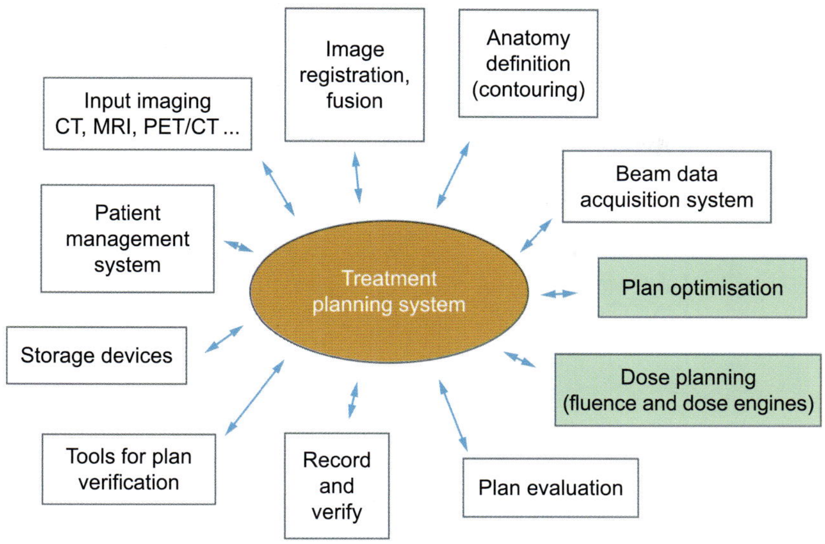

Fig. 12.34 The treatment planning system as the hub of radiotherapy. *CT*, Computed tomography; *MRI*, magnetic resonance imaging; *PET/CT*, positron emission tomography–computed tomography.

on the tolerances for this testing; these being primarily dependent on the location where the dose is being evaluated.[91]

Patient-Specific Quality Assurance

A standard set of tests is typically executed to provide confidence that the equipment and software can be clinically used safely. Traditionally, for treatment planning, there has been a secondary check on the MUs or dose being computed by the TPS. With PSQA, one refers to the checks that are carried out to confirm that the treatment is delivered as planned for each individual patient.

These additional checks incorporate some experimental verification of the plan, and this has been the role of in vivo dosimetry, such as TLDs and solid-state detectors to measure entry and exit dose at specific locations on surfaces and from these to derive an estimate of the dose at a midline in the patient.[92,93] Designing and maintaining an in vivo dosimetry program necessitates sufficient resources in RT physics and is time-consuming. The application of in vivo dosimetry using a single detector to measure dose in modulated plans (IMRT or VMAT) is not straightforward, because a large number of corrections to the detector reading are needed to account for its response in fields that differ considerably from the irradiation geometry used at calibration.[94–96]

The verification of treatment plans can be classified into different categories or levels. The first level is what is widely known as *pretreatment verification*. Here, one checks that the treatment unit delivers the treatment as planned without the presence of the patient. With this approach, changes in the delivered dose distribution because of changes in the patient are not checked, and any changes in data transfer or machine output at the time of patient treatment are also not checked. Pretreatment verification is carried out either by delivering the plan on a phantom using one-dimensional or two-dimensional detector systems, or on the portal imager. With two-dimensional detectors and portal imagers, special software is used to evaluate and compare the fluence or dose delivered to the detector/images against that calculated by the planning system.

The second level in PSQA is to perform checks during patient treatment. Here, one records and then reviews the changes in machine parameters such as MLC leaf positions and gantry angle saved in machine log files. The dose can be recalculated on the planning CT using the parameters from the log files. It is also possible to use transmission detectors mounted on the LINAC head, which record the fluence exiting the machine during treatment. In this way, it is possible to also record changes in beam output during treatment and calculate the influence of this on the dose distribution. In both of these cases, changes in the patient anatomy during treatment are not taken into consideration.

The third level in PSQA is true in vivo dosimetry, referred to as *transit dosimetry* (Chapter 14). The dose delivered to the patient is confirmed and compared against the planned dose. There are several ways to address this. The general concept is to record the fluence through the patient during treatment on the MV portal imager and compare this with the calculated fluence on the imager (in vivo transit dosimetry). An alternative method is a back-projection approach and uses the fluence exiting the patient to reconstruct the dose on the planning CT or the cone beam CT instead. The possibility to compute the delivered dose to the Cone Beam Computed Tomographs (CBCT) allows changes in the internal anatomy during treatment to be included in the calculation and more easily identified during verification. There are several commercial products aiming to provide solutions to PSQA based on the above or similar concepts.

Ultimately, to evaluate the success of a patient's radiotherapy treatment, it is important to know the dose delivered from the treatment and not only that the planned dose is deliverable. The integration of efficient and fast PSQA solutions in the radiotherapy chain, perhaps as part of the tools available on TPSs, is a necessity if adaptation of treatment plans during the course of radiotherapy is to become routine practice.

REFERENCES

1. ICRU (International Commission on Radiation Units and Measurements). Prescribing, recording, and reporting photon beam therapy. ICRU report no. 50. Bethesda, MD: ICRU; 1993.
2. ICRU (International Commission on Radiation Units and Measurements). Prescribing, recording, and reporting proton beam therapy. ICRU report no. 78. Bethesda, MD: ICRU; 1993.
3. ICRU (International Commission on Radiation Units and Measurements). Prescribing, recording, and reporting photon-beam intensity-modulated radiation therapy (IMRT). ICRU report no. 83. Bethesda, MD: ICRU; 1993.
4. ICRU (International Commission on Radiation Units and Measurements). Prescribing, recording, and reporting photon beam

therapy (Supplement to ICRU Report 50). ICRU report no. 62. Bethesda, MD: ICRU; 1999.
5. ICRU (International Commission on Radiation Units and Measurements). Prescribing, recording, and reporting electron beam therapy. ICRU report no. 71. Bethesda, MD: ICRU; 2004.
6. ICRU (International Commission on Radiation Units and Measurements). Prescribing, recording, and reporting of stereotactic treatments with small photon beams. ICRU report no. 91. Bethesda, MD: ICRU; 2017.
7. Bentzen SM, Constine LS, Deasy JO, et al. Quantitative analyses of normal tissue effects in the clinic (QUANTEC): an introduction to the scientific issues. *Int J Radiat Oncol Biol Phys.* 2010;76(3 Suppl):S3–S9.
8. Marks LB, Yorke ED, Jackson A, et al. Use of normal tissue complication probability models in the clinic. *Int J Radiat Oncol Biol Phys.* 2010;76(3 Suppl):S10–S19.
9. Benedict SH, Yenice KM, Followill D, et al. Stereotactic body radiation therapy. Report of the AAPM Radiation Therapy Committee Task Group 101. *Med Phys.* 2010;37:4078–4101.
10. Grimm J, Marks LB, Jackson A, Kavanagh BD, Xue J, Yorke E. High dose per fraction, hypo-fractionated treatment effects in the clinic (HyTEC): an overview. *Rad Onc Biol Phys.* 2021;110(1): 1–10.
11. Timmerman R. A story of hypofractionation and the tables on the wall. *Rad Onc Biol Phys.* 2022;112(1):P4–P21.
12. Reft C, Alecu R, Das IJ, et al. Dosimetric considerations for patients with HIP prostheses undergoing pelvic irradiation. Report of the AAPM Radiation Therapy Committee Task Group 63. *Med Phys.* 2003;30(6):1162–1182.
13. Kruis MF. Improving radiation physics, tumor visualisation, and treatment quantification in radiotherapy with spectral or dual-energy CT. *J Appl Clin Med Phys.* 2022;23(1):e13468.
14. McCollough CH, Boedeker K, Cody D, et al. Principles and applications of multienergy CT: Report of AAPM Task Group 291. *Med Phys.* 2020;47(7):e881–e912.
15. Davis AT, Palmer AL, Nisbet A. Can CT scan protocols used for radiotherapy treatment planning be adjusted to optimize image quality and patient dose? A systematic review. *Br J Radiol.* 2017;90(1076):20160406.
16. Hurkmans CW, Scheepers E, Springorum BGF, Uiterwaal H. Influence of radiotherapy on the latest generation of pacemakers. *Radiother Oncol.* 2005;76(1):93–98.
17. Hurkmans CW, Knegjens JL, Oei BS, et al. Management of radiation oncology patients with a pacemaker or ICD: a new comprehensive practical guideline in The Netherlands. Dutch society of radiotherapy and oncology (NVRO). *Radiat Oncol.* 2012;7:198.
18. Olch AJ, Gerig L, Li H, Mihaylov I, Morgan A. Dosimetric effects caused by couch tops and immobilization devices: report of AAPM task group 176. *Med Phys.* 2014;41(6):061501.
19. Keall PJ, Mageras GS, Balter JM, et al. The management of respiratory motion in radiation oncology report of AAPM task group 76. *Med Phys.* 2006;33(10):3874–3900.
20. Batista V, Gober M, Moura F, et al. Surface guided radiation therapy: an international survey on current clinical practice. *Tech Innov Patient Support Radiat Oncol.* 2022;22:1–8.
21. Freislederer P, Batista V, Ollers M, et al. ESTRO-ACROP guideline on surface guided radiation therapy. *Radiother Oncol.* 2022;173:188–196.
22. Jonsson J, Nyholm T, Soderkvist K. The rationale for MR-only treatment planning for external radiotherapy. *Clin Transl Radiat Oncol.* 2019;18:60–65.
23. Owrangi AM, Greer PB, Glide-Hurst CK. MRI-only treatment planning: benefits and challenges. *Phys Med Biol.* 2018;63(5): 05TR01.
24. Keall PJ, Glide-Hurst CK, Cao M, et al. ICRU Report 97: MRI-guided radiation therapy using MRI-linear accelerators. *J ICRU.* 2022;22(1):1100.
25. Das IJ, McGee KP, Tyagi N, Wang H. Role and future of MRI in radiation oncology. Br J Radiol. 2019;92(1094):20180505.
26. Ahnesjö A, Aspradakis MM. Dose calculations for external photon beams in radiotherapy. *Phys Med Biol.* 1999;44(11): R99–R155.
27. Karlsson M, Ahnesjö A, Georg D, Nyholm T, Olofsson J, eds. *Physics Booklet Nr 10: Independent Dose Calculations Concepts and Models.* Brussels: European Society for Therapeutic Radiology and Oncology; 2010.
28. Aspradakis MM. *IPEM Report 103: Small Field MV Photon Dosimetry.* York, UK: Institute of Physics and Engineering in Medicine; 2010.
29. Aspradakis MM, Lambert GD, Steele A. Elements of commissioning step-and-shoot IMRT: delivery equipment and planning system issues posed by small segment dimensions and small monitor units. *Med Dosim.* 2005;30(4):233–242.
30. International Commission on Radiation Units and Measurements (ICRU). *ICRU Report 91: Prescribing, Recording, and Reporting of Stereotactic Treatments with Small Photon Beams.* Bethesda, MD: ICRU; 2017.
31. Bush K, Gagne IM, Zavgorodni S, Ansbacher W, Beckham W. Dosimetric validation of Acuros XB with Monte Carlo methods for photon dose calculations. *Med Phys.* 2011;38(4): 2208–2221.
32. Han T, Followill D, Mikell J, et al. Dosimetric impact of Acuros XB deterministic radiation transport algorithm for heterogeneous dose calculation in lung cancer. *Med Phys.* 2013;40(5):051710.
33. Mohan R, Chui CS. Use of fast Fourier transforms in calculating dose distributions for irregularly shaped fields for three-dimensional treatment planning. *Med Phys.* 1987;14(1):70–77.
34. Seco J, Verhaegen F. *Monte Carlo Techniques in Radiation Therapy.* Boca Raton, FL: CRC Press; 2016.
35. Verhaegen F, Seuntjens J. Monte Carlo modelling of external radiotherapy photon beams. *Phys Med Biol.* 2003;48(21): R107–R164.
36. Mackie TR, Bielajew AF, Rogers DWO, Battista JJ. Generation of photon energy deposition kernels using the EGS Monte Carlo code. *Phys Med Biol.* 1988;33(1):1–20.
37. Nyholm T, Olofsson J, Ahnesjo A, Karlsson M. Photon pencil kernel parameterisation based on beam quality index. *Radiother Oncol.* 2006;78(3):347–351.
38. Ahnesjö A, Andreo P, Brahme A. Calculation and application of point spread functions for treatment planning with high energy photon beams. *Acta Oncol.* 1987;26(1):49–56.
39. Boyer A, Mok E. A photon dose distribution model employing convolution calculations. *Med Phys.* 1985;12(2):169–177.
40. Mackie TR, Scrimger JW, Battista JJ. A convolution method of calculating dose for 15-MV x rays. *Med Phys.* 1985;12(2): 188–196.
41. Ahnesjö A. Collapsed cone convolution of radiant energy for photon dose calculation in heterogeneous media. *Med Phys.* 1989;16:577–592.
42. Bourland JD, Chaney EL. A finite-size pencil beam model for photon dose calculations in three dimensions. *Med Phys.* 1992;19(6): 1401–1412.

43. Tillikainen L, Helminen H, Torsti T, et al. A 3D pencil-beam-based superposition algorithm for photon dose calculation in heterogeneous media. *Phys Med Biol.* 2008;53(14):3821–3833.
44. Ulmer W, Pyyry J, Kaissl W. A 3D photon superposition/convolution algorithm and its foundation on results of Monte Carlo calculations. *Phys Med Biol.* 2005;50(8):1767–1790.
45. Dutreix A, Bjärngard BE, Bridier A, Mijnheer B, Shaw JE, Svensson H. *Monitor Unit Calculation For High Energy Photon Beams, in Physics for Clinical Radiotherapy, Booklet No. 3.* Leuven/Apeldoorn: Garant Publishers, N. V.; 1997.
46. Zhu TC, Ahnesjö A, Lam KL, et al. Report of AAPM therapy physics committee task group 74: in-air output ratio, Sc, for megavoltage photon beams. *Med Phys.* 2009;36(11):5261–5291.
47. Stern RL, Heaton R, Fraser MW, et al. Verification of monitor unit calculations for non-IMRT clinical radiotherapy: report of AAPM task group 114. *Med Phys.* 2011;38(1):504–530.
48. Gibbons JP, Antolak JA, Followill DS, et al. Monitor unit calculations for external photon and electron beams: report of the AAPM Therapy Physics Committee Task Group No. 71. *Med Phys.* 2014;41(3):031501.
49. Brahme A. Design principles and clinical possibilities with a new generation of radiation therapy equipment. A review. *Acta Oncol.* 1987;26(6):403–412.
50. Brahme A. Optimization of stationary and moving beam radiation therapy techniques. *Radiother Oncol.* 1988;12(2):129–140.
51. American Association of Physicists in Medicine (AAPM). *AAPM Report No. 50: Basic Applications of Multileaf Collimators.* 2001.
52. Boyer AL, Li S. Geometric analysis of light-field position of a multileaf collimator with curved ends. *Med Phys.* 1997;24(5): 757–762.
53. Boyer AL, Ochran TG, Nyerick CE, Waldron TJ, Huntzinger CJ. Clinical dosimetry for implementation of a multileaf collimator. *Med Phys.* 1992;19(5):1255–1261.
54. Mackie TR, Holmes T, Swerdloff S, et al. Tomotherapy: a new concept for the delivery of dynamic conformal radiotherapy. *Med Phys.* 1993;20(6):1709–1719.
55. Carol MP. A system for planning and rotational delivery of intensity-modulated fields. *Int J Imag Syst Tech.* 1995;6:56–61.
56. Bragg CM, Conway J, Robinson MH. The role of intensity-modulated radiotherapy in the treatment of parotid tumors. *Int J Radiat Oncol Biol Phys.* 2002;52(3):729–738.
57. Clark CH, Mubata CD, Meehan CA, et al. IMRT clinical implementation: prostate and pelvic node irradiation using Helios and a 120-leaf multileaf collimator. *J Appl Clin Med Phys.* 2002;3(4):273–284.
58. Carol MP. A system for planning and rotational delivery of intensity-modulated fields. *Int J Imaging Syst Technol.* 1995;6:56–61.
59. Mackie TR, Holmes T, Swerdloff S, et al. Tomotherapy: a new concept for the delivery of dynamic conformal radiotherapy. *Med Phys.* 1993;20(6):1709–1719.
60. Mackie TR. History of tomotherapy. *Phys Med Biol.* 2006;51(13): R427–R453.
61. Otto K. Volumetric modulated arc therapy: IMRT in a single gantry arc. *Med Phys.* 2008;35(1):310–317.
62. Plowman PN. A review of total body irradiation. *Br J Radiol.* 1988;22:135–144.
63. Schmitt D, Blanck O, Gauer T, et al. Technological quality requirements for stereotactic radiotherapy: Expert review group consensus from the DGMP Working Group for Physics and Technology in Stereotactic Radiotherapy. *Strahlenther Onkol.* 2020;196(5):421–443.
64. Pinnaduwage DS, Srivastava SP, Yan X, et al. Small-field beam data acquisition, detector dependency, and film-based validation for a novel self-shielded stereotactic radiosurgery system. *Med Phys.* 2021;48(10):6121–6136.
65. van Herk M, McWilliam A, Dubec M, Faivre-Finn C, Choudhury A. Magnetic resonance imaging-guided radiation therapy: a short strengths, weaknesses, opportunities, and threats analysis. *Int J Radiat Oncol Biol Phys.* 2018;101(5):1057–1060.
66. Ng J, Gregucci F, Pennell RT, Nagar H, Golden EB, Knisely JPS, Sanfilippo NJ, Formenti SC. MRI-LINAC: a transformative technology in radiation oncology. *Front Oncol.* 2023;13: 1117874.
67. Aspradakis MM, Byrne JP, Palmans H, et al. *Small field MV photon dosimetry. IPEM technical report 103.* York, UK: Institute of Physics and Engineering in Medicine (IPEM); 2010.
68. Andreo P. The physics of small megavoltage photon beam dosimetry. *Radiother Oncol.* 2018;126(2):205–213.
69. IAEA (International Atomic Energy Agency). *Dosimetry of small static fields used in external beam radiotherapy.* Technical Report Series No. 483. Vienna, Austria: IAEA; 2017.
70. SABR UK Consortium. *Stereotactic Ablative Body Radiation Therapy (SABR): a resource.* Version 6.1. 2019. https://www.sabr.org.uk/wp-content/uploads/2019/04/SABRconsortium-guidelines-2019-v6.1.0.pdf
71. Hogstrom KR, Mills MD, Meyer JA, et al. Dosimetric evaluation of a pencil-beam algorithm for electrons employing a two-dimensional heterogeneity correction. *Int J Radiat Oncol Biol Phys.* 1984;10(4):561–569.
72. Hogstrom KR. Treatment planning in electron beam therapy. *Front Radiat Ther Oncol.* 1991;25:30–52 discussion 61-33.
73. Neuenschwander H, Mackie TR, Reckwerdt PJ. MMC: a high-performance Monte Carlo code for electron beam treatment planning. *Phys Med Biol.* 1995;40(4):543–574.
74. Kawrakow I, Fippel M, Friedrich K. 3D electron dose calculation using a voxel based Monte Carlo algorithm (VMC). *Med Phys.* 1996;23(4):445–457.
75. McKenzie AL. A simple method for matching electron beams in radiotherapy. *Phys Med Biol.* 1998;43(12):3465–3478.
76. Paganetti H. Range uncertainties in proton therapy and the role of Monte Carlo simulations. *Phys Med Biol.* 2012;57(11): R99–R117.
77. Willoughby TR, Starkschall G, Janjan NA, Rosen II. Evaluation and scoring of radiotherapy treatment plans using an artificial neural network. *Int J Radiat Oncol Biol Phys.* 1996;34:923–930.
78. Hernandez V, Saez J, Pasler M, Jurado-Bruggeman D, Jornet N. Comparison of complexity metrics for multi-institutional evaluations of treatment plans in radiotherapy. *Phys Imaging Radiat Oncol.* 2018;5:37–43.
79. Andratschke N, Willmann J, Appelt AL, et al. European Society for Radiotherapy and Oncology and European Organisation for Research and Treatment of Cancer consensus on re-irradiation: definition, reporting, and clinical decision making. *Lancet Oncol.* 2022;23(10):e469–e478. https://doi.org/10.1016/S1470-2045(22)00447-8.
80. Bentzen SM, Dörr W, Gahbauer R, et al. Bioeffect modeling and equieffective dose concepts in radiation oncology—terminology, quantities and units *Radiother Oncol.* 2012;105(2):266–268. https://doi.org/10.1016/j.radonc.2012.10.006.
81. West N, Covington E, Vasquez Osorio E, et al. Consistency in reirradiation scenarios: terminology, tissue recovery in calculations, units and reporting. *Radiother Oncol.* 2024. https://doi.org/10.1016/j.radonc.2024.110587.

82. Nenoff L, Amstutz F, Murr M, et al. Review and recommendations on deformable image registration uncertainties for radiotherapy applications. *Phys Med Biol.* 2023;68(24):24TR01.
83. Das IJ, Cheng CW, Watts RJ, et al. Accelerator beam data commissioning equipment and procedures: report of the TG-106 of the Therapy Physics Committee of the AAPM. *Med Phys.* 2008;35(9):4186–4215.
84. International Atomic Energy Agency (IAEA). *Commissioning and Quality Assurance of Computerized Planning Systems for Radiation Treatment of Cancer.* Technical Report Series No. 430. Vienna: IAEA; 2004.
85. Low DA, Moran JM, Dempsey JF, Dong L, Oldham M. Dosimetry tools and techniques for IMRT. *Med Phys.* 2011;38(3):1313–1338.
86. Bruinvis IAD, Keus RB, Lenglet WJM, et al. *NCS Report 15: Quality Assurance of 3-D Treatment Planning Systems for External Photon and Electron Beams.* Netherlands Commission on Radiation Dosimetry; 2005.
87. Fraass B, Doppke K, Hunt M, et al. American Association of Physicists in Medicine Radiation Therapy Committee Task Group 53: Quality assurance for clinical radiotherapy treatment planning. *Med Phys.* 1998;25(10):1773–1829.
88. International Atomic Energy Agency (IAEA). Commissioning of Radiotherapy Treatment Planning Systems: Testing for Typical External Beam Treatment Techniques. IAEA-TECDOC-1583. Vienna: International Atomic Energy Agency; 2008.
89. Mijnheer B, Olszewska A, Fiorino C et al, eds. *Quality Assurance of Treatment Planning Systems – Practical Examples for Non-IMRT Photon Beams.* Brussels: European Society for Therapeutic Radiology and Oncology; 2004.
90. Smilowitz JB, Das IJ, Feygelman V, et al. AAPM Medical Physics Practice Guideline 5.a.: Commissioning and QA of treatment planning dose calculations: megavoltage photon and electron beams. *J Appl Clin Med Phys.* 2016;17(1):14–35.
91. Venselaar J, Welleweerd H, Mijnheer B. Tolerances for the accuracy of photon beam dose calculations of treatment planning systems. *Radiother Oncol.* 2001;60:191–201.
92. American Association of Physicists in Medicine (AAPM). *Diode In Vivo Dosimetry for Patients Receiving External Beam Radiation Therapy.* Report No. 87. College Park, MD: AAPM; 2005.
93. Huyskens D, Bogaerts R, Verstraete J, et al. Practical guidelines for the implementation of in vivo dosimetry with diodes in external radiotherapy with photon beams (entrance dose). *Physics for Clinical Radiotherapy.* Booklet No. 5. Brussels: ESTRO; 2001.
94. Higgins PD, Alaei P, Gerbi BJ, Dusenbery KE. In vivo diode dosimetry for routine quality assurance in IMRT. *Med Phys.* 2003;30(12):3118–3123.
95. Kadesjo N, Nyholm T, Olofsson J. A practical approach to diode based in vivo dosimetry for intensity modulated radiotherapy. *Radiother Oncol.* 2011;98(3):378–381.
96. Nijsten SM, Mijnheer BJ, Dekker AL, Lambin P, Minken AW. Routine individualised patient dosimetry using electronic portal imaging devices. *Radiother Oncol.* 2007;83(1):65–75.

13

Networking, Data, Image Handling and Computing in Radiotherapy

John Sage

CHAPTER OUTLINE

INTRODUCTION

Technology is so much fun, but we can drown in our technology. The fog of information can drive out knowledge.

Daniel Boorstin

Computers permeate every aspect of modern radiotherapy. With their application, we can deliver ever more intricate treatments. However, every technological innovation comes at a cost: in equipment, maintenance and added complexity. With care, these costs can be kept in balance and benefits to the patient achieved.

Computing in radiotherapy has developed as computers have grown more powerful. In 1965, Gordon Moore, cofounder of the computing giant Intel, predicted that microchip complexity would increase exponentially for at least 10 years.[1] In fact, Moore's law still holds today, with processors doubling in complexity approximately every 2 years. Moore's law typifies the growth in all aspects of computing. Hard disk drive capacity nearly doubles each year while the cost per gigabyte nearly halves.[2]

This growth has consequences for radiotherapy. The useful lifetime of any item of computer software or hardware is going to be fairly short. Commonly, the longest warranty period available for a computer server is 5 years, compared with 10 years for a linear accelerator. This growth also needs to be considered when planning for long-term needs. It will be more costly to purchase 5 years' worth of data storage immediately than it will be to buy half now and half in 2 years' time, at a quarter of the cost.

History

For many decades, radiotherapy was developed without computers. Isodose planning and linear accelerators came before the use of computers. In the 1960s, the first investigations were made into using computers for radiotherapy. Such use required access to one of the small number of large mainframe computers, probably at a university, because personal computers were not invented until the 1970s. The first widespread use of computers was for calculating isodose distributions, replacing laborious manual calculations. In the late 1970s, the first use was made of computed tomography (CT) data for radiotherapy planning. This required a magnetic tape reader connected to the planning system to read the CT scanner tapes.

As networking technology became available, it was possible to connect computers together directly. However, CT scanners still used different file formats. In 1985, the American College of Radiology and the National Electrical Manufacturers Association created a standard for medical images, called *ACR-NEMA*. In the third version, in 1991, the standard was developed to specify how systems should communicate directly. To mark this change, a new name for the standard was used: *Digital Imaging and Communication in Medicine*, or *DICOM 3.0*.

Networking and computing capability have continuously driven radiotherapy development, from the first simple electronic checking of the LINAC beam settings in the 1980s to advanced systems which allow real-time updating of the beam to respond to patient position. Similarly, the use of digital imaging continues to expand, with magnetic resonance imaging (MRI) at the point of treatment now in routine clinical use.

Such a wealth of information creates a problem in how the information is organised and best used. Oncology information systems manage data flow within a single centre. The next boundary to be overcome will be the pooling of information across whole populations. This will allow clinical collaboration between practitioners for rare cancers and facilitate the continuous learning systems that we are just beginning to see emerge.[3]

Benefits and Hazards of Computerisation

The more advanced techniques that we practise would not be possible at all without the assistance of computers. Intensity modulated radiotherapy (IMRT) would be totally unfeasible without computers or data communication. Even simple techniques are enhanced by the use of computers. If data are transferred directly between computers, there is less chance of human error. The use of record and verify systems has certainly reduced the number of random human errors at the point of treatment delivery.[4]

Ultimately, the hazards of computerisation relate to our increased dependence on computer systems and the faulty assumption that they are reliable. Computers and networks do fail. A radiotherapy department that is reliant on a system can be crippled if that system is the victim of component failure, a virus or even theft.

As systems become more complicated, they are harder to check for errors. It should never be assumed that the computer is correct. Furthermore, computers do not remove the risk of human error altogether. Proper use of a system relies on operators performing tasks correctly. If they do not, incorrect information can be passed down the line and used at a later stage. Where errors do occur in computerised systems, they may affect a series of patients or a single patient for every fraction of their treatment.[5]

To reduce these risks, we need to reverse the assumption that the computer is reliable. Key checks should be made during system testing and for individual treatments. Is the isocentre correct? Is the patient reference position correct? Where there are multiple data sets, has the correct one been used for the treatment? When every plan had to be calculated and delivered manually, each person involved had to fully understand the technique and the treatment. Now that the treatment can be delivered at the touch of a button, that level of understanding is critical to detect errors.

NETWORKING

Networks are commonly described as having a number of layers. In one of the simpler descriptions, the Transmission Control Protocol (TCP) and Internet Protocol (IP) model, four layers are described.[6] To understand these layers, we draw a comparison with the postal system (Table 13.1).

TABLE 13.1 The Four Network Layers of the TCP/IP Model

Layer	Network	Postal
Link	The infrastructure of cables, switches, modems and so on which allow information to be moved from one place to another	The infrastructure of vehicles and sorting offices which allow post to be moved around
Network	The addressing system which allows a single computer to be identified and for data to be routed to it	The addressing system which allows post to be directed to the correct destination
Transport	The process of packing the data and sending it into the network; also the process of receiving data from the network	Taking letters to the post office to send and picking up received letters
Application	Defining the data to be sent and interpreting any data received	Writing and reading your post

TCP/IP, Transmission Control Protocol/Internet Protocol.

Link Layer: Physical Infrastructure

In a very large network, such as a hospital, there will be a large number of switches controlling and routing the flow of data in the hospital. In such a large network, the computers may be organised into subnetworks, or *subnets*. Access between subnets is controlled by gateways which can prevent unauthorised access between areas (Fig. 13.1).

Network Layer: Addressing

When you type 'www.estro.org' into a web browser, how does your computer connect to the computer that contains the home page of the European Society for Therapeutic Radiotherapy and Oncology (ESTRO)? Each domain name is registered to a computer address, called an *IP address*, which consists of four numbers. Your computer initially sends a request to a directory to find out the correct IP address. Then, it sends a request to that IP address to retrieve the correct web page.

In a private network, such as a hospital, computers are still referenced using an IP address. Special ranges of numbers are reserved for use in private networks to avoid confusion with internet traffic. On

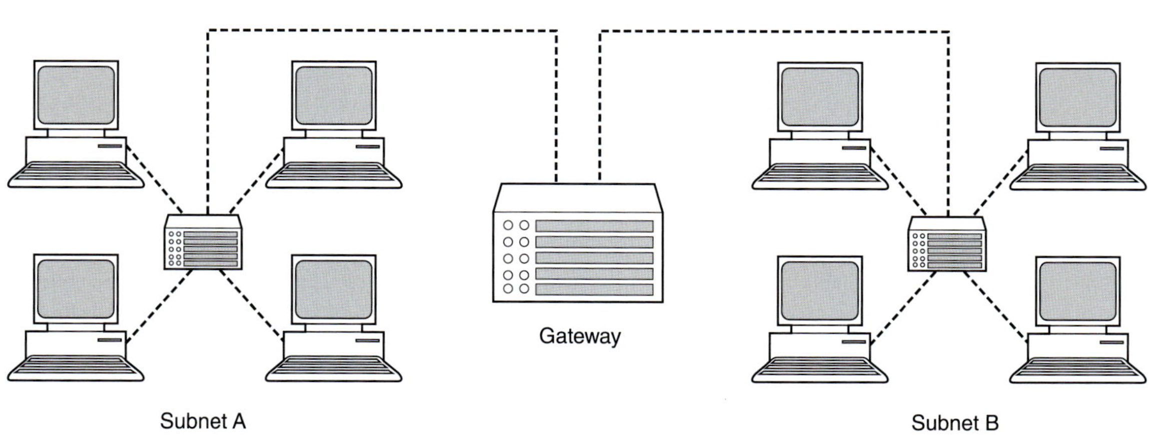

Fig. 13.1 Two subnets separated by a gateway.

```
Windows IP Configuration
Ethernet adapter Local Area Connection:
  Connection-specific DNS suffix  . : hospital.nhs.uk
  IP Address . . . . . . . . . . . : 192.168.123.45
  Subnet mask. . . . . . . . . . . : 255.255.255.0
  Default Gateway  . . . . . . . . : 192.168.123.1
```

Fig. 13.2 Sample output from ipconfig.

```
Pinging 192.168.123.1 with 32 bytes of data:
Reply from 192.168.123.1: bytes=32 time<1ms TTL=255
Reply from 192.168.123.1: bytes=32 time<1ms TTL=255
Reply from 192.168.123.1: bytes=32 time<1ms TTL=255
Reply from 192.168.123.1: bytes=32 time<1ms TTL=255
Ping statistics for 192.168.123.1:
    Packets: sent = 4, Recieved = 4, Lost = 0 (0% loss)
Approximate round trip times in milli-seconds:
    Minimum = 0ms, Maximum = 0ms, Average = 0ms
```

Fig. 13.3 Sample output from ping.

many Windows computers, it is possible to see the network configuration by typing the command 'ipconfig' at a command prompt.[1] If you do this and your computer is attached to a network, you will see something like that shown in Fig. 13.2.

This tells us that our computer is in the network domain hospital, nhs.uk. The first two numbers of the IP address are among those reserved for private networks. That tells us this computer cannot be seen by the internet. The second two numbers in the IP address will be unique for this computer within the hospital. The subnet mask describes the range of IP addresses that are in our local subnet; in this case, the IP addresses 192.168.123.1 through 192.168.123.255. The default gateway is the IP address of the computer or switch that our computer must go through to access the network outside the local subnet, such as the internet.

Transport Layer: Send and Receive

The simplest form of data transport is the *ping*, which is used for the testing of data connections. If you still have a command prompt open on your computer, type 'ping 192.168.123.1', replacing the IP address here with the IP address of your gateway (Fig. 13.3).

Your computer has just packaged a data packet and sent it into the network addressed to the gateway. On receipt, the gateway sends a return package back to your computer. The ping command is often one of the first tools used when testing a network connection. A successful ping proves that both the link layer and the network layer are working correctly.

There are a lot of different potential connections that a computer can make. In the preceding example, how did the gateway know that this single data packet came from a ping request and that it should send a return message? Also, how can a computer make multiple connections of different types without them getting confused? Each computer has a whole series of network 'ports'. When a computer receives a data packet addressed to port 7, it knows that this is a ping request and responds accordingly, whereas requests for web pages are normally addressed to port 80. Imagine having a whole series of slots outside your house and the postal worker sorting them out for you into bills, junk mail and so on.

Application Layer: The Program

The final layer is the program itself, which is often the hardest part. Just because you can send a letter to anywhere in the world, it doesn't mean that the recipient will be able to understand what you have written.

Network Security

On 12 May 2017, about one-third of NHS trusts in England were disrupted by the WannaCry virus, resulting in the cancellation of thousands of patient appointments and operations.[7] Radiotherapy departments were not immune, although for many the subsequent lockdown and emergency network restrictions had a greater impact than the initial attack. Because the modern radiotherapy department is so reliant on the network, it is important to protect it against various hazards. There is also a legal requirement to protect patient data and often a minimum security level which must be reached to connect to the hospital network. These are summarised in Fig. 13.4.

Most modern medical devices are network connected, and this brings particular challenges. The requirement for device manufacturers to strictly control and test any change in the device design conflicts with the need to continuously update computer systems to maintain security. It is important to obtain from equipment providers detailed plans on how network security will be maintained over the equipment's lifespan.

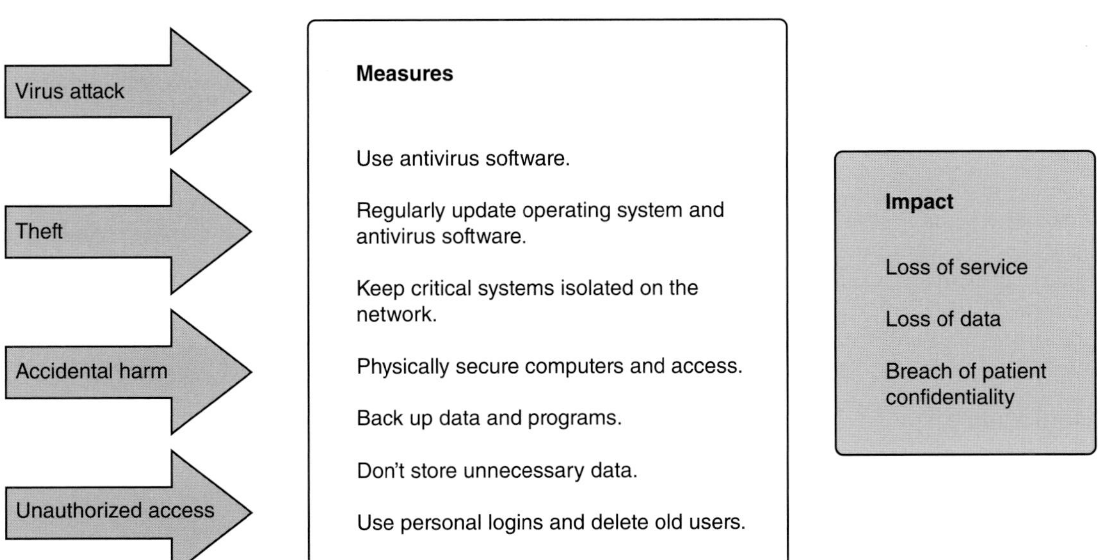

Fig. 13.4 Potential impact of network hazards and measures to mitigate them.

Hardware Failure Security: Redundancy, Virtualisation and the Cloud

A further risk arises from the potential for hardware failure. A computer system is a collection of hardware components: disks, memory, processors, boards and the like. All of these components have a lifetime and can fail. The failure of an oncology information system could mean the total stop of all activity in the radiotherapy department until the problem is fixed. All critical systems should be designed with redundancy, where spares of each critical component automatically come into use in the event of any failure.

The greatest level of protection from physical hardware failure can perhaps be found in cloud computing. In cloud systems, each individual computer does not physically exist as a unique piece of hardware at all. The computers exist as virtualised systems, sharing an allotment of resources from a much larger pool of computing hardware. Redundancy can be created with multiple copies of an entire computer system. Because the computing resource is provided across a large number of physical systems, the failure of one of those systems does not impact the functioning of the virtual system.

The use of commercial cloud systems for healthcare and government systems is encouraged as long as certain conditions are met for housing the data.[8] The increased robustness and cost efficiency of cloud deployment does need to be weighed against the increased reliance on an external internet connection. As with any system, contingency measures need to be in place in the event of a total network failure.

DICOM

As described previously, DICOM stands for Digital Imaging and Communication in Medicine and is produced by the National Electrical Manufacturers Association in the United States. DICOM is a constantly evolving standard with a number of working parties and regular releases.[9]

DICOM is often mistakenly considered a data file format. While there is a file format within DICOM, it is primarily a data transfer protocol, a means to move medical images between systems. DICOM aims to be a complete specification for such transfer and specifies requirements over all the network layers.

The second common misconception about DICOM is that two DICOM-compliant devices will communicate correctly. This mistake is the root cause of a great deal of anxiety. Given the huge variety of medical imaging equipment, DICOM is not prescriptive. There is a great deal of variation possible within the standard. Where there is variation, DICOM provides us with a common language to describe the functionality of a system and check whether two systems are compatible.

DICOM Services

DICOM connections are not always about the transfer of images from one computer to another. A connection may be to print an image, send a worklist to a scanner or find patient images. Each of these possibilities is called a *service class*. Furthermore, in any transaction, there will be a *service class provider (SCP)* and a *service class user (SCU)*. Therefore a server may offer the storage class as SCP and a number of systems may send images to it as SCU.

DICOM Communication

To establish a DICOM connection, we need two critical pieces of information: (1) the IP address of the computer we wish to connect to and (2) which network port the DICOM program is monitoring. Port 104 is reserved for use by DICOM programs and is normally the correct port. However, this is not always the case; a single computer may run several DICOM servers on different ports. With these two pieces of information, we are able to establish communication with the DICOM server, but this does not necessarily mean that the connection will be successful.

The security of DICOM servers varies widely. Some will communicate with any system that has the correct address and port. This makes system setup easy, but security will be poor. Others will make further checks. Each DICOM program has a name, called an *application entity title (AET)*. Most servers will refuse a connection to a system that does not call it by the correct name. Furthermore, many servers will check the AET of the requesting system against a list of known AETs.

Upon connection, the two systems perform what is known as a *handshake*. They swap credentials and determine whether the action which is being requested is supported and whether to continue with the action. Then, information is exchanged and the association is closed.

DICOM Data Objects

One key problem in sending data between imaging systems is defining the exact meaning of the information sent. DICOM solves this through the use of a data dictionary. Each possible piece of information about the image, called a *data element*, is catalogued and given a code. The exact definition of the information for each code is contained in the DICOM Standard.[9]

Any *data object*, such as a radiotherapy plan or a CT image, will consist of a collection of data elements relevant to that object. The DICOM standard details which data elements are mandatory for a given object and which are optional. Another new term, the *service-object pair (SOP)*, is used to describe the application of a particular service class to a data object. We may talk about a general *SOP class*, such as CT image storage, or even a particular *SOP instance*, one specific stored CT image.

The diagram in Fig. 13.5 shows an example of a minimal CT object. Each row of the diagram shows the entry for each of the separate data elements. For each data element there is a two-number code which relates that element to the DICOM data dictionary. The data elements are grouped by the first number. In this example, Group 0008 is the identity group and contains all the elements which help to uniquely identify this object. Group 0010 is the patient demographics group, Group 0018 is the CT parameters group and so on. The last of all of the data elements contains the actual image data itself.

One special class of data element, the *unique identifier (UID)*, consists of a long numeric code. This code must be truly unique and may not be reused. In Fig. 13.5 there are three kinds of UID. The values for the SOP class UID are defined in the DICOM Standard and each code describes the object. In this case, this is the code for a stored CT image. The SOP instance UID is the unique code for this object. No other DICOM object in the world may have the same UID. In this way a DICOM server can tell if it is sent the same image twice and can disregard one of them. The study instance UID is the unique code for this study for this patient. All images in this study will contain the same study instance UID, and a DICOM server can use this to correctly group images together.

DICOM Conformance

Whereas the CT object in Fig. 13.5 is a valid CT object according to the standard, it contains very little information and would probably be rejected by many DICOM servers. This is the problem. By allowing manufacturers to choose which data elements are contained in the data object, the standard creates room for incompatibility. It becomes very important for manufacturers to describe exactly how their system behaves, which data elements are important and which are ignored.

The DICOM standard specifies a common format for such descriptions, the *DICOM conformance statement*. It should be possible to determine whether two systems will be able to successfully

```
0008 0008 Image Type                      ORIGINAL\PRIMARY\AXIAL
0008 0016 SOP ClassVID                    1.2.840.10008.5.1.4.1.1.2
0008 0018 SOP Instance VID                1.2.345.6.789.8.76.5.4321.0.10
0008 0020 Study Date                      20021011
0008 0060 Modality                        CT
0008 0090 Referring Physician             DR
0008 1030 Study Description               SAMPLE CT SCAN

0010 0010 Patient Name                    Walter/Miller
0010 0020 Patient ID                      01234

0018 0050 Slice Thickness                 5
0018 0060 KVP                             130
0018 5100 Patient Posistion               HFS

0020 000d Study Instance VID              1.2.345.6.789.8.76.4.4321.0
0020 0010 Study ID                        123
0020 0013 Image Number                    10
0200 0020 Patient Orientation             L\P
0020 0032 Image Position Patient          -200\-500\-40
0020 0037 Image Orientation               1\1\0\0\1\0

0028 0004 Photometric Interpretation      MONOCHROME2
0028 0010 Rows                            512
0028 0011 Columns                         512
0028 0030 Pixel Spacing                   0.9\0.9

7fe0 0010 Pixel Data                      _
```

Fig. 13.5 A minimal stored computed tomography DICOM object.

communicate by comparing their DICOM conformance statements. In practice, these documents are quite long and an incompatibility might be difficult to spot.

DICOM and Connectivity

Because standards alone do not guarantee connectivity, the Integrating Healthcare Enterprise – Radiation Oncology (IHE-RO) initiative[10] takes a more direct approach. IHE-RO teams, built from the clinic and industry, publish profiles which specify more closely how to apply the DICOM standard to radiotherapy data. At 'connectathon' events, manufacturers come together to send data between systems to demonstrate the success, or not, of any interoperability.

RADIOTHERAPY DATA

Data Storage

Data storage essentially comprises a number of switches, which are on or off. The smallest size of data storage is one switch, called a *bit*, which can store a 1 or a 0. More bits are used to store larger numbers. If 8 bits are used, a number from 0 to 255 can be stored, called a *byte*. A kilobyte (kB) is equal to 1024 bytes. A megabyte (MB) is equal to 1024 kB, a gigabyte (GB) is equal to 1024 MB and a terabyte (TB) is equal to 1024 GB.

Image Quality

There is a trade-off between the quality of the image and the space it takes up. For reference, a standard CT slice uses 512 kB. To illustrate this section, a test image is used which also requires approximately 512 kB, shown in Fig. 13.6A.

Dimensions and Scale

Many images are two dimensional. We frequently also use three-dimensional data sets consisting of a series of two-dimensional images. A CT series might comprise 50 slices at 5-mm spacing, requiring 25 MB. Time sequences can also be considered as a series of two-dimensional frames. As the number of points increases in any dimension, so does the image size. In Fig. 13.6B the test image is shown at one-eighth of the resolution. Now the image only requires 8 kB of storage, 64 times less. Much of the detail is lost at this resolution.

The *bit depth* describes the number of shades of grey between the maximum and minimum possible values. In medical imaging, most images are either 8-bit, with 256 levels of grey, or 16-bit, with 65,536 levels of grey. It is widely accepted that a person cannot discriminate between more than 256 shades of grey. However, a user may interrogate 16-bit images by changing the contrast window to examine different grey levels more clearly. Fig. 13.7A shows the loss in contrast from a reduced bit depth in the test image.

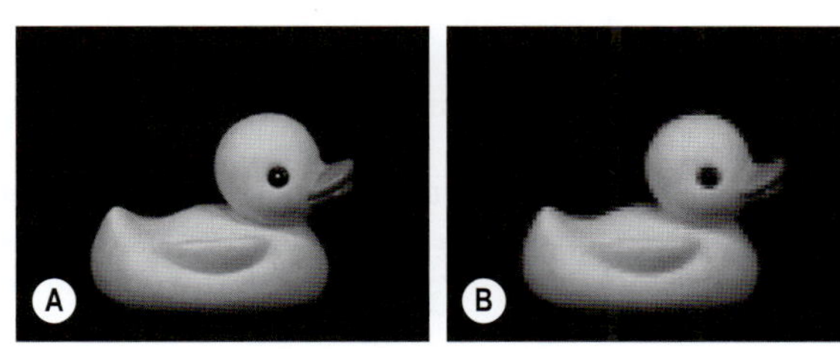

Fig. 13.6 (A) Test image. (B) Test image at reduced resolution.

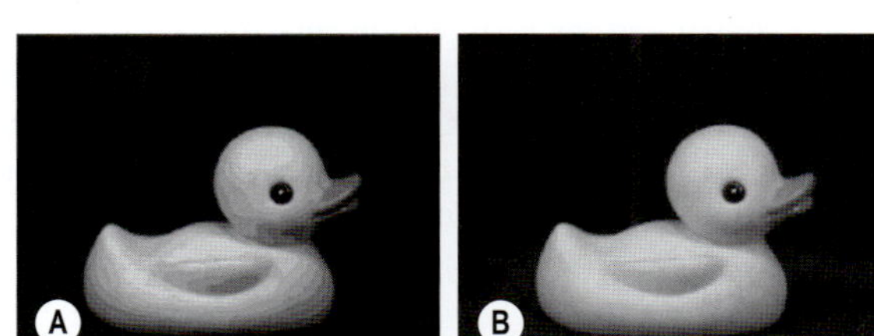

Fig. 13.7 (A) A 4-bit image showing significant degradation for only 50% space savings. (B) A compressed image taking up just 2% of the original space, but differences are visible.

Compression of Data

There are two kinds of compression. *Lossless compression* reduces the size of the data, generally to about half, without any alteration of the data. *Lossy compression* has greater ability to reduce the size of the data but at the expense of some degradation of the data, as shown in Fig. 13.7B. Lossy schemes can achieve much greater compression with an almost undetectable reduction in image quality. However, they are often considered inappropriate for medical applications where any subtle change might affect patient treatment.

Radiotherapy Data Types

Given the huge range of definitions found between different manufacturers, it will be easiest to consider these in the context of the range of data objects defined within DICOM. Within radiotherapy, these fall into two groups: general image data types and those data types specific to radiotherapy, commonly referred to as *DICOM RT*.

Tomographic Images

In radiotherapy, CT images are used extensively, with MRI and positron emission tomography (PET) becoming more widespread. All of these are well defined in DICOM. However, many radiotherapy systems will still only accept images with a simple transverse imaging geometry. As the use of three-dimensional images increases, it is anticipated that manufacturers will increase the range of acceptable imaging geometries. This also includes tomographic verification images, such as cone beam CT.

Planar Images

Ideally, all planar images in radiotherapy should be presented as true RT images, described in the 'RT Image' section. However, many manufacturers have not implemented this and still use one of several DICOM data objects appropriate for simple planar images.

Curves, Annotations and Overlays

There is scope in DICOM to store and send any annotation that has been made on an image. Some manufacturers use these to attach additional information to an image, such as anatomical outlines. Any use of these which is more than just the simple display of annotation tends not to be transferable across manufacturers.

RT Structure Set

The RT structure set describes anatomical outlines that have been defined on tomographic data. It is used for the transfer of target volumes and organs at risk (OARs) between planning systems. The structure set object specifically references the UID of each image on which it was defined. In this way a system can check that it does not load a structure set onto the wrong set of images.

RT Plan

The RT plan contains all the required information to deliver a radiotherapy treatment. It is possible for an RT plan to describe an external beam or a brachytherapy treatment. If the RT plan was created using target volumes from a CT data set, it will reference the UID of the RT structure set from which it was defined.

RT Dose

The RT dose object contains the result of the dose calculation. There may be a single dose object for each calculated slice or a full three-dimensional calculation in a single object. Dose objects may also contain dose volume histograms.

RT Image

The RT image data type is used for all radiotherapy planar images. There are several differences between an RT image and a standard planar image. RT images contain much more precise details about the imaging geometry and explicitly specify the type of RT image, digital reconstructed radiograph (DRR), portal image and so on. RT images also allow the aspects of the RT plan which are relevant to that beam to be attached to the image, such as gantry angle, jaw positions and beam shaping.

RT Treatment Summary

The RT treatment summary is less widely used and is often overlooked. It contains a record of the treatment that was delivered.

DATA BURDEN

The build-up of patient data can represent a serious problem for the radiotherapy department. Without care, it is possible for a system such as the planning system to fill up completely, with a risk of system failure, loss of data and disruption to the service. The additional build-up of data is often an unforeseen side effect of service development. For example, a patient verified using cone beam CT will have a greatly increased data use over one verified using portal images.

Measures can be taken to manage the radiotherapy data burden:

- Avoid increases in patient data for which there is no clinical benefit, such as inappropriate dose grid size or unnecessary imaging.
- Practise good housekeeping. Delete any patient plans or images which are not used clinically.
- Consider whether data are being stored multiple times. Identical CT data may be being stored on the CT scanner, the virtual simulator, the planning system and a central disk.
- Assess data requirements for any new technique and ensure that facilities are in place.
- Monitor the rate of data build-up and the capacity of clinical systems. Investigate any unforeseen increase in data and any system regularly greater than 80% full.
- Plan future data requirements.

With fewer data sets being stored, there is also a reduced risk of patient mistreatment as a result of an incorrect data set being used.

Table 13.2 demonstrates the total data storage commitment for an example lung patient. In this example the greatest storage commitment is by far the cone beam CT verification images, because of the finer resolution in the craniocaudal axis and the number of such images acquired. With temporal images such as four-dimensional CT (4DCT) and dynamic MR images, this data burden will be significantly increased again.

Data Backup

It is critical that the data are not lost in the event of a failure of the system on which they are stored. To achieve this, the data should be

TABLE 13.2 Data for an Example Lung Patient

Item	No.	Format	Memory
Planning CT	120	512 × 512 × 16 bit	60 MB
CT outlines	1		3 MB
Treatment plan	1		100 kB
Dose distribution	2	200 × 200 × 200 × 32 bit	61 MB
Cone beam verification	24	410 × 410 × 162 × 16 bit	1247 MB
		Total	1371 MB

CT, Computed tomography.

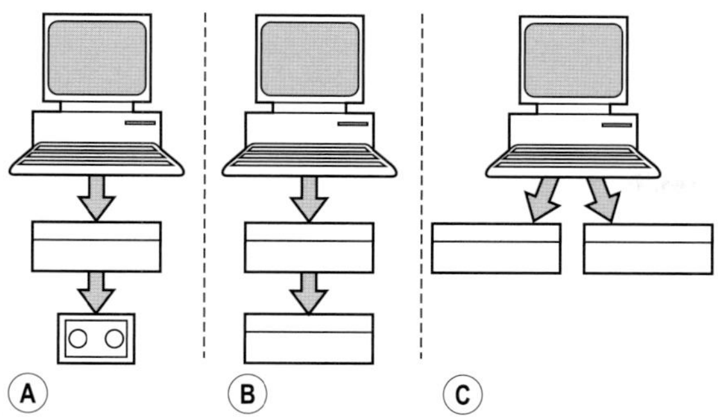

Fig. 13.8 Backup schemes: (A) backup to tape; (B) backup to disk; (C) mirrored disks.

copied to a second location. There are many ways in which this can be achieved. In Fig. 13.8A the data are written by the computer to a hard disk. Overnight, an automatic program copies the data to a digital tape. The scheme shown in Fig. 13.8B is similar except the data are copied overnight to a second hard disk drive. This has the advantage that the copies can be retrieved without any time delay. In Fig. 13.8C the data are written immediately to two separate independent disk drives. This scheme is known as *drive mirroring*.

It is important to ensure that backups performed by any method can actually be read. It has been known for systems to be backed up every night, but when actually required, the tapes were useless. As the number of computer systems and the amount of data in a department grow, backup can be a significant technical problem.

Data Archive

As patient data are acquired, computer systems may become full, and old data should be transferred to an archive to release storage capacity. Archive is very similar to backup and the two are often confused, but they fulfil very different roles. Backup is very short term in scope. Data today are stored in case of a catastrophe tomorrow. Archival is long term in scope. Archived data will need to be kept for years. It is important that sufficient records are kept to enable the data to be located in the future. Furthermore, one must have the means to read the data. It is pointless storing patient data if it can only be read by a planning system that is no longer available.

If data are archived to a physical medium such as tape or CD, the long-term life of the medium will need to be considered. As the archive grows, the number of media being stored will grow and may take up a significant amount of space. Because disk storage is so cheap, it is feasible to create a hard disk archive and simply purchase new disk storage when it fills up. Some systems are now being written with this in mind and have no archive facility. All of the data are available all of the time.

Data Protection

Patients' rights with regard to their data are set out in laws such as the Data Protection Act (UK, 2018).[11] The data holder has a responsibility to undertake good stewardship, ensuring that data are accurate and safe from loss or misuse. Organisations should be open about what patient data are held for what purposes and then limit use or sharing of the data to those purposes. Generally, if patient data are to be used for research, explicit consent should be obtained. There are situations where data can be used for research without consent, for example, historical data analysis, but expert advice should be taken to ensure that use is legal, fair and justifiable.

Data Use and the FAIR Principles

All the data being produced can be of immense value in research and in developing automated systems. The FAIR principles[12] aim to ensure that data collected can actually be of use to researchers. FAIR is a mnemonic of the following four principles:

- **Findable:** A detailed description of the data should exist in a searchable source. This could be achieved with an academic publication describing the data or an entry in a data repository archive.
- **Accessible:** The data should be readable by humans and computer programs and any approval process for access well described and functional.
- **Interoperable:** The terms and fields used in the data should be standardised using ontologies[13]; formal representations of information in a given scientific domain, which should themselves conform to the FAIR principles.
- **Reusable:** Sufficient information should be given about the acquisition and processing of the data to allow researchers to conduct meaningful research. The license terms under which the data may be reused should be clearly stated.

Increased adherence of these principles has led to a growth of repositories such as the Cancer Imaging Archive.[14]

ARTIFICIAL INTELLIGENCE AND DEEP LEARNING

At the time of this writing, there is an explosion in the development of artificial intelligence (AI) in radiotherapy. This is driven by the convergence of the coming of age of AI technology, the availability of radiotherapy data and post-COVID pressures on radiotherapy capacity.

One could conceivably try to build an AI by writing a vast number of rules for a task, say, identifying flowers. Such a mechanistic approach is doomed to fail given the subtle differences between flowers, and it does not mimic the development of intelligence in the natural world. A human would learn the names of flower by seeing the flowers and being told what they are many times over. In modern AI, this process is mimicked using deep learning (DL).

Imagine building a system to identify flowers with a phone camera. The process begins with a deep neural network, as shown in Fig. 13.9. This is formed of layers of connected virtual switches, called *nodes*, designed to mimic the connections of neurons in the brain, which span from an input to an output. The input layer would be the camera image and the output layer would be the identification label. The network is deep because there are a large number of layers.

To train the network requires a large set of training data with input images and the known result for each. In our example, this would be images of flowers with the correct names. In training mode, both the input image and output result are presented to the network and all connections that positively link the two are strengthened. Over a large number of training images, the connections which reliably link an image of a flower to the correct label are strengthened. In use, a fresh input image is applied to the input layer of the network, and the prediction of the network can be read at the output layer.

This greatly simplified description of DL helps us to understand some of its characteristics. Primarily, DL is a statistical technique. The network learns patterns that link the inputs to the outputs consistently. Outlier cases may not be handled well, and presenting an unusual case to a DL system can produce unexpected results. It follows that the quality of any DL system is highly dependent on the quality and scope of the training data. The inputs in the training data should be broad, covering any variations in presentation that the system will encounter in use. The known outputs for the training data must be consistently generated to avoid the DL learning spurious variation in the results. Despite the label of AI, DL doesn't reason. It does not apply rules or protocols and cannot explain the rationale for its choices. It learns patterns in training data which are applied to new data. It may be that the combination of rules and learning will come with the next generation of AI.

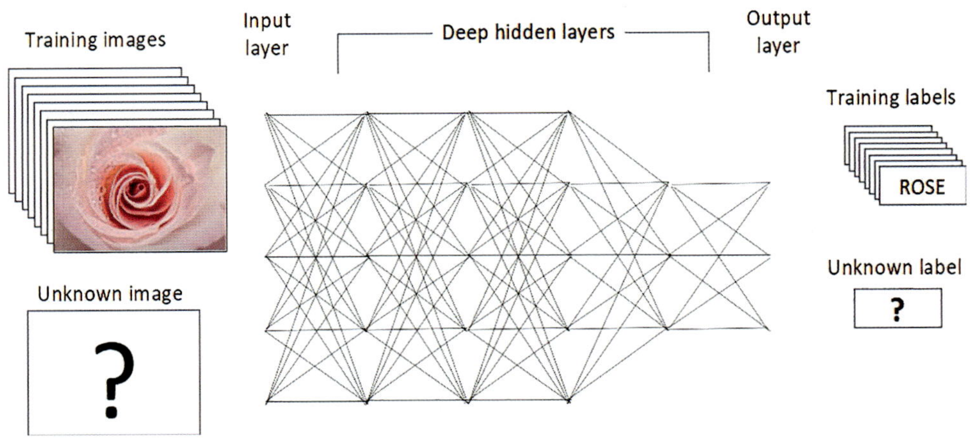

Fig. 13.9 A conceptual diagram of a deep learning system.

SOFTWARE DEVELOPMENT

Frequently, there comes a time when available products do not meet the immediate need and a centre must consider in-house developed software. Even the simplest spreadsheet can be considered software and should be developed with care. One of the worst series of radiation therapy incidents, the Therac 25 incidents, had poor software design and testing as the root cause.[15]

Detailed advice on the management and validation of software projects is available. One excellent example is 'General Principles of Software Validation; Final Guidance for Industry and FDA Staff', which is available online.[16] Of particular relevance is the 'Software Is Different From Hardware' section which details a series of reasons why care must be applied to software development. Even the simplest software program may be classed as a medical device and potentially be subject to legal control. Advice is available through the Medical and Healthcare products Regulatory Authority (MHRA).[17]

A software development project can be considered as having five main areas of effort, which are shown in Fig. 13.10. Frequently, the only area of effort which has allocated resources is the actual computer programming itself, with all other effort taking place on an ad hoc basis. This approach is inefficient, as the software will need constant reworking as the specification changes during the project. This approach is also unsafe, as it often leads to software coming into use without proper documentation and with only superficial testing and training. In the safer approach shown, only 20% of the effort is actually spent on computer programming.

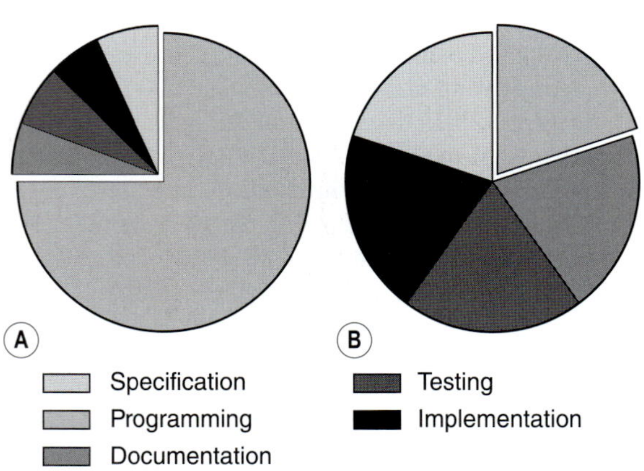

Fig. 13.10 Division of effort in software development projects. (A) What is often perceived as required. (B) A much more realistic and safe approach.

In the specification and design work area, it is important to clearly describe the requirements for the project. This will include the functionality and any technical requirements. Important decisions such as the programming language to be used should not be left solely to the programmer, as this will affect the ability of a centre to support the software in the future. This phase should also include a risk assessment of the impact of software failure and consequently any safety requirements. A framework for keeping adequate clinical safety documentation for software development is available through NHS Digital.[18]

Documentation is vital to maintaining a safe software system, not just user manuals but clear technical documentation and descriptions of the operation of the computer code itself. It is not sufficient for all documentation to be written retrospectively, as important details can be forgotten. Testing can also be undertaken throughout software development and should be done by both the programmer and a second party. The testing program should relate closely to the system specification and especially the risk assessment.

Finally, the implementation of the system needs to be planned with various 'what if' scenarios considered and all training, technical and user, undertaken in a timely manner. Ideally, the whole project will be managed by an individual or a small team who will be able to sign off on the project when all aspects are complete. Various software quality assurance systems exist[19,20] and should be considered for critical software projects. However, the principals outlined here should be applied to all software projects, large or small.

CONCLUSION

This simple introduction to the use of computers in radiotherapy will, regrettably, by the very nature of the subject, be out of date almost instantly. It is important to obtain up-to-date guidance on specific aspects. The field of radiotherapy computing overlaps traditional work boundaries. There are frequently problems with IT professionals who don't fully understand the requirements of radiotherapy as much as radiotherapy professionals who don't fully understand the technicalities of IT. Out of this situation, a new breed is rising: radiotherapy computing and information specialists. Such people will be extremely important to ensure that we continue to reap the benefits of computerised radiotherapy.

REFERENCES

1. Moore G. Cramming more components onto integrated circuits. *Electronics Magazine*. 1965.
2. Walter C. Kryder's law. *Sci Am*. 2005:7–25.

3. Lustberg T, van Soest J, Jochems A, et al. Big data in radiation therapy: challenges and opportunities. *Br J Radiol.* 2016;90(1069): 20160689.
4. Muller-Runkel R, Watkins S. Introducing a computerized record and verify system: its impact on the reduction of treatment errors. *Med Dosim.* 1991;16(1):19–22.
5. Patton G, Gaffney DK, Moeller JH. Facilitation of radiotherapeutic error by computerized record and verify systems. *Int J Radiat Oncol Biol Phys.* 2003;56(1):50–57.
6. Cerf V, Kahn R. A protocol for packet network intercommunication. *IEEE Transact Commun.* 1974;COM-22(5):637–648.
7. National Audit Office, Department of Health. *Investigation: WannaCry cyber attack and the NHS.* HC 414 Session 2017–2019, April 25, 2018. https://www.nao.org.uk/wp-content/uploads/2017/10/Investigation-WannaCry-cyber-attack-and-the-NHS.pdf
8. Gov.UK. *Guidance: Cloud guide for the public sector.* Updated November 29, 2023. https://www.gov.uk/government/publications/cloud-guide-for-the-public-sector/cloud-guide-for-the-public-sector
9. DICOM website. https://www.dicomstandard.org
10. American Association of Physicists in Medicine. IHE-RO. https://www.aapm.org/IHERO/
11. Data Protection Act 2018, c. 12. https://www.legislation.gov.uk/ukpga/2018/12/contents/enacted
12. Kalendralis P, Sloep M, van Soest J, Dekker A, Fijten R. Making radiotherapy more efficient with FAIR data. *Phys Med.* 2021;82: 158–162.
13. Phillips MH, Serra LM, Dekker A, et al. Ontologies in radiation oncology. *Phys Med.* 2020;72:103–113.
14. Clark K, Vendt B, Smith K, et al. The cancer imaging archive (TCIA): maintaining and operating a public information repository. *J Digit Imag.* 2013;26:1045–1057.
15. Leveson N. *Safeware: System Safety and Computers.* Reading, Massachusetts, USA: Addison-Wesley; 1995.
16. US Food and Drug Administration. *Guidance document: general principles of software validation. Guidance for Industry and FDA Staff.* Washington, DC; 2002. January. https://www.fda.gov/regulatory-information/search-fda-guidance-documents/general-principles-software-validation.
17. Gov.UK. *Guidance: medical devices: software applications (apps),* August 8, 2014; updated July 1, 2023. https://www.gov.uk/government/publications/medical-devices-software-applications-apps
18. NHS England. *Clinical safety documentation.* https://digital.nhs.uk/services/clinical-safety/documentation
19. ISO/IEC 25010:2011. Systems and software engineering: systems and software quality requirements and evaluation (SQuaRE), System and Software Quality Models. ISO; 2011.
20. TickITplus website. http://www.tickitplus.org

14

Quality Control

Phil Sharpe and Kevin Young

CHAPTER OUTLINE

INTRODUCTION

Quality control (QC) is the process of conducting measurements to demonstrate that any piece of equipment is performing to a satisfactory level. Throughout Europe, the need for such measurements to protect individuals against the dangers of ionising radiation in relation to medical exposure is set out in Article 8 of the European Commission (EC) Directive 93/47/Euratom.[1] In the United Kingdom, the essential requirement for QC is specified in the statutory Ionising Regulations for Medical Exposure (IRMER).[2] The level of performance is set out in both national and international standards and includes what professional bodies have identified as the best practice which can be achieved. For example, the International Electrotechnical Commission (IEC) Standard IEC60601,[3] which is the general standard for medical devices, contains parts which relate to the performance[4] and safety[5] of radiotherapy equipment as well as diagnostic x-ray equipment and electrical equipment. Several publications also specify performance criteria including the International Commission for Radiation Protection (ICRP),[6] the International Atomic Energy Agency,[7] the American Association of Physics in Medicine (AAPM)[8] and in the United Kingdom, the Institute of Physics and Engineering in Medicine (IPEM).[9]

The hazards of radiation to normal tissue and the risk of oncogenesis[10] complicate the use of radiation in cancer treatment. From clinical experience and radiobiological studies, the acceptable variation in delivered dose is estimated to be ±5%, and this puts into perspective the seriousness of the 25% overdose that occurred at Exeter in 1987 because of incorrect dose measurement.[11] In addition to inadequate QC or absence of QC, accidents have occurred because of safety failures and human error. Systems of QC measurements endeavour to ensure safe and effective treatment.

The Quality Control Required

Effective QC fulfils two complementary roles: it demonstrates satisfactory performance or it detects a problem with the equipment which needs to be addressed. The boundary between the two is the tolerance within which performance is considered to be satisfactory.

QC was historically developed to ensure that equipment can perform within a specific tolerance. The tests take place prospectively with regards to the clinical use of the equipment and may be referred to as *prospective quality control (PQC)*. PQC alone does not demonstrate that the correct treatment delivery has been achieved, and the limitations of PQC became apparent with the increasing complexity of treatment machines.

With the introduction of dynamic therapy involving multileaf collimator (MLC) shape, MLC movement, gantry rotation and dose-rate modulation, ensuring accuracy in treatment delivery by solely checking machine performance could not realistically be done prospectively. However, it is possible to ensure accuracy of the dose delivery for a specific patient treatment with a unique combination of machine operations, referred to as *patient-specific quality control (PSQC)*. Not only does PSQC verify the performance of the machine; it also verifies that patient data acquisition, such as computed tomography (CT) scanner, dose prediction and dose measurement data, is also performing satisfactorily.

The EC Directive[1] requirements for PQC are clear and essential. They apply to the following aspects:

- *Following installation* of equipment, acceptance requires testing to ensure that the specification has been met.
- *Post repair*, it is necessary to ensure that the performance has been restored.
- *Post intervention*, such as with beam control adjustment, it is necessary to ensure that performance is restored.
- *Following machine upgrade*, there is a need to undertake PQC checks.
- *Following planned maintenance*, there is a need to undertake PQC checks.

In addition to these, the following can be added:

- PSQC variation from expected results.
- Interlocks. These are a major aspect which requires PQC, as they ensure the safety of treatment delivery. Beam characteristic interlocks such as flatness monitors are related to the performance of the beam and thus need to be checked in conjunction with performance measurements.

Commitment to Quality Control

The important requirement of QC, both patient specific and prospective, is borne out in the timescale of the detection of the 25% overdose at Exeter in 1987. Although patient early skin reactions were noticed, this did not prompt any measurement of delivered dose, and the official report[11] states:

> *...it is seen that even a person whose treatment had started as early as mid February would not necessarily have shown any abnormal signs until about mid-May.*

An underdose may well go on for a much longer period of time, such as when an approximate underdose of 20% continued for a number of years at Stoke-on-Trent[12] during the late 1970s and early 1980s. Measurements can reveal problems much more quickly than clinical indications will reveal them.

The difficult decision to be made is what to check, how often to check, how to judge measurement results and what action to take. In this respect, PSQC simplifies the complete QC process as it provides an overall assurance that a treatment is satisfactory. Although it does not eliminate the need for PQC, it removes the need to make any judgment about the clinical significance of a specific aspect of the performance of the equipment.

It is essential that the staff group responsible for equipment performance and technical checks as opposed to the clinical delivery of the treatment embrace the QC requirements for modern radiotherapy.

Safety, Position and Dose

The magnitude of the physical dose along with its delivery to the correct location represent, in addition to safety, the three critical aspects of effective radiotherapy. In considering the various components in the radiotherapy process, namely, data acquisition, dose prediction, treatment delivery and dose measurement, each component can be associated with both physical dose and position or a combination of both. For example, the calibration of CT number is related to dose prediction, whereas movement accuracy of the scanner and processing of the image matrix is a positional aspect. PSQC provides a combined assessment of dose and positional accuracy, whereas PQC can be used to measure specifically a physical dose or a positional aspect.

Frequency, Tolerances and Failure Trends

There is no clear relationship by which the frequency of checks and the tolerances applied can be easily and systematically identified. This is in part attributed to the unknown pattern of failure which can be anything from a linear deterioration in its simplistic form to a catastrophic event unpredictable from any trend analysis. This complexity is explored in the previous edition of this book.[13]

For a linear failure trend with a tolerance of ±3%, the variation in dose can be up to ±3%. If something is wrong with the machine for longer or shorter than the total number of fractions, that affects how close the variation in treatment dose will get to ±3%.

Although PQC can be readily used for postrepair purposes, this makes the choice of frequency for PQC difficult unless the deterioration of a performance parameter is explicitly known.

This problem is largely overcome with the use of PSQC, as it will be performed regularly, even if done on a sample basis, for example, when 1 in 10 prostate patient treatments are checked. It therefore provides an overview of overall treatment machine performance as well as associated imaging, dose prediction and dose measurement performance. It provides virtually continuous confidence in the treatment being delivered.

MEASUREMENT AND UNCERTAINTY

Measurement error can be characterised by two quantities: accuracy and precision. *Accuracy* is how close a given set of measurements are to their true value and *precision* is how close the measurements are to each other. Accuracy can be related to a systematic error in measurement and precision is related to random errors (Fig. 14.1).

Measurement of any parameter will not determine the value exactly, and instead we make multiple measurements from which the 'best estimate' is obtained. The variation in the multiple measurements is attributed to differences in the measurement process, measurement equipment and statistical fluctuation of the parameter being measured. Calculation of the mean value, M, of the multiple measurements is the best estimate, whereas the variation in the multiple measurements is the uncertainty of the best estimate.

Typically, we can assume that the multiple measurements fall in a normal distribution with mean M and a standard deviation, σ (Fig. 14.2).

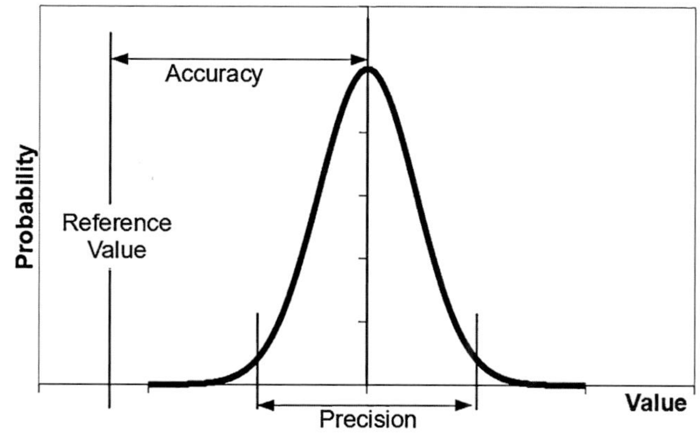

Fig. 14.1 Concept of accuracy and precision.

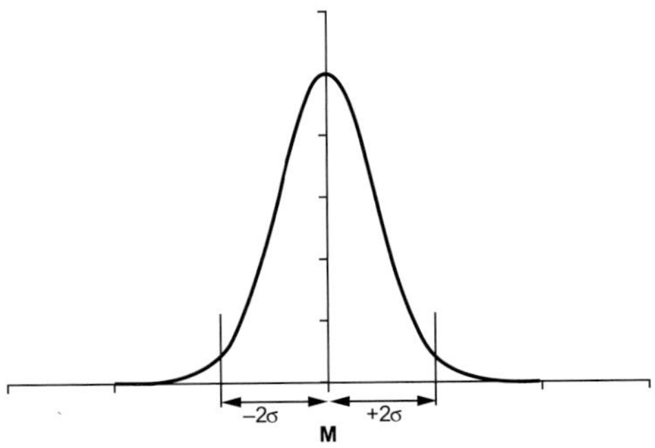

Fig. 14.2 Normal distribution of a measurement with mean M and standard deviation σ.

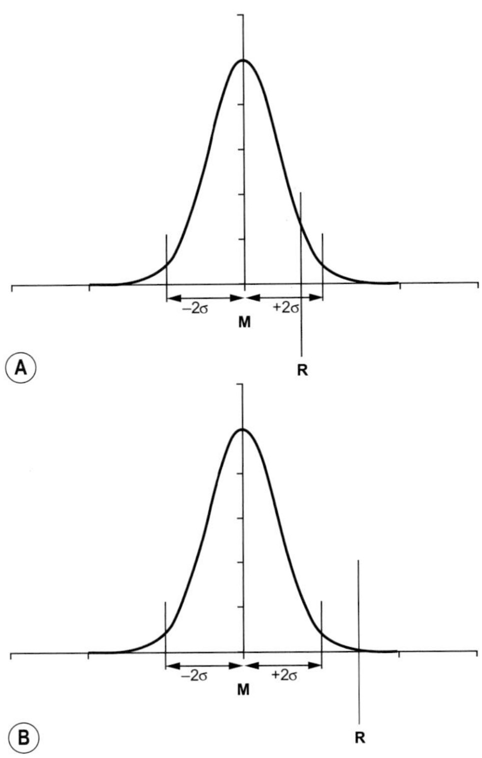

Fig. 14.3 Conceptual relationship of a reference value *R*, to a measurement *M*. (A) *R* lies within $\pm 2\sigma$ of *M*. (B) *R* lies outside $\pm 2\sigma$ of *M*.

In a normal distribution, approximately 95% of measurements will lie between $\pm 2\sigma$. Hence there is a 5% probability that the true value does not lie within $\pm 2\sigma$ of the best estimate *M*, and this can be used to consider the significance of a measurement with regards to a reference value *R*.

Null Hypothesis

This aspect of statistical analysis provides the method by which we can evaluate a measurement *M*, with standard deviation σ, with respect to a reference value *R*. The null hypothesis (H_0) is that *M* is not different from *R*, and the normal distribution can be used to determine with what confidence this can be assumed. In Fig. 14.3A the reference value *R* lies within $\pm 2\sigma$ of the best estimate *M*, whereas in Fig. 14.3B *R* lies beyond $\pm 2\sigma$ of *M*. This can also be stated as having 95% confidence that *R* belongs to *M* in Fig. 14.3A and therefore in Fig. 14.3B only being 5% confident that *R* belongs to *M*. Hence, at a 95% confidence level, the measurement *M* can be judged to be within adequate agreement of *R* and H_0 applies, or the measurement *M* can be judged that it is not within adequate agreement and H_0 is rejected.

Combining Variances and Tolerances

The *variance* is the standard deviation squared, σ^2. The variance therefore is attributed to differences in the measurement process, measurement equipment and fluctuation of the parameter being measured. The general method to determine an overall variance is to assume contributing variations are independent and combine them, as in Eq. (14.1), a combination known as *quadrature*:

$$\text{Total variance} = (\sigma_{\text{Total}})^2 = (\sigma_1)^2 + (\sigma_2)^2 + (\sigma_3)^2 + \cdots + (\sigma_n)^2 \quad \textbf{(14.1)}$$

As an example, let the measurements from a given technique have a standard deviation of 0.5% and the intrinsic fluctuation of the parameter also be 0.5%. These values can be combined in quadrature to determine σ_{Total} as follows:

$$(\sigma_{\text{Total}})^2 = (0.5)^2 + (0.5)^2 = 2 \times 0.25 = 0.5 \quad \textbf{(14.2)}$$

This results in $\sigma_{\text{Total}} = 0.707\%$, and this gives $\pm 2\sigma = \pm 1.4\%$.

It therefore follows that if a number of parameters have an associated tolerance, the overall tolerance can also be determined by combining the individual tolerances in quadrature.

This can be illustrated by considering the factors used to calculate the dose delivered, as shown in Eq. (14.3):

$$\text{D} = \text{M.O.W.T.S.C} \quad \textbf{(14.3)}$$

where D is the dose; M is the number of monitor units (MUs); the terms O, W, T and S represent output, wedge, tray and source to surface factors; and C is the machine calibration factor in Gy/MU.

The assumption that the variation in the factors is independent and as suggested above should be combined in quadrature leads to the overall variance being written as:

$$\begin{aligned}(\text{Total tolerance})^2 &= (\sigma_{\text{Total}})^2 \\ &= (\sigma_{\text{O}})^2 + (\sigma_{\text{W}})^2 + (\sigma_{\text{T}})^2 + (\sigma_{\text{S}})^2 + (\sigma_{\text{C}})^2 \quad \textbf{(14.4)}\end{aligned}$$

If the aim was to deliver a dose within a total tolerance of ±3% and the calibration factor C was maintained to within ±1%, the maximum tolerance on O, W, T and S would each be ±1.4%, if they were all taken as equal and the total tolerance maintained. This type of consideration enables realistic tolerances to be set, and based upon known performance results it can also indicate the overall performance which can be expected.

Setting a Tolerance to Achieve a Performance Level

The distribution associated with any measurement indicates that there is a 50% chance that the true value is above the mean measurement and a 50% chance that the true value is below the mean measurement. Hence, if the mean measurement is exactly on the tolerance value, there is as much chance that it is in tolerance as there is that it is out of tolerance. For the measured value to be considered to be in tolerance with 95% confidence, the tolerance must be reduced by an amount related to the standard deviation of the measurement.

Hence, if a measurement M can be made with standard deviation σ_{Total} and the aim is for performance to remain within $\pm P$, the tolerance should be set at $T = P - 2 \times \sigma_{\text{Total}}$. For example, if the performance requirement is ±3.0% and the measurement has a standard deviation of ±0.5%, the tolerance should be set to $\pm(3.0 - 2 \times 0.5)\%$. So, using a tolerance of ±2.0% will ensure that performance is maintained within ±3.0%.

PERFORMANCE IMPROVEMENT

Setting a tolerance is an important aspect of maintaining performance. An overall tolerance in dose delivery is set based on known clinical outcomes and complications. However, it does not help to improve performance. Simply working to a tolerance range of $\pm T\%$ means that it is as good for the performance to be $-T\%$ from a target value as it is for it to be 0% or $+T\%$ from the target value. Clearly, this is not the case, and it would be desirable for the performance to be closer to the required performance far more than not—that is, for the measurement difference from the reference value to be minimised.

The Taguchi technique[14] is an example of how performance can be improved and driven towards the ideal zero variation from the required performance. The technique uses a loss of performance parameter based upon a quadratic sum, as follows:

$$\text{Loss} = K \cdot [(\sigma_{\text{Total}})^2 + (1/N \cdot \Sigma\sigma_n)^2] \quad \textbf{(14.5)}$$

where K is a constant and N is the number of contributing uncertainties, σ_n, to the overall uncertainty, σ_{Total}.

For the example expressed in Eq. (14.4):

$$1/N \cdot \Sigma\sigma_n = 1/5 \cdot (\sigma_O + \sigma_W + \sigma_T + \sigma_S + \sigma_O) \quad \textbf{(14.6)}$$

which is the mean standard deviation for the parameters.

This loss parameter can be used to improve performance by intervention, by reducing the variation from nominal targets, σ_n.

An example from industrial production which illustrates the benefit of this technique concerns the production of Sony TV sets in Japan and the United States. The Japanese plant applied the Taguchi methodology and the US plant relied on a simple tolerance of $\pm T\%$ for colour density. A nonparametric assessment of customer satisfaction on a scale of A for Excellent to D for Unacceptable revealed a striking contrast between the US and Japanese manufactured TV sets, as shown in Fig. 14.4.

It can be clearly seen that whereas the Japanese satisfaction level was concentrated around Excellent, the US satisfaction level was uniform across the colour density range. For the US TV sets, this was due to the greater number of Unacceptable responses than Excellent responses.

Although the overall target for performance such as ±5% is set by clinical indications, improvement techniques such as Taguchi can provide a way for QC to improve performance towards an optimal minimal variation.

MAINTENANCE AND CATASTROPHES

Not all aspects of equipment performance can be maintained. Catastrophes are unpredicted events that lead to absolute failure of a part or process. These are inevitable and are usually because of component failure or human error. Although some devices and components can be replaced or action taken based upon the monitoring of a performance parameter, not everything can be maintained. The best possible provision needs to be made for catastrophes, with provisions for enabling routine treatment to continue while the equipment is repaired.

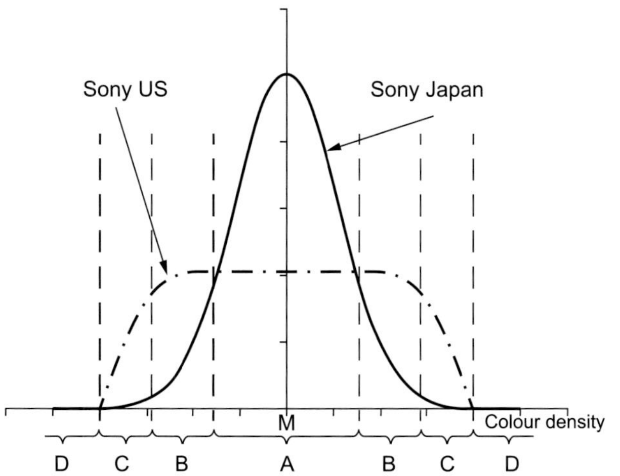

Fig. 14.4 Comparison between basic tolerance band (Sony US) and improvement method (Sony Japan) production techniques.

MONITORING TRENDS AND CORRECTIVE ACTION

Monitoring of performance parameters can be achieved by reviewing the data collected from QC measurements. These measurements can be used to examine trends in performance and, if possible, used as predictors of performance deterioration, enabling the scheduling of adjustments or corrective action.

One routinely used but simple trend technique is when a double tolerance level is set against which to monitor the variation of a parameter. For example, say these levels are $\pm a\%$ and $\pm b\%$, where $b > a$. Results outside $\pm b\%$ are considered to require immediate attention, whereas results outside $\pm a\%$ but within $\pm b\%$ can be allowed to occur on a number of subsequent occasions before action is taken.

There are three major categories of monitoring: immediate, short term and long term. Each method provides different but appropriate means by which to evaluate and maintain performance.

Immediate Monitoring

An immediate effect on performance is determined from the performance response to changing a control parameter. Using this approach, the optimum tuning of a circuit or system can be determined. The monitoring can involve measuring parameters within the machine, such as current or voltage, as well as external parameters, such as beam characteristics like beam uniformity and energy.

Long-Term Monitoring

Many parameters alter slowly as components age or as performance deteriorates. To correct and compensate for the changes, including component replacement, long-term data trends provide an indication as to when action is required. This could, for instance, be for a parameter which requires continuous adjustment to remain within specification, or it may indicate when the end of life of a component is expected so as to schedule a replacement component and minimise treatment interruption and delays by ensuring that components are available if required and preparation is done in adequate time. As with immediate monitoring, the parameters may be internal—that is, measured from the machine—or they could be from the beam characteristics and measured using other external equipment such as beam flatness or symmetry. Inevitably, data can be difficult to record, log and process. Any systems which will assist with the recording and processing of these data are valuable.

Short-Term Monitoring

In contrast to immediate and long-term monitoring, short-term endeavours to monitor performance of the machine during at least one treatment day. Only internal parameters of the machine are recorded during the day for subsequent processing. But these can be used in conjunction with daily measurements of the beam, such as those made when the machine is run up before treatment that day. By analysing such data, it is again possible to identify deterioration in performance and to schedule adjustments.[15] Analysis of this wealth of data is currently being ignored in modern radiotherapy. This is in contrast to, for example the aero industry where parameters monitored during a flight are used to indicated maintenance and adjustment needs of an aircraft.

THE RADIOTHERAPY PROCESS

QC has a role throughout the radiotherapy process because of the significant technology involved at every stage. Three distinct aspects can be identified with QC: dose, position and safety. All of these aspects contribute to ensuring effective treatment delivery.

The radiotherapy process can be considered to consist of the distinct aspects of acquisition, analysis and delivery, and any piece of equipment can be involved in any or all of these aspects. For example, the CT scanner will acquire positional and image data which will be used in the dosimetric analysis for treatment planning and the delivery verification analysis of portal dosimetry.

Acquisition

Patient information that is not determined from clinical examination and physiological and biochemical testing is almost entirely obtained through imaging. The focus of the information is the CT scan which forms the basis for dose prediction. This is supplemented by magnetic resonance imaging (MRI) and positron emission tomography (PET) imaging, the use of which relies on accurate image registration to ensure accurate target localisation and associated margins. Ultrasound can also be used on occasion.

In brachytherapy, localisation of radioactive sources or applicators is readily achieved with a C-arm radiographic device and with CT supplemented by MRI.

Analysis

The manipulation of large CT data sets enables accurate delineation of target regions and organs at risk (OARs) in a virtual environment, permitting the clinical staff to make informed choices concerning the efficacy of treatment in terms of the balance between treatment and risk to the patient.

Dose prediction remains a significant part of the analysis to determine an adequate dose distribution in the target while sparing critical tissue. With the increasing use of intensity modulated radiotherapy (IMRT), the analysis is an automated process, also referred to as *inverse planning*. The automated process is governed by guidance parameters set and adjusted by operators skilled in the use of the processing software.

Delivery

The final part of the process following acquisition and analysis is treatment delivery. The uncertainty of the first two aspects will have an impact on the final delivery. The majority of radiotherapy treatment delivery takes place with linear accelerators. However, proton treatment machines, kilovoltage machines, radionuclide therapy, brachytherapy afterloading machines and implants with their associated equipment must also be considered.

PATIENT-SPECIFIC QUALITY CONTROL

Increased complexity in treatments such as intensity modulated arc therapy has prompted the need for more PSQC. No longer can PQC—that is—routine periodic checks, completely cover all the aspects of a treatment machine used for IMRT. Radiotherapy departments are becoming more focused on the patient pathway from referral through to treatment, involving a multidisciplinary team that combines different staff groups communicating together in a patient-led environment. Running parallel to that, QC now focuses on a patient's individual treatment, encompassing the whole procedure from CT scan to treatment, rather than individual tests for each stage.

A modern intensity modulated arc therapy treatment contains multiple segments, variable dose rates and varying gantry speeds, all combined into one or more continuous treatment arcs. The complexity of this means that from a practical point of view, the beams cannot be split into single segments or individual gantry angles for analysis. Therefore a test that can measure the sum of all these individual aspects is required.

TABLE 14.1 Six Aspects of a CT Scanner That Require Quality Control

1	Patient alignment lasers
2	Couch movement
3	Slice thickness
4	Image size
5	Image geometry
6	Hounsfield numbers for range of materials

The increased complexity of treatments has given rise to QC equipment explicitly designed for such patient-specific checks. A phantom or device that can be scanned, planned and treated using an individual patient's plan ensures a more robust QC procedure to cover all aspects of the patient pathway. The practical side of the PSQC and equipment is discussed further in the 'Practical Patient-Specific Quality Control' section.

RADIOTHERAPY TECHNOLOGY

Consideration of the radiotherapy process in the previous section indicates that treatment is dependent upon the equipment used throughout the process and thus on the QC of that equipment. Detailed QC is available from several sources, for example, IPEM 81[9] for all categories of equipment used, so here we consider some general aspects and principles which should be applied.

Planning Imaging

The purpose of QC for the CT scanner is twofold: (1) to ensure that patient alignment with respect to the scanner is appropriate and accurate; and (2), to ensure that any patient density information is appropriate for dosimetry calculations. Table 14.1 lists areas of consideration which are typical but not comprehensive.

Whereas the CT image data set forms the basis for dose prediction, the MRI and PET images aid volume localisation for target and critical organ delineation. Hence MRI and PET registration with the CT image data needs to be checked to ensure that geometric alignment is accurate and that volume sizes and dimensions are not transferred inaccurately from one to the other.

C-arm radiographic devices often provide the imaging facilities essential for dose prediction in brachytherapy treatment as well as source position verification during treatment. For dose prediction, the geometric accuracy of the system needs to be checked with routine QC. In addition, safe levels of radiation exposure and satisfactory imaging performance should also be included in a QC program.

Virtual Simulation

The basis for accurate treatment simulation lies with the performance of the CT scanner. However, QC checks of the virtual simulator facility ensure that the manipulation of the CT data sets does not introduce any geometric distortions which could compromise the perception of the alignment of the treatment machine to the patient. Although it can be argued that there will be no changes once software is initially verified through customer acceptance and system commissioning, there is still a need for adequate QC to follow software upgrades or hardware changes. Also, because the data set originates from the CT scanner, periodic checks will verify whether the process of data handling between the systems is satisfactory.

Dose Prediction

Dose prediction accuracy is dependent upon the calculation algorithm, geometrical resolution and the application of stored electron density

TABLE 14.2 Seven Aspects of Orthovoltage Machines That Require Quality Control

1	Focal spot to applicator alignment
2	Applicator dimensions and orthogonality
3	Large field uniformity
4	Beam energy
5	Dose variation with tube angle
6	Dose linearity and reproducibility
7	Absolute dose

TABLE 14.3 Five Aspects of Brachytherapy Machines That Require Quality Control

1	Source position autoradiograph
2	Dummy source agreement with autoradiograph
3	Timer
4	Air kerma rate measurement
5	Absorbed dose of simulated treatment

data to apply to CT images. As with virtual simulation, there is a need for QC following software and hardware upgrades as well as routinely checking data transfer integrity with the CT scanner.

Kilovoltage Machines

Kilovoltage treatment machines require mechanical, radiation field and dosimetry checks. One fundamental aspect is the alignment of the focal spot to the mechanical alignment of collimators and applicators. Once this is accurately established and verified, accurate mechanical alignment of applicators and attachments will ensure adequate performance. Table 14.2 lists checks for an orthovoltage kV machine which are typical but not comprehensive.

Afterloading Brachytherapy Machines

Machines providing high, medium and low dose rates all require QC checks for safety and performance. With this type of equipment, the mechanical aspects concern the positional accuracy of the radiation source or sources and assurance that dummy source indicators used for planning radiographs accurately reflect the source positions. Finally, of course, measurement of the absolute dose delivered will check source activity, timer and positional accuracy in combination. Table 14.3 lists checks that are typical but not comprehensive.

Megavoltage Machines

Besides ensuring the satisfactory operation of safety interlocks, there are many aspects concerning the performance of these machines that require routine QC. These aspects concern mechanical and optical alignment, radiation beam performance and the radiation beam's alignment to the machine's optics and mechanics. The relative dose distribution within the beam has associated properties of uniformity and symmetry that require checking for various orientations of the treatment gantry. Both the mechanical-optical and radiation performance checks are prerequisites to ensuring accurate dose delivery for prospective QC. In patient-specific QC, all three components are integrated in the measurement and so have no differentiation as to what may be causing a variation. There may be multiple energy beams to check, whether electrons, photons or protons. QC needs to be performed for all energies and modes. Table 14.4 lists checks that are typical (not comprehensive) for a linear accelerator.

TABLE 14.4 Twelve Aspects of Linear Accelerators That Require Quality Control

1	Isocentre determined by the radiation beam
2	Isocentre indicators (e.g. distance meter)
3	Light field size, symmetry and x-wires
4	Patient alignment lasers
5	Radiation beam symmetry with gantry angle
6	Radiation field size
7	Radiation field alignment to optical field
8	Couch isocentric and vertical movement
9	Beam energy
10	Dose variation with gantry angle
11	Dose linearity and reproducibility
12	Absolute dose

Linear Accelerators With Magnetic Resonance Imaging

In terms of megavoltage linear accelerators with in-built MRI capability, the MRI LINAC presents a significant challenge due to electronmagnetic influences between the two systems. Although the machines are designed to minimise the effect of one on the other, electron trajectories and energy deposition are influenced by the MRI magnetic field, and the linear accelerator beam and control magnets have an effect on the geometric image performance of the MRI. Both systems need to be checked, and guidance and experience in this regard are steadily being accumulated.[16,17]

Patient Positioning

Besides patient laser alignment systems, there are active systems which use stereotactic cameras and kV imaging systems to monitor patient position at treatment setup and during treatment delivery. For such systems, QC is required to ensure that detected displacements are accurate and that the relationship of the system reference point to the LINAC reference point or isocentre is accurate.

Treatment Verification

Treatment verification systems monitor machine setup parameters, patient positioning parameters and dose delivery parameters which are measured or determined from a variety of devices and techniques. Some examples are cone beam CT, portal imaging and in vivo dose measurements. Some aspects of QC are required to make sure that performance parameters crucial for satisfactory operation of these devices are checked and verified. In particular, treatment systems rely on the automatic detection of inappropriate settings before irradiation, especially with conformal and intensity modulated techniques when delivery is complex. The high complexity of treatment delivery now also benefits from an automated record of the treatment.

Computer Systems and Networking

Computer systems handle critical data across the entire radiotherapy process. QC of the computer systems and networks aims to verify that the data transferred remain accurate. It can also identify the limitations in the system and monitor them. For example, resolution changes may occur within image sets as they are processed after acquisition. The integrity of the treatment requires that treatment data can be stored, accessed and transferred correctly.

Measurement Equipment

An important requirement for QC is that appropriate, accurate and precise measurement is used, and it is essential to ensure that the measurement equipment continues to operate satisfactorily. All equipment, from a ruler and spirit level used in mechanical checks to calibrated ionisation chambers and electrometers used for absolute dose measurements, requires QC.

PRACTICAL PATIENT-SPECIFIC QUALITY CONTROL

The increased complexity of treatments involving intensity modulated arcs consisting of multiple small segments of dose per beam means each treatment can be highly individualised. Therefore some form of patient-specific QC is required to ensure treatment accuracy.

The two stages within the patient process that can be used to perform patient-specific QC are:

- Pretreatment QC: Measurements taken and processed before the start of treatment
- On treatment verification: Measurements taken and processed either online during treatment or offline after treatment (this is discussed in detail in Chapter 11)

A range of technology and techniques are used in patient-specific QC. These involve absolute and relative dose measurements and predictions with comparisons between results to demonstrate the satisfactory delivery of the treatment or to identify problems which need to be addressed before treatment is given. In the following sections, an overview is given of these techniques and equipment.

Phantom-Based Measurements

These measurements require some form of phantom that can be imaged on the CT scanner and the image set imported into the treatment planning system (TPS). Patient-specific plans can then be applied to the phantom and the dose distribution calculated; this is known as a *QA plan*.

With the phantom set up on the treatment machine, the treatment plan is delivered. There must be some dose measurement devices within the phantom at known positions. The measured dose distribution can then be compared to the predicted dose distribution from the planning system, thus verifying treatment accuracy. The simplest method is the application of the treatment plan to a water-equivalent uniform density block of material, for example, solid water or Perspex. Single or multiple dose points can be measured using an ion chamber within the phantom and compared with the expected result from the planning system. A single cumulative dose point makes this method limited in respect to checking the whole plan. Multiple measurement points are better but very time-consuming when done manually. There are various commercially available devices that can be used.

Dosimetric Arrays

Dosimetric arrays comprise a phantom consisting of multiple dosimeters uniformly distributed in a solid geometric body in either two- or three-dimensional arrangements. The treatment plan can be delivered to the array, and the measured dose can be compared to that of the QA plan produced by the planning system. The most common forms of dosimeter used are small volume ion chambers or diodes.

Two-Dimensional Array

A two-dimensional array has the advantage of allowing a measurement in a single plane which is generally quicker to measure than in three dimensions but has limited resemblance to the actual plan dose distribution. The array can be set on the treatment couch for fixed-gantry measurements or held in a jig that rotates with the gantry for arc treatments; see Fig. 14.5.

Three-Dimensional Array

A three-dimensional array enables the user to measure a dose distribution within a volume which has a closer resemblance to the original treatment plan distribution than that acquired in a plane on the two-dimensional array. The dosimeters in the three-dimensional array shown in Fig. 14.6 are arranged in a cross structure, with the device placed on the treatment couch and aligned to the machine isocentre.

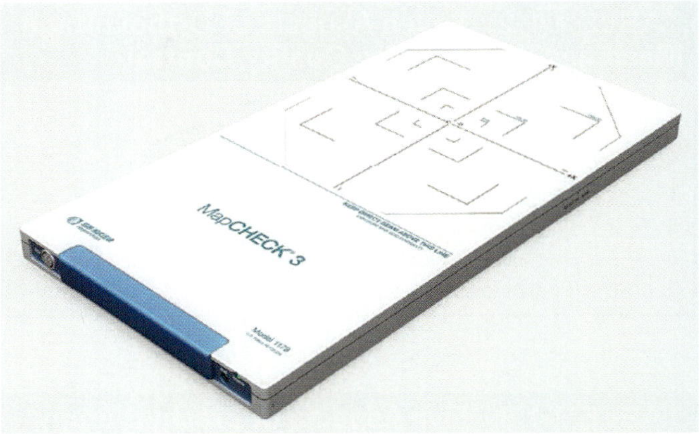

Fig. 14.5 A two-dimensional measurement array. (Courtesy Sun Nuclear, a Mirion Medical Company.)

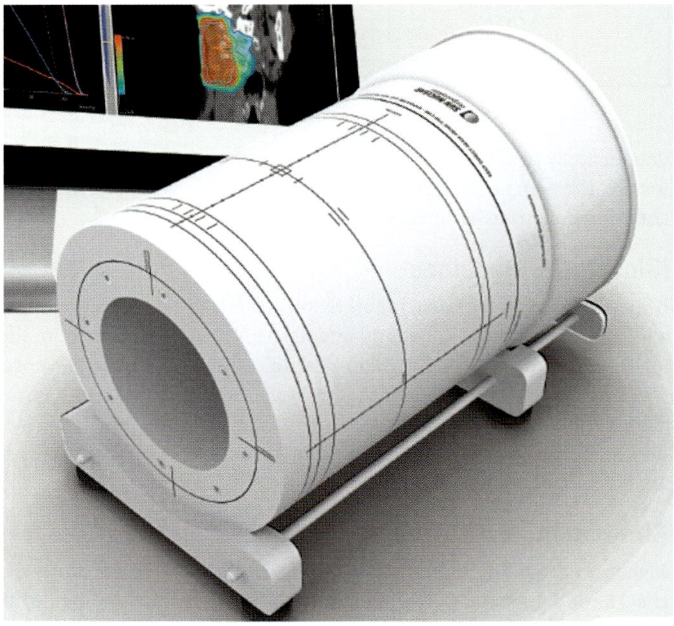

Fig. 14.6 A three-dimensional measurement array. (Courtesy Sun Nuclear, a Mirion Medical Company.)

The treatment is given to the array, and software provided by the manufacturer is used to reconstruct the measured dose distribution. Comparison to the QA plan dose distribution is then determined, with the typical comparison parameter being the gamma index.

Gamma Index

A series of measurement points throughout the two-dimensional plane or three-dimensional volume are compared with the QA plan and evaluated using a combination of dose difference and distance to agreement. The *dose difference* is the comparison of the dose from the QA plan to the dose measured at specific points. The *distance to agreement* is the shortest distance between a dose point in the QA plan and the same measured dose within the measured data. A combination of these is used in gamma index analysis to produce an index accommodating both dose deviation and spatial deviation. Each point of the dose distribution that lies within a range given by defined criteria, for example, ±3% dose and ±3 mm spatially, is classed as passing. Each point that does not lie within the defined range is classed as failing. It is common to set a threshold proportion of points, typically 95%, that need to pass. Compliance indicates an acceptable dose distribution.

Transit Dosimetry

Transit dosimetry or electronic portal imaging device (EPID)–based in vivo dosimetry (IVD) is a feature of modern radiotherapy and its function is to detect treatment error, facilitate treatment adaption and record the dose to the patient.

Initially, EPIDs were developed for patient setup verification imaging (Chapter 11). However, the EPID also has dosimetric characteristics suitable for IVD verification. From the early 2000s, the current generation of amorphous silicon flat-panel technology has become universal on newly acquired LINACs (Chapter 10).

The primary layers of an amorphous silicon EPID detection structure consist of:

- A build-up or interaction layer which is normally copper
- A scintillating phosphor layer which is normally gadolinium oxysulfide
- A photo-diode matrix with a support material of amorphous silicon

The dosimetric response of the EPID differs from an ion chamber for several reasons, including the high atomic number (Z) of the materials and the inherent beam energy spectrum. All transit dosimetry systems use the image signal from the transmission energy fluence that is incident on the detector panel. The factors influencing the signal are

- Fluence of the beam incident on the patient
- Attenuation of the beam fluence within the patient
- Scatter of the fluence within the patient
- Response of the EPID detection system

There are two basic systems in transit dosimetry. The first, the *forward system*, is to predict the signals measured at the EPID, and the second, the *back projection system*, is to predict doses within the patient based upon the signals measured.

Forward System

In the forward system, the aim is to predict reference EPID image signals and compare these with the measured portal image signals. The predicted signals are determined using the treatment plan, planning CT and beam model. The disadvantage of this method is that the comparisons are nonintuitive and not readily related to clinical metrics such as patient dose volume histograms. An alternative forward system is to predict the dose absorbed in a slab of water at the location of the EPID.

Back Projection System

In the back projection system, a point dose or dose distribution is estimated within the patient from the measured EPID image signals. The planning CT scan is typically used to model fluence interactions through the patient. However, if a cone beam CT scan is acquired immediately prior to treatment, the prediction more accurately reflects the dose delivered for that fraction, as it accounts for current patient anatomy and setup.

There are two methods of back projection: direct and indirect. *Direct back projection* calculates a primary fluence by correcting for the effect of the EPID and patient scatter. The primary fluence is back-projected through the patient model and combined with dose deposition kernels to determine the dose distribution. There have been various solutions put forward to compensate for suboptimal density inhomogeneity corrections with this approach.

With *indirect back projection*, a primary fluence is calculated by correcting for the effect of the EPID and patient scatter. The primary fluence is then back-projected to obtain an incident fluence which is used with a conventional beam model to calculate the patient dose distribution.

The advantages of back projection systems are that the dose distributions can be visualised and compared through the use of dose volume histograms and gamma index maps.

Table 14.5 lists and compares the systems of transit dosimetry.

Independent Software Verification

Patient-specific QA can be performed using software to calculate doses within the patient at multiple points, either applied to the patient's original CT planning scan or geometrically calculated using the beam parameters relative to the plan isocentre and patient source to surface distances (SSDs). This is a quicker method for patient-specific QC but is further removed from the original plan. It is a useful method of QC verification for tried and tested techniques that have been shown to have low failure rates. A suitable tolerance, for example, ±3%, can be applied to these initial QA checks with the failures being sent on for a more comprehensive QC using a dosimetric array or phantom on the linear accelerator.

Secondary Treatment Planning System

For centres fortunate enough to have more than one TPS, patient-specific QC can be performed by exporting the plan and CT scan to the second system and recalculating the dose distribution. The advantage of this is that the second TPS has its own independent dose algorithm which allows comparison of dose with that produced with the original plan algorithm for OARs and target volumes. QC should be as independent as possible from the original calculation to minimise user influence upon said test if possible. Exporting from the record and verify system back to the second TPS allows a check on the original plan export, further enhancing QC robustness.

Patient-Specific Quality Control Implementation

The implementation of IMRT is usually undertaken initially on one particular treatment site to risk-assess the possible errors. Once this has been done, it can be expanded to other sites in parallel with associated PSQC. The initial QC is usually done with the more comprehensive methods of

TABLE 14.5 Transit Dosimetry System Comparison

System	Comparison Location	Prediction	Measurement
Forward: Dose	EPID plane	Predicted dose to a water slab	Dose at the EPID
Forward: Image	EPID plane	Predicted portal image greyscale values	Image at the EPID
Back projection: Direct	Within patient model	Treatment planning system dose distribution	Dose distribution in patient directly from a model of back projection through the patient
Back projection: Indirect	Within patient model	Treatment planning system dose distribution	Dose distribution in patient calculated using an incident fluence from back projection through the patient

EPID, Electronic portal imaging device.

phantom or array measurements, thus ensuring a more complete check of the IMRT program in its infancy and allowing a reduction in PSQC as confidence and auditing of the system are progressed.

The increased demand for complex treatments means the equipment is in regular use, putting greater pressure on QC resources. For example, phantoms incorporating dosimeters and devices acquiring dose measurements during treatment require robust QC to monitor their accuracy and consistency.

Regular audits of PSQC may indicate changes in the treatment process which will need further investigation to isolate the possible problem. As well as individual patient tests, it is also recommended to have a standard QA plan that can be run on every treatment machine periodically (e.g. monthly) for intercomparison; this allows monitoring of both individual machine performance and QC equipment performance.

Patient-specific QC has now become a common method for checking plan delivery accuracy in the modern radiotherapy centre. With NHS targets for IMRT treatments increasing every year, it becomes ever more important for a robust and independent system to be in place within the department.

GETTING THINGS IN BALANCE

QC more often than not will demonstrate adequate performance of the equipment being checked. However, there are three aspects which need to be balanced when dealing with a problem:

- Clinical effect because of the problem
- Resources, including manpower and equipment to correct the problem
- Component availability to correct the problem

All problems can be considered to be a balance between the three, and this can assist in determining how to deal with a problem (Fig. 14.7). The clinical effect really relates to the performance of the equipment and making a judgment about how clinically significant it will be to treat the patient with the performance compromised to a known extent. The resource required consists of the man-hours required and the skill and expertise available to restore the performance. The component availability relates to whether a component is affordable or available from stores or, conversely, whether it is too expensive or inappropriate to keep on the shelf at the hospital and therefore requires ordering.

The balance can be illustrated by considering two extremes: (1) high clinical impact and minimal component cost and (2) very high component cost coupled with insignificant clinical impact (Fig. 14.8).

On the one hand, if clinical significance is small and the resource or component availability is large, the work can be scheduled for an

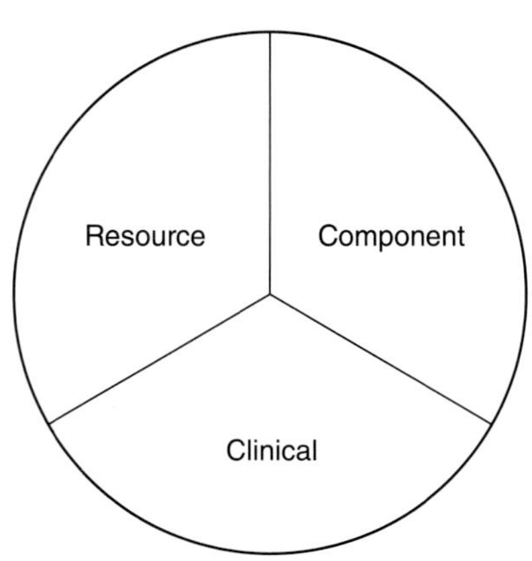

Fig. 14.7 The three aspects to be considered in equipment problems and restoring performance.

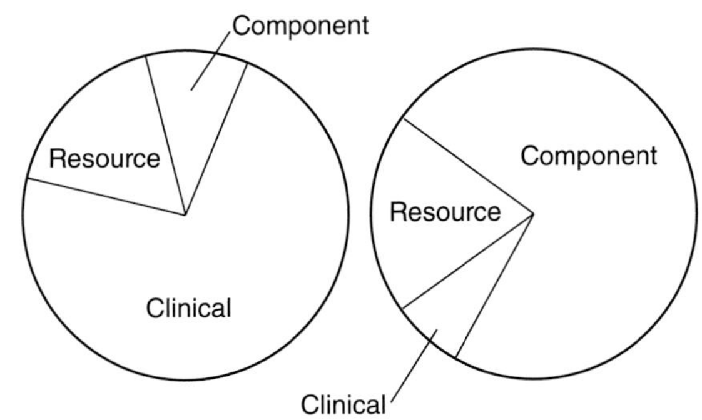

Fig. 14.8 Illustration of the contrast in split between the three aspects to be considered for two extreme equipment problems.

appropriate time such as a planned preventive maintenance (PPM) slot. However, if the clinical significance is large, an immediate repair will be appropriate.

There are no unambiguous solutions to the numerous situations between the two extremes. In reality the skill, knowledge and insight of the scientists and technicians involved in the work will be a determining factor in the exact repair schedule.

QC coupled with planned maintenance forms an essential component in ensuring that safe and effective radiotherapy is achieved.

QUALITY CONTROL SCHEDULING FOR MEGAVOLTAGE MACHINES

The scheduling of routine QC should be chosen to suit local circumstances. For many types of equipment, this can be accommodated within normal working hours. However, in the case of treatment machines, this may not be possible because of patient demand and a lack of treatment capacity. Suitable guidance as to the frequency of tests is available from the British Standards Institution (BSI)[5] and IPEM (in IPEM 81).[9] Both provide guidance for checks to be conducted on a monthly to yearly frequency. The BSI document does not specify weekly checks, though an estimate of the total annual time for the suggested checks is approximately the same. Based upon typical times for the QC, they amount to between 117 and 128 hours per year, respectively (for the two guidance documents), which is roughly in line with a practice that requires 1 to 2 hours per week and one-half day per calendar month and a practice that requires 120 hours. If this time is taken from the normal working day, it amounts to only about a 5% loss from the typical treatment unit.

With the increasing number of treatment machines and treatment complexity in a centre, the time and resources for treatment machine QC increase and scheduling techniques are required to accommodate them. On-board QC systems can alleviate this (discussed in the next section). However, paradoxically the increased treatment complexity has led to the need for PSQC which, in providing an overall assurance of adequate dose delivery, reduces the need for direct machine QC checks or PQC. If an integrated view of PQC and PSQC is taken, this can lead to a reduction in the QC resource required.[18]

ON-BOARD QUALITY CONTROL FOR MEGAVOLTAGE MACHINES

One of the linear accelerator suppliers, Varian, provides an on-board QC facility. This is dependent upon the performance of the MV and kV imaging systems as well as the isocentre alignment indicators. Known as Machine Performance Check (MPC), it learns a baseline which is subsequently tracked within set tolerances. MPC enables beam output, uniformity and symmetry to be checked as well as geometric checks on the MLC performance, gantry, collimator and couch positions using an MPC phantom. Relearning the baseline is operator dependent and is independent of machine adjustments. MPC is readily available on the machine, enabling a rapid and efficient check of the machine. While it has been in use at radiotherapy centres for several years, the balance between MPC and independent checks with output monitors, beam profile scanners, absolute dose and water tank measurements is under review as more experience is gained.[19]

CONCLUSION

QC and planned maintenance are a requirement of IRMER.[2] It is obviously the case that QC will require time that would otherwise be used for patient treatment. A general understanding among staff of the importance of QC and its influence on patient treatment quality is required to mitigate any pressure to substitute QC time with patient treatment time in a target-driven environment. The importance of QC is highlighted by the fact that previous incidents have shown that appropriate measurement of a physical parameter could have averted incorrect treatment,[11] sometimes over a lengthy period before clinical indicators indicated a problem.

It is important to put the checks on performance into context. This can be done in relation to the dose distribution planned for a patient when the ICRU 50[20] criteria of a dose variation between +7% and −5% across the target is sought. The performance of the machine can compromise this because of several factors. For example, a nonuniform beam because of energy change or a tilted beam because of incorrect steering could change delivered dose by ±6%. In addition, the variation of the factors used to calculate the monitor units in combination with the dose calibration of the machine could also change delivered dose by ±6%. Geometric misalignment between the radiation beam and the beam indicators can result in dose differences, particularly in regions of high dose gradient such as wedged or modulated fields. It is worth bearing in mind that, typically within 5 mm of a radiation field's geometric edge, a 1-mm positional discrepancy can result in a dose variation of up to 10%.

A random combination of these many error sources throughout the treatment cannot be guaranteed not to occur. The performance variation which might result therefore, without adequate QC and planned maintenance, could well cause significant variation from the dose prediction planned for the treatment.

A comprehensive system of QC for all the equipment used in radiotherapy will ensure that accurate and reproducible treatment is being delivered.

REFERENCES

1. Council Directive 93/47/Euratom. *Off J Eur Commun.* 1997;L180:22–27.
2. UK Statutory Instruments. The Ionising Radiations Regulations 2017. Statutory Instrument 1999 No. 3232. HMSO.
3. BSI (British Standards Institution). BS EN 60601-1:2006+A2:2020. *Medical electrical equipment. General requirements for basic safety and essential performance.* London, UK: BSI; 2021.
4. BSI (British Standards Institution). *BS EN 60976. Medical electrical equipment. Particular requirements for the safety of electron accelerators on the range 1 MeV to 50 MeV.* London, UK: BSI; 1998.
5. BSI (British Standards Institution). *BS EN 60601-2-1. Medical electrical equipment. Medical electron accelerators. Functional performance characteristics.* London, UK: BSI; 1998:2007.
6. Protection of the Patient in Radiation Therapy. London, UK: ICRP Publication; 1985;44.
7. Thwaites DI, Mijnheer BJ, Mills JA. Quality assurance of external beam radiotherapy. In: Podgorsak EB, ed. *Radiation Oncology Physics: A Handbook for Teachers and Students.* Vienna, Austria: IAEA; 2005:407–450.
8. Klein EE, Hanley J, Bayouth J, et al. Task group 142 report: quality assurance of medical accelerators. *Med Phys.* 2009;36:4197–4212. http://doi.org/10.1118/1.3190392.
9. IPEM (Institute of Physics and Engineering in Medicine). *Physics Aspects of Quality Control in Radiotherapy.* 2nd ed. York, UK: IPEM; 2018 IPEM Report 81.
10. Amemiya K, Shubuya H, Yoshomura R, Okada N. The risk of radiation induced cancer in patients with squamous cell carcinoma of the head and neck and its results of treatment. *Br J Radiol.* 2005;78:1028–1033.
11. The Exeter District Health Authority. The report of the committee of enquiry into overdoses administered in the Department of Radiotherapy in the period February to July 1988. https://depositedpapers.parliament.uk/depositedpaper/2206108/details
12. West Midlands Health Authority. Second report of the Independent Enquiry into the conduct of isocentric radiotherapy at the North Staffordshire Royal Infirmary.
13. Mills JA. Quality control. In: Symonds P, ed. *Walter and Miller's Textbook of Radiotherapy.* UK: Elsevier; 2012:211–221.
14. Karna SK, Sahai R. An overview on Taguchi method. *Int J Eng Math Sc.* 2012;1:11–18.
15. Sharpe P. Data Mining for Radiotherapy Linear Accelerators. MSc Thesis. 1999. Coventry University.
16. van Zijp HM, van Asselen B, Wolthaus JWH, et al. Minimizing the magnetic effect in MR-linac specific QA-tests; the use of electron dense materials. *Phys Med Biol.* 2016;61(3):N50–N59. http://doi.org/10.1088/0031-9155/61/3/N50/meta.
17. Tanadini-Lang S, Budgell G, Bohoudi O, et al. An ESTRO-ACOP guideline on quality assurance and medical physics commissioning of online MRI guided radiotherapy systems based on a consensus expert opinion. *Radiat Oncol.* 2023;181:109504–109511. http://doi.org/10.1016/j.radonc.2023.109504.
18. Mills JA, Colligan SC. Megavoltage quality control, resources and demand: a pragmatic review. *Br J Radiol.* 2016;89:20150709. http://doi.org/10.1259/bjr.20150709.
19. Liebig T, Chief Radiotherapy Engineer, Exeter. Personal communication; 2023.
20. ICRU (International Commission on Radiation Units and Measurements). Prescribing, recording and reporting photon beam therapy. ICRU Report No. 50. Washington, DC: ICRU; 1993.

15

Quality Management in Radiotherapy

Karen Waite, Jody Deacon-Viney and Helen Baines

CHAPTER OUTLINE

INTRODUCTION

There are many well-documented theories and approaches to quality and quality management in healthcare.[1] Approaches to quality have seen a shifting emphasis and have evolved from being reactive to being proactive through the following stages:

1. Inspection and remedial action
2. Identifying improvements and taking steps to prevent mistakes
3. Doing things differently—that is, modernisation, including taking a systems approach

The current emphasis is focused on continual improvement, safety and risk management. These changes are reflected in the history of quality in radiotherapy (RT)[2,3] such that the interpretation of quality has widened and can now be applied to every aspect of the service, incorporating many local, professional and national standards. It is not possible to cover every aspect of quality in detail in a single chapter. Therefore this chapter aims to provide an overview of quality and quality management and their significance to RT, outline the requirements of the international quality standard ISO 9001,[4] signpost readers to further information on a number of quality initiatives and promote an integrated approach to quality management in oncology centres in the United Kingdom.

There are also many different definitions and perceptions of quality and several terms associated with quality that are important to describe from the outset. Quality may be defined as fitness for purpose or conformance to requirements, but it is more than this:

> *Quality is the degree to which a set of inherent characteristics of an object fulfils requirements.*[5]

In other words, it is the degree to which a product or service satisfies the requirements of the user. Some definitions do not take costs into account. However, quality is about meeting customer requirements, stated or implied, while also keeping costs to a minimum.

Another often used term is *quality control (QC)*, which is a procedure or set of procedures intended to ensure that a manufactured product or performed service adheres to a defined set of criteria or meets the requirements of the client or customer. In RT, QC applies not only to controlling the performance of the equipment but also to controlling the performance of RT processes.

Quality assurance (QA) refers to 'the part of quality management focused on providing confidence that quality requirements will be fulfilled'.[5]

QA incorporates risk assessment: that is, determining what might go wrong or what is critical to get right, and then planning the process and putting procedures in place to ensure that a reliable service is provided. Aspects to be included should be operational, including legislative and educational requirements; physical and technical checks to verify correct functioning of equipment; and clinical aspects, including patient care and management. This can be achieved through activities such as documentation, training and ongoing review of existing processes.

Quality management (QM) is 'management with regard to quality', where management is 'the coordinated activities to direct and control an organisation'.[5] The underpinning philosophy—that is, to get the process and the service right the first time—applies to all parts of the organisation and involves managing all functions and activities to achieve quality.

A *quality system (QS)* is the organisational structure, responsibilities, procedures, processes and resources which must be in place to implement QM.

A *quality management system (QMS)* is part of a management system with regard to quality, where a *management system* is a set of interrelated or interacting elements of an organisation to establish policies, objectives and processes to achieve those objectives.[5]

There are a number of documented approaches to quality, including total quality management (TQM), continuous quality improvement (CQI), the European Foundation for Quality Management (EFQM)[6] model and business process reengineering. From these different approaches, it is possible to identify a number of key recurring themes:

- Management commitment
- Staff involvement
- Identification of clear requirements or standards
- Identification of clear processes, broken down into identifiable steps
- A focus on the prevention of problems
- Recognition that quality is a continual process

The steps to achieving any quality initiative must include the following stages:

- Analysis of the current service
- Identification of recommendations for change

TABLE 15.1 Chronology of Quality Development in Radiotherapy in the United Kingdom

Year	Event
1988	Exeter: Overdose, 207 patients affected.
1988	Thwaites Report: Detailed root cause of Exeter incident.
	DoH working party, chaired by Professor Bleehen, to investigate the application of quality assurance to radiotherapy to reduce the probability of incidents occurring in other centres.
1982–1991	Stoke: Underdose, 1045 patients affected.
1991	Bleehen Report: Quality assurance in radiotherapy (QART).[12] Took the form of a quality standard and provided a formal system for managing quality in radiotherapy. It was based on the predecessor of ISO 9001[4] (Quality Standard BS 5750, Part 2, 1987, a quality standard which was generic to a range of industries and services and thus open to a degree of interpretation and translation).
	DoH funded two pilot sites, Bristol and Manchester, to implement a quality system to see if it was feasible and to prepare manuals that would serve as examples to other radiotherapy departments.
1994	Stoke: Report from investigation.
1994	Sample documents from two pilot sites published and DoH recommendation for all departments to develop their own quality management system.[13]
1994	BS EN ISO 9001:1994 replaced BS5750.
2000	BS EN ISO 9001:2000 replaced BS EN ISO 9001:1994. Increased emphasis on a process approach and continual improvement.
2006	Incident at Beatson Oncology Centre.[14]
2008	BS EN ISO 9001:2008 replaced BS EN ISO 9001:2000.
2008	Publication of *Towards Safer Radiotherapy*.[11]
2015	BS EN ISO 9001:2015 replaced BS EN ISO 9001:2008. Continued focus on leadership, process approach and improvement. Increased emphasis on risk management.
2016	Edinburgh: Report into unintended exposure September 2015.[15]
2017	MPACE (Medical Physics and Clinical Engineering) accreditation pilot; assessment against BS 70000. See Box 15.1.

DoH, Department of Health.

BOX 15.1 Medical Physics and Clinical Engineering (MPACE) Accreditation

In 2017, UKAS (UK Accreditation Service) launched the pilot phase of accreditation called MPACE (Medical Physics and Clinical Engineering). The aim was to introduce a system for assessing competence for medical physics and clinical engineering departments based on the BS 70000 standard. It also went one step further than other quality standard certification organisations, as MPACE also assesses whether a service is fit for purpose. The initiative followed the iCEPSS project (Improving Clinical Engineering and Physical Science Services) carried out by IPEM, NHS England, the Academy for Healthcare Science (AHCS) and UKAS, which started in 2013. Technical experts, stakeholders and volunteers from healthcare services worked together to establish a set of criteria for assessment considering the appropriate quality standards and the scope of the accreditation. In radiotherapy physics, this includes treatment planning and delivery, particularly the quality assurance, calibration, maintenance and commissioning procedures as well as IT systems and medical devices. The pilot for radiotherapy physics ended in 2019 and has successfully completed accreditation of a number of centres. This national accreditation system remains voluntary, but it is hoped that it will help the United Kingdom to provide a high-quality medical physics and clinical engineering service, which is important given the significant reliance that modern healthcare has on scientific and technical services.

- Implementation of change
- Evaluation of the impact of change

The main aim of quality in RT is safe and effective treatment. In addition to ensuring that all treatments are optimised, a QS should ensure that all possible measures are taken to prevent inappropriate exposures from occurring.

HISTORY OF QUALITY IN RADIOTHERAPY

There are a number of well-documented RT incidents[7–11] which have occurred both in the United Kingdom (Table 15.1) and internationally. These have led to hundreds of patients receiving incorrect doses of radiation which, in turn, may have led to the possibility of the treatment intent being compromised or causing unnecessary and distressing acute and late side effects of treatment. Subsequent outcomes in the United Kingdom have included key reports which have contributed to the development of QMSs in RT.

It is notable that, throughout numerous reported incidents, a number of recurring themes can be identified as contributing factors. These include:

- Lack of communication, especially at staff group interfaces
- Training, competency and supervision issues
- Lack of up-to-date procedures, protocols and documentation
- No independent check or calibration
- Inadequate identification of clear responsibilities

It is of the utmost importance that the RT community shares information and learns from past mistakes.[11,16] Departments should also search for, correct, monitor and learn from their own incidents. Departments open themselves up to risk if there are workload or time pressures or if there is an insufficiency in:

- Attention to detail, alertness or awareness
- Procedures or checks
- Resources, for example, qualified and well-trained staff
- Coordination, communication and clear responsibilities

All of these factors are encompassed by ISO 9001:2015[4] and should be incorporated into a department's QMS. These are areas that should be kept under regular review with a view to achieve continual improvement.

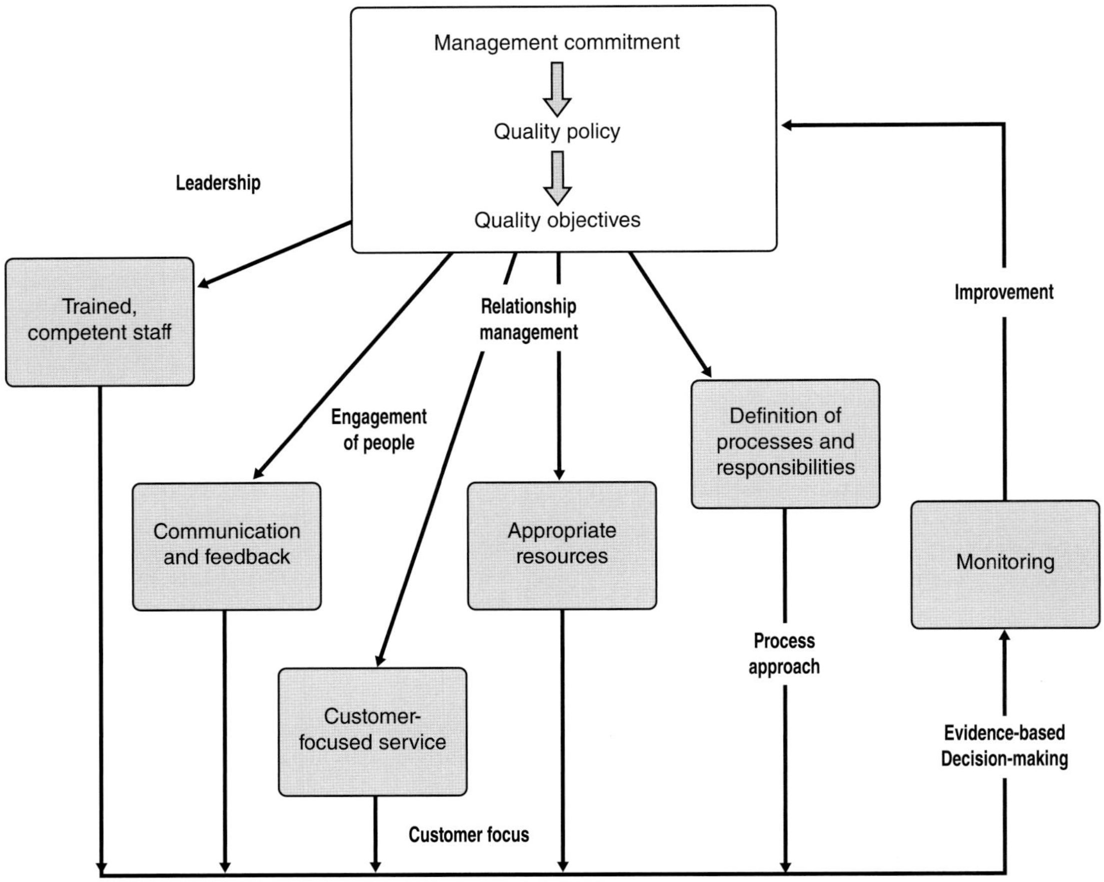

Fig. 15.1 Key quality management principles underpinning ISO 9001:2015.

QUALITY MANAGEMENT SYSTEMS

A QMS is a set of interrelated or interacting processes which provide a framework for an organisation to manage its activities to achieve its quality policy and quality objectives. Management system standards, such as the ISO 9000[5] family of documents (see the section titled 'The ISO 9001 Standard') provide a model to follow in setting up and operating a QMS. The ISO 9001:2015[4] requirements are based on seven QM principles, the key elements of which are illustrated in Fig. 15.1.

Customer Focus

A service should understand and strive to meet and exceed the current and future needs and expectations of its customers. In RT, this would include not only external customers such as patients, carers and healthcare commissioners whose respective requirements and expectations may well be different from each other, but also internal customers such as sections within oncology, for example mould room and RT physics staff.

Leadership

Management is responsible for creating a positive, engaging environment in which quality can flourish. The department's management team must establish a clear vision and a quality policy with linked objectives which are specific, measurable, achievable and realistic and which incorporate other initiatives, all of which must be communicated to all staff.

Engagement of People

All staff should be fully involved in the service and encouraged to use all of their abilities to the benefit of the department. They should be supported to achieve competence and participate in continual improvement to benefit themselves and the service.

Process Approach

Quality should be process driven: that is, all resources and activities should be managed as a process, giving consideration to both inputs and outputs.

Improvement

Systems, such as audit, should be in place for continual measurement, review and improvement of a department's processes and service. Departments should be able to react to changes in internal and external parties' needs and expectations and use them as opportunities for improvement.

Evidence-Based Decision-Making

All decisions should be evidence based, supported by appropriate data and information including key performance indicators. For example, there should be appropriate data collated to support future service planning and developments, including reflecting on previous implementations, current resources and risk assessment.

Relationship Management

Any interested party, for example customer, supplier or partner organisation, has an effect on quality, and a healthy relationship between a department and its interested parties, both internal and external, enhances the ability of both to ensure that a high level of quality is maintained.

THE ISO 9001 STANDARD

The International Organization for Standardization (ISO) provides the ISO 9000 family of documents, which are an international standards code of practice for QMSs. It is designed to be generic so that it is independent of any specific industry and therefore applicable to both manufacturing and service industries, including healthcare.

It consists of:

- ISO 9000:2015[5] Quality management systems—Fundamentals and vocabulary, published by ISO in 2015
- ISO 9001:2015[4]Quality management systems—Requirements, the current ISO standard for QMS
- ISO 9004[17]: Managing for the sustained success of an organization—A QM approach, published in 2018

The standards themselves are subject to a review program to ensure that they remain relevant. ISO 9001:2000[18] was introduced in 2000. It was withdrawn in 2012 following the publication of ISO 9001:2008,[19] which included only minor amendments. That was also withdrawn, following the publication of ISO 9001:2015,[4] which has an increased emphasis on leadership, improvement and risk management. In 2024 there was a further addition to ISO 9001:2015 relating to climate change, the organisation must consider whether climate change is a relevant issue and considered when implementing the management system.[39]

The scope of a department's QMS defines the activities and is determined by the department. There are variations between oncology departments: some include just RT treatment, whereas others include planning, dosimetry, medical physics, chemotherapy, clinical trials and clerical areas. ISO 9001:2015[4] is the standard against which a department is assessed. It specifies the requirements a QMS must meet but not how the department should meet them.

The ISO 9001:2015[4] standard comprises 10 clauses, listed in Box 15.2.

The Introduction to the standard describes the potential benefits of implementing a QMS, identifies the seven QM principles which are reflected throughout the requirements and outlines the process approach based on the Plan-Do-Check-Act cycle, as illustrated in Fig. 15.2, as well as being risk-based and forward thinking. It also identifies its

BOX 15.2 The Clauses of ISO 9001:2015[4]

1. Scope
2. Normative References
3. Terms and Definitions
4. Context of the Organization
5. Leadership
6. Planning
7. Support
8. Operation
9. Performance Evaluation
10. Improvement

relationship with other management system standards. Clause 1, Scope, states that the standard specifies requirements which an organisation's QMS should fulfil. Clause 2, Normative References, and Clause 3, Terms and Definitions, give reference to the document ISO 9000:2015,[5] which is necessary for the interpretation and application of the ISO standard. The remaining clauses, 4 to 10, described subsequently, contain the requirements against which departments are assessed.

Clause 4, Context of the Organization

Clause 4 changed in the 2015 version to begin with the importance of defining the purpose and strategy of the department. The department needs to consider internal issues, such as culture, and external issues, such as legal requirements (Clause 4.1). It needs to determine interested parties, both internal and external, such as patients, carers, suppliers and healthcare authorities, and what their needs and expectations are (Clause 4.2). The information determined through Clauses 4.1 and 4.2 underpins subsequent requirements, such as Clause 6, Planning. A number of methodologies are available to support this, such as a PESTLE

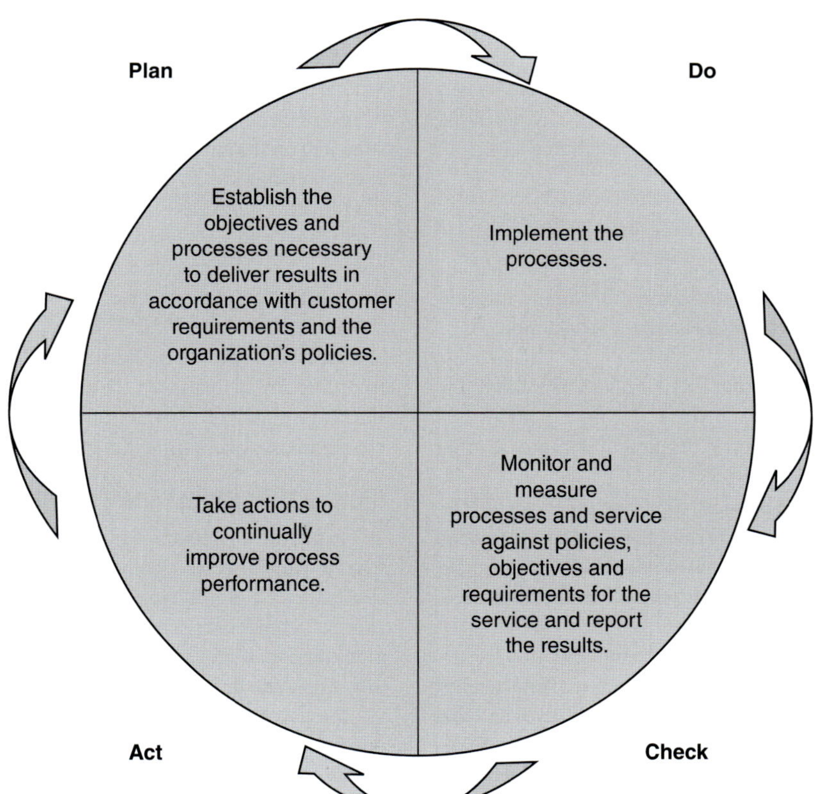

Fig. 15.2 The Plan-Do-Check-Act cycle applied to ISO 9001:2015.

(political, economic, social, technological, legal, environmental) analysis.[20] Given the potential wide-reaching nature of their service objectives, the department must produce a clear scope of what is and isn't covered in its QMS. This clause also requires a department to define its processes and their interactions. The 2015 version no longer requires specific procedures, instead requiring documented information throughout the requirements, with specific requirements detailed in Clause 7.5.

Clause 5, Leadership

The management team is required to demonstrate leadership and commitment and is accountable for the effectiveness of the QMS. In addition to general requirements such as a process approach, risk-based thinking, continual improvement, an integrated approach to the QMS requirements and the department's processes, and the availability and effective allocation of resources, there are specific requirements linked to a commitment to meeting customer requirements and enhancing customer satisfaction; establishing, maintaining and communicating a documented quality policy and objectives which reflect the vision of the department; and ensuring a clear organisational structure with well-defined responsibilities and authorities.

Clause 6, Planning

The management team is responsible for implementing a risk-based culture within the department, determining the risks and opportunities that will impact its ability to achieve intended results. To accomplish this, it needs to assess the internal and external issues that will affect it together with the needs of interested parties. Actions should be identified, communicated, implemented, monitored and evaluated for their effectiveness. Examples of risks could include not having sufficient capacity to achieve waiting time targets, or not being able to implement a best practice because of obsolete equipment. Examples of opportunities might include implementing new techniques through participation in clinical trials, or networking with other departments. A department should have documented quality objectives, consistent with the quality policy, that are specific, measurable, achievable and relevant. These objectives should be monitored, communicated and updated as required. When changes to the QMS are required, they should be carried out in a planned way with consideration to who is responsible, available resources, timing and any consequences which may arise.

Clause 7, Support

Sufficient resources are essential for an effective QMS. The management team is responsible for determining and providing adequate resources to implement, maintain, monitor and continually improve the effectiveness of the QMS and enhance customer satisfaction.

Examples include:

- Human resources, for example, sufficient numbers of trained and competent staff
- Infrastructure, for example, buildings, treatment machines, other equipment and IT and support services
- The work environment including physical, social and psychological factors, for example, health and safety, local rules and radiation protection
- Monitoring and measurement, for example, patient satisfaction surveys or dose measuring instruments, with calibration traceable to a national standard
- Knowledge, for example, information on current legislation

There are specific requirements which cover defining competencies: ensuring that staff are aware of the quality policy and objectives and that they understand their role and how their performance may affect the QMS, internal and external communication and documented information. A department should maintain documented information as specified by ISO 9001:2015[4] as it determines what is necessary for the QMS to be effective.

This may include:

- Procedures and work instructions
- Clinical protocols
- Process flowcharts
- Equipment maintenance records
- Internal audit documents
- Patient survey results
- Forms
- Data
- Reference documents

All documents within the QMS should be subject to a robust method of document control, have adequate protection from accidental changes or loss, be stored securely and be easily retrievable. It is vital to ensure that a document is identifiable, available, current and relevant to the area in which it is used. Systems should be in place to prevent previous versions from being accessed. Documentation also includes records such as patient records, training records and equipment maintenance records which provide evidence of activities performed. Departments must ensure that they incorporate any legislative, national[21] and local requirements into their documentation management processes.

Clause 8, Operation

This is the largest clause and includes requirements for providing a service from initial planning through the design, production and delivery stages to achieve consistency and meet intended requirements. A department needs to consider and review the requirements for its service including, for example, customer feedback, performance targets and legislation. Where the department processes include design and development, there are specific requirements which must be met from planning the development through to validating the output. When dealing with external providers, such as treatment machine manufacturers, departments need to establish controls to ensure that externally provided products conform to required standards and do not adversely affect the quality of their service. This may be achieved by performing QA, for example, QC or safety checks of the end product or checks along the pathway. General requirements relating to service delivery include the provision of controlled conditions, such as taking actions to minimise the risk of human error. There are also requirements to ensure identification and traceability throughout, such as identification of patients and equipment, and to ensure that any changes to service provision are managed effectively. Checks must be in place at identified points of a process to detect any problems or faults, prevent errors and ensure that requirements have been met through, for example, independent treatment plan checks. Documentation must be kept to ensure confidence in the implementation of the service, and outputs must be continually reviewed against requirements. Finally, processes must be in place for identifying any problems, such as complaints, preventing them from escalating and recording any actions taken. There should also be provision to use concessions, permitting use of a nonconforming product or service with special conditions in place, such as for off-protocol treatments.

Clause 9, Performance Evaluation

To ensure the effectiveness of its QMS, a department needs to consider what it can measure and how to evaluate its performance. Requirements include monitoring customer satisfaction, for example, by using surveys, complaints, compliments and user groups. Also, data such as clinical incidents, machine down time, waiting time and other key indicators can be used to measure, monitor and analyse performance.

The department should have a program of internal audits to demonstrate whether the QMS:

- Meets the requirements of ISO 9001:2015[4]
- Meets the requirements of the department
- Is implemented, effective and maintained

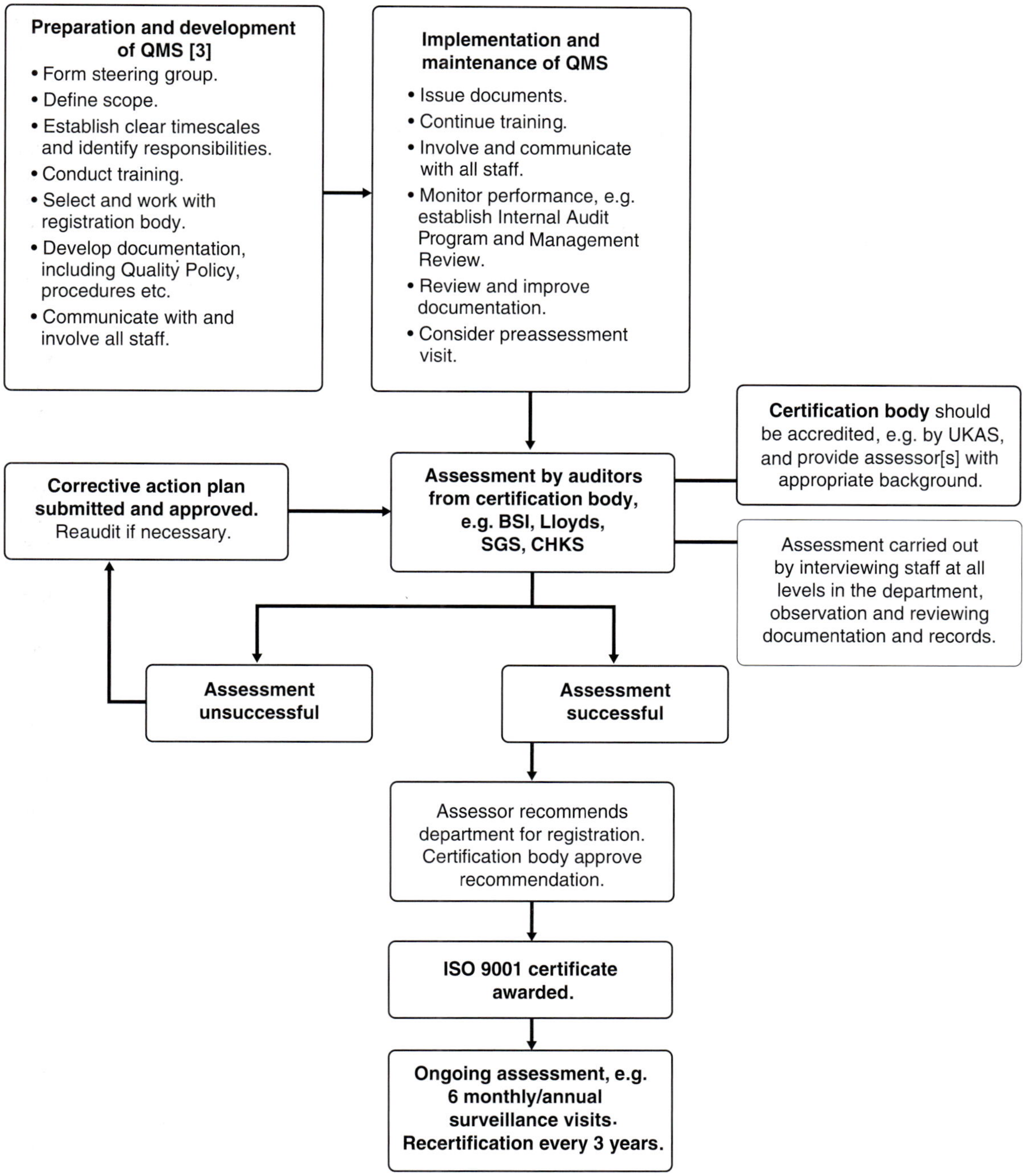

Fig. 15.3 The route to ISO 9001 registration.

Documented management reviews must take place at planned intervals. The management team should review information on performance and effectiveness, such as audit results, nonconformities and key performance indicators, to determine the suitability, effectiveness and adequacy of the QMS and whether it meets the direction and requirements of the department. The team should also consider provision of resources, improvement opportunities and any changes required to the QMS.

Clause 10, Improvement

Continual improvement is key to achieving departmental objectives and ensuring customer satisfaction. It can range from corrective action to innovation. Departments should take actions and opportunities that lead toward continual improvement. Examples include:

- Implementation of new evidence-based techniques
- Replacement of obsolete equipment
- Improvements to the environment
- Identifying the causes of incidents, nonconformities, audit findings and complaints and implementing appropriate action to prevent recurrence
- Identifying potential nonconformities and taking action to reduce the risk of occurrence

Further reading on ISO 9000[5] should include the standards themselves. In addition, there are many textbooks which interpret how to apply the requirements.[20] Fig. 15.3 illustrates the process of implementing QMS through to ongoing surveillance visits.

THE RADIOTHERAPY PROCESS

ISO 9000:2015[5] defines a process as 'A set of interrelated or interacting activities that use inputs to deliver an intended result.' ISO 9001:2015[4] follows a process-based approach and requires systematic identification and management of the department's processes and the interaction between them. To adopt a process-based approach, an RT department should identify each process carried out and consider the following questions:

- What are the inputs?
- What are the outputs?
- How are they measured?
- What are the critical interfaces with other processes?
- Have responsibilities been clearly identified?

Processes are best illustrated with a diagram or flowchart. An example relating to the treatment process is shown in Fig. 15.4. It is important to remember that a process can be defined at many levels. A core process, such as treatment, will be made up of a number of sub-processes. Fig. 15.5 illustrates an example of the interaction between a department's core processes. For each process, consider the following key elements of the ISO 9001 requirements in addition to the list already mentioned:

- Are resources allocated effectively?
- Is the work environment suitable for the task?
- Are staff trained and competent?
- Are training records up-to-date?
- How do you know if your customers' expectations have been fulfilled?
- How are complaints or other problems resolved?
- How could potential improvements be identified?
- What are the arrangements for ensuring that calibration equipment remains within specification?
- Are identification and traceability, for example, of equipment and patients, maintained throughout the process?

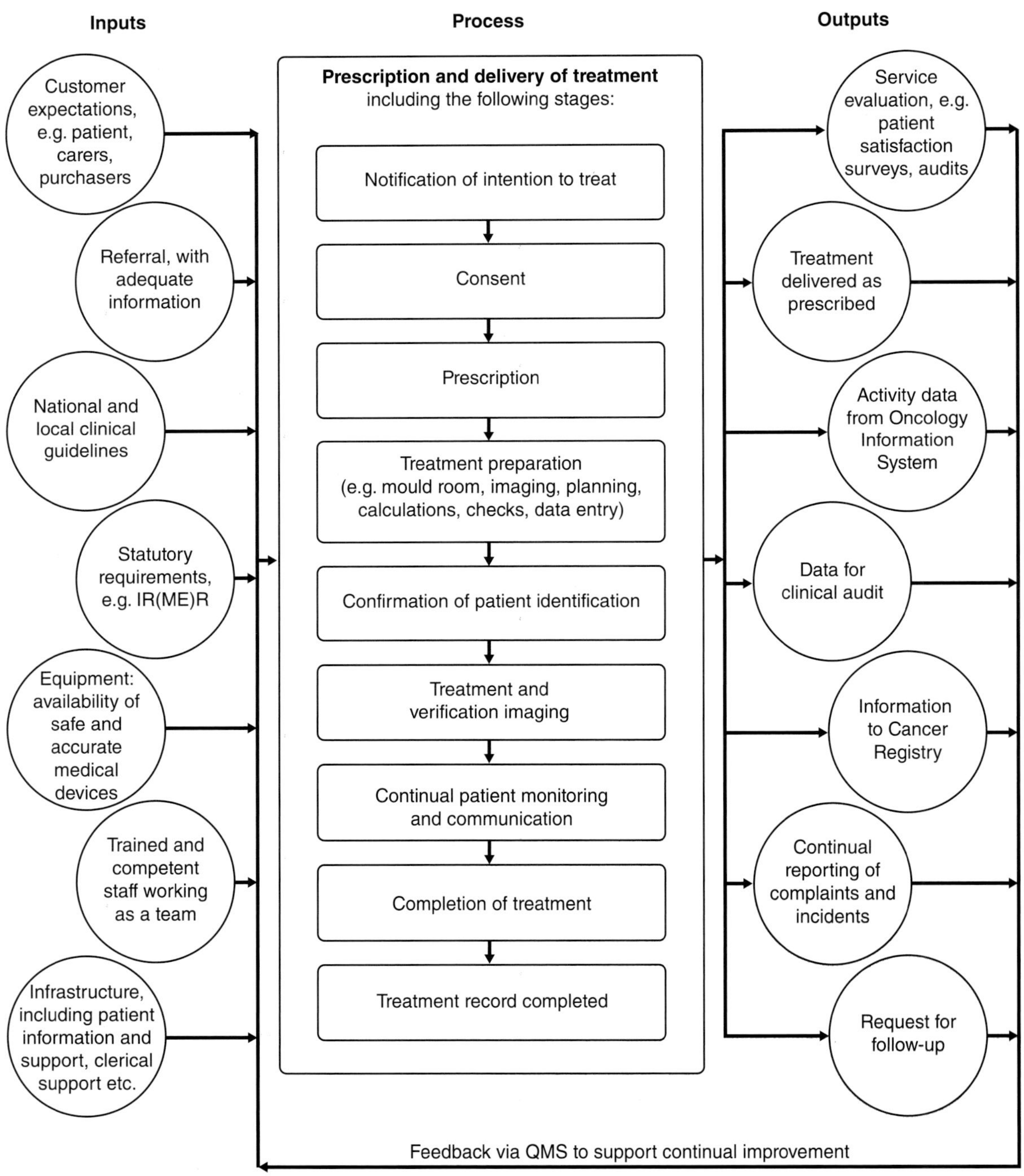

Fig. 15.4 The radiotherapy process.

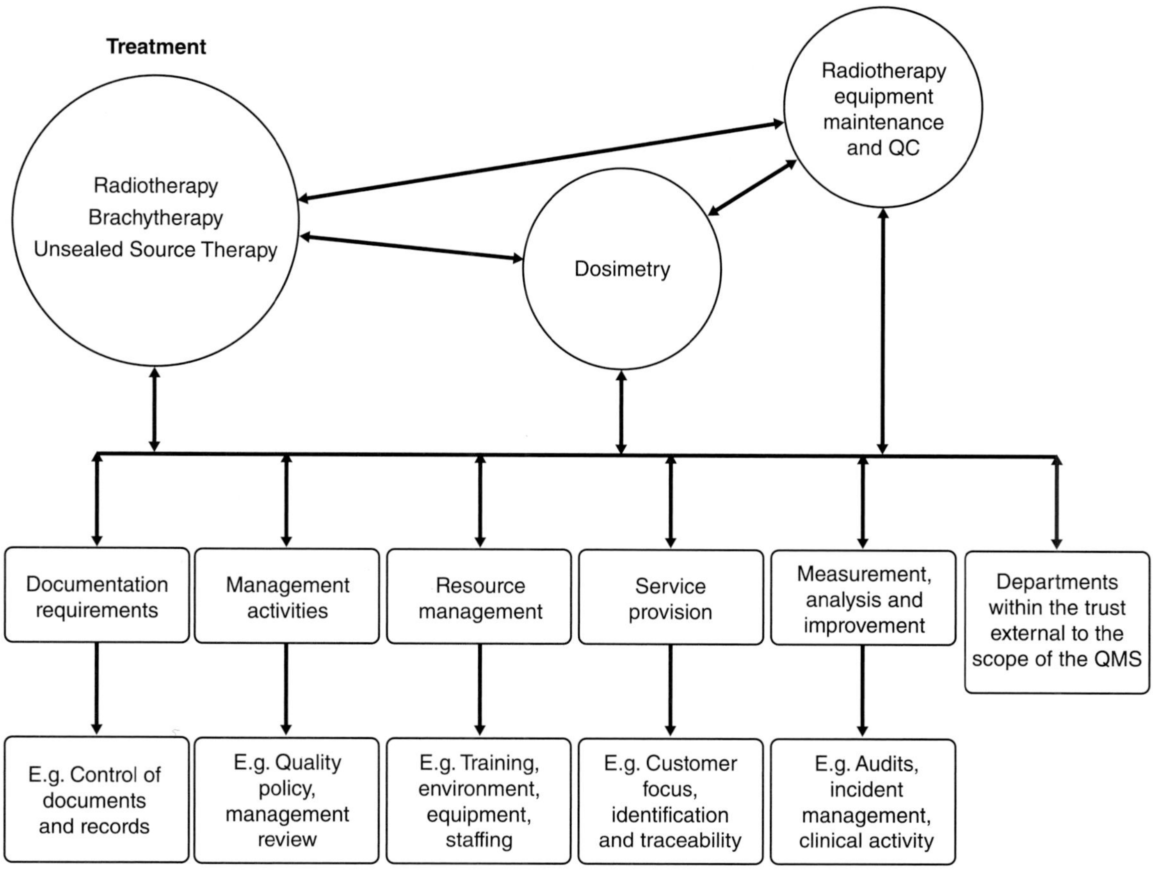

Fig. 15.5 The interaction of processes in a radiotherapy department. *QC*, Quality control; *QMS*, quality management system.

QUALITY IN THE NATIONAL HEALTH SERVICE

Quality may be measured in a number of ways, and there are a number of historical and current standards, measures, targets and improvement initiatives within the National Health Service (NHS), both generic and specific to cancer services. Previous examples of this include clinical governance and the National Cancer Peer Review. Table 15.2 lists a number of other initiatives and documents that have contributed to the development of quality and safety throughout the NHS and in RT departments. Many of these complement each other or have common characteristics and should not be considered in isolation. They reflect the same principles that underpin QMS, together with the current NHS focus on clinical effectiveness, patient experience and safety, which are the three core dimensions of quality. They are all designed with the same ultimate objective: to improve the patient experience, whether this is by, for example, improving treatment outcome, reducing waiting times, reducing the risk of incidents, improving communication with patients or improving patient facilities. Meeting such standards gives an indication that an acceptable level of quality has been achieved and allows intercomparison. Obviously, getting the right measure of quality is important. For example, waiting times measure the speed of throughput for patients but have no bearing on the standard of treatment delivered. This chapter has discussed the principles of QMS, but this is only part of developing and maintaining a quality service. An effective QMS should be a tool to help implement, integrate and measure any new initiative introduced into a department. In England, hospitals are regulated by the Care Quality Commission (CQC) (Box 15.3), and an effective QMS will ensure an integrated approach to incorporating all the requirements addressed during a CQC inspection. The following paragraphs on risk management, clinical incidents, audit and patient-focused care give more detail on some of the most important areas where a robust QMS can ensure smooth interfaces between different initiatives.

RISK MANAGEMENT

Patient and staff safety is foremost in all NHS trusts, and risk-based thinking is a key concept throughout the requirements ISO 9001:2015.[4] Risk can be defined in many ways; an example is 'the effect of uncertainty'.[5] Although RT is widely recognised as one of the safest specialities in healthcare, there is also the potential for severe patient harm when incidents do occur. There are two international documents which address managing the risks in RT. The first,[10] published by the World Health Organization (WHO) in 2008, reviews previous incidents and outlines a risk profile for RT, identifying 10 stages in the RT pathway, the key risks associated with each stage and potential interventions to improve safety. The second,[24–26] published by the European Commission in 2015, focuses on two main approaches: proactive risk assessment and reactive analysis of events. Risk assessment includes the initial identification and evaluation of a risk, quantifying the risk by taking account of both the likelihood and the consequences, and deciding appropriate action to mitigate the risk. In simple terms, risk management aims to reduce the risks to patients, thereby improving patient safety. Effective risk management should be integrated into all activities throughout the RT process and is supported by QMS requirements such as effective communication, staff competency and audit. Methods of risk prevention range from physical measures such as interlocks and computerisation to human-orientated measures such as documented procedures and competency standards which are recognised as less effective due to

TABLE 15.2 Overview of Quality Initiatives in Oncology and the National Health Service

Item	Year	Initiative, Publication or Requirement	Comment	Further Information (Correct as of May 2025)
1	2008	*Towards Safer Radiotherapy*	A joint report published by the British Institute of Radiology, the Institute of Physics and Engineering in Medicine, the National Patient Safety Agency, the Society and College of Radiographers and The Royal College of Radiologists. The report includes recommendations for improving safety in radiotherapy, including the implementation of an externally assessed QMS.	https://www.rcr.ac.uk/our-services/all-our-publications/clinical-oncology-publications/towards-safer-radiotherapy/
2	2008	World Health Organization (WHO) Radiotherapy Risk Profile. Technical Manual	Comprises two parts: the first is an international review of patient safety measures in radiotherapy practice and the second sets out WHO's Radiotherapy Risk Profile and analyses the radiotherapy process, from patient assessment to treatment verification and monitoring.	https://cdn.who.int/media/docs/default-source/patient-safety/radiotherapy/090715-who-radiotherapy_risk_profile.pdf?sfvrsn=ec752b08_3
3	2008	High Quality Care for All NHS Next Stage Review Final Report	The final report from Lord Darzi's review. This is a review of the way the NHS delivers healthcare, looking at how it can become fairer, more personalised, effective and safe, setting out immediate and longer-term priorities to ensure a patient-centred, high-quality health service.	https://www.gov.uk/government/uploads/system/uploads/attachment_data/file/228836/7432.pdf
4	2009	Care Quality Commission	A public body formed from three former organisations, including the Healthcare Commission, with a role to ensure that care services, including hospitals, provide safe, effective and high-quality care	http://www.cqc.org.uk/
5	2010	Implementing *Towards Safer Radiotherapy*: Guidance on reporting radiotherapy errors and near misses	Provided guidance on reporting radiotherapy errors to the National Patient Safety Agency (NPSA) and on the classification of these errors which are analysed by the HPA (now PHE) (see 20 for updated guidance)	https://www.england.nhs.uk/patient-safety/monthly-data-patient-safety-incident-reports/ https://www.npsa.org.uk/
6	2011	Improving Outcomes: A Strategy for Cancer	The government's commitment to improving health outcomes, including a section on providing radiotherapy services which are equitable, high quality, safe, timely, protocol-driven, quality controlled and focused on patients' needs	http://www.legislation.gov.uk/ukpga/2012/7/contents/enacted https://www.gov.uk/government/publications/health-and-social-care-act-2012-fact-sheets
7	2012	Health and Social Care Act	Recognised the need for modernisation in the NHS. Six key policy areas included clinically led commissioning and a greater voice for patients. Nine key themes included improving the quality of care.	http://www.legislation.gov.uk/ukpga/2012/7/contents/enacted https://www.gov.uk/government/publications/health-and-social-care-act-2012-fact-sheets
8	2013	Report of the Mid Staffordshire NHS Foundation Trust Public Inquiry	Referred to as the Francis Report.[22] This details the failings in care at the Mid Staffordshire NHS Foundation Trust.	https://www.gov.uk/government/publications/report-of-the-mid-staffordshire-nhs-foundation-trust-public-inquiry
9	2013	A promise to learn – a commitment to act: Improving the Safety of Patients in England	Known as the Berwick Report.[23] This followed the Francis Report to address areas of improvement needed in patient safety in England.	https://www.gov.uk/government/uploads/system/uploads/attachment_data/file/226703/Berwick_Report.pdf
10	2013	National Institute for Health and Care Excellence (NICE)	Became a nondepartmental government body. It provides evidence-based guidance, develops quality standards and provides a range of information services.	https://www.nice.org.uk/
11	2014	'Hello my name is ...' campaign	A campaign founded by Dr Kate Granger, MBE, to highlight the importance of communication and patient-centred care	https://hellomynameis.org.uk/

(continued)

TABLE 15.2 Overview of Quality Initiatives in Oncology and the National Health Service—con't

Item	Year	Initiative, Publication or Requirement	Comment	Further Information (Correct as of May 2025)
12	2014	Patient Safety Collaboratives (PSC)	A national safety initiative set up to underpin a culture of safety, continuous learning and improvement. Fifteen regional PSCs are funded and supported by NHS Improvement to facilitate improvements across the NHS.	https://www.england.nhs.uk/wp-content/uploads/2020/08/Patient_Safety_Collaboratives-1.pdf
13	2015	Culture change in the NHS	Update on the progress made since Mid Staffordshire 2013	https://www.gov.uk/government/publications/culture-change-in-the-nhs
14	2015	The NHS Constitution for England updated	Establishes the values and principles of the NHS, including the rights of patients, the public and staff	https://www.gov.uk/government/publications/the-nhs-constitution-for-england
15	2015	NHS Complaints guidance updated	Advice on how patients can give feedback or make a complaint about healthcare services	https://www.gov.uk/government/publications/the-nhs-constitution-for-england/how-do-i-give-feedback-or-make-a-complaint-about-an-nhs-service
16	2015	Radiation Protection No. 181. General guidelines on risk management in external beam radiotherapy (European Commission, 2015)	EU guidance on how to reduce accidental or unintended radiation doses of patients in radiotherapy	https://op.europa.eu/en/publication-detail/-/publication/01f57fc8-73f2-4bfc-93fa-9eec0b2c8d3c
17	2015	The Q Community	A network supported by the Health Foundation and NHS Improvement to facilitate shared learning, experience and development of sustainable improvement initiatives	https://q.health.org.uk/
18	2015	Achieving world-class cancer outcomes: A strategy for England, 2015–2020.	An independent report with 96 recommendations across the cancer pathway, including a national radiotherapy equipment replacement program	http://www.cancerresearchuk.org/sites/default/files/achieving_world-class_cancer_outcomes_-_a_strategy_for_england_2015-2020.pdf
19	2016	Cancer Strategy Implementation Plan: Achieving World Class Cancer Outcomes	The NHS five-year plan for delivering improved cancer services in England, including prevention, diagnosis, patient experience and high-quality modern services	https://www.england.nhs.uk/wp-content/uploads/2016/05/cancer-strategy.pdf
20	2016	Development of learning from radiotherapy errors, PHE	The introduction of additional taxonomies (causative factors and safety barriers) for the classification of radiotherapy errors	https://www.gov.uk/government/publications/development-of-learning-from-radiotherapy-errors
21	2014	Learning from Excellence	Initiative based on the concept of learning from examples of good practice	http://learningfromexcellence.com/
22	2016	BS70000:2017	A new British standard for medical physics, clinical engineering and associated scientific services in healthcare, with requirements for quality, safety and competence	https://shop.bsigroup.com/ProductDetail/?pid=000000000030323397
23	2017	MPACE (formerly iCEPSS)	UKAS pilot for Medical Physics and Clinical Engineering accreditation scheme	See Box 15.1. https://www.ukas.com/accreditation/standards/mpace/
24	2019	Adult External Beam Radiotherapy Services Delivered as Part of a Radiotherapy Network	Document that sets out the clinical, service and quality requirements and standards for the delivery of external beam radiotherapy to which all providers of radiotherapy must comply. It also identifies designated networks and member departments.	https://www.england.nhs.uk/wp-content/uploads/2019/01/External-Beam-Radiotherapy-Services-Delivered-as-Part-of-a-Radiotherapy-Network-Adults.pdf Additional information on radiotherapy commissioning: https://www.england.nhs.uk/commissioning/spec-services/npc-crg/group-b/b01/
25	2019	NHS Long Term Plan (LTP) ambitions for cancer	The government's commitment to improving cancer services in England over the next 10 years	https://www.england.nhs.uk/cancer/strategy/

EU, European Union; *HPA*, Health Protection Agency; *iCEPSS*, Improving Clinical Engineering and Physical Science Services; *MBE*, Member of the British Empire; *MPACE*, Medical Physics and Clinical Engineering; *NHS*, National Health Service; *PHE*, Public Health England; *UKAS*, United Kingdom Accreditation Service.

BOX 15.3 Care Quality Commission (CQC)

The CQC is the independent regulator of healthcare in England. It is their role to:

- Register hospitals
- Monitor, inspect and rate their services
- Take action to protect people who use the services
- Speak with an independent voice, publishing views on major quality issues in health and social care

They carry enforcement powers, such as fines, public warnings or closure, if standards are not being met.

Inspection visits are carried out by a team of people and take place over a number of days. An inspection is carried out by:

- Meeting and talking to people, including staff in all roles and patients, both as individuals and in focus groups
- Observation, including day-to-day practice and the general environment
- Checking records and data

The inspection team use Key Lines of Enquiry (KLOEs), prompts and sources of evidence to answer core questions. The five questions in use are:

- **Is it safe?** Does the hospital ensure that all patients are protected from abuse and avoidable harm? For example, are medicines safely secured and medical devices compliant? Are there effective measures in place for infection control, safeguarding, duty of candour and incident reporting and learning?
- **Is it effective?** Does the hospital ensure that all patients receive the care, treatment and support they need to achieve the best possible outcomes and quality of life? Is the service provided in accordance with NICE guidance, national guidelines, legislation and local and national audit, and are outcomes monitored, for example, with mortality reviews?
- **Is it caring?** Does the hospital ensure that all patients are treated with kindness, compassion, dignity and respect? For example, do they support patients to maintain independence and request support from other teams where needed (e.g. dementia service, pain management, alcohol liaison)? Are patients involved in decision-making, and does the service seek patient participation and feedback?
- **Is it responsive to people's needs?** Does the hospital ensure that the care, treatment and support it provides meet the needs of all patients? For example, is there evidence of personalised care and an awareness of patients' needs and choices, and are there effective systems in place to respond to concerns and complaints?
- **Is it well-led?** Do the leaders and managers provide vision, direction and energy with clear responsibilities and accountabilities and do the systems in place support the delivery of high-quality, patient-centred care? Is there evidence of good governance and of learning, improvement and innovation? Is there an open and fair culture? Are risk and performance managed effectively?

Following an inspection, informal feedback will be given at the end of the visit with a detailed report published later. For each core hospital service assessed, each key question will receive a rating: Inadequate, Requires Improvement, Good or Outstanding. The service will also receive an overall rating.

Detailed information about inspections and KLOEs is available on the CQC website: https://www.cqc.org.uk

their dependence on human behaviours.[25] Effective risk management should also identify latent threats which may lie dormant for months before an error actually occurs or the risk is detected.

Examples of risk management throughout the RT process include:

- A strict equipment maintenance program and rigorous QC checks (see Chapter 14)
- Active, independent checks at a number of stages within the treatment process to provide an effective error prevention system[26]
- Audits of existing checking processes to ensure that they are effective and any redundant checks are eliminated
- Reducing manual tasks, such as the transfer of data, wherever possible
- Methods to reduce the risk of involuntary automaticity, where staff carry out checks automatically and see or hear what they expect to see, rather than what is actually written or said
- Ensuring that a supervising member of staff is not responsible for checking a task for which they have provided supervision
- Peer review of target volume definition[27]
- A study of incidents and near misses including prominent causes,[28,29] contributory factors and the risk of accidental or unintended exposures[30]

CLINICAL INCIDENTS

In 2016, NHS Improvement took over statutory patient safety functions including operating the National Reporting and Learning System (NRLS) and developing advice and guidance for the NHS on reducing risks to patients. Health organisations should be open in reporting incidents and should implement local systems which are nonpunitive. There are a number of tools available for use in managing clinical incidents, such as incident decision trees,[31] root cause analysis and the London Protocol for systems analysis of clinical incidents. There is a long history of incident reporting in RT both in the United Kingdom and internationally,[10,32,33] including systematic incidents affecting multiple patients and random errors affecting an individual.

Historically there has been:

- No unified approach
- No standard definitions for the terminology in use
- No defined classifications, such as level of impact, source or root cause

This has made it difficult to compare error rates and to define any standards. Examples of current international systems include Safety in Radiation Oncology (SAFRON)[34] and the Radiation Oncology Safety Information System (ROSEIS).[16] A UK multidisciplinary working party including representation from the Royal College of Radiologists (RCR), the Institute of Physics and Engineering in Medicine (IPEM), the Society of Radiographers (SoR), the British Institute of Radiology (BIR) and the National Patient Safety Agency (NPSA) was established in 2006, and in 2008 it published a report[11] containing recommendations for a national system to support the reporting, analysis and learning from RT incidents. The Health Protection Agency (HPA), now Public Health England (PHE), implemented a taxonomy for severity and pathway classification dedicated to RT and developed a UK-wide voluntary RT reporting system. There is now established data analysis and feedback through PHE.[35,36] The coding was extended in 2016 to include reporting and analysis of safety barriers and causative factors and in 2018 was extended again to include methods of detection.

All RT departments should operate a system for defining, recording, analysing and learning from RT incidents including near misses. Local incident reporting should include a full objective description of the event, how it was detected, any identified causes and contributing factors, the severity of consequences, the risk of recurrence and preventive actions to avoid future occurrence.

Major incidents are reportable to various agencies under different regulations, including:

- NHS Improvement. All patient safety incidents should be reported via the National Reporting and Learning System (NRLS).

- CQC. Under IR[ME]R,[30] any incident in which a person has been exposed to levels of ionising radiation significantly greater or lower than those generally considered to be proportionate in the circumstances should be reported.
- Health and Safety Executive (HSE). Under the Ionising Radiations Regulations 2017,[37] any incident where a person has received an overexposure as a result of work with ionising radiation carried out by that employer should be reported.
- Medicine and Healthcare Products Regulatory Agency (MHRA). Under the Medical Devices Regulations 2002, incidents and faults relating to medical equipment should be reported. Device Bulletin DB2011(01) gives further advice.
- HSE. Under the Reporting of Injuries, Diseases and Dangerous Occurrences Regulations (RIDDOR), any work-related accident resulting in death or specified injuries should be reported.

Action following an incident should be considered carefully by departments, including disclosure to the patient and Duty of Candour[38] as well as support for staff involved.[11] Communicating honestly and sympathetically with patients and their families is a vital component in dealing effectively with errors or mistakes. An apology can be an expression of regret and sympathy and not necessarily an admission of guilt.

AUDIT

Audit is a key requirement of ISO 9001:2015.[4] It is also a recommendation or requirement of other standards, regulations and guidance such as IR(ME)R[30] and *Towards Safer Radiotherapy.*[11] There are many definitions of audit, but ISO 9000:2015[5] defines it as:

> *A systematic, independent and documented process for obtaining objective evidence and evaluating it objectively to determine the extent to which the audit criteria are fulfilled*

where 'audit criteria' are a set of policies, procedures or requirements used as a reference against which 'objective evidence' is compared, and 'objective evidence' is data verifying or supporting the existence of something.

Types of audit include:

- Clinical audit, which is typically used in the healthcare setting (Box 15.4)
- Internal audit, which is used by departments to monitor their QMS and is conducted by employees of the department
- External audit, which is an objective check of a department's QMS conducted by an independent external auditing organisation

All audits are cyclical in nature (Fig. 15.6) and have the same key features. Audits are a valuable tool for ensuring continual improvement. Many departments will have a clinical audit program that is developed independently to the QMS internal audit program. Whereas clinical audits may focus more on outcomes, such as the effect on health or on patient experience, QMS audits aim to verify processes, particularly at the interfaces, highlight any areas of concern and identify areas for potential improvement. An integrated approach to both QMS and clinical audits could encompass a range of audit projects and provide a comprehensive audit program.

It is important to distinguish audit from research. In the most simplistic terms, research tells us the most effective way to do things and how to achieve the best results, and audit tells us if we are doing that.

BOX 15.4 Clinical Audit

Clinical audit, initially termed *Medical Audit,* was introduced to the National Health Service (NHS) through the 1989 white paper, 'Working for Patients'. It has continued to evolve and is now well established in the NHS, forming a key component of the clinical governance framework.

Clinical audit is defined by the Health Quality Improvement Partnership (HQIP) as:

> *a quality improvement cycle that involves measurement of the effectiveness of healthcare against agreed and proven standards for high quality, and taking action to bring practice in line with these standards so as to improve the quality of care and health outcomes.*

Clinical audits should be patient focused. They can be conducted at a local level or nationwide. Healthcare professionals use clinical audits to measure their clinical practice against standards. It provides a framework to identify opportunities for improvement to the quality of patient care in a collaborative and systematic way. A good clinical audit will identify or confirm any problems and then lead to changes that should result in improved patient care.

At a national level, HQIP on behalf of NHS England manage and commission the National Clinical Audit and Patient Outcomes Programme (NCAPOP). The data collected from NCAPOP audits provide NHS providers with reports on compliance and performance, helping to improve patient care. The National Institute for Health and Care Excellence (NICE) use the results of national clinical audits to measure compliance to NICE guidelines.

More guidance on clinical audit is available from the Health Quality Improvement Partnership (HQIP).

PATIENT-FOCUSED CARE

The National Institute for Health and Care Excellence (NICE) recommends that the patient should be given the opportunity to make informed choices about their care and treatment, supported by healthcare professionals. This is referred to as patient-centred care and is about an individual being able to take an active role in their healthcare. The Mental Capacity Act 2005 exists for those unable to make such decisions.

However, patient-focused care is not just about involving the patient themselves in their care choices; it is also about recognising the need to put the patient first. This was one of the key changes recommended by the 2013 Francis Report,[22] which highlighted the need for all staff to take an active role in QM and for this to be encouraged by senior management. ISO 9001:2015[4] follows on this need for a culture change to promote accountability and empowerment in the organisation.

Following the Francis and Berwick Reports,[22,23] there has been a push for NHS organisations to be more open to the public about how their services are performing. NHS England, alongside the DoH, Health and Social Care Information Service, CQC and Public Health England, developed the MyNHS online tool that provides transparent performance data and encourages accountability and improvement.

There is a long history of patient and public participation in the United Kingdom, with national policies making it clear that all NHS cancer services are responsible at a local level for developing user involvement in service evaluation, planning and delivery. Patient reported outcome measures (PROMs) are about reviewing treatment in a way that is relevant to the patient by looking at quality of life and patient perceptions. In practical terms, the development of patient and carer input can be achieved in various ways including questionnaires, complaint monitoring, focus groups, interviews, websites, newsletters, workshops, user involvement training programs, suggestion boxes, facilitating support groups, patient liaison services and user councils. Patient reported experience measures are about reviewing treatment through patient feedback. A recent resource rolled out in 2013 following the Francis and Berwick Reports[22,23] is the Friends and Family Test, which provides feedback on patient experience data from patients on

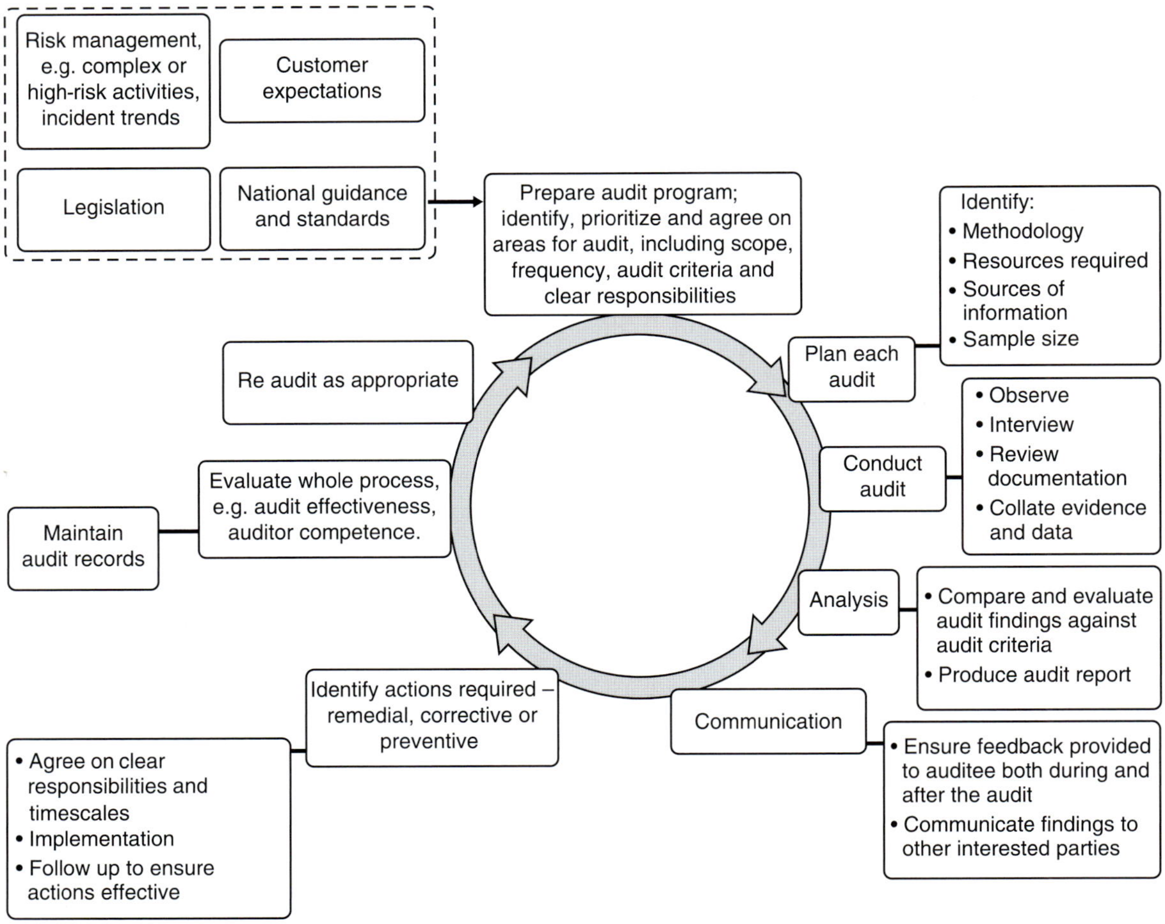

Fig. 15.6 The audit cycle.

a local and national level. There is also the National Cancer Patient Experience Survey (NCPES), which started taking place annually in England in 2010.

It is important to include the patient perspective in establishing how the overall patient experience can be improved. In addition to offering the latest techniques, this may simply include adequate parking provision, a comfortable waiting area and effective communication and provision of information. In today's world, patients' expectations have increased, as has their intolerance of failure or complications. The most common complaints concern delays, incorrect treatment, morbidity, perception of professional competence and efficiency of a process.

IMPLEMENTATION OF NEW TECHNOLOGY AND NEW TECHNIQUES

The development of technology and techniques in RT continues to progress rapidly. Introducing any new development, equipment, software or change in procedure, however small, carries with it the risk of error[25] and must be managed carefully with full evaluation of safety issues and training competencies[11] and with final approval by the appropriate authority. Satisfactory management can include, for example:

- Setting up specialist multidisciplinary groups to fully evaluate all implications and inviting feedback from all staff groups involved
- Visiting/liaising with other departments who already use the technique/technology
- Carrying out a full risk assessment of implementing the new technique/technology
- Developing clear guidelines as to when and how new techniques/technology may be used
- A review of the number of staff and training needs

Fig. 15.7 illustrates how the principles of ISO 9001[4] can be applied to the safe introduction of new techniques or technology. It is vital that attention is paid to the recurrent themes identified in error reporting as outlined in this chapter, such as provision of adequate training and assessment of competency.

CONCLUSION

The NHS has undergone many changes, with a current priority being to raise the quality of care with a focus on safety, treatment effectiveness and patient experience. High-quality care is a continuously moving target with the constant development of new techniques and technology together with challenges such as increased costs, staff shortages, lack of resources and increasing patient expectations. The concept and requirements of a QMS have also undergone a number of changes since it was first introduced to RT in the United Kingdom as QART[12] in the 1990s. It is now more customer focused, with an increased emphasis on leadership, improvement and risk management. Departments must build on the QMS framework and processes they have in place to manage both developments and challenges.

A culture of continuous improvement and a multidisciplinary approach will generate service-wide problem identification.[3] It may be argued that a QMS is costly to implement and maintain and that there is a risk of running a system without addressing vital quality issues. However, if a system has management commitment and is run

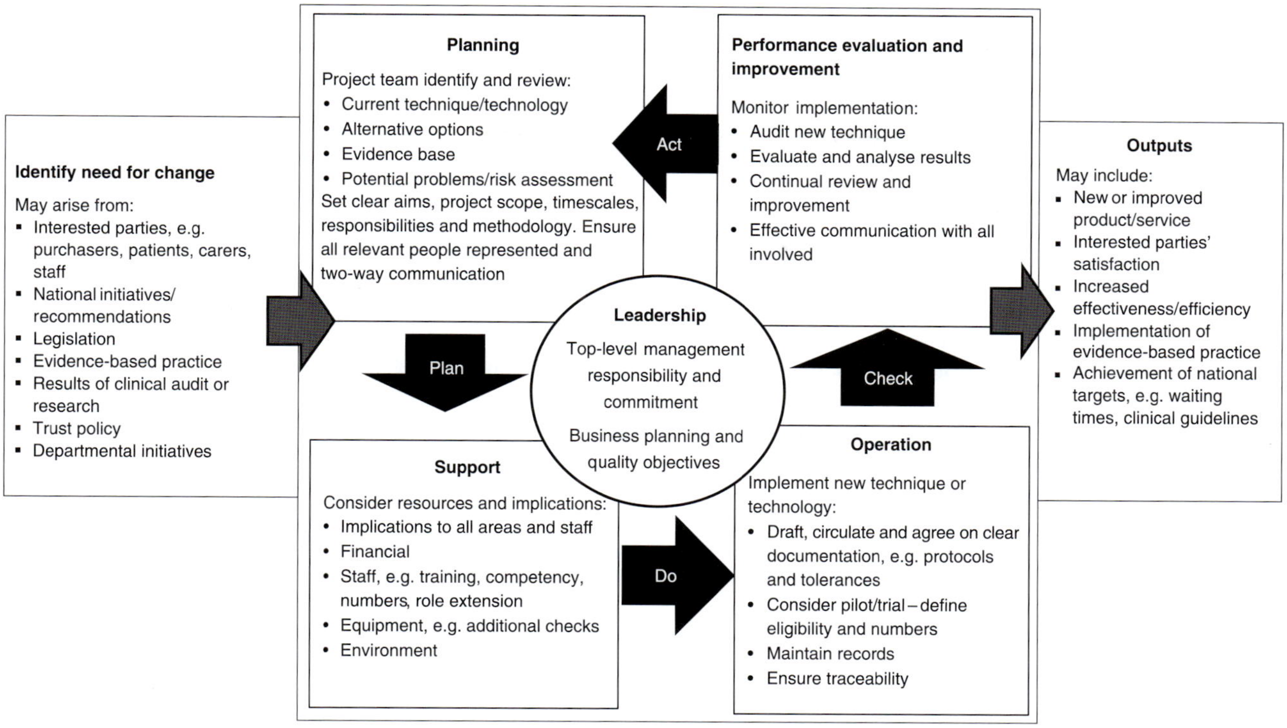

Fig. 15.7 Principles of ISO 9001:2015 applied to the introduction of new techniques or technology.

effectively, although it may not prevent disasters or eliminate human error, it will:

- Reduce a department's exposure to the common elements behind disasters.
- Ensure that a department has systems in place to prevent problems from escalating into disaster.
- Provide the tools to react quickly to put things right.
- Minimise the risk of major errors and reduce the frequency of minor errors to ensure safe and effective treatment.[3]

Historically, the ISO quality requirements have received criticism for being too generic, because it is up to the organisation to set some of its own standards. To provide a QMS effectively and gain the most benefit, oncology and RT departments should implement the ISO 9001:2015[4] requirements in such a way as to provide a framework which ensures an integrated approach to the numerous quality standards, legislation, targets, reports, recommendations and initiatives that they are required to fulfil. A QMS is not just about achieving certification. It is about ensuring that the best possible treatments and standards of care are provided within the resources available.

REFERENCES

1. Health Foundation. Quality improvement made simple. 2021. Accessed May 12, 2025. https://www.health.org.uk/publications/quality-improvement-made-simple
2. Pawlicki T, Mundt AJ, Dunscombe P, Scalliet P. *Quality and safety in radiotherapy*. Boca Raton, Florida, USA: CRC Press; 2010.
3. Kehoe T, Rugg L-J. From technical quality assurance of radiotherapy to a comprehensive quality of service management system. *Radiother Oncol.* 1999;51(3):281–290.
4. ISO (International Organization for Standardization). *Quality Management Systems – Requirements (ISO 9001:2015.* Geneva, Switzerland: ISO; 2015. https://www.iso.org/obp/ui/#iso:std:iso:9001:ed-5:v1:en.
5. BSI (British Standards Institution). *BS EN ISO. 9000:2015. Quality Management Systems – Fundamentals and Vocabulary.* London, UK: BSI; 2015.
6. Coucke P, Boga D, Lenaerts E, Delgaudine M. From reporting incidents in a radiation therapy department to enterprise risk management (ERM) based on the European Foundation for Quality Management philosophy (EFQM). *Int J Healthc Manag.* 2014;7(2):127–131.
7. IAEA (International Atomic Energy Agency). *Radiation Protection and Safety in Medical Uses of Ionizing Radiation.* Vienna, Austria: IAEA; 2006. Specific Safety Guide No. SSG-46. https://www-pub.iaea.org/MTCD/Publications/PDF/PUB1775_web.pdf.
8. Valentin J. Prevention of accidental exposures to patients undergoing radiation therapy. ICRP Publication 86. *Ann ICRP.* 2001;30(3):7–70.
9. IAEA (International Atomic Energy Agency). *Lessons Learned From Accidental Exposures in Radiotherapy.* Vienna: Austria: IAEA; 2000. IAEA Safety Report Series No. 17. http://www-pub.iaea.org/MTCD/Publications/PDF/Pub1084_web.pdf.
10. WHO (World Health Organization). *Radiotherapy Risk Profile. Technical Manual.* WHO Press; 2008. https://cdn.who.int/media/docs/default-source/patient-safety/radiotherapy/090715-who-radiotherapy_risk_profile.pdf?sfvrsn=ec752b08_3.
11. Royal College of Radiologists, Society and College of Radiographers, Institute of Physics and Engineering in Medicine, National Patient Safety Agency, British Institute of Radiology. *Towards Safer Radiotherapy.* London, UK: Royal College of Radiologists; 2023. Accessed May 12, 2025. https://www.rcr.ac.uk/our-services/all-our-publications/clinical-oncology-publications/towards-safer-radiotherapy/
12. ROSEIS (Radiation Oncology Safety Education Information System). Accessed May 12, 2025. https://www.estro.org/Advocacy/ROSEIS
13. Department of Health. *Quality Assurance in Radiotherapy: A Quality Management System for Radiotherapy.* London, UK: HMSO; 1994.
14. AAPM (American Association of Physicists in Medicine). *Unintended Exposure of a Patient During Radiotherapy Treatment at*

the Beatson Oncology Centre. Alexandria, VA: AAPM; 2023. Glasgow in January 2006. https://www.aapm.org/government_affairs/documents/glasgowEvent10-06.pdf.

15. Scottish Government. Unintended Overexposure of a Patient During Radiotherapy Treatment at the Edinburgh Cancer Centre, in September 2015. Publication – Progress Report. Scottish Government. July 8, 2016. http://www.gov.scot/Publications/2016/07/8854
16. BSI (British Standards Institution). *BS EN ISO 9004:2018. Quality Management – Quality of an Organisation – Guidance to Achieve Sustained Success*. London, UK: BSI; 2018.
17. ISO (International Organization for Standardization). *Quality Management Systems – Requirements*. Geneva, Switzerland: ISO; 2000 (ISO Standard No. 9001:2000). https://www.iso.org/standard/21823.html.
18. ISO (International Organization for Standardization). *Quality Management Systems – Requirements*. Geneva, Switzerland: ISO; 2008 (ISO Standard No. 9001:2008). https://www.iso.org/standard/46486.html.
19. Hoyle D. *ISO 9000 Quality systems handbook – updated for the ISO9001:2015 standard*. 7th ed. Abingdon, Oxfordshire, UK: Routledge; 2017.
20. IGA (Information Governance Alliance). Records Management Code of Practice for Health and Social Care 2016. Cheshire, UK: IGA. Published August 4, 2021, updated August 7, 2023. Accessed May 12, 2025. https://www.gov.uk/government/publications/records-management-code-of-practice-for-health-and-social-care
21. Malicki J, Bly R, Bulot M, et al. Patient safety in external beam radiotherapy – Guidelines on risk assessment and analysis of adverse error-events and near misses: introducing the ACCIRAD project. *Radiother Oncol*. 2014;112(2):194–198.
22. European Commission. *General Guidelines on Risk Management in External Beam Radiotherapy*. Luxembourg City, Luxembourg: European Commission; 2015. Radiation Protection No. 181. Accessed May 12, 2025. https://op.europa.eu/en/publication-detail/-/publication/01f57fc8-73f2-4bfc-93fa-9eec0b2c8d3c
23. European Commission. *Technical Supplement to Radiation Protection No. 181*. Luxembourg City, Luxembourg: European Commission; 2015. https://www.radioterapiaitalia.it/wp-content/uploads/2015/12/RP181web.pdf
24. Royal College of Radiologists. *Radiotherapy Target Volume Definition and Peer Review, Second Edition – RCR Guidance*. London, UK: Royal College of Radiologists; Accessed May 12, 2025. https://www.rcr.ac.uk/our-services/all-our-publications/clinical-oncology-publications/radiotherapy-target-volume-definition-and-peer-review-second-edition-rcr-guidance/
25. Elnahal S, Blackford A, Smith K, et al. Identifying predictive factors for incident reports in patients receiving radiation therapy. *Int J Radiation Oncol Biol Phys*. 2016;94(5):993–999.
26. Chang DW, Cheetham L, te Marvelde L, et al. Risk factors for radiotherapy incidents and impact of an online electronic reporting system. *Radiother Oncol*. 2014;112(2):199–204.
27. UK Statutory Instruments. The Ionising Radiation (Medical Exposure) Regulations 2017. 2017 No. 1322. http://www.legislation.gov.uk/uksi/2017/1322/contents/made
28. Meadows S, Baker K, Butler J. The incident decision tree. *Clin Risk*. 2005;11(2):66–68.
29. Holmberg O, McClean B. Preventing treatment errors in radiotherapy by identifying and evaluating near misses and actual incidents. *J Radiother Pract*. 2002;3(1):13–25.
30. Pawlicki T, Coffey M, Milosevic M. Incident learning systems for radiation oncology: development and value at the local, national and international level. *Clin Oncol*. 2017;29(9):562–567.
31. IAEA (International Atomic Energy Agency). Safety in Radiation Oncology (SAFRON). Accessed May 12, 2025. https://www.iaea.org/resources/rpop/resources/databases-and-learning-systems/safron
32. Gov.UK. Safer Radiotherapy: Error Data Analysis. Published July 30, 2014; updated January 31, 2025. Accessed May 12, 2025. https://www.gov.uk/government/publications/safer-radiotherapy-error-data-analysis-report; 2018
33. Findlay Ú, Best H, Ottrey M. Improving patient safety in radiotherapy through error reporting and analysis. *Radiography*. 2016;22:S3–S11.
34. UK Statutory Instruments. Health and Safety. *The Ionising Radiation Regulations 2017. 2017 No. 1075*. London, UK; 2017. http://www.legislation.gov.uk/uksi/2017/1075/pdfs/uksi_20171075_en.pdf.
35. CQC (Care Quality Commission). *Regulation 20: Duty of Candour*. London, UK: CQC; 2015. https://www.cqc.org.uk/sites/default/files/2022-12/20220722-duty-of-candour-pdf-version-FINAL-2.pdf.
36. Mid Staffordshire NHS Foundation Trust Public Inquiry. *Report of the Mid Staffordshire NHS Foundation Trust Public Inquiry: Executive Summary (HC 947)*. The Stationery Office; 2013. https://assets.publishing.service.gov.uk/government/uploads/system/uploads/attachment_data/file/279124/0947.pdf.
37. Berwick D. A promise to learn – a commitment to act: improving the safety of patients in England. *HSC 2901213*. Department of Health and Social Care; 2013.
38. Bleehen Report. *Quality Assurance in Radiotherapy: A Quality Management System for Radiotherapy*. London, UK: Department of Health; 1994 PL/CMO (94).7.
39. ISO (International Organisation for Standardisation), IAF/ISO Joint Communiqué on the addition of Climate Change considerations to Management Systems Standards, February 2024. https://committee.iso.org/files/live/sites/jtcg/files/news/Joint%20ISO-IAF%20Communique%20re%20Climate%20Change%20Amds%20to%20ISO%20MSS%20Feb%202024a.pdf

SECTION 2

16

Epidemiology of Cancer and Screening

Thankamma V. Ajithkumar

CHAPTER OUTLINE

THE CANCER PROBLEM

Globally in 2022, 20 million new cancer cases were diagnosed and 9.7 million deaths occurred. In many countries, more than 25% of deaths are attributable to cancer. Cancer is also a significant public health problem in developing countries, matching its effect in industrialised nations.

It is predicted that 35 million new cases of cancer will be diagnosed in 2050. This increase will mainly be as a result of steadily ageing populations in both developed and developing countries and also to current trends in smoking prevalence and the growing adoption of unhealthy lifestyles. However, there is clear evidence that healthy lifestyles and public health action by governments and health practitioners could stem this trend and prevent as many as one-third of cancers worldwide.

Lung cancer is the most common cancer (2.5 million new cases; 12.4% of the total new cases), followed by breast cancer (2.3 million cases; 11.6%), colorectal cancer (1.9 million cases; 9.6%) and prostate cancer (1.5 million cases; 7.3%). The number of cases of other cancers are as follows: stomach, 968,000; liver, 865,000; thyroid, 821,000; cervical, 661,000; bladder, 613,000; non-Hodgkin lymphoma, 553,000; oesophageal, 510,000; pancreas, 510,000; leukaemia, 487,000; uterine, 420,000; melanoma, 331,000; nervous system, 321,000; and Hodgkin lymphoma, 82,409. Mesothelioma (30,618) and vaginal cancers (18,800) are uncommon.

In developed countries, the probability of being diagnosed with cancer is more than twice as high as in developing countries. However, in rich countries, some 50% of cancer patients die of the disease, whereas in developing countries, 70% of people are diagnosed with late-stage incurable tumours, pointing to the need for much better detection programs. The main reasons for the more significant cancer burden of affluent societies are the earlier onset of the tobacco epidemic, earlier exposure to occupational carcinogens, and Western nutrition and lifestyle. With increasing wealth and industrialisation, however, many countries undergo rapid lifestyle changes that will significantly increase their future disease burden.

Cancer in the United States

Cancer, after heart disease, is the second leading cause of death. It is estimated that in 2022, 1.9 million Americans will receive a new diagnosis of invasive cancer and over 0.6 million Americans will die of this disease. The most common cancers among males are prostate, lung and colorectal and among females are breast, lung and colorectal. For both sexes, these cancers made up over 50% of newly diagnosed cases.

Mortality from the four most common cancer killers—lung, breast, prostate and colorectal—has been in decline since the late 1990s. Overall, cancer incidence in males decreased from the early 1990s until around 2013, then stabilised through 2018. However, cancer incidence rates in females were relatively stable through the mid-2010s but have ticked up slightly (0.2% per year) in recent data years. The steep decline in lung cancer rates in males and the relative stability of rates in females are steps in the right direction, and further progress will require the rigorous application of strategies known to be effective in reducing tobacco use. Death rates from breast cancer are falling despite a gradual, long-term increase in the rate of new diagnoses. This has been attributed to the successful implementation of more effective adjuvant treatment and the increased use of mammography screening. However, higher rates of late-stage disease exist in some population groups, such as females who lack health insurance and recent immigrants.

Prostate cancer death rates have been declining since 1994; the incidence rate has dropped rapidly between 2007 and 2014 due to decreased detection of tumours by screening. However, the incidence of local-stage disease has increased by 4% per annum since 2013, and the proportion of distant metastases was increased to 8.2% in 2018. Colorectal cancer death rates have been declining since the 1970s, with steeper declines beginning in the mid-1980s. This is probably a result of improving surgical techniques and, more recently, the introduction of adjuvant treatment regimens.

Cancer in Europe

In Europe, cancer accounts for 20% of disease-related mortality. There were 3.5 million new cancer cases and 1.6 million cancer deaths in Europe in 2022. The most common cancers are breast (523,000 cases; 13% of all cancer cases), colorectal (500,000 cases; 13%), lung (470,000 cases; 12%) and prostate (450,000 cases; 12%). Among males, the top five cancers were prostate, lung, colorectal, bladder and kidney. Among females, the most common cancers were breast, colorectal, lung, endometrium and melanoma. In terms of mortality, it is estimated there were 1.9 million cancer deaths, with the leading causes being lung (319,970 deaths), colorectal (203,482 deaths), breast (122,384 deaths) and pancreas (116,763 deaths). As the European population ages, these numbers will increase even if the age-specific rates remain constant. Lung, colorectal, stomach and breast cancers account for nearly half of all cancer deaths in Europe and point very clearly to the priorities for cancer control action.

EPIDEMIOLOGY OF CANCER

Terminology

Epidemiology is the study of disease occurrence, distribution and causes across populations. It can be divided into three main components: descriptive, analytical and experimental.

Descriptive epidemiology deals with the variation in frequency (incidence or mortality) of a disease over space and time and in relation to age, gender and socioeconomic status. Analytical epidemiology studies the relationship between potentially causal risk factors (e.g. cigarette smoking, asbestos, ionising radiation) or their proxies and disease development. Experimental epidemiology involves observing the effects of controlling relevant adverse risk factors (e.g. stopping cigarette smoking) or promoting possible preventive factors (e.g. beta-carotene).

The *incidence rate* of any disease is the total number of new cases occurring over a given period (1 year) among a given number of people (usually 100,000 for cancer). This differs from the *prevalence rate*, which is the number of cases of a particular disease alive at a given time. A statement should qualify this as to how far back in time cancer patients are considered to be at risk from their disease—this is often taken as referring to cancers diagnosed within the previous 5 years. The *mortality rate* is the number of deaths attributed to cancer in a given period (1 year) among a given number of people (usually 100,000 for cancer).

Crude incidence or *death rates* are defined as the total number of cancers or deaths divided by the total population. Crude rates are of limited value because they do not take into account the differing proportions of people in particular age groups between populations. The crude rate for a specific population may exceed that of another country simply because it contains a higher proportion of older adults. The age-standardised incidence or death rate accounts for the effect of age distribution on rates by attributing a weighting system to each age-specific rate. A choice of weighting systems exists—the two most common are the world-standardised population and the European-standardised population. When comparing cancer incidence rates in countries with very different proportions of older adults (e.g. those in the developing world versus those in the developed world), the world standard is recommended. This is known as the World Standardised Rate (WSR). For comparison of countries with more similar proportions of older adults, the European standard is preferable. This is known as the European Standardised Rate (ESR).

An alternative method of expressing relative incidence or mortality is the *standardised incidence ratio (SIR)* or the *standardised mortality ratio (SMR)*. This is an overall measure of incidence (mortality) which compares the observed number of cases (deaths) in a particular population with the expected number of cases (deaths) that would have been anticipated in a standard population (e.g. national) if the age-specific incidence (death) rates were the same. This is usually expressed as a ratio of 100 if the observed and expected rates are the same and greater than 100 if the rate in the population of interest is higher than that for the standard (national) rate. SIRs help to compare cancer incidence between socioeconomic or particular occupational groups.

SURVIVAL AND CURE OF CANCER

What do we mean by 'cure' for a cancer patient? Technically, it is when the survival for that patient is the same as that for the general population from which they originate—their 'excess' risk of death becomes zero. Thus it makes sense to talk of a 'cure', for example, of a small basal cell carcinoma treated by surgery or radiotherapy where recurrence or persistent disease is uncommon. However, for other cancers, particularly breast cancer, the possibility of local or distant recurrence remains for many years after the tumour has been successfully removed surgically. This likelihood increases substantially for larger tumours with nodal involvement and adverse histological features. Thus survival rates are quoted as a measure of success but should be qualified by the length of follow-up, usually 5 years.

Five-year survival is often interpreted as a cure. Although this is true of many tumours, it is not true of breast cancer, as suggested previously. For breast cancer, 10-, 20- or even 30-year survival figures are more appropriate endpoints because of the long-term pattern of relapse and death from the disease. Survival may be with or without evidence of cancer. For this reason the terms *disease-free* and *recurrence-free survival* are commonly used to define the treatment outcome. These results require an elaborate system of clinical follow-up. Yet, it is only from detailed analysis of this kind that we can derive a sound knowledge of both the natural history of cancer and treatment effects. Survival data are commonly presented and plotted graphically as curves that allow the comparison of different treatments for different stages of disease over time.

In studies of patients treated for cancer, a variety of ways are used to describe their survival. *Crude survival rate* refers to the percentage of patients alive a given number (n) of years after treatment. This is invalid unless all the patients have been followed up for at least n years. More often, a sizeable proportion of patients have been followed up for a shorter time than n years, and the life table or Kaplan–Meier method is more appropriate. This method uses information from all the patients for the time intervals they have been followed. Thus someone in the study for 1 year will contribute to the first-year survival estimate, those in for 2 years will contribute to the first- and second-year survival estimates and so on. There is an underlying assumption that all patients are subject to the same time-specific probability of dying from a particular cancer whether or not they have been followed for all or part of the study's follow-up period. This method can be used for calculating survival rates for all causes of death (*overall survival rate*) or death from cancer (*cancer-specific survival rate*). Patients who die from causes other than the cancer of interest (i.e. from intercurrent disease) are considered to have been withdrawn from the study at the point in time that their death occurred.

An alternative method for dealing with the problem of intercurrent deaths or mortality from natural causes of the patients studied is to examine *relative* or *net survival*. This is the ratio of the overall survival for a population with cancer to that of a comparable population (generally matched for age, gender and socioeconomic status) of people without cancer. Net survival is the method used to calculate the most commonly reported publicly available cancer survival statistics.

Outcome of Palliative Care

Survival figures are essential for estimating the success of treatment aimed at cure but are of limited value in assessing the effects of palliative treatment. The main aim of palliative treatment is the relief of distressing symptoms. Palliative radiotherapy or chemotherapy may sometimes restrain tumour growth sufficiently to prolong the patient's life for a few months or sometimes years. In this case a better measure of survival would be the median survival time. This is calculated by ranking the survival times in ascending order and choosing the middle value.

EPIDEMIOLOGY AND THE PREVENTION OF CANCER

The principal role of epidemiological studies in cancer has been identifying risk factors, assessing their likelihood of being causative agents and, ultimately, whether their avoidance offers a practical solution for reducing the cancer burden. Most of the research has been directed at identifying factors associated with an increased cancer risk. Still, it is equally legitimate to try to identify factors associated with a decrease in risk. One often misunderstood concept, particularly by the general media, is that epidemiological studies' findings indicate causal effects. Epidemiological studies will only ever identify associations.

Criteria for Causality

After individual epidemiological studies of cancer have been summarised and the quality assessed, a judgment is made concerning the strength of evidence that the agent or exposure in question is carcinogenic for humans. Several criteria are considered: a strong association (a large relative risk) is more likely to indicate causality than a weak one. Associations that are replicated in several studies of the same design or using different epidemiological approaches or under other circumstances of exposure are more likely to represent a causal relationship than isolated observations from single studies if the risk of the disease increases with the amount of exposure; this is considered to be a strong indication of causality demonstration of a decline in risk after cessation of, or reduction in, exposure in individuals or whole populations also supports a causal interpretation. However, a carcinogen may act upon more than one target organ, and the specificity of an association (an increased occurrence of cancer at one anatomical site or of one morphological type) adds plausibility to a causal relationship where an increase in exposure in a population and an increase in the incidence of cancer is apparent. There must be a sensible latency (20+ years for solid tumours, 3+ years for blood-borne cancers) between the timings of the two increases. There is evidence from animal models of a link between the exposure and the occurrence of the cancer. There is a biological mechanism in humans for a link between exposure and cancer bias, and confounding can be ruled out as a possible explanation for the association.

These criteria don't need to hold for a judgment that causality exists. One area of controversy that concerns public health is the impact of chronic low levels of exposure to known carcinogens. Two examples would be the impact of ionising radiation on the general population and leukaemia risk and the effect of inhaling secondhand tobacco smoke among nonsmokers and lung cancer risk. In both cases the first criterion listed above would not be expected to hold; the relative risks are likely to be low because the level of exposure is (relatively) low. In these circumstances a more appropriate interpretation would be that the level of risk should be compatible with an acceptable extrapolation from the dose-response relationship observed for higher levels of exposure.

Such studies have played a significant role in establishing occupational hazards in several industries (e.g. bladder cancer in aniline dye workers) and the link between lung cancer and smoking.

Epidemiology can assist in the prevention of cancer in several ways. First, it can show differences in cancer incidence in different populations and correlate them with differences in the prevalence of a potential causal factor. Second, it can test a hypothesis about the relationship between the occurrence of the disease and an aspect of the affected individual's constitution or exposure to some environmental factor. Third, it can test the validity of a causal relationship by seeing whether the disease can be prevented or its incidence reduced by changing the prevalence of the suspected agent. An excellent example of the latter is the reduction in lung cancer observed among doctors since they gave up smoking cigarettes.

AETIOLOGY AND SCREENING

Lung Cancer

Tobacco

Lung cancer is currently still the highest single cause of death from any cancer in the world, as well as being the most common incident cancer (excluding nonmelanoma skin cancer). It was, however, a rare disease at the start of the 20th century. Still, exposures to new aetiological agents, particularly tobacco, and an increasing lifespan led to enormous increases in the number of cases. Although smoking had been used throughout the world for many centuries, the 20th-century pandemic was a result of the introduction of manufactured cigarettes on a mass scale. Its addictive properties led to sustained exposure to inhaled carcinogens. Scientists in Nazi Germany conducted some of the earliest research on the links between smoking and lung cancer, but their results were generally dismissed as propaganda. In the early 1950s, case-control studies in Britain and the United States suggested a strong association. Three major cohort studies were initiated at that time—UK doctors, US veterans and the American Cancer Society volunteers—and their findings corroborated the earlier observations as well as identifying other cancers and causes of death as also being strongly linked to cigarette smoking. An increase in the risk of lung cancer (relative to a nonsmoker) is consistently evident at the lowest level of daily consumption. It is at least linearly related to increasing consumption.

The risk of lung cancer in males who smoke 15 to 24 cigarettes per day is 26 times higher than in nonsmokers. The relative risk of lung cancer for all levels of smoking ranges from 7.5 for light smokers (<15/day) to 26 for heavy smokers (≥25/day) as compared with lifelong nonsmokers. These levels of risk are higher than previously observed, highlighting the fact that earlier analyses have underestimated the full effect of persistent cigarette smoking.

Smoking cessation is by far the most effective means of reducing the risk of lung cancer among active smokers. Lung cancer risk shows a steady upwards trend from never-smokers through later ages at cessation to continuing smokers. Thus there is substantial protection even for those who stop at 55 to 64 years of age and progressively greater protection for those who stop earlier (up to 90% reduction in those stopping between 25 and 34 years of age).

On a global scale, the rise in cigarette consumption in developing countries, and currently, 80% of the world's tobacco users, live in low- and middle-income countries. Going on the current worldwide smoking patterns, whereby about 30% of young adults become smokers, there will be about 7 million lung cancer deaths worldwide unless there is widespread cessation. Convincing the next generation not to start smoking remains a significant public health imperative. The recent popoularity of electronic cigarettes or 'vaping' has been heralded by some as a welcome alternative to smoking. Despite the rapid uptake of vaping, there remain some uncetainities and concerns, as these devices still introduce harmful chemicals into the lungs. Research into the effects of e-cigarettes is still in early stages, and the long-term impact on lung cancer is still very much unknown.

Passive Smoking

The question as to whether involuntary smoking poses a significant risk of lung cancer has received considerable scientific interest since 1980. Involuntary (or passive) smoking is exposure to secondhand tobacco smoke, which is a mixture of exhaled mainstream smoke and sidestream smoke released from the smouldering cigarette and diluted with ambient air. Involuntary smoking involves exposure to the same numerous carcinogens and toxic substances that are present in tobacco smoke produced by active smoking, which is the principal cause of lung cancer. This implies that there will be some risk of lung cancer from exposure to secondhand tobacco smoke.

More than 50 studies, based on over 7300 nonsmoking lung cancer cases, have examined the association between involuntary smoking and the risk of lung cancer in never-smokers, especially spouses of smokers. Most showed an increased risk, especially for persons with higher exposures. In a metaanalysis of 55 studies, the pooled relative risk (RR) for lung cancer for never-smoking females exposed to secondhand tobacco smoke from spouses was 1.27 (95% CI = 1.17–1.37). In another metaanalysis of 22 studies that assessed the effect of secondhand tobacco smoke exposures at work, the relative risk for lung cancer among exposed nonsmokers was 1.24 (95% CI = 1.18–1.29), and among those workers classified as highly exposed to secondhand tobacco smoke at work, it was 2.01 (95% CI = 1.33–2.60) compared to those with no exposure at work. Interestingly, an association has also been shown between exposure to environmental tobacco smoke in infancy and the risk of lung cancer in adulthood among 60,182 lifelong nonsmokers who participated in the EPIC (European Prospective Investigation Into Cancer and Nutrition) study.

Asbestos

It has been known for many years that asbestos exposure is a major cause of lung cancer. In 1999, a metaanalysis of 69 cohort studies found an SMR of 163 for lung cancer, but a substantial heterogeneity existed, largely attributable to the different cumulative exposures to asbestos in various cohorts. These cohorts comprised workers from multiple industries—mining, textile and manufacturing, insulation, asbestos-cement factories and shipyards—and risk was closely related to the level of exposure in the different industries. The type of asbestos was also observed to be relevant, with chrysotile fibres being considered less carcinogenic than amphiboles.

Asbestos dust and cigarette smoke are both causes of lung cancer. What is less clear is the effect of the combination of the two carcinogenic agents. Initially, two hypotheses existed about the way asbestos and cigarette smoking interact. In one, it is assumed that asbestos produces the same additional risk in males who smoke cigarettes as in those who do not (additive hypothesis); in the other, it is assumed that asbestos produces an effect that is proportional to the impact of the other agent (multiplicative hypothesis). Which hypothesis is best explained by the available data remains debated.

One often quoted study by Hammond et al. estimates relative risks of 1, 5, 11 and 53 for no asbestos exposure and never smoked, asbestos-exposed and never smoked, and any asbestos exposure and never smoked and exposed to both, respectively. These results favoured the multiplicative model but have not proven generalisable to other studies. Indeed, a recent analysis of the Quebec chrysotile miners and millers cohort concluded that an additive model provided the best fit to their data but cautioned that there seems no good reason to believe that interactions should conform to any simple theory.

The situation concerning mesothelioma is far simpler in that asbestos exposure is a causal factor, but cigarette smoking is not. The disease is rapidly fatal, with most of those affected dying within 18 months of diagnosis. There is a long latent period between first asbestos exposure and diagnosis of mesothelioma that is seldom less than 15 years and often exceeds 60 years. In all, 85% of deaths are among males, and the risk is highest in occupations with substantial asbestos exposure. Shipyard workers have been a particularly susceptible group in that considerable exposures were to be found during the 1940s and 1950s and into the 1960s when ships were being repaired, and the merchant fleet was being rebuilt after World War II.

Although mesothelioma is almost exclusively a result of inhalation of asbestos fibres, this is not exclusively an occupational disease: in some areas of Turkey, environmental exposure to erionite is associated with high incidence of mesothelioma; domestic exposure and increased risk has been observed among the wives of South African Cape miners who brought home contaminated workclothes for cleaning; finally, fibre concentrations in the lungs of (nonmining) residents near the chrysotile mines in Quebec are up to 10 times higher than in the average Canadian. The latter raises the critical question of whether this level of exposure represents an increased risk of the disease. The answer to this question is almost certainly yes, as there appears to be no evidence that a threshold level exists below which there is no excess risk. There might exist a background level of mesothelioma occurring in the absence of asbestos exposure. Still, there is no proof of this, and this 'natural level' is probably lower than one case per million per year.

Radon

Underground miners exposed to radioactive radon and its decay products are at an increased risk of lung cancer. Indoor radon exposure has been associated with a marginal increase in the risk of lung cancer.

Chemoprevention

Chemoprevention is defined as the reduction of the risk of cancer development through the use of pharmaceuticals or micronutrients. There has been consistent evidence that high intake of fruit and vegetables is associated with some reduction in risk of lung cancer. Thus it has been suggested that micronutrients and macronutrients present in our diet may act as cancer-inhibiting substances. Epidemiological studies have verified that beta-carotene is inversely related to lung cancer risk, and several randomised controlled intervention trials have been undertaken. None of these trials showed a reduction in lung cancer incidence or mortality, even in high-risk populations. On the contrary, a recent metaanalysis of eight studies (167,141 participants) suggests that beta-carotene supplements lead to an increased risk of lung cancer (RR = 1.16, 95% CI = 1.06–1.26), an effect more noticeable among smokers and asbestos workers (RR = 1.21, 95% CI = 1.08–1.35). Our understanding of the mechanism by which relatively short-term intake of retinoids and carotenoids affects the development of cancer in large populations is insufficient to use this approach as a specific lung cancer control procedure.

Screening

Given the high incidence of advanced disease at presentation and mortality of lung cancer, screening has been investigated as a means to improve mortality. Screening using chest x-rays and sputum cytology has not been shown to reduce lung cancer mortality. Low-dose computed tomography (CT) screening in high-risk populations has been shown to reduce lung cancer mortality, although at the cost of significant false-positive diagnoses and likely overdiagnosis. Ongoing studies are assessing the harms, benefits and cost-effectiveness of this intervention in populations at varying levels of risk. In the United Kingdom, a national targeted lung cancer screening program uses CT scans to detect cancer in people 55 to 74 years of age who have a smoking history.

Colorectal Cancer

Incidence rates for cancer of the colon vary significantly across the world. The highest estimated incidence rates are in Australia and New Zealand and the lowest in Western Africa. Studies of migrants suggest that environmental factors rather than ethnic or genetic factors play a significant role in its aetiology. Most studies have involved migrants moving from low-risk to high-risk areas such as from China and Japan to Hawaii or the rest of the United States, or southern Europeans moving to North America or Australia. In general, the risk in migrants approximates that of the new country, with rates increasing with increasing duration of stay, presumably as their lifestyles merge with that of the host country.

Over time, the incidence of colon cancer has been rising, slowly in high-risk areas but more rapidly in areas where the risk was formerly low. These changes have been accompanied by changing ratios between the subsites within the bowel at which tumours occur, with left-sided tumours (of the descending and sigmoid colon and rectum) becoming more frequent.

The risk of colorectal cancer is closely related to diet and other lifestyle factors. International comparisons have suggested increased risks with increased intakes of dietary fat and a decreased intake of cereal grains and dietary fibre. Analytical studies within populations have shown that a deficiency of vegetables and fruits and a sedentary lifestyle are associated with increased risk. However, attempts to identify independent roles for specific macronutrients have proved unsuccessful, except for the overconsumption of energy. Thus dietary associations with colon cancer are characterised as typical of the Western diet without being able to tie in any specific components. There is rapidly growing evidence, however, to link the risk of colorectal cancer to the microbiome of the intestinal tract. The microorganisms living in the gut shape their environment and the body's inflammatory response, influencing tumour growth and spread. As dietary and lifestyle factors can strongly influence the gut microbiota, understanding these relationships may prove hugely informative in understanding the aetiology of this disease.

Although the vast majority of colorectal cancer cases occur sporadically in the general population, several specific disease groups—Crohn's disease, ulcerative colitis and familial polyposis—are subject to increased risks. For example, whereas colorectal cancer in ulcerative colitis only accounts for 1% of all colorectal cancer cases, it accounts for one-sixth of all deaths in ulcerative colitis patients. The overall prevalence of colorectal cancer in any ulcerative colitis patient is estimated to be 3.7%. However, there is general agreement that the colorectal cancer risk is highest in those with extensive disease of long duration. Overall, incidence rates build to cumulative probabilities of 2% by 10 years, 8% by 20 years and 18% by 30 years.

Screening

Colorectal cancer is one of the few internal cancers amenable to *secondary prevention*, or prevention by detecting preclinical lesions. The precursor of advanced colorectal cancer is either an adenomatous polyp or a flat neoplastic area. To prevent premature death, people 50 to 74 years of age are the main focus of attention.

Screening programs for the disease can be undertaken in several ways. These can include a one-off flexible sigmoidoscopy at around age 55. Although such screening can and does identify cancers, its principal aim is to remove precancerous lesions and reduce the incidence and mortality of the disease. A large randomised trial has shown this strategy to be effective. Other screening approaches based on direct exposure to diagnostic tests include colonoscopy, CT colonography or flexible sigmoidoscopy at 5- or 10-year intervals. Such tests are, however, expensive and so potentially more cost-effective programs using faecal occult blood tests (FOBTs) or the more sensitive faecal immunochemical tests (FITs) to limit these diagnostic tests to those people at higher risk of having some underlying relevant bowel pathology are commonly deployed. These initial screening tests detect blood in stool samples, as bleeding within the gastrointestinal tract can indicate the presence of a tumour. If blood is found, the individuals would be encouraged to undergo a diagnostic test, most commonly a colonoscopy, to determine if a tumour or other relevant pathology was present. Again, randomised trials have shown such screening to reduce colorectal cancer mortality, and evaluations of national screening programs in the United Kingdom and elsewhere suggest it positively impacts cancer outcomes. In the United Kingdom, the bowel cancer screening program targets people 50 to 74 years of age and uses FIT.

Breast

Breast cancer is the most common cancer in females worldwide. Although the majority of cancers exhibit a consistently increasing rise in incidence rates with age, breast cancer is an exception. It demonstrates how the frequency of a disease can be a function of the duration of exposure rather than age per se. Among premenopausal females, the incidence risk doubles with each decade of age. After menopause (generally amongst females in their 50s), the incidence rate remains relatively steady (sometimes called Clemmensen's hook). After that, it rises again but at a shallower gradient than is observed for premenopausal females. Examining the shape of age-specific incidence curves can indicate causal factors, particularly those that change over a person's lifetime, such as hormonal factors. Thus, for breast cancer, it would seem to suggest that the factors related to premenopausal breast cancer may well be different from those which cause postmenopausal breast cancer. Add to this the observation that the incidence of premenopausal breast cancer has remained stable over time. In contrast, postmenopausal breast cancer rates have been slowly but steadily increasing over time, and it may well be that premenopausal and postmenopausal breast cancer should be considered as two separate diseases in aetiological terms.

Reproductive factors have been consistently related to (postmenopausal) breast cancer, in that early age at first full-term pregnancy and high parity are associated with lower levels of the disease. Furthermore, risk is increased in females who have early menarche or who have late menopause. Obesity, related to various alterations in plasma levels of total and bioavailable sex steroids, is also a strong risk factor. Because circulating levels of sex steroids are regulated by a range of factors, including insulin and insulin-like growth factors, this may provide the link between many observations regarding excessive energy intake and increased risk of cancer.

The oestrogen excess hypothesis stipulates that risk depends directly on breast tissue exposure to oestrogens. Oestrogens increase breast cell proliferation and inhibit apoptosis in vitro, and in experimental animals, they cause increased rates of tumour development when administered. This theory is consistent with the epidemiological evidence showing an increase in breast cancer risk in postmenopausal females who have low circulating sex hormone–binding globulin and elevated total and bioavailable oestradiol.

Oral contraceptives, in the form of oestrogen-progestogen combinations, were introduced in the early 1960s and rapidly found widespread use in most developed countries. Preparations of oral contraceptives have undergone substantial changes over time, reducing the potency of the oestrogens, adding in different progestogens and using biphasic and triphasic pills. A slight increase in risk has been observed in current and recent users of combined oral contraceptives (a relative risk of about 1.2). Still, this association is unrelated to the duration of use or type and dose of preparation, and 10 years after cessation of use, the excess risk disappears. Causation has not been established, and one suggestion has been that it could be the result of detection bias as a result of the increased attention to the occurrence of breast abnormalities in females regularly visiting their doctor for contraceptive prescriptions.

Hormone replacement therapy (HRT) is used to treat the symptoms of menopause, and during the 1990s, up to one-third of all menopausal females in the United States and many European countries used HRT for some period. A small increase in breast cancer risk is correlated with a longer duration of oestrogen replacement therapy use in current and recent users. The increase seems to cease several years after use has stopped. Initially, there appeared to be no difference in breast cancer risk between long-term users of all HRT and users of oestrogens alone. However, two recent studies have suggested that HRT may pose a greater risk than oestrogens alone.

A second oestrogen-progestogen hypothesis postulates that compared with exposure to oestrogens alone (as in postmenopausal females not using any exogenous hormones), the risk of breast cancer is increased further in females who have elevated plasma and tissue levels of oestrogens in combination with progestogens. This theory is supported by observations that postmenopausal females using oestrogen-plus-progestogen preparations for HRT have a more significant increase in risk than females using oestrogens alone.

Screening

No practical strategies exist which can be recommended for the prevention of breast cancer, and so considerable effort has been aimed at developing methods of early detection. Mammography can detect *preclinical cancer*, before it is palpable or before it causes symptoms. Tumours detected and treated at an early stage would be expected to be associated with a better survival rate than those detected symptomatically. However, as some breast cancers are characterised by early systemic dissemination, the actual effectiveness of screening is not at all apparent. In this context, several large randomised trials were undertaken to evaluate its effectiveness on a population basis. The analysis of these trials has shown that in females 50 to 69 years of age, mammography screening can reduce mortality from breast cancer by 25% to 30%. For females in the age group 40 to 49 years, screening efficacy is significantly less. The UK Age trial showed that yearly mammographic screening, starting at 40 years of age, reduces breast cancer mortality at 10 years of follow-up (relative rate 0.75 (95% CI = 0.58–0.97); $p = 0.029$). However, there was no significant reduction in death after 10 years of follow-up.

The only accurate measure of the success of a screening program is an associated reduction in mortality. Survival rates can theoretically improve without extending the length of life by the simple expedient of bringing forward the date of diagnosis, whereas the date of death remains the same. This is known as *lead-time bias*. Analysis of trial data suggests that screening brings forward the date of diagnosis by an average of about 3 years, but this will vary considerably on an individual basis depending on how long the tumour remains in the screen-detectable phase. This raises a second phenomenon known as *length-time bias*. The argument is based on the well-founded assumption that tumours grow at varying speeds in different females. Therefore slow-growing tumours will remain in the screen-detectable window longer than fast-growing tumours. Hence a screening program tends to pick up slow-growing tumours disproportionately more than fast-growing ones. If slow-growing tumours are also more amenable to cure, survival rates will tend to be artificially inflated as they will include a larger proportion of better-prognosis tumours.

The majority of developed countries have now established national or subnational screening programs. Eligible age ranges vary; the repeat interval varies; some use single-view mammography, others use two-view; and independent double reading of mammograms is recommended but not always adhered to. One of the side effects of the introduction of national breast screening programs has been the necessity to overhaul the referral and management pathway for breast cancer generally. Now, designated surgical units provide specialist expertise to manage breast cancer, particularly in those females with impalpable tumours; pathologists and oncologists with a special interest in breast cancer and clinical nurse specialists combine to form a multidisciplinary team for the management of the disease.

The effectiveness of routine national breast screening programs has been questioned. There is general agreement that the extent of the reduction in mortality has been lower than that experienced in the trial situation. Under optimal conditions with a high compliance rate, a mortality reduction of 20% appears achievable. In reality, this may be more in the region of 10% to 15% on current data. One of the major problems in assessing the reduction in mortality due to screening now is that other factors have come into play which were not operating when the trials were being conducted. Before the late 1980s, no decline in mortality had been seen, but then a smooth downturn occurred in Europe, North America and Australia. These changes accelerated in the early 1990s, but the fall occurred too soon after the widespread availability of mammography to be a consequence of it. More likely, the success of adjuvant therapy based on tamoxifen and chemotherapy was the major cause of this trend. Thus the concurrent changes in improved adjuvant therapy, better and more focused surgical services, protocol-driven management and a better awareness of breast cancer and its symptoms among the general population make it almost impossible to isolate the contribution that breast screening is now making. However, there is no denying the fact that more females are being diagnosed with smaller tumours and consequently can safely be offered conservation surgery rather than radical mastectomy.

Stomach

On a global scale, mortality from stomach cancer is second only to lung cancer. The areas with the highest incidence rates are Eastern Asia, the Andean regions of South America and Eastern Europe. There is marked geographical variation in incidence between countries and among different ethnic groups within the same locale. Migration studies show that the risk of cancer changes within two generations when people move from high-incidence to low-incidence areas. For example, Japanese immigrants to the United States retain their original risk, whereas subsequent generations share the incidence of the host country. No matter what level of incidence, there has been a general decline worldwide. In most European countries, it has fallen by more than 60% during the past 50 years.

Dietary risk factors include inadequate intake of fresh fruits and vegetables, high salt intake and consumption of smoked or cured meats or fish. There is good evidence that food refrigeration also protects against this cancer by facilitating year-round consumption of fruit and vegetables and probably by reducing the need for salt as a preservative. Vitamin C, contained in vegetables, fruits, and other foods of plant origin, is probably protective, as are diets high in whole-grain cereals, carotenoids and allium compounds.

Conditions that cause an excessive rate of cell proliferation in the gastric epithelium, thus increasing the chance of fixation of replication errors induced by dietary and endogenous carcinogens, include *Helicobacter pylori* infection, gastric ulcer, atrophic gastritis and autoimmune gastritis associated with pernicious anaemia. Gastritis is associated with increased production of oxidants and reactive nitrogen intermediates, including nitric oxide. There is increased expression of the inducible isoform of nitric oxide synthase in gastritis. Gastritis and atrophy alter gastric acid secretion, elevate gastric pH, change gastric flora and allow anaerobic bacteria to colonise in the stomach.

Screening

About 80% of Western patients with stomach cancer present with advanced tumours. Screening for early disease by x-ray (photofluoroscopy), followed by gastroscopy and biopsy of suspicious findings, has been widely used in Japan since the 1960s. It is a costly approach to prevention, and the results have been controversial. With the background incidence now falling substantially, screening has not been considered a national priority in most other countries.

Prostate

Prostate cancer is the third most common cancer in males worldwide. In the majority of developed and developing countries, prostate cancer is the most commonly diagnosed neoplasm affecting males beyond middle age. In recent times, incidence rates of prostate cancer have been influenced by the diagnosis of latent cancers whose presence has been suggested by screening of asymptomatic individuals. In the United States, for example, the introduction of screening using prostate-specific antigen (PSA) testing has led to an enormous increase in the diagnosis of prostate cancer, making it by far the most commonly diagnosed cancer in males.

The distribution of mortality rates is less affected than incidence by the effects of early diagnosis of asymptomatic cancers. It is thus a more reliable way of comparing rates of the disease. High rates are found in North America, Northern and Western Europe, Australia, New Zealand and the Caribbean. The difference between China and the United States is 26-fold, and within the United States, Black populations have higher rates than White populations, who in turn have rates considerably higher than populations of Asian origin.

The causes of prostate cancer are not well understood. The development of this malignancy is a multistep process associated with a long natural history. The initiation of preneoplastic lesions and microscopic cancer is probably influenced by environmental factors, which implies a case for lifestyle causes and primary prevention. The strong association of race, familial and geographic patterns and the weak link of many of the risk factors proposed suggests a significant role for genetic-environmental interactions in determining disease patterns. The role of hormones, particularly androgens, is essential given the impact of orchidectomy on progression. Genetic polymorphisms in the androgen receptor may be more critical than any imbalance of hormones in the circulation. A diet characteristic of Asian countries, essentially a low-fat intake with consequent low body weight and an intake of relatively high levels of phytoestrogens, may provide the means of restraining the growth and progression of prostate cancer.

Screening

Secondary prevention of prostate cancer is feasible but subject to controversy because the capacity to detect early disease must inevitably result in the overtreatment of some individuals, with substantial costs both to individuals and to society, in exchange for decreased prostate cancer mortality. PSA testing is widely used for the early detection of prostate cancer. Elevated levels of PSA are closely, but not definitely, associated with the presence of a tumour. Using a cutoff level of 4 ng/mL for normality, 25% of patients diagnosed with prostate cancer will have levels below this value. Of males with moderately raised levels (4–10 ng/mL), 25% will have cancer, but this rises to 60% when PSA levels are greater than 10 ng/mL. It should be combined with a digital rectal examination to improve the sensitivity of the PSA analysis. This will provide an assessment of the volume of the gland because PSA is also released into the bloodstream of patients with benign prostatic hyperplasia and other prostatic diseases. Additionally, different age-specific reference values for the cutoff threshold are of value: 2.5 ng/mL for age group 40 to 49 years and 3.5 ng/mL for age group 50 to 59 years. Any patient who asks for a PSA test should be counselled about the risks and benefits of the procedure and its outcome.

Some national authorities have recommended screening for the detection of prostate cancer starting at the age of 50 for males with at least a 10-year life expectancy. However, randomised studies have produced conflicting results regarding the benefits and harms of screening. Prostate cancer diagnosis has been shown to increase with screening. However, prostate cancer–specific mortality was only reduced in some studies, and overall mortality was unchanged. The general expectation that the earlier detection of prostate cancer inevitably provides a unique chance for a cure has to be balanced against the apparent prevalence of overdiagnosing and treating a disease which may never become symptomatic during a person's lifetime.

Cervix

Cancer of the cervix is the fourth most common cancer among females worldwide, with about 660,000 new cases diagnosed each year. Some 80% of cases of cervical cancer occur in developing countries where, in many regions, it is the most common cancer among females. The highest incidence rates are in South America, the Caribbean, sub-Saharan Africa, and South and Southeastern Asia.

Incidence and mortality have declined markedly in the past 40 years in Western Europe, the United States, Canada, Australia and New Zealand. These are mainly about extensive screening programs based on exfoliative cervical cytology, typically using the Papanicolaou (Pap) smear. Nevertheless, in several countries, notably the United Kingdom, Australia, New Zealand and Central Europe, there have been increases in risk in younger females, probably due to changes in exposure to risk factors. These changes are most evident for adenocarcinomas, which share, to some extent, the same aetiological agents of squamous cell carcinomas but for which cytological screening is ineffective in countering the increase in risk.

Molecular studies have shown that certain human papillomavirus (HPV) types are the central cause of cervical cancer and cervical intraepithelial neoplasia (CIN), the preinvasive state. It is now clear that the well-established risk factors associated with sexual behaviour, such as multiple sexual partners and early age of starting sexual activity, reflect the probability of being infected with HPV. HPV DNA has been detected in virtually all cervical cancer specimens. The association of HPV with cervical cancer is equally strong for the two main histological types: squamous cell carcinoma and adenocarcinoma. Over 100 HPV types have been identified, and about 40 can infect the genital tract. Twelve of these have been classified as high risk, and two of these (HPV 16 and 18) are responsible for most HPV-related cancers. However, because only a small fraction of HPV-infected females will eventually develop cervical cancer, there must be other exogenous or endogenous factors which, acting in conjunction with HPV, influence the progression from cervical infection to cervical cancer. In assessing the role of these cofactors, it should be recognised that HPV is very much the dominant effect. Cofactors which have been identified as being associated with an increased risk include high parity, smoking and long-term use of oral contraceptives.

Screening

Population-based cervical cancer screening programs using the Pap smear were first implemented in 1949 in British Columbia. Pap smear screening programs have since been introduced in many developed countries. The evidence supporting this is predominantly nonrandomised, being based on the trends in the incidence of or mortality because of cervical cancer in relation to screening intensity and the risk of cervical cancer in individuals with regards to their screening history. For example, national programs were established in Finland, Iceland and Sweden; in Denmark, programs covered about 40% of the female population, and in Norway, only 5%. In Iceland, cervical cancer mortality fell by 80% between 1965 and 1982, compared with 50% in Finland, 34% in Sweden, 25% in Denmark and 10% in Norway. Similarly, cancer registry–based studies have shown a reduction in the age SIRs compared with before screening, with reductions of at least 25% in 11 of the 17 populations studied and the largest effect occurring in those 45 to 55 years of age.

Cytological screening has been carried out using liquid-based cytology supplemented by HPV testing. In randomised studies, HPV-based screening provides 60% to 70% greater protection against invasive cervical cancer than cytology alone. In the United Kingdom, cervical cancer cytological screening targets females 25 to 64 years of age.

HPV vaccination is a cost-effective intervention to reduce the incidence of cervical cancer. The HPV vaccination was introduced in England in 2008, and the results after a total of 13.7 million years of follow-up showed a 34% relative reduction in the incidence of cervical cancer for females 16 to 18 years of age, 62% for females 14 to 16 years or age and 87% for females 12 to 13 years of age. In the United Kingdom, the HPV vaccine is recommended for children 12 to 13 years of age and people at high risk of HPV. Even though HPV vaccination is effective, more than 25% of countries do not have a national HPV vaccination program. More alarmingly, low- and middle-income countries, where 90% of new cases of cervical cancer are diagnosed, have limited access to HPV vaccination and screening.

Oesophagus

Cancer of the oesophagus is the 11th most frequent cancer worldwide. About 600,000 new cases occur each year, of which over 80% are in developing countries. Although squamous cell carcinomas arise frequently in many developing countries, adenocarcinomas are essentially tumours of more developed, industrialised nations. Differences between the incidence of oesophageal cancer in distinct geographical areas are more extreme than observed for any other cancer, with the high incidence being seen in an oesophageal cancer belt stretching from Northern Iran to North Central China, Southeast Africa and parts of South America.

Consumption of tobacco and alcohol, associated with low intake of fresh fruit, vegetables and meat, is causally associated with squamous cell carcinoma of the oesophagus worldwide. In developed countries, about 90% of squamous cell cancers are attributable to tobacco and alcohol, with a multiplicative increase in risk when individuals are exposed to both factors. Risk factors for oesophageal cancer in developing countries vary by region, however, with oral consumption of opium by-products an important factor in the Caspian Sea area, betel chewing in Southeast Asia, drinking of scalding hot beverages such as mate in South America and environmental factors including nitrosamines, contamination with fungi and deficiency of vitamins A and C in parts of China.

In contrast to squamous cell carcinoma, the most important risk factor for oesophageal adenocarcinoma is gastrooesophageal reflux disease, which results in the premalignant condition Barrett's oesophagus. Obesity is another significant risk factor, with smoking playing a less significant role in adenocarcinoma. Given the strong relationship between Barrett's oesophagus and oesophageal adenocarcinoma, some countries have implemented routine surveillance for patients with known Barrett's oesophagus. Randomised data supporting this are, however, lacking.

Melanoma

There are about 325,000 new cases of melanoma worldwide each year. It occurs predominantly in White populations (Caucasians) living in countries where there is high-intensity ultraviolet radiation, but this malignancy afflicts, to some degree, all ethnic groups. Assessed in relation to skin colour, melanoma incidence falls dramatically as skin pigmentation increases, and the disease is very rare in dark-skinned people. The highest incidence of melanoma occurs in Australia, where the population is predominantly Caucasian and there is an average of 6 hours of bright sunlight every day of the year and an essentially outdoor lifestyle. The lifetime risk of developing melanoma in Australia is 4% to 5% in males and 3% to 4% in females.

Dark-skinned people have a low risk of melanoma in Africa and South America; the sole of the foot, where the skin is not pigmented, is the most frequently affected site in this context of a low incidence. Asians have a low risk of melanoma despite their paler skin; naevi in Asian people, although common, are predominantly of the acral-lentiginous type, which has low malignant potential. Many countries observe significant increases in incidence and mortality in both genders.

It is estimated that 80% of melanoma is caused by ultraviolet damage to sensitive skin: skin that burns easily, fair or reddish skin, multiple freckles and skin that does not tan and develops naevi in response to early sunlight exposure. Prevention of melanoma is based on limiting exposure to ultraviolet radiation, particularly in the first 20 years of life.

Ultraviolet radiation is particularly hazardous when it involves sporadic intense exposure and sunburn. Most damage caused by sunlight occurs in childhood and adolescence, making this the most important target group for prevention programs. Established but rare risk factors include congenital naevi, immunosuppression and excessive use of solaria. Although melanoma may occur anywhere on the skin, the majority of melanoma in males is on the back, whereas in females, the majority is on the legs. The difference in site incidence is not entirely explained by differential exposure to ultraviolet light.

Head and Neck

Cancers of the oral mucosa, oropharynx, larynx and hypopharynx can be considered together because there are similarities in epidemiology, treatment and prognosis. The geographic patterns and trends in incidence for these cancers vary depending upon the anatomical subsites concerned, a phenomenon that is often explicable by the influence of risk factors such as tobacco use and alcohol consumption. These cancers are high in the Indian subcontinent, Australia, France, South America (Brazil) and Southern Africa. Cancers of the mouth and anterior two-thirds of the tongue generally predominate in developing countries, whereas pharyngeal cancers are common in developed countries and in Central and Eastern Europe.

Smoking and drinking are the major risk factors for head and neck cancer in developed countries, in the Caribbean and in South American countries. These risk factors have a joint multiplicative or synergistic effect on laryngeal and oropharyngeal cancers. Smoking is estimated to be responsible for about 41% of laryngeal and oral/pharyngeal cancers in males and 15% in females worldwide, and these proportions vary among different populations. Tobacco smoking has also been found to be an important risk factor for nasopharyngeal cancer in otherwise low-risk populations, while reverse smoking (in which the lit end of the cigarette is placed in the mouth so that an intense heat is experienced) is a risk factor for cancer of the hard palate. In the Indian subcontinent, chewing tobacco in the form of betel quid (a combination of betel leaf, slaked lime, areca-nut and tobacco with or without other condiments), bide (a locally hand-rolled cigarette of dried temburni leaf containing coarse tobacco), smoking and drinking locally brewed crude alcoholic drinks are the major causative factors. Oral snuff use is an emerging risk factor for oral cancer, particularly among young males in the United States.

Infection with Epstein-Barr virus has long been recognised as being important in the aetiology of nasopharyngeal cancer. This virus is not found in normal epithelial cells of the nasopharynx but is present in all nasopharyngeal tumour cells and even in dysplastic precursor lesions. It has also been recognised that HPV infection (transmitted sexually or perinatally) is associated with an increased risk of head and neck squamous cell carcinoma development, with an estimated 40% of oropharyngeal tumours attributable to HPV. Notably, HPV-related tumours carry a markedly better prognosis. Recent data suggest that HPV vaccination in adolescent males can prevent head and neck cancers.

Lymphoma

Lymphoma covers a heterogeneous group of neoplasms of lymphoid tissue. Traditionally, lymphomas have been categorised as either Hodgkin lymphoma (HL) or non-Hodgkin lymphoma (NHL). These distinct entities having different patterns of behaviour and response to treatment.

Geographically, NHL is most common in developed countries, although in the developing world, there are areas of moderate to high incidence in some Middle Eastern countries (Saudi Arabia, Israel) and in parts of sub-Saharan Africa. Much of the latter's high rate is because of the high incidence of Burkitt's lymphoma, an aggressive subtype of NHL.

NHL incidence rates have risen dramatically in the past few decades, particularly in developed countries, including Western Europe, North America and Australia. In part, this reflects better diagnosis and changing classification systems, but this is by no means the complete explanation. The increasing trend is also not explained entirely, because of the fact that NHL is a complication of acquired immune deficiency syndrome (AIDS) (occurring in up to 5% to 10% of AIDS cases in developed countries). In contrast to incidence, mortality rates have, in general, been declining as a consequence of improvement in therapy.

In developed countries, HL incidence reaches a peak in young adults, whereas in developing countries, HL occurs mainly in children and the elderly. In developed countries, incidence has fallen over the past 20 years.

Patients with human immunodeficiency virus (HIV)/AIDS or who have received immunosuppressant therapy have a higher risk of developing NHL. Viral infection such as HIV-1, human T-cell leukaemia virus type 1 (HTLV-1) and Epstein-Barr virus (EBV) are also associated with NHL. Infection of the stomach with *H. pylori* is associated with gastric lymphoma. There is also an increased risk of NHL among persons with a family history of lymphoma or haematological cancer.

A subtype of HL cases, the mixed cellularity type, has been linked to EBV. Overall, around 45% of cases may be attributable to EBV. The presence of EBV in tumours seems also to be related to age and socioeconomic circumstances. EBV is involved in the aetiology of Burkitt's lymphoma, especially in cases in tropical Africa, where over 95% of tumours contain the virus. The proportion of EBV-positive tumours is much less in the sporadic cases of HL occurring in Europe and North America. The singular geographic distribution of Burkitt's lymphoma is not explicable on the basis of EBV alone; however, because infection by the virus is ubiquitous, suspicion has fallen upon intense malarial infection as predisposing to Burkitt's lymphoma in the presence of EBV infection. The risk of HL is also increased in patients with HIV infection.

Leukaemia

Leukaemias comprise about 2.5% of all incident cancers worldwide, with about 474,500 new cases occurring annually. A relatively high incidence is evident in the United States, Canada, Western Europe, Australia and New Zealand, whereas rates are generally low in most African and Asian countries, where rates are less than half those in the former group. The trends in overall incidence of leukaemia have generally been stable or slowly increasing. However, a substantial reduction in death rates from leukaemias, particularly in childhood, has been observed since the 1960s, thanks to advances in treatment and consequent improvement in survival.

Leukaemia peaks in incidence in the first 4 years of life, predominantly due to acute lymphoblastic leukaemia (ALL), the most common paediatric malignancy, accounting for nearly 25% of all such diseases. After infancy, rates of leukaemia steeply decline with age, with the lowest incidence at ages 15 to 25, after which there is an exponential rise up to age 85.

The usual form of the disease in adults is acute myeloid leukaemia (AML), accounting for 70% of all cases. The more differentiated or chronic forms of leukaemia are predominantly adult diseases, rarely occurring before the age of 30, and then increasing progressively in incidence with age. Chronic myelogenous leukaemia (CML) accounts for 15% to 20% of all cases of leukaemia. For patients over age 50, chronic lymphocytic leukaemia (CLL) is the dominant type of leukaemia.

The cause of most leukaemias is not known. A range of risk factors have been predominantly, although not exclusively, associated with particular leukaemia subtypes. Ionising radiation (nuclear bombs, medical procedures) and occupational exposure to benzene are associated with acute myeloid leukaemia.

Leukaemia (mainly acute myeloid) may occur in a small proportion of cancer patients treated with chlorambucil, cyclophosphamide, melphalan, thiotepa, treosulphan or etoposide, as well as certain combination chemotherapy. Leukaemia has followed induction of aplastic anaemia by the antibiotic chloramphenicol. Certain risk factors, such as Down syndrome, have been identified for childhood leukaemia but, generally, the causes of the disease are not known. Some studies have shown a risk of childhood leukaemia with exposure to high-level residential extremely low frequency electromagnetic fields, but causality has not been established.

Infection with the virus HTLV-1 has been established as a cause of leukaemia. This virus is responsible for adult T-cell leukaemia, a disease mainly observed in tropical countries and Japan, and rarely in the United States and Europe. In experimental animals, particularly in mice, there are many retroviruses which can cause a variety of leukaemias, but such retroviruses have not been identified in humans.

REDUCING THE RISKS OF DEVELOPING CANCER

Based largely on our current knowledge of the aetiology of cancer, it has been estimated that 40% of malignancies are preventable. To put the environmental causes of cancer in perspective, the estimated attributable fraction of the population of worldwide cancer cases they relate

TABLE 16.1 Major Causes of Cancer

Factor	Type of Cancer	Percent (%) Population Attributable Fraction
Smoking	Lung Mouth and oropharynx Oesophagus Stomach Cervix Leukaemia	21
Alcohol	Mouth and oropharynx Oesophagus Breast	5
Low fruit and vegetable intake	Oesophageal Stomach Colorectal Lung	5
Indoor smoke from household use of solid fuels	Lung	<0.5
Urban air pollution	Lung	1
Overweight and obesity	Colorectal Breast	2
Physical inactivity	Colorectal Breast	2
Unsafe sex	Cervix	3

to has been summarised for some common cancers in Table 16.1. Similarly, Table 16.2 presents a summary by the International Agency for Research on Cancer (IARC) of human carcinogens that relate to some common cancers. The striking feature is the high proportion as a result of dietary factors and smoking. Changing dietary habits could potentially reduce the risk of cancer, possibly by one-third. The main cancers involved are those of the stomach, colon, rectum and breast. A number of initiatives, such as the European Commission's 10-point code, have been produced to summarise ways in which the risk of cancer can be reduced.

Reducing Tobacco Smoking

Every country should give high priority to tobacco control in its fight against cancer as, unchecked, smoking will cause more than 10 million deaths from cancer (mostly lung cancer) in the next decade. Additionally, with passive smoking now implicated as a cause of lung cancer, as well as being a contributing factor in increasing coronary heart disease, the emphasis has now moved to what action public health policymakers should advocate and what legislation the government should enact to reduce not only smoking but also involuntary smoking. Many countries worldwide have now imposed bans on smoking in public places and working environments to protect workers' health. One of the additional benefits of such restrictions has been a reduction in the rate of active smoking among the population at large. Further measures taken by governments around the world include making health warnings mandatory on commercial tobacco products, banning advertising of tobacco, increasing taxation, reducing tar content in cigarettes, regulating and enforcing plain packaging of tobacco and setting up clinics for smokers to help them break the habit. As a result of these interventions and ongoing public health campaigns, smoking rates are declining internationally and lung cancer incidence is falling in many countries. Worryingly, smoking rates in the Eastern Mediterranean and African regions are continuing to increase.

TABLE 16.2 International Agency for Research on Cancer Carcinogenic Agents

Cancer Site	Carcinogenic Agents With Sufficient Evidence of an Association With Cancer
Oral cavity	Alcoholic beverages Betel quid with tobacco Betel quid without tobacco Human papillomavirus type 16 Tobacco, smokeless Tobacco smoking
Salivary gland	X-radiation, gamma radiation
Tonsil	HPV type 16
Pharynx	Alcoholic beverages Betel quid with tobacco Human papillomavirus type 16 Tobacco smoking
Nasopharynx	Epstein-Barr virus Formaldehyde Salted fish, Chinese-style Tobacco smoking Wood dust
Nasal cavity and paranasal sinus	Isopropyl alcohol production Leather dust Nickel compounds Radium-226 and its decay products Radium-228 and its decay products Tobacco smoking Wood dust
Larynx	Acid mists, strong inorganic Alcoholic beverages Asbestos (all forms) Tobacco smoking
Digestive tract, upper	Acetaldehyde associated with consumption of alcoholic beverages
Oesophagus	Acetaldehyde associated with consumption of alcoholic beverages Alcoholic beverages Betel quid with tobacco Betel quid without tobacco Tobacco, smokeless Tobacco smoking X-radiation, gamma radiation
Stomach	*Helicobacter pylori* Rubber production industry Tobacco smoking X-radiation, gamma radiation
Colon and rectum	Alcoholic beverages Tobacco smoking X-radiation, gamma radiation Processed meat (consumption of)
Lung cancer	Acheson process, occupational exposures associated with aluminium production Arsenic and inorganic arsenic compounds Asbestos (all forms) Beryllium and beryllium compounds Bis(chloromethyl)ether; chloromethyl methyl ether (technical grade) Cadmium and cadmium compounds Chromium (VI) compounds

(*continued*)

TABLE 16.2 International Agency for Research on Cancer Carcinogenic Agents—con't

Cancer Site	Carcinogenic Agents With Sufficient Evidence of an Association With Cancer
	Coal, indoor emissions from household combustion
	Coal gasification
	Coal-tar pitch
	Coke production
	Engine exhaust, diesel
	Hematite mining (underground)
	Iron and steel founding
	MOPP (vincristine-prednisone-nitrogen mustard-procarbazine mixture)
	Nickel compounds
	Outdoor air pollution
	Painting
	Particulate matter in outdoor air pollution
	Plutonium
	Radon-222 and its decay products
	Rubber production industry
	Silica dust, crystalline
	Soot
	Sulfur mustard
	Tobacco smoke, secondhand
	Tobacco smoking
	Welding fumes
	X-radiation, gamma radiation
Melanoma	Solar radiation
	Ultraviolet-emitting tanning devices
	Polychlorinated biphenyls
Breast	Alcoholic beverages
	Diethylstilbestrol
	Oestrogen-progestogen contraceptives
	Oestrogen-progestogen menopausal therapy
	X-radiation, gamma radiation
Cervix	Diethylstilbestrol (exposure in utero)
	Oestrogen-progestogen contraceptives
	Human immunodeficiency virus type 1
	Human papillomavirus types 16, 18, 31, 33, 35, 39, 45, 51, 52, 56, 58, 59
	Tobacco smoking

The rise of e-cigarettes as a means to reduce smoking remains controversial. It is unclear currently what the long-term effects of vaping are, although it is very likely to be considerably safer than cigarettes. Opinion is divided between those who feel the shift towards vaping is a public health good (reducing disease both in active and passive smokers) and those who think vaping may (1) encourage smoking in younger age groups, (2) not result in the levels of cessation advertised and (3) cause many users of e-cigarettes never to transition completely away from tobacco (with no evidence that reducing cigarette smoking without quitting is beneficial). At an individual level, although evidence does not support e-cigarettes being more effective than other strategies for tobacco cessation, it should be considered as an option.

Modifying Alcohol Consumption

After smoking, alcohol is the second most important cause of cancer. It may be responsible in some countries for up to 10% of deaths from cancer. Cancers of the mouth, larynx, pharynx, oesophagus, liver, colorectum, breast and stomach are certainly caused in part by alcohol. For several tumours, the risk rises with the quantity consumed to more than tenfold for lifelong nondrinkers. Alcohol and tobacco smoking act as synergistic carcinogens (i.e. the combined effect is greater than that of either alone). This combination accounts for the very high incidence of these tumours in France, where they are often multifocal. Alcohol probably acts as a cocarcinogen rather than a carcinogen (i.e. it promotes rather than initiates carcinogenesis). Spirits may have a slightly stronger carcinogenic effect than other alcoholic beverages.

Any policy on moderating the consumption of alcohol has to take account of a number of facts. First, many people find it pleasurable. Second, moderate amounts (2–3 units/day) protect against coronary thrombosis, although heavy drinking has other undesirable social consequences (e.g. violent behaviour and road accidents). Third, its carcinogenic effects are largely in conjunction with smoking tobacco. Thus the risk of cancer induction by alcohol in nonsmokers is relatively small.

HPV Vaccination

With increasing awareness of the role of HPV in cancers of the cervix, head and neck, anus, vagina, vulva and penis, a number of countries have implemented vaccination programs. The vaccines used provide immunity to the HPV genotypes primarily responsible for cancer (16 and 18) and, in some cases, other additional genotypes (e.g. HPV 6 and 11, which result in genital warts). Early observational studies report reductions in high-grade cervical intraepithelial neoplasia alongside marked reductions in genital warts. Although vaccination programs have initially been aimed at young females, a number of countries are now moving to provide vaccination for all teenagers. The cost-effectiveness of these programs varies between jurisdictions and as such differing approaches exist.

Ultraviolet Light

Exposure to ultraviolet light has been increasing with the reduction of the ozone layer, caused by chemical pollution. An increase in the incidence of all forms of skin cancer can be expected. The principal culprits are chlorofluorohydrocarbons (CFCs). These are components in, for example, aerosol sprays, refrigerants and solvents for cleaning electronic equipment. However, to put the contribution of commercial sources of CFCs into context, one volcano in Antarctica emits 100 tons of chlorine every month, substantially more than the combined output of CFCs from deodorants over the same period. Nitrogen oxides from vehicle exhaust fumes also deplete the ozone layer. International agreements have been reached, aimed at eliminating the use of CFCs.

Occupational Exposure

A wide variety of occupations are known to carry the risk of exposure to carcinogens. It is estimated that 4% of all cancer deaths are attributed to occupational carcinogens. The IARC classifies 129 agents as carcinogenic (group 1), 96 as probably carcinogenic (group 2A) and 321 as possibly carcinogenic (https://monographs.iarc.who.int/agents-classified-by-the-iarc/). These included industrial processes, industrial chemicals, pesticides, laboratory chemicals, drugs, food ingredients, and tobacco smoking and related stimulants. Drugs and industrial chemicals represent the largest risks. There are many other occupations where an agent is thought to be carcinogenic to workers, but a causal link has not been established. Of these, exposure to asbestos dust, aromatic amines and the products of burning fossil fuels are the most common. Measures to prevent occupational exposure include labelling of products as carcinogenic and prohibiting the marketing and use of certain substances, for example, the four aromatic amines (naphthylamine, 4-aminobiphenyl, 4-nitrodiphenyl and benzidine) and blue asbestos (crocidolite).

It is thought that preventive methods are likely to have little impact on mortality from occupational cancers in the near future. The detection of tumours at an early stage by screening is likely to have a greater effect on mortality. Screening of urine by cytology among workers in the dyestuff and rubber industries has long been practised.

Diet

Diet influences carcinogenesis in various ways: carcinogens may be eaten, food substances may be converted to carcinogens once ingested, and dietary components may modify how the body metabolises and responds to carcinogens. The only component of food that has been found to be strongly linked to the development of cancer is aflatoxin. This is a product of the fungus *Aspergillus fumigatus*, which often contaminates damp cereals in tropical countries. It causes primary liver cancer, although the data are unclear because there is a high incidence of hepatitis B, itself associated with liver tumours, in the same group of patients.

Bracken fern containing nitrates is suspected of causing oesophageal cancer, particularly among the Japanese. Salted fish is implicated in the aetiology of nasopharyngeal cancer, possibly as a cocarcinogen with the Epstein-Barr virus.

Diet may also be indirectly related to carcinogenesis. One example is fibre, which seems to have a protective effect against colorectal cancer. A second is obesity, which is associated with an increased incidence of cancer of the breast, endometrium, colon, kidney, gallbladder and oesophagus, amongst others. A third is vitamin A (retinol) and its derivatives, retinoids, which may inhibit the full malignant transformation of cells and prevent tumour formation.

Dietary measures likely to reduce the risk of cancers are:

- High-fibre diet
- Reducing saturated fats
- Plenty of fresh fruit and vegetables (owing to the presence of antioxidants such as vitamin E)
- Maintaining a healthy body weight through a combination of diet and exercise

Ionising Radiation

The whole spectrum of sources of ionising radiation, both natural and manmade, has been calculated to contribute 1.5% of all fatal cancers. Table 16.3 shows the sources of radiation exposure in the United Kingdom.

It is estimated that exposure to radon gas from domestic buildings may be responsible for 1% of lung cancer in Europe. Concentrations of radon gas in excess of 400 Bq/m^3 (about 1 in 1000 homes) will expose the occupants to 20 mSv per year. The lifetime risk of fatal cancer from this exposure is about 10%. The carcinogenic risks of ionising radiation have been revised upwards since 1988. Current estimates of risk are two to five times higher. However, it is unclear whether these revised estimates apply to very low levels of exposure to natural background radioactivity.

TABLE 16.3 Estimated Annual Dose of Ionising Radiation Received by a Member of the General Public

External terrestrial radiation	0.4 mSv
Cosmic radiation	0.3 mSv
Ingestion of naturally occurring radioactive substances	0.3 mSv
Inhalation of radon progeny	2.4 mSv
Use of ionising radiation and radioactive substances in medicine (mainly diagnostic x-rays)	1.5 mSv
Fallout from nuclear weapons testing	<0.01 mSv
Nuclear power plants	<0.01 mSv
Reactor accident in Chernobyl	<0.02 mSv
Use of radioactive materials and ionising radiation in industry, in research and at home	<0.01 mSv
Occupational exposure	<0.01 mSv

The role of ionising radiation in the causation of cancer is mainly derived from occupational exposure. Early evidence came from the development of lung cancer among miners at Joachimsthal in the Czech Republic and Schneeberg in Germany. Lung disease has been known to occur among these workers since the 16th century. It was subsequently appreciated that the disease was lung cancer because of radioactive radon gas in the mines.

The main source of evidence of the effects of ionising radiation in humans are the survivors of the atomic bombs dropped on Hiroshima and Nagasaki in 1945. The incidence of acute and chronic leukaemia was significantly raised within a radius of 1.5 km from the epicentre. The highest incidence occurred 6 to 8 years afterwards. For cancers other than leukaemia, the latent period was longer (15–20 years) among victims who received 1 Gray (Gy) or more; indeed, the incidence is still higher over 50 years later.

It is assumed that there is no threshold below which ionising radiation cannot induce cancers. Indeed, children who received only 0.01 to 0.02 Gy in utero when their mothers were irradiated had an additional 1 in 2000 risk of cancer. At low doses, the risk of developing cancer is probably proportional to dose, although much uncertainty remains.

Reducing the levels of radon gas in domestic buildings requires several measures. First, systematic surveys are needed to identify buildings that pose a hazard. Alterations to the floors and installation of extractor fans can also reduce levels of radon gas.

POLLUTION

Atmospheric pollution has been suspected to be carcinogenic ever since the incidence of lung cancer was found to be higher in cities than in the country. The combustion products of coal are known to contain carcinogenic hydrocarbons. However, because the atmosphere is polluted by a wide variety of substances, often in small quantities, the assessment of carcinogenic risk is very difficult. The situation is further complicated by the contribution to atmospheric pollution of tobacco smoking. In the past, pollution probably accounted for about 1% of cancers. Atmospheric pollution in the United Kingdom is now falling, with stricter rules on the burning of fossil fuels. The evidence suggests that the current burning of fossil fuels, arsenic and asbestos will contribute to much less than 1% of future cancers.

Chemoprevention

The oral cavity, lung and colon have been the most common primary sites subject to attempts at chemoprevention. Beta-carotene, synthetic retinoids, calcium and a variety of vitamins reduce the risk of developing oral cancer. A trial of alpha-tocopherol and beta-carotene showed no protective effect against the development of lung cancer.

Among patients in China at high risk of oesophageal or stomach cancer, treatment with vitamin and mineral supplements reduced the incidence and mortality of these tumours. These populations have a 20% incidence of oesophageal dysplasia.

Trials of adjuvant tamoxifen have shown a reduction in the risk of contralateral breast cancer. Trials are ongoing to determine whether tamoxifen can prevent the disease among females at high risk on the basis of their strong family history of the disease. Antioxidants, for example, vitamins A and E, are thought to act by reducing DNA damage early in the process of carcinogenesis. It seems most likely that chemoprevention with such agents should occur early in life if they prove to be effective. The cost-effectiveness of chemoprevention needs to be carefully considered.

Preventive treatment may have to be continued for several decades, which may prove very expensive when compared with the number of lives saved.

CONCLUSION

The negative impact of cancer on individuals and communities can be greatly reduced through cancer control programs. Although the scope of cancer control extends from prevention and screening to management of disease, rehabilitation and palliative care, successful prevention can make a huge contribution to reducing the global cancer load, and, compared with the other strategies, at a relatively low cost. Because this involves changes in lifestyle for many individuals, it is critical that medical and public health professionals engage with populations in embracing healthy living as a shared goal.

ACKNOWLEDGMENT

The author would like to acknowledge the contributions of Katie Spencer, David Hole (deceased), Paul Symonds and Eva Morris, authors of this chapter in the previous edition.

FURTHER READING

Bray F, Laversanne M, Sung H, et al. Global cancer statistics 2022: GLOBOCAN estimates of incidence and mortality worldwide for 36 cancers in 185 countries. *CA Cancer J Clin*. 2024;74(3): 229–263.

Doll R, Peto R, Boreham J, Sutherland I. Mortality from cancer in relation to smoking: 50 years observations on British doctors. *Br J Cancer*. 2005;92(3):426–429.

Hammond E, Selikoff I, Seidmant H. Asbestos exposure, cigarette smoking and death rates. *Ann N Y Acad Sci*. 1979;330:473–490.

International Agency for Research on Cancer. Global cancer observatory. Accessed 5 May 2024. http://gco.iarc.fr/en

Siegel RL, Miller KD, Fuchs HE, Jemal A. Cancer statistics, 2022. *CA Cancer J Clin*. 2022;72(1):7–33.

Thomas GA, Symonds P. Radiation exposure and health effects—is it time to reassess the real consequences? *Clin Oncol*. 2016;28: 231–236.

Vineis P, Wild CP. Global cancer patterns: causes and prevention. *Lancet*. 2014;383:549–557.

17

Biological and Pathological Introduction

John R. Goepel and Abhik Mukherjee

CHAPTER OUTLINE

INTRODUCTION

Radiotherapy is used almost exclusively for the treatment of cancer and related conditions. It is thus very important to have a reasonable understanding of this disease. This chapter contains an outline of the basic characteristics of cancer cells and the conditions that can cause cancer. There is consideration of the natural history of untreated cancer and of the ways that different types of cancer are named and classified.

GROWTH: PROLIFERATION, DIFFERENTIATION AND APOPTOSIS

Growth is the process of increase in size and maturity of tissues from fertilisation through to the adult. When normally controlled, the different parts of the body attain their correct size and specialist functions and their relationship to one another. Furthermore, throughout life, these attributes continue despite the need for replacement and repair. This is all a reflection of accurate control of the timing and extent of cellular proliferation, cell-to-cell orientation and organisation, and differentiation. *Differentiation* is the process of a cell taking on a specialised function; this is usually associated with a change in its microscopic appearance. It is also usually a one-way commitment, with relative or complete loss of the ability to continue proliferating. Also important is the ability to delete cells which are no longer needed by a process called *apoptosis* or *programmed cell death*. This is used in the development of the foetus and in maintaining or adjusting the size of a structure in the adult. Apoptosis is also used to delete defective cells.

Growth Disorders

Hypertrophy is an increase in the size of an organ due to an increase in the size of its constituent cells. For example, the left ventricle of the heart becomes hypertrophic if it has to work harder because of hypertension. An inherited cause of cardiac hypertrophy is hypertrophic cardiomyopathy.

Hyperplasia is an increase in size because of an increase in the number of cells. The adrenal cortex will become hyperplastic if there is excessive adrenocorticotrophic hormone to stimulate it. However, it will return to normal if the stimulus is reduced again. Hyperplasia is also seen in other benign proliferative diseases such as in the breast, commonly, usual-type ductal hyperplasia; however, when there is atypia in the cells (atypical ductal hyperplasia), there is an increase of future malignancy, and patients may require additional follow-up.

Metaplasia is a change from one type of tissue to another. Smoking induces a change of the bronchial lining from the usual respiratory mucosa to a squamous epithelium, with resultant loss of mucus-producing and ciliated cells. It is also potentially reversible. An important metaplastic lesion in the context of cancer is Barrett's metaplasia, where there is a change of oesophageal squamous mucosa to intestinal-type mucosa, commonly induced by gastrooesophageal reflux disease. It predisposes to a higher risk of oesophageal adenocarcinoma and is managed by surveillance protocols for any developing dysplasia.

Neoplasia (literally a new growth), in contrast, is an irreversible process once initiated: it is the main subject of this chapter. It is also called *cancer* or a *tumour*, although the latter is sometimes used to denote any swelling.

NEOPLASIA

A *neoplasm* can be defined as a lesion resulting from the autonomous or relatively autonomous abnormal growth of cells which persists after the initiating stimulus has been removed—that is, cell growth has escaped from normal regulatory mechanisms. The abnormality affects all aspects of cell growth and apoptosis to varying degrees. Proliferation continues unabated, irrespective of the requirements of the organ in which the neoplasm is situated. This, combined with loss of control of the normal relationships between cells, often results in the new tumour cells replacing and insinuating themselves between the adjacent normal tissues, a process called *invasion*. Loss of differentiation accompanies and often correlates with failure of proliferation control and invasiveness. Failure of apoptosis may also be a major contribution to the survival of abnormal cells.

Benign and Malignant Neoplasms

Neoplasia is not a single disease, but rather, a common pathological process with a multitude of different varieties and clinical outcomes. Neoplasms are categorised as benign or malignant mainly based on their capability of distant spread (metastases). Benign tumours remain localised, with generally relatively little effect on the patient. In contrast, malignant tumours are locally destructive, may spread to other parts of the body and ultimately result in the death of the patient. Fig. 17.1 and Table 17.1 show some of the differences between benign and malignant neoplasms. Further aspects of the classification of tumours are discussed later in this chapter.

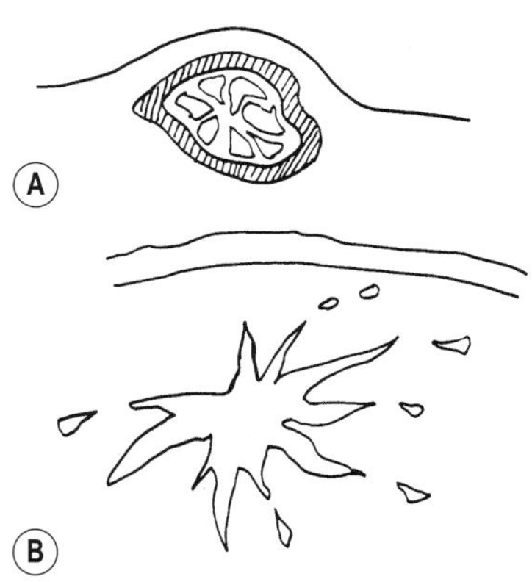

Fig. 17.1 The difference between a benign tumour (A) contained by a definitive capsule and a malignant tumour (B) actively invading the tumour bed.

TABLE 17.1 Characteristics of Neoplasms

Feature	Benign	Malignant
Growth rate	Slow	Variable, may be rapid
Margin	Encapsulated	Invasive
Local effect	Little	Destructive
Differentiation	Good	Variable, may be poor
Metastases	No	Frequently
Usual outcome	Good	Fatal

The term *cancer* (Latin/Greek for 'crab') is very ancient, and there are several explanations for its usage. Some say it reflects the tenacious grip the disease has on its victim; some say that it describes the radiating prominent veins that may surround an advanced superficial tumour. Others contend that it describes the irregular infiltrative profile of some tumours, for example, of the breast. Suffice it to say that *cancer* is a common colloquial term that is generally applied to any malignant neoplasm.

Although the behaviour of tumours, particularly malignant ones, may seem very odd, it can generally be explained by the excessive or inappropriate expression of genes that are present in all cells. The tumour continues to be dependent upon an adequate blood supply (although many acquire the capacity to induce new vessels, a process termed *angiogenesis*). Also, many of those which arise from hormone-dependent tissues (e.g. breast, prostate) continue to show a degree of dependence on those hormones. This can be exploited to therapeutic advantage by giving antihormonal therapy.

CARCINOGENESIS

The causes of cancer are numerous and mechanisms of its production complex, but some of the principles will be presented. There are two avenues of thought to follow: one at the molecular and genetic levels and the other concerned with causative associations. It is not always easy to relate these to each other. Underlying the mechanistic approach is the assumption that cell behaviour is controlled by the genes expressed (which ones, and how strongly), bearing in mind that these can be influenced by chemical messages relayed from outside the cell. Every cell contains the entire genetic code but only expresses those genes appropriate to its own situation. In cancer, this has gone wrong, particularly with respect to proliferation, differentiation or apoptosis. We can generalise to say that multiple abnormalities need to have occurred between normality and cancer and that this reflects a multistep process. Only those cells capable of division are at risk of transforming into a neoplasm. This excludes terminally differentiated cells such as circulating red cells, the uppermost keratinised cells of the skin and adult voluntary muscle and nerve cells.

Initiation

This describes the first step towards neoplasia. It reflects a change at the molecular level of how a cell can function, escaping in some small way from a control mechanism. Nothing can be seen microscopically at this stage. Substances that can initiate neoplasia are called *initiators* or *carcinogens* and possess the capability to cause mutations. These include either directly acting chemical initiators such as nitrogen mustard or benzoyl chloride, or those which require metabolic activation, for example, polycyclic aromatic hydrocarbons.

Promotion

No more will come of the initiated cell unless it continues to divide. Further abnormalities of cell function (i.e. gene expression) arise over a period of time. Substances that enhance this process are called *promoters*, which unlike initiators may not be inherently mutagenic.

Progression

Neoplasms are clonal—that is, they are derived from a single cell. For this to happen, a cell and its progeny must acquire and sustain a growth advantage over other cells throughout succeeding cell divisions. This eventually results in visible alterations at the microscopic level. Not all the daughter cells will be identical, giving rise to differences between individual cells or subclones; this is called *pleomorphism*. In the process of evolution, a subclone of tumour cells may gain selective advantage due to their metastatic potential or resistance to therapy.

Cancer Stem Cells

Within the tumour cell population there exists a cohort of cells that are biologically distinct in that they have the capacity to self-renew and differentiate into the tumour cell population: these are cancer stem cells (CSCs). CSCs have been characterised in a wide variety of tumours including leukaemias and skin, colon and breast cancers. CSCs may remain dormant and cause recurrence and metastases. Exterminating this population would effectively destroy the tumour as it would eliminate the root cause of the cancer. However, in other schools of thought (stochastic models), all cells are equipotent to suffer mutations, self-renew or differentiate into tumours based on both genetic and epigenetic influences, resulting in tumour heterogeneity. However, current research brings these schools of thought together; it is envisaged that there is plasticity allowing cells to transit between CSC and non-CSC states. Given these complexities, it may be more worthwhile to modulate stem cell–niche functions rather than target treatments solely to intrinsic CSC features.

Clinical Cancer

After passing through the phenomena of initiation, promotion and progression, the neoplasm finally becomes manifest as a clinically significant tumour. Unless removed, it will continue to progress with a general tendency towards further loss of growth restraint and acquisition of the capacity to spread to other parts of the body (metastasise).

Oncogenes and Tumour Suppressor Genes

The function of a cell is critically dependent on the expression of its genes. In cancer, it has been observed that there may be (1) inappropriate levels of expression of otherwise normal genes and (2) abnormalities of genes. Although copying of the genetic code from one cell generation to another is very accurate, it is not perfect. An abnormal copy or mutation may give rise to a protein with excessive function or reduced function, or it may fail to produce a protein at all, resulting in no function. Alternatively, it may be the control of the gene which is altered so that there is increased or decreased expression resulting in excess or deficient protein product and hence function. An *oncogene* is an altered gene which contributes to cancer development when its expression is increased. The normally functioning counterparts of these genes (protooncogenes) are often concerned with control of cell proliferation. An activating mutation transforms it into an oncogene. Examples include RAS, MYC, EGFR and so on.

In contrast, tumour suppressor genes are those which, when totally absent or nonfunctioning in a cell, permit the emergence of neoplasia—that is, their presence prevents neoplasia. Given that all normal cells will have two copies of each gene (one on each chromosome pair), the development of neoplasia by this means requires loss or mutation of both copies. Examples of tumour suppressor genes include Rb, p53, PTEN and so on.

It must be stressed that clinical cancer does not reflect a solitary abnormality of one of these genes, but rather, the final result of a combination of several errors of function. The gradual accumulation of multiple genetic defects is typified by the progression of a benign polyp in the colon to a cancer over about 10 years. Indeed the adenoma carcinoma sequence has been characterised in great detail in the Vogelstein model of colorectal carcinogenesis.

Defective DNA Repair Mechanisms

How is it that a cell can acquire so many abnormal genes? The explanation in several situations is that there is failure of the screening of the cell's genetic code for abnormalities, or there is defective repair of incidental genetic damage. The protein p53 (termed the guardian of the genome) is important in assuring the integrity of the genome and is frequently defective in cancer cells. Similarly, the failure of DNA repair can result in much more rapid accumulation of mutations, the mutator phenotype. An inherited defect in DNA repair makes an individual prone to cancer. Accumulating DNA damage causes mutations to arise during DNA synthesis, resulting in malignancies. Common known germline mutations that lead to an increased risk of cancer include, among others, defects in BRCA1/2 and the ataxia-telangiectasia mutated (ATM) gene, which result in defective homologous recombination and/or nonhomologous end-joining (NHEJ) processes of DNA repair and have been observed in both solid (breast, ovarian) and haemopoietic malignancies (leukaemia and lymphomas). Another common example of faulty DNA repair is exemplified by deficiencies in the DNA mismatch repair (MMR) system that normally corrects for errors in insertion, deletion and misincorporation of bases during DNA replication or damage repair. Inherited mutations in the MMR proteins (viz. MLH1, PMS2, MSH2 and MSH6) cause microsatellite instability (MSI) with an abnormal length of microsatellite repeats. This is seen in hereditary nonpolyposis colorectal cancers (HNPCCs or Lynch syndrome), predominantly affecting the right colon, and Muir-Torre syndrome (MTS), which predisposes to sebaceous carcinomas of the skin. DNA mismatch repair defects are also observed in some sporadic colorectal tumours, but unlike germline defects as in HNPCC, the defect ensues from epigenetic mechanisms that reduce DNA repair gene expression, for example, methylation of the MLH1 promoter that silences MLH1.

Defective Apoptotic Mechanisms

Defective apoptosis has several consequences with regard to cancer. Inappropriately increased expression of BCL-2, which inhibits apoptosis, is a major reason for cell accumulation in some tumours, for example, follicular lymphoma. Failure of apoptosis may contribute to survival of defective cells and to cell survival in abnormal environments such as during invasion and metastasis. Finally, many cancer treatments rely on induction of apoptosis to kill tumour cells, so these will be less effective if apoptosis is defective. The apoptotic machinery is complex and depends on the critical balance between BCL-2 and its dimerising partners, which may be pro- (e.g. with BAD) or antiapoptotic (e.g. with BAX), as well as the concerted activity of a group of enzymes called *caspases*, which may suffer mutations in cancers.

Blood Vessels

The development of cancer cells into a clinically important mass requires establishing a blood supply, a process called *angiogenesis*. New capillaries form under the influence of vascular endothelial growth factors (VEGF); platelets are the main source of VEGF in the blood. VEGF may be secreted directly by tumour cells, particularly when stimulated by hypoxia but also when tumours abnormally express a range of other oncogenes, for example, epidermal growth factor receptor (EGFR) and HER2. HER2 is important in many breast cancers and is a therapeutic target for trastuzumab (Herceptin). Drugs available to target angiogenesis include the anti-VEGF antibody bevacizumab (Avastin), often used to treat colorectal cancer, whereas other small molecule tyrosine kinase inhibitors (e.g. sunitinib, sofarenib etc.) act by inhibiting VEGF receptors. Tumours also develop new lymphatic channels (*lymphangiogenesis*), detectable by lymphatic channel markers (such as D2-40/podoplanin), and in some cancers such as breast cancer, lymphovascular invasion has been shown to be the major route of metastases rather than blood vascular invasion. In general, both blood vascular and lymphovascular invasion confer poor prognosis in a wide variety of neoplasms.

Heredity and Cancer

The great majority of common tumours do not seem to have any relationship to hereditary factors. However, some rare tumours do and have led to an understanding of tumour suppressor genes. The pioneering work of Knudson on families of patients with multiple retinoblastomas (a tumour of the eye) indicated first that there must be two genetic events (Knudson's two-hit hypotheses). In due course, it became clear that one defective gene was inherited by the patient, whereas its corresponding gene on the opposite chromosome became defective, or was lost, in some cells during the growth of the eye. With both retinoblastoma (Rb) genes now defective, the cells proceeded to neoplasia.

It is apparent that a minority of common tumours run in families because of the same sort of mechanism. For example, breast cancer kindreds may be passing on mutations in the BRCA-1 or BRCA-2 genes and may also be associated with carcinoma of the ovary or colon. In familial adenomatous polyposis, a defective APC gene results in adenomas and colon cancers, whereas as mentioned earlier, in HNPCC, one of a number of mismatch repair genes or abnormal hypermethylation is involved, giving rise to colon cancer by a different molecular biology route. These issues are discussed in further detail in the relevant sections about breast cancer or colon cancer. An inherited risk of malignancy, however, does not imply that it is certain that a cancer will arise in a particular individual.

Physical Agents

Ionising Radiation

There is no doubt that ionising radiation can cause cancer. Knowledge of radiation effects has come from evidence following exposure to the atom bomb and the Chernobyl accident, which caused an increased incidence of thyroid carcinoma and radiation-related breast cancers. Direct damage to DNA (i.e. the chemical basis of genetic information) and damage mediated via ionisation of water can result in mutation of genes. The damage is randomly scattered throughout the genetic code but can include sites critical to the development of cancer by the usual sequence of initiation, promotion and so on. Traditionally, it has been thought that radiation causes a somatic mutation in a normal cell. The earliest event is probably genomic instability. Subsequently, there is a multistep sequence of genetic events. This typically results in an interval of many years between exposure and clinical cancer. The source of radiation does not matter from the point of view of causing cancer, although it will affect the sites at risk.

Ionising radiation can lead to loss of tumour suppressor genes and activation of protooncogenes. A *protooncogene* is a normal gene which, when altered by mutation, becomes an oncogene that can contribute to the development of cancer. Oncogenes may also be activated as a result of point mutations. Gene amplification can lead to activation and overexpression of a protooncogene. It had previously been thought that mutagenesis only occurred in normal cells traversed by radiation particles. However, normal cells can undergo change without such damage by virtue of what is termed the *bystander effect*. The mechanism of this bystander effect is not clear, but it could be as a result of secretion of factors (as yet unidentified) from irradiated cells that influence the survival of adjacent nonirradiated cells.

The dose at which carcinogenesis occurs may be tissue specific. Actively proliferating tissues within or adjacent to the irradiated volume (e.g. in the pelvis), and having a high capacity for proliferation not inhibited by radiation, will carry a risk of radiation-induced malignancy at lower doses than in slowly turning-over tissues such as connective tissue.

Industrial Exposure. Early workers using x-rays unknowingly induced tumours and other radiation damage in their hands. Today, diagnostic and therapeutic radiation also carry this risk to patients and staff alike, necessitating stringent safety regulations. Some mine workers are exposed to high levels of radon, which is inhaled and may cause lung cancer (a risk increased by cigarette smoking). Radon-induced lung cancer has been linked to mutations of p53, a tumour suppressor gene. This mutation differs from those seen in lung cancer induced by smoking. Another industrial association was with the painters of luminous watch dials. These ladies pointed their brush with their lips, thereby taking in minute quantities of radium. Some of the material remained near the jaw, whereas some was absorbed and passed to bone marrow, where the alpha emissions resulted in bone necrosis, tumours and marrow failure. In all cases, there was the usual long time delay between exposure and clinical cancer.

Atomic bomb survivors have been followed up very carefully. There has been an excessive number of cases of leukaemia, mainly 7 to 12 years after exposure, and also a larger number of other cancers from about 20 years later onwards.

Ultraviolet Light. The shorter wavelengths of solar ultraviolet light, UVB, are capable of damaging the DNA of various skin cells, resulting in mutations and eventually cancers. Melanin pigment protects against UV penetration to the deeper layers of cells. The common tumours, basal cell and squamous cell carcinomas, seem to result from chronic overexposure; malignant melanoma correlates better with acute and intense exposure.

Chemicals

Coal Tars, Oils and Cigarette Smoke

Percival Pott, in 1775, described carcinoma of the scrotal skin in chimney sweeps and attributed it to the soot. Similarly, mule-spinners in mills developed tumours because of the oil that soaked their clothing and, even today, motor mechanics are at risk from lubricating oils. However, the greatest problem at present from this group of chemicals is cigarette smoke. This contains many known *carcinogenic* substances, including benzo[a]pyrene, a potent carcinogen also present in coal tars. Not only do smokers have a very greatly increased incidence of lung cancer; they also have a higher risk of cancer at several other sites, such as the bladder. Chemicals that are able to cause tumours are called *direct carcinogens*, but most require metabolism to the active chemical and so are called *procarcinogens*.

Aniline Dyes and the Rubber Industry

Workers in the chemical industry, particularly those involved in making dyes, were found to develop bladder cancer. A similar risk was noted in the rubber-processing industry. The chemical implicated, β-naphthylamine, needs to be metabolised in the kidney, thus releasing the active ingredient into the urine.

Asbestos

Many particulate minerals are now recognised as carcinogenic, including asbestos. The blue asbestos (crocidolite) particles used for insulation are easily inhaled when very small but are then retained within the lung. Over a period of decades, they may then cause tumours of the pleura (malignant mesothelioma); they also correlate with bronchial cancer, particularly if associated with smoking. Asbestos-related fatalities therefore have compensation implications for families.

Hormones

Are endogenous chemicals such as hormones carcinogenic? There is no doubt that hormone levels are important in hormonally responsive organs and their cancers. Whether the hormone is actually carcinogenic or simply contributes to the process of carcinogenesis by promoting cell proliferation is debatable; the latter is more probable. The relationship between oestrogens and endometrial cancer is discussed in Chapter 28. Oestrogens in breast cancers and androgens in prostate cancers play major roles, and hence hormonal manipulation is an important therapeutic tool in such cancer treatment.

Viruses and Cancer

As viruses contain genetic material and gain access to the inside of cells, they have long been suspected of having a role in carcinogenesis. This speculation has been fuelled by finding close similarity between some viral genes and oncogenes. Viruses are clearly responsible for a variety of tumours in several species, such as leukaemias in mice and cats and sarcomas in chickens. In humans, common skin warts are self-limiting benign tumours caused by a virus. Over recent years, these human papilloma (wart) viruses (HPVs) have been found to be a large family of related organisms, some of which correlate closely with cancer of the uterine cervix and a subset of anal, penile, vulvar, vaginal and oropharyngeal cancers. Similarly, Epstein-Barr virus, which is very widespread and causes infectious mononucleosis, is closely associated with tumours such as Hodgkin lymphoma, Burkitt's lymphoma (a high-grade non-Hodgkin lymphoma) and nasopharyngeal carcinoma. Within mesenchymal malignancies, HHV8, the Kaposi's sarcoma–associated herpesvirus (KSHV), is associated with all varieties of Kaposi's sarcoma, whether human immunodeficiency virus (HIV) related, endemic or sporadic.

Infectivity and Cancer

Some patients, or their relatives, worry that cancer may be infectious. It is possible to allay these fears and assure them that this is not the case. The association with viruses mentioned above is a rare sequel to agents widely present in the community; the cancer cannot be passed on.

Immunity and Cancer

The immune system exists to detect and eliminate foreign substances, from isolated molecules to whole organisms. This is effected by antibodies and cells, principally lymphocytes. In the development of a tumour, it is quite possible for new or inappropriate antigens to be generated, provoking an immune response. There are several examples of rare and common tumours with evidence of an immune response, evidenced by the presence of numerous lymphocytes within and around the tumour. Indeed, subcategories of immune cells in the tumour microenvironment are being increasingly recognised for their complex roles in tumour development and progression. These include not only a variety of lymphocytes (CD3 and CD8 positive protective cytotoxic T cells; CD4 positive helper T cells, including the cancer-promoting Th2 and Th17 cells and regulatory T cells, Tregs, which may secrete immunosuppressive cytokines; immunity promoting effector B cells and immune inhibiting regulatory B cells) but also macrophages, (both classical-activated proinflammatory M1 and alternative activated antiinflammatory M2 macrophages), neutrophils including immunosuppressive myeloid cells, mast cells and so on. When in contact with tumour cells, the immune population secretes cytokines, which may either potentiate or abrogate the immune environment and contribute to tumour containment/progression. Histopathology reports of common tumours such as colorectal, breast, melanomas and seminoma of the testis may therefore include a comment on the density of tumour-infiltrating lymphocytes. Studies of patients have correlated the density of lymphocytes with survival, often showing an advantage to those with an immune response. With malignant melanoma of the skin, there is slightly more evidence to suggest a significant favourable immune response in some patients. Microscopic examination sometimes shows areas of apparent regression within the primary growth. There are also some patients with advanced melanoma who respond to stimulation of their immune system against the tumour (immunotherapy).

Despite a few encouraging observations, it is obvious that a large proportion of clinical cancer is beyond the capability of the patient's immune system. In some cases, there is evidence that tumour cells may simply evade it. This is achieved by multiple mechanisms such as local immune evasion, induction of tolerance, and disruption of the T lymphocyte signalling pathways. In developing neoplasms, there might indeed be a selection pressure of less immunogenic apoptosis-resistant cells, a process termed *immune editing*. Indeed, developing immunotherapeutic approaches now seek to either stimulate immune effector mechanisms in tumours (e.g. interferon and aldesleukin) or attempt to counteract inhibitory pathways (e.g. checkpoint inhibitors). A further advancement in the field is CAR (chimeric antigen receptor)-T-cell therapy. In simple terms, this involves incorporation of a new gene into the patient's T cells to equip them to better detect and kill malignant cells. B-cell acute lymphoblastic leukaemia, diffuse large B-cell lymphoma and primary mediastinal B-cell lymphoma are some neoplasms where this therapy is being implemented.

Immune Surveillance

The normal immune system actively seeks foreign material, apparently screening everything against its memory bank to distinguish self from nonself. This may allow the detection and elimination of some cancers before they are clinically established. For example, renal transplant patients require drugs to suppress their immune response for the new kidney to survive. These patients have many more skin tumours than would otherwise be expected, possibly as a result of loss of immune surveillance. Patients with AIDS suffer from a wide range of tumours, but this does not necessarily imply that loss of immune surveillance is the key event. Many patients with defects of the immune system (as a result of either disease or treatment) have an increase in tumours of lymphocytes, but this is probably a different phenomenon.

Injury and Cancer

For injury to be acceptable as a cause of cancer, three factors must be considered: (1) the injury would need to be severe enough to have caused tissue damage; (2) there must be evidence that the site was previously normal and the tumour arose at the site of injury; and (3) the time interval must be long enough to be plausible, generally several years. The mechanism is presumably via a nonspecific induction of cell division as part of the repair process, rather than anything actually carcinogenic. There are a few instances that fulfil these criteria, but the usual circumstance is simply that the injury draws attention to a preexisting tumour.

PRECANCEROUS LESIONS

There are a number of conditions in which there is an increased risk of the subsequent development of cancer. Some are disorders that are not of themselves neoplastic but carry a risk of cancer. Others are more like a halfway house in which the process of development towards cancer is recognisable as neither normal nor cancer. Some are benign tumours that may change to be malignant. In none is the development of cancer inevitable, although the risk and timescale vary greatly. Some examples include the following:

- Undescended testis is an abnormality of development: it carries a high risk of neoplasia.
- Paget's disease of bone, a condition of middle to late adult life, has a risk of osteosarcoma, a tumour otherwise seen in adolescence.
- Solar/actinic keratosis is a warty skin lesion as a result of sun exposure; it may progress to cancer.

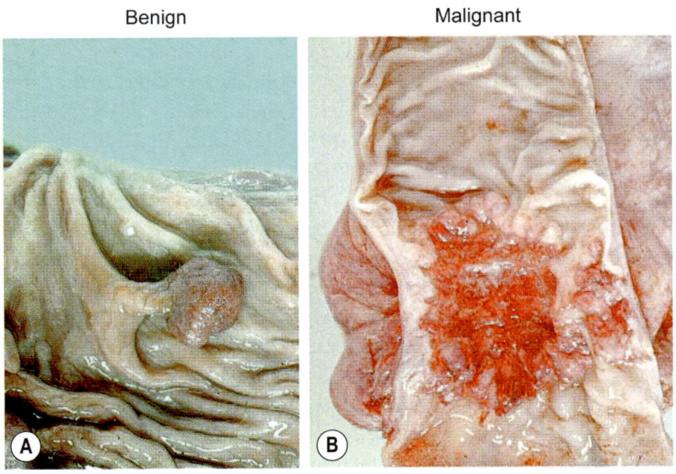

Fig. 17.2 Benign (A) and malignant (B) colorectal tumours.

- Leukoplakia, a whitish patch in the mouth or vulva, is a descriptive term including several conditions. Some run the risk of cancer later.
- Erythroplakia, a fiery reddish patch in the mouth, is a morphological appearance that has strong relationships to cancers in the oral cavity.
- Barrett's metaplasia, a change in the squamous epithelium of the oesophagus to intestinal-type epithelium, increases the risk of dysplasia and subsequent carcinoma.
- Dysplasia may be detected at several sites (e.g. stomach, colon, urothelium), and indicates a microscopic abnormality of cells with some, but not all, features of malignancy. Carcinoma-in-situ may be seen on a surface (e.g. cervix) or within the lumen of a duct (intraductal carcinoma of the breast). This has all the microscopic features of cancer, but the cells are still confined to their normal anatomical limits—that is, they have not invaded.
- Adenomatous polyp of the large intestine (Fig. 17.2A) is a benign tumour. However, it may develop into a malignant tumour. In the condition, familial adenomatous polyposis, there are so many polyps (thousands) that malignancy (Fig. 17.2B) becomes inevitable, often at an earlier age. In addition to the malignant potential of adenomas, it is now becoming apparent that large hyperplastic polyps of the right colon and those with a serrated morphology (sessile serrated lesions) can also progress to cancer but by a different molecular pathway.

An important consideration is that the detection of some of these conditions allows surgical intervention before cancer becomes established.

Field Change

Although an individual tumour arises from a single cell, within the vicinity of that cell there are often other cells partway through carcinogenesis. Removal of the tumour or of its precursor lesion may be followed by the local development of further lesions. This is regarded as a field change across the whole area. An example would be the appearance of cancer on the tongue following removal of one from the buccal mucosa. Common alterations in areas of field changes include mutations, aberrant methylation leading to reduced gene expression (e.g. DNA repair genes) and altered protein profiles.

NATURAL HISTORY AND SPREAD OF CANCER

As stated earlier, benign tumours remain localised, often separated from surrounding tissue by a capsule. The tumour has relatively little effect on the adjacent structures, unless it arises in a particularly critical site, and surgical removal is curative. In contrast, malignant tumours show a capacity to invade, frequently recur after surgery, spread to other sites and result in the death of the patient. The initial or primary site of tumour growth thus gives rise to separate secondary tumours, or metastases. Some tumours, such as basal cell carcinoma of the skin, have an intermediate behaviour; they invade locally but do not give rise to metastases.

In summary, spread may occur in several ways (Fig. 17.3):

- By local invasion
- By lymphatic vessels
- By blood vessels
- Across cavities

Local Invasion

As the tumour invades, adjacent tissues are displaced and destroyed to be replaced by tumour. The tumour margin is ill-defined and irregular. Surgical removal therefore needs to include a generous extent of normal tissue. Failure to do so results in some tumour being left behind which proliferates and gives rise to *local recurrence*. Radiotherapy is frequently used after surgery to prevent this situation. The invasion often follows anatomical tissue planes; it may be temporarily halted by some dense structure such as bone, until this is also eroded. Certain anatomical sites may be more prone to local recurrence, such as the nonperitonealised resection margin in the lower rectum.

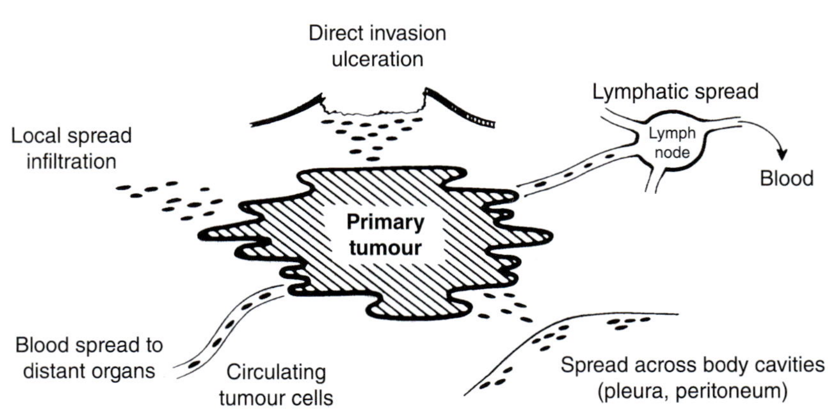

Fig. 17.3 Metastasis or secondary spread. Tumours can spread by a variety of routes including local spread, spread through the lymphatics via the blood and across cavities. (Reproduced from Calman KC, Smyth JF, Tattersall MHN. *Basic principles of cancer chemotherapy*. London, New York: Macmillan; 1980.)

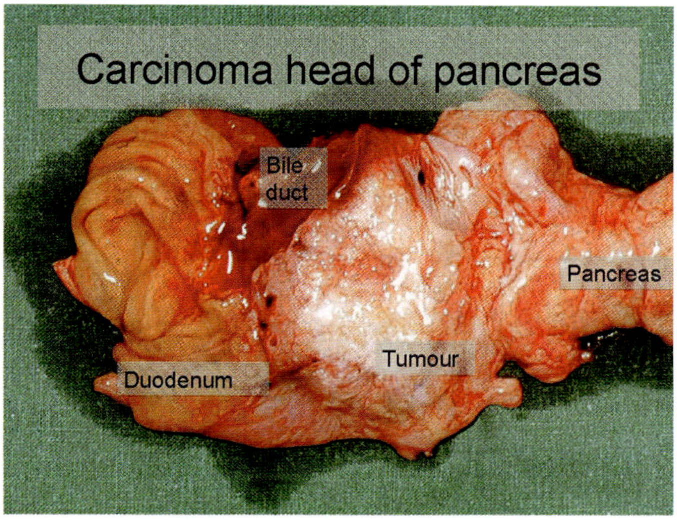

Fig. 17.4 Carcinoma of head of pancreas.

Functional Effects

The effects a tumour produces will depend upon the site involved; a knowledge of anatomy and physiology allows prediction of many symptoms. Thus a tumour in the head of the pancreas will soon obstruct the bile duct so that the patient becomes jaundiced (Fig. 17.4). A tumour of the left lung may obstruct its bronchus, with resultant pneumonia from infection of retained secretions. Further local invasion of this mass will compress the recurrent laryngeal nerve and the patient's voice will be altered. Further growth may obstruct the superior vena cava passing through the mediastinum, causing discoloration (cyanosis) and swelling of the face and arms (superior vena caval obstruction syndrome). If the cervical sympathetic chain is involved, this may manifest as Horner's syndrome (with droopy eyelids, less sweating on the face and constriction of the pupil).

A tumour just beneath the skin can so stretch it and impair its nutrition that it breaks down to form an ulcer. This is then liable to infection or bleeding. Pain and weakness will occur when peripheral nerves are affected, for example, Pancoast tumour at the apex of the lung invading upwards to compress nerves to the arm and hand.

The extent of local invasion dictates the extent of surgery necessary to remove it and, indeed, may render the tumour inoperable if critical structures are involved. However, the usual reason why a tumour is 'inoperable' is because of metastatic disease. Sometimes it is worth debulking the tumour, but surgery alone is insufficient to cure the patient.

Metastasis

The hallmark of tumour cells is the ability to spread to distant sites of the body (metastases). The molecular events leading to the development of metastases are thought to follow either a linear or a parallel mode of progression. The models differ in the relative timing of emergence of the metastatic precursor clone in the primary tumour, arising and disseminating late in the linear model, just before clinical detection of the primary, whereas in the parallel model, the metastatic clone is thought to evolve alongside and disseminate early from the primary. In the first model, the genetic divergence between the primary and secondary is small whereas it is substantial in the latter. In fact, the latter theory postulates that dissemination of metastasis may occur in multiple waves even before the primary tumour is clinically detectable. Different clones of metastases may even seed at different sites through different routes of spread. The major routes of metastases of tumours and clinical implications thereof are explained below.

By Lymphatic Vessels

Invasive tumours readily penetrate the thin wall of lymphatics. Then, fragments of tumour are carried downstream to lodge in one or more local lymph nodes. If the tumour cells survive this journey and proliferate in the node, they form a *metastasis*, or secondary tumour. Further dissemination may proceed to other lymph nodes along the chain, for example, from pelvic to paraaortic to supraclavicular nodes. Some primary tumours remain tiny, yet have massive nodal deposits. If the node capsule is breached by tumour, the whole mass becomes fixed to surrounding structures. In some tumours, such as breast cancers or melanomas, it may be possible to identify the first lymph node/s (sentinel node/s) draining the region of the cancer and evaluate whether these are involved or not, with a view to modifying the treatment plan based on the involvement status of these nodes. In other tumours, such as colorectal cancer, involvement of the lymph node at the site of arterial ligation (the high-tie lymph node) forms part of the synoptic pathology report and may imply poorer prognosis. Knowledge of propensity of spread of tumours to some lymph node groups may guide treatment planning. The classical dog leg field of radiation used in the treatment of testicular seminomas is based on the tenet that this field includes the lymph nodes (paraaortic and ipsilateral pelvic) most likely to be involved by this malignancy.

By Blood Vessels

Thin-walled blood vessels are similarly at risk of tumour invasion, and again, fragments of tumour float passively downstream. (Single tumour cells are generally destroyed by nonspecific defence mechanisms in the blood.) These then lodge in the next capillary bed, where they may develop into metastases. Although this can happen in any tissue, the liver, lungs and bone (Fig. 17.5) are by far the most frequent sites for secondaries.

Across Cavities (Transcoelomic)

Access to the pleura enables tumour cells to seed themselves around the pleural cavity, forming numerous further deposits or seedlings. These may be associated with secretion of fluid into the cavity, with resultant impairment of respiration. An identical process may occur in the peritoneum; the fluid accumulation is called *ascites*. Malignant cells may settle on the ovaries (Krukenberg tumours) or all over the omentum and peritoneum (Fig. 17.6). Related to this, some intracranial tumours, such as medulloblastoma of the cerebellum, may disseminate

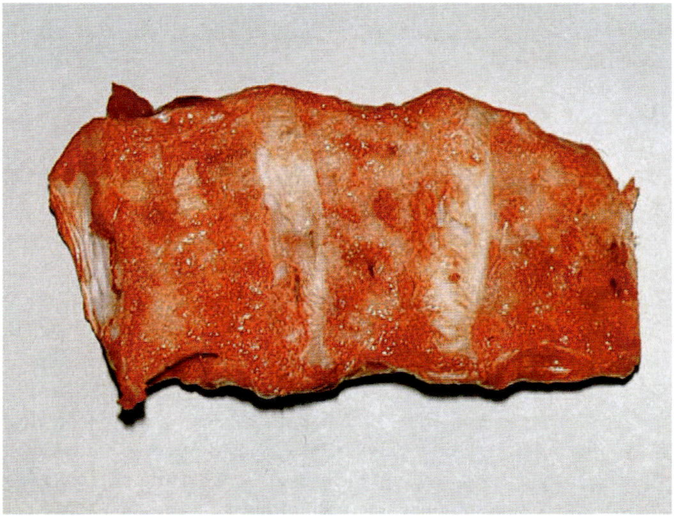

Fig. 17.5 Bone metastatic carcinoma.

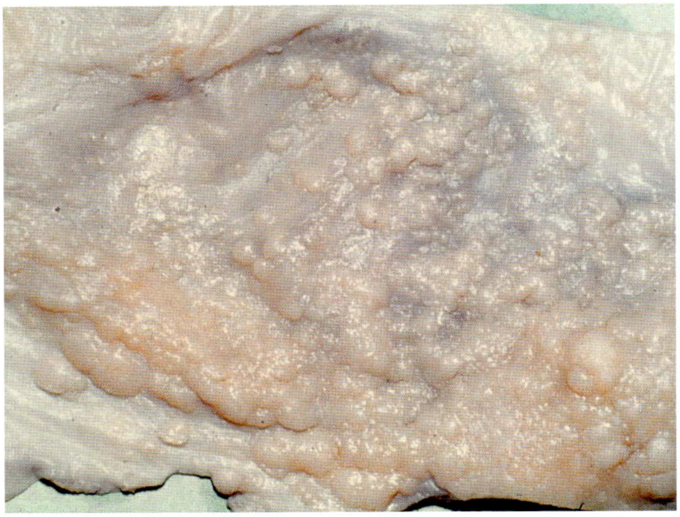

Fig. 17.6 Peritoneal deposits of metastatic carcinoma.

by the cerebral spinal fluid (CSF), seeding over the surface of the brain and down the spinal canal (see Chapters 31 and 34). Indeed, radiation treatment often preempts and abrogates this possibility by inclusion of spinal fields during treatment planning.

Implantation

Occasionally, cells may be implanted in the scar by the surgeon's knife while removing a tumour, or through a pleural or abdominal paracentesis drainage site.

Functioning Tumours

Many tumour cells continue certain cell functions related to their tissue of origin but, in some, this has a profound effect on the patient. Tumours of endocrine glands typically produce an excess of their hormone. The problem is that the tumour is no longer responsive to the usual control of secretion. Thus an adrenal cortex tumour will produce steroids despite switching off its pituitary drive, and Cushing syndrome will result.

In other circumstances, the hormone production is quite inappropriate for the tumour site. Many lung tumours produce substances that mimic the function of parathyroid hormone, antidiuretic hormone or adrenocorticotrophic hormone. Again, it is not subject to the normal control of secretion, and the clinical consequences may be severe. Some of the other effects that tumours may have, such as profound weight loss (cancer cachexia), could be caused by tumour-derived proteolytically generated peptides.

Cause of Death From Cancer

As the word *malignant* implies, death is the natural consequence of untreated cancer. Sometimes the tumour will have grown locally and spread in a predictable manner. In other cases, the primary site remains undetected despite widespread metastatic deposits. Some tumours show relentless progression and run their course in a few months; others take many years, with long intervals of apparent dormancy.

Many patients with locally advanced or metastatic cancer become bedridden and die from bronchopneumonia, inanition and/or metabolic disturbance. Sometimes there may be liver failure because of numerous liver secondaries. Often the actual cause of death is unclear. It is important to consider carrying out a postmortem examination if there is reasonable doubt about the cause of death. Patients with cancer are still at risk of nonneoplastic conditions such as coronary artery disease. This is particularly likely in patients who smoke. Indeed, smoking may have given rise both to the primary tumour (e.g. in the lung, oral cavity or pharynx) and to ischaemic heart disease.

It is important to make a judgment as to whether the patient died from cancer or from an unrelated condition, because this influences cancer mortality statistics. Where a patient has remained disease free from cancer for more than 5 years, and the cause of death is said to be cancer, this conclusion should be questioned. However, late relapses can occur after 5 years, in breast cancer, for example. Alternatively, a new primary may develop, especially in head and neck cancer.

STAGING OF CANCERS

It is of the greatest practical importance in many cases to estimate the extent of the spread of a tumour at the time of initial diagnosis. This process is called *staging*. Staging often influences the choice of treatment and can provide valuable information on prognosis. Staging may include clinical, pathological, radiological and biochemical information. This enables similar groups of patients to be compared between different oncology centres nationally and internationally. A number of staging classifications are in use. The simplest and oldest classification is:

Stage 1: Tumour confined to the organ of origin
Stage 2: Local lymph nodes invaded
Stage 3: Distant nodes invaded, or local spread beyond the organ of origin
Stage 4: Blood-borne metastasis present

This classification is still used with some cancers, although often with slight modification to bring in subcategories, as with the International Federation of Gynecology and Obstetrics (FIGO) system for cervical cancer. The Union for International Cancer Control (UICC) has worked towards international agreement on the staging of many tumours, coding them on the TNM system (described next).

TNM Classification

The TNM staging system provides an internationally accepted common language platform for clinicians to communicate the extent of cancer and hence aids treatment planning, prognostication and monitoring response to treatment. This includes a succinct summary of the extent of malignancy in the patient and includes a description of the primary tumour (T), nodal spread (N) and distant metastases (M).

The mandatory parameters included are as follows:

T: Size or direct extent/depth of invasion of the primary tumour
- Tx: Tumour cannot be assessed
- Tis: Carcinoma in situ
- T0: No evidence of tumour
- T1, T2, T3, T4: Depending on increasing size or extent of the primary tumour (with T4 often signifying involvement of adjacent structures)

N: Degree of involvement of regional lymph nodes
- Nx: Lymph nodes cannot be assessed
- N0: No evidence of regional lymph node metastasis
- N1: Regional lymph node metastasis present; at some sites, tumour spread to closest or limited number of regional lymph nodes
- N2: Tumour spread to an extent between N1 and N3 (all sites may not have N2)
- N3: Tumour spread to more distant or greater number of regional lymph nodes (N3, not for all sites)

M: Presence/absence of distant metastasis
- M0: No distant metastasis
- M1: Spread to distant organs (beyond lymph nodes)

Given the increase in tumour burden with the increasing value of numerical qualifiers, T1N0M0 would represent a very early cancer,

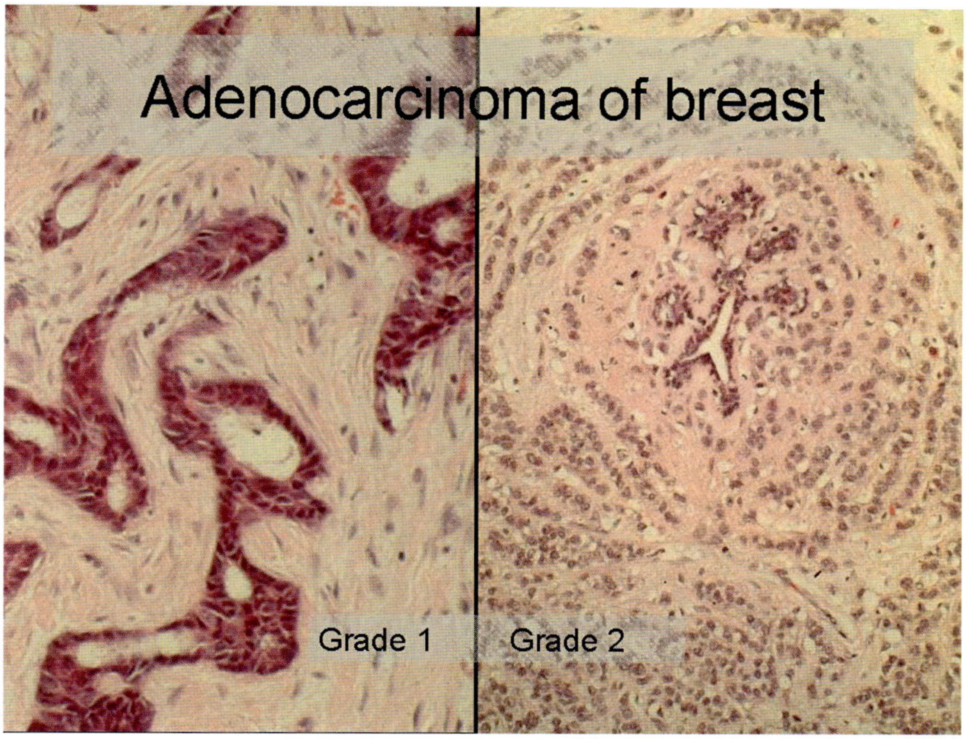

Fig. 17.7 Adenocarcinoma of breast (grade 1 and grade 2).

whereas T4N3M1 indicates a very advanced cancer. The details of how to categorise a tumour may vary between sites; the TNM classification for breast cancer is shown in Table 27.4.

Other nonmandatory parameters that are now being increasingly used as adjuncts to the basic TNM parameters include G (1–4) for the grade of differentiation, S (0–3) for various levels of serum tumour markers, R (0–2) for the completeness of surgical excision at margins, L (0–1) for lymphovascular invasion and V (0–2) for blood vascular (typically venous) invasion.

The clinical staging may differ from the pathological staging. For example, a tumour in the breast may be measured clinically as 2 cm in diameter and thus be staged as T1. However, when actually measured directly in the mastectomy specimen, it might be 3 cm in maximum diameter and thus be pathologically T2 (abbreviated as pT2). Most staging classifications are based on the clinical extent of spread. The overall stage gets a prefix p if this has been pathologically determined and y if the assessment is after chemotherapy/radiation. These designations help to facilitate discussion at multidisciplinary team meetings to assess inconsistencies between clinical/radiological/pathological staging and the response to neoadjuvant treatment.

Radiological information may influence staging. For example, in carcinoma of the cervix, the presence of an obstructed kidney on ultrasound or other investigation (in the absence of a nonneoplastic cause) automatically indicates stage 3B.

The staging of testicular cancer is an example in which tumour biochemical information (the presence of the serum tumour markers lactate dehydrogenase, alpha-fetoprotein and human chorionic gonadotrophin) is included. S0 signifies markers are at normal levels; S1 slightly raised markers; S2 moderately raised markers; and S3 very high levels of markers.

HISTOLOGICAL GRADING: DIFFERENTIATION

In an effort to predict the future course of a tumour, an estimate is made of how malignant it is for a particular site and type of tumour. Generally speaking, the closer a tumour cell resembles its normal counterpart—that is, the better it is differentiated—the more orderly and slower its growth. Thus histological examination allows tumour grading on the basis of the extent of differentiation. Attention is given to the nucleus (how abnormal it is and how often mitosis is observed) and the cytoplasm (the extent to which normal structures are seen). In cancers such as breast cancer, the grading scheme also includes the proportion of cancer cells still retaining glandular/tubular differentiation (Figs. 17.7 and 17.8). In others, such as pancreatic neuroendocrine tumours, the proliferative fraction, as determined by Ki67 immunohistochemistry or the mitotic count, helps to determine the grade. The Ki67 index is currently based on at least 500 cells in areas of hot spots and is expressed as follows: less than 3%, grade 1; 3% to 20%, grade 2; greater than 20%, grade 3. Mitoses are counted in approximately 10

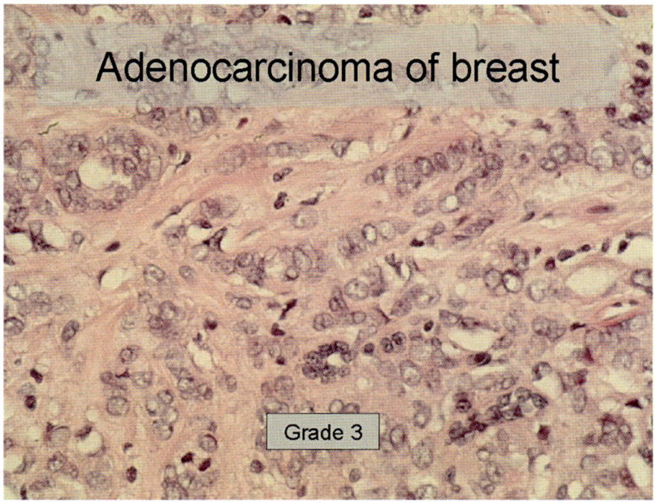

Fig. 17.8 Adenocarcinoma of breast (grade 3).

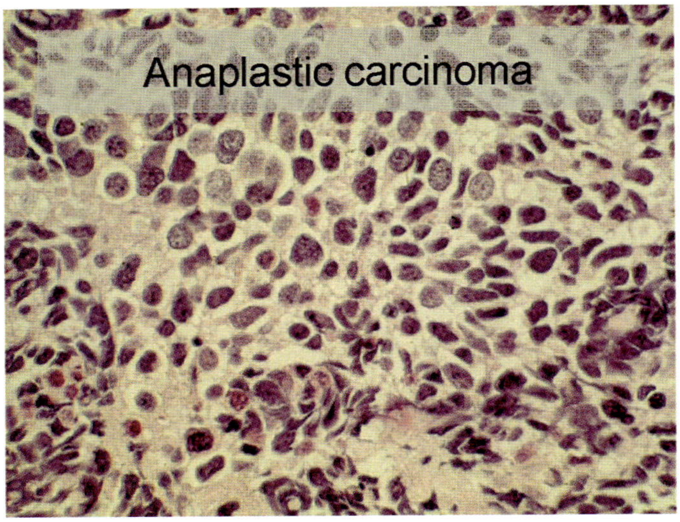

Fig. 17.9 Histological features of an anaplastic carcinoma.

high power fields (hpf), adjusted per microscope specifications, each hpf being 0.2 mm^2 with at least 50 consecutive fields evaluated at hot spots.; the cutoffs are grade 1, less than 2/10 hpf; grade 2, 2–20/10 hpf; grade 3, greater than 20/10 hpf. The final grade is determined by the worse of the Ki67 index or mitotic count. The grading system used for sarcomas, the French Federation of Cancer Centers Sarcoma Group (FNCLCC) system, incorporates necrosis as a parameter in addition to differentiation and mitoses.

For most of the common tumours, the pathologist divides them into descriptive categories: well differentiated, moderately differentiated and poorly differentiated. Undifferentiated tumours lack sufficient features to allow more than a broad classification, as do anaplastic tumours (Fig. 17.9) (see the 'Classification of Neoplasm' section).

Limitations of Grading

First, assessment of grading has an element of subjectivity, and there may be a variation between pathologists in assigning pleomorphism and hence grades across different categories. Also, Ki67 assessment, where required, may be prone to errors of subjective quantification. Indeed, new technology such as digital pathology helps to overcome such errors. Biologically, some tumours show a tight correlation between histological grading and behaviour, such that treatment is guided by this information. Cancer of the bladder is one of these. However, the tumour stage is of overriding importance. Some tumours (e.g. pancreatic islet) have a high variable rate of clinical progression but uniform histology; grading in this circumstance is misleading if attempted. Other tumours vary considerably from one microscopic field to another: in general, the outlook will depend upon the worst areas, but these could be missed without adequate sampling. Finally, the organ of origin is important: a well-differentiated cancer of the skin carries an excellent prognosis, whereas in the lung it may not.

GROWTH RATE OF CANCERS

As indicated in the 'Carcinogenesis' section, there is usually a considerable time between initiation of a tumour and its clinical detection. Part of this time is taken by the process of becoming a cancer cell and part by growing to a sufficient size to be found. The latter can be measured as the time taken for it to double in diameter, its *doubling time*. A mass 1 mm in diameter would represent about one million cells: this could result from one cell, and each of its subsequent daughter cells, dividing 20 times. A word of caution is needed before theorising further. Once a tumour exceeds about 2 mm, it is essential for it to have its own blood supply: this, together with other supporting structures, is the *tumour stroma*. In some tumours the stroma is very scanty, whereas in others it constitutes the majority of the mass. (The character of the stroma also influences what the tumour feels like on palpation; most breast cancers are hard because of abundant, dense stroma.) Thus calculations about how many cancer cells there are in a tumour of a certain size will be incorrect if they ignore the stroma. With the advent of molecular diagnostics, which often require a minimum tumour load to be present to achieve the limit of detection, accurate assessment of the number of tumour cells in a pathology sample is becoming more important.

Another consideration is that the clinical growth of a tumour will be the result of the balance between cell proliferation and loss. It will be influenced too by the growth fraction or proportion of cancer cells actually proliferating. Many cancer cells in a tumour cease to proliferate as they differentiate, or produce nonviable daughter cells. Furthermore, if the vascularity of the stroma is inadequate, there will be necrosis.

Although a cancer produces an expanding mass, this is a reflection of loss of control of growth. The actual rate at which individual cancer cells divide may be slower than comparable normal tissues. If there is a very sudden increase in the size of a tumour, it will probably reflect internal hemorrhage or fluid accumulation. (On the other hand, a slow-growing mass which begins to grow faster may have changed from benign to malignant.)

Observation of established clinical cancers has shown that doubling times vary widely but average about 2 months. Leaving aside the question of whether this is true for the first 20 doublings to reach a 1-mm size, it would require about a further 10 doublings (i.e. 20 months) to reach a 1-cm diameter, at which point it might be detectable. Many tumours are 2 cm or more in diameter before they produce symptoms, so a considerable time has elapsed between the first emergence of a clone of cancer cells and the clinical disease. In comparison with that, the remainder of its course, if unchecked, is liable to be over after five or so more doublings. Metastatic deposits may be disseminated during the preclinical period, only to appear after removal of the primary. If the doubling time is considerably more than 2 months, the whole process takes on a much longer timescale.

Bearing these matters in mind, there is no fixed length of disease-free interval that equates with a cure. However, for practical purposes, 5 years disease free is tantamount to cure for many of the common tumours, with breast cancer as a notable exception. The earlier detection of a cancer at a minute size increases the possibility of removal before metastases develop, even if the tumour has been around for a long time. Prolonged postoperative survival in these patients may simply reflect earlier diagnosis rather than longer survival, a phenomenon called *lead-time bias*.

Spontaneous Regression of Cancer

Occasionally, a tumour may regress and disappear without treatment, although the original diagnosis could have been erroneous. Most of the reported cases are renal cell carcinoma, malignant melanoma and gestational choriocarcinoma. In all these instances, immunological mechanisms are thought to be responsible. Some cases of lymphoid tumours fluctuate in size, and may temporarily disappear, only to return later. In some cases of neuroblastoma, a primitive tumour of nerve cells, there is subsequent differentiation and growth ceases.

CLASSIFICATION OF NEOPLASMS

Table 17.2 lists examples of tumour nomenclature. In general, the names are built up from one part to describe the tissue type and

TABLE 17.2 Types of Neoplasms

Type	Benign	Malignant
Epithelial		Carcinoma
Squamous	Papilloma	Squamous cell carcinoma
Transitional	Papilloma	Transitional cell carcinoma
Basal cell	Papilloma	Basal cell carcinoma
Glandular	Adenoma	Adenocarcinoma
Mesenchymal		Sarcoma
Smooth muscle	Leiomyoma	Leiomyosarcoma
Striated muscle	Rhabdomyoma	Rhabdomyosarcoma
Fat	Lipoma	Liposarcoma
Blood vessels	Angioma	Angiosarcoma
Bone	Osteoma	Osteosarcoma
Cartilage	Chondroma	Chondrosarcoma
Hematological		Lymphoma
Lymphoid tissue		Hodgkin lymphoma
		Non-Hodgkin lymphoma
Plasma cell		Multiple myeloma
White blood cells		Leukaemia
Intracranial and neural		
Supporting cells		Glioma
Meninges	Meningioma	
Cerebellum		Medulloblastoma
Retina		Retinoblastoma
Sympathetic nerve	Ganglioneuroma	Neuroblastoma
Pigment cells of		
Skin or eye gonad	Mole or nevus	Malignant melanoma
Germ cells	Dermoid cyst mature teratoma (Fig. 17.10)	Malignant teratoma
		Seminoma
Placenta	Hydatidiform mole	Choriocarcinoma

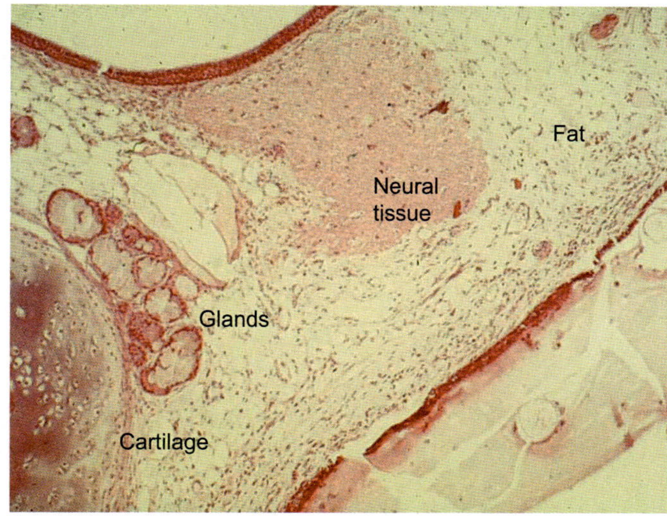

Fig. 17.10 Microscopic features of a mature teratoma.

another to indicate its behaviour. All end in *oma* to denote a lump, a suffix almost restricted to neoplasms, although a few other terms are in use, such as *hematoma* for an accumulation of blood. Most malignant tumours fall into the following broad categories:

- Carcinoma
- Sarcoma
- Lymphoma

The majority of tumours arise from epithelium (surface lining cells). Benign tumours are called *papilloma* (Fig. 17.11) or *adenoma*; malignant tumours are called *carcinoma*, often with a prefix to give the cell type. Carcinoma is Latin/Greek for 'crab' but is used in a more restricted sense than cancer and applied only to epithelial malignancy, which makes up 75% of cancer.

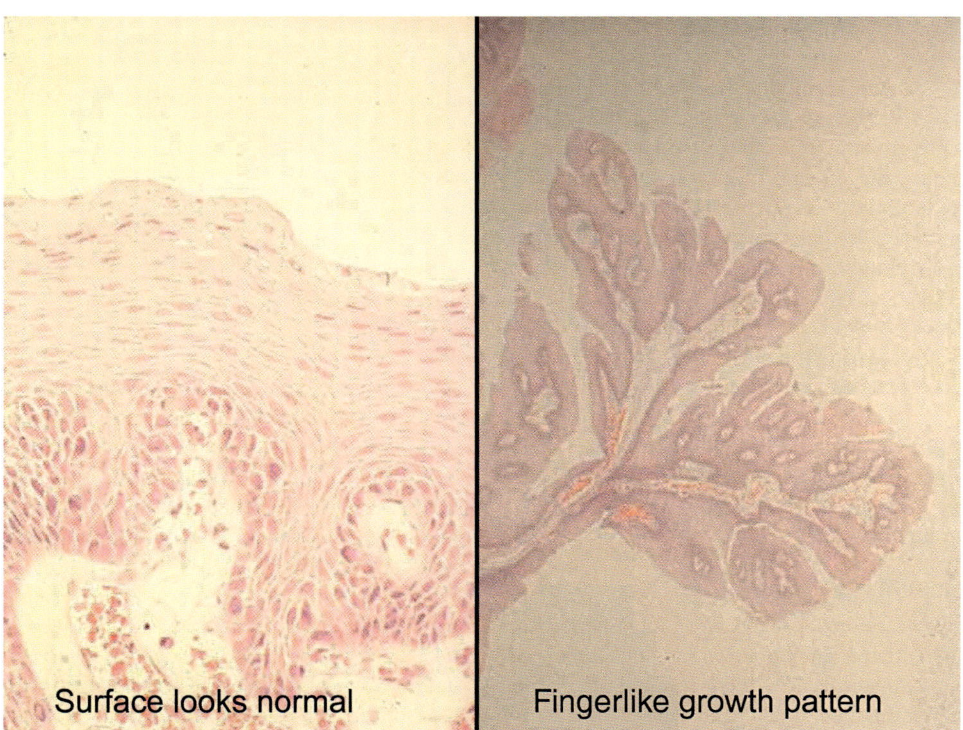

Fig. 17.11 Squamous papilloma.

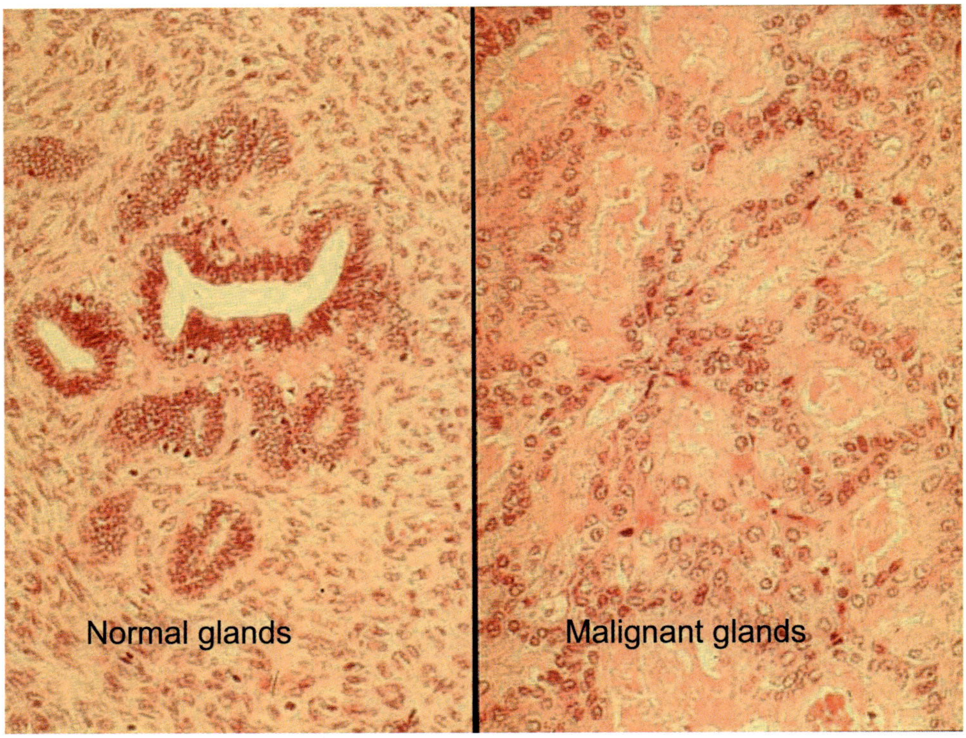

Fig. 17.12 Adenocarcinoma of endometrium.

Squamous epithelium lines the skin, where it is called *epidermis*, the upper aerodigestive tract (mouth, pharynx, larynx, oesophagus), anus, vagina and cervix. It is present in the bronchi if there is metaplasia. Transitional cell epithelium (or urothelium) lines the renal pelvis, ureters and bladder.

Glandular (secretory) epithelium lines the gut from stomach to rectum and forms the related secretory glands (salivary, pancreas, biliary tract and liver), endocrine glands (pituitary, thyroid, parathyroids and adrenals), kidneys, ovarian surface, endometrium (Fig. 17.12) and breast (Figs. 17.7 and 17.8).

Sometimes the tumour name is combined with a description of shape or function. If a cyst is formed, it may be cystadenoma or cystadenocarcinoma, both of which are common in the ovary. Mucin-secreting variants would be mucinous cystadenoma.

Sarcoma denotes any tumour of mesenchymal origin (supporting structures). They are much less frequent than carcinoma. Metastasis from sarcomas is generally blood-borne, and few give rise to lymph node secondaries (Fig. 17.13).

Lymphomas are malignant tumours of lymphoid cells; many are classified as Hodgkin lymphoma, leaving the remainder as non-Hodgkin lymphoma. Some are closely related to leukaemias (tumours of white blood cells).

There are many tumours that do not easily fit the guidelines mentioned, such as ovarian and testicular teratomas (refer to Fig. 17.14); some are shown in Table 17.2 and others are referred to elsewhere in this book under the relevant organ.

Undifferentiated Tumours

Some tumours lack obvious features to allow their identification or classification. An undifferentiated carcinoma or sarcoma cannot be ascribed to any subcategory. An anaplastic tumour could be carcinoma, lymphoma or sarcoma. Because these different categories have major therapeutic consequences, it is important to attempt a more detailed diagnosis. Simple microscopy can now be supplemented by special staining procedures, many of which involve detecting cell components with antibodies. The presence of the leukocyte common antigen (CD45), B-cell (CD20) marker or T-cell (CD3) marker would indicate a lymphoma, whereas finding broad spectrum cytokeratins (AE1/3, MNF116, CAM5.2) would suggest a carcinoma (Fig. 17.15). Positivity for only mesenchymal markers (smooth muscle actin, desmin) would indicate a sarcoma, whereas positivity for melanocytic markers (S100, HMB45, MelanA) would indicate a malignant melanoma. After initial panel probe to determine the basic cell lineage, additional immunohistochemistry proves helpful, especially in metastatic tumours/cancers of unknown primary, such as CDX2 positivity in gastrointestinal cancers, GATA3 for breast/urothelial cancers, TTF1 for lung and thyroid cancers, PAX8 for gyanecological malignancies and PAX2 for renal cancers. Synaptophysin and chromogranin A help to identify tumours with

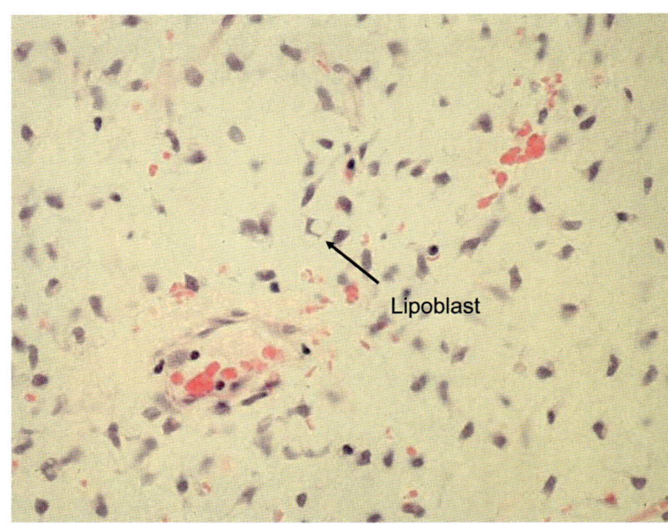

Fig. 17.13 Myxoid liposarcoma.

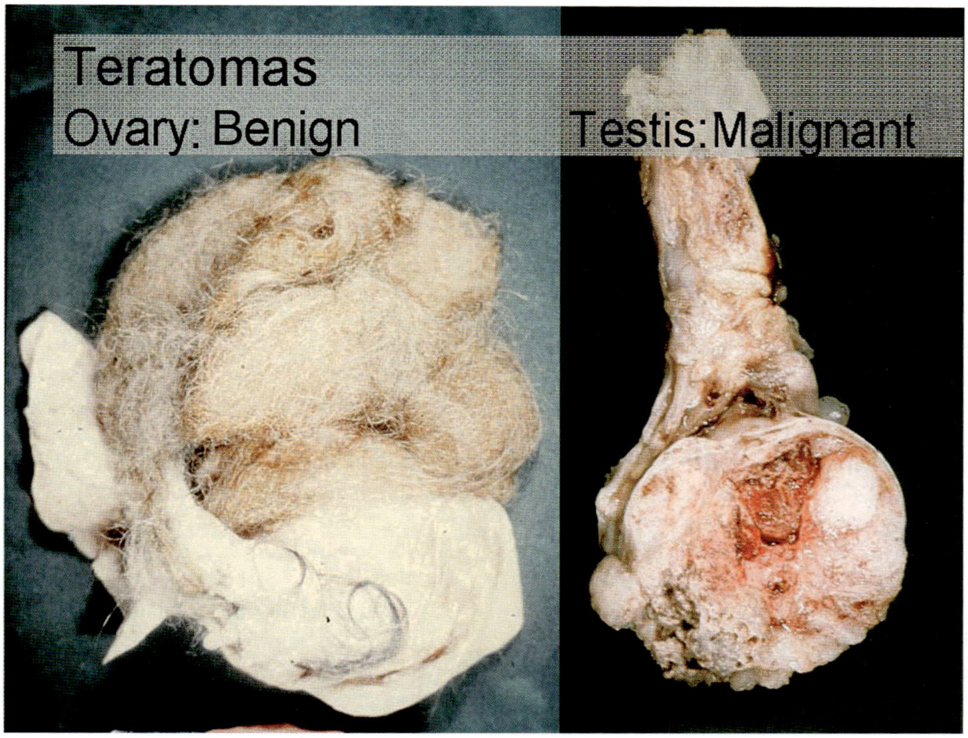

Fig. 17.14 Teratomas: ovary benign, testis malignant.

neuroendocrine differentiation. Indeed, immunostaining approaches have superseded other techniques such as electron microscopy in undifferentiated tumour diagnosis. Because tumours have deranged genetic function, there are other approaches of help, such as cytogenetics, which depend upon finding characteristic abnormalities of the chromosomes. These are most often loss or gain of part or the whole of a chromosome, or translocations in which two chromosomes break and are rejoined with the fragments on the wrong chromosome, for example, the classic t(9;22) in chronic myelogenous leukaemia.

Most oncology centres arrange for many of their patients' tumours to be reviewed before treatment. Diagnosis and classification of rare or undifferentiated tumours form a considerable part of such work.

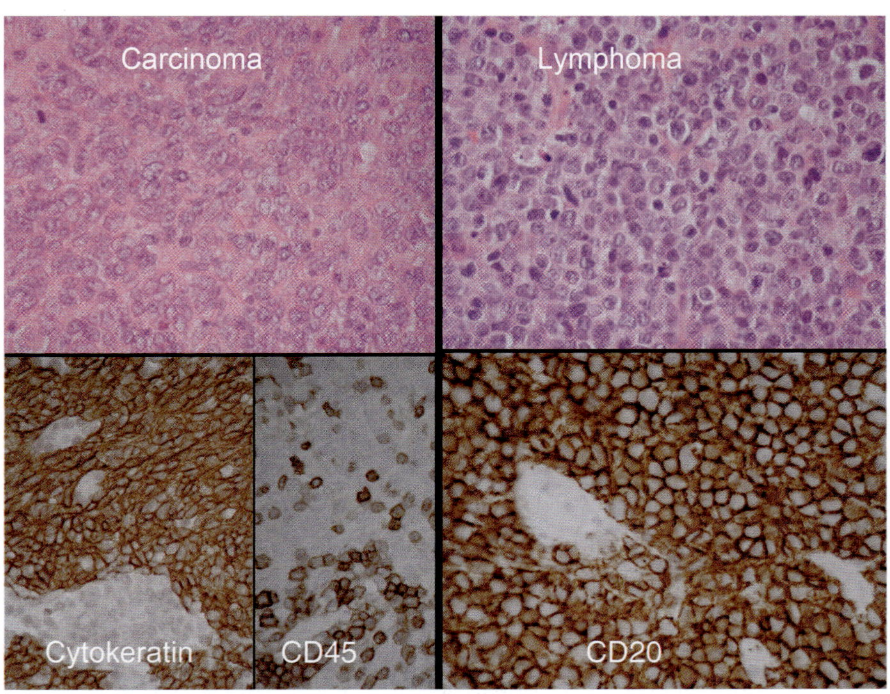

Fig. 17.15 Immunocytochemistry to distinguish lymphoma from carcinoma. (Carcinoma positive for cytokeratin; lymphoma for CD20. CD45 staining only tumour infiltrating lymphocytes in the carcinoma.)

CURRENT ADVANCES IN PATHOLOGY GUIDING PATIENT MANAGEMENT

Molecular Pathology

The molecular pathology revolution has been transformational for oncology. With humble origins, looking at specific proteins by immunohistochemistry, with development of sequencing techniques that are high throughput (next-generation sequencing), the template requirement has shifted to DNA and RNA samples. Hence it is important for clinicians to appreciate the importance of template quality and tumour cellularity in samples to ensure that interpretation is permissible within the limit of detection of the test. The applications of molecular testing affect all aspects of patient management, ranging from prevention, diagnosis and prognostication to prediction of therapeutic efficacy. For example, MMR immunohistochemistry/MSI testing helps in screening for Lynch syndrome in colorectal/endometrial cancers, and IDH1/2 mutation analysis helps to classify gliomas. Several pathological parameters apart from their prognostic value also guide patient management, for example, hormone receptor status in breast cancers (antioestrogens for HER-positive tumours and trastuzumab for HER2-positive tumours). With advances in molecular therapeutics, there is a demand for companion diagnostics to tailor therapy for patients. Examples (see Table 17.3 for examples in some common solid malignancies) include assessing for Ras mutations in colorectal cancers, the presence of which precludes treatment with EGFR tyrosine kinase inhibitors; ALK-EGFR mutations in non-small cell lung cancers for sensitivity to EGFR inhibitors such as Erlotinib and Gefitinib; c-kit mutations in gastrointestinal mutations guiding imatinib treatment; or BRAF mutations in melanomas guiding treatment with BRAF inhibitors, vemurafenib and dabrafenib. Some tests such as OncotypeDx integrate the activity of a panel of genes to figure out the risk of recurrence to guide further chemotherapy in early-stage oestrogen receptor–positive breast cancer or radiation treatment in DCIS (ductal carcinoma in situ). Newer approaches such as testing for circulating tumour DNA now allow screening for early detection of cancer or its recurrence. Immunomodulation is another burgeoning field where pathology is increasingly playing a crucial role in patient selection for therapy. Apart from cancer vaccines utilising cancer antigens to activate the immune response, strategies have been developed to diminish regulatory T cells (CD25-targeted antibodies) which suppress the immune response, and use antibodies against immune-checkpoint molecules such as CTLA-4 and PD1. Immunohistochemical analysis of the programmed death receptor 1 (PD1) and its ligand (PDL-1), for example, in non-small cell lung cancer, is helping to choose patients for treatment with drugs targeting PD-1 (pembrolizumab, nivolumab etc.) or PD-L1 (atezolizumab, durvalumab etc.). With further understanding of the tumour-associated immune response and their modulators, PD-1/PDL-1 testing has gained leverage in additional tumours such as gastrooesophgeal, pancreatic, bladder, breast and so on. Liquid biopsies investigating for circulating tumour DNA/tumour cells for mutational analysis and monitoring for response and recurrence are exciting avenues of research, and technological advances such as chromogenic multiplexing is unravelling the spatiotemporal nuances of tumour biology.

TABLE 17.3 Examples of Common Molecular Pathology Test Requests in Common Malignancies[a]

Type of Cancer	Gene Screened	Rationale
Colorectal cancer	KRAS, BRAF, NRAS	Anti-EGFR therapy contraindicated in RAS mutant tumours
	NTRK1/2/3	*NTRK* fusion–positive cancers may respond to TRK inhibitors, such as larotrectinib or entrectinib.
Non-small cell lung cancer	EGFR	With EGR mutations, treatment with tyrosine kinase inhibitors may be possible, for example, gefitinib, afatinib, erlotinib etc.
	ALK, ROS1, RET, MET (Ex14 skipping), KRAS	Guides response to drugs such as crizotinib (ALK, ROS), ceritinib (ALK), entrectinib (ROS1), tepotinib (MET), selpercatinib (RET), sotorasib (KRas)
	NTRK1/2/3	*NTRK* fusion–positive cancers may respond to TRK inhibitors.
Melanoma	BRAF, KIT, NRAS	Vemurafenib treatment feasible for unresectable or metastatic melanoma harbouring BRAF V600 mutation Melanomas with KIT mutations may respond to tyrosine kinase inhibitors (imatinib and sorafenib). NRAS mutant melanoma: may benefit from immunotherapy
	NTRK1/2/3	*NTRK* fusion–positive cancers may respond to TRK inhibitors.
Gastrointestinal stromal tumour	KIT, PDGFRA	KIT/PDGFRA inhibitors indicated for treatment of GISTs (e.g. imatinib, sunitinib etc); Avapritinib indicated for multiresistant PDGFRA D842V mutation
	NTRK1/2/3	*NTRK* fusion–positive cancers respond to TRK inhibitors.
Breast cancer	PIK3CA	Hormone receptor status positive, HER2-negative, locally advanced or metastatic breast cancer patients with PIK3CA mutations may be treated with alpelisib.
	NTRK1/2/3	*NTRK* fusion–positive cancers may respond to TRK inhibitors, such as larotrectinib or entrectinib.
Cholangiocarcinoma	IDH1	IDH mutations found in a proportion of intrahepatic cholangiocarcinoma may be treated with IDH inhibitors such as ivosidenib.
	FGFR2, NTRK1/2/3	Chonagiocarcinomas with FGFR2 fusions may be treated with inhibitors such as pemigatinib and infigratinib. *NTRK* fusion–positive cancers respond to TRK inhibitors.
Glioma	MGMT methylation	MGMT methylation presence in glioblastomas are associated with a better response to alkylating chemotherapy.
	NTRK1/2/3	*NTRK* fusion–positive cancers respond to TRK inhibitors.
Thyroid cancer	BRAF	BRAF V600E mutant anaplastic thyroid cancer may be amenable for treatment with Dabrafenib (RAF inhibitor) + Trametinib (MEK inhibitor).
	NTRK1/2/3, RET	*NTRK* fusion–positive cancers may respond to TRK inhibitors. Follicular cell–derived thyroid cancers or medullary thyroid cancers may be treated with Selpercatinib or Pralsetinib if they harbour RET mutations or fusions.

[a]DNA-based tests are usually used for single nucleotide variation detection, while RNA is used for testing fusions.

With the advent of sophisticated techniques and improved bioinformatics support, more and more actionable targets will be further characterised and prove integral to the multidisciplinary dialogue and patient management.

Digital Pathology

Like several other disciplines, the digital revolution is also being experienced in pathology, driving changes in pathology workflows. Advantages include speeding up the diagnostic pathway, improving turnaround times for reporting, telepathology, facilitation of peer consultation, easing of multidisciplinary meeting delivery and providing novel tools for pathology education. The transformation has been aided by industry-led advances in scanner technology. In addition, image analysis, computational pathology and artificial intelligence-based algorithms are in development for both diagnostic and research usage; indeed, clinical grade algorithms for cancer detection (e.g. Paige Prostate for prostate cancer) have started gaining regulatory approval. The developments in the field are envisaged to be transformational for routine diagnostics, and integration of clinical, radiological and classical/molecular/digital pathology data will revolutionise clinical big data mining initiatives in the future. However, challenges of cost, infrastructure, variability and quality control will need to be carefully addressed to maximise benefits from technological advances.

FURTHER READING

Batlle E, Clevers H. Cancer stem cells revisited. *Nat Med.* 2017;23: 1124–1134.

Baxi V, Edwards R, Montalto M, Saha S. Digital pathology and artificial intelligence in translational medicine and clinical practice. *Mod Pathol.* 2022;35(1):23–32.

Brierley JD, Gospodarowicz MK, Wittekind C. *The TNM classification of malignant tumours.* 8th ed. Chichester: Wiley-Blackwell; 2016.

Costa AC, Santos JM, da Costa RMG, Medeiros R. Impact of immune cells on the hallmarks of cancer: a literature review. *Crit Rev Oncol Hematol.* 2021;168:103541.

Curtius K, Wright NA, Graham TA. An evolutionary perspective on field cancerization. *Nat Rev Cancer.* 2018;18(1):19–32.

Dietel M. Molecular pathology: a requirement for precision medicine in cancer. *Oncol Res Treat.* 2016;39(12):804–810.

Fearon ER, Vogelstein B. A genetic model for colorectal tumorigenesis. *Cell.* 1990;61(5):759–767.

Haverkos HW. Viruses, chemicals and co-carcinogenesis. *Oncogene.* 2004;23(38):6492–6499.

Luch A. Nature and nurture—lessons from chemical carcinogenesis. *Nat Rev Cancer.* 2005;5(2):113–125.

Turajlic S, Swanton C. Metastasis as an evolutionary process. *Science.* 2016;352(6282):169–175.

Vanneman M, Dranoff G. Combining immunotherapy and targeted therapies in cancer treatment. *Nat Rev Cancer.* 2012;12: 237–251.

Wenzel C, Herold S, Wermke M, Aust DE, Baretton GB. Routine molecular pathology diagnostics in precision oncology. *Dtsch Arztebl Int.* 2021;118:255–261.

Williams D. Radiation carcinogenesis: lessons from Chernobyl. *Oncogene.* 2008;27:S9–S18.

18

Molecular, Cellular and Tissue Effects of Radiotherapy

Thankamma V. Ajithkumar

CHAPTER OUTLINE

INTRODUCTION

One of the most frequently used and successful modalities in the clinical treatment of cancer is the local eradication of a patient's tumour using radiotherapy (RT). In addition, external beam RT is often used to palliate cancer-associated symptoms, such as treating pain or spinal cord compression, shrinking tumour masses or relieving bleeding. The local treatment of a patient's tumour via external beam RT is accomplished by (1) the precise and focused delivery of radiation to kill both tumour and locally metastatic cancer cells by conforming and modulating the delivered radiation dose to the target volume and (2) exploiting the differences in the response of tumour and normal tissue to irradiation. Through largely empirical studies, this has previously led to curative external beam RT protocols of typically around 2 to 3 Gray (Gy) being delivered in daily fractions to the tumour site over 4 to 7 weeks, with the exact dose and fractionation schedule depending on the clinical situation and the tolerance of the irradiated normal tissue. Indeed, in many instances, the likelihood of normal tissue damage limits the total dose that can be delivered to the tumour site. Overall, however, the exact basis for the success of RT in eliminating cancers is still poorly understood, appearing to depend on differences in intrinsic sensitivity, ability to proliferate, and repair capacity between both normal and malignant tissues.

In the past few decades, radiobiology has gone some way to providing explanations and reasoning for these empirically derived schedules. In contrast, many of the advances in RT have been achieved by the optimisation of treatment delivery schedules and technological improvements in the physical targeting of dose; biological discoveries, particularly those investigating the molecular and cellular response to irradiation, continue to point the way towards new and more effective methods/protocols of treatment. Indeed, there is every hope that this biological information will improve RT efficacy, both in terms of superior targeted treatments and better patient selection.

This chapter aims to describe some of the pertinent molecular and cellular principles and phenomena that underpin current radiation treatment practice, relate this to outcomes observed in the clinic and provide insight into possible future developments and potential pitfalls in RT and radiobiology research. This is a vast field, so this chapter concentrates mainly on the molecular, cellular and tissue radiobiology of low linear energy transfer (LET) x-ray irradiation. Only a brief mention of other radiations, such as proton irradiation, will be made, because this modality is covered in detail in Chapter 10 of this book.

IONISING RADIATION, FREE RADICAL GENERATION AND SUBCELLULAR RADIOGENIC DAMAGE

Radiations interact with matter by transferring energy to the molecules of the absorbing material. Indeed, radiations of wavelengths less than 10^{-6} cm have sufficient photon energy to eject orbital electrons from the atoms of the absorber's molecules, leading to their ionisation. Because the most abundant molecule in a cell is water, a key product of this initial process is an ionised water molecule ($H_2O^{\bullet+}$); these radical cation species then interact with other water molecules to form hydroxyl radicals ($^{\bullet}OH$) (Fig. 18.1A). The initially ejected electrons (e^-) may possess sufficient energy to cause further ionisations until their energy dissipates. They become solvated to give an aqueous electron (e^-_{aq}) and/or combine with other species, such as protons (H^+) or molecular oxygen (O_2), to generate reducing species such as hydrogen atoms ($H^{\bullet}$) or superoxide ($O_2^{\bullet-}$). Ionising radiation is nondiscriminatory in that all molecular species in a cell

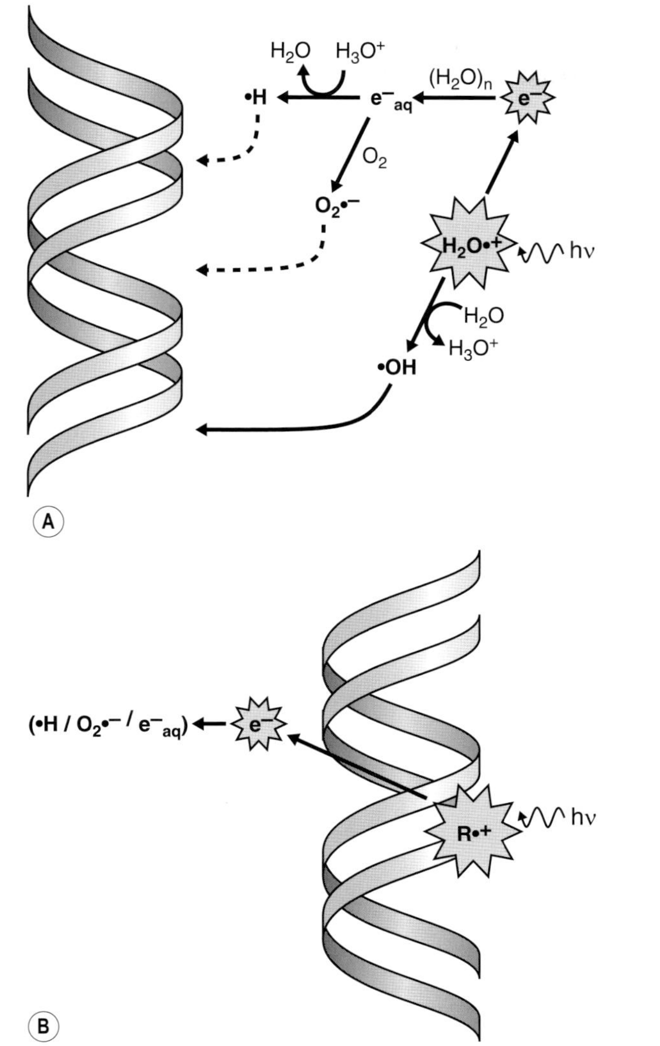

Fig. 18.1 The (A) indirect and (B) direct effects of ionising radiation. In the indirect effect, radiation interacts with water to produce hydroxyl free radicals (•OH) which, in turn, react with the DNA, producing damage. In the direct effect, the radiation interacts directly with the DNA to produce damage. Although both direct and indirect effects damage DNA, it is suggested that only indirect events happen within 2 nm of the DNA. Indirect effects dominate for low linear energy transfer ionising radiations. (The • *(dot)* refers to an unpaired electron of a free radical, and the *dashed lines* reflect the lower reactivity of the reducing species with DNA, as compared with the high reactivity of •OH.)

are prone to damage. However, DNA is a key molecular target for the deleterious effects of ionising radiation in cells. •OH radicals are highly reactive and will react with the DNA bases by addition reactions, whereby the •OH radicals add to the double bonds of DNA bases to form base radical adducts and by abstraction reactions, whereby the •OH radicals abstract hydrogen atoms from the deoxyribose moieties of the DNA sugar-phosphate backbone to form carbon-centred sugar radicals. Via these mechanisms, •OH radicals, together with the less reactive reducing species, are said to damage DNA via the so-called *indirect* effect (see Fig. 18.1A), whereby the initial ionisation event happens in a molecule near the ultimate target molecule. Radiation can also directly ionise the DNA, leading to direct damage of the DNA's bases or sugar-phosphate backbone ($R^{+\bullet}$) (see Fig. 18.1B). However, the distinction between direct and indirect damaging effects is not always clear, as electrons and radical cations produced in the DNA and DNA-associated water may lead

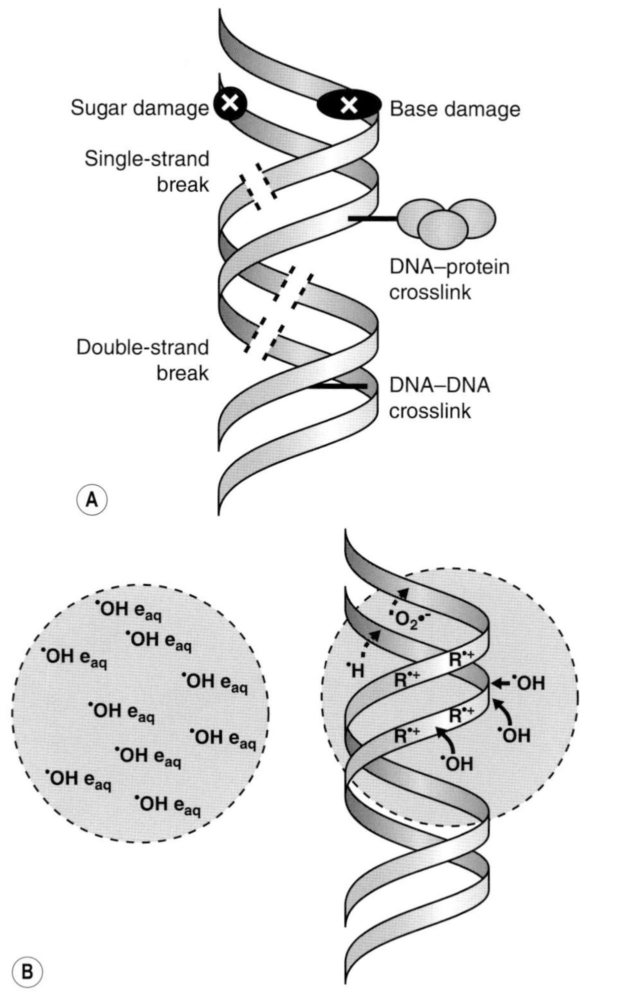

Fig. 18.2 (A) The types of damage produced by radiation. (B) The concept of multiply damaged sites (MDSs) is produced by a cluster of ionisations that impinge on DNA and its local environment. Energy deposition for x-rays is not uniformly absorbed but deposited in discrete events of high energy sufficient to generate a number of ion pairs. Should this happen in pure water, it will generate locally several •OH + e^- pairs; however, should these events overlap the DNA, both the direct and indirect effects will contribute to MDS formation.

to further ionisations/oxidations in the DNA macromolecule and its surrounding microenvironment.

Through directly and indirectly induced base radical adducts and deoxyribose radicals, radiation causes a wide range of damage in DNA, including strand breaks (both single- and double-strand breaks (DSBs)), base or sugar damage and cross-links between macromolecules (i.e. DNA–DNA or DNA–protein cross-links) (Fig. 18.2A); the frequency of these DNA lesions is shown in Table 18.1. In general, it is considered that the DNA DSB is the most responsible for the lethal effects of radiation; evidence for this is as follows:

- Under various experimental conditions, the relative level of induced or unrepaired DSBs best correlates with cell killing.
- A single DSB is lethal to yeast.
- Enzymatically produced DSBs (produced by inserting DNA restriction enzymes into cells) give the same pattern of chromosome damage and lethality as radiation.
- Microbeam irradiation has shown the cell nucleus to be the most radiation-sensitive site in the cell.
- The extreme radiosensitivity of some mutant cell lines is because of defects in DSB repair.

TABLE 18.1 Types and Frequency of Radiation-Induced Damage

Type of Damage	Approximate Number/Gy/Cell
DNA double-strand breaks	40
DNA single-strand breaks	1000
DNA–protein cross-links	150
DNA–DNA cross-links	30
Base damage	2000
Sugar damage	1500

However, not all DSBs are the same, because the chemical nature of the strand break ends and the separation between the constituent single-strand breaks can vary considerably, as can the proximity of other types of lesions. Indeed, the influence of the proximity of induced base lesions has been shown to affect the reparability of damage, and this is relevant because low LET radiations (x-rays and γ-rays) can produce multiple ionisations in localised isolated events (previously termed *spurs* and *blobs*). When these isolated events occur close to and/or overlapping the DNA molecule (see Fig. 18.2B), several lesions may be formed within a region of a few base pairs, producing so-called *multiply damaged sites* (MDS), as described by Ward.

On a larger scale, radiation damage to chromosomes and chromatids leading to aberrations involving breakage and rejoining of chromosome/chromatid fragments (e.g. translocations and ring formations) is observed in many irradiated cells (Fig. 18.3). Because these events appear to correlate radiation-induced cell killing, such damage is considered an important aspect of the radiation-induced effects in many cells. Furthermore, chromosome damage may be a very sensitive indicator of low-dose/environmental radiation exposure in an individual.

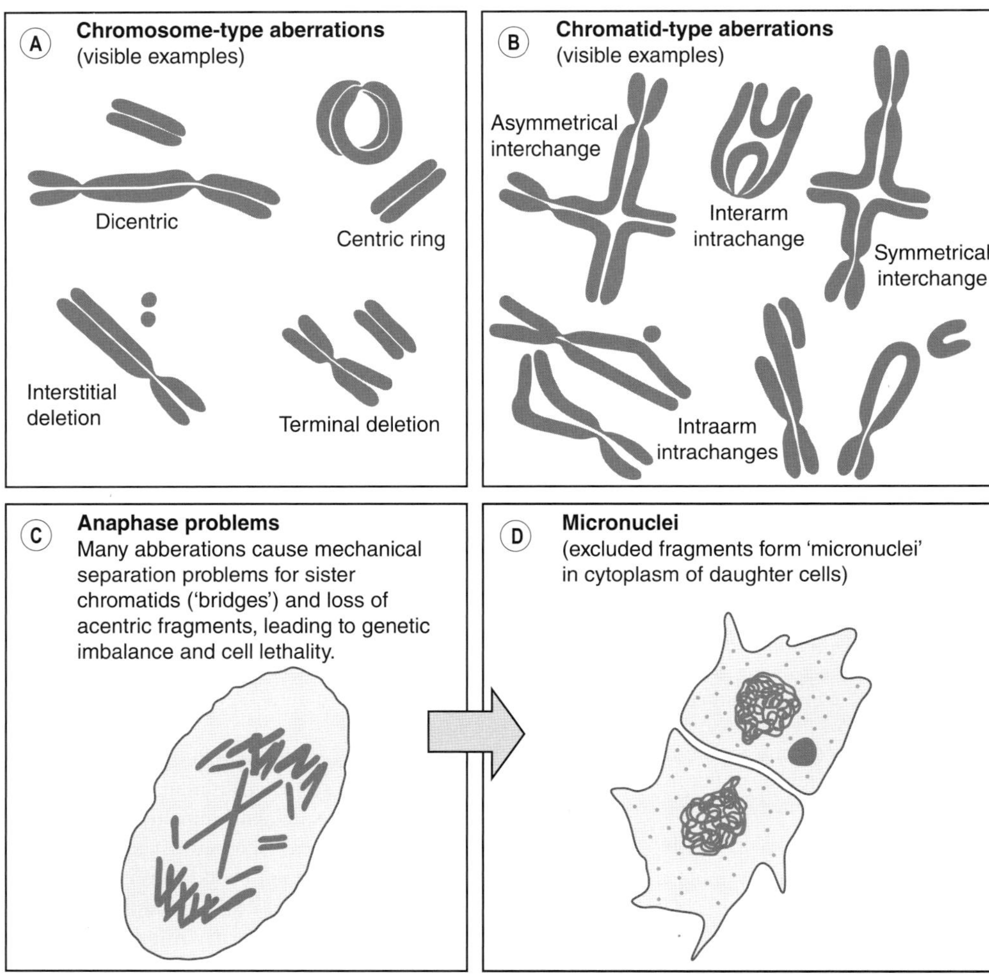

Fig. 18.3 Some examples of radiation-induced chromosomal structural changes, solid stained. (A) *Chromasome-type* aberrations—all breaks and rejoins affect both sister chromatids at the same locus. Only forms that produce acentric fragments are visible with solid staining. However, much-hidden damage is present, some of which is transmitted to future cell generations. (B) *Chromatid-type aberrations*—all breaks and rejoins affect only one of the sister chromatids at any one locus. Compared with chromosome-type changes, many more forms are visible with solid staining, but hidden damage still occurs. The observed frequencies always vary with postirradiation sampling time, so there is never a fixed yield to set against a given exposure dose. Ionising radiation can produce both types; the type recovered at first postirradiation division depends upon the duplication status of the target chromatin, with chromosome types arising from prereplicated chromatin. (C) Many forms lead to mechanical separation problems at anaphase (intercell bridges), and acentric fragments are usually excluded from the daughter nuclei, leading to micronuclei in their cytoplasm. (D) The exclusion of any visible fragment means the loss of many megabases of DNA. These bridges and fragments are the primary cause of cell lethality and genetic imbalance. (Courtesy Dr John Savage.)

RECOVERY, DNA DAMAGE REPAIR AND DAMAGE SIGNALLING

Recovery

Much of the DNA damage induced in cells is subject to repair (see later), with initial evidence coming from recovery studies, such as split dose and delayed plating experiments. For the former, the effect of a radiation dose was less if it was split into two fractions delivered a few hours apart, which was attributed to the sublethal damage recovery (SLDR) or Elkind repair. For the latter, it was observed that cells irradiated in a nongrowing state and left in this state for increasing periods showed enhanced survival. This has been termed *potentially lethal damage recovery (PLDR)*. Both SLDR and PLDR are practical in that they reflect the decrease in cell kill when RT is prolonged using lower dose rates, fractionated (SLDR), or delivered to a tissue in a nonproliferative state (PLDR). Both are believed to have a basis in DNA repair capacity, although there is some evidence that they do not reflect the same repair processes. It has been suggested that some resistant tumours owe their resistance to substantial PLDR, although this is controversial.

TABLE 18.2 Pathways Involved in the Repair of DNA Damage

Repair Pathway	Type of Lesion	Involved in Radiosensitivity?
Base excision repair	Base damage, abasic site, single-strand base	Yes
Homologous recombination repair	Double-strand break	Yes
Nonhomologous end joining	Double-strand break	Yes
Nucleotide excision repair	Cross-links, dimers, bulky adducts	?
Transcription-coupled repair	Base damage, dimers, bulky adducts	?
Mismatch repair	Mismatched bases	?

From Gordon Steel G. *Basic Clinical Radiobiology*, 3rd Edition. With permission of Hodder Education.

Double-Strand Break Repair and Damage Signalling

One of several DNA repair pathways (Table 18.2), mostly alone but potentially in combination, repairs each type of radiation-induced DNA damage. Of particular significance to the deleterious biological effects of radiation is the repair of DNA DSBs. Consequently, intricate damage response pathways have evolved to repair DSBs. Two principal DSB repair pathways that employ mostly separate protein complexes have been recognised: homologous recombination repair (HRR) (Fig. 18.4A) and nonhomologous end joining (NHEJ) (see Fig. 18.4B). Briefly, DSB repair by HRR requires an undamaged template molecule that contains a homologous DNA sequence, typically on the sister chromatid found in the S and G2 phases of the cell cycle, during which the genome is being duplicated (S phase) or has been duplicated (G2 phase). This form of DNA repair is error-free but takes longer than NHEJ. In contrast, NHEJ of two double-stranded DNA ends, which may occur in all phases of the cell cycle, does not require an undamaged

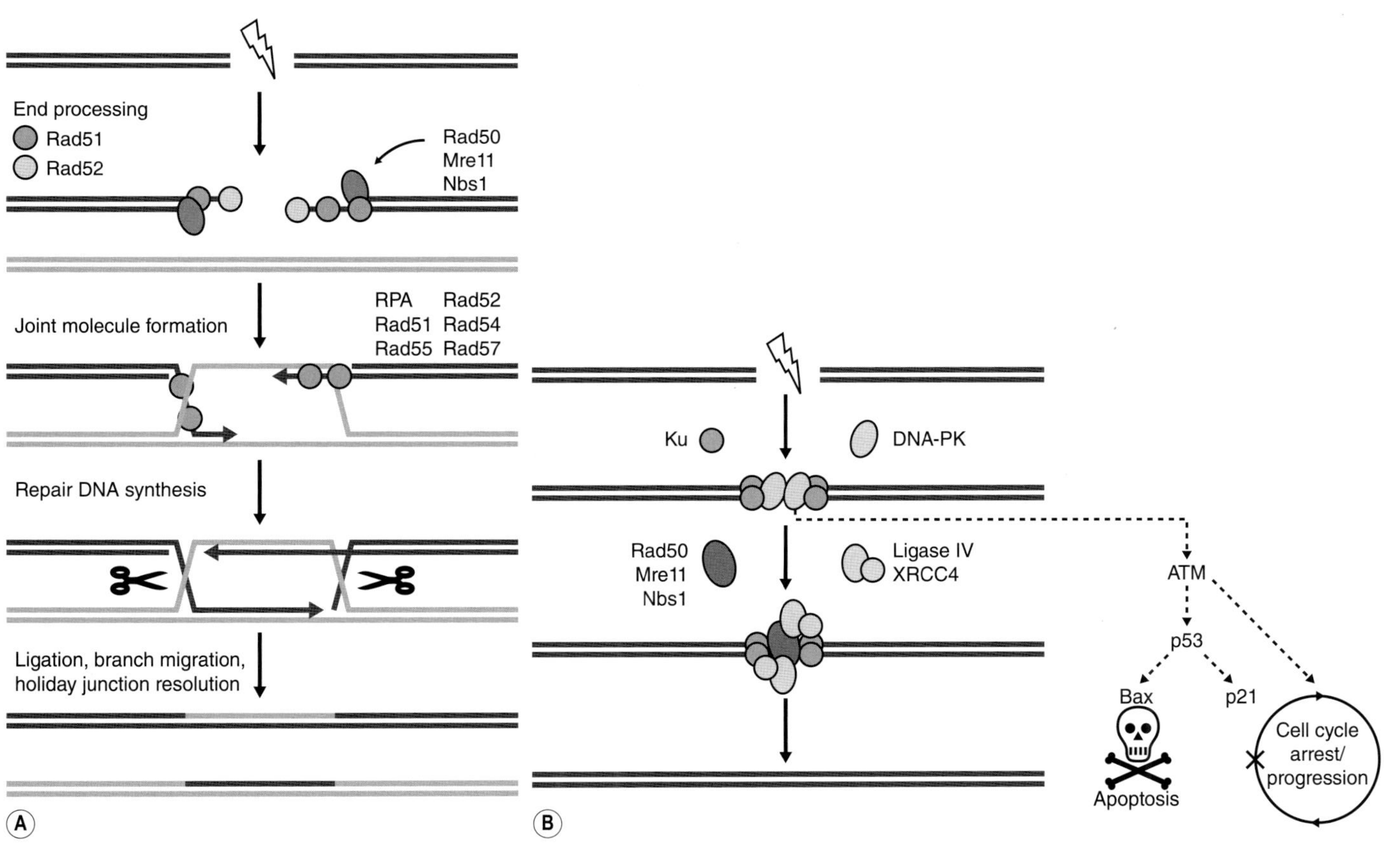

Fig. 18.4 DNA double-strand break repair; (A) homologous recombination repair (HRR) and (B) nonhomologous end joining (NHEJ). NHEJ is potentially error-prone and occasionally may rejoin the wrong ends (particularly at high doses) to give translocations. HRR uses a nondamaged homologous template and is therefore considered error-free.

partner and does not rely on extensive homologies between the recombining ends. It is likely that the balance between NHEJ and HRR in the removal of DSBs depends on the type and location of the lesion. Of note, however, is that NHEJ, unlike HRR, may rejoin the wrong ends to generate translocations (i.e. has reduced fidelity of repair) and may not restore the original DNA sequence if sequence information is lost from both DNA strand ends. Still, NHEJ is considered the dominant DSB repair pathway in mammalian cells. Further studies have uncovered additional mechanisms of DSB rejoining that use end resection and microhomology-mediated end joining to generate deletions. One such process is alternative NHEJ (Alt-NHEJ), which occurs predominantly when immediate NHEJ is compromised.

Both NHEJ and HR DSB repair are facilitated by the sequential recruitment and assembly of a variety of DNA repair proteins and cofactors to the sites of DNA damage in a highly choreographed process (see Figs. 18.4A and B). Patterns are now emerging that allow for the recognition of critical molecules and pathways linking DNA damage and DNA damage repair to classical outcomes of radiation exposure and pointing the way towards targets for improved outcomes. Many cancers have known DNA damage repair (HHR) and/or DNA damage response (p53) deficiencies but survive high levels of treatment-induced DNA damage via alternate/backup pathways; however, the selective targeting/inhibition of these alternate/backup pathways via inhibitors of specific repair enzymes or response mediators renders the cells highly sensitive. This is the concept of synthetic lethality, with, for example, poly ADP ribose polymerase (PARP) inhibitors of DNA single-strand break repair significantly enhancing cytotoxicity in BRCA/HRR deficient cells; several PARP inhibitors are now in clinical trials in combination with RT.

An ongoing question, which is now the focus of extensive research, is the extent to which variation in the level of expression/activity of DNA repair enzymes plus enzymes and proteins involved in downstream signalling influences the outcome of RT. Given the highly ordered nature of the described protein machines, small structural changes introduced by single amino-acid changes in individual proteins may alter the activity of the complex significantly. Indeed, there is increasing evidence that mild reductions in DNA repair capacity, assumed to be the consequence of common genetic variation in the human population (polymorphisms), affect cancer predisposition and, by inference, may modulate the response to radiation treatment.

Epigenetic Radiation Signalling Mechanisms

Although nuclear DNA has traditionally been considered the key target for the biological effects of ionising radiation, numerous studies have revealed several nongenomic epigenetic targets that influence a cell's response to ionising radiation. Radiation-induced damage to cytoplasmic, mitochondrial and membrane structures; changes in redox balance; and protease activity have been suggested to mediate cellular responses to ionising radiation. These include ceramide production from plasma membrane–derived sphingomyelin and activation of numerous signalling pathways, including inflammatory-type pathways, mediated by proinflammatory cytokines, for example, tumour necrosis factor α (TNF-α) and cytokine IL-1, and other cytokines and cytokine receptors, plus cell adhesion molecules and proteases/antiproteases. These responses play an important role in tissue recovery and remodelling following irradiation (see later). Another example of epigenetic radiation–induced signalling includes the expression of epidermal growth factor receptor (EGFR), which has a prosurvival effect on the cancer cell. Pharmacological inhibition of this pathway leading to cell sensitisation can be achieved with EGFR-binding antibodies or small molecule inhibitors of the EGFR tyrosine kinase, for example, gefitinib (Iressa) and erlotinib (OSI 774, Tarceva).

Another factor to consider is the bystander effect, an intercellular signalling pathway now described in several studies. These responses appear to be cell-type dependent, and they consist of broad cellular changes, including gene activation, induction of genomic instability, differentiation and changes in apoptotic potential. This appears to be mediated, at least in part, by diffusible substances because the effect occurs when bystander cells are physically separated from the irradiated cells. Although the diffusible substance remains to be identified, contenders include nitric oxide and/or cytokines being released to mediate membrane-dependent signalling events and possibly even exosomes; cell-derived vesicles that are present in many and perhaps all eukaryotic fluids, including blood exosomes secreted from tumour cells, which can deliver signals to surrounding cells and have been shown to regulate myofibroblast differentiation. Consequently, the entire tumour microenvironment may need to be taken into account when considering the consequences of cancer cell irradiation.

RADIATION-INDUCED CELL KILLING

As already mentioned, the objective of RT is to kill cancer cells while limiting damage to the surrounding normal tissue. This is achieved in part by exploiting the differences in the response of tumour and normal tissue to irradiation. One of the best-known and most studied differences between tumours and normal tissue is the manifestation of hypoxia in tumours.

Tumour Hypoxia, Oxygen Effect and Reoxygenation

Solid tumours need to develop their own blood supply through angiogenesis to grow. However, the formation of this neovasculature tends to shadow tumour growth; consequently, the nutrient and oxygen demands of a growing tumour can exceed the capacity of the host's blood supply. Furthermore, the chaotic nature of tumour vasculature coupled with the limited diffusion of oxygen in a highly proliferating tumour (see later) results in areas of chronic and sustained hypoxia and nutrient deprivation. In addition, areas of acute reversible hypoxia are also found, which may result from physiological defects in the new vessels (leading to a temporary closure of blood vessels), transient flow instability or changes in fluid pressure.

The relevance of hypoxia to the radiation treatment of cancer stems from laboratory studies that have demonstrated that cells irradiated in the absence of oxygen are considerably more resistant to the lethal effects of radiation than those irradiated in oxygen (Fig. 18.5). This is partly because of molecular oxygen reacting with the induced DNA radicals to produce chemically irreparable peroxy radicals (Fig. 18.6A). Thus, in effect, oxic cells suffer more DNA damage. The degree of sensitisation by oxygen is often quoted as an *oxygen enhancement ratio (OER)*, which is the ratio of doses needed to produce a given biological effect in the presence and absence of oxygen (see Fig. 18.5). For most cells and tissues, the OER has a value of around 2.0 to 3 (*ca.* 2 at clinically relevant doses).

Numerous studies have linked hypoxia to poor RT outcomes. The number of hypoxic cells is an important factor following the irradiation of human tumours. Direct and indirect clinical studies have shown this. One of the most important studies was by Tomlinson and Gray in 1955. They examined sections of human bronchogenic carcinoma specimens and showed that there were cords of viable cells close to blood vessels. By contrast, 150 to 180 μm from blood vessels, there were areas of necrosis. The width of the viable tissue (150–180 μm) was equal to the calculated diffusion distance of oxygen from blood vessels, beyond which cells could not survive. They postulated that radioresistant hypoxic cells were present within the areas of necrosis.

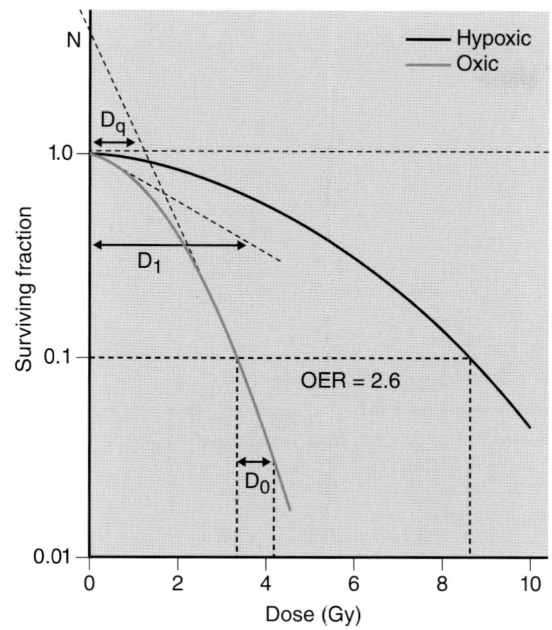

Fig. 18.5 Survival curves (and derived measures) for mammalian cells exposed to low linear energy transfer radiation under oxic or hypoxic conditions. Because the initial and final slopes depend on the presence of oxygen, the oxygen enhancement ratio is 2.5 to 3.0 for high dose–related effects (2.6 for 10% survival in the figure) but is typically less for lower dose–related effects. *OER*, Oxygen enhancement ratio. (From McBride, Doughert and Milas 2002, with permission of John Wiley & Sons.)

It is possible to measure oxygen tensions in accessible tumours, such as carcinoma of the cervix, by directly inserting Eppendorf electrodes into the tumour. The degree of hypoxia within tumours has been correlated to clinical outcome; tumours with large areas of hypoxia tend to persist after RT, whereas those better-oxygenated tumours are more likely to be controlled.

In addition to its effects on DNA damage, laboratory studies have shown that hypoxia can trigger genetic mechanisms that may give tumour cells additional survival advantages. Hypoxia induces the expression of several genes, particularly genetic programs under the control of hypoxia-inducible factor 1 (HIF-1). HIF-1 is recognised as a key mediator of gene expression in hypoxic tumours. The range of its downstream target genes is extensive. Some of these (i.e. vascular endothelial growth factor (VEGF), erythropoietin and TNF-α) are aimed at increasing angiogenesis and oxygen delivery, driving tumour growth. HIF-1–regulated mechanisms also control the acidity of tumour tissue and may further enhance tumour growth and radioresistance. Hypoxia can induce apoptosis by a mechanism dependent on a drop in extracellular pH. Although, intuitively, this process would be expected to reduce the tumour cell population, it can provide a selective pressure for the emergence of apoptotic-resistant subclones (see Fig. 18.6B). In this way, hypoxia may be selected for cells with p53 mutations (because cells expressing wild-type p53 tend to undergo apoptosis more readily), and these tumours will have an antiapoptotic, more malignant phenotype. For these reasons, large areas of hypoxia may be a marker of an intrinsically more aggressive tumour; indeed, hypoxic cervical cancers have a poorer prognosis than well-oxygenated tumours when treated with surgery.

Initially, hypoxic cells may become more oxygenated during a fractionated course of RT. Following a fraction of RT, more radiosensitive aerobic cells in a tumour will be killed, and the surviving fraction will be more hypoxic. If sufficient time is allowed before the next fraction of radiation, some of the tumour cells will oxygenate through the process of reoxygenation, and if this is efficient, the presence of hypoxic cells will not overtly affect the response of the tumour. However, the speed of reoxygenation varies widely, occurring within a few hours in some tumours and several days in others.

In the past, patients were irradiated in hyperbaric oxygen chambers, breathing oxygen at three atmospheric pressures to reduce the number of hypoxic cells in a tumour. Breathing in hyperbaric oxygen is advantageous in some tumours (locally advanced head and neck cancer) but not in others (cervical cancer). However, because of the dangers of fire, explosion and fits within the hyperbaric oxygen chamber, this treatment has fallen into disrepute.

A class of electron-affinity drugs that mimics the damage-fixating radiosensitising effects of oxygen, the nitroimidazoles, were evaluated as radiosensitisers. It was postulated that such agents would diffuse out of the tumour blood supply and, unlike oxygen, which is rapidly metabolised by tumour cells, could diffuse further and reach the more distant hypoxic cells, thus sensitising them. The drug misonidazole produced impressive results in treating mouse tumours, but neurotoxicity prevented this drug from being of clinical value in patients. Nimorazole has been shown to increase locoregional control in patients with advanced head and neck cancer in a Danish study, but this drug is not in widespread use. However, the reduction in the toxicity of the sensitising compounds and the ability to identify tumours with significant hypoxic fractions has restored faith in the potential for this approach. One potentially fruitful opportunity for further development in this area centres on recognising that cells can react to hypoxia by switching on specific genes, such as glucose transporter 1 (GLUT-1) and carbonic anhydrase 9 (CA 9). This will not only allow the identification of hypoxic cells but may allow the specific targeting of hypoxic cells in gene therapy approaches. In addition, the use of drugs that are specifically activated in hypoxic areas, namely tirapazamine, nitroimidazoles, and carbogen, has also been studied. Unfortunately, many hypoxia modifiers are not proven to be clinically useful. Current research focuses on DDR, HIF, immunotherapy and FLASH RT. Studies have shown alterations in the DDR in hypoxic cells, and therefore ATR and PARP inhibitors should be explored in hypoxic tumours such as head and neck cancer. Hypoxia may alter tumour immunosurveillance, and thus there is a potential role for a combination of immunotherapy with RT. Intuitively, such approaches will benefit patients with hypoxic tumours more, necessitating biomarkers that reflect oxygenation status. Tissue biomarkers have shown utility in many studies as gene expression markers (see later). Further significant advances have been made in the noninvasive measurement of tumour hypoxia with positron emission tomography (PET), magnetic resonance imaging (MRI) and other imaging modalities.

The Cell Cycle and Sensitivity to Irradiation

The radiosensitivity of cells varies throughout the cell cycle. Most cells are more vulnerable in the G2/M phase of the cell cycle (because the cells have less time to repair radiation-induced damage before the cells divide) and are least vulnerable in late S phase (possibly attributed to an increased opportunity for homologous recombination). Within the tumour, individual cells are in different phases of the cell cycle. If their cell division could be synchronised in some way so that they would be in a sensitive phase of the cell cycle during treatment, this would increase the effectiveness of RT. Although it is possible to synchronise the population of cells in culture, it has not proved possible in clinical practice. Several drugs have been used to try to produce a cell cycle block, leading to increased killing by radiation by synchronisation. Taxanes and nucleoside analogues (e.g. gemcitabine) appear to have similar effects.

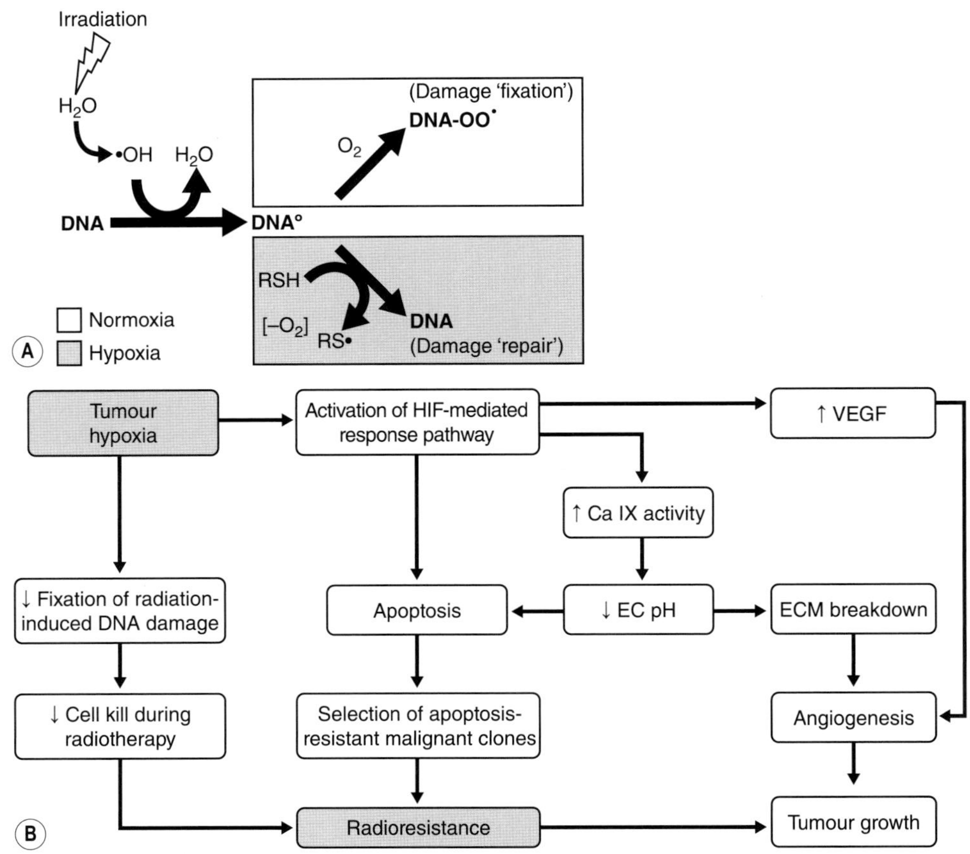

Fig. 18.6 (A) The pivotal role of oxygen in the fixation of radiation-induced DNA damage. Ionising radiation generates hydroxyl free radicals (•OH) that lead to the formation of DNA-centred radicals (DNA•). In the presence of oxygen, this damage becomes fixed. However, under hypoxic conditions, endogenous thiols (RSH) are able chemically to repair this damage (by donating hydrogen), effectively contributing to radioresistance. (B) Schematic diagram showing the role of hypoxia in causing radioresistance. In addition to its physical effects on the 'fixation' of radiogenic DNA damage, hypoxia triggers specific patterns of gene expression, mediated by HIF-1α. Ca IX is pivotal in this response, causing acidification of the extracellular space and promoting extracellular matrix breakdown and apoptosis, which, in turn, may provide a selective pressure to favour apoptosis-resistant subclones. *ECM*, Extracellular matrix; *HIF*, hypoxia-inducible factor; *VEGF*, vascular endothelial growth factor.

Patterns of Cell Death After Irradiation

Historically, radiation has been considered to kill cells mainly by mitotic cell death in which proliferating cells undergo a general breakdown (i.e. necrosis, see later) when they attempt to divide with radiation-damaged chromosomes. This holds true for many cells, but it is clear that some cells, notably those of some normal tissues, die via the morphologically distinct mechanism of apoptosis. The differences between apoptotic and necrotic cells are listed in Table 18.3. Cells lethally injured by radiation typically execute one or more divisions before dying. The number of divisions depends on the size of the radiation dose, but after a dose of 2 Gy, two or three attempts to divide may be made. The progeny of these cells may all die, or a proportion may survive and contribute to the reproductive (clonogenic) pool. In the *interphase death* process, cells die before they divide, and cells die 2 to 6 hours after irradiation. These tend to be radiosensitive cells such as lymphocytes, spermatogonia and hair follicles; only relatively low radiation doses are required.

TABLE 18.3 A Comparison of Some of the Morphological Features of Apoptosis and Necrosis

Necrosis	Apoptosis
Cells swell.	Cells shrink.
Mitochondria dilate, and other organelles dissolve.	Organelles retain definition for a long time.
Plasma membranes rupture.	Cells dissociate from surrounding cells.
Nuclear changes are unremarkable.	Chromatin condensation and regular DNA degradation occur.

Apoptosis is an important mechanism of normal tissue homeostasis and is a form of programmed cell death. It is a mechanism for eliminating cells that have sustained high levels of potentially deleterious, irreversible damage. It is now recognised as being the outcome of a sequence of biochemical signals, usually requiring the involvement of p53 gene products that ultimately result in the activation of a series of enzymes (caspases) that degrade cellular proteins and DNA endonucleases that cut DNA in regularly repeated regions that are not protected by nucleosomal proteins. The latter results in DNA fragmentation into multiples of 80 to 100 base pairs, producing a characteristic ladder pattern when the DNA is separated in an agarose gel. The significance of this is that apoptosis is under specific genetic control; therefore susceptibility to radiation-induced apoptosis may be amenable to manipulation. Apoptotic cells undergo phagocytosis by neighbouring cells, and inflammation is not induced. Within a few hours, there was no trace of the dead cell. For this reason, apoptosis was underestimated in the past as a source of cellular loss. The frequency by which cells undergo apoptosis varies in different tumour types. For example, lymphomas have a high incidence of spontaneous and treatment-induced apoptosis, whereas high-grade gliomas do not.

Necrosis is a pathological process, not a component of normal tissue haemostasis, and may occur in tumours because of prolonged nutrient and oxic deprivation. It involves the loss of membrane integrity and increased cell size, with the release of lysosomal enzymes and a subsequent inflammatory response. Necrosis can follow vascular injury, changes in the pattern of perfusion through the tumour, or maybe the mode of death of cells that lack an adequate apoptotic pathway.

Models of Radiation Cell Survival

Because radiation-induced cell killing is exponential rather than arithmetic, it is traditionally illustrated as the logarithm of survival plotted against linear dose. A typical survival curve produced by low LET radiation (x- or γ-rays) is shown in Fig. 18.5. There are two components to this curve. First, there is an initial slope (designated D_1) and shoulder. Then, the curve becomes steeper and straighter at higher doses as survival decreases exponentially with the dose. Cell killing is measured in the exponential part of the curve by using the value D_0, which is the dose sufficient to reduce the survival fraction by 37% (1/e). In doing so, the radiation induces, on average, one lethal event per cell. The size of the shoulder is regarded as giving an indication of the repair capacity of the cell and can be quantified by the quasithreshold dose D_q.

Several mathematical models have been developed to describe cell survival curves, including the multitarget equation, the multitarget with single hit equation and the linear quadratic equation. The oldest, the multitarget theory, presumed that the cell contained several critical targets, all of which had to be deactivated to bring about lethality. However, studies with human tumour cells indicate that the initial shoulder is not absolutely flat, so the simple multitarget equation is inappropriate. The linear quadratic model is a better description of cell killing, particularly at lower doses (also see Chapter 5). This assumes that radiation can produce both nonrecoverable and repairable lesions. Nonrepairable damage is the alpha component (represented as αD on a logarithmic scale). It is induced linearly by 'single hit' mechanisms, whereas the beta component (βD^2) describes the quadratic cell inactivation by the accumulation and possible interaction of repairable damage induced by multiple hits. When plotting cell survival, alpha-type damage is represented by a straight line and beta damage by a curve (Fig. 18.7). The ratio of alpha to beta (α/β) is the dose at which single and multihit mechanisms contribute equally to cell killing: that is, $\alpha D = \beta D^2$.

The α/β ratio defines survival curve characteristics and classifies cellular and tissue responses to RT. Acute/early responding tissues, which express radiation damage days or weeks after irradiation, have high α/β values of 7 to 20 Gy (typically around 10 Gy) (see Fig. 18.7). Well-oxygenated tumours have even higher ratios. In contrast, late-responding tissues, which express radiation damage months to years after RT, have low α/β values of between 0.5 and 6 Gy (typically ≈ 3 Gy). The survival curves of cells in late-responding tissues are significantly more curved than those with high α/β ratios. Late-responding tissues, such as the spinal cord, are much more sensitive to changes in fraction size than acute-responding tissues, such as skin or the mucosa of the mouth. Generally, tumours have α/β ratios similar to acute-responding tissues.

Two clinically important exceptions are breast and prostate cancer. In the case of both tumour types, larger treatment doses per fraction (hypofractionation) will deliver a higher biological dose to the tumour while reducing or maintaining the same biological dose to normal tissues compared with a standard fraction of 2 Gy. The α/β ratio in prostate cancer has been estimated to be as low as 1.5. In a trial using

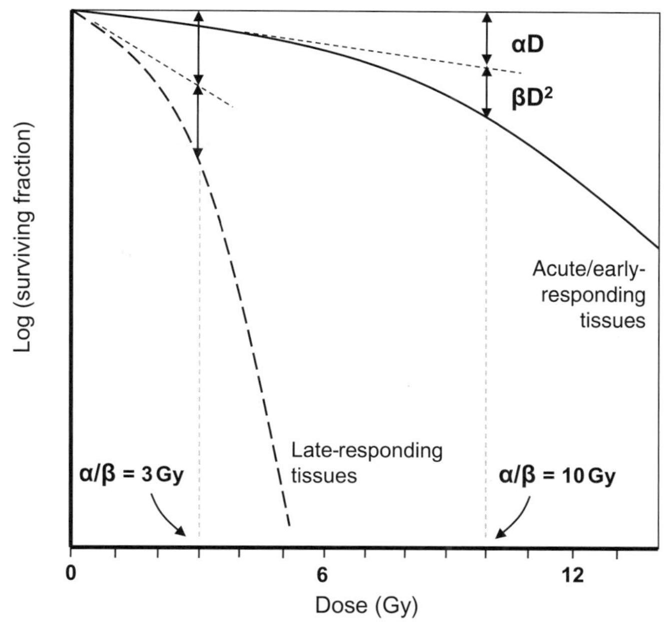

Fig. 18.7 Dose-response relationships for early- and late-responding tissues. The relationship for late-responding tissues is more curved than for early-responding tissues, which in the linear-quadratic formula translates into a larger α/β ratio for early rather than for late effects.

intensity modulated RT (IMRT) (the CHHiP trial), a regimen of 60 Gy in 20 fractions was shown to produce slightly better clinical or biochemical freedom from prostate cancer recurrence at 5 years (90.6% versus 88.3%) compared with 74 Gy in 37 fractions, with a very similar incidence of late effects. A 2017 metaanalysis of three conventional versus hypofractionated noninferiority trials in 5484 males with prostate cancer has shown a statistically significant improved disease-free survival (hazard ratio 0.869 95%, confidence interval 0.66–1.07, $P = .047$) without any increase in late toxicity. The ultimate form of hypofractionated RT is the current PACE trial, where males suffering from low/intermediate risk of prostate cancer are being treated stereotactically with a dose of 36.25 Gy given in 5 fractions in 1 week.

Breast cancer, in many cases, has a low α/β ratio. Previously, the START trials showed that a schedule of 40 Gy in 15 fractions was as effective as 50 Gy in 25 fractions with less breast shrinkage, telangiectasia, fibrosis and breast oedema. Recently, the FAST-forward trial has shown that 26 to 27 Gy in 5 fractions over 1 week is as effective as 40 Gy in 15 fractions.

These values can be used to calculate isoeffect relationships in RT, and calculations of parameters such as the biologically effective dose (BED) are important when manipulating fractionation regimens. The BED, in effect, is the dose required to produce a given biological effect when the radiation is given as an infinitely large number of very small fractions or as a single dose at an extremely low dose rate. For a given treatment, the BED can be calculated if the α/β ratio of the dose-limiting tissue and the tolerance dose (TD) for a given fractionation regimen are known. Using the BED, the relationship between TD and dose per fraction can be worked out for new fractionation regimens. Attempts to introduce biological mechanisms into the models have led to the lethal, potentially lethal damage and repair saturation models, although the actual mechanisms are rudimentary and poorly defined.

RADIATION EFFECTS IN NORMAL AND MALIGNANT TISSUE

As mentioned previously, both DNA and epigenetic sites are important initiators of radiation-induced signalling responses following exposure.

Indeed, many of the effects seen at the tissue level in the clinic (i.e. recovery and remodelling) are the manifestation of these pathways. Cellular responses to irradiation include induction of early response genes (e.g. V-jun avian sarcoma virus 17 oncogene homologue (JUN), v-fos FBJ murine osteosarcoma viral oncogene homologue (FOS) and early growth response 1 (EGR1)), which can bind to specific DNA sequences to modulate the expression of other genes. Also, intermediate and late genes are induced, such as TNF-α, platelet-derived growth factor (PDGF), transforming growth factor (TGF) β and fibroblast growth factor 2 (basic) (bFGF), which are involved in premature terminal differentiation of fibroblasts by ionising radiation and therefore mediate fibrosis as a late response to RT. In addition, a growing body of evidence supports the hypothesis that chronic oxidative stress drives the progression of radiation-induced late effects. Some of the pathways that mediate these effects are now revealed, but their importance remains the subject of debate and the focus of continued research. What follows is a brief description of the effects of radiation at a tissue level.

Acute Responses of Normal Tissue

Following large single x-ray treatment, such as a single fraction of 10 Gy to treat bone metastasis, cytokines and proteases, products of cell signalling and from cell killing (apoptosis and necrosis) are released from the irradiated tissue and interact with normal macrophages and lymphocytes. This may bring about both erythema of treated skin within hours and oedema and may be the source of nausea and vomiting associated with RT. The acute effects of RT are usually seen in tissues with a high cellular turnover rate, such as gastrointestinal mucosa, skin, bone marrow and mucosa of the upper aerodigestive tract. These effects are usually seen after 2 to 3 weeks during a fractionated course of radical RT lasting 4 to 7 weeks.

Acute reactions are a result of cellular loss. A good model is the acute reaction in the skin, especially if the patient is treated with kilovoltage radiation. After about 14 days, hair loss (epilation) occurs. This is followed by erythema. If the dose is high enough, dry desquamation may be followed. As the skin is shed, there is a serous exudate, referred to as *moist desquamation*. Healing depends on the initial recovery of the skin stem cells, which usually regenerate most of their number before differentiating to restore function. This process is typically completed within a few weeks. A similar effect is seen within the mucosa of the upper aerodigestive tract. Following RT, cells are lost from the mucosa, leading to a characteristic radiation reaction. Initially, there is erythema of the mucosa followed by mucosal cell loss. This denuded area is covered by a white membrane containing inflammatory exudate and dead cells. In the normal mucosa, only about 15% of stem cells undergo cellular division to replace normal cell loss. Most are in the cell cycle's resting phase (G0). After about 10 to 12 days into a standard course of RT, virtually all surviving stem cells are dividing to replace cells loss from RT. Usually, within a few weeks of completing a standard dose of RT, the mucosa has healed, but if a very high dose has been given sufficiently to destroy the stem cell pool, the patient may be left with a persisting area of ulceration within the treated area.

Subacute Reactions of Normal Tissue

Some tissues, such as neural tissue, have a much longer normal turnover time than skin or oral mucosa. The effects of radiation may not be seen until several months after treatment. A typical example is Lhermitte's syndrome following irradiation of the spinal cord. A few weeks after treatment, the patient complains of electric shocks radiating down to fingers and toes, especially if they flex their neck. This is a result of partial temporary demyelination of the spinal cord. There is often a 9-to-18-month interval before late effects are seen in cell populations with a slow proliferation rate, such as nervous tissue, kidney, blood vessels, subcutaneous tissue and bone or cartilage. Initially, damage to the slowly proliferating vascular endothelium was thought to be the common cellular injury linking most late effects. Undoubtedly, damage to blood vessels is important, but, for example, with late demyelination of the brain, there is also loss of oligodendrocytes and, subsequently, neurons and damage to small blood vessels. Similarly, there is a loss of renal tubular cells and vascular injury in the kidney. Cell loss is rapid in late-responding tissues, such as jejunal mucosa, and there may be evidence of radiation-induced cell loss within 24 hours of irradiation. By contrast, there may be no histological evidence of cell depletion in the kidney for many months after RT. If a high enough radiation dose has been given to destroy all the clonogenic tubular cells, the tubules will not regenerate. If one or more tubular clonogenic cells per nephron survive, the tubule may regenerate over several months.

The Effect of Radiotherapy on Tissues

All tissues have different cellular populations and may undergo acute and late damage. A typical example is the effects on skin and subcutaneous tissue. If the radiation dose is moderate, any acute reaction may settle without late effects. However, if there has been a marked depletion of the epidermal proliferating cell compartment, the skin may be thin (atrophic) and white owing to the loss of pigment-producing cells. There may also be permanent loss of hair. The tissues of the dermis may be replaced with fibrous tissue, which may lead to the thickening of the subcutaneous tissues and loss of elasticity. The thickening of tissues around joints, such as the shoulder, may lead to a marked reduction in movement. The walls of arteries may be replaced by fibrous tissue, leading to narrowing of the lumen and thrombosis. This is often followed by compensating dilation of skin capillaries, leading to telangiectasia of the skin. These red blood vessels on the skin surface may be very disfiguring. Ultimately, perhaps following a minor insult such as trauma or infection, the skin may necrose, leading to a nonhealing ulcer.

The Tolerance of Normal Tissues

The dose that can be given to tumours is limited by the tolerance of normal tissues. The TD depends on the overall radiation dose, fraction size and time between fractions. Overall treatment time and the volume irradiated are lesser factors, but the type of radiation used is also very important. Megavoltage x-rays spare the skin compared with kilovoltage (250–300 kV). Absorption in bone and cartilage is also much less with megavoltage x-rays, and there is less risk of necrosis. The tolerance of organs that have rapidly proliferating cells may be quite low. RT tolerance also depends on the hierarchical structure of organs. Based on the architecture of the functional subunits, organs in the body can be serial, parallel or serial-parallel. Serial (tubular) organs are those in which functional subunits (FSUs) are arranged serially, and all FSUs must be preserved to maintain the function of the organ. Serial organs may lose function completely if even a few FSUs receive a dose above the TD (dose effect). Examples are the spinal cord, optic nerve and chiasm. In parallel organs, such as in the lungs and kidney, FSUs are arranged in parallel. The function of parallel organs is affected only if a proportion of FSUs are damaged by a dose above the TD (volume effect). Some organs' functional units are arranged in a serial and parallel architecture. A typical example is the heart, where the coronary arteries have a parallel structure and the myocardium has a serial structure.

Acute reactions settle with simple medical measures (see Chapter 35). The late effects are most feared, as target organ damage can be severe, and the capacity for recovery is usually small. Such injuries are challenging to treat surgically, as the blood supply to heavily irradiated tissues is very poor. The frequency of late effects depends upon the site and the stage of the tumour.

RT, when used either as a primary treatment with or without chemotherapy or as an adjuvant, aims to achieve maximal possible tumour

TABLE 18.4 QUANTEC Recommendation on Tolerance Doses for Conventional Radiotherapy

Organ	Endpoint (% risk)	TOLERANCE DOSE		
		Dmax (Gy)	Dmean (Gy)	Dose/Volume
Brain	Symptomatic necrosis (<5)	72	-	-
Brainstem	Necrosis or cranial nerve palsy (<5)	<64	-	D1-10cc ≤59 Gy D100 <54 Gy
Spinal cord	Grade ≥2 myelopathy (<0.2)	50	-	-
Optic apparatus	Optic neuropathy (<3)	<55	<50	-
Retina	Blindness (<1)		<50	-
Cochlea	Hearing loss (<15)	-	≤45	-
Salivary glands	Dry mouth (<20)	-	<20	
Mandible	Radionecrosis (5)	70		
Pharyngeal constrictors	PEG tube dependent (<5)	-	<50	-
Larynx	Grade ≥2 laryngeal oedema	-	<44	V20 <27%
Brachial plexus	Brachial plexopathy (<5)	<60	-	-
Lungs	Symptomatic pneumonitis (5)		7	V20 <22%
	Symptomatic pneumonitis (10)		13	V20 <31%
	Symptomatic pneumonitis (20)		20	V20 <40%
Oesophagus	Grade ≥3 oesophagitis (<10)	74	34	V50 <30%
Heart	Cardiac mortality (<1)			V25 <10%
	Pericarditis (<15)			V30 <46%
Liver	Radiation-induced liver disease (5)		Normal liver ≤28; diseased liver ≤30	
Kidney	Renal dysfunction (<5)		<18	
Stomach	Ulceration			D100 <50 Gy
Spleen	Hyposplenism			D100 <10 Gy
Small bowel (individual loops)	Late obstruction/ulceration (<5)			V50 <5%
	Acute grade ≥3 toxicity (<10)			V15 <120 cc
Rectum				V50 <50%, V60 <35%, V65 <25%, V70 <20%, V75 <15%
Bladder			D100 <65	V65 ≤50%, V70 ≤35%, V75 ≤25%, V80≤15%
Penile bulb			<50	
Femoral head				D100 <52 Gy

control with acceptable late toxicities. It is debatable what is considered acceptable. The concepts of minimal and maximal tissue tolerance TDs were introduced in the early 1970s. The minimal tissue tolerance (also called tolerance dose 5/5; TD5/5) is the radiation dose that would result in a 5% risk of severe complications within 5 years, and the maximal TD (TD50/5) is the dose that would result in a 50% risk of severe complications within 5 years. These concepts are applied to the whole and partial organ volumes receiving conventional treatment with 1.8 to 2 Gy per fraction. In the early 1990s, Emami et al. published a set of normal tissue TDs; however, this was before the routine use of three-dimensional conformal RT or IMRT. Based on available dose-volume data, the Quantitative Analyses of Normal Tissue Effects in the Clinic (QUANTEC) group revised the recommendations on TDs for adults in 2010. The maximum dose to any point (Dmax) for serial organs should not exceed the recommended dose. For parallel organs, the TD is generally a mean dose and/or a dose based on different volumes of organ irradiated. Table 18.4 gives the recommended TDs for conventional (1.8–2 Gy per fraction) fractionated RT.

As mentioned earlier, hypofractionated RT (>2 Gy per fraction) has been increasingly used based on a recent understanding of clinical radiobiology and advances in RT techniques and delivery. However, the QUANTEC recommendations for conventional fractionation are not suitable for hypofractionation. The American Association of Physicians in Medicine recently published the report 'High Dose per Fraction, Hypofractionated Treatment Effects in the Clinic (HyTEC)' to derive TDs for hypofractionated regimens. Other groups are developing similar consensus and guidelines for TDs. Table 18.5 summarises the recommended TDs for hypofractionated RT by the UK SABR consortium and HyTEC. The variability in recommendations emphasises the lack of complete understanding of radiation tolerance.

Retreatment

The conventional belief is that heavily irradiated tissue will not tolerate a retreatment. Recent reports of successful outcomes following reirradiation to radical RT refute this perception. Factors governing the possibility of further therapy include the amount of cell depletion, the time elapsed since the previous treatment, the dose given and the fraction size used. This topic is discussed in detail in Chapter 19.

Response of Tumours to Radiation

Tumours may have numerous mitoses visible on histological examination, but they only grow slowly. A classic example is the slow-growing basal cell carcinoma of the skin. In this tumour, virtually all cells produced following cell division are lost by apoptosis and necrosis, and only a small number of the progeny of the dividing tumour adds to the tumour mass. In most carcinomas, over 90% of cells are lost in this way and are referred to as the *cell loss factor*. The potential volume doubling time (i.e. the time to go from a volume of 2 to 4 cm^3) in many tumours

TABLE 18.5 **Recommended Tolerance Doses for Hypofractionated Radiotherapy Based on the UK SABR Consortium and HyTEC**

	1-FRACTION		3-FRACTIONS		5-FRACTIONS	
OAR (toxicity)	**UK**	**HyTEC**	**UK**	**HyTEC**	**UK**	**HyTEC**
Brain (necrosis)	V12 ≤10 cm^3	V12 ≤5 cm^3	-	V20 ≤20 cm^3	-	V24 ≤20 cm^3
Optic apparatus (neuropathy)	Dmax <8 Gy	Dmax <10–12 Gy	Dmax <15 Gy	Dmax <20 Gy	Dmax <22.5 Gy	Dmax <25 Gy
Lungs (grade ≥2 toxicity)	-	-	V20 <10%	Mean dose ≤8 Gy V20 <10–15%	V20 <10%	Mean dose ≤8 Gy V20 <10–15%
Liver (grade ≥3 toxicity)			Dose to ≥700 cm^3 <19.2 Gy	Mean ≤13 Gy	Mean dose <15.2 Gy; V10 <70%	Mean ≤18 Gy for 6 fractions
Bladder (grade ≥2–3 toxicity)	-	-	Dmax <28.2 Gy	-	Dmax <18.3 Gy	Vprescription dose <5–10 cm^3 (4–5 fractions)
Rectum (grade ≥3 toxicity)	-	-	Dmax <28.2 Gy	-	Dmax <32 Gy	Dmax <35–38 Gy for 4–5 fractions
Spinal cord (myelopathy)	Dmax <14 Gy	Dmax <12.4–14 Gy	Dmax <21.9 Gy	Dmax <20.3–23.1 Gy	Dmax <23 Gy	Dmax <25.3–28.8 Gy

is on the order of 60 days. Without cell loss, tumours have the potential to grow much faster than this. Mitotic count, S-phase count and bromodeoxyuridine labelling index would suggest that, in many tumours, they have a potential doubling time of 3 to 8 days. Although the growth potential of many tumours is extremely rapid, owing to the high cell loss factor, they grow much more slowly in practice.

Cell loss factors may influence the rate of tumour regression during RT. Tumours with a high spontaneous cell loss factor will regress more rapidly during therapy, regardless of whether the tumour was growing quickly or slowly before treatment. However, the number of clonogenic tumour cells that survive radiation treatment will govern the ultimate outcome. Classically, only one clonogenic cell needs to survive; the tumour will then regrow. Many squamous cancers have high loss fractions and regress quickly. By contrast, the cell loss factor in prostatic cancer is much smaller, and these tumours shrink much more slowly after a lethal dose of radiation.

The growth fraction is the number of cells in the cycle. In solid tumours, this is usually less than 20% of the cells. Tumours with a high growth fraction may shrink more rapidly than those with a smaller growth fraction; however, unless all clonogenic cells are sterilised, these tumours may also rapidly regrow. Tumour growth fraction and repopulation may be increased following radiation treatment. Experiments have shown that there can be rapid regrowth of the clonogenic population of the tumour even while the tumour mass is regressing.

Overall Treatment Time

Local control in cervical cancer has been shown to decrease if the overall treatment time (external beam plus brachytherapy) exceeds 56 days. This is because of the repopulation of tumour cells during RT. Data, particularly from the Danish DAHANCA studies where patients with head and neck cancer were treated 5 or 6 days a week, have shown that a dose of 0.6 Gy per day is required to compensate for tumour repopulation between fractions, including weekend breaks. Reducing overall treatment time to 3 weeks may be one reason why 40 Gy in 15 fractions in the START trial was as effective as 50 Gy in 25 fractions. Gaps in RT treatment schedules should be avoided if possible, especially in patients with rapidly proliferating tumours such as head and neck cancer.

Modification of Fractionation Patterns

Repopulation during fractionated treatment is one reason why tumours persist after RT. This may be overcome by giving two or three treatments daily. A fraction size of less than 2 Gy is normally given to reduce the late effects in tissues, although acute reactions may be enhanced. Interfraction intervals should be as long as possible, but there should be at least 6 hours between treatments. The use of fraction sizes less than 2 Gy is usually referred to as *hyperfractionation*, and treatment schedules shorter than standard treatments are usually called *accelerated treatment*. Patients with well- or moderately well-differentiated tumours seem to have the greatest capacity for repopulation during RT and seem to be the group most likely to benefit from accelerated treatment, as shown in the CHART trials.

OTHER RADIATION MODALITIES

Heavy Particle Radiotherapy

Neutrons were perceived as a solution to the hypoxic cell problem, as hypoxic cells were more sensitive to neutrons than conventional x- or γ-rays in experimental systems. However, neutron irradiation was no more effective in practice than conventional fractionated photon RT. Moreover, many trials had to be abandoned because of the severity of severe late effects associated with neutrons. This treatment is no longer used.

By contrast, treatment with protons is intuitively more promising. The relative biological effect of protons is similar to x-rays, and the physical characteristics of a proton beam have potentially marked depth-dose advantage in treating some tumours. The dose-depth curve for protons in tissue is entirely different to those of photons (x- and γ-rays). Protons increase their rate of energy deposition as they slow down, increasing penetration and finally stopping and releasing an intense burst of ionisation called the *Bragg peak*. The beam has sharp edges with little side scatter, and the dose falls to zero after the Bragg peak at the end of the particles' range. By selecting proton beams of suitable proton energy, it is possible to release most of the proton's energy within the tumour if the Bragg peak is superimposed over the tumour-bearing area. Chapter 37 gives a detailed account of the application of proton beam therapy.

DRUG–RADIOTHERAPY COMBINATIONS

Chemoradiotherapy (CRT, CRTx) is the combination of chemotherapy and RT to treat cancer. Chemoradiation can be concurrent (together) or sequential (one after the other). The chemotherapy component can be or include a radiosensitising agent. Chemoradiotherapy, as a neoadjuvant therapy before surgery, is effective in various cancers. However, apart from combining traditional cytotoxic chemotherapy with

RT, little progress has been made in identifying and defining optimal targeted therapy and RT combinations to improve the efficacy of cancer treatment. Several novel agents could potentially improve clinical outcomes in combination with RT. However, the evaluation of appropriate novel drug–RT combinations should be prioritised early during the clinical development of new drugs with a solid scientific rationale based on understanding mechanisms of action and a clear line of sight to registration for the combination based on clinical need.

FUTURE DIRECTIONS

With many of the advances in RT being realised via technological improvements in the physical targeting of radiation, work is continuing to deliver superior instruments. Theoretically, precision RT techniques such as VMAT, IMRT, and Tomotherapy can cause a larger volume of normal tissue to be exposed to lower doses and increase the number of monitor units by a factor of 2 to 3, increasing the total-body exposure because of leakage radiation. Both factors could increase the risk of second cancers, with IMRT estimated to approximately double the incidence of second malignancies compared with conventional RT, from about 1% to 1.75% for patients surviving 10 years. The numbers may be even larger for more prolonged survival (or for younger patients), but the ratio should remain the same. Globally, we have extensive experience delivering image-guided radiation therapy (IGRT) and adaptive RT. At the beginning of this century, there were only a limited number of proton therapy facilities worldwide. As of 2023, 106 centres can provide proton therapy, and an additional 60 centres are setting up the facility. The meteoric adoption of hypofractionation and stereotactic ablative radiotherapy (SABR) in various common and uncommon cancers poses competition to conventionally fractionated proton beam therapy regarding patient convenience. Currently, the scope of proton therapy lies in smaller, more efficient delivery units and focused applications, particularly in children, teenagers and young adults and in adult tumours where there is a clear dose response for the clinical outcome (e.g. chordoma and chondrosarcoma). In the future, new indications may be established among the more common cancers, perhaps postoperative breast treatment or liver cancer, not just paediatrics. When that happens, Britain should expand its proton network cautiously, following the evidence and using newer single-room systems linked with high-performing academic cancer centres.

There is massive enthusiasm for FLASH technology and its potential use in clinics. FLASH-RT delivers ultrahigh dose–rate RT (>40 Gy per second) to the target. The ultrahigh dose rate contributes to oxygen depletion in normal tissues, thereby inducing radioresistance, leading to better sparing of the normal tissue. This, thus, potentially improves the therapeutic ratio.

An important future aim of molecular/biologic studies in RT is to increase the therapeutic ratio to increase tumour control and/or decrease late effects by predicting outcomes individually to select the most appropriate treatment for each patient. Also, molecular/biological studies should enable the development of new combined-modality treatments such as RT and concurrent biological therapies or chemotherapy in a scientifically rational manner. The advent of 'omic' technologies holds great promise for developing molecular studies in RT. Gene expression arrays (cDNA and oligonucleotide arrays) allow investigation of large numbers of patients' genes and show variation in gene expression among tumours with similar histological features. Proteomic technologies may also have a role in investigating radiosensitivity as they can provide a more accurate indicator of protein function than gene expression arrays by considering posttranslational modifications.

In summary, radiobiology has reached a stage where specific molecular and cellular pathways and responses are related to the various outcomes of RT. Such studies are exposing new potential targets for therapeutic manipulation of radiation responses. The well-established efficacy of RT and the accumulated knowledge of many decades of treatment provide a robust platform on which to launch novel approaches to extend its usefulness and increase its effectiveness. Combined with the molecular evaluations of the probability of tumour cure and normal tissue complication, as well as the more precise delivery of the dose, the future of radiobiology in RT research looks bright.

ACKNOWLEDGMENT

We greatly acknowledge the valuable contributions of George DD Jones and Paul Symonds to this chapter in the previous edition.

FURTHER READING

Connell PP, Kron SJ, Weichselbaum RR. Relevance and irrelevance of DNA damage response to radiotherapy. *DNA Repair (Amst)*. 2004;3:1245–1251.

Diez P, Hanna GG, Aitken KL, et al. UK 2022 consensus on normal tissue dose-volume constraints for oligometastatic, primary lung and hepatocellular carcinoma stereotactic ablative radiotherapy. *Clin Oncol Clin Oncol (R Coll Radiol)*. 2022;34(5):288–300.

Emami B, Lyman J, Brown A, et al. Tolerance of normal tissue to therapeutic irradiation. *Int J Radiat Oncol Biol Phys*. 1991;21(1): 109–122.

Grimm J, Marks LB, Jackson A, Kavanagh BD, Xue J, Yorke E. High dose per fraction, hypofractionated treatment effects in the clinic (HyTEC): an overview. *Int J Radiat Oncol Biol Phys*. 2021;110(1):1–10.

Hanna GG, Murray L, Patel R, et al. UK consensus on normal tissue dose constraints for stereotactic radiotherapy. *Clin Oncol (R Coll Radiol)*. 2018;30(1):5–14.

Li S, Shen L. Radiobiology of stereotactic ablative radiotherapy (SABR): perspectives of clinical oncologists. *J Cancer*. 2020;11(17):5056–5068.

Mangoni M, Borghesi S, Aristei C, Becherini C. Radiobiology of stereotactic radiotherapy. *Rep Pract Oncol Radiother*. 2022;27(1):57–62.

Marks LB, Yorke ED, Jackson A, et al. Use of normal tissue complication probability models in the clinic. *Int J Radiat Oncol Biol Phys*. 2010;76(3 Suppl):S10–S19.

Milano MT, Marks LB, Olch AJ, et al. Comparison of risks of late effects from radiation therapy in children versus adults: insights from the QUANTEC, HyTEC, and PENTEC efforts. *Int J Radiat Oncol Biol Phys*. 2024;119(2):387–400.

Muirhead R, Jones B. (Eds.). Re-irradiation. *Clin Oncol*. 2018; 30:65–136.

Sharma RA, Plummer R, Stock JK, et al. Clinical development of new drug-radiotherapy combinations. *Nat Rev Clin Oncol*. 2016;13(10): 627–642.

Symonds P, Jones GDD. FLASH radiotherapy: the next technological advance in radiation therapy? *Clin Oncol (R Coll Radiol)*. 2019; 31(7):405–406.

Symonds P, Jones D. (Eds.). Advances in clinical radiobiology. *Clin Oncol*. 2013;25:567–624.

Symonds P, Jones D. (Eds.). Advances in clinical radiobiology (part 2). *Clin Oncol*. 2014;26:241–308.

Ward JF. Complexity of damage produced by ionizing radiation. *Cold Spring Harb Symp Quant Biol*. 2000;65:377–382.

West C, Huddart R. (Eds.). Biomarkers and imaging for precision radiotherapy. *Clin Oncol*. 2015;27:545–618.

Willers H, Dahm-Daphi J, Powell SN. Repair of radiation damage to DNA. *Br J Cancer*. 2004;90:1297–1301.

19

Principles of Management of Patients With Cancer

Pete Bridge, John Rodgers and Thankamma V. Ajithkumar

CHAPTER OUTLINE

INTRODUCTION

The diagnosis of a malignancy is only the beginning of the journey for a patient with cancer, and throughout this time, decisions about how to best manage and care for the patient have to be addressed. Before seeing the oncologist, the majority of patients will have been given their diagnosis, most frequently in the outpatient department rather than a hospital ward. The importance of this event cannot be overemphasized, and the manner of communicating this information is pivotally important.

Consultation

When patients meet their oncologist for the first time, the presence of a family member or friend can be helpful because they can provide emotional support, assist in recall of the conversation and ask supplementary questions. This can be important at a time when patients will be trying to understand their condition and what the future may hold for them. There is little doubt that the majority of patients with cancer want as much information as possible. This often includes the elderly and the incurable. The first, sometimes initially unspoken, question is 'Is it curable?' and after that, 'Is it treatable?' At some point, most patients want to know their options for treatment and the side effects of possible treatments. Absorbing this information can be traumatic, and often patients cannot take in this complex web of information in one consultation. Support nurses or other healthcare professionals who are present in the clinic can provide useful reinforcement and clarification of patients' questions. Often the oncologist needs to cover the ground more than twice.

This whole process involves relaying information that can severely alter a patient's view of their future and is challenging for the person providing the information and for the patient. A useful guide in this process is the 10-step approach to giving bad news (Table 19.1). This model advocates good preparation, finding out what patients want to know, allowing denial and listening to concerns. It also recognises the importance of encouraging the ventilation of feelings and the significant role played by relatives.

The most important decision at this time is whether the patient should be treated radically, with cure as the aim of treatment. Radical treatment, however, may be associated with treatment-induced morbidity and, occasionally, mortality, and it is therefore vital to ensure that it is the appropriate route to be taking. Unfortunately, a number of patients will be unsuitable for a radical approach to treatment, and palliation will be the appropriate option.

The next question is which is the best treatment modality or modalities for that particular patient. Clearly, the patient needs to have been fully investigated before such a decision can be made, and usually this investigation will have been conducted before referral to the oncologist. However, supplementary investigations may need to be carried out. These may include examination under anaesthesia, endoscopy and appropriate radiological investigations such as computed tomography (CT), magnetic resonance imaging (MRI) or isotope bone scans. Because the diagnosis of cancer can possibly have dire implications, all patients should have histological proof of the diagnosis, if this is possible, especially if radical treatment is planned. To make appropriate management decisions, the clinician must take into account tumour and patient factors (listed later).

Frequently, the patient's management may have been discussed in a multidisciplinary team (MDT) meeting in which the patient's pathology and radiological investigations will have been reviewed. The decision is usually made about whether cure is possible and the appropriate treatment modality. However, only one or two members of the treating team may have met the patient at this stage, and decisions made at the MDT meeting may not survive the consultation with the patient and oncologist. When discussing treatment options, the patient's wishes are paramount. However, in practice, the majority of patients will accept the careful reasoned advice of their doctors. Very occasionally, patients ask for radical treatment when this is futile. Somewhat more frequently, such requests come from relatives. However, a doctor is not obliged to provide a treatment that they conscientiously feel is not in the patient's best interest.

TABLE 19.1 Ten Steps to Breaking Bad News

	Step	Action
1	Prepare.	Know all the facts before the meeting, find out who the patient wants present and ensure privacy and chairs to sit on.
2	What does the patient know?	Ask for a narrative of events by the patient (e.g. 'How did it all start?').
3	Is more information wanted?	Test the waters, but be aware that it can be very frightening to ask for more information (e.g. 'Would you like me to explain a bit more?').
4	Give a warning shot.	For instance, 'I'm afraid it looks rather serious'; then allow for a pause for the patient to respond.
5	Allow denial.	Denial is a defence and a way of coping; allow the patient to control the amount of information.
6	Explain (if requested).	Narrow the information gap, step by step; detail will not be remembered, but the *way* you explain will be.
7	Listen to concerns.	Ask 'What are your main concerns at the moment?' and then allow space for expression of feelings.
8	Encourage ventilation of feelings.	This is the *key* phase in terms of patient satisfaction with the interview because it conveys empathy.
9	Summarise the meeting and create a plan.	Summarise concerns, plan treatment, and foster hope.
10	Offer availability.	Most patients need further explanation and support (adjustment takes weeks or months) and benefit greatly from a family meeting.

FACTORS GOVERNING CLINICAL DECISIONS

Tumour Factors

Organ of Origin

The organ in which the cancer develops is an important factor affecting both outcome and treatment. Complete surgical removal of brain tumours is usually impossible, as a complete excision would normally damage vital parts of the brain, leading to either death or an unacceptable neurological deficit. Similarly, the brain is sensitive to ionising radiation, which limits the dose of radiotherapy (RT) that can be given. However, in other sites, such as the kidney, a complete organ can be removed with impunity.

Histological Type

Identification of the precise histological type of a tumour governs both treatment and prognosis. For instance, basal cell and squamous carcinomas arising from the epidermis of the skin have a good prognosis and the treatment is straightforward. By contrast, melanomas arising from pigment-producing cells (melanocytes) have a much more serious outlook.

Degree of Differentiation

The pathologist can grade the degree of differentiation. Well-differentiated tumours look like the tissue of origin, and poorly differentiated tumours may look primitive and do not look like the tissue from which they arise. For instance, well-differentiated thyroid cancer has a good prognosis and is relatively easily treated by such measures as surgical excision and radioiodine. Anaplastic thyroid cancers spread rapidly and respond poorly to any treatment.

Tumour Staging

Where possible, tumours should be staged using the international T, N and M classifications. *T* stands for primary tumour stage, which is usually decided based on the tumour size. *N* stands for the presence or absence of lymph node metastases, the usual method of spread in carcinomas and some sarcomas. *M* represents the presence or absence of distant metastases. In practice, other staging systems have been developed and are referred to in the preceding chapters.

Tumour Size

In general, the larger the tumour, the lower the chance of cure by either surgery or RT. It may not be possible to completely excise a large tumour. Similarly, a large tumour treated by RT contains more clonogenic tumour cells (cells capable of forming colonies of cells following RT) and an increased proportion of radioresistant hypoxic cells. Stage IB carcinoma of the cervix describes a tumour confined to the cervix, but this stage is subdivided into stage IB1 (<4 cm) and IBb2 (>4 cm). By and large, stage IB1 tumours are treated by radical hysterectomy and stage IB2 by chemoradiotherapy.

Locoregional Spread

Spread to regional lymph nodes usually indicates a poorer prognosis and the need for more aggressive therapy. Patients with squamous carcinoma of the head and neck with spread to regional lymph nodes may be treated by a radical neck dissection along with primary RT or surgical excision of the affected organ. As the spread to lymph nodes in breast cancer is often associated with occult distant spread, such patients usually receive adjuvant chemotherapy following surgery.

Distant Metastases

The presence of distant metastases may suggest that attempts to completely remove the primary tumour are futile, as is the case in lung cancer. However, such metastases may be chemosensitive and a high probability of cure may be possible. A typical case is testicular teratoma, where high cure rates are seen following cisplatin-based chemotherapy.

Tumour Site

The tumour site may determine the treatment modality. For instance, the skin on the back of the hand or the shin does not tolerate RT well. There is an increased risk of skin necrosis at these sites compared with elsewhere in the body. Surgery is often the preferred treatment for basal cell or squamous carcinoma in these areas. However, small basal cell carcinomas on the eyelid are often better treated by RT than surgery.

Operability

Many factors must be taken into account before deciding to treat the patient by radical surgery. A patient may have additional illnesses that may make the risks of surgery or anaesthesia extremely high (see later). The size of the tumour or involvement of adjacent structures may prevent complete removal of the cancer. The site of origin must also be taken into account together with the chance of complications following surgery and the functional result. Removal of inguinal lymph nodes is an important part of the treatment of carcinoma of the vulva. However, groin wounds are slow to heal and may become infected, especially in elderly people. The high risk of complications may be a contraindication for this type of surgery in the very elderly. Functional and cosmetic results are extremely important in head and neck surgery. Before the decision is made to remove a cancer, it must be possible to reconstruct the appropriate part of the upper aerodigestive tract and guarantee reasonable function and cosmesis.

Pathological Examination of the Excised Tissue

At first, surgery may be planned as the sole method of treatment modality. However, pathological examination of the excised tissue may change this decision. If the pathologist finds that the tumour extends to surgical margins, the chance of tumour recurrence is very high indeed. Postoperative RT may then be required. Radiation treatment may also be required depending on the degree of spread within the organ. The chance of microscopic spread to the pelvic lymph nodes is associated with the degree of differentiation of endometrial cancer and the degree of spread into the myometrium. Following simple hysterectomy, patients with poorly differentiated tumours and/or deep spread into the myometrium are often offered postoperative RT to reduce the chance of pelvic recurrence.

Patient Factors

Age/Performance Status

As a general rule, patients up to 75 years of age tolerate surgery or radical RT well. However, the biological age of the patient needs to be considered in addition to the chronological age. A fit patient in their 80s will tolerate RT well, but younger patients with serious general medical conditions may find treatment side effects intolerable. Many elderly patients may have chronic medical problems, such as chronic obstructive airway disease or ischaemic heart disease. These comorbid conditions may increase the risks of surgery to an unacceptable degree. Similarly, they may affect outcome after RT. Patients with poor pulmonary function are not suitable for radical treatment for lung cancer. The lung may become fibrosed around the irradiated tumour. This will have no effect in a fit patient, but the loss of even a small amount of lung function may cause respiratory failure in someone with chronic obstructive airway disease. Patients with ischaemic heart disease may have poor normal tissue perfusion. This may increase the number of radioresistant hypoxic cells within the tumour and also affect the ability of normal tissue to repair damage following radiation treatment.

Performance status (Tables 19.2 and 19.3) provides a crude but very effective method for judging response to treatment, especially with chemotherapy. Poor performance status is associated with shorter life expectancy. Patients with performance status 3 (in bed more than 50% of the time) are often not suitable for radical treatment. A paradox is that, although these patients have marked symptoms and the most to gain from chemotherapy, they are the group least likely to respond to this treatment. The highest response rates are seen in those with performance status 0 or 1.

TABLE 19.2 Karnofsky Performance Status Scale (Allows Patients to Be Classified as to Their Functional Impairment)

100	Normal, no complaints
90	Normal activity, minimal signs or symptoms
80	Normal activity with effort, some symptoms
70	Caring for self, unable to work
60	Needs occasional assistance but able to cater to most needs
50	Needs considerable assistance and frequent medical care
40	Disabled, needs special care
30	Severely disabled, needs hospital care
20	Very ill, in hospital, needs supportive care
10	Moribund
0	Dead

TABLE 19.3 Union for International Cancer Control Performance Status Scale

Grade	
0	Able to carry out normal activity
1	Able to live at home with tolerable symptoms
2	Disabling symptoms, but less than 50% of the time in bed
3	Severely disabled, greater than 50% of the time in bed, but able to stand
4	Very ill, confined to bed

Patient Preference

Patient preference should be taken into account. For instance, Stage IB carcinoma of the cervix can be treated equally well by radical surgery or RT. By and large, younger and fitter patients are offered radical hysterectomy, and older patients or those with obesity tend to be treated by RT. However, the individual patient may have a preference for one modality or the other.

Chance of Cure

Decision-making is easy if the chance of cure is high. A typical case is a T1 larynx cancer, which carries a chance of cure better than 90%. The side effects of RT to the larynx are tolerable even in the very elderly. By and large, patients with a 30% or better chance of cure are offered radical treatment. In more advanced disease with a poorer outlook, a lot depends on the patient's age and fitness. For instance, a T4 carcinoma of the bladder carries a 10% to 25% chance of cure. A fit middle-aged male may be offered intensive chemotherapy before removal of the bladder and construction of an ileostomy, whereas the right treatment for an unfit elderly male may be palliative RT to suppress symptoms from the bladder cancer.

TREATMENT MODALITY

Increasing use of multimodality treatment has rather blurred the once clear-cut rules for treatment by the various modalities. A brief summary of the main modalities available for management follows.

Surgery

Surgery, traditionally, was important for establishing the diagnosis and finding the extent of spread of the cancer. Increasingly, diagnosis is made without operation using sophisticated imaging techniques such as in vivo nuclear magnetic resonance (NMR) spectroscopy or positron emission tomography–computed tomography (PET/CT) scanning. Histological proof may be obtained by fine needle or tru-cut biopsy. Radical surgery is still the treatment of choice for many adenocarcinomas, particularly those arising in the stomach, colon, thyroid and kidney.

Palliative Surgery

Before palliative surgery, the risks and benefits to the patient need to be carefully measured and the patient's potential life expectancy needs to be taken into account. Surgery is particularly useful in dealing with obstruction of an organ. A classical case is colonoscopy for the relief of large bowel obstruction due to colon cancer. However, palliative surgery may be inappropriate in patients with multiple small bowel obstructions. This is often the case in ovarian cancer, where the risks of surgery outweigh the benefits. Advanced fungating breast tumours are much less common than they were 25 years ago, but surgery offers a rapid method of relieving the unpleasant odour and bleeding associated with such tumours. The pinning of the broken bone, which is often followed by palliative RT, may relieve pain following a pathological fracture.

Surgical Methods

Traditional open operations are being replaced by less invasive keyhole techniques. Many patients with colon cancer are now treated laparoscopically. A telescope (laparoscope) connected to a video camera plus a light source is introduced through a small abdominal incision. The abdomen is distended by insufflating CO_2 gas. Instruments can be inserted through another small incision and are guided using the video camera. The advantages of this method are that (1) there is less pain postoperatively, (2) haemorrhage is reduced because smaller incisions are used and (3) healing and recovery time are shortened. Disadvantages are a lack of depth perception through the laparoscope and a limited range of motion of the instruments introduced into the abdomen. In some cases, especially in advanced colon cancer, the operation may be converted to an open laparotomy so that the surgeon can get a better view and therefore a better understanding of the complete picture. It may also be easier to mobilise and completely resect the tumour.

The current ultimate form of keyhole surgery is robotic laparoscopic surgery. In Britain the most commonly used device is the Da Vinci robot, which costs more than £1 million. There are two parts to the robot. The first is the patient unit, which has four arms: one arm holds the laparoscope and the others hold surgical instruments. The second is the control unit, which is where the surgeon sits. The control unit is remote from the patient and has a screen showing a magnified three-dimensional view of the operative field, allowing the surgeon to manipulate the instruments more smoothly and with better control compared with using the human hand. Robots are increasingly used in gynaecological surgery to treat cervix and endometrial cancer and to perform radical prostatectomies. Direct evidence is lacking that this form of expensive surgery is superior, because of a lack of clinical trials comparing robotic surgery with older techniques.

Chemotherapy

Chemotherapy can be given as the sole source of treatment when there is a high chance of cure. Only a small number of tumours are highly chemosensitive, and these include the lymphomas, testicular teratoma and choriocarcinoma. Chemotherapy frequently cures children with Wilms tumours, rhabdomyosarcomas and acute lymphoblastic leukaemia. Chemotherapy may be given before RT or surgery to reduce the tumour's size. This is often referred to as *neoadjuvant treatment*. Increasingly, RT and chemotherapy are given together. This is of proven value in the treatment of carcinoma of the cervix, squamous carcinoma of the anus, carcinoma of the oesophagus and head and neck cancer. Clinical trials are continuing involving other tumour sites, particularly in lung cancer. Chemotherapy may be of palliative value only in advanced breast cancer or carcinoma of the colon, but in the treatment of small-volume disease following surgery, adjuvant chemotherapy may improve cure rates. Chemotherapy improves 10-year survival in node-positive breast cancer by about 10%. A similar survival advantage is seen following adjuvant chemotherapy in Dukes stage C colon cancer. For more information, please see Chapter 20.

Hormone Therapy

Hormone therapy plays an increasingly important role in the treatment of a range of cancers that are hormone sensitive. This therapeutic approach aims to either block the production of specific hormones or interfere with their actions, thus impeding cancer cell growth. Commonly used in breast and prostate cancers, hormone therapy is designed to target hormone receptors on cancer cells. In breast cancer, for instance, hormone receptor–positive tumours can respond to drugs such as tamoxifen or aromatase inhibitors, which block oestrogen receptors, hindering the hormone's ability to promote cancer cell proliferation. Similarly, in prostate cancer, where testosterone drives tumour growth, androgen deprivation hormone therapy has a valuable role to play in reducing risk of recurrence, slowing growth and relieving symptoms and rates of spread in metastatic disease. While hormone therapy can be effective, its success depends on factors such as the type of cancer, hormone receptor status and individual patient characteristics. Side effects to hormone therapy are varied and include hot flashes, fatigue, mood swings, sexual dysfunction in males, osteoporosis and cardiovascular issues. Both genders may experience weight gain and altered lipid profiles. For more information about hormone therapy, please see Chapter 20.

Immunotherapy

There is significant interest in research and continuing advancement in the role of immunotherapy for cancer treatment. Immunotherapy works by stimulating the body's immune system to recognise and destroy cancer cells. This makes it much more targeted and able to attack cancer cells alone. Checkpoint inhibitors are a common form of immunotherapy; these work by blocking proteins that inhibit immune responses, such as PD-1 and CTLA-4. By doing so, these inhibitors unleash the immune system to better recognise and eliminate cancer cells. Another approach involves CAR-T cell therapy, where a patient's T cells are genetically modified to express chimeric antigen receptors, enabling them to target specific cancer proteins. Immunotherapy developments are helping with the management of malignancies that were traditionally challenging to treat, and immunotherapy is being used across a range of tumours, including melanoma, lung and kidney cancers.

While immunotherapy represents a groundbreaking advancement, it is not without challenges. Response rates can vary among patients, and immune-related adverse events may occur, impacting on the skin, gastrointestinal tract or endocrine system. Ongoing research aims to refine and expand the use of immunotherapy, exploring combination approaches with other treatments to enhance efficacy. Immunotherapy is a rapidly evolving treatment that represents a paradigm shift in cancer treatment, enabling a targeted and personalised approach that harnesses the body's natural defences.

Radiotherapy

Radical Radiotherapy

The decision to treat the patient by radical RT depends on the tumour and patient factors previously discussed. The precise regimen will depend on the potential radiosensitivity of the tumour, the size of the treatment volume and the proximity of dose-limiting critical tissues. Seminoma of the testes is among the most radiosensitive tumours. The doses required to control small-volume disease in the paraaortic lymph nodes are 25 to 30 Gray (Gy) in 15 fractions over 3 weeks. By contrast, large lymph nodes containing metastatic squamous carcinoma may not be controlled by doses as high as 70 Gy given in 35 fractions over 7 weeks.

What governs radiation dose is the tolerance of the surrounding normal tissues. The small bowel is the most sensitive tissue in the abdomen and pelvis, and the chance of serious small bowel damage rises steeply with doses exceeding 50 Gy given in 25 fractions over 5 weeks. Radiation damage to the spinal cord can be catastrophic, leading to permanent paralysis. In the treatment of tumours in the head and neck, oesophagus and bronchus, care must be taken to restrict the spinal cord dose to 45 to 50 Gy in 25 fractions over 5 weeks.

The side effects of radical RT may be marked. For instance, the mucositis associated with treatment of head and neck cancer may prevent the patient swallowing and may require nasogastric or percutaneous endoscopic gastrostomy (PEG) feeding. However, acute side effects are normally self-limiting and settle in a few weeks with the help of simple supportive measures. This is a probability of late radiation damage that limits the dose to the tumour. In the treatment of breast cancer, the incidence of serious late effects should be vanishingly small and certainly less than 0.5% of those patients treated. As the life-threatening nature of the tumour increases, the patient and the oncologist may be persuaded to take greater chances. Serious damage is seen in the larynx following treatment for a T3 (fixed vocal cord) tumour in 1% to 3% of patients. In patients with inoperable cervical cancer, the only realistic chance of cure is chemoradiotherapy. Some of the highest complication rates associated with RT are seen following the treatment of cervical cancer. On average, 6% of patients require surgery to try to correct late damage following treatment.

Palliative Radiotherapy

Palliative treatments can make up between one-third and one-half of the workload of any department. The aim of such treatment is to relieve local symptoms in advanced cancer. An important part of the treatment is that there should be minimal upset. Treatment should be simple and a minimum number of fractions should be used. Symptomatic relief should be rapid.

Up to 80% of patients with bone metastases have significant pain relief within 3 weeks of a single radiation treatment of 8 to 10 Gy. Pain relief will be complete within half of these patients. Other important indications for palliative RT are the relief of haemoptysis, cough, dyspnoea and mediastinal obstruction in lung cancer. These symptoms can be suppressed in between 50% and 80% of patients by a course of RT lasting up to 1 week, with minimal side effects.

However, some symptoms require longer RT treatments. Tumours involving nerves, such as the brachial plexus (Pancoast tumours from the apex of the lung) or the lumbosacral plexus, produce pain of a very unpleasant quality that is difficult to relieve with opiate analgesia. Relief of such neuropathic pain may require 4 to 5 weeks of RT treatment. Typically, neuropathic pain from advanced rectal cancer can be relieved in two-thirds of patients with doses of 45 to 50 Gy given over 4 to 5 weeks. RT can prolong life in some patients with incurable tumours. Randomised controlled trials have shown that the average survival of patients with glioblastomas of the brain following optimal surgery and RT is only 1 year. However, 6 weeks of RT increases a patient's survival by, on average, 9 months compared with treatment with surgery and best supportive care. When making the decision to offer a patient 6 weeks of RT, one needs to balance life expectancy that is taken up by the RT treatment and the associated fatigue with the survival benefit associated with a treatment which is unlikely to cure the patient. Elderly or more infirm patients are probably better treated by a simple scheme of 30 Gy given in 6 fractions 3 times per week over 2 weeks rather than 60 Gy given in 30 fractions.

Brachytherapy

The use of brachytherapy where gamma ray–emitting sources are implanted directly into the tumour or are placed in body cavities such as the uterus and vagina adjacent to malignant tissue is becoming uncommon. Brachytherapy is still an essential part of radical RT regimens for cervical cancer, but treatment elsewhere by interstitial sources in diseases such as prostate and head and neck is decreasing or has ceased entirely, being replaced by surgery, newer forms of RT or combinations of radiation and chemotherapy.

Intensity Modulation

Traditionally, external beam radiotherapy (EBRT) was given by square or rectangular plain or wedged fields. The majority of patients treated radically receive intensity modulated radiotherapy (IMRT). In IMRT, treatment is delivered by a linear accelerator equipped with multileaf collimators (MLCs), thin tungsten columns which move independently to form shapes that fit precisely around the tumour. This allows a high dose to be given to the tumour with sparing of vulnerable normal tissue. In particular, IMRT can create concave shapes, which is particularly helpful in the treatment of head and neck cancer, allowing treatment of tumour-containing structures such as lymph nodes but with sparing of the spinal cord. The majority of patients with pelvic cancers such as cervical, rectal and prostate cancer are treated with IMRT with lower doses to small and large bowel and reduced acute and late bowel damage. Patients with breast cancer benefit from IMRT treatments as unwanted high-dose areas can be eliminated, and if a boost is required to the excised tumour bed, this can be included in the IMRT plan rather than a localised electron treatment at the end of photon therapy. One theoretical disadvantage of IMRT is owing to the fact that multiple beams are used and more normal tissue is irradiated, albeit at a low dose. Although this low-dose irradiation does not cause increased acute side effects, it may increase the risk of second radiation-induced cancers developing 20 or more years after successful IMRT treatment.

Stereotactic Methods

The use of stereotactic RT which precisely delivers RT in a highly focused manner is increasing, and its use is likely to increase further in the next decade. The term *stereotactic* means the three-dimensional localisation of a point in the body, usually relating to a fixed external reference frame or other fixation devices and requiring highly accurate imaging to locate the lesion to be treated. Stereotactic treatment, sometimes called *stereotactic ablative radiotherapy (SABR)*, when used in the treatment of small nonsmall cell lung cancer can give equivalent cure rates to those seen after surgery. The use of this modality is increasing in the treatment of prostate cancer, and if phase III clinical trials fulfil the promise of phase II pilot studies, this may become the treatment of choice in prostate cancer with only five daily treatments leading to cure with a low incidence of acute and late side effects. The palliative use of SABR is increasing, especially in the treatment of cerebral metastases, and it may become the treatment of choice for bone metastasis, especially vertebral lesions.

Britain now has the first of two planned proton facilities. There are established indications in the treatment of children, especially the treatment of brain tumours, owing to the sparing of normal brain in proton therapy. The indications in adults are less well defined and the majority of proton treatments in the United States are for prostate cancer, where there is no evidence of superiority of protons over other modalities. Proton therapy must be evaluated in careful, well-planned clinical trials.

Image-Guided Radiotherapy

Contemporary EBRT techniques are characterised by highly conformal plans delivered by modern linear accelerators using IMRT and volumetric modulated arc therapy (VMAT). By directing dose precisely to the intended target, applying steep dose gradients and thereby sparing critical surrounding tissues, the aim is to improve the therapeutic ratio via dose escalation and hypofractionation. In addition, adaptive radiotherapy (ART) has become increasingly important as a means to deliver radiation as effectively as possible. This process of incremental complexity and sophistication has been facilitated not only through advanced planning approaches and delivery systems but also by the development of image-guided radiotherapy (IGRT). Many of these recent developments, such as ultrahypofractionated treatment regimens, would be impossible without IGRT as a key driver to ensure that very high doses of RT are delivered accurately to the intended target, while avoiding organs at risk (OARs) throughout the treatment course.

TABLE 19.4 Current Imaging Modalities: Advantages and Disadvantages

Modality	Advantages	Disadvantages
MV portal imaging	Fast acquisition Can be used for in vivo dosimetry	Negligible soft-tissue contrast 2D imaging; paired images are necessary to calculate 3D position
kV planar imaging	Fast acquisition Reduced dose compared to megavoltage Higher-quality images compared to megavoltage	Low soft-tissue contrast 2D imaging; therefore paired images are necessary to calculate 3D position
Cone beam computer tomography	3D images with reasonable soft-tissue contrast	Increased imaging dose to patient; longer acquisition time compared to 2D kV
Ultrasound	Nonionising Potential for intrafractional guidance	Limited vendor support
Electromagnetic transponders	Real-time monitoring during treatment delivery	Requires implantation prior to treatment
Surface-guided radiation therapy	Nonionising Monitoring patient throughout treatment	Most appropriate for superficial target localisation
Magnetic resonance imaging	Nonionising Superior soft-tissue contrast Ability to image in real time during treatment Daily online adaptive planning	Resource intensive Longer treatment times limit throughput Limited treatment field size

2D, Two-dimensional, *3D*, three-dimensional; *kV*, kilovoltage; *MV*, megavoltage.

Historically, two-dimensional radiographic images produced from either cobalt or LINAC megavoltage (MV) beams have been used to verify patient position using skeletal anatomy. Technology for image guidance has developed and diversified to include numerous IGRT modalities, as seen in Table 19.4. Despite these advances, two-dimensional MV portal imaging remains commonly used for breast treatments, although cone beam computed tomography (CBCT) is being utilised increasingly often. The development of gantry-mounted CBCT in the late 1990s was the most influential factor in encouraging the rapid evolution of IGRT.

Although introduced in the late 1990s, and despite a plethora of competing modalities, CBCT remains the workhorse of IGRT, responsible for image guidance for the majority of treatment areas and techniques. CBCT image acquisition generally takes from 1 to 4 minutes and can be three dimensional or four dimensional. Once acquired, the CBCT image is overlaid and registered with the plan reference image, usually via a rigid algorithm. This aligns the images and provides a displacement vector to correct setup error in three translational planes via automated table shifts. Rotations are only mitigated with treatment couches capable of six degrees of freedom. Prior to treatment delivery, images are assessed by trained radiographers to determine whether the alignment of target volumes and critical normal tissues is appropriate.

However, patients are not static entities, and image review often proves more complex than a simple process of eliminating setup error. Frequently, there are variations between the position and shape of relevant planned anatomy to that seen on treatment. Such variations can be physiological in nature; changes in bladder, rectal or gastric filling (Fig. 19.1); bowel mobility and peristalsis (Fig. 19.2); variable lung presentations caused by pleural effusion, atelectasis, collapse or reexpansion (Fig. 19.3); contour changes, oedematous swelling, weight loss and weight gain (Fig. 19.4); tumour progression or regression (Fig. 19.5); changes in respiratory motion; and gross displacements in patient position, such as spinal flexion and flattening. Tumour lesions can quite simply displace from their planned location. These can be isolated or complex and multifactorial, random or systematic.

Invariably, achieving accurate assessment of such changes can be problematic. Radiographers responsible for IGRT review have to identify, quantify and assess whether such changes can be mitigated sufficiently via simple couch shifts to allow safe and accurate treatment delivery or whether differences are significant enough in terms of plan dosimetry, tumour coverage or critical tissue toxicity to require escalation. This analysis has to be made within a reasonable time frame so as to limit the prospect of intrafraction motion. Subjectivity and variance are inevitable during the process. Therefore it is essential that radiographers are sufficiently trained and supported by site-specific protocols and clinician-directed IGRT decision-making frameworks. This has become increasingly important with the expansion of more complex plans encompassing multiple clinical target volumes (CTVs) and multiple dose levels, while the use of ultrahypofractionated ablative treatments means confident, informed judgments on OAR positions is fundamental.

Ultimately, the purpose of IGRT should be to improve patient outcomes, whether that means reducing OAR toxicity or improving overall survival. IGRT directly reduces geometric uncertainty during RT delivery. It might be expected that its introduction would lead to better outcomes. However, robust clinical evidence to support this assertion has proven to be elusive. The introduction of IGRT has been gradual, and during this time many other developments have been introduced. Therefore quantifying the contribution of IGRT alone amongst many confounders can be demanding. In addition, IGRT is ubiquitous in RT. Designing randomised controlled trials to establish differences in an IGRT arm to another without, or with less frequent, image guidance may be ethically challenging. However, from a pragmatic perspective, IGRT has enabled new treatment options, such as ultrahypofractionated RT. Primary lung SABR, for example, provides similar local control and lung cancer survival rates to those of surgery and would not be possible without IGRT (Chen et al., 2018).

Adaptive Radiotherapy

Adaptive RT is a process by which anatomical variations that have been deemed significant can be addressed by amending the patient's treatment plan. The most frequent method is offline ART, meaning new plan preparation such as contouring and optimisation occurring outside the online treatment workflow with the intent of replacing the original with a new optimised plan. In the meantime, treatment may be halted, or it may continue, following the original plan.

Other types of ART exist, but ultimately, online adaptive radiotherapy (OART) represents the next paradigm shift in RT. The recent development of hybrid magnetic resonance linear accelerators to deliver MR-guided adaptive radiotherapy (MRgART) has not only delivered exquisite soft-tissue information, real-time imaging and the prospect

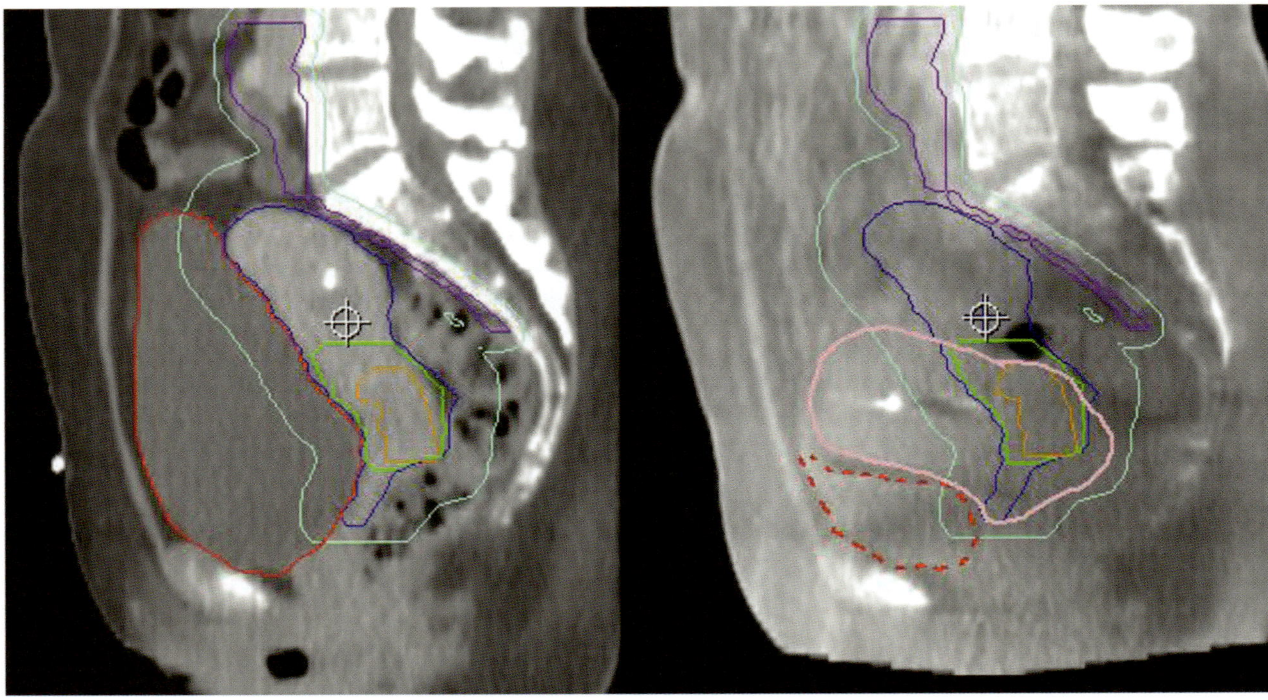

Fig. 19.1 Smaller bladder allowing uterus to displace forwards out of planning target volume (PTV). This demonstrates the influence of bladder volume on target position. On the planning computed tomography image *(left)*, a full bladder *(red)* pushes the uterus posteriorly *(dark blue)* and displaces the bowel away from high-dose regions. On the verification cone beam computed tomography image *(right)*, an empty bladder *(dashed red)* allows the uterus *(pink)* to displace anteriorly/inferiorly beyond the PTV *(light blue)*. The bowel also drops into the PTV.

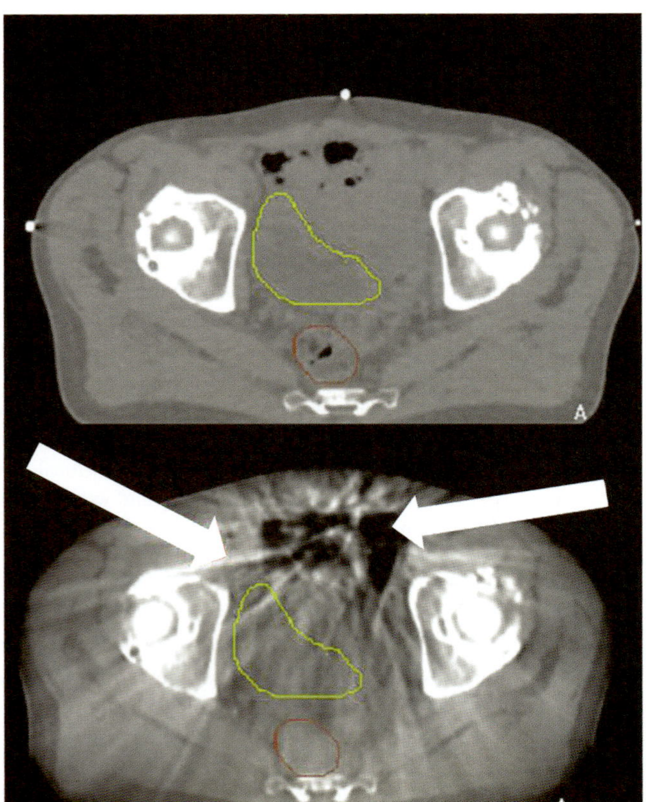

Fig. 19.2 Small bowel peristalsis contributing to streak artefacts on a cone beam computed tomography scan. Streak artefacts *(red arrow)* are caused by bowel gas peristaltic motion *(white arrow)*, resulting in deterioration in image quality.

of functional imaging to become integrated within IGRT but also has resulted in the ability to alter the RT plan online based on daily variations detected in patient anatomy. This combines deformable registration, automatic anatomical contouring, plan optimisation, evaluation and quality assurance (QA) within a single treatment workflow (Fig. 19.6).

The positive experience with MRgART has been tempered by several limitations which may hinder rapid widespread adoption. These include the expense of the equipment and a complex treatment workflow that has proven to be resource intensive and time-consuming. This means that while MRgART is likely to prove highly capable at delivering ultrahypofractionated treatment to mobile, deformable targets that are difficult to see on CBCT and are close to radiosensitive critical structures, it is unlikely to replace the traditional RT IGRT workflow for a majority of treatment sites.

Recently, online adaptive systems have emerged that employ CBCT images for OART. The Varian Ethos (Varian Medical Systems, Palo Alto, CA) and the Elekta Evo (Elekta AB, Stockholm, Sweden) both use machine learning and artificial intelligence (AI) to detect and contour normal tissue structures on the CBCT while propagating target structures from the planning CT to the CBCT image. A synthetic CT is generated, and automated planning is carried out to produce an adapted plan based on the anatomy of the day. This can be selected for treatment, or a reference plan can be used.

While this technology is still nascent, and contemporary CBCT OART workflows may extend treatment times compared to standard workflows, it provides the very real and enticing prospect of online adaptive radiotherapy supplanting IGRT and becoming routine for many treatment sites.

Reirradiation

Over the past two decades, the outcomes of cancer have significantly improved due to advances in surgical and RT techniques and the

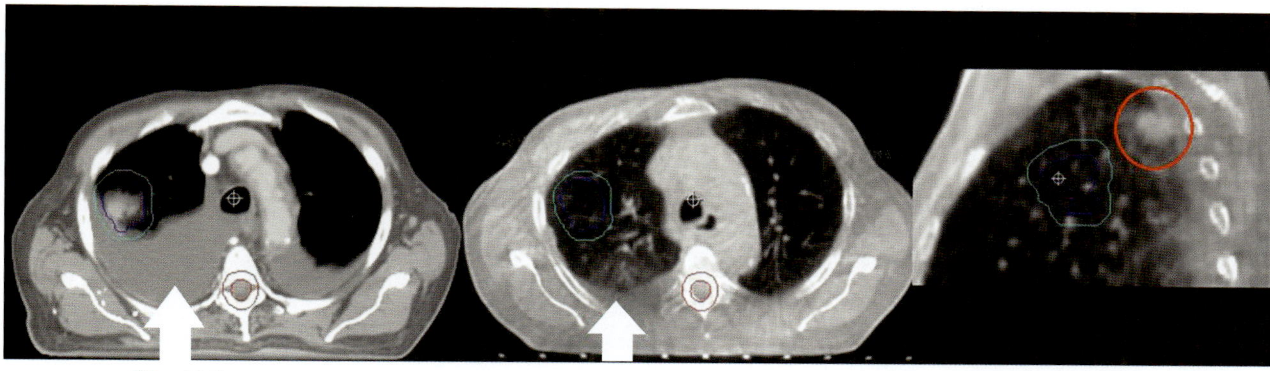

Fig. 19.3 Resolution of pleural effusion causing displacement of the target lesion. The patient was planned with a large, apparently stable, pleural effusion *(right-hand arrow)*. Cone beam computed tomography midway through treatment demonstrates rapid resolution of effusion *(middle arrow)*, causing significant displacement of the tumour *(right-hand red circle)* out of the planning target volume *(light blue contour in all images)*.

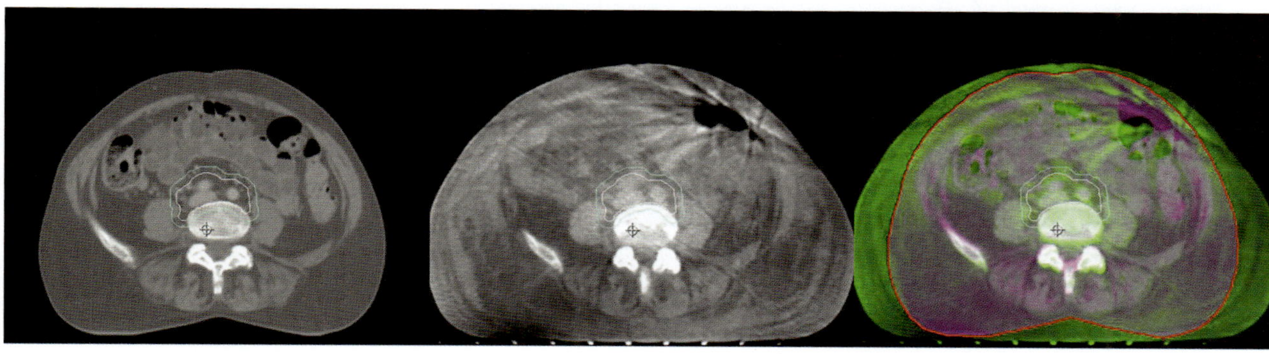

Fig. 19.4 Significant contour change detected on a cone beam computed tomography (CBCT) scan, requiring that the patient be replanned. Rapid weight gain due to steroids was detected on day 1 of treatment. The image on the left is the original treatment planning scan, the centre image is the CBCT localisation image. The image on the right shows the CBCT verification image overlaid upon the treatment planning image *(red contour)*. The increase in the patient contour on the CBCT is show in *green*. The patient underwent a replan during treatment.

routine clinical use of novel systemic therapies. However, patients still present after initial curative or adjuvant RT with locoregional recurrences. Rarely, some patients may develop second neoplasms (e.g. second primary in lung, and head and neck region). Curative or palliative reirradiation is an option depending on the type of recurrence and stage.

Traditionally, reirradiation has been used at least 1 to 2 years after a previous course of RT. However, with the increasing availability of high-precision RT techniques, reirradiation is considered as early as 3 to 6 months after the last course of RT. Reirradiation can be delivered

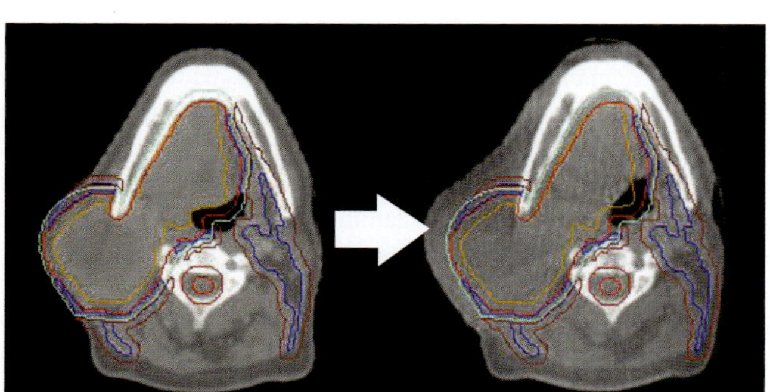

Fig. 19.5 An example of disease progression in a head and neck patient. The *arrow* highlights an increase in tumour volume displacing tissue well beyond the planning target volume *(pale blue contour)* on the verification CBCT image on the right. Original CT planning image is show on the left. The patient was replanned during treatment.

using imaged-guided brachytherapy, IMRT/VMAT/tomotherapy or particle beam therapy. To minimise radiation side effects, reirradiation target volumes tend to be smaller (e.g. no CTV margins, treating only residual volume after salvage surgery or chemotherapy).

Studies have shown encouraging clinical outcomes with reirradiation for recurrent tumours of the brain, head and neck, pelvis and thorax. A recent ESTRO and EORTC consensus has broadly categorised a second or further courses of RT as reirradiation and repeat organ irradiation. Reirradiation is a new course of RT either to the previously irradiated volume, irrespective of toxicity concerns (type 1), or to the previously nonoverlapping irradiated volume where the cumulative dose raises toxicity concerns (type 2) (see Andratschke et al., 2022). When the new course of RT is delivered to a target volume within the same organ (e.g. contralateral lung) but without overlap of irradiated volumes and concern for toxicity from cumulative doses, it is considered repeat-organ irradiation. This definition of reirradiation helps to distinguish it from repeat irradiation, which denotes reirradiation to a different organ with neither an overlap of irradiated volumes nor any concern for toxicity from cumulative doses.

Planning and QA processes for reirradiation follow the same principles as any radical RT course, as described in Chapter 12. However, reirradiation in the palliative setting is less complex, as the intent for treatment is short-term palliation rather than long-term disease control with acceptable late toxicities. While there is great enthusiasm for the clinical use of reirradiation, there is a vast knowledge gap in tissue recovery and the usefulness of existing mathematical

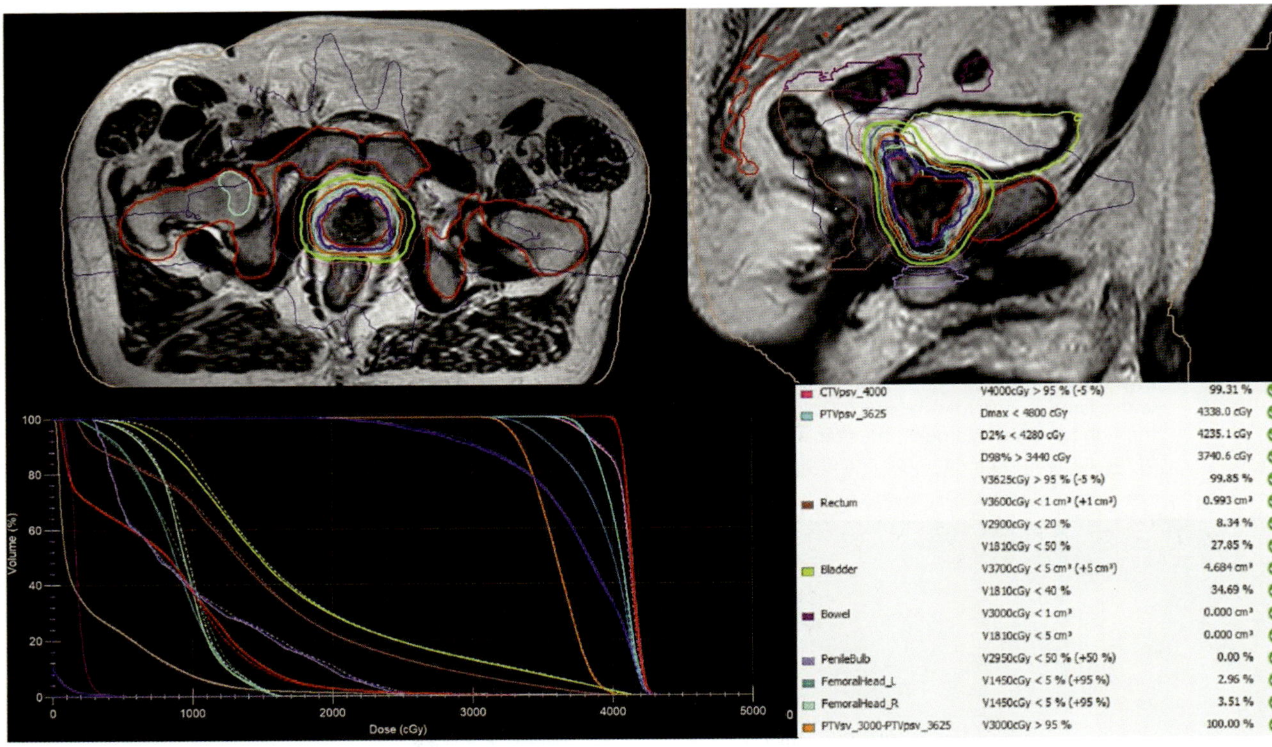

Fig. 19.6 Elekta Unity online planning interface. *Top left:* Axial view through planning scan. *Top right:* Sagittal view through planning scan. *Bottom left:* Dose volume histogram comparing treatment plan and reference plan. *Bottom right:* Treatment and reference plan comparison using the traffic light system.

models of radiation damage and recovery to guide reirradiation. In the current literature, the incidence of significant RT side effects after reirradiation is lower than expected, suggesting partial or complete recovery between courses of RT. It is widely appreciated that concurrent chemotherapy, salvage surgery, infection and inflammation may affect reirradiation tolerance. There are limited data on individual reirradiation tolerance for individual OARs. A few experimental and clinical studies evaluated adult spinal cord reirradiation tolerance. Patients who receive a cumulative EQD22 of 75 Gy with an interval of ≥6 months and EQD22 of both courses <51 Gy to the spinal cord have an estimated 3% risk of radiation myelopathy (see Doi et al., 2021). A cumulative EQD22 above 75 Gy, a time interval of <6 months between primary and reirradiation or an EQD22 >51 Gy for individual courses increases the estimated risk of myelopathy to 25%. A cumulative EQD22 <75 Gy to the optic apparatus is also reported to be safe (Stiefel et al., 2021). A PENTEC review (Ajithkumar et al., 2024) suggests that in children/AYA with recurrent brain tumours, reirradiation with a total EQD22 of about 112 Gy is associated with an approximate 5% to 7% incidence of brain/brainstem necrosis after a median follow-up of 1.6 years. Fig. 19.7 shows a reirradiation for a recurrent anaplastic ganglioglioma (WHO grade III). The right optic nerve received a cumulative EQD22 of 95.5 Gy. A potentially higher risk of right optic neuropathy was discussed with and accepted by the patient. Unfortunately, 6 months after reirradiation, the patient developed spinal-only metastases.

The total dose, fractionation and techniques for reirradiation are dictated by perception and estimates of tissue recovery and reirradiation tolerance, the availability of advanced RT techniques and the confidence the RT team has gained from increasing experience. However, whether there is an optimal dose–response relationship between reirradiation and clinical outcome and whether any technique is better is unknown. Nevertheless there is an ongoing international effort to derive the optimal workflow, capture prospective data and standardise clinical guidelines for reirradiation to gain an in-depth understanding of the safety and efficacy, tissue recovery and tolerance dose of critical organs in the future.

Complementary Therapies

Complementary therapies do not offer patients an alternative approach to established treatments such as surgery, chemotherapy and RT; rather, as the name suggests, they are designed to complement existing treatments. These therapies are diverse and varied and include self-help approaches such as relaxation, meditation, visual therapies and touch therapies, such as aromatherapy, massage and reflexology, as well as more established practices of homeopathy and acupuncture.

Although debate continues about the efficacy of many therapies, it has to be acknowledged that increasingly, patients express an interest in their use and reports have indicated that up to one-third of patients with cancer have used complementary therapies. This debate is ongoing, and as demands for conventional reliable evidence for efficacy increase and research continues, the aim must be an acknowledgment among health professionals that patients will continue to search these therapies out. This means that we must be informed and open to dialogue with patients and their families. This is of particular importance because some therapies patients may engage in may be viewed as more 'alternative' treatments, which could possibly result in a tension with orthodox treatment and, indeed, there is growing concern among clinicians that sometimes their use can interfere with conventional treatments such as chemotherapy and produce harmful effects. Two therapies that are now known to be toxic and should be discouraged are Laetrile, a concentrated form of amygdalin found in raw nuts and berries that breaks down in the body into cyanide, and Iscador, extracted from mistletoe, which has been shown to worsen survival in disseminated melanoma.

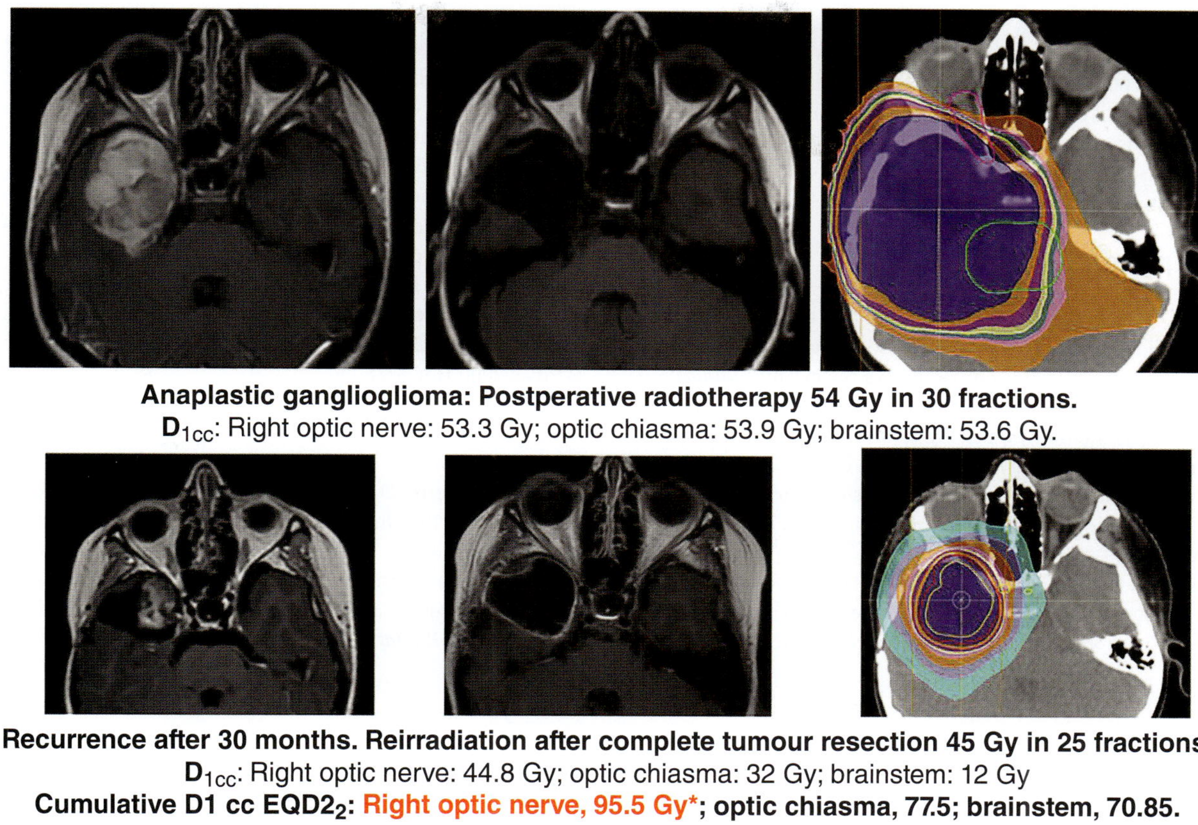

Fig. 19.7 A reirradiation for a recurrent anaplastic ganglioglioma (WHO grade III).

It should be recognised that the reasons given by patients for seeking out complementary therapies are varied and often relate to the perception that they are 'natural' and holistic, and that they will improve quality of life and help to relieve the symptoms of both disease and the effects of treatment. They offer the patient a sense of personal involvement in their own care and often the feeling that they are taking some control of their disease. In addition, this form of treatment tends to foster a feeling of psychological empowerment, because patients feel it allows them to cope better with their illness. So, although the reasons for seeking out complementary therapies are highly individual and may not be based on the same philosophical approach shared by many clinicians, they surely have to be regarded as personally valid for patients. Thus the aims for health professionals should first be to encourage disclosure by patients if they are using complementary therapies, and then to try and provide high-quality information and opportunity for discussion that empowers patients to make their own decisions.

CLINICAL TRIALS

Progress in the treatment of cancer is largely dependent on well-conducted clinical trials. In the United Kingdom, the National Cancer Research Network (NCRN) requires trusts to enter at least 12% of their patients into approved trials. Clinical trials must be conducted according to good clinical practice (GCP), which is an international ethical and scientific quality standard for designing, conducting, recording and reporting trials that involve the participation of human subjects. In brief, GCP acts to ensure that the safety of patients participating in a trial is protected and the drugs or interventions developed are safe for patients in the future. The data generated in the trial must be valid and reproducible and seen by the greater public to be credible. Trial activity is backed by a raft of legislation, in particular, the set of ethical principles on human experimentation listed in the 1964 Declaration of Helsinki. Trials involving investigational medicinal products are governed by Medicines for Human Use (2004) Regulations. RT trials are governed by either the medical devices regulations or the overarching GCP principles.

To carry out a trial, the chief investigator must secure funding and a sponsor who has overall responsibility for the proper conduct of the trial. Sponsors may be universities or a National Health Service (NHS) trust. Ethics committee and organisational research and development department approval must be obtained. Any patient entering a study must be supplied with written material about the trial and must be given time to absorb this and ask questions before signing a consent form. Consent is commonly obtained by a GCP-trained doctor, but a suitably trained nurse or radiographer can obtain informed consent.

RT trials follow a similar pattern to medicinal product research. Phase I trials are essentially toxicity and dose-finding studies. Phase II studies are designed to evaluate efficacy. Patients in phase I studies often have very advanced cancers with limited therapeutic choices. A recent example is a Canadian study of stereotactic RT used to retreat vertebral metastases in patients who already have had conventional EBRT.

Single fractions were associated with a greater degree of postradiotherapy vertebral body collapse when compared with fractionated treatments. This phase I study provided the data for the ongoing Canadian clinical trials SC.24 phase II trial in patients receiving initial treatment for vertebral metastases who are randomised to either 20 Gy in 5 fractions using conventional EBRT, or 24 Gy given in 2 fractions stereotactically.

A very well-planned ongoing UK phase III trial is Prostate Advances in Comparative Evidence (PACE), a randomised evaluation trial for males suffering from localised prostate cancer; it may answer the question of whether surgery is superior to RT and which is the best RT technique. In total, 1700 males will be recruited into this study. If surgery is an option, they will be randomised to either laparoscopic prostatectomy or 5 fractions of stereotactic RT. If surgery is not an option, they will be randomised to either conventional high-dose EBRT or stereotactic treatment.

FURTHER READING

Ajithkumar T, Avanzo M, Yorke E, et al. Brain and brain stem necrosis after reirradiation for recurrent childhood primary central nervous system tumors: a PENTEC comprehensive review. *Int J Radiat Oncol Biol Phys*. 2024;119(2):655–668.

Andratschke N, Willmann J, Appelt AL, et al. European Society for Radiotherapy and Oncology and European Organisation for research and treatment of cancer consensus on re-irradiation: definition, reporting, and clinical decision making. *Lancet Oncol*. 2022;23(10):e469–e478.

Chen H, Laba JM, Boldt RG, et al. Stereotactic Ablative Radiation Therapy Versus Surgery in Early Lung Cancer: A Meta-analysis of Propensity Score Studies. *Int J Radiat Oncol Biol Phys*. 2018 May 1; 101(1):186–194. doi: 10.1016/j.ijrobp.2018.01.064. Epub 2018 Feb 3. PMID: 29619964.

Department of Health. *The NHS Cancer Plan*. HMSO; 2000.

Doi H, Tamari K, Oh RJ, Nieder C. New clinical data on human spinal cord re-irradiation tolerance. *Strahlenther Onkol*. 2021;197(6):463–473.

Kaye P. *Breaking Bad News: A Ten Step Approach*. EPL Publications; 1996.

Meredith C, Symonds P, Webster L, et al. Information needs of cancer patients in West Scotland; cross sectional survey of patients' views. *Br Med J*. 1996;313:724–726.

National Cancer Institute. https://www.cancer.gov/

National Institute for Health Research. https://www.nihr.ac.uk/

NHS Executive. *Improving the Quality of Cancer Services*. NHS Executive; 2000 *HSC/021*.

Nieder C, Willmann J, Andratschke NH. Prospective randomized clinical studies involving reirradiation: update of a systematic review. *Strahlenther Onkol*. 2023;199(9):787–797.

Stead M, Cameron D, Lester N, et al. Strengthening clinical cancer research in the United Kingdom. *Br J Cancer*. 2011;104:1529–1534.

Stiefel I, Schröder C, Tanadini-Lang S, et al. High-dose re-irradiation of intracranial lesions: efficacy and safety, including dosimetric analysis based on accumulated EQD2Gy dose EQD calculation. *Clin Transl Radiat Oncol*. 2021;27:132–138 Apr.

20

Chemotherapy and Hormones

Oyeyemi O. Akala and Harriet S. Walter

CHAPTER OUTLINE

INTRODUCTION

Chemotherapy is the use of cytotoxic (cell poisoning) drugs to control tumour growth. Over the past 30 years, there have been significant advances in the management of several solid tumours and haematological malignancies, such as testicular teratoma, the leukaemias, childhood cancers and choriocarcinoma. Over 70% of childhood cancers are now curable and the cure rate for teratoma is over 95%. More recently, chemotherapy in combination with immunotherapies and other targeted therapies has dramatically altered outcomes even in those presenting with metastatic disease. However, when we consider treatment with chemotherapy alone, many common tumours fail to respond, such as nonsmall cell lung cancer, colorectal cancer and melanoma. These tumours often present in the metastatic setting. Despite intense research, chemotherapy for these tumours remains palliative in intent rather than curative. One of the major drawbacks of cytotoxic agents is that they affect all rapidly dividing cells and do not discriminate between normal tissues and tumours, hence the toxicity of chemotherapy. We are now entering an exciting era in oncology, with new targeted and immunotherapy treatments becoming available. These novel agents are designed to exploit our increased understanding of molecular oncology and will hopefully be more successful in overcoming drug resistance and reducing the side effects of treatment. They are often used in combination with chemotherapy.

Hormone therapy is another systemic treatment for cancer. It may involve inhibiting the production of endogenous hormones or introducing synthetic ones. There are now many different hormone preparations available and they play a vital role in the treatment of tumours such as prostate and breast cancer.

General Indications for Chemotherapy

There are four main ways in which chemotherapy can be used in the treatment of cancer. First, it is used as the primary treatment for patients with advanced cancers for which no alternative treatment exists. This is sometimes called palliative chemotherapy and is essentially used to palliate the symptoms of cancer, control or reduce the volume of disease and prolong survival. Adjuvant chemotherapy is the use of cytotoxic drugs after the primary tumour has been controlled by either surgery or radiotherapy. Here, the rationale is to eradicate subclinical micrometastatic disease and reduce the risk of recurrence. Examples of this would be in the treatment of bowel and breast cancer. Neoadjuvant (or primary) chemotherapy is used to debulk the primary tumour in an attempt to make the definitive treatment, for example, surgery, successful. An example of this is neoadjuvant therapy of large primary tumours of the breast so that conservative local surgery rather than mastectomy is made possible. The fourth setting is to use chemotherapy directly into the tumour site, for example, into the blood supply of liver metastases from colorectal cancer.

Development and Testing of Anticancer Agents

Cytotoxic therapies have been discovered in a variety of ways. First, some drugs have been developed de novo based on distinct properties that should confer antitumour effect. Alternatively, a range of compounds are produced and then screened against a selection of resistant tumour cell lines. Those with significant activity are then taken forward. Once this first-generation drug is discovered, analogues with superior pharmacological properties (e.g. less toxicity, more convenient administration) are synthesised. Of course, one should not forget the past serendipitous discovery of drugs, such as cisplatin. Once an agent has been shown in its preclinical assessment to have sufficient activity against animal tumours, with acceptable toxicity, it can be considered for clinical evaluation. There are three phases of clinical assessment. However, often the first two phases are now conducted within the same trial to reduce time for drug development.

Phase I Studies

In *phase I* studies, the main aim is to establish the maximum tolerated dose and the safety of the agent under investigation. Such studies are often performed with the informed consent of patients for whom standard therapy has no role. The starting dose is determined by preclinical data and is usually one-tenth of the lethal dose (LD_{10}) in rodents. In phase I studies, pharmacokinetic studies (how the body handles the drug, for example by metabolism) and pharmacodynamic studies (assessing the impact of the drug on the physiology of the body) are conducted. Historically, phase I studies were completed in patients for whom no further standard chemotherapy options were available. Nowadays, particularly when the tumour type is rare or when the outcomes are very poor, these studies may be carried out in patients as part of their first-line treatment. This provides a much better signal readout for benefit compared with heavily pretreated patients and increases the chances of future phase II studies to be successful. Furthermore, with the era of targeted therapies, we are able to select patients who are more likely to respond.

Phase II Studies

Once a drug is found to have acceptable side effects, it is taken forward into *phase II studies* to study its efficacy in a specific tumour type. The type selected is usually ascertained from the responses to therapy seen in the cell lines and sometimes ascertained from activity demonstrated in the phase I setting. The main outcome is to achieve a response rate which is at least comparable with the standard agent in that setting. Now there is a trend to randomise some phase II studies so that either the drug can be compared with the standard or two different dose schedules can be studied. Gaining these data as early as possible in a drug's development obviously enables the pharmaceutical company to withdraw a drug as soon as possible if activity is disappointing or, alternatively, to fast-track drugs that have impressive potential.

Phase III Studies

In *phase III studies*, the new drug is compared against the gold standard in a randomised fashion. The main endpoint is survival, but toxicity data are collected, as are quality of life and health economic data. The cost-effectiveness of the drug has to be assessed and deemed to be acceptable before the drug can be licensed and marketed. In this era of agents targeting specific molecular aberrations in tumours, two other types of studies are increasingly used. In *umbrella studies*, patients with the same type of cancer are assigned to different treatments/arms of a study based on their mutations. In *basket studies*, patients with a variety of cancers which share a single genomic alteration are assigned to a treatment/arm that is expected to be active. In the United Kingdom, the National Cancer Research Institute has a portfolio of studies that are peer reviewed and of the highest standard possible. The United Kingdom is divided geographically into research networks to coordinate the delivery of clinical studies to ensure that patients who are eligible for these studies can be referred appropriately. The rates of recruitment to clinical studies do vary network to network, but there is evidence that where centres recruit high numbers, survival outcomes for patients increase, even if they were nontrial participants. Therefore clinical trials help to raise the standard of cancer care.

Assessing Tumour Responses

It is essential that there is standardisation of how tumours are measured and responses defined so that studies can be interpreted accurately. A number of different response criteria are available, but the system used most commonly now is RECIST (Response Criteria in Solid Tumours, updated to version 1.1 in 2008). In this system, the lesions are measured in one dimension, the longest diameter (LD). A *complete response* is defined as eradication of all known disease based on two assessments at least 4 weeks apart. A *partial response (PR)* represents a reduction of at least 30% in the sum of the LD of target lesions maintained for at least 4 weeks. *Progressive disease (PD)* represents an increase of 20% or more in the sum of the LD of lesions or the development of new lesions. *Stable disease (SD)* occurs when the measurements are either not good enough for a PR but also not bad enough for a PD. RECIST has been modified into iRECIST, used in cancer immunotherapy trials to reflect the difference in response to immunotherapy treatments as compared with chemotherapeutic agents. In neurooncology, the RANO (Response Assessment in Neuro-Oncology) criteria are used in assessing central nervous system (CNS) tumours.

Evaluation of Targeted Therapies

With the advent of targeted therapies such as antiangiogenic treatment and epidermal growth factor inhibition, it has become apparent that there are difficulties in assessing these agents using conventional study design endpoints. This is because the classical endpoint of the maximum tolerated dose may not actually be the biologically active dose. Moreover, these agents may be cytostatic rather than cytotoxic. This means that stabilisation of disease is the best response that can be expected and the classical endpoint of reduction in tumour volume is not reached. It is therefore imperative that the actual target of these drugs is known and that assays are incorporated into the study design as some 'surrogate' endpoints. An example of this would be the studies that investigated the activity of trastuzumab, the HER2/erb-b2 growth factor inhibitor, in breast cancer. Here, assays were carried out in tumour biopsies to ensure that the HER2 receptor was indeed being targeted. It is now increasingly common for new agents to have a specific molecular diagnostic associated with them; for example, patients with lung cancer to be treated with the anaplastic lymphoma kinase (ALK) inhibitor crizotinib must have positive ALK expression demonstrated in their tumour biopsy sample.

PRINCIPLES OF CYTOTOXIC THERAPY

To understand the rationale of cytotoxic chemotherapy, it is important to recognize the features of tumour growth. The asymmetric sigmoidal growth curve, the *Gompertz growth curve* (Fig. 20.1), describes the natural history of tumour growth. By the time a tumour is clinically detectable, the majority of its growth has already occurred. In the early exponential phase of growth, the rates of tumour cell growth and tumour cell loss are proportional to the tumour cell burden at any point. The fact that most anticancer agents are more toxic to proliferating cells and most tumours are in a relatively slow phase of growth when diagnosed (i.e. they lie high and towards the plateau of the Gompertz growth curve) explains the limited effectiveness of chemotherapy for many cancers. The reason for tumour cytoreduction (e.g. by surgery) before chemotherapy is to bring the tumour to a lower point

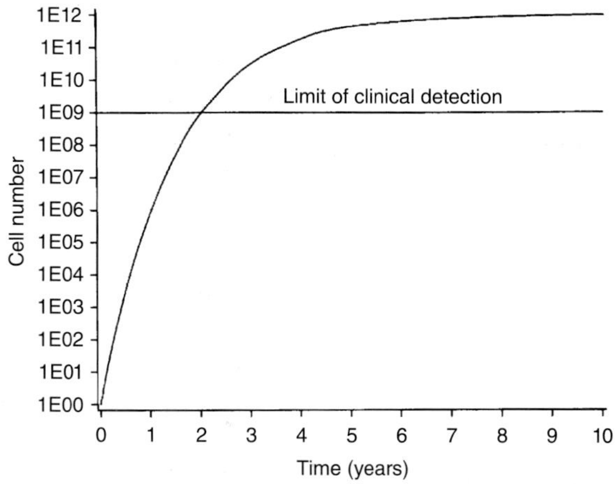

Fig. 20.1 Gompertz growth curve.

on the growth curve when the growth fraction of the tumour rises. The concept of moving the tumour down the Gompertz curve underpins the rationale of adjuvant chemotherapy.

Unfortunately, it is not only the proliferating cells that must be eradicated by chemotherapy but also the small population of clonogenic cells, mainly in the G_0 phase. This explains some of the inherent problems of tumour chemoresistance. Cytotoxic drugs prevent cell division by inhibiting DNA replication. Unfortunately, these agents are not specifically acting against malignant cells and damage both normal and malignant proliferating cells. A careful balance has to be kept between toxicity to the tumour and to the patient's normal tissues. What distinguishes normal and malignant cells is the failure of the malignant cell, unlike normal cells, to recover from cytotoxic damage. It is the exploitation of these differences that underpins the role of targeted therapies.

Drug Resistance

A variety of host factors influence the response to chemotherapy. These include the growth fraction of the tumour, the availability of the drug to the tumour and drug resistance. Resistance to chemotherapy may be intrinsic or acquired. Some tumours are intrinsically chemoresistant and show no response to treatment de novo. In other tumours, there is an initial response followed by relapse due to acquired resistance. Acquired resistance may have a variety of mechanisms, including:

- Changes in the cell membrane impeding drug transport (e.g. of methotrexate)
- DNA repair of drug-induced lesions (e.g. caused by cisplatin)
- Utilisation of alternative metabolic pathways (e.g. 5-fluorouracil)
- Increased production of a target enzyme (e.g. dihydrofolate reductase binding to methotrexate)
- Modification of the target enzyme, enabling it to recognize the difference between true and false metabolites (e.g. 6-mercaptopurine)

The multiple drug resistance gene (*MDR1*) encodes P-glycoprotein. The latter is a membrane-associated efflux pump that is widely found in normal cells and serves to protect them from drug-induced damage. Normally, P-glycoprotein is found in very low levels; however, cancer cells can overexpress *MDR1* and so confer resistance to a variety of chemotherapeutic agents. In addition, *p53*, the 'guardian' of the genome and an important mediator of apoptosis (programmed cell death), may mutate and give rise to chemoresistance in a number of solid tumours.

The reasons for drug resistance are not fully understood. It is common to find that a tumour responds to a particular drug or combination of drugs for a period of time and then ceases to do so. It is thought that within many tumour populations there are genetically determined drug-resistant cells. When the chemosensitive cells have been killed, the resistant population may proliferate. Drug resistance to repeated exposure to a single agent will usually result in cross-resistance to other compounds of the same class of drugs. This is probably due to common transport mechanisms and pathways of metabolism as well as intracellular cytotoxic targets. However, cancer cells that have become resistant to one class of drugs may retain sensitivity to another class of drugs. Most drugs have a variety of mechanisms of drug resistance.

Some drugs which show excellent cell kill in vitro fail to do so in vivo. There may be multiple reasons for this. For example, if the tumour is in a sanctuary site such as the CNS, the drug does not cross the blood–brain barrier and is therefore ineffective. There is also evidence that some tumours exhibit drug resistance that is partly due to host factors which modify the pharmacokinetics of the anticancer agent in vivo. Chemotherapy is most effective in killing proliferating cells. While the growth fraction is high in many chemosensitive tumours such as the lymphomas and testicular teratomas, it is relatively low in many common tumours such as colorectal cancer. Finally, in parts of the tumour, the blood supply tends to be poor. Not only does this result in an inadequate concentration of drug reaching the tumour, but the hypoxia also reduces the growth fraction.

Selection and Scheduling of Chemotherapy Agents

In an attempt to improve the curative potential of chemotherapy, agents with proven anticancer properties against a particular tumour but with different mechanisms of action and, as far as possible, nonoverlapping toxicities are combined. This is known as *combination chemotherapy*. For example, in treating breast cancer, three agents—cyclophosphamide, methotrexate and 5-fluorouracil (known as CMF)—all have activity against breast cancer as single agents. However, their response rate as a combination (around 40%) is two- to threefold that of their response rates as single agents. Thus the overall response is at least additive if not synergistic.

Most schedules of chemotherapy administer the drugs on an intermittent basis to take advantage of the growth kinetics of malignant cells and normal tissues. After each pulse, the normal and malignant cell populations decline due to killing of cells in mitosis. The lowest level of the blood count is known as the *nadir*. However, whereas the bone marrow recovers to its previous level, the malignant cell population does not. With each subsequent course, this difference is accentuated. If the interval between pulses is too short, toxicity may prevent the delivery of further pulses on schedule. Conversely, if the interval is too long, the tumour may regrow between courses. The total dose that can be administered is therefore limited by the tolerance of normal tissue, particularly the bone marrow. The crucial nadir blood count is the *neutrophil value*, with *neutropenia* being defined as an absolute neutrophil count of less than 0.5×10^9/L, or less than 1.0×10^9/L and 'falling', the interpretation of which requires some knowledge of chemotherapy regimens and expected patterns of myelosuppression. Neutropenic sepsis in patients on chemotherapy is regarded as a medical emergency and requires prompt intervention with intravenous antibiotics; failure to do this can result in death. Toxicity is often cumulative and may be irreversible. For example, the major dose-limiting toxicity of the anthracycline doxorubicin is cardiotoxicity.

High-Dose Chemotherapy

Higher than conventional doses of chemotherapy can be delivered if the primary organ toxicity is to the bone marrow and there is minimal toxicity to other organs. Dose intensity is recognised to be important, particularly in chemosensitive tumours. Bone marrow toxicity can be overcome by autologous bone marrow transplantation. Normal bone marrow is harvested from the patient before high-dose chemotherapy.

It is then returned to the patient at the time of chemotherapy to support the bone marrow through the period of neutropenia and thrombocytopenia. While high-dose strategies have been extremely useful in haematological malignancies, the results from similar approaches in solid tumours have been disappointing.

ROUTE OF ADMINISTRATION

The route of administration is governed by the solubility, chemical stability and local irritant properties of the agent. The simplest route, and the one that patients prefer, is the oral route. Patients can take their tablets at home, with intermittent outpatient visits to monitor treatment. Unfortunately, many cytotoxic drugs are unstable and inactivated in the stomach, rendering them ineffective. Intravenous injection is the most common route of administration of cytotoxic agents because it gives direct access to the systemic circulation. It can be done by delivery of a bolus dose or by infusion. Continuous infusions can be given (e.g. 5-fluorouracil) linked to a battery-operated pump worn around the patient's waist. The risks of intravenous administration are the introduction of infection and damage to the tissues around the site of administration if extravasation occurs.

It is possible to administer intraperitoneal chemotherapy, for example in ovarian cancer. However, the drug absorption is variable and there are concerns about adverse effects, such as the development of adhesions. Intraarterial administration has the advantage of delivering the drug in high concentrations to the tissue supplied by the artery. Its limitations are the complexity of administration and the difficulty in correctly identifying the arterial supply of the tumour. Its main use is in the infusion of chemotherapeutic agents into the hepatic artery of patients with liver metastases from colorectal cancer. Intrathecal injection is used to deliver drugs in high dose into the CNS. Many cytotoxic drugs do not cross the blood–brain barrier and are therefore unable to kill tumour cells within the CNS. Methotrexate is the agent most commonly given by this route, for example when the meninges are involved in lymphoma.

SIDE EFFECTS OF CHEMOTHERAPY

The main normal tissues damaged by cytotoxic therapy are those with rapidly dividing cell populations: the bone marrow, the gastrointestinal epithelium, the hair and the germ cells of the testis. By contrast, there is little effect on nonproliferating tissues, such as skeletal muscle and nervous tissue. The most common side effects of individual cytotoxic drugs are shown in Table 20.1. The most dramatic improvement in the management of side effects was with the development of the 5-hydroxytryptamine ($5HT_3$) antagonist antiemetics. More recently the neurokinin-1 antagonists (NK_1), such as aprepitant, have improved the emesis of patients undergoing highly emetogenic chemotherapy. Typical antiemetic regimens are shown in Table 20.2. Other drugs that have improved drug delivery have been the recombinant growth factors for red (erythropoietin) and white cells (human granulocyte colony-stimulating factor (G-CSF)). These agents stimulate the release of progenitor cells from the bone marrow and are useful in the treatment and prevention of anaemia and neutropenia.

CLASSIFICATION OF CYTOTOXIC DRUGS

The available agents may be divided into a few broad groups on the basis of their mechanism of action:

- Alkylating agents
- Antimetabolites
- Mitotic inhibitors
- Topoisomerase inhibitors
- Miscellaneous
- Hormones

Some cytotoxic drugs act only on particular phases of the cell cycle (cell-cycle specific), while others act throughout the cycle (cell-cycle nonspecific).

Alkylating Agents

The main antitumour action of alkylating agents is the binding of an alkyl chemical group (R-CH2) to DNA, so inhibiting its synthesis. They also bind to RNA and other cell proteins, but these reactions are much less cytotoxic. The majority of alkylating agents have two available alkyl groups with which they can bind with DNA. Cross-linking may occur between a single strand of DNA or between two separate strands. Alkylating agents with this capacity to cross-link are called *bifunctional* and are more cytotoxic than alkylating agents with only one available alkyl group for binding to DNA.

The intravenous alkylating agents are nearly all vesicants and are irritant to the skin and other tissues if they extravasate out of the vein. In general, they do cause nausea and vomiting but this is usually controlled with antiemetics. They all cause myelosuppression, alopecia and temporary amenorrhoea. Nitrosoureas are a group of similar drugs whose main mode of action is alkylation. Specific examples of alkylating agents and nitrosoureas with specific side effects and main uses are shown in Table 20.3.

Trabectedin is an alkylating agent that is licensed for use in soft-tissue sarcoma. Its discovery is of interest; in the 1960s, the National Cancer Institute carried out a wide-ranging program of screening plant and marine organism material. As part of that program, extract from the sea squirt *Ecteinascidia turbinata* was found to have anticancer activity, and a semisynthetic analogue, trabectedin, was synthesised. The compound binds to DNA in the minor groove and interacts with DNA repair mechanisms, causing DNA double-strand breaks.

Antimetabolites

Antimetabolites are structurally similar to normal metabolites involved in nucleic acid synthesis. They are divided into three groups: folate, purine and pyrimidine antagonists. They substitute for their normal purine and pyrimidine counterparts in metabolic pathways, resulting in abnormal nuclear material that fails to function normally or bind to enzymes, so inhibiting protein synthesis.

Folate Antagonists

Methotrexate is the classical example of a folate antagonist. A number of cofactors are necessary for the synthesis of purines and pyrimidines. The reduction of folic acid is essential for the production of these cofactors. A key reaction in this process is the reduction of dihydrofolic acid to tetrahydrofolic acid by means of an enzyme, *dihydrofolate reductase*. Methotrexate is structurally similar to folic acid and has a much greater affinity for dihydrofolate reductase than does folic acid. Methotrexate therefore binds preferentially to dihydrofolate reductase and inactivates it. As a result, tetrahydrofolates cannot be made and purine and pyrimidine synthesis is inhibited. Methotrexate can be given orally, intravenously or at low dose intrathecally (Fig. 20.2).

The metabolic block on the activity of dihydrofolate reductase can be bypassed by administering an intermediate metabolite, folinic acid (also known as leucovorin). Folinic acid is a tetrahydrofolate which provides an alternative source for continuing nucleic acid synthesis. The cytotoxic action of methotrexate and its toxicity can be diminished by administrating folinic acid. This is termed *folinic acid rescue* and is particularly useful after high-dose methotrexate therapy has been used. The main side effects of methotrexate are on the bone marrow

TABLE 20.1 Side Effects of Treatment

	Alopecia	Gastrointestinal Toxicity	Neurotoxicity	Cardiotoxicity	Urological Toxicity	Myelotoxicity	Skin Changes	Lung Toxicity	Allergic Reactions
Cyclophosphamide	+	+			+	+			
Ifosfamide	+	+	++		++	+	+		
Chlorambucil		+				+	+		
Thiotepa		+				+	+		
Busulphan		+			+	+	+	+	+
Procarbazine		+	+			+		+	+
CCNU		+				+		+	
BCNU		+				+		+	
Dacarbazine		++				+	+		+
Mitoxantrone		+		+		+			
Temozoamide	+	+				+	+	+	
Mitomycin C		+				+			
Melphalan		+				+	+	+	+
Methotrexate		+	+		+	+	+		
6-Mercaptopurine		+				+	+		
Fludarabine		+			+	++		+	
5-Fluorouracil		+		+		+	+		
Cytosine arabinoside		+				+	+	+	
Gemcitabine		+				++	+		+
Vincristine		+	++			+	+		
Vinblastine		+				+			
Vinorelbine	+	+	+			+			
Paclitaxel	++	+	++			+	+		+
Docetaxel	++	++	+			+	+		+
Doxorubicin	++	+		++		++	+		
Epirubicin	+	+		+		+	+		
Actinomycin D	+	+				+	+		+
Bleomycin	+						+	++	+
Cisplatin		+	+		++	+			
Carboplatin		+	+		+	+			
Oxaliplatin		+	++			+			+
Etoposide	+	+				++	+		+
Topotecan	+	+				+			
Irinotecan	+	++			+	+			
Asparaginase		+				+			+
Hydroxyurea		+				+	+		

+, Minor toxicity; ++, moderate to high toxicity.

TABLE 20.2 Typical Antiemetic Regimens

Grade of Emesis	Antiemetic Protocol
Low	Metoclopramide 20 mg intravenously if required Metoclopramide 10–20 mg orally 3 times daily as needed
Moderate	$5HT_3$ antagonist orally and dexamethasone 8 mg orally then Metoclopramide 20 mg 3 times daily Dexamethasone 4 mg twice daily Both for 3 days
High	$5HT_3$ antagonist orally and dexamethasone 8 mg orally, NK1 antagonist orally then $5HT_3$ antagonist orally for 1 day NK1 antagonist orally for 2 days Dexamethasone 4 mg twice daily for 3 days Metoclopramide 20 mg twice daily as needed

Second-line antiemetics
Acute emesis: Give the antiemetic protocol for next grade of emesis. If already at 'high', give metoclopramide regularly, consider alternative antiemetics. Add in aprepitant 125 mg orally pre chemotherapy and 80 mg orally for 2 days post chemotherapy.
Delayed emesis (>24 hours post chemotherapy) Consider lengthening course of steroids, add in aprepitant and consider alternative antiemetics.
Anxiety component: Add Lorazepam 1 mg orally or sublingually twice daily as needed. This can be started 1–2 days prior to chemotherapy.
Alternative antiemetics Domperidone rectally 30–60 mg 4–8 hourly as needed.
Haloperidol 1.5 mg twice daily as needed, Cyclizine 50 mg twice daily as needed or regularly, or levomepromazine 6 mg 4 times daily as needed.

and gastrointestinal tract. The nadir of the white count is at 10 days. Anorexia, nausea and vomiting are the first symptoms, followed 4 to 6 days later by oral and pharyngeal mucositis and diarrhoea. Conjunctivitis may occur as a result of accumulation of the drug in tears. Renal failure may complicate high-dose therapy. Liver damage (ranging from elevated liver enzymes to cirrhosis) and lung injury (mainly fibrosis) may complicate prolonged therapy. Alopecia is uncommon. Methotrexate is used most commonly in non-Hodgkin lymphoma, acute lymphoblastic leukaemia, breast cancer and choriocarcinoma. Over the past 10 years, new antifolates have been developed, including pemetrexed. This is a multitargeted pyrrolopyrimidine-based antifolate. When polyglutamated, it targets a number of folate-dependent enzymes, for example DHFR and TS. It has activity in a number of tumour types including nonsmall cell lung cancer and mesothelioma.

Purine Antagonists

The purine antagonist 6-mercaptopurine inhibits a number of enzymes involved in the synthesis of the purine bases adenine and guanine, which thus inhibits the synthesis of DNA. It is normally given orally and used in the treatment of leukaemia. The main toxicity is on the bone marrow (leucopoenia and thrombocytopaenia) and the liver. The nadir for white count and platelets is at 15 days.

Raised serum bilirubin is the most common feature of liver toxicity. This usually returns to normal on withdrawing the drug.

Another purine antagonist, 6-thioguanine, is an analogue of guanine. It may be given orally or intravenously but is now very rarely used in practice.

Fludarabine is a more recently developed antipurine. It is an adenosine analogue and is currently the most active single agent in the treatment of chronic lymphatic leukaemia (CLL). It is also active in the treatment of lymphomas. Its main limiting side effect is myelosuppression, which can be very severe.

Pyrimidine Antagonists

5-Fluorouracil (5-FU) is a fluoropyrimidine that inhibits DNA synthesis by inhibiting the main enzyme in pyrimidine synthesis and thus the formation of cytosine and thymine. In addition, it is erroneously incorporated into RNA instead of uracil and inhibits RNA synthesis. 5-FU is metabolised intracellularly in a number of steps to the active fluorodeoxyuridine monophosphate (FdUMP), which then forms covalent bonds with thymidylate synthase and its cofactor, 5,10-methylene tetrahydrofolate, creating a complex which inhibits the formation of thymidine from deoxyuridine monophosphate (dUMP), so inhibiting DNA synthesis (see Fig. 20.2). One problem with 5-FU is that elevated dUMP levels may overcome the inhibition of thymidylate synthase, thereby causing chemoresistance. Specific thymidylate synthase

TABLE 20.3 Summary of Alkylating Agents and Nitrosoureas

Name	Route of Administration	Main Use	Nadir	Specific Side Effects
Cyclophosphamide	Orally or intravenously	Non-Hodgkin lymphomas, breast, ovary, sarcomas	9–15 days	Haemorrhagic cystitis due to the urinary metabolites of the drug, treated with Mesna
Ifosfamide	Intravenously	Sarcomas	5–10 days	As above Encephalopathy Nephrotoxicity
Chlorambucil	Orally	Low-grade lymphoma	8–15 days	Gastrointestinal upset
Melphalan	Orally or intravenously	Myeloma	14–21 days	Mucositis
Thiotepa	Intravenously	High-dose therapy	28 days	Myelosuppression
Busulfan	Orally	Chronic myeloid leukaemia	28 days	Lung fibrosis Prolonged myelosuppression
Procarbazine	Orally	Brain tumours Hodgkin lymphoma	28+ days	Central nervous system toxicity
CCNU (Lomustine)	Orally	Brain tumours, lymphomas	28+ days	Delayed myelosuppression
BCNU (Carmustine)	Intravenously	High dose, lymphomas	28+ days	Pulmonary fibrosis Delayed myelosuppression
DTIC	Intravenously	Melanoma	21 days	Myalgia
Temozolomide	Orally	Brain tumours	10–14 days	Myelosuppression
Mitomycin C	Intravenously	Gastric, breast	14–28 days	Prolonged neutropenia

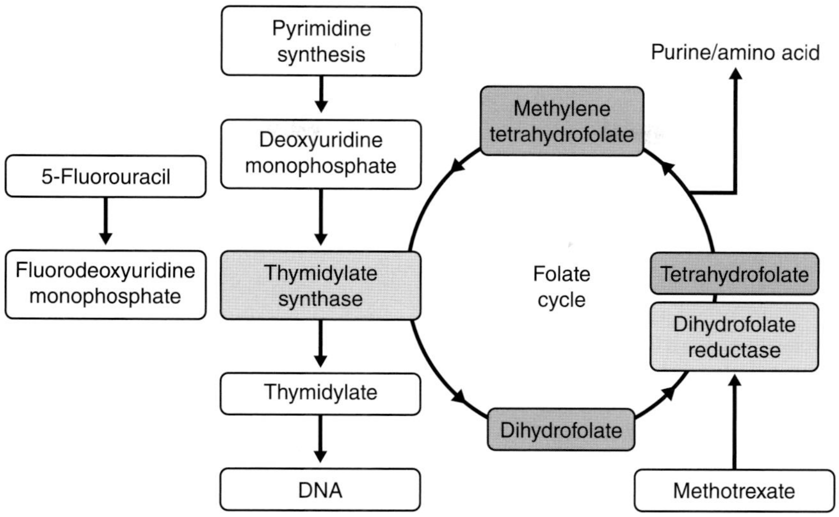

Fig. 20.2 Enzymatic pathway for 5-fluorouracil and methotrexate.

inhibitors, such as raltitrexed, have therefore been developed. Unfortunately, despite initially encouraging results, raltitrexed has not been as useful against colorectal cancer as predicted. In reality, it appears only to have a role in treating patients with cardiac problems as it has a safer cardiac profile than 5-FU.

Historically, it was only possible to give 5-FU intravenously as the oral bioavailability of 5-FU was too unpredictable. The development of the oral fluoropyrimidines tegafur/uracil (UFT) and capecitabine have overcome this. In particular, capecitabine is an interesting compound as it was formulated to be preferentially activated in the tumour. Capecitabine is metabolized to 5-FU in a three-step enzymatic reaction with tumour-selective generation of 5-FU through exploitation of the higher level of thymidine phosphorylase in tumour compared with normal tissue. The pharmacokinetics of orally administered capecitabine essentially mimics a continuous infusion rather than bolus 5-FU. To be able to prescribe an oral formulation of 5-FU is an enormous advantage as, understandably, patients prefer to take tablets and the potential risk of central line complications is avoided.

The main toxicities of 5-FU are to the gastrointestinal tract (diarrhoea, nausea and vomiting) and myelosuppression. The severity of the toxicity depends on the scheduling of 5-FU. For example, it is well recognised that giving 5-FU as a continuous infusion over 48 hours (de Gramont schedule) produces fewer side effects than giving the drug once every day for 5 days every month (Mayo schedule). Rarely, if a patient has genetic deficiency of the dihydropyrimidine dehydrogenase, very severe toxicity can result, including neurological effects. 5-FU is widely used in a number of tumours, especially those of the gastrointestinal tract. A recently developed compound in this class is trifluridine/tipiracil (LONSURF), which is an oral combination drug for the treatment of metastatic colorectal cancer. It consists of trifluridine, a nucleoside analogue, and tipiracil, a thymidine phosphorylase inhibitor.

Cytosine arabinoside is an analogue of deoxycytidine. It is a competitive inhibitor of the enzyme DNA polymerase. Its principal action is as a false nucleotide competing for the enzymes which are responsible for converting cytidine to deoxycytidine and for incorporating deoxycytidine into DNA. It can be given by intravenous or subcutaneous routes and is used mainly in acute leukaemias. The main side effects are bone marrow suppression, nausea, vomiting and diarrhoea.

Gemcitabine is a second-generation pyrimidine analogue. It is metabolised by nucleotide kinases intracellularly to the active diphosphate and triphosphate and inhibits DNA synthesis. Side effects include nausea and vomiting, myelosuppression, flulike symptoms, rashes and oedema. Gemcitabine is the standard therapy for pancreatic tumours and also is used in nonsmall cell lung cancer.

Mitotic Inhibitors

There are two major classes of mitotic inhibitors, the vinca alkaloids and the taxanes. The vinca alkaloids are naturally occurring or semisynthetic compounds found in the periwinkle plant (*Vinca rosea*): vincristine, vinblastine and vinorelbine. They inhibit formation of the microtubule spindle on which the chromatids line up during metaphase in mitosis and therefore prevent cell division. They are all given intravenously and, despite being similar in structure, have differing side effects. Vincristine is used in lymphomas, leukaemias and breast cancer. It is vesicant locally and neurotoxicity is the main dose-limiting toxicity. This presents in the form of a sensorimotor peripheral neuropathy (paresthaesiae in fingers, muscle cramps, paralytic ileus, constipation). Vinblastine is also a sclerosant, but myelosuppression, especially thrombocytopenia, is the main dose-limiting toxicity. Neurotoxicity is less severe than with vincristine. It is used mainly in lymphoma, testicular teratoma and nonsmall cell lung cancer. Vinorelbine is the most recently discovered vinca alkaloid and causes less alopecia and neuropathy than the older agents. It can, however, cause significant constipation. It also has the advantage of being available for intravenous and oral administration.

The taxanes are an important class of anticancer drugs in the field of oncology. Although they also have an effect on the formation of the microtubule spindle, they differ from the vinca alkaloids because they promote the assembly of the microtubule's spindle and inhibit its disassembly. Paclitaxel is an extract from the bark of the Pacific yew. Initially, its development was hampered by the limited supply of the primary source and also its poor solubility in water. With the development of docetaxel, the semisynthetic analogue from the needles of the tree, the supply was no longer threatened. The most important antitumour activity of these drugs has been seen in breast and ovarian cancer, although they are also used in other solid tumours such as gastrooesophageal cancer and cancer of unknown primary. The latest semisynthetic analogue to be developed is Cabazitaxel, which is licensed for use in males with castration-resistant prostate cancer.

All drugs are given intravenously and there has been a great deal of work involved in optimising the scheduling. Despite being closely related, there are some differences in their toxicity profiles. Both have myelosuppression as one of the major limiting side effects, with the nadir occurring at days 8 to 10 post infusion. A relatively rare but important side effect of paclitaxel is a hypersensitivity reaction with dyspnoea, urticaria and hypotension. Patients therefore receive prophylactic steroids and H2 inhibitors as premedication. Paclitaxel also produces a peripheral neuropathy characterised by sensory symptoms in a glove and stocking distribution. This can be permanent. A newcomer to the field is ABRAXANE, a novel nanoparticle albumin–bound paclitaxel. It has fewer hypersensitivity reactions and is licensed for use in metastatic breast cancer.

Docetaxel is characterised by a unique fluid retention syndrome with the development of oedema and weight gain. As with paclitaxel, a premedication is used. Skin toxicity may occur, and this produces a widespread itchy erythematous rash and nail changes characterised by discolouration, ridging and onycholysis (the nails lift up from the nail bed). Liver toxicity can occur if patients with impaired liver function are not given a dose reduction. Stomatitis and diarrhoea are more common with docetaxel. All taxanes cause alopecia.

A new approach to selectively delivering mitotic inhibitors to cancer cells has been achieved with the development of trastuzumab emtansine. This is an antibody–drug conjugate consisting of the monoclonal antibody trastuzumab (Herceptin) linked to the mitotic inhibitor emtansine (DM1). Trastuzumab is a targeted therapy (see later in this chapter) that binds to the HER2/neu receptor on cancer cells. The conjugate thereby allows delivery of the toxin (DM1) specifically to these tumor cells and kills them.

TOPOISOMERASE INHIBITORS

Topoisomerases are enzymes involved in the coiling and uncoiling of DNA. There are two types. Topoisomerase I inhibitors bind to double-stranded DNA and cause a single-strand break in DNA. The camptothecin analogues topotecan and irinotecan are topoisomerase I inhibitors. Topoisomerase II exists as alpha and beta isoenzymes. They undergo covalent bonding to complementary strands of DNA and cleave both strands. Topoisomerase II inhibitors prevent the relegation of DNA cleaved by topoisomerase II and produce protein-linked breaks in DNA. Epipodophyllotoxins are examples of topoisomerase II inhibitors. The anthracyclines inhibit both type I and type II topoisomerases and therefore will be discussed in this section too.

Camptothecin was the first topoisomerase I inhibitor to be discovered. Its further development was hindered by toxicity, and it was not until its analogues, topotecan and irinotecan, were developed that the usefulness of this group of drugs became apparent. Topotecan was the first camptothecin analogue approved for clinical use and is now used in ovarian cancer and small cell lung cancer. It can be given intravenously or orally, with the latter being far more convenient. The major side effects are neutropenia and nausea and vomiting. Interestingly, although the neutropenia can be profound, the nadir is very short lived and therefore is seldom complicated by sepsis.

Irinotecan is a semisynthetic derivative of camptothecin. Its active metabolite, SN-38, binds to the topoisomerase I enzyme–DNA cleaved complex and prevents religation, thus causing double-strand breaks. SN-38 is mainly cleared by the liver and the drug can only be used with caution in patients with abnormal liver function. Irinotecan has a role in the treatment of colorectal cancer and is active in patients with 5-FU–resistant disease. The major side effects are diarrhoea and myelosuppression. These can occur concurrently with fatal outcome if the diarrhoea is not controlled correctly. Irinotecan is also used in the management of upper gastrointestinal malignancies.

Etoposide (VP16) is the most widely used epipodophyllotoxin. Like 5-FU, it is a good example of a schedule-dependent drug as it is more effective given over 5 days than on 1 day. It can be given orally or intravenously and the dose-limiting toxicity is bone marrow suppression. The nadir is at about 16 days. Nausea, vomiting and anorexia are relatively minor but more marked if etoposide is given orally. Alopecia is also common, as is mucositis. Etoposide is used mainly in Hodgkin disease, non-Hodgkin lymphoma, small cell lung cancer and testicular teratoma.

Daunorubicin, doxorubicin (Adriamycin) and epirubicin are the principal anthracycline antibiotics. They are produced from different strains of fungi (*Streptomyces*). The mechanisms of their cytotoxic action are not fully understood. They induce formation of topoisomerase–DNA complexes and prevent the enzyme from completing the religation of the ligation–religation reaction. In addition, they insert part of their planar structure between two adjacent base pairs (intercalation), causing single- and double-strand breaks. They also can undergo chemical reduction to form free radicals.

Doxorubicin and epirubicin are given intravenously and the main toxicity is to the bone marrow, gastrointestinal tract and heart. The nadir of the white count is at 10 days. Epirubicin causes slightly less vomiting than the other two anthracyclines. Daunorubicin and doxorubicin and, to a much lesser extent, epirubicin cause cumulative cardiotoxicity and there is a maximum recommended total dose. Acute cardiac toxicity is manifest by arrhythmias and abnormalities of electrical conduction. The chronic effect is a cardiomyopathy (pericarditis and congestive cardiac failure), and thus anthracyclines should be avoided if there is previous history of cardiac failure or ischaemic heart disease. Their use is widespread in lymphoma, breast cancer, sarcomas, lung cancer, Wilms tumour and acute myelogenous leukaemia (daunorubicin).

In an attempt to improve the antitumour effect of doxorubicin, a liposomal preparation called doxil (Caelyx in the United Kingdom) has been developed. Essentially, the doxorubicin molecule has been formulated in a fat 'bubble'. The body's reticuloendothelial system fails to recognise the molecule as being foreign, hence the term 'stealth liposome', and therefore the drug has a longer half-life. The side effects of doxil are generally less than for doxorubicin, except for the development of a hand-foot syndrome called palmar-plantar erythrodysaesthesia. It is used in breast cancer and ovarian cancer.

Miscellaneous

Platinum Analogues

The platinum drugs are widely used in a variety of tumours, such as testicular teratoma and seminoma, ovarian, cervical, nonsmall cell lung cancer and osteosarcoma. Cisplatin and carboplatin inhibit DNA synthesis in a similar way to alkylating agents. They form cross-linkages (adducts) between a pair of their chlorine atoms and the guanine molecules of opposing DNA strands (interstrand linkages), but they differ in that they also bind to bases on the same DNA strand (intrastrand linkages). Both drugs are administered intravenously and are predominantly excreted in the urine. Cisplatin causes severe nausea and vomiting, which can be prevented with 5-HT$_3$ antagonists and with aprepitant, the NK-1 antagonist. In addition, cisplatin causes renal impairment, and therefore it is essential that pre- and posttreatment hydration be used. The peripheral nerves and auditory nerves are sensitive to cisplatin, and patients may develop high-frequency hearing loss and peripheral neuropathy. Carboplatin has the advantage of much less emesis, ototoxicity, nephrotoxicity and neurotoxicity. The dose-limiting toxicity is to the bone marrow, particularly to platelets. Unlike the other chemotherapy agents, carboplatin is dosed depending on the renal function of the patient rather than the patient's body surface area.

Oxaliplatin is the most recent platinum analogue to be licensed. It is a third-generation platinum compound and differs from the other platinum drugs by having a large 1,2-diaminocyclohexane (DACH) ligand in its structure. It is thought that the presence of the DACH group renders the molecule nonrecognizable by the mismatch repair process. This means that the DNA repair mechanisms that are responsible for platinum resistance are not so effective. Oxaliplatin therefore is useful in tumours where cisplatin has failed and also in colorectal cancer, a tumour type not classically treated by platinum agents. Oxaliplatin does not have the nephrotoxicity associated with carboplatin, although it does have a striking neurotoxicity. Patients develop a peripheral neuropathy with cumulative drug exposure. They also develop an acute neuropathy that is characterised by cold-induced tingling (paraesthesia) in the fingertips and toes after infusion. This can also affect the throat on drinking cold drinks and the patient develops a feeling of choking. Oxaliplatin is usually administered with 5-FU chemotherapy, as in combination, they are synergistic.

Nonanthracycline Antibiotics

Actinomycin D is a highly toxic drug which is only given intravenously. It is used in the treatment of some sarcomas and causes significant myelosuppression, oral ulceration, nausea, vomiting, diarrhoea, alopecia and skin rashes.

Bleomycin intercalates with DNA strands, causing single- and double-strand breaks. It inhibits DNA synthesis and, to a lesser degree, RNA synthesis. It is usually given intravenously, although it can be given intramuscularly, subcutaneously or intrapleurally (for pleural effusions). The main toxicity is to the lung, and progressive fibrosis occurs causing nonproductive cough and dyspnoea. Respiratory complications of general anaesthesia are increased. Occasionally, patients have an immediate life-threatening anaphylactic reaction, although fever and chills are more common. Skin changes are common with pigmentation, erythema and thickening of the nail bed. There is little myelosuppression and so it is often used in combination with other agents. The main use of bleomycin is in the treatment of testicular teratoma, although it is also used in lymphoma.

Enzymes

Asparaginase is used mainly in the treatment of leukaemia. It is an enzyme that degrades asparagine, an essential amino acid for protein and nucleic acid synthesis. Tumour cells, unlike their normal counterparts, have no or little asparagine synthetase, the enzyme necessary for making asparagine. When asparagine levels fall, both protein and nucleic acid synthesis are inhibited. It is used in the treatment of acute leukaemias and the most common side effect is a hypersensitivity reaction.

Hormones

There is a group of cancers where the mainstay of treatment is hormone therapy. These include breast, prostate and endometrial tumours. In recent years, an increase in the understanding of the molecular biology of hormone receptors has greatly improved the treatment of these cancers, in particular, breast cancer. Remissions may last for years, and symptomatic benefit may be substantial and even dramatic during this period. While the administration of hormones avoids the morbidities particular to surgery, radiotherapy and cytotoxic chemotherapy, side effects are seen, some of which are unacceptable (e.g. masculinising effects of androgens in females with breast cancer) and can be dangerous (e.g. cardiovascular morbidity from diethylstilbestrol for prostate cancer). A careful balance has to be struck between toxicity and benefit in tumour control. There are five main areas that will be discussed:

- Antioestrogens
- Aromatase inhibitors
- Gonadotrophin-releasing hormone analogues
- Antiandrogen therapy
- Female hormones

Antioestrogens

Tamoxifen is the most important synthetic antioestrogen preparation. First, it blocks the oestrogen stimulation of breast cancer cells by competitive binding to oestrogen receptors (ER). It also has weak oestrogenic action, raising levels of sex hormone–binding globulin, which binds to freely circulating oestrogen and so reduces the amount of free oestrogen available to bind to ER. The binding of oestrogen to ER reduces the synthesis of growth factors and stimulates the production of progesterone receptors. Tamoxifen is used in females whose breast tumour cells are found on immunohistological staining to express oestrogen or progesterone receptors. It is indicated as adjuvant therapy in early breast cancer in pre- and postmenopausal females and also in recurrent and advanced breast cancer.

The oestrogenic properties of tamoxifen are responsible for both its activity and toxicity. In general, tamoxifen is tolerated well; however, females do experience significant hot flushes and also an increase in incidence of endometrial cancer. On a more positive note, tamoxifen can prevent cardiovascular events and also osteoporosis in postmenopausal females. In an attempt to overcome the negative aspects of tamoxifen, other selective oestrogen receptor modulators (SERMs) have been developed. These include those that are tamoxifen-like including toremifene, fixed ring compounds such as raloxifene and selective oestrogen receptor downregulators (SERDs) such as fulvestrant. There has been a significant amount of work carried out to further understand the mode of action of these compounds and this information will inform the use of these compounds both as chemoprevention agents and as therapy for early and advanced breast cancer. More recently, complete oestrogen receptor blockade is being evaluated in ongoing metastatic breast cancer clinical trials.

Aromatase Inhibitors

Aromatase inhibitors play an important role in the endocrine management of adjuvant, advanced and recurrent ER-positive breast cancer. The earliest of these aromatase inhibitors was aminoglutethimide, a drug now considered to be outdated due to the development of selective aromatase inhibitors with superior side-effect profiles. In postmenopausal females, oestrogen synthesis occurs peripherally (e.g. adrenals and fat) as the enzyme aromatase converts androstenedione to estrone. Aromatase inhibitors block this conversion and are therefore extremely valuable drugs for postmenopausal females with breast cancer. In premenopausal females, oestrogen synthesis is governed by gonadotrophin-releasing hormone stimulating the ovary. Aromatase inhibitors are therefore only useful in premenopausal females who have been oophorectomized. There are a number of first-, second- and third-generation aromatase inhibitors available, as shown in Table 20.4. Common toxicities of these drugs include nausea, headache, hot flushes and weight gain. Unlike tamoxifen, aromatase inhibitors may decrease bone density and predispose to osteoporosis. Although clear molecular differences exist between these two types of aromatase inhibitors, significant clinical differences have not been forthcoming from the studies to date. There may be some non-cross resistance between the groups as switching from one to another can confer a modest improvement

TABLE 20.4 Summary of Aromatase Inhibitors

Generation	Nonsteroidal	Steroidal
First	Aminoglutethimide	Testolactone
Second	Fadrozole	
Third	Anastrozole Letrozole	Exemestane

in outcome. A Cochrane analysis has found that in metastatic breast cancer, aromatase inhibitors show a survival benefit compared to other endocrine therapy, although there are limited data available to identify which individual aromatase inhibitor has the greatest efficacy.

Gonadotrophin-Releasing Hormone Analogues

Downregulation of the gonadotrophin-releasing hormone (GnRH) receptors in the pituitary is achieved by the application of continuous secretion of GnRH analogues. These analogues of the naturally occurring hypothalamic luteinising hormone-releasing hormone (LHRH) initially cause a transient surge of gonadotrophin (LH) secretion, or 'tumour flare'. However, with continuous exposure to these analogues, the LHRH receptors in the pituitary become desensitised, resulting in a reduction in the secretion of gonadotrophins. They therefore cause a 'medical oophorectomy' in females and a 'medical orchidectomy' in males. The advantage of this medical suppression of gonad function with GnRH analogues is that the process is reversible.

Goserelin is the most commonly used agent and is about 100 times more potent than naturally occurring GnRH. It is given as a subcutaneously injected capsule on either a monthly or 3-monthly basis for prostate cancer or premenopausal breast cancer. Obviously, the symptoms are what would be expected from sex hormone withdrawal, with menopausal symptoms in females and lack of libido in males. Gynaecomastia is uncommon. However, in general, they are very well tolerated. An alternative GnRH analogue is degarelix (Firmagon), which is a synthetic derivative of the natural GnRH hormone. It therefore competes with natural GnRH for binding to GnRH receptors in the pituitary gland, and the reversible binding blocks the release of LH and FSH from the pituitary, leading to a rapid suppression of testosterone. Its fast rate of action combined with lack of tumour flare are clearly advantageous.

Antiandrogen Therapy

The initial approach to treat males with prostate cancer is to reduce androgen levels with androgen deprivation therapies including antiandrogens and GnRH analogues. Flutamide is a nonsteroidal antiandrogen and is a pure androgen antagonist used in males with prostate cancer. One of its important metabolites, hydroxyflutamide, is thought to be responsible for its cellular action. It blocks the binding of dihydrotestosterone to its receptor, so inhibiting the action of androgen. It is often used in combination with GnRH analogues. The side effects include gynaecomastia and/or breast tenderness, nausea, diarrhoea and tiredness. Bicalutamide is another nonsteroidal antiandrogen that binds to androgen receptors and therefore inhibits androgen stimulation. Again, it is used in prostate cancer, usually in conjunction with a GnRH analogue to reduce a 'flare reaction'.

Cyproterone acetate is a progestogenic antiandrogen and has two actions. First, it reduces the production of testosterone in the testis by inhibiting the secretion of the pituitary gonadotrophins. Second, it competes with androgen receptors, from which it displaces testosterone. It is used in prostate cancer to suppress the tumour flare with initial GnRH analogue therapy, and when GnRH analogues are contraindicated or poorly tolerated. Side effects include liver dysfunction, impotence and fluid retention.

When males no longer respond to androgen deprivation therapy, the disease is called *castration-resistant prostate cancer*. There are a number of further oral drugs that target the androgen pathway: abiraterone, enzalutamide, apalutamide and darolutamide. CYP171A is a member of the cytochrome P450 family and is responsible for the conversion of pregnelonone and progesterone to their 17α metabolites. In addition, it can convert 17α-hydroxypregnelonone and 17α-hydroxyprogesterone to the androgens androstenedione and dihydroepiandrostenedione. Abiraterone binds CYP17A1 irreversibly and prevents the formation of androgens in the adrenal gland and peripheral tissues of castrate and noncastrate males. Enzalutamide is a drug that blocks the androgen receptor in a number of ways, preventing the binding of androgen to the receptor, preventing the transfer of the androgen receptor to the nucleus and then inhibiting the association of the receptor with nuclear DNA. Similarly, apalutamide and darolutamide also block the androgen receptor through a number of mechanisms. While these androgen receptor antagonists have transformed the treatment of prostate cancer, there are no direct head-to-head comparisons between the three as of yet to help guide clinical decision-making.

Female Hormones (Oestrogens and Progestogens)

Synthetic rather than naturally occurring oestrogens (these are metabolized in the liver), such as diethylstilbestrol, are sometimes used in the treatment of prostate cancer. The side effects from these agents are significant, in particular, risk of cardiovascular disease and nausea and vomiting. With the advent of the antiandrogens, the use of these hormones is now declining.

Progestogens, such as medroxyprogesterone and megestrol, are occasionally used in the treatment of advanced breast cancer and also in endometrial cancer. Their mechanism of action is not completely understood, but probably the most important effect is its antiestrogenic action and less important its direct cytotoxic action. Side effects include weight gain, fluid retention, increased blood clotting and risk of thrombosis and vaginal bleeding.

Targeted Therapies

The real highlight in oncological research over the past 10 years has been the incorporation of targeted therapies into clinical practice. There has been a phenomenal increase in the understanding of the cellular and molecular events in carcinogenesis. By focusing on the differences between normal and malignant tissue, we can target pathways and receptors unique to cancer cells, thus avoiding the blunderbuss, universal killing of dividing cells of conventional cytotoxics. Molecular events that distinguish malignant from normal cells are activation of oncogenes (e.g. RAS, erb-b2), inactivation of tumour suppressor genes (e.g. p53) and activation of immortality genes (e.g. telomerase). At the cellular level, for a tumour cell to grow and divide it needs its own blood supply (angiogenesis) and the ability to migrate through local tissue (tumour invasion and migration).

Leading the way in this field was the development of imatinib. Nearly all patients (90%) with chronic myeloid leukaemia have a specific genetic abnormality called the Philadelphia chromosome. This is a genetic mutation where reciprocal translocation between chromosomes 9 and 22 results in the production of the oncogene BCR-ABL. Investigators developed the agent imatinib mesylate (STI571), which specifically inhibits the receptor kinase of BCR-ABL. The results of the clinical trials were truly impressive; complete haematological responses were seen in patients with chronic myeloid leukaemia who failed to respond to conventional agents. Moreover, not only is imatinib an oral drug, but the patients had mild side effects, particularly when compared to their previous cytotoxic-induced toxicity. Results of this kind were really unprecedented in oncology and warranted the accelerated approval of imatinib for clinical use. The development of imatinib therefore represents a paradigm for the development of targeted therapies. Currently there are 68 FDA-approved kinase inhibitors for cancer therapy, with hundreds in development. In addition, there are 27 monoclonal antibodies licensed for use in cancer therapy. Key groups of targeted therapies include:

- Epidermal growth factor receptor (EGFR) inhibitors
- RAS-RAF-ERK (MAPK) and PI3 kinase inhibitors
- Vascular endothelial growth factor (VEGF) inhibitors

- Protease inhibitors
- Poly ADP ribose polymerase (PARP) inhibitors
- CDK4/6 inhibitors

Epidermal Growth Factor Receptor

EGFR (ERBB1) and ERBB2 (HER2) are overexpressed or amplified in many malignancies including nonsmall cell lung, breast, head and neck, pancreas and colorectal cancers. Licensed anti-EGFR therapies include monoclonal antibodies (cetuximab, panitumumab, trastuzumab and pertuzumab) and oral small-molecule inhibitors of the TK activity (gefitinib, erlotinib and lapatinib).

Trastuzumab (Herceptin) is a humanized anti-HER2 (ERBB2) monoclonal antibody that has been approved for mono- or combination therapy (with paclitaxel) for females with HER2 overexpressing breast cancer and HER2-positive gastric cancer. Pertuzumab (Perjeta) is a monoclonal antibody used in combination with trastuzumab and docetaxel for the treatment of metastatic HER2-positive breast cancer. It is the first-in-class HER dimerisation inhibitor, which means it inhibits the dimerisation of HER2 with other HER receptors, thereby preventing the signalling pathway in the cell and subsequent proliferation. Cetuximab (Erbitux) is a chimeric IgG1 antibody and is licensed for use in combination with irinotecan-containing chemotherapy in patients with metastatic colorectal cancer with wild-type RAS mutation status. This treatment is complicated by a unique rash which is acneiform—indeed, there is a suggestion that the rash may actually be a predictive biomarker of response to cetuximab. Other side effects include diarrhoea and infusion reactions. Panitumumab (Vectibix) is a fully human IgG2 monoclonal antibody that binds to the ectodomain of EGFR. It is also licensed for use in RAS wild-type colorectal cancer.

Gefitinib (IRESSA) is a tyrosine kinase inhibitor (TKI) which blocks the binding of the adenosine triphosphate to the intracellular domain of EGFR. Only patients with activating EGFR mutations respond well to the drug, and therefore gefitinib is only approved for use in metastatic nonsmall cell lung cancer with activating mutations of the EGFR-TK. The most common side effects seen with gefitinib are rash, diarrhoea and fatigue. Erlotinib (Tarceva) is another EGFR TKI and is licensed for use in nonsmall cell lung cancer and pancreatic cancer. Lapatinib (Tykerb) is a dual-specific TKI targeting both EGFR and HER2. It is licensed for use in combination with capecitabine chemotherapy in patients with metastatic breast cancer who have progressed after trastuzumab and other chemotherapy. Afatinib (GILOTRIF) is an inhibitor of (EGFR) and erb-b2 (HER2) and is used in patients with EGFR mutation–positive nonsmall cell lung carcinoma. Osimertinib (TAGRISSO) is a third-generation EGFR TKI which is used to treat locally advanced or metastatic nonsmall cell lung cancer, with a T790M mutation in EGFR. This mutation may be de novo or acquired following first-line treatment with other TKIs, such as gefitinib and afatinib.

Signalling Through RAS-RAF-ERK and PI3K-AKT

Both of these pathways are major downstream signals for the EGFR family members, and RAS-regulated pathways interact at multiple points, including with the PI3K-AKT-mTOR pathway, and with c-MYC. The PI3K-Akt-mTOR pathway is activated in many cancers and therefore is a good target for therapy. Temsirolimus (Torisel) is the first-in-class mTOR inhibitor licensed for use in metastatic renal cancer. It is administered intravenously, unlike everolimus (Afinitor), which is an oral mTOR inhibitor used in renal cell cancer, breast cancer and some neuroendocrine tumours. Both compounds are relatively well tolerated, with pneumonitis, asthenia, rash, anemia, nausea, anorexia and hyperglycemia being documented but not usually severe.

It has not been possible to develop a drug to target RAS. However, the BRAF protein kinase, which is downstream in the pathway, has been successfully directly targeted with the oral small-molecule inhibitors vemurafenib (Zelboraf) and dabrafenib (TAFINLAR). Overall, 6% of human cancers contain activating mutations in BRAF13 and like RAS mutations, BRAF mutations are very oncogenic. Just as RAS-mutated cells are dependent on MEK, it is also the case that cells with the activating BRAF mutation V600E are dependent on MEK and thus ERK signalling for cell survival and proliferation. Vemurafenib and dabrafenib and the MEK inhibitor trametinib (Mekinist) are now approved for the treatment of BRAF-mutated melanoma, clinically validating the possibility of targeting the RAS/RAF/MEK pathway to achieve meaningful benefit for patients.

Vascular Endothelial Growth Factor Signalling Pathway

Angiogenesis is known to be pivotal in tumour progression and metastasis and as VEGF is the driving force behind angiogenesis, it is not surprising that it has been the target of many approaches. Agents have been developed that target the VEGF ligand, blocking its interaction with the VEGF receptors (bevacizumab) and agents that directly block the receptor (TKIs such as sunitinib). Bevacizumab (Avastin) is a recombinant humanized monoclonal antibody to VEGF-A. It is licensed for use in metastatic colorectal, breast, nonsmall cell lung and renal cancer. The side-effect profile of bevacizumab includes hypertension (a classical effect of VEGF inhibitors), thromboembolic events (both arterial and venous) and gastrointestinal perforation. Aflibercept (ZALTRAP) is a recombinant fusion protein consisting of VEGF-binding portions from the extracellular domains of human VEGF receptors 1 and 2 that are fused to the Fc portion of the human IgG1 immunoglobulin. It is used in the treatment of metastatic colorectal cancer and has a similar side-effect profile to Avastin but with more neutropenia demonstrated.

Because VEGF mediates its angiogenic effect through several tyrosine kinase receptors, many VEGF TKIs have been tested. Sorafenib (Nexavar) is licensed for use in renal cell and hepatocellular cancer, and sunitinib (SUTENT) is licensed for use in renal cell cancer and gastrointestinal stromal tumor. Numerous other TKIs are in clinical studies. Some are highly selective, targeting only specific VEGF receptors, whereas others are more 'promiscuous' and target other kinases such as PDGF and EGFR. Despite being 'targeted' therapies, these drugs do have significant side effects including neutropenia, fatigue, rashes, diarrhoea and stomatitis.

Proteasome Inhibitors

These drugs, exemplified by bortezomib (Velcade), prevent degradation of various proteins in the proteasome. Bortezomib was the first selective proteasome inhibitor and is licensed in patients with refractory or relapsed multiple myeloma. It is believed to be effective in myeloma by interfering with normal function of the NF-kB signalling pathway, thus reducing tumour cell replication and angiogenesis and promoting apoptosis. Other drugs in the class include carfilzomib (Kyprolis) and ixazomib (NINLARO). Both are used to treat myeloma and the latter is the first orally available proteasome inhibitor.

PARP INHIBITORS

DNA damage and its repair, or lack of, are responsible for the formation of mutations, which cause nearly all cancers. Healthy cells defend themselves against the potential negative effects of DNA damage through the DNA damage response (DDR). In this process, DNA damage is recognised, the cell cycle pauses and DNA repair mechanisms start, with the result of genomic integrity and fidelity. PARPs are critical enzymes in repairing DNA damage, specifically single-strand breaks. If single-strand breaks are not repaired before DNA is replicated, double-strand breaks occur during that process, which results in cell death. Therefore PARP inhibitors have for some time been studied as anticancer therapies. However, it was only with the application of the genetic concept of synthetic lethality that real progress was made in getting the agents into the clinic. This concept is based on the idea that a defect in either one of two genes has little effect on the cell, but a simultaneous combination of defects in both genes results in death. Thus, for example, tumor cells with inactivating mutation of the BRCA DNA-repair genes, which in itself is not lethal, will be killed if they are also exposed to PARP inhibitors. So far, four agents—olaparib (Lynparza), rucaparib (Rubraca), niraparib (ZEJULA) and talazoparib (TALZENNA)—are available with varying licensing in BRCA mutant ovarian, breast and prostate cancers. Generally, the agents are well tolerated; nausea and fatigue are relatively common, with grade 3 and 4 events being seen more rarely. Patients are therefore able to take them for prolonged periods, unlike many cytotoxic agents, although the accumulation of a number of grade 2 toxicities may lead to dosing interruptions.

CDK4/6 INHIBITORS

Even before the publication of Hanahan and Weinberg's seminal paper 'The Hallmarks of Cancer', targeting the cell cycle was a key anticancer strategy. Only recently, with the development of CDK4/6 inhibitors, has this approach come to fruition. CDK4 and CDK6 are cyclin-dependent kinases that control the transition between the G1 and S phases of the cell cycle. CDK4/6 activity is usually deregulated and overactive in cancer cells. A major target of CDK4 and CDK6 during cell-cycle progression is the retinoblastoma protein (Rb). When Rb is phosphorylated, its growth-suppressive properties are inactivated. Selective CDK4/6 inhibitors 'turn off' these kinases and dephosphorylate Rb, resulting in a block of cell-cycle progression in mid-G1. This causes cell-cycle arrest and prevents the proliferation of cancer cells. Estrogen receptor–positive breast cancer is particularly dependent upon CDK4 for proliferation. Therefore the combination of a CDK4/6 inhibitor and antioestrogen therapy works synergistically in ER-positive breast cancer. Palbociclib (IBRANCE) and ribociclib (KISQALI) are both licensed for use in ER-positive metastatic breast cancer in combination with aromatase inhibitors. Abemaciclib (Verzenio) is licensed both in the adjuvant and metastatic settings. Toxicities are manageable, although patients need to be carefully monitored for neutropenia, diarrhoea, liver dysfunction and QTc prolongation.

THERAPEUTIC ANTIBODIES

In addition to the antibodies discussed in the previous section, rituximab (MabThera) is a chimeric monoclonal antibody targeting the CD20 antigen found on normal B cells and B-cell lymphomas. It is licensed for use for follicular lymphoma, diffuse large B-cell lymphoma and CLL and has remarkably improved the outlook for these patients. It can be administered either as monotherapy or in combination with chemotherapy such as the 'CHOP' regimen. Iodine 131 tositumomab (Bexaar) and 90Y ibritumomab tiuxetan (Zevalin) are both radiolabelled CD20-targeted antibodies. They are licensed for use in some refractory lymphomas but their costs are prohibitive. Obinutuzumab and ofatumumab are also available for use in CLL.

Alemtuzumab (previously known as CAMPATH) is a humanised monoclonal antibody targeting the CD52 antigen found on B lymphocytes. Its previous license was for use in patients with B-cell CLL who are unable to receive the chemotherapy drug fludarabine, although now rarely used. One of its primary indications now is for use in T-cell prolymphocytic leukaemia or in 17p-deleted CLL. It is associated with significant haematological toxicity, especially neutropenia. There are also some bispecific antibodies now licensed for use in diffuse large B-cell lymphoma such as epcoritamab and glofitamab.

Lenalidomide is an immunomodulating drug that is licensed for patients with advanced multiple myeloma (MM). It is a potent analogue of thalidomide and works in a number of ways: inhibiting proliferation of certain haematopoietic tumour cells (including MM plasma tumour cells and those with deletions of chromosome 5), enhancing T-cell– and Natural Killer (NK) cell–mediated immunity, inhibiting angiogenesis and inhibiting production of proinflammatory cytokines (e.g. TNF-α and IL6) by monocytes. In studies, the most concerning side effects of treatment were venous thromboembolic events and myelosuppression. Not surprisingly, there is also a significant risk of teratogenicity and therefore patients or their partners must not get pregnant while on treatment.

ANTIBODY–DRUG CONJUGATES

Antibody–drug conjugates (ADCs) are an emerging class of therapeutic agents. The basic components of an ADC include a target-specific antibody, a linker and a cytotoxic payload. Once the antibody binds to its target antigen, the ADC becomes internalised into the tumour cells, the linker breaks down and the payload is released with lethality. This way, ADCs are highly specific with low toxicity in comparison with traditional chemotherapeutics.

There are currently approximately 100 ADCs in clinical trials across different tumour types. Areas of recent success include breast and urothelial cancers. Trastuzumab emtansine (Kadcyla) and trastuzumab deruxtecan (ENHERTU) are both licensed for use as a standard of care in advanced HER2-positive breast cancers. The approval for trastuzumab emtansine was subsequently expanded to include patients with adjuvant HER2-positive breast cancer with signs of residual disease postoperatively. Sacituzumab govitecan (TRODELVY) is a newer ADC licensed in metastatic triple-negative breast cancers based on data from the ASCENT trial that demonstrated superior survival outcomes over standard chemotherapy options.

In 2019 the FDA granted accelerated approval for Enfortumab vedotin (PADCEV) in the treatment of advanced urothelial malignancies that had progressed after two prior lines of treatment. Other ADCs such as Brentuximab vedotin (ADCETRIS) and Polatuzumab vedotin (POLIVY) are licensed for use in lymphomas.

IMMUNOTHERAPY

In recent years, there has been an explosion of activity in the area of immunotherapy. Some extraordinary responses to these therapies have been realised in tumour types such as melanoma, renal cell and nonsmall cell lung cancer. Essentially the main premise of immunotherapy approaches in cancer treatment is to stimulate the patient's immune system to attack the tumour. This can be achieved by immunising the patient with a cancer vaccine, administering therapeutic antibodies or, with greatest recent success, manipulating immune checkpoints and pathways.

Immune Checkpoint Inhibitors

The two main targets currently for manipulating the immune checkpoint mechanism are cytotoxic T-lymphocyte–associated molecule-4 (CTLA-4) and programmed cell death receptor-1 (PD-1) or programmed cell death ligand-1 (PD-L1). Ipilimumab (Yervoy) was the first-in-class anti–CTLA-4 antibody to be licensed for the treatment of melanoma, nonsmall cell lung carcinoma, small cell lung cancer, bladder and metastatic hormone-refractory prostate cancer. Some exceptional responses were seen, especially in melanoma, although there was quite marked variation in response. In addition, unique side effects were seen due to nonspecific immunological activation; immune-related adverse events (irAEs). These include skin, gastrointestinal, liver and endocrine toxicities, often requiring specific management strategies not usually adopted in more 'typical' cytotoxic reactions. For some, the irAEs were fatal and for others the adverse event persisted even when the causative agent was stopped. Completely new algorithms have had to be developed to manage these compounds safely, for example using high-dose steroids and then infliximab for the treatment of immune-related colitis.

Antibodies that disrupt the PD-1 pathway include those that target PD-1, nivolumab (OPDIVO), pembrolizumab (Keytruda) and those that target PD-L1 atezolizumab (TECENTRIQ) and avelumab (Bavencio). Due to durable responses and reduced toxicity, these agents are licensed for use in urothelial cancer, nonsmall cell lung cancer, Merkel cell cancer and head and neck squamous cancer. Interestingly, in 2017 pembrolizumab was licensed for use by the FDA, not based on a specific tumour type, but rather a specific genetic alteration: mismatch repair deficiency or microsatellite instability. Generally speaking, these agents are less toxic than CTLA-4 inhibitors. However, there is a lag phase prior to response which on average is 2 months. Therefore, to use these drugs safely, patients need to be well enough to tolerate this wait. Also, when monitoring responses, the standard RECIST criteria can be misleading as occasionally there can be pseudoprogression seen on CT scans. This is borne out by the fact that in one analysis of patients with melanoma on ipilimumab surviving 4 years or more, 25% had never achieved more than progression of disease as measured by RECIST. Hence, as previously described, the iRECIST criteria were introduced to address such problems.

Emerging Immune Checkpoint Inhibitors

In an attempt to overcome resistance mechanisms and to improve treatment response rates, combination therapies of immune checkpoint inhibitors (ICIs) have been introduced, such as the ipilimumab-nivolumab doublet in metastatic melanoma. Although such combinations lead to improved response rates, this is often at the expense of more severe grade toxicities.

Possibly the next most evaluated checkpoint after CTLA4 and PD1 is lymphocyte activating gene 3 (LAG3). LAG3 is another immune checkpoint protein expressed on the surface of activated T cells and negatively regulates T-cell function. The LAG3 inhibitor relatlimab has been evaluated in combination with nivolumab (Opdualag) and is currently approved by the FDA and EMA as first-line treatment for advanced metastatic melanoma, based on clinical trials that showed improved survival outcomes.

Currently in the field of immunotherapy, further clinical studies are ongoing studying agents such as bispecific antibodies which combine recognition of antigen-binding sites on tumour cells with engagement of effector immune cells. There are more antibody–drug conjugates in development and of course numerous combination studies trying to combine immunotherapies with cytotoxics, radiotherapy and also different classes of immunotherapies. Combinations are particularly challenging due to the adverse event profiles and establishing safe but biologically effective doses when the adverse event may arise later in the course of treatment and outside the stand window of testing in a classical phase I study. Major enthusiasm at the moment is around the utility of chimeric antigen receptor (CAR) T cells. Typically, these are synthetically engineered T-cell receptors with an extracellular domain that recognises a tumour cell antigen and an intracellular domain that activates T cells. In practice, T cells are removed from the patient, genetically engineered and reinfused. To date, some significant clinical results have been seen using this technique in patients with haematological malignancies. For example, anti-CD19 CAR T cells have been approved for treatment in lymphoma (Axicabtagene ciloleucel, marketed as YESCARTA) and tisagenlecleucel (Kymriah) in B-cell acute lymphoblastic leukaemia. Translating these successes into the management of solid tumours remains the subject of much ongoing research. Many other targets and effector cells are thus being explored.

There is no doubt that major progress has occurred in the management of patients with anticancer agents. This is both in the supportive care of patients undergoing toxic treatment and the development of innovative therapies. We cannot, however, afford to be complacent. Even with extraordinary early responses with immunotherapy, eventually the hope of cure is thwarted by development of resistance. Precision medicine approaches are again limited by resistance pathways, tumour heterogeneity and the availability of drugs which have been licensed on the basis of a tissue biopsy rather than genetic aberration. Toxic effects can be very burdensome to patients, and finally the costs of these drugs are prohibitive. In the next decade, we will continue to see great innovation, but we need to ensure that these approaches are affordable and continue to benefit patients. Making cancer a chronic disease that is treatable rather than a fatal disease is acceptable as long as the therapy is acceptable for the quality of life of patients.

FURTHER READING

Bardia A, Hurvitz SA, Tolaney SM, et al. Sacituzumab govitecan in metastatic triple-negative breast cancer. *N Engl J Med*. 2021;384(16):1529–1541.

Brock A, Huang S. Precision oncology: between vaguely right and precisely wrong. *Cancer Res*. 2017;77(23):6473–6479.

Brufsky A. Long-term management of patients with hormone receptor-positive metastatic breast cancer: concepts for sequential and combination endocrine-based therapies. *Cancer Treat Rev*. 2017;59:22–32.

Cai L, Li Y, Tan J, Xu L, Li Y. Targeting LAG-3, TIM-3, and TIGIT for cancer immunotherapy. *J Hematol Oncol*. 2023;16(1):101.

Chau CH, Steeg PS, Figg WD. Antibody–drug conjugates for cancer. *Lancet*. 2019;394(10200):793–804.

Corona SP, Ravelli A, Cretella D, et al. CDK4/6 Inhibitors in HER2-positive breast cancer. *Crit Rev Oncol Hematol*. 2017;112:208–214.

Devita VT, Lawrence TS, Rosenberg SA, Depinho RA, Weinberg RA. *Cancer Principles and Practice of Oncology*. 10th ed. Lippincott Williams; 2016.

Downing A, Morris EJA, Corrigan N, et al. High hospital research participation and improved colorectal cancer survival outcomes: a population-based study. *Gut*. 2017;66:89–96.

Eisenhauer EA, Therasse P, Bogaerts J, et al. New response evaluation criteria in solid tumours: revised recist guideline (version 1.1). *Eur J Cancer*. 2009;45:228–247.

Gougis P, Wassermann J, Spano JP, Keynan N, Funck-Brentano C, Salem JE. Clinical pharmacology of anti-angiogenic drugs in oncology. *Crit Rev Oncol Hematol*. 2017;119:75–93.

Ke X, Shen L. Molecular targeted therapy of cancer: the progress and future prospect. *Front Lab Med*. 2017;1:69–75.

Komura K, Sweeney J, Inamoto T, Ibuki N, Azuma H, Kantoff P. Current treatment strategies for advanced prostate cancer. *Int J Urol*. 2018;25(3):220–231. https://doi.org/10.1111/iju.13512.

Lancet Oncology Editorial. Calling time on the immunotherapy gold rush. *Lancet Oncol*. 2017;18:981.

Lee P, Yeoh Y, Low TY. A recent update on small-molecule kinase inhibitors for targeted cancer therapy and their therapeutic insights from mass spectrometry-based proteomic analysis. *FEBS J*. 2023;290(11):2845–2864.

Lopez JS, Banerji U. Combine and conquer: challenges for targeted therapy combinations in early phase trials. *Nat Rev Clin Oncol*. 2017;14(1):57–66.

Manasanch EE, Orlowski RZ. Proteasome inhibitors in cancer therapy. *Nat Rev Clin Oncol*. 2017;14:417–433.
Michaud LB, Buzdar AU. Complete estrogen blockade for the treatment of metastatic and early stage breast cancer. *Drugs Aging*. 2000;16(4):261–271.
Ohmoto A, Yachida S. Current status of poly(ADP-ribose) polymerase inhibitors and future directions. *Onco Targets Ther*. 2017;10:5195–5208.
Perry MC. *The Chemotherapy Source Book*. 54th ed. Lippincott Williams; 2012.
Peters C, Brown S. Antibody–drug conjugates as novel anti-cancer chemotherapeutics. *Bioscience Rep*. 2015;35(4):e00225.
Seidel JA, Otsuka A, Kabashima K. Anti-PD-1 and anti-CTLA-4 therapies in cancer: mechanisms of action, efficacy, and limitations. *Front Oncol*. 2018;8:86.
Seymour L, Bogaerts J, Perrone A, et al. iRECIST: guidelines for response criteria for use in trials testing immunotherapeutics. *The Lancet Oncology*. 2017;18(3):e143–e152.
Shastry M, Gupta A, Chandarlapaty S, Young M, Powles T, Hamilton E. Rise of antibody-drug conjugates: the present and future. *Am Soc Clin Oncol Educ Book*. 2023;43:e390094.
Velasquez M, Bonifant C, Gottschalk S. Redirecting T cells to hematological malignancies with bispecific antibodies. *Blood*. 2018;131(1):30–38.
Vidal N, Rivas JG, Fernández L, et al. The past, present, and future of non-metastatic castration-resistant prostate cancer (nmCRPC): a narrative review. *Precision Cancer Medicine*. 2022;5. DOI: 10.21037/pcm-21-34
Wang X, Huang S, Zhang Y, Zhu L, Wu X. The application and mechanism of PD pathway blockade for cancer therapy. *Postgrad Med J*. 2018;94:53–60.
Wu P. Small-molecule kinase inhibitors: an analysis of FDA-approved drugs. *Drug Discov Today*. 2016;21(1):5–10.
Younes A, Ansell S, Fowler N, et al. The landscape of new drugs in lymphoma. *Nat Rev Clin Oncol*. 2017;14:335–346.
Zheng H-C. The molecular mechanisms of chemoresistance in cancers. *Oncotarget*. 2017;8(35):59950–59964.

21

Skin and Lip Cancer

Thankamma V. Ajithkumar

CHAPTER OUTLINE

INTRODUCTION

Skin cancer is the most common human cancer. It can be divided broadly into two types: melanoma and nonmelanoma. Keratinocyte-derived skin cancers are a group made up of squamous and basal cell carcinoma. A further group of much less common skin tumours, arising from the skin appendages, are primary cutaneous lymphoma, Kaposi sarcoma and Merkel cell tumours.

Keratinocyte skin tumours, particularly basal cell carcinomas, are the most common skin cancers. Their true numbers are often underreported because they do not have to be counted as new cancers in many cancer registries.

Basal cell carcinomas are very common and relatively benign. However, melanomas and squamous cell carcinoma of the skin carry a significant mortality, as do much less common Merkel cell tumours, skin lymphomas and Kaposi sarcoma (KS). In the United Kingdom, more than 16,700 people are diagnosed with malignant melanoma each year with 2300 deaths. By comparison, there are approximately 156,000 new cases of nonmelanomatous skin cancer (NMSC) and 920 deaths.

The incidence of both melanoma and keratinocyte skin cancers is increasing decade by decade, and further increases can be expected as the population ages.

KERATINOCYTE SKIN TUMOURS

Keratinocyte skin tumours from epidermal keratinocytes. The incidence of both squamous cell carcinoma (SCC) and basal cell carcinoma (BCC) is related to increased lifetime sun exposure.

Aetiology

The following factors can all be involved in developing keratinocyte skin tumours, but these cancers are more common in people with white skin. Skin pigmentation protects against the development of these tumours so that, at one extreme, albinos have a much-increased risk of skin cancer, whereas NMSC is rare in people with black skin.

Ultraviolet Radiation

Excessive exposure to ultraviolet B (UVB) from sunlight and ultraviolet A (UVA) from sunbeds has been implicated as an aetiological factor. BCCs are common in Caucasians living in Australia and the United States. It is estimated that 3.6 million new BCCs will be diagnosed in the United States each year. The incidence is highest in the southern and southwestern states.

Premalignant Skin Lesions

Lesions such as actinic keratosis (Fig. 21.1) or Bowen disease (Fig. 21.2) are known for their potential to develop into SCC. These lesions are found on sun-exposed parts of the body. Bowen disease is squamous carcinoma in situ and, in about 5% of cases, develops into invasive squamous cancer. Actinic keratoses do carry an increased risk of developing SCC, but only a small minority, approximately 1 in 1000, go on to become skin cancers.

Topical Carcinogens

Direct skin contact with chemicals such as tar, pitch or nonsolvent refined mineral oils are a potential cause of SCC.

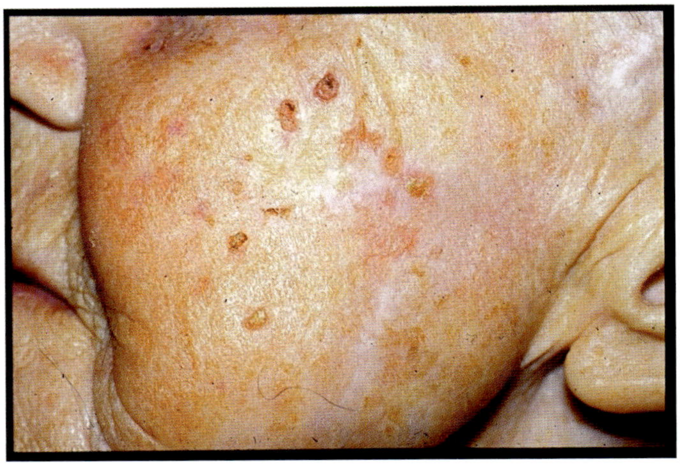

Fig. 21.1 Actinic keratosis with a background of sun-damaged skin.

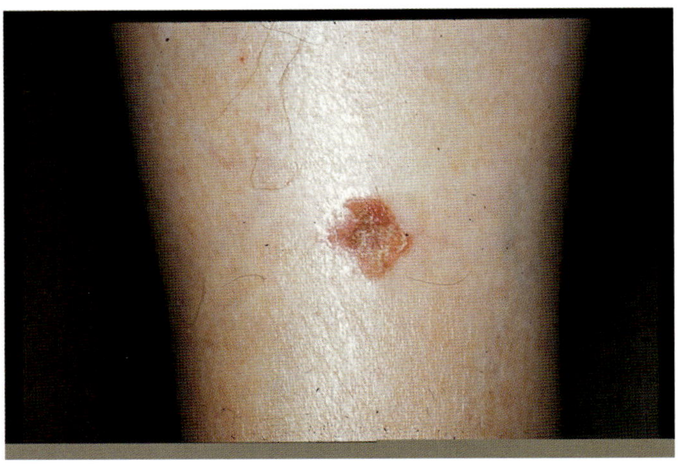

Fig. 21.2 Bowen disease on a limb. Note the colour and the superficiality of the lesion.

Ingested Carcinogens

These are becoming less common, but previously, it was relatively common to include arsenic in proprietary 'tonics'. Arsenic can cause multiple skin tumours, both SCCs and basal cell, as well as premalignant skin changes (Fig. 21.3).

Psoralen Ultraviolet A Treatment for Psoriasis

Psoralen UVA (PUVA) (Fig. 21.4) is an effective treatment for psoriasis. In this treatment, a drug (psoralen) is given before exposing the patient to UVA. However, this treatment does increase the chance of developing a keratinocyte-originating tumour, particularly a squamous cancer. The risk increases with the cumulative dose of UVA.

Immunosuppression

This is most commonly seen now in patients who have had organ transplants, and the normal ratio of SCC to BCC is reversed, with SCC becoming more common than BCC. Twenty years after a kidney transplant 50% of patients listed in the Oxford transplant register had either a squamous or basal cell skin tumour.

Basal Cell Naevus Syndrome (Gorlin Syndrome)

Basal cell naevus syndrome (BCNS) is an uncommon autosomal dominant genetic abnormality having a familial syndrome, with patients at increased risk of developing multiple BCCs at a relatively young age.

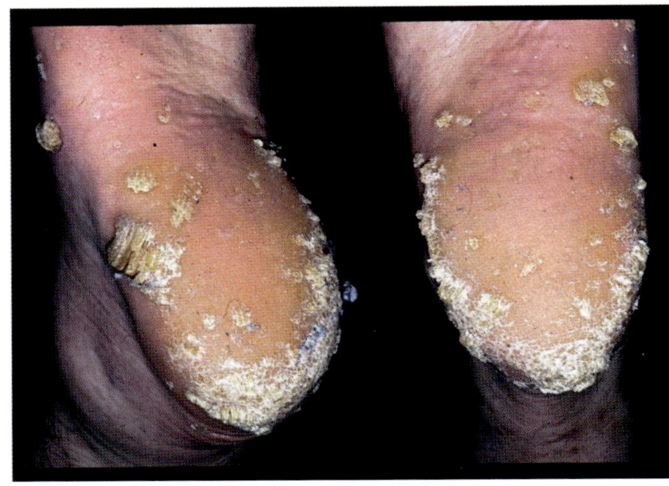

Fig. 21.3 Thick keratoses which developed following the ingestion of arsenic as a constituent of a 'tonic'.

There are also other skeletal and skin abnormalities, such as tiny pinpoint lesions on the palms known as *palmar pitting* (Fig. 21.5), dental cysts, frontal bossing, bifid ribs and calcification of the falx. These other abnormalities may well be picked up by chance when the patient is being investigated for other problems. Radiotherapy (RT) is contraindicated in patients with the syndrome, as it is thought that giving RT can initiate the development of BCCs. Medulloblastoma is also more common in patients with BCNS. It is important to exclude BCNS before RT is given to children with medulloblastoma because of the risk of radiation-induced multiple BCCs at the treatment site.

Xeroderma Pigmentosa

Xeroderma pigmentosa (Fig. 21.6) is a very rare, autosomal recessive genetic condition in which the repair of DNA after damage by UV exposure is defective. These patients can develop SCC or BCC of the skin or Bowen disease in childhood after minimal sun exposure.

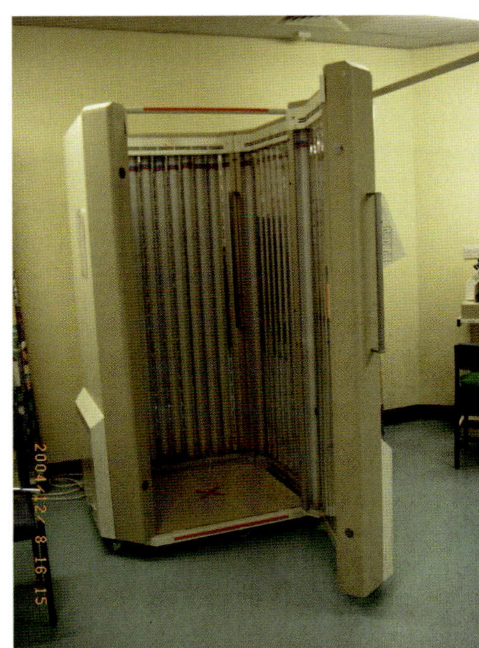

Fig. 21.4 A typical ultraviolet A (UVA)–generating machine used in psoralen UVA treatments. Note the tubes used to produce the UVA.

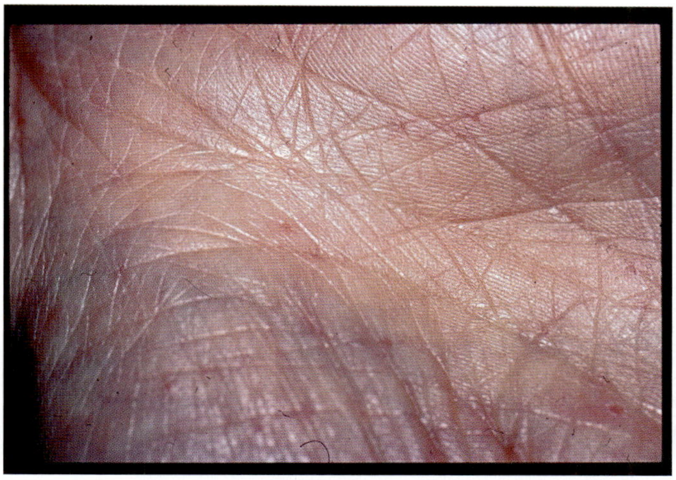

Fig. 21.5 The very subtle palmar pitting found in Gorlin syndrome.

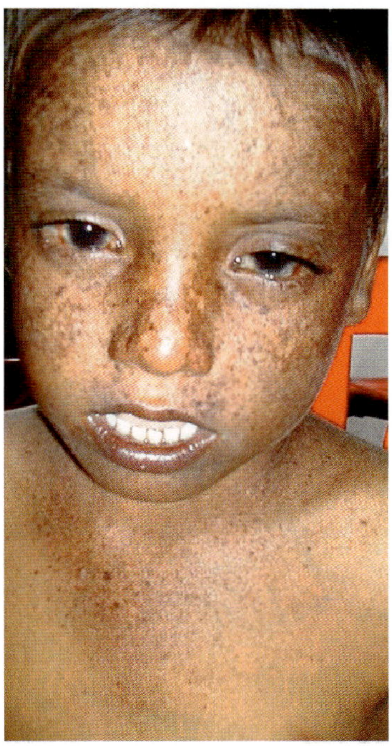

Fig. 21.6 This patient shows the characteristic signs of skin damage at an early age, found in xeroderma pigmentosa. There are also cataracts present, which can also be found in this condition.

Although very uncommon, xeroderma pigmentosa has provided great insight into the mechanism of skin cancer development.

Chronic Trauma

Forms of chronic ulceration (Fig. 21.7), direct thermal damage or previous burn scars can all predispose to the development of SCC of the skin.

Age

These skin cancers are essentially a disease of the elderly, reflecting accumulated UV skin damage. As the population ages, the incidence of skin cancer is steadily increasing.

Ionising Radiation

In the early days of RT, ionising radiation was used to treat a variety of benign skin diseases. Many years after treatment, basal cell or squamous

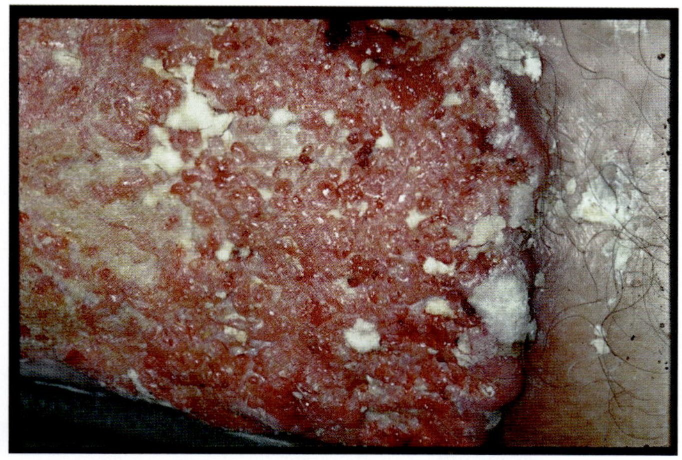

Fig. 21.7 Marjolin ulcer. Here, a carcinoma has developed in a long-standing area of damaged skin on the leg.

lesions appeared in the irradiated skin. The maximum effects were seen in children treated for ringworm.

Basal Cell Carcinoma

BCC is the most common skin cancer in White populations, three to four times as common as SCC. As the name suggests, these tumours arise from cells in the basal cell layer of the epidermis. They are more common in the elderly. Because the main cause of these tumours is UV exposure, they are more common on sun-exposed sites (Fig. 21.8A).

There are several clinical subtypes, the most characteristic being nodular BCC (see Fig. 21.8B). This presents as a characteristic pearly papule or nodule, classically with the rolled translucent edge and telangiectasia. The centre of this lesion often ulcerates and becomes crusted. The lesion may appear as if it is about to heal but then can progress into further cycles of growth, breakdown, crusting and regression. These lesions will not, however, disappear without active treatment.

There are other clinical subtypes as well as the classical nodular BCC including superficial, micronodular, sclerosing, infiltrating and pigmented variants. Diagnosis of these variants may be difficult without a biopsy. It is rare for a BCC to metastasise, but it can occur and is more frequent with long-standing large lesions, which have often been neglected for years.

The most common site for BCC is in a butterfly distribution in the central face. Elsewhere, tumours are more common on sun-exposed areas of the skin. If untreated, tumours invade deep tissues, including bone, leading to extensive ulceration and deformity over several years in patients who have not sought medical help (see Figs. 21.8C–E).

A typical example of a BCC at the left nasolabial fold before and 6 weeks after being treated with RT is shown in Figs. 21.8F and G.

Squamous Cell Carcinoma of the Skin

SCC is the second most common skin cancer after BCC, and the incidence of this tumour is rising as a result of increased exposure to UV radiation because there seems to be a direct association between the development of these tumours and hours of sun exposure. These tumours can enlarge and cause local destruction and metastasise, initially to regional nodes, which should be checked clinically when the patient first presents.

Following treatment for SCC, a full 5-year follow-up is required as they can recur locally, in lymph nodes or even with distant metastases. This is in contrast to BCCs, where patients can be discharged from follow-up as soon as the treatment side effects have settled.

Well-differentiated SCCs produce keratin and the presence of keratin on the surface of a tumour is the characteristic feature of SCCs. The best example of this is SCC producing a keratin horn, although these

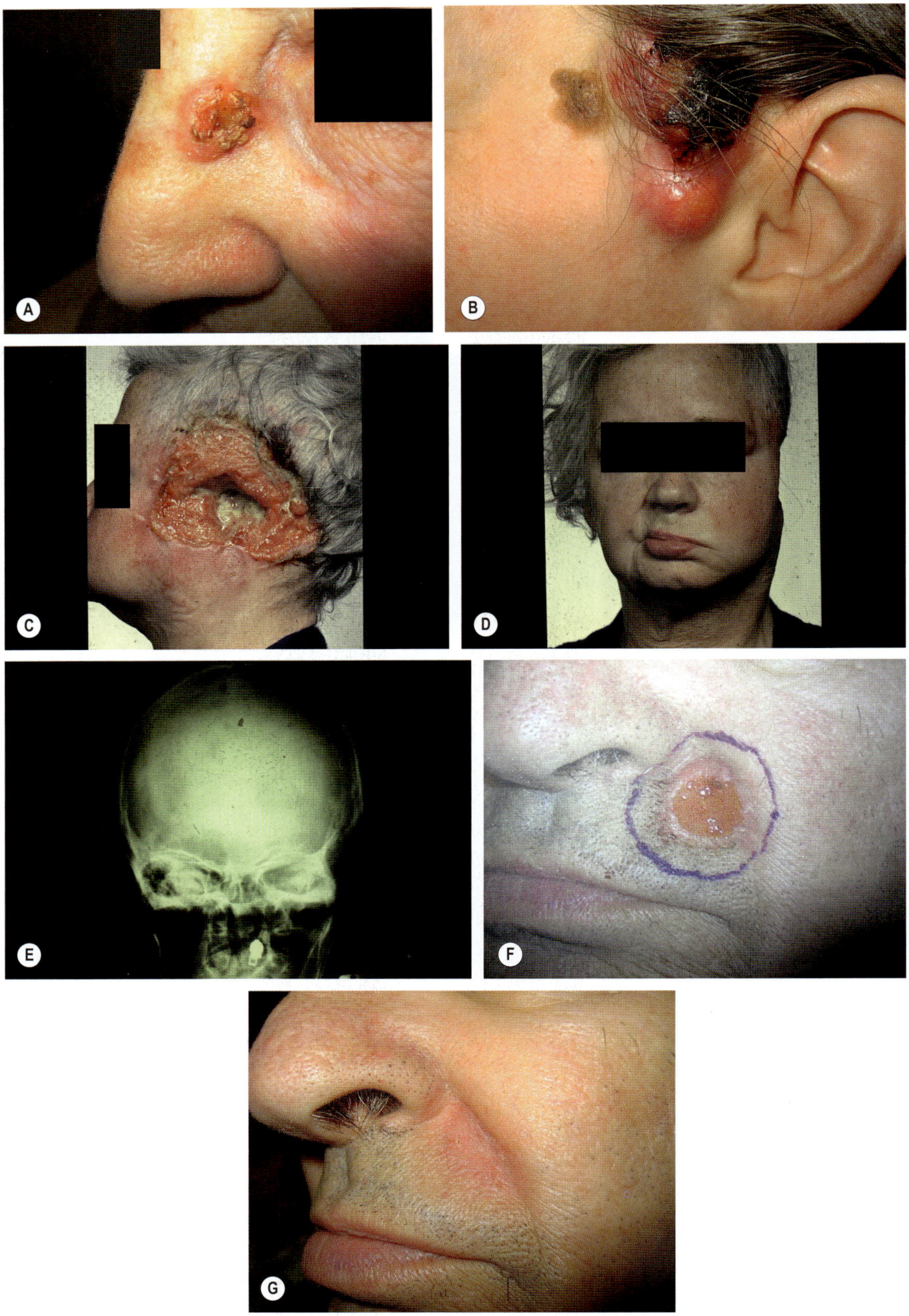

Fig. 21.8 (A) A typical basal cell carcinoma (BCC), with a pearly appearance to the edge and central ulceration. (B) A nodular BCC. (C–E) An advanced BCC. Note the local soft-tissue destruction (C), the left seventh nerve palsy (D) and the bone loss because of erosion by this tumour (E). (F, G) A typical example of a BCC at the left nasolabial fold before and 6 weeks after being treated with radiotherapy.

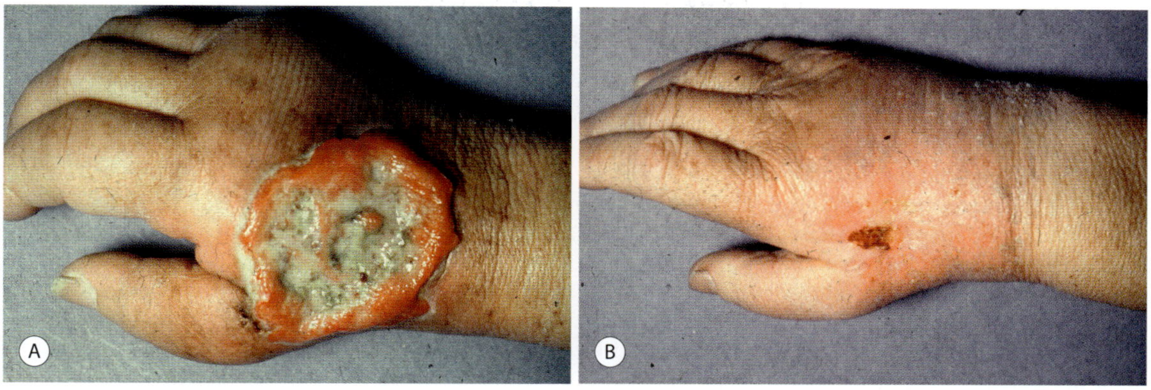

Fig. 21.9 (A) An extensive squamous cell carcinoma of the back of the hand before radiotherapy and (B) 4 weeks after treatment.

can also result from a benign cause, such as actinic keratosis or a viral wart. Poorly differentiated and hence more aggressive SCCs are often less distinctive and present as a nodule or ulcer (Fig. 21.9A). SCC may develop within Bowen disease or actinic keratosis.

A typical SCC before and 4 weeks after RT is shown in Figs. 21.9A and B.

Cancer of the Lip

Cancer of the lip is predominantly a malignancy affecting elderly males. The lower lip is affected more frequently than the upper lip by a factor of 10. Almost all lower lip cancers are SCCs. It is rare to find BCCs on the lip vermilion, but they can arise from skin immediately adjacent. BCC develops most commonly on the skin close to the upper rather than the lower lip.

These malignancies are more common in fair skinned, weather-beaten outdoor workers. Sun exposure is one important factor but there may be others, such as pipe smoking, as cumulative UV exposure does not always correlate with some of the higher-risk occupational groups prone to developing this cancer. As with squamous carcinoma of the skin, transplant patients are at a higher risk of developing lip SCC.

Clinically, premalignant changes leading to carcinoma of the lip may precede the development of a mass or ulcer within the lip. This then enlarges, involving more of the lip. Spread to the submental or submandibular nodes is possible, especially with larger or poorly differentiated lesions, but spread to other neck nodes early on is uncommon. Classically, 5% of lip cancers have palpable nodes at diagnosis and 5% subsequently develop nodal metastases after successful treatment of the primary.

Management of Cancer of the Lip

Initially, a pathological diagnosis needs to be made with an incisional biopsy. The treatment options can be discussed with the patient. For early tumours involving only the vermilion of the lip, the tumour can be removed with a lip shave and the oral mucosa advanced to replace the area removed. Superficial early tumours may be associated with other areas of premalignant change. This technique allows for these areas of premalignant change to be removed at the same time and sent for histological evaluation to exclude other areas of carcinoma in situ or frank invasive change. With larger lesions, the tumour can be removed surgically using a 'V' or 'W' incision. Here, the amount of functional tissue loss may make RT more appropriate.

Electron beam radiotherapy (EBRT) is usually given with wax and lead behind the lip to protect the rest of the mouth and take advantage of the backscatter effect. Dose/fractionation regimens used include 55 Gray (Gy) in 20 fractions or 66 Gy in 33 fractions. The cosmetic result is usually very good, as the lip has an excellent blood supply and healing usually occurs quickly and completely.

Keratoacanthoma

Keratoacanthomas are benign but can be very difficult to distinguish from SCC of the skin. They present as a rapidly growing nodule with a central keratin plug. The central plug detaches, and the residual lesion resolves (Figs. 21.10A and B). Keratoacanthomas are problematic in that they cannot be differentiated from SCC of the skin by biopsy alone and, in the growth phase, the pathologist will usually call them an SCC. As a result, although benign, they are often excised to avoid missing a rapidly growing squamous cell cancer.

Treatment of Nonmelanoma Skin Cancer

As can be seen from the list later in this chapter, there are several ways to treat keratinocyte skin tumours.

Few randomised studies have been conducted on different treatment modalities for BCC and SCC primary treatment, but Mohs micrographic surgery (MMS) gives the lowest short- and long-term recurrence rate for BCC and probably for SCC. One of the few randomised controlled trials in skin cancer treatment, which was carried out in the Netherlands, has shown a lower, but not statistically significant, recurrence rate after MMS compared with conventional excision. Operative costs were higher for the Mohs methodology. However, MMS is the preferred treatment option for ill-defined tumours and tumours arising in unhealthy or diseased skin, where MMS achieves 100% clear margin with minimal tissue resection.

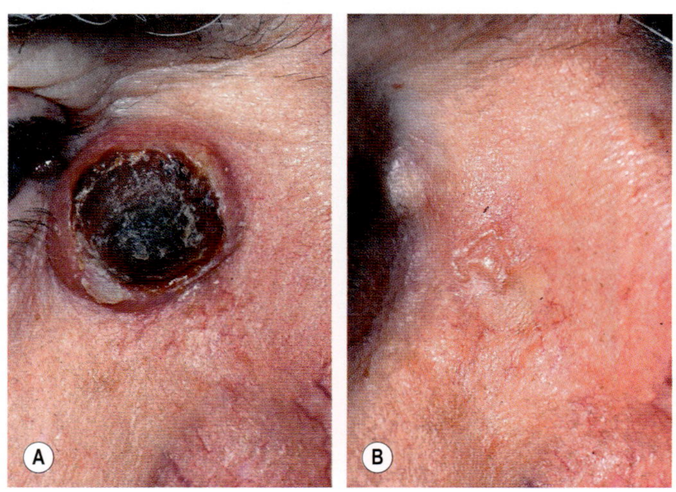

Fig. 21.10 (A) Keratoacanthoma in its rapidly developing stage. The central keratin plug is obvious. This lesion has developed in a matter of a few weeks. (B) Keratoacanthoma in its healing stage. This is the same lesion as in (A), 3 months later. The keratin plug was discharged spontaneously and complete healing rapidly ensued.

Patients with these tumours should be seen in the multidisciplinary skin cancer clinic where a treatment plan can be formulated for the individual patient. Often, the decision as to which treatment is given is based not on the historical evidence of the efficacy of that particular treatment but on the size and site of the skin lesion; the age, fitness and wishes of the patient; and the local resources and distances from the local hospital and cancer centre. In general, surgery or RT are equally effective in eradicating early-stage disease. RT is often avoided in younger patients on the basis that long-term cosmesis is usually better with surgery. As time passes, the surgical scar becomes less obvious, whereas the hypopigmentation produced by RT can become more prominent. RT is also often not given in situations where it yields a lower cure and/or worse cosmesis or function than surgery. These situations include large lesions involving cartilage, bone, tendons or joints and lesions arising in areas of poor vascular supply (e.g. lower leg, dorsum of hand, feet) and in areas likely to result in repeated pressure or trauma such as the elbow.

Curettage and Electrolysis

This is the simplest approach, but it is usually only suitable for small, previously untreated, well-defined BCCs less than 10 mm in diameter on noncritical sites (Figs. 21.11A–D).

Cryosurgery With Liquid Nitrogen

This technique is used more for BCCs than SCCs. Two to three days after treatment, oedema, blister formation, sloughing, and crust formation can occur. It has the advantage of being done in the outpatient clinic and can be useful in the frail elderly patient, where surgery is best avoided, and when the patient does not wish to travel to their local RT centre (Fig. 21.12).

Surgical Excision

Pathological evidence of complete removal is the main advantage of surgical excision, but for some morphoeic BCCs this may give a false reassurance with subsequent recurrence. For these tumours, MMS gives a higher rate of complete excision. The main disadvantage of surgical excision is that, in some sites, primary skin closure may be impossible and flap closure or skin grafting is required. The cosmetic results may be poor, especially in areas such as the tip of the nose.

Photodynamic Therapy

In photodynamic therapy, a cream containing a porphyrin precursor is placed on the skin. The tumour metabolises this precursor to porphyrin. The porphyrin is then activated by exposure to red light, and in the process, free radicals are produced that destroy the tumour.

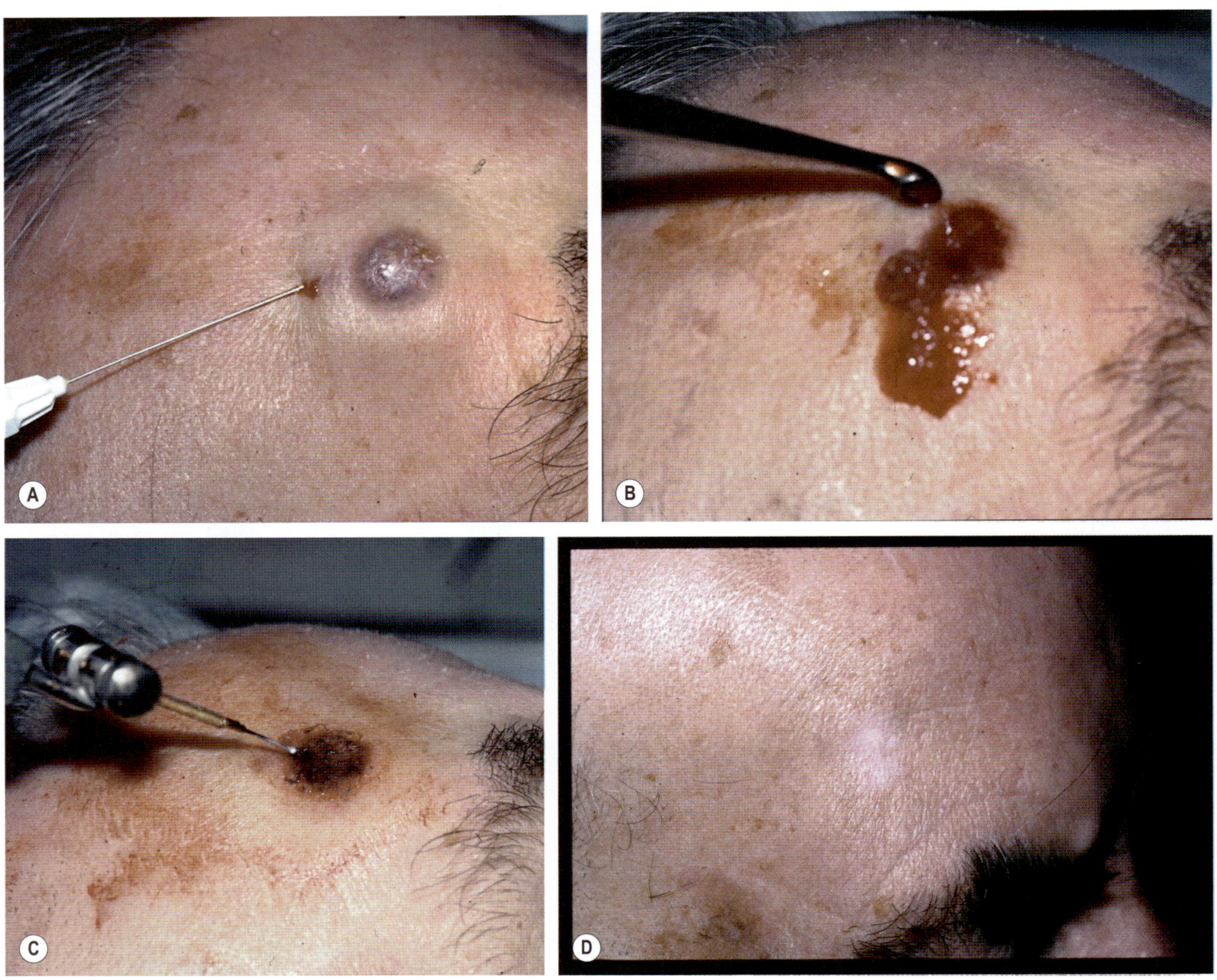

Fig. 21.11 (A) An area being prepared for curettage, with local anaesthetic being given. (B) The tumour is curetted out. (C) Further curettage is performed at the tumour's base. (D) The result at 2 years following curettage.

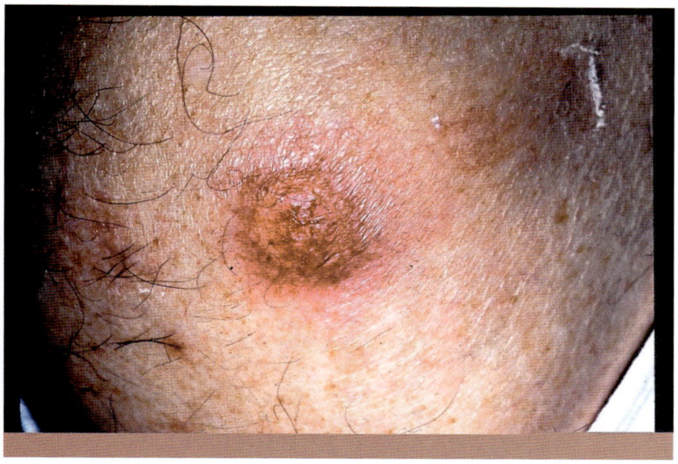

Fig. 21.12 The appearance of an area of skin 1 week after cryosurgery.

Photodynamic therapy is partially effective and still being developed. It is mainly reserved for large superficial truncal BCCs.

Mohs Micrographic Surgery

MMS uses repeated excisions at the tumour site until there is no histological evidence of any remaining tumour. It gives the highest cure rate but is also resource intensive. The interval between excisions depends on whether frozen sections or fixed tissue are examined by the pathologist. Frozen sections enable the surgeon to do several excision stages in 1 day. Inevitably, the time taken to fix and examine paraffin-embedded sections results in the excision stages being spread over several days (Figs. 21.13A–G).

Imiquimod

Imiquimod is a cream that can be applied on 'low-risk' BCCs as an alternative to surgery or RT. It is a form of local immunotherapy that releases interferons into the skin. In a UK multicentre trial comparing 5% imiquimod applied for 6 or 12 weeks to surgical excision, by 5 years the local control rate was 97.7% for those receiving surgery compared with 82.5% for imiquimod.

Medical Treatment of Basal Cell Carcinomas

Vismodegib is an inhibitor of the smoothen homologue oncogene (SMO), which is part of the hedgehog signalling pathway responsible for the uncontrolled proliferation of basal cells in BCCs. Vismodegib is an oral preparation that is indicated for the treatment of locally advanced BCC unsuitable for surgery and/or RT, including people suffering from Gorlin syndrome or metastases. Metastases from basal cell tumours are rare. Two phase II studies gave similar results with durable responses. In the ERIVANCE study, the complete response rate (CR) was 20.6% with a partial response (PR) rate of 22.2%. In the STEVIE trial, the CR rate was 33.4% with a PR rate of 35.1%. The median duration of response was 23 months for local advanced lesions and 13.9 months for metastasis.

Patients, predominantly elderly, often find the side effects of vismodegib (altered or decreased taste, decreased appetite, fatigue, muscle and

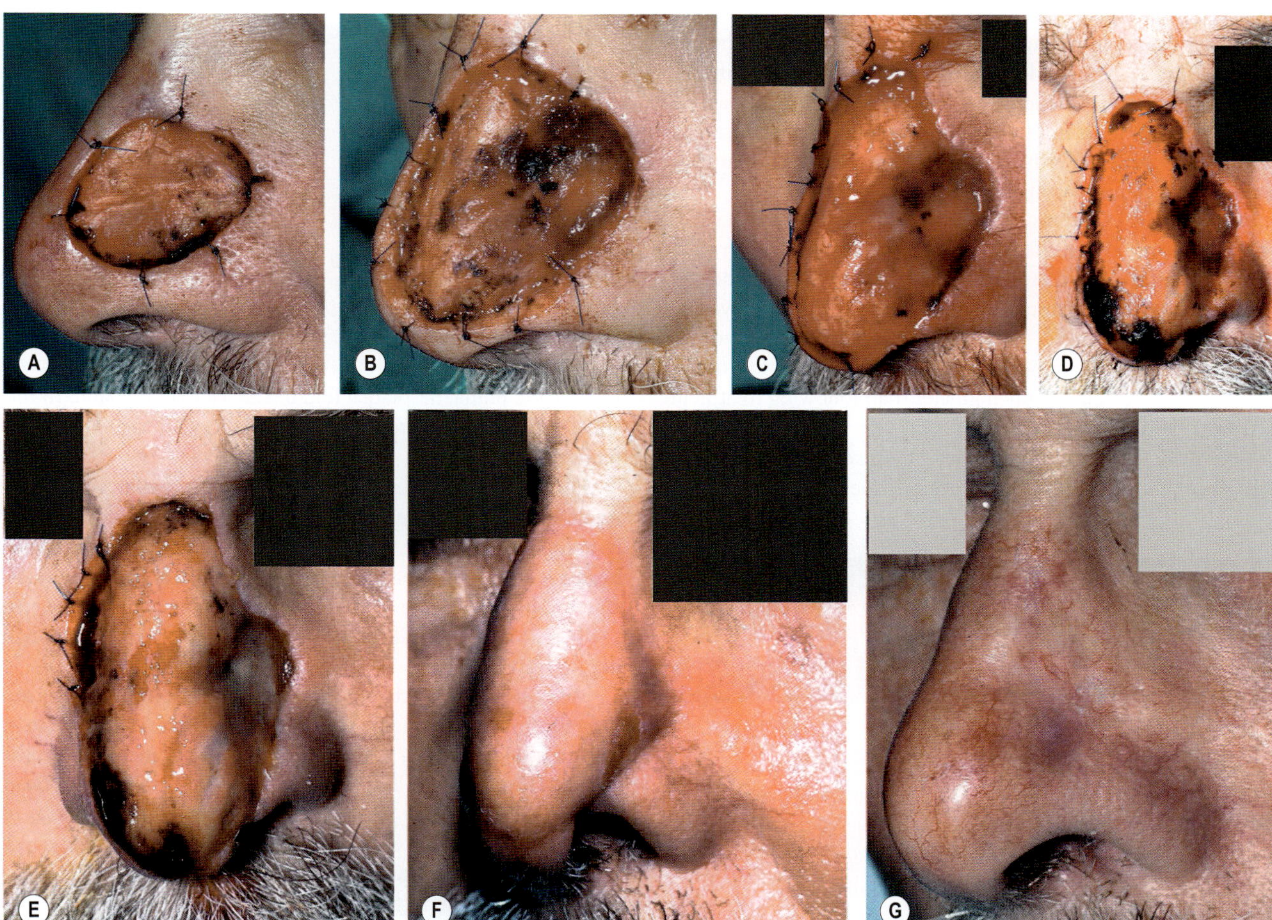

Fig. 21.13 (A–G) Series of clinical photographs showing Mohs micrographic surgery, with the initial incision, the further wider excisions and the final result.

joint pain) intolerable and ask to discontinue the medication. In the United Kingdom, the National Institute for Health and Care Excellence (NICE) has not recommended vismodegib, and permission for its use has been withdrawn 'because of the uncertainty in the evidence and because it is not cost effective' (https://www.nice.org.uk/guidance/TA489/chapter/1-recommendations). Pembrolizumab, with or without vismodegib, is being tested in the same patient population. A number of studies are evaluating the role of immunotherapy using checkpoint inhibitors for BCC. The UK phase II IMPACT trial is evaluating the role of cemiplimab (anti-PD1) in locally advanced inoperable BCC, which can be treated with RT.

Radiotherapy for Keratinocyte Skin Cancers

RT is particularly useful in treating tumours of the central face, around the nose and eyes, where surgical treatment may give a relatively poor cosmetic result or more loss of function than with RT. There is a relative contraindication for giving RT to certain sites, such as the pinna, with its underlying cartilage; the back of the hand, with its tendons lying superficially; and the anterior shin where there is a relative lack of underlying subcutaneous tissue. These sites can even be treated in appropriate patients if due consideration is given to the skin condition, site of treatment and treatment volume, total dose and fractionation.

When giving RT around the eye, treating the lateral upper eyelid may damage the lacrimal gland and ducts, leading to a permanently dry eye. Lesions at the medial canthus can also occlude the lacrimal drainage system. However, if the lacrimal duct is uninvolved by cancer and is patent before RT begins, it is more likely than not to remain patent after RT.

The RT dose used for treating skin malignancies varies from centre to centre and dose/fractionation schedules have developed empirically over the years. In general, the more fractions used, the better the late cosmetic result (Table 21.1). In addition to efficacy in curing the tumour, other factors, such as late cosmetic effects and convenience to the patient, are also important. Some elderly, frail patients will trade off the cosmetic outcome against convenience if they can visit the RT treatment centre for fewer visits without compromising the probability of cure.

RT can be given to these skin cancers using either superficial or deep x-ray beams, usually in the range of 50 to 300 kV, or with electron beams. The latter are used where rapid falloff of the depth dose is required to spare underlying normal tissue. If the skin tumour overlies cartilage or bone, low-voltage x-rays are absorbed disproportionately, owing to the high atomic number of bone compared with soft tissue, and the risk of radionecrosis is much greater than following treatment with electrons.

Electron Beam Treatment. Sites where the use of electron therapy beams may be indicated in preference to superficial x-ray beams include the pinna, nasolabial fold or the back of the hand. In the latter site, the use of an electron beam may reduce damage to the underlying tendon sheaths.

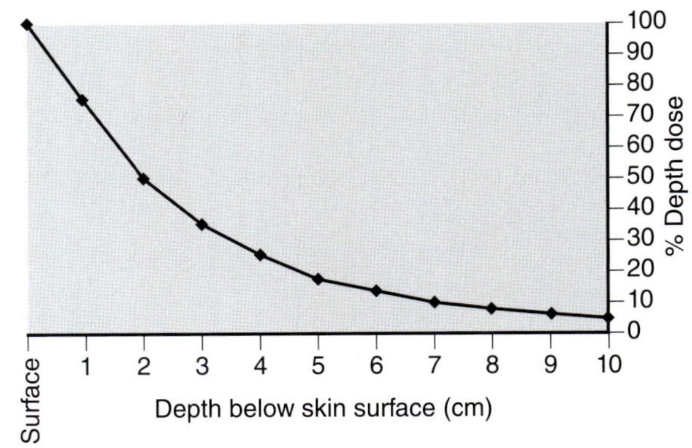

Fig. 21.14 The exponential falloff of dose at depth as a superficial x-ray beam penetrates tissue.

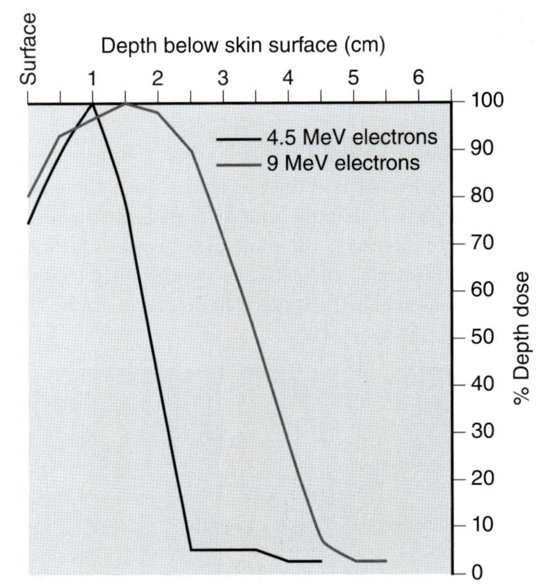

Fig. 21.15 Diagram showing how two electron beams of different energies interact with matter, delivering different doses at depth, depending on their energy. *MeV*, Megaelectron volt.

Electron beams are also used to irradiate larger areas of skin, either treating larger single epithelial skin tumours or when treating skin lymphomas. As can be seen in Figs. 21.14 and 21.15, superficial x-ray beams lose energy exponentially through matter (see Fig. 21.14), and electron beams reach a peak (at a depth proportional to the energy of the beam) and then fall off rapidly, delivering very little radiation at depth (see Fig. 21.15).

When using an electron beam on superficial tumours, the aim is to have the tumour within the 90% isodose (see Fig. 21.15) and to achieve this for some tumours, bolus may be needed to increase surface dose. Electron beams have a larger penumbra and have a different beam profile to superficial x-ray beams. Low-energy electron beams as used in treating skin tumours show isodoses coming together at depth, and this requires that a larger margin of normal tissue is included at setup, for example, 1.5 cm instead of 1 cm.

Electron Backscatter. Electron beams also have the advantage of being able to use the physical phenomenon of backscatter (Fig. 21.16A). If electrons encounter lead, a proportion will be scattered back towards

TABLE 21.1 Examples of Superficial Radiotherapy Fractionation Regimens for Treating Basal Cell Carcinoma and Squamous Cell Carcinoma of the Skin

Total Dose (Gy)	Number of Fractions/Interval	Indication
18–20	1/1 day	For field size <3 cm
32.5–35	4–5/1 week	Lesions <4 cm
45	10/2–3 weeks	Any size
50	15–20/3–4 weeks	Any size
55	20/4 weeks	Any size
60	30/6 weeks	Large area or areas of poor radiation tolerance

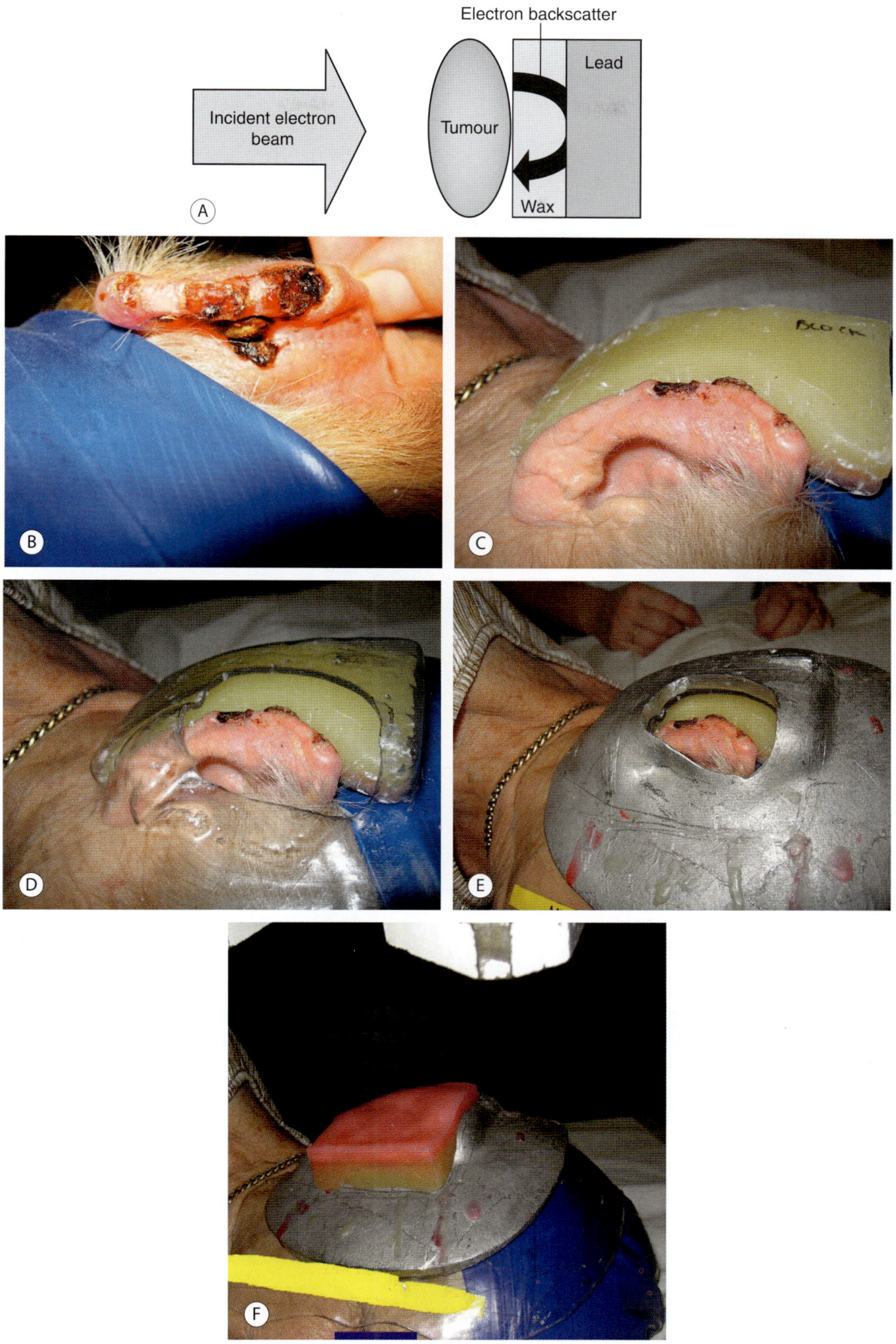

Fig. 21.16 (A) A simplified diagrammatic representation of the electron backscatter effect. By choosing different thicknesses of the lead and wax used, both the amount of backscatter and how many backscatter electrons are absorbed by the wax can be controlled, improving the homogeneity of dose over the tumour volume. (B–F) Use is made of the electron backscatter effect in treating a squamous cell carcinoma on the pinna of the ear. (B) The lesion. (C) Wax and lead are placed behind the ear, in the thicknesses required for maximal affect. (D) A Perspex cutout is placed over the ear, giving the treated electron field volume. An alloy cutout is placed over this (E) to tailor the electron beam to the treatment volume. (F) More wax bolus is applied to increase the percentage depth dose at the skin surface.

(*continued*)

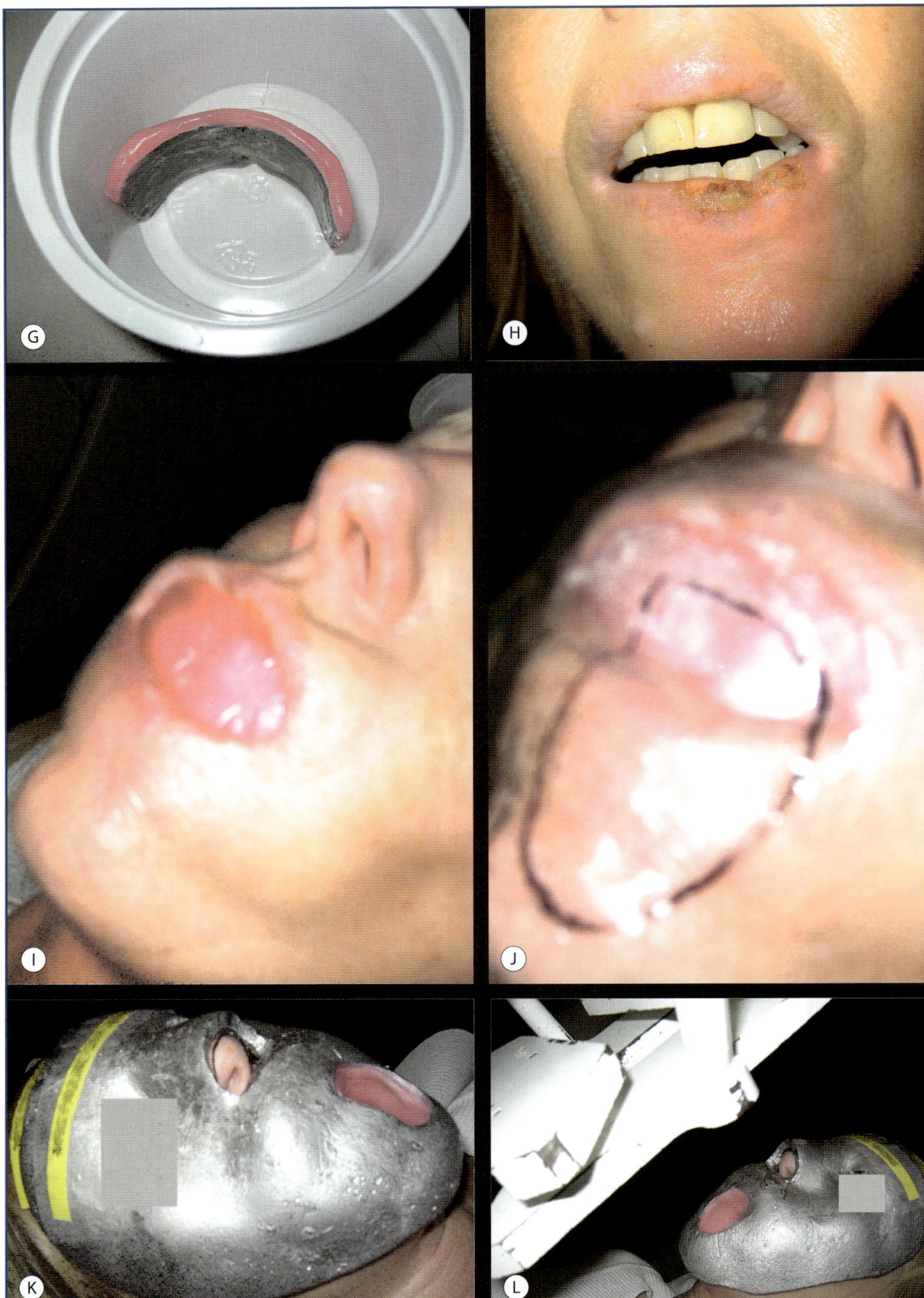

Fig. 21.16—Cont'd (G–L) The process of treating a lower lip cancer with electrons. A wax and lead insert is made, the treatment volume is marked out with it inserted and a Perspex mask is fitted over this. An alloy cutout is then placed on top. In this case, it is large, not to protect the whole face but because it is less likely to fall off during treatment. Further wax is used to increase the surface electron dose at the lip. Finally, the treatment reaction on the last day of treatment after 55 Gy in 20 fractions is shown.

the direction of the incident beam, and by placing wax in front of the lead, some of the backscatter electrons will be absorbed in the wax. By choosing the thickness of the lead and the wax carefully, the degree of backscatter can be modified. This allows greater homogeneity within the treated area. However, the amount of backscatter is difficult to measure and its contribution to irradiating the tumour volume changes with every individual patient setup. Electrons are scattered in many directions, not just at 180 degrees to the incident beam, and may contribute to dose outside the treatment volume. Therefore, by placing wax in front of the lead, some of these backscattered electrons will be absorbed in the wax. Backscatter thus has both positive and negative potential effects (see Figs. 21.16B–F, which illustrate an SCC of pinna treated by electrons).

One of the most common treatment sites for the use of backscatter to clinical advantage is when a cancer of the lower lip is treated with electrons. Wax and lead are put behind the lip. The lead helps to protect the oral cavity from the electron radiation beam. By varying the thickness of the wax for each individual patient, depending on how thick the lip and tumour are and, consequently, how wide the target volume needs to be, the degree of backscatter can be modified, giving greater homogeneity in dose across the tumour.

Figs. 21.16G–L show a wax and lead block being used for a lower lip cancer, with the area to be treated marked out in Fig. 21.16I.

Superficial X-ray Treatment. Most small BCCs on the face can easily be treated using x-ray energies of 90 to 120 kV. A lead cutout is placed around the lesion, with a margin of 5 mm if a BCC and 10 mm if an SCC (Figs. 21.17A and B). If the lesion is an irregular shape, a lead cutout may need to be specifically made, tracing the area to be treated with adequate margin onto a piece of lead, which is then cut out. If the treated site is close to the eyes, an external or internal eye shield is used to keep radiation dose to the eye to a minimum (Fig. 21.18).

Each fraction takes only a few minutes to deliver, and the patient should be warned that the reaction will start with erythema, followed by ulceration, over which a crust forms. Healing occurs underneath this crust, which detaches a few weeks after treatment. A second or even a third crust can form if it is detached prematurely or inadvertently knocked off.

After the acute reaction has settled down, late changes may develop with the possibility of hypopigmentation and telangiectasia.

Comparison of Outcome for Different Modalities in the Treatment of Basal Cell Carcinomas

In 2018, Drucker and colleagues published a systematic review and metaanalysis of 40 randomised and 5 nonrandomised trials comparing different modalities used to treat basal cell lesions. Estimated recurrence rates were excision (3.8%), MMS (3.8%), curettage and diathermy (6.9%) and EBRT (3.5%). Recurrence rates were higher for cryotherapy (22.3%), curettage and cryotherapy (19.3%), imiquimod (14.1%) and dynamic phototherapy using methylaminolevulinic acid (18.8%) or aminoaminolevulinic acid (16.6%).

MELANOMA

The incidence of melanoma is rising worldwide, but successful public education programs have reduced mortality in countries such as Australia.

Aetiology

Melanoma is much more common in White races and is related to UV radiation exposure. There is evidence that episodes of sunburn before the age of 15 increase the risk of developing melanoma.

Approximately 50% of melanomas arise in preexisting moles and 50% on otherwise normal skin.

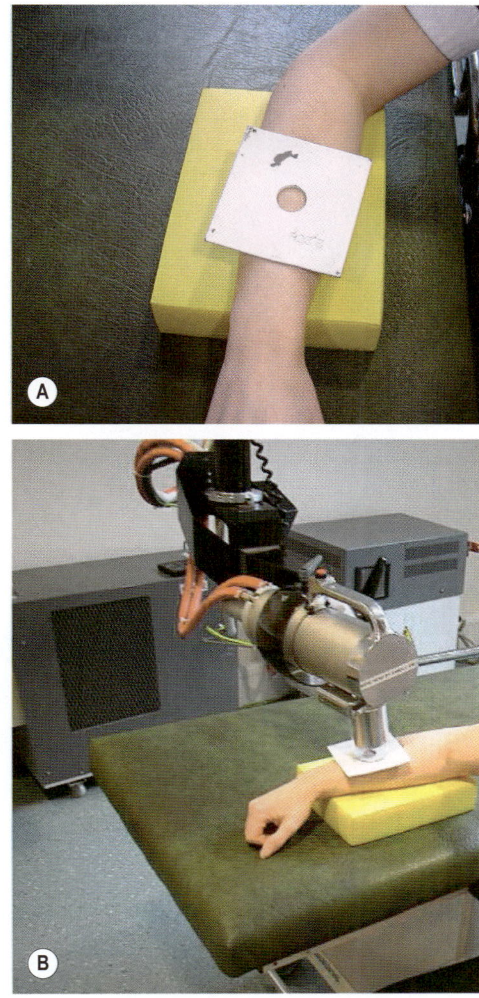

Fig. 21.17 (A) A typical example of a lead cutout used in treating small skin tumours with a superficial x-ray machine. (B) A superficial x-ray machine being set up with a volunteer.

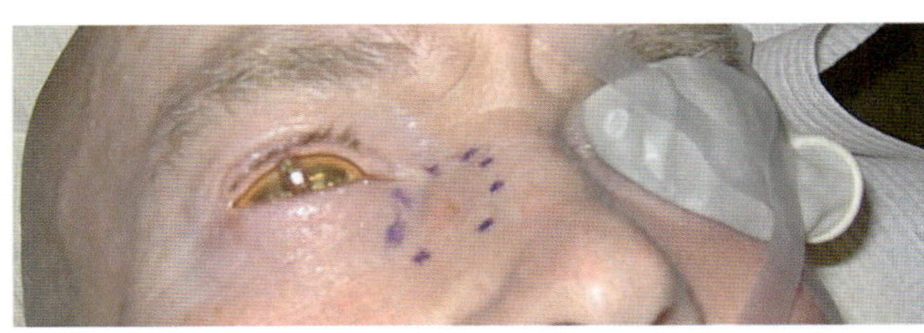

Fig. 21.18 If eye shields are required, either an external shield as shown covers this patient's left eye or an internal gold shield can be inserted under the eyelid after anaesthetising the conjunctiva with local anaesthetic, as shown with the right eye.

Subtypes of Melanoma

As with other skin tumours, there are several types of melanoma.

Superficial Spreading

Superficial spreading (Fig. 21.19) is the most common, representing 60% to 70% of all cases. It appears as a flat, pigmented lesion which may be related to a naevus. As the name implies, it initially grows outwards before invading downwards. Consequently, patients may present with a better prognosis if they seek help while the lesion is still in its horizontal or 'radial' growth phase, which may last for many months or even years.

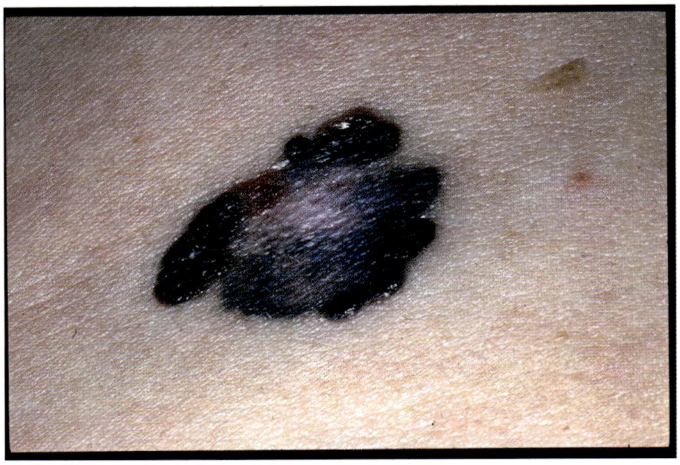

Fig. 21.19 Superficial spreading melanoma.

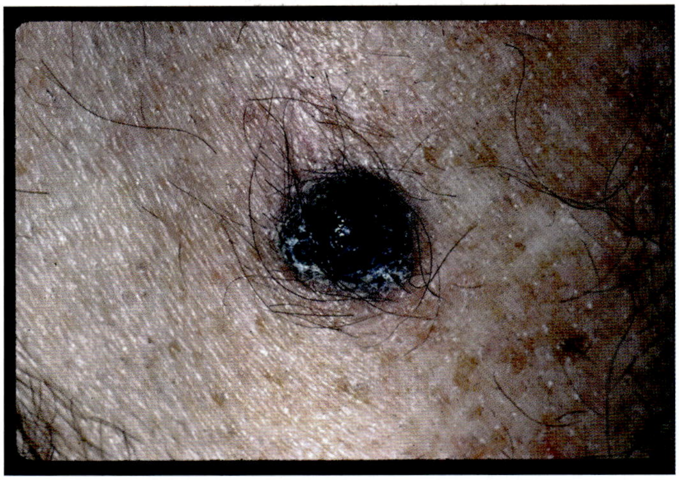

Fig. 21.20 Nodular melanoma.

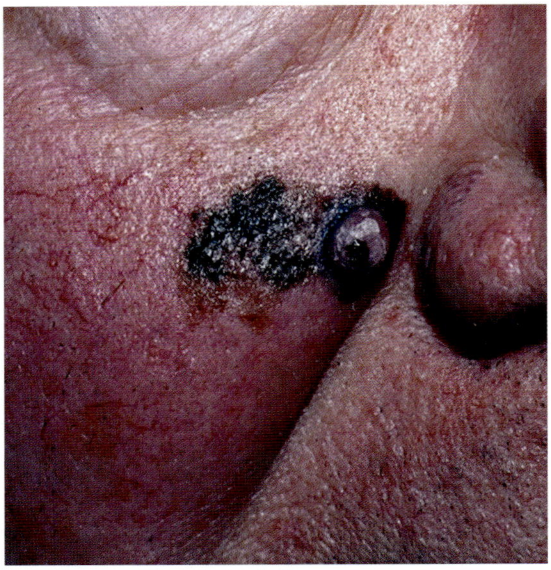

Fig. 21.21 Lentigo maligna melanoma.

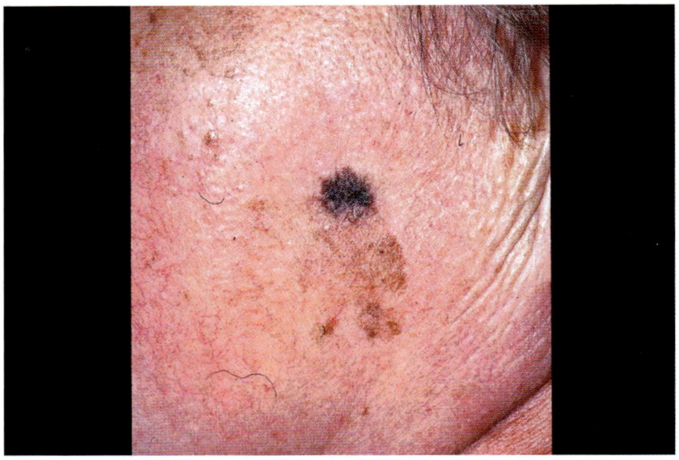

Fig. 21.22 Lentigo maligna, from which lentigo maligna melanoma can develop.

Nodular Melanoma

Nodular melanoma (Fig. 21.20) is less common, making up 15% to 20% of all cases. It appears clinically as a papule or nodule, usually pigmented, which represents the malignancy in the vertical growth phase from early in its natural history. This gives a worse prognosis at presentation. The clinical course is more rapid than with superficial spreading lesions.

Lentigo Maligna Melanoma

Lentigo maligna melanoma (Fig. 21.21) makes up 5% to 15% of melanomas. It is most commonly found in the skin of the nose or the cheek in the elderly and develops within a premalignant pigmented lesion known as *lentigo melanoma* (Fig. 21.22), which can be present for several years. This lesion eventually enlarges, undergoes malignant change and may develop a central pigmented nodule. RT is favoured in elderly patients with significant comorbidities and in situations where surgery might result in unacceptable functional and cosmetic results. RT achieves an excellent tumour control of >90% with a recurrence rate of 7% at a mean time of 45.6 months. There is an ongoing Australia and New Zealand Melanoma Trials Group study (RADICALS) comparing imiquimod versus RT in this group of patients.

Acral Lentiginous Melanoma

Acral lentiginous melanoma (Fig. 21.23) is much less common, comprising only 5% to 10% of melanomas, and is seen more frequently in pigmented skin. It can occur on the palms, sole of the foot or characteristically, beneath nails. There may be a relatively long radial growth phase. In some cases of subungual melanoma, suspicion may be raised by the extension of the pigmentation onto the skin of the proximal nail fold (Hutchinson sign).

Note that not all melanoma presents as pigmented lesions, and a nonpigmented 'amelanotic melanoma' (Fig. 21.24A) can cause diagnostic confusion until it is biopsied.

Diagnosis

Clinically, there should be suspicion that a melanoma may be developing. There are three cardinal features to look out for when considering the possibility of malignant change in an existing mole:

- Increase in diameter
- Change of colour
- Change in shape: becoming asymmetrical or developing border irregularity

This is the basis of the ABCDE method: Asymmetry, Border, Colour, Diameter, Evolving—changing in size, shape or colour.

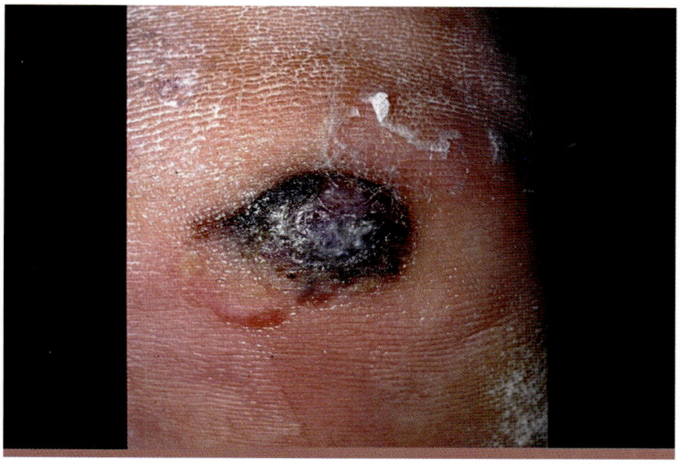

Fig. 21.23 Acral melanoma on the heel.

Moles greater than 6 mm are more likely to be malignant. Dermatoscopic examination using an amplified illuminated image is a helpful adjunct to clinical examination.

Melanoma TNM Staging

The TNM 2018 Classification of Malignant Tumors, 8th edition, was introduced at the beginning of 2018. These classifications can be gathered together into stage groupings so that each stage can bring together several TNM classes. Mitotic rate and Clark levels are no longer used for prognostic purposes.

Stage and Prognosis

In summary, the stage and subsequent prognosis depend on tumour thickness and the presence or absence of ulceration. The finding of nodal spread shows the melanoma has already metastasised and ultimate survival depends on the number of nodes involved by melanoma and the quantity of tumour in the lymph nodes (macroscopic or microscopic). Distant spread to the liver, lungs or brain carries a grave prognosis, with average survival times of 3 to 12 months depending on the metastatic site. Patients with metastases confined to the skin can often survive surprisingly long.

Five-year survivals based on the American Joint Committee on Cancer, 8th edition, are shown in Table 21.2 for stages I to III. For stage IV, there has always been a tail to the survival curve and today it would level out at just under 20% survival, but the present survival figures and prognostic forecasting are almost certainly obsolete, being based on patient information from the era before the introduction of targeted agents and immunotherapy. We are going through a seismic change in melanoma treatment, possibly even curing some patients with metastatic disease, who were previously incurable. The survival graphs have not had enough time to incorporate these changes as yet, and the real-world situation may well not be reflected in older survival graphs.

TABLE 21.2 Five-Year Survival Rates for Stage Groups

Melanoma Stage	Five-Year Survival %
IA	99
IB	97
IIA	94
IIB	87
IIC	82
IIIA	93
IIIB	83
IIIC	69
IIID	32

From Gershenwald JE, Scolyer RA. Melanoma staging: American Joint Committee on Cancer (AJCC) 8th edition and beyond. *Ann Surg Oncol.* 2018;25:2105-2110. Correction: https://doi.org/10.1245/s10434-018-6689-x

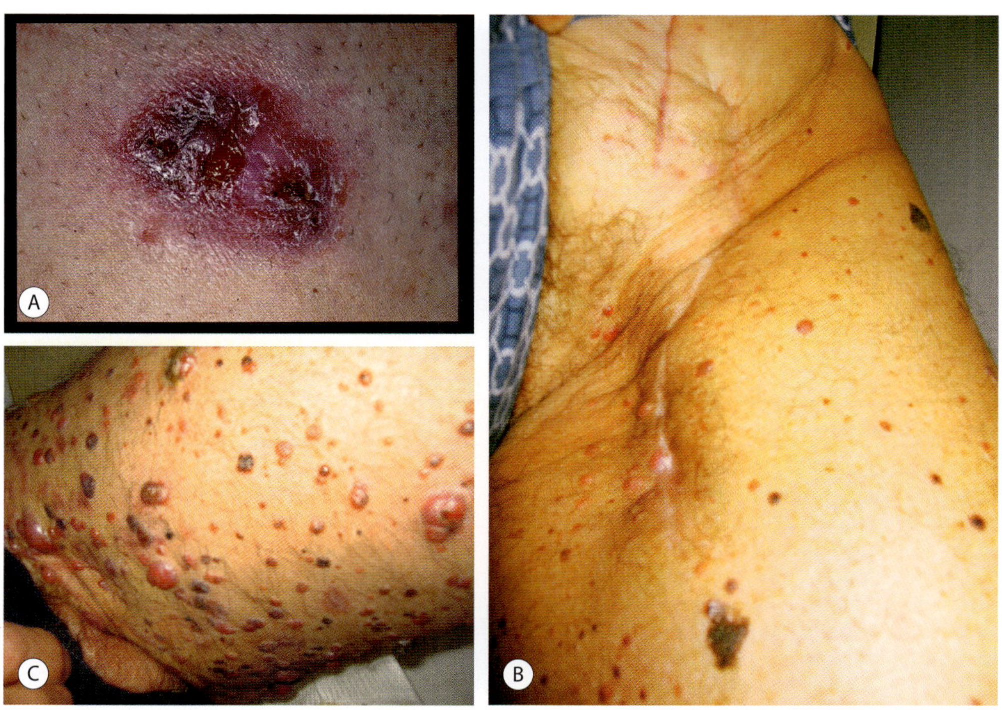

Fig. 21.24 (A) An amelanotic melanoma, which is not markedly pigmented. (B) Malignant melanoma in transit metastases. (C) The same patient 4 months later.

Melanoma TNM Classification AJCC, 8th Edition, January 2018

T Category	Criteria/Thickness	Criteria/Ulceration Status
TX	Primary tumour thickness cannot be assessed (e.g. diagnosis by curettage)	Not applicable
T0	No evidence of primary tumour (e.g. unknown primary or completely regressed melanoma)	Not applicable
Tis	Melanoma in situ	Not applicable
T1	≤1.0 mm	Unknown or unspecified
T1a	<0.8 mm	Without ulceration
T1b	<0.8 mm	With ulceration
T1b	0.8–1.0 mm	With or without ulceration
T2	>1.0–2.0 mm	Unknown or unspecified
T2a	>1.0–2.0 mm	Without ulceration
T2b	>1.0–2.0 mm	With ulceration
T3	>2.0–4.0 mm	Unknown or unspecified
T3a	>2.0–4.0 mm	Without ulceration
T3b	>2.0–4.0 mm	With ulceration
T4	>4.0 mm	Unknown or unspecified
T4a	>4.0 mm	Without ulceration
T4b	>4.0 mm	With ulceration

EXTENT OF REGIONAL LYMPH NODE AND/OR LYMPHATIC METASTASIS

N Category	Number of Tumour-Involved Regional Lymph Nodes	Presence of In-Transit, Satellite and/or Microsatellite Metastases
NX	Regional nodes not assessed (e.g. SLN biopsy not performed, regional nodes previously removed for another reason) **Exception:** Pathological N category is not required for T1 melanomas; use cN.	No
N0	No regional metastases detected	No
N1	One tumour-involved node or in-transit, satellite and/or microsatellite metastases with no tumour-involved nodes	One tumour-involved node or in-transit, satellite and/or microsatellite metastases with no tumour-involved nodes
N1a	One clinically occult (i.e. detected by SLN biopsy)	No
N1b	One clinically detected	No
N1c	No regional lymph node disease	Yes
N2	Two or three tumour-involved nodes or in-transit, satellite and/or microsatellite metastases with one tumour-involved node	Two or three tumour-involved nodes or in-transit, satellite and/or microsatellite metastases with one tumour-involved node
N2a	Two or three clinically occult (i.e. detected by SLN biopsy)	No
N2b	Two or three, at least one of which was clinically detected	No
N2c	One clinically occult or clinically detected	Yes
N3	Four or more tumour-involved nodes or in-transit, satellite and/or microsatellite metastases with two or more tumour-involved nodes, or any number of matted nodes without or with in-transit, satellite and/or microsatellite metastases	Four or more tumour-involved nodes or in-transit, satellite and/or microsatellite metastases with two or more tumour-involved nodes, or any number of matted nodes without or with in-transit, satellite and/or microsatellite metastases
N3a	Four or more clinically occult (i.e. detected by SLN biopsy)	No
N3b	Four or more, at least one of which was clinically detected, or presence of any number of matted nodes	No
N3c	Two or more clinically occult or clinically detected and/or presence of any number of matted nodes	Yes

M CRITERIA

M Category	Anatomic Site	LDH Level
cM0	No evidence of distant metastasis	Not applicable
cM1	Evidence of distant metastasis	Any
cM1a	Distant metastasis to skin, soft tissue including muscle and/or nonregional lymph node	Not recorded or unspecified
cM1a(0)	Distant metastasis to skin, soft tissue including muscle and/or nonregional lymph node	Not elevated
cM1a(1)	Distant metastasis to skin, soft tissue including muscle and/or nonregional lymph node	Elevated
cM1b	Distant metastasis to lung with or without M1a sites of disease	Not recorded or unspecified
cM1b(0)	Distant metastasis to lung with or without M1a sites of disease	Not elevated
cM1b(1)	Distant metastasis to lung with or without M1a sites of disease	Elevated
cM1c	Distant metastasis to non-CNS visceral sites with or without M1a or M1b sites of disease	Not recorded or unspecified
cM1c(0)	Distant metastasis to non-CNS visceral sites with or without M1a or M1b sites of disease	Not elevated
cM1c(1)	Distant metastasis to non-CNS visceral sites with or without M1a or M1b sites of disease	Elevated

M Category	M CRITERIA Anatomic Site	LDH Level
cM1d	Distant metastasis to CNS with or without M1a, M1b or M1c sites of disease	Not recorded or unspecified
cM1d(0)	Distant metastasis to CNS with or without M1a, M1b or M1c sites of disease	Not elevated
cM1d(1)	Distant metastasis to CNS with or without M1a, M1b or M1c sites of disease	Elevated
pM1	Evidence of distant metastasis, microscopically proven	Any
pM1a	Distant metastasis to skin, soft tissue including muscle and/or nonregional lymph node, microscopically proven	Not recorded or unspecified
pM1a(0)	Distant metastasis to skin, soft tissue including muscle and/or nonregional lymph node, microscopically proven	Not elevated
pM1a(1)	Distant metastasis to skin, soft tissue including muscle and/or nonregional lymph node, microscopically proven	Elevated
pM1b	Distant metastasis to lung with or without M1a sites of disease, microscopically proven	Not recorded or unspecified
pM1b(0)	Distant metastasis to lung with or without M1a sites of disease, microscopically proven	Not elevated
pM1b(1)	Distant metastasis to lung with or without M1a sites of disease, microscopically proven	Elevated
pM1c	Distant metastasis to non-CNS visceral sites with or without M1a or M1b sites of disease, microscopically proven	Not recorded or unspecified
pM1c(0)	Distant metastasis to non-CNS visceral sites with or without M1a or M1b sites of disease, microscopically proven	Not elevated
pM1c(1)	Distant metastasis to non-CNS visceral sites with or without M1a or M1b sites of disease, microscopically proven	Elevated
pM1d	Distant metastasis to CNS with or without M1a, M1b or M1c sites of disease, microscopically proven	Not recorded or unspecified
pM1d(0)	Distant metastasis to CNS with or without M1a, M1b or M1c sites of disease, microscopically proven	Not elevated
pM1d(1)	Distant metastasis to CNS with or without M1a, M1b or M1c sites of disease, microscopically proven	Elevated

Clinical Stage Groups

When T is...	*And N is...*	*And M is...*	*Then the stage group is...*
Tis	N0	M0	0
T1a	N0	M0	IA
T1b	N0	M0	IB
T2a	N0	M0	IB
T2b	N0	M0	IIA
T3a	N0	M0	IIA
T3b	N0	M0	IIB
T4a	N0	M0	IIB
T4b	N0	M0	IIC
Any T, Tis	≥N1	M0	III
Any T	Any N	M1	IV

Management of Melanoma

It is important to have a high level of suspicion if there is any change in a pigmented skin lesion. Change in size or shape, degree or homogeneity of pigmentation, ulceration or bleeding in a pigmented lesion should lead to referral to the local melanoma screening clinic.

A suspicious mole should be excised with a margin of 2 mm. Shaving a suspected melanoma is contraindicated because this will not allow the true Breslow thickness to be measured and results in incomplete excision. The pathology report should give details on the depth of invasion in millimetres (the Breslow thickness), ulceration and/or regression, mitotic rate, deep and peripheral margin status, presence or absence of microstellitosis, presence of pure desmoplasia and presence of lymphovascular, angiolymphatic and perineural invasion. These are all prognostic factors. If regression is present, this may obscure the dermoepidermal junction, and the given Breslow depth may be an underestimate.

If melanoma is discovered, the patient should then undergo a definitive wider local excision. If the tumour was 1 mm Breslow thickness or less, another lateral excision margin of 1 cm is taken, down to the deep fascia. Tumours greater than 1.0 mm thick are normally excised with a 2-cm lateral margin down to deep fascia.

Pathological Stage Groups

When T is...	*And N is...*	*And M is...*	*Then the stage group is...*
Tis	N0	M0	0
T1a	N0	M0	IA
T1b	N0	M0	IA
T2a	N0	M0	IB
T2b	N0	M0	IIA
T3a	N0	M0	IIA
T3b	N0	M0	IIB
T4a	N0	M0	IIB
T4b	N0	M0	IIC
T0	N1b, N1c	M0	IIIB
T0	N2b/c, N3b/c	M0	IIIC
T1a/b, T2a	N1a, N2a	M0	IIIA
T1a/b, T2a	N1b/c, N2b	M0	IIIB
T2b, T3a	N1a/b/c, N2a/b	M0	IIIB
T1a/b, T2a/b, T3a	N2c, N3a/b/c	M0	IIIC
T3b, T4a	Any N ≥ N1	M0	IIIC
T4b	N1a/b/c, N2a/b/c	M0	IIIC
T4b	N3a/b/c	M0	IIID
Any T, Tis	Any N	M1	IV

Thicker, more advanced melanomas carry a higher risk of occult positive lymph nodes. Prophylactic node dissection to identify those with occult metastases has not improved survival and is associated with a high potential complication rate, including wound infection and lymphoedema. Patients who require node dissection can be identified by the sentinel biopsy technique. Trials are still being performed on the technique of sentinel lymph node biopsy (SLNB), where the first node that drains the area of the primary tumour is identified by injecting both a blue dye and a radioactive marker close to the site of the primary tumour bed. The theory that underlies the concept of SLNB suggests that these markers are then taken up by the local lymphatics and identify the first or sentinel draining node. This node is then sampled surgically and, if tumour free, it is thought it is unlikely there is tumour in further nodes. Only one randomised trial has an endpoint of melanoma-specific survival following SLNB. In this trial, 2001 patients were randomised to either observation or SLNB after wide local excision. Both the interim and final results were negative, with a 10-year melanoma-specific survival rate of 81.4% in the sentinel node group and 78.3% in the nodal observation group ($P = .18$).

If the sentinel node is positive, active nodal basin surveillance with imaging (ultrasound or other modalities) is preferred over complete lymph node dissection (CLND). In the German DeCOG-SLT trial containing 473 patients, there was no difference in 3-year distant metastases-free survival following ultrasound-based follow-up (77%) compared with immediate lymph node dissection (74%). Similar results were seen in the larger American MSLT-II trail containing 1934 patients. The 3-year melanoma-specific survival was the same in 86% in both the observation arm and the immediate lymph node dissection group. However, in patients with a high risk of additional nodal disease, those with head and neck melanoma or those who can't comply with imaging surveillance, CLND may be considered.

Patients with clinically detected stage IIIB to IIIC melanoma or nodal disease on imaging are treated with CLND.

Adjuvant Systemic Treatment for Melanoma

Melanoma is largely resistant to standard cytotoxic chemotherapy. There is no role for adjuvant cytotoxic chemotherapy to destroy micrometastases because it used to treat patients with colorectal or breast cancer. There is, however, rapidly emerging evidence that drugs that stimulate the patient's own immune system can improve survival in patients with a high risk of recurrence after surgery. Immune checkpoints are negative regulators of the immune response. One of the immune checkpoints most successfully targeted is the PD-1 receptor found on the surface of T lymphocytes. In health, PD-1 acts to regulate excessive immune responses and this is manipulated by tumours to evade immunological action against the cancer. Antibodies that block the PD-L1/PD-1 (programmed cell-death ligand 1or 2) reduce tumour downregulation of the antitumour immune response and increase the cytotoxic response of antitumour-specific T cells. The most common anti–PD-1 drugs in current clinical use are pembrolizumab and nivolumab. A more toxic antibody is ipilimumab, which is a human monoclonal antibody against cytotoxic T-cell–associated protein (CTLA-4).

To date, there have been several trials of immunotherapy as adjuvant treatment showing a survival advantage with this treatment. In the European Organisation for Research and Treatment of Cancer (EORTC) 1325 trial, pembrolizumab was compared with a placebo in patients with fully resected stage III disease. The 1-year recurrence-free survival was 74.5% in the pembrolizumab group compared with 61% in those receiving a placebo. In the CheckMate 238 study, patients with completely resected stage IIIb/IIIc or stage 1V disease were randomised to receive either ipilimumab or nivolumab. The 12-month recurrence-free survival was 70.5% in the nivolumab group compared with 60.8% in the ipilimumab group. Toxicity was considerably greater in the ipilimumab group. Little data at present indicate the superiority of pembrolizumab over nivolumab as adjuvant treatment. In the United Kingdom, nivolumab and pembrolizumab are approved adjuvant treatments for completely resected stage III melanoma.

Another approach to adjuvant therapy is to take advantage of a mutation in the BRAF oncogene that can be therapeutically exploited. Between 40% and 50% of melanomas have a mutation in the BRAF oncogene. This encodes a protein (activated threonine kinase) which is important for melanoma cell proliferation. Combining a BRAF pathway inhibitor (dabrafenib) with an inhibitor (trametinib) of another growth pathway, Mek, in patients with completely resected stage III melanoma exhibiting either a BRAF V600 E or 600 K mutation produced superior 3-year relapse-free survival compared with a placebo in the COMBI-ADD trial. The 5-year relapse-free survival was 52% in the combination arm compared with 36% in the placebo group ($P = .001$). In the United Kingdom, dabrafenib with trametinib is an option for adjuvant treatment for resected stage III BRAF V600 mutation-positive melanoma.

Adjuvant Radiotherapy for Melanoma

In patients with resected stage III melanoma, only one randomised prospective phase III trial (ANZMTG 01.2/TROG 02.01) reported less nodal relapse (21% versus 36%, $P = .023$), with no improvement in overall or relapse-free survival with adjuvant RT compared with observation alone. Also, patients on observation who developed isolated lymph node relapse (24%) treated with surgery or RT had similar outcomes as that of the adjuvant RT group. There were significantly higher rates of lower limb oedema in the RT group (15% versus 7.7%, $P = .014$). Although RT does reduce local recurrence, this effect may be dwarfed by the increase in survival seen in adjuvant immunotherapy trials. Therefore adjuvant RT is not offered routinely for patients with resected stage III melanoma. It may be considered in carefully selected groups of patients when the reduction in the risk of local recurrence outweighs the risk of side effects. The commonly used dose fractionation is 48 Gy in 20 fractions over 4 weeks.

In patients with desmoplastic melanoma who had a resection margin of less than 8 mm, adjuvant RT (48 Gy in 20 fractions) improves local control (17% local recurrence with RT compared with 24% without RT at 5 years).

Management of Unresectable, Metastatic and Recurrent Melanoma

In-transit metastases may present in a limb (Figs. 21.24B and C). These represent the disease in cutaneous lymphatics between the primary site and local draining nodes. They can erupt and involve widespread areas of skin as small erythematous or pigmented macules and nodules. In-transit metastases can be very problematic and distressing to the patient, especially if they break down or coalesce into larger masses. Patients who develop this condition can be referred to one of a few specialised units around the United Kingdom which offer isolated limb perfusion (ILP), a technique in which the circulation in a limb is isolated and chemotherapy is given to the limb alone, without significant amounts of drug entering the general circulation. This technique can give considerable palliative benefit and, in some patients, a complete response may be achieved with all the nodules and papules disappearing. If in-transit metastasis affects the skin of the trunk, the area cannot be isolated and systemic chemotherapy is required.

Patients may develop blood-borne metastasis, most commonly in the liver, lungs, brain or bone. Systemic therapies using immunotherapy and biologically targeted agents are the standard of care for unresectable stage III and untreated stage IV disease. The checkpoint inhibitor immunotherapy drugs used in melanoma are antiprogrammed cell death protein 1 (PD-1) antibodies (e.g. nivolumab and pembrolizumab) and the anticytotoxic T-lymphocyte–associated antigen (CTLA) 4 antibody ipilimumab. Ipilimumab blocks CTLA4, present on cytotoxic T lymphocytes, and results in an active immune response to melanoma cells. Vemurafenib is a B-raf enzyme inhibitor which can cause cell death in melanomas which show a V600E B-raf mutation. This mutation is characterised by glutamic acid replacing valine at position 600 on the B-raf protein. Vemurafenib is only effective in melanomas with this mutation. Other drugs with similar mechanisms of action are also being developed.

Immunotherapy offers the possibility of increased survival in patients with metastatic disease, especially those without BRAF mutations. Ipilimumab was the first systemic treatment to show prolonged survival in patients with metastatic disease entered into randomised clinical trials. A pooled analysis of 12 studies of patients with advanced melanoma showed a 3-year survival of 26% and a survival up to 10 years in about 20% of all patients. Ipilimumab was associated with considerable toxicity. Skin rashes were seen in 47% to 68% of patients. The most important toxicities were colitis, leading to diarrhoea, with a grade 3/4 incidence in 8% to 23%, and hepatitis, with a grade 3/4 incidence in 3% to 7% of patients. The checkpoint inhibitors, nivolumab and pembrolizumab, have shown superior overall survival and progression-free survival with less toxicity than ipilimumab. In the KEYNOTE-006 trial, the overall survival at 33 months was 50% in the pembrolizumab group compared with 39% in the ipilimumab group.

Combining ipilimumab with an anti–PD-1 drug is clinically advantageous. In the CheckMate 067 trial, the median OS was 72.1 months with ipilimumab and nivolumab combination compared with 36.9 months with nivolumab alone and 19.9 months with ipilimumab alone. In the United Kingdom, for patients suitable for immunotherapy, nivolumab in combination with ipilimumab is the treatment of choice, and if the combination is unsuitable or unacceptable, single-agent pembrolizumab or nivolumab is offered. If immunotherapy is unsuitable or contraindicated, alternatives for patients with BRAF V600 mutated melanoma are either a combination of trametinib with dabrafenib or encorafenib with binimetinib.

Immunotherapy can affect almost all visceral organs, causing the common muscle aches and pains of myositis, immune-based hepatitis, colitis, carditis, pneumonitis and several forms of endocrinopathy, including, commonly, hypothyroidism and the rare but potentially fatal sudden-onset type 1 diabetes or pituitary failure. The side effects, especially immune hepatitis and endocrinopathies, can develop several weeks after starting treatment and, in some cases, even after immunotherapy has been discontinued. Careful recurrent assessment of patients on immunotherapy is therefore essential.

Any evidence of further local, regional or metastatic melanoma requires that the patient be restaged to define the extent of the recurrence. If there is only local recurrence at the primary site, further surgery should be considered. This may be appropriate even if another locoregional or metastatic disease is present to achieve local control. If regional lymph nodes are involved, a nodal block dissection may be indicated, depending on the extent and fixity of the nodal disease, the extent of other diseases and patient factors such as performance status, frailty, comorbidities present and the potential functional loss and changes in quality of life (both positive and negative) that extensive surgery may bring. In selected cases, adjuvant RT may improve local control after surgery.

Role of Radiotherapy in Recurrent, Inoperable and Metastatic Melanoma

RT is useful for brain, bone and cutaneous metastases. Malignant melanoma is often said to be 'radioresistant', and it is true that melanoma cells can sustain more sublethal damage than other cancer cell lines. However, this may be countered by using regimens using a higher dose per fraction and treating less frequently, for example, 3 times per week rather than 5 times per week. Cutaneous metastasis can be treated by relatively small electron fields, restricting both the field size on the skin and the depth treated.

Standard palliative doses bring about pain relief in at least one-third of those with bone metastases using, for example, 20 Gy in 4 fractions, or a single 8-Gy fraction. *Stereotactic radiosurgery (SRS)*, in which brain metastases are treated individually with a very narrow margin, can bring about useful shrinkage in brain metastases, and more and more patients are being treated with this modality instead of with whole brain RT (WBRT). With the latter dose, fractionation is usually 30 Gy in 10 fractions or 6 fractions treated on alternate days using 6-MV beam energy, but with SRS, single doses of up to 21 Gy can be given to individual brain metastases, depending on volume in cubic centimetres (cc) and the number of metastases to be treated. If more than three metastases are to be treated, fractionated schedules using 21 Gy in 3 fractions or 25 Gy in 5 fractions are used again; depending on the number and volume in cc of the metastases to be treated, there are also studies ongoing of using SRS with WBRT and with immunotherapy, based on the theory that SRS should cause melanoma cell breakdown, exposing more antigen for an enhanced immune response.

CUTANEOUS LYMPHOMAS

Primary cutaneous lymphomas are uncommon tumours. The majority are T-cell lymphomas, with less than 25% being B-cell. They are more common in males. Their aetiology is unknown, but a viral association has been suggested.

Within the primary cutaneous T-cell lymphomas, mycosis fungoides are the most common type and are usually present in males over 60 years of age. There is a range of clinical presentations varying from erythematous cutaneous patches, which may show very slow progression, to thickened plaques or nodular tumours over several years (Fig. 21.25).

The development of lymphadenopathy or visceral organ involvement worsens prognosis markedly and the development of large abnormal circulating T cells, the so-called Sézary cells, in the peripheral blood in association with lymphadenopathy and erythroderma is diagnostic of Sézary syndrome. Patients with this condition are also at greater risk of developing other SCCs of the skin and internal malignancies, especially lung cancer.

There is a wide range of treatments for cutaneous T-cell lymphomas. Topical chemotherapy with nitrogen mustard, carmustine or PUVA all have high response rates for early disease. For thicker plaques, total skin electron therapy is effective (Figs. 21.26A–E). Systemic chemotherapy is indicated for more advanced disease. There are studies in progress evaluating immunotherapy with interferon or interleukin, monoclonal antibody therapy, photopheresis and new combination chemotherapy regimens.

Primary cutaneous B-cell lymphomas are rare and include a wide variety of subtypes, including primary cutaneous follicular centre cell lymphoma and marginal zone B-cell lymphoma. In general, these lymphomas have a more indolent course. They are more likely to be

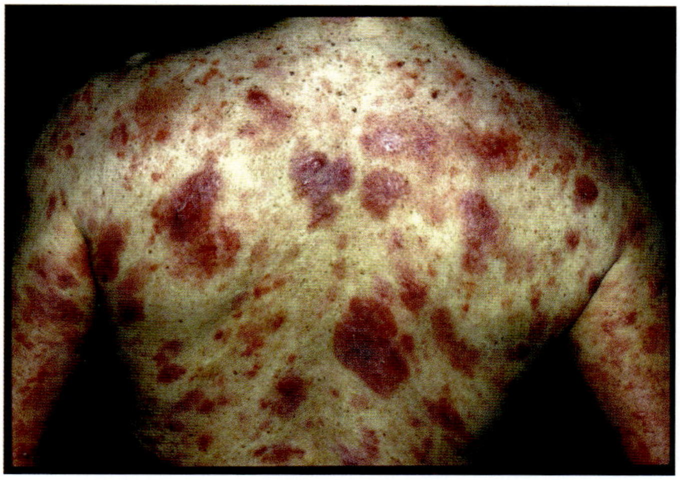

Fig. 21.25 Mycosis fungoides, with patches, plaques and nodules.

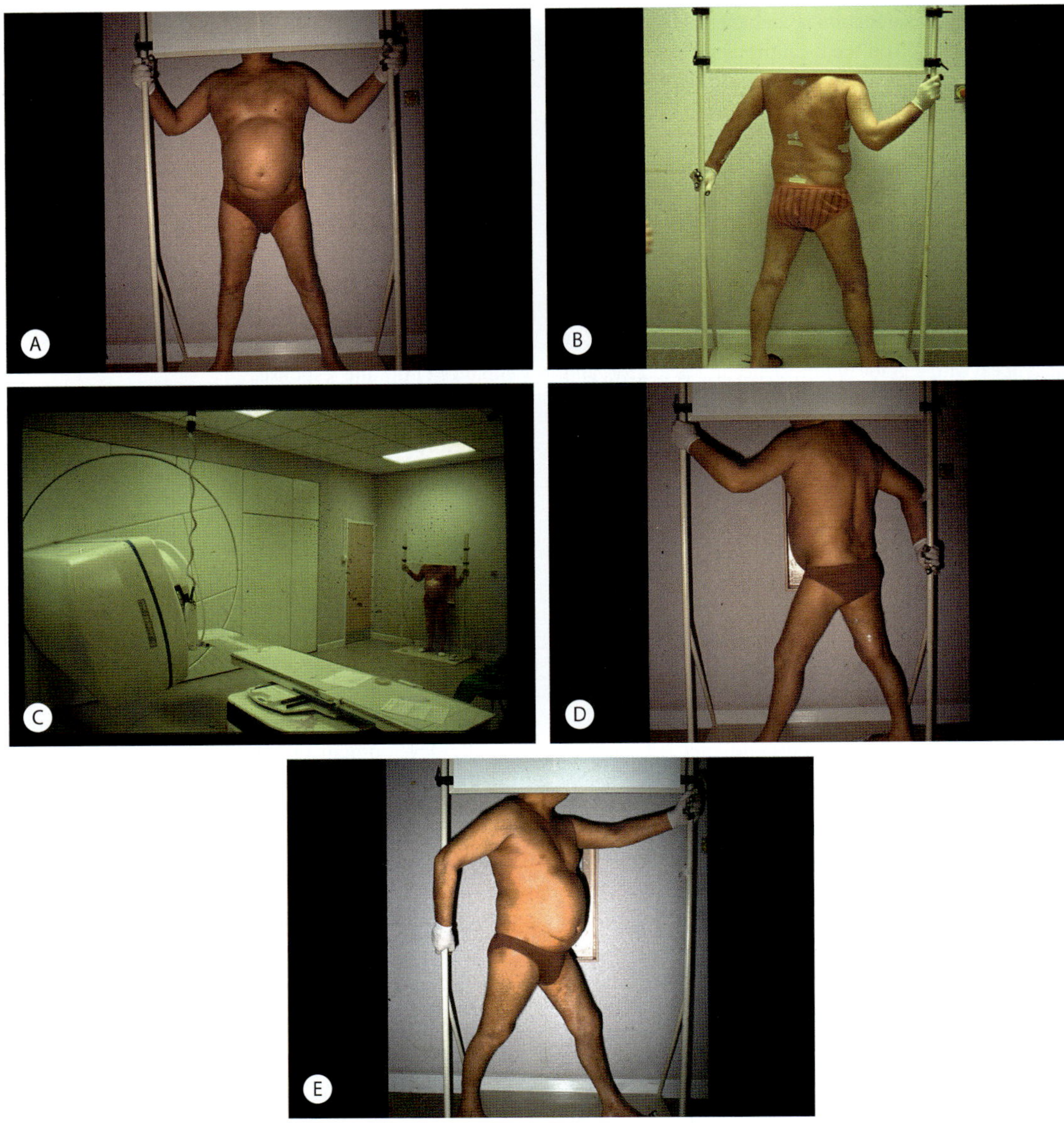

Fig. 21.26 (A–E) Total skin electrons being used to treat cutaneous lymphoma.

managed by local RT presenting as a solitary mass or systemic chemotherapy if they have spread. Secondary cutaneous lymphomas may also affect the skin.

MERKEL CELL TUMOURS

These tumours represent neuroendocrine carcinoma of the skin. They tend to affect the elderly, often presenting as a painless nodule in the head and neck or on a limb. They may respond well to initial treatment but go on to recur locally or to develop metastatic spread. They are treated with wide local excision where possible, with postoperative RT (50 Gy in 20–25 fractions), or RT alone (60 Gy in 30 fractions), if inoperable. Chemotherapy is used for advanced local or recurrent disease, using agents similar to those used in small cell lung cancer, such as carboplatin and etoposide combination. Initially, tumours may respond to chemotherapy but almost inevitably recur. The main differential diagnosis of MCT is small cell carcinoma, which has metastasised to the skin. Cytokeratin 20 is useful in differentiating between these two possibilities histologically. The JAVELIN MERKEL 200 study reported a 40% response rate and a median OS of 20.3 months with Avelumab, an anti–PD-L1 monoclonal antibody, in patients with treatment-naïve metastatic MCT.

SKIN SARCOMA

Primary sarcomas of the structures of the skin or subcutaneous tissues are uncommon but may present as a diagnostic problem. They often have no defining clinical characteristics and most often present as a skin or subcutaneous nodule. These tumours can arise from a range of connective tissue cell precursors, including vascular nerve and muscle tissues with a wide range of pathological types and subtypes, often not easy to diagnose even with adequate histological material.

The most important pathological diagnosis is to decide if the tumour is benign or malignant, with the potential to recur or metastasise. If the tumour is benign and has been excised completely, no further intervention is required.

True malignant sarcomas affecting the skin, for example, angiosarcoma, can carry a poor prognosis. These vascular malignancies (Fig. 21.27A) present with an erythematous or vascular nodule, which can then ulcerate or go on to form several other nodules. They can metastasise early, and wide surgical excision is the treatment of choice. They are also associated with developing in areas of postmastectomy lymphoedema, either in the chest wall or arm, often a decade after initial surgery. This phenomenon is known as Stewart-Treves syndrome.

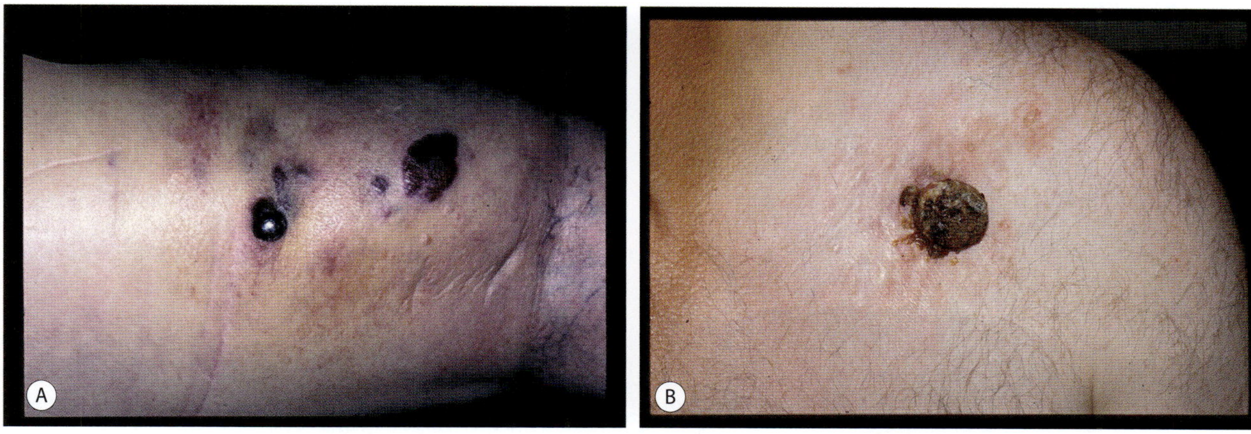

Fig. 21.27 (A) Angiosarcoma. (B) Dermatofibrosarcoma protuberans.

Other malignant variants of sarcoma which can develop from skin structures include malignant fibrous histiocytoma, malignant peripheral nerve sheath tumours and clear cell sarcoma, which is a malignancy derived from melanocytes. These are all uncommon and initial treatment for all is wide surgical excision.

As well as the skin sarcomas with true metastatic potential, there are also connective tissue tumours that can affect the skin, showing local invasion and having the potential for local recurrence if inadequately excised. Metastases are very rare. The most common example in this group would be dermatofibrosarcoma protuberans (see Fig. 21.27B). These tumours can be difficult to diagnose pathologically, especially in their early stages, when histologically they may appear to be benign. They have a long natural history, with local recurrences stretching over years. The can dedifferentiate and become more aggressive clinically and more malignant histologically. If this occurs, there is a greater risk of metastasis.

KAPOSI SARCOMA

This is a particular form of vascular sarcoma which is derived from endothelial cells. It has become much more prevalent with the increased incidence of acquired immune deficiency syndrome (AIDS). KS has several variants including classical KS and epidemic KS, both associated with human herpes virus type 8. There are also types associated with immunosuppressive treatment and African KS.

Before the AIDS epidemic, classical KS was a rare disease, affecting elderly males, usually of Italian or East European Jewish descent, who developed the pigmented patches and nodules around the lower leg or ankle (Figs. 21.28A–C). These tumours develop slowly, but patients are at risk of developing a second malignancy, often non-Hodgkin lymphoma. Most patients are treated with relatively low doses of RT, such as 8 Gy in 1 fraction, which may be repeated.

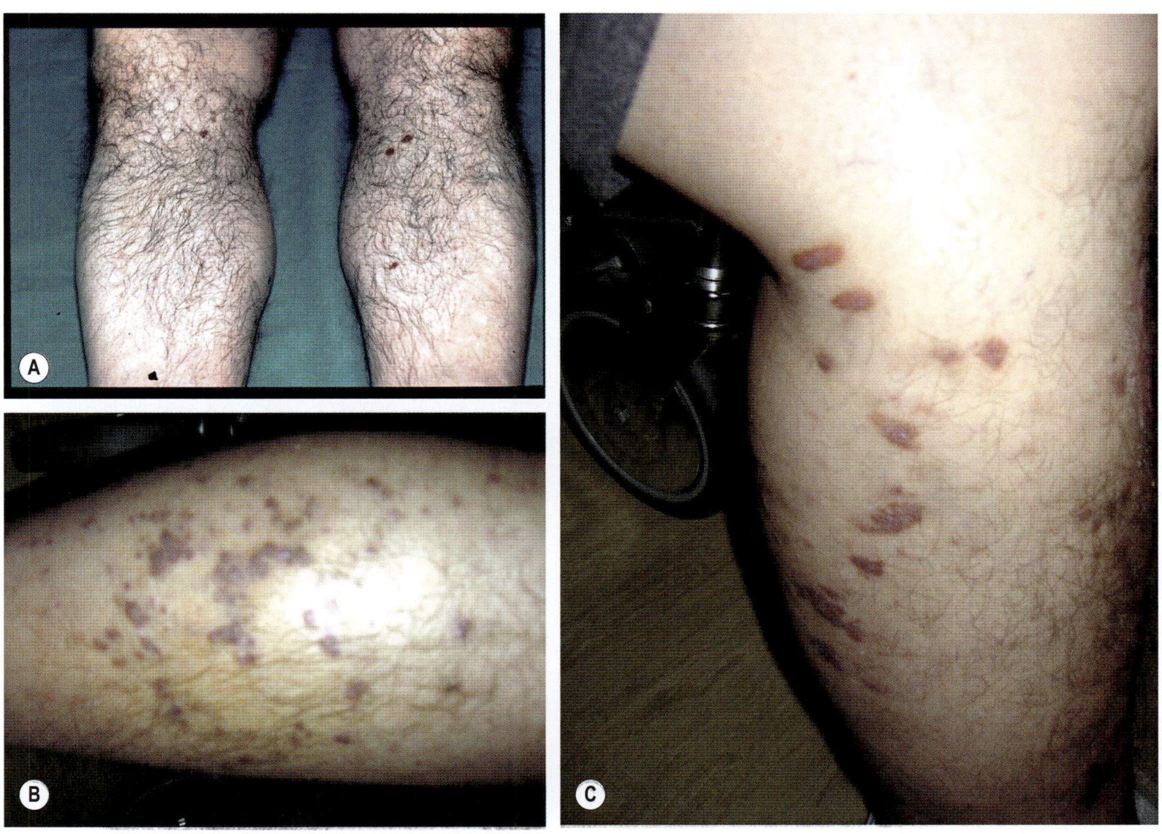

Fig. 21.28 (A–C) Kaposi sarcoma.

Epidemic KS develops in approximately 20% to 25% of patients with AIDS, although there was a much higher incidence in AIDS patients when the epidemic first started. Since the introduction of highly active antiretroviral treatment (HAART), the incidence of age-related KS has been reduced. Patients with this variant are more likely to develop disseminated disease. Chemotherapy is used to treat KS using agents such as liposomal doxorubicin or a taxane. These tumours can be exquisitely sensitive to RT: great care must be taken in treating sites such as the oral mucosa or considerable morbidity can be caused. There have been a variety of dose schedules used, all giving relatively low total doses for the management of this condition, such as 6 Gy in 1 fraction, using a low-energy electron beam, for a single or a few cutaneous lesions, or 12 Gy in 3 fractions. There is a suggestion that using slightly higher fractionated doses, such as 20 to 30 Gy in 10 to 15 fractions, may produce a longer-lasting response for individual lesions.

SKIN APPENDAGE TUMOURS

These are also known as *adnexal tumours*. They arise from skin structures including the hair follicle, sebaceous glands or sweat glands. There is a wide range of benign skin appendage tumours which occasionally undergo malignant transformation. They most often appear as smooth nondistinctive masses which are diagnosed not by their clinical appearance but on biopsy histopathology. There are multiple pathological subtypes (Figs. 21.29A and B).

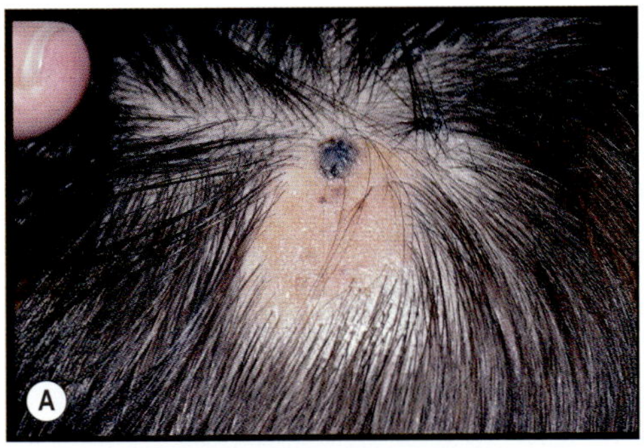

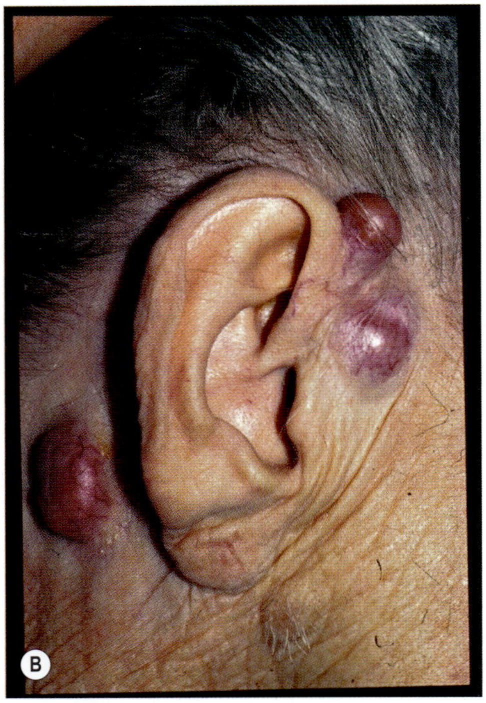

Fig. 21.29 Skin appendage tumours. (A) A sebaceous naevus with an associated basal cell carcinoma. (B) A multiple cylindroma, with a typically noncharacteristic appearance.

Sebaceous carcinoma is an example of an uncommon potentially metastatic skin appendage tumour. These classically occur on the eyelid, diagnosed on biopsy. Surgery is the treatment of choice. Sweat gland carcinoma gives a similar indistinct clinical picture. These tumours usually present as an odd-looking BCC or SCC, with the diagnosis again not being made until excision biopsy has been done. Surgery is again the treatment of choice.

Paget disease of the breast or nipple is a malignant condition in or around the skin of the nipple. It can also occur outside the breast, when it is known as extramammary Paget disease, with the most common extramammary site being the vulva. This condition is thought to arise from epithelial cells in an apocrine duct and looks like eczema. It can give rise to pruritus and ulceration and may spread to local regional nodes and even metastasise systemically.

FURTHER READING

Chang AS, Tran DC, Cannon JGD, et al. Pembrolizumab for advanced basal cell carcinoma: an investigator initiated, proof-of-concept study. *Jam Acad Dermatol*. 2019;80(2):565–566.

Chapman PB, Hauschild A, Robert C. Improved survival with vemurafenib in melanoma with BRAF V600E mutation. *N Engl J Med*. 2011;364:2507–2516.

Drucker AA, Adam GP, Rofeberg V, et al. Treatments of primary basal cell carcinoma of skin; a systematic review and network meta-analysis. *Ann Intern Med*. 2018;169:456–466.

Dummer R, Hauschild A, Santinami M, et al. Five-year analysis of adjuvant dabrafenib plus trametinib in stage III melanoma. *N Engl J Med*. 2020;383(12):1139–1148 17.

Eggermont A, Blank C, Mandala M, et al. Adjuvant pembrolizumab versus placebo in resected stage 111 melanoma. *N Engl J Med*. 2018; 378:1789–1801.

Fogarty GB, Hong A, Economides A, Guitera P. Experience in treating lentigo maligna with definitive radiotherapy. *Derm Res Pract*. 2018;2018:7439807.

Frampton JE, Basset-Seguin N. Vismodegib: a review in advanced basal cell carcinoma. *Drugs*. 2018;78:1145–1156.

Gauci ML, Aristei C, Becker JC, et al. Diagnosis and treatment of Merkel cell carcinoma: European consensus-based interdisciplinary guideline—update 2022. *Eur J Cancer*. 2022;171:203–231.

Gershenwald JE, Scolyer RA. Melanoma staging: American Joint Committee on Cancer (AJCC) 8th edition and beyond. *Ann Surg Oncol*. 2018;25:2105–2110.

Gershenwald JE, Scolyer RA, Hess KR, et al. Melanoma staging: evidence-based changes in the American Joint Committee on Cancer eighth edition cancer staging manual. *CA Cancer J Clin*. 2017;67(6):472–492.

Henderson MA, Burmeister BH, Ainslie J, et al. Adjuvant lymph-node field radiotherapy versus observation only in patients with melanoma at high risk of further lymph-node field relapse after lymphadenectomy (ANZMTG 01.02/TROG 02.01): 6-year follow-up of a phase 3, randomised controlled trial. *Lancet Oncol*. 2015;16(9):1049–1060.

Hennequin C, Rio E, Quéro L, Clavère P. Radiation therapy of cutaneous cancers. *Cancer Radiother*. 2022;26(1–2):397–403.

Hersh E, Weber J, Powderly J, et al. Long-term survival of patients (pts) with advanced melanoma treated with ipilimumab with or without dacarbazine. *J Clin Oncol*. 2009;27:9038.

Kamath P Darwin E, Arora H, Nouri K. A review on imiquimod therapy and discussion on optimal management of basal cell carcinomas. *Clin Drug Invest*. 2018;38(10):883–899.

Kaufman HL Russell JS, Hamid O, et al. Updated efficacy of avelumab in patients with previously treated metastatic Merkel cell carcinoma after 1 year of follow-up: JAVELIN Merkel 200, a phase 2 clinical trial. *J Immunother Cancer*. 2018;6(1): 7–14.

Long GV, Hauschild A, Santinami M, et al. Adjuvant dabrafenib plus trametinib in stage 111 BRAF-mutated melanoma. *N Engl J Med*. 2017;377:1813–1823.

Morton DL, Thompson JF, Cochran AJ, et al. MSLT group sentinel node biopsy or observation in melanoma. *N Engl J Med*. 2014;370(19): 1307–1817.

Robert C, Schacter J, Long G, et al. KEYNOTE-006 investigators. Pembrolizumab versus ipilimumab in advanced melanoma. *N Engl J Med*. 2015;372(26):2521–2532.

Shadendorf D, Hodi FS, Robert C, et al. Pooled analysis of long-term survival data from phase II and phase III trials of ipilimumab in unresectable or metastatic melanoma. *J Clin Oncol*. 2015;33(17): 1889–1894.

Stelzer KJ, Griffin TW. A randomised prospective trial of radiation therapy for AIDS-associated Kaposi's sarcoma. *Int J Radiat Oncol Biol Phys*. 1993;27:1057–1061.

UK NICE Guideline. Melanoma. https://www.nice.org.uk/guidance/ng14/update/ng14-update-1/documents/draft-guideline-4

Veness MJ, Delishaj D, Barnes EA, Bezugly A, Rembielak A. Current role of radiotherapy in non-melanoma skin cancer. *Clin Oncol (R Coll Radiol)*. 2019;31(11):749–758.

Weber J, Mandala M, Del Vecchio M, et al. Adjuvant nivolamab versus ipilimumab in resected stage III or IV melanoma. *N Engl J Med*. 2017;377(19):1824–1835.

Wolchok JD, Chiarion-Silini V, Gonzalez R, et al. Overall survival with combined nivolumab and ipilimumab in advanced melanoma. *N Engl J Med*. 2017;377:1345–1356.

Wolchok JD, Chiarion-Sileni V, Gonzalez R, et al. Long-term outcomes with nivolumab plus ipilimumab or nivolumab alone versus ipilimumab in patients with advanced melanoma. *J Clin Oncol*. 2022;40(2):127–137 10.

22

Head and Neck Cancer—General Principles

Christopher D. Scrase

CHAPTER OUTLINE

INTRODUCTION

Head and neck cancer is a rather inaccurate term for describing cancers of the upper aerodigestive tract, because tumours of the facial skin and the brain are not conventionally included. They are a diverse group comprising oral cancers; cancers of the oropharynx, larynx, nasopharynx and hypopharynx; and cancers of the paranasal sinuses, salivary glands and ear (Fig. 22.1). Worldwide, there are more than 500,000 cases per year. In England and Wales, the overall incidence is approximately 11 cases per 100,000 per year, although there are regional variations, giving rise to about 12,000 new cases per year. The incidence is increasing at present (see the 'Aetiology' section). Although the treatment for these areas is often highly specialised, the areas also have many features in common with regards to investigation, diagnosis and management. Perhaps more than any other anatomical site, the concept of a multidisciplinary team is paramount in head and neck cancer, and it is essential that the team members are involved as early as possible to provide the best outcome in terms of tumour control, maintaining function and acceptable cosmesis. Radiotherapy (RT) and chemotherapy are now widely used, either as primary therapy or as postoperative treatments.

DEMOGRAPHICS

Head and neck cancers make up 3% to 4% of all new cancers in the United Kingdom and are thus the eighth most-seen cancer. Overall, 70% of all head and neck cancers in the United Kingdom occur in males and 30% occur in females. Between 1993 and 1995 and 2017 and 2019, age-standardised incidence rates of head and neck cancer increased by 35%, with a larger increase in females than in males. The majority of head and neck cancers present beyond the fifth decade, reflecting cell DNA damage accumulating over time, with an average age of onset of 60 years. Cancers of the head and neck are more commonly found in people from the lower social classes, and this is multifactorial, with higher incidences of smoking and alcoholism, late presentation, poor oral hygiene, inadequate diet and so on. These cancers are linked to delayed diagnosis and worse outcome.

AETIOLOGY

Of head and neck cancers in the United Kingdom, 46% to 88% are preventable. The most important risk factor in the development of head and neck cancers is tobacco. Smoking or chewing tobacco is associated with 85% to 90% of head and neck malignancies. Alcohol intake has also been shown to cause an increase in this group of cancers. There is also a synergistic effect of combining alcohol and tobacco with regards to developing cancers in this site. There is a clear increase in the incidence of second malignancy of the head and neck and other sites (lung, oesophagus) in persistent smokers.

Other risk factors in head and neck cancers have been suggested, including poor oral hygiene, dental disease and trauma from badly fitted dentures, although direct causation has not been demonstrated. Viral infections have

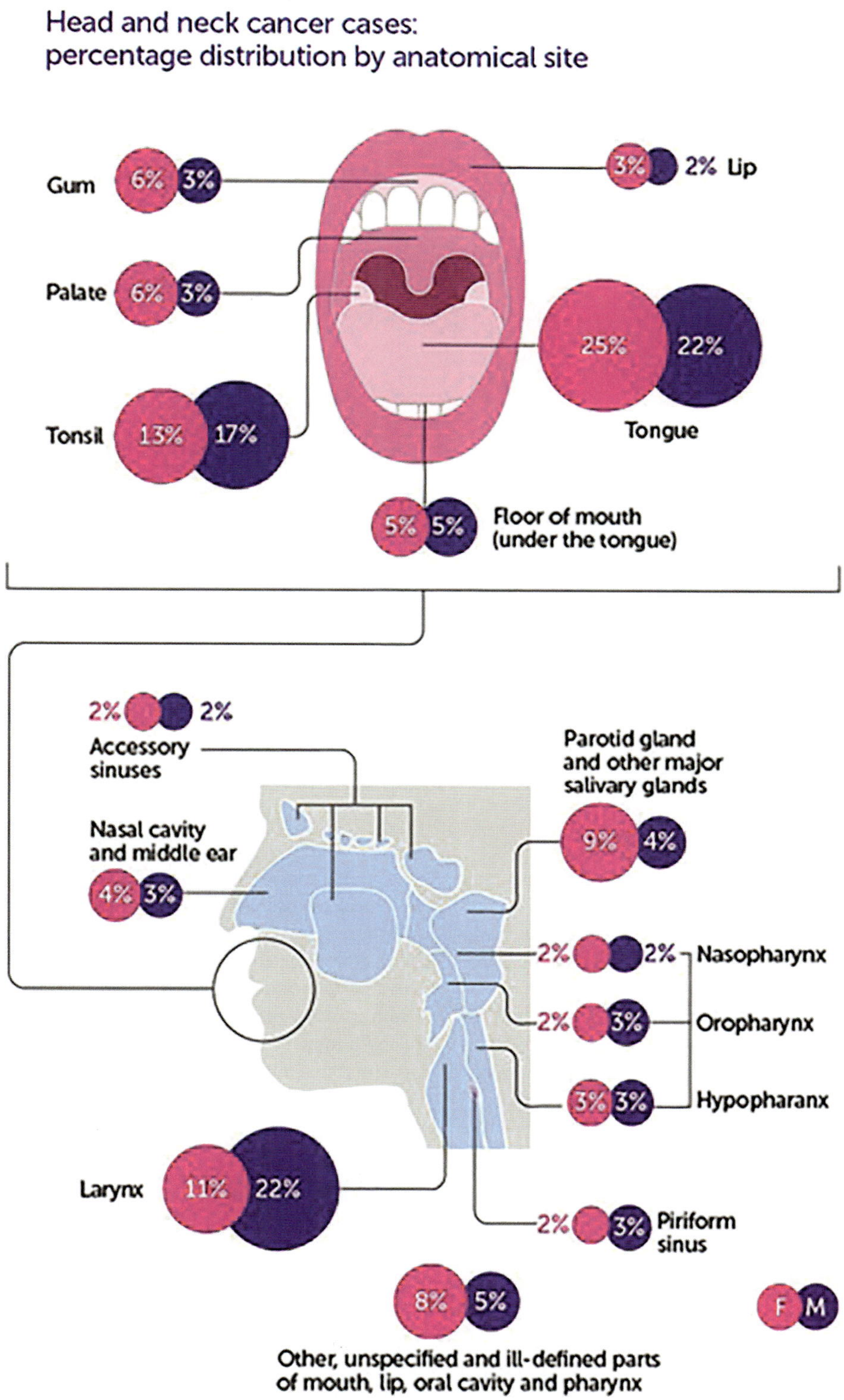

Fig. 22.1 Head and neck cancer (C00–C14, C30–C12) 2016 to 2018. Distribution of cases diagnosed by anatomical site, United Kingdom. (From Cancer Research UK, 2026, Head and neck cancers risk, Cancer Research UK.)

also been investigated for a role in the aetiology of head and neck cancers. There is a very strong association with Epstein–Barr virus infection and nasopharyngeal cancer. There is an increasing incidence of human papilloma virus (HPV)-associated oropharyngeal tumours worldwide. Such tumours develop in younger patients and have an inherently better prognosis. Immunosuppression is known to be a risk factor for malignancy, and this includes cancers of the head and neck. Syphilis is a recognised risk factor too, and it is of significance given the resurgence of cases.

Premalignant conditions also exist, which predispose for the development of head and neck cancers. These are most commonly seen in

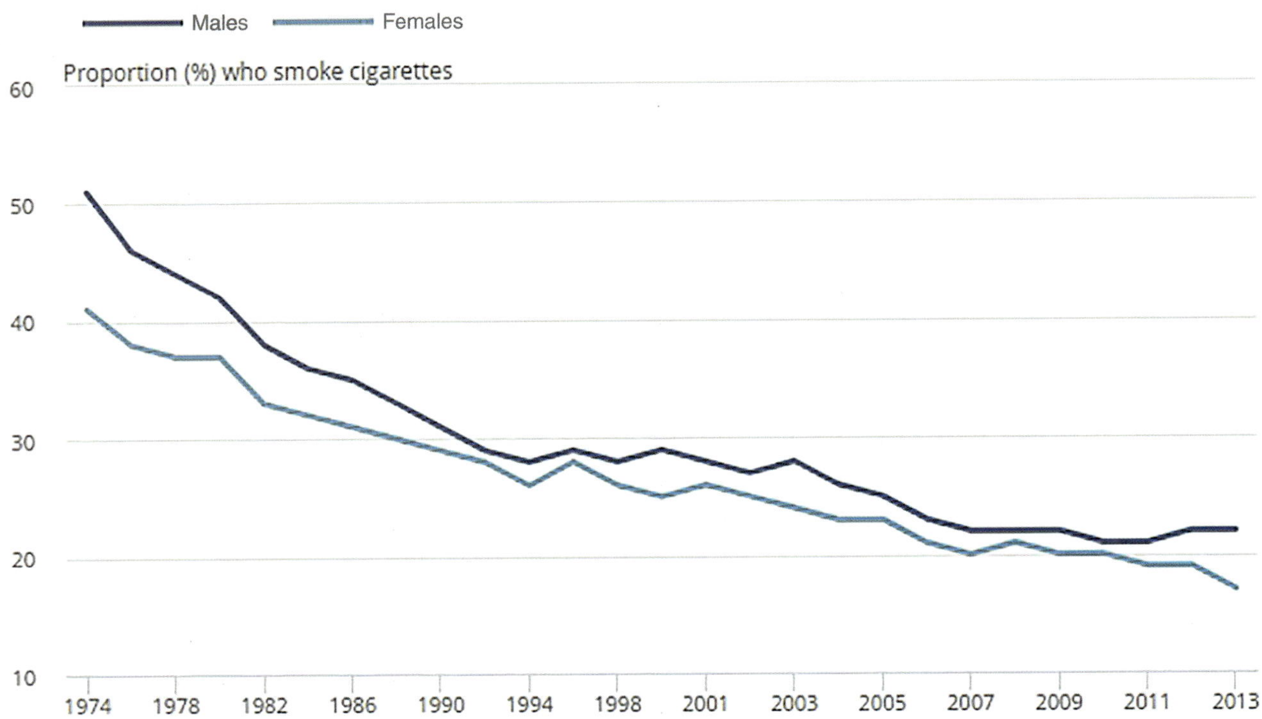

Fig. 22.2 Cigarette smoking prevalence: 1974 to 2013. Proportion of population who smoke cigarettes, by gender, Great Britain. (Data for 2012 onwards: Office for National Statistics. Opinions and lifestyle survey. https://www.ons.gov.uk/peoplepopulationandcommunity/healthandsocialcare/healthandlifeexpectancies/compendium/opinionsandlifestylesurvey/2015-03-19)

the oral cavity and include leucoplakia (white patches), which carries an approximately 5% risk of progressing to invasive malignancy, and, more sinisterly, erythroplakia. Regular specialist follow-up is therefore essential. Lichen planus with dysplastic features can also become malignant and requires monitoring.

Radiation exposure is also a risk factor for developing head and neck cancers. A previous history of RT treatment should be sought in newly diagnosed patients. Radiation exposure will also have an impact on any future RT treatment options.

PREVENTION AND EARLY DIAGNOSIS

When diagnosed early, head and neck cancer has quite a good chance for cure, but at present there is no established screening program. It has been shown that targeted education in the primary sector with general practitioners and dentists has had some impact on early referral for oral cancers. This is important, as patients presenting with advanced disease have a poorer prognosis.

Tobacco cessation is also an important factor in preventing head and neck cancers. The prevalence of cigarette smoking has fallen in Great Britain by nearly 50% in males and females over the past 40 years. The gender gap in cigarette smoking prevalence has also narrowed in recent years (Fig. 22.2). Aggressive treatment of premalignant conditions is important in reducing the incidence of invasive cancer. One can envisage, in perhaps a generation's time, a positive impact on HPV-related cancers in nonsmokers subsequent to the HPV vaccination program.

TUMOUR TYPES

The majority (>90%) of cancers of the head and neck are squamous cell carcinomas (SCCs) arising from mucosal cells. They are usually graded into well, moderately or poorly differentiated on the basis of their histological assessment (mitoses, pleomorphism). Poorly differentiated tumours tend to metastasise to lymph nodes more frequently than well-differentiated lesions. The remainder are made up of small numbers of adenocarcinoma, lymphoma (these are treated by a different team in most institutions), sarcoma, melanoma and various salivary gland tumours (mucoepidermoid, adenoid cystic, acinic tumours). It is essential that a histological diagnosis is confirmed before treatment to ensure correct management and that a specialist head and neck pathologist is part of the multidisciplinary team.

PRESENTATION

The majority of cases of head and neck cancer present symptomatically. The symptoms therefore depend on the primary site and the adjacent structures that may be involved. This may be a visible lesion in the oral cavity—leucoplakia, erythroplakia or nonhealing ulcer—or may relate to a swelling or mass in the oropharynx, hypopharynx or larynx. There may be hoarseness, difficulty swallowing, discomfort or pain on eating, referred aural pain, trismus or cranial nerve palsies. The onset of these symptoms is an indication for urgent referral to a head and neck department. More nonspecific symptoms of weight loss, anorexia or generalised discomfort can also be seen in this group of patients.

A common presentation of head and neck cancer is with lymph node metastases in the neck. The histology may be confirmed by fine needle aspiration (FNA) or biopsy. A thorough search for a potential primary tumour is required, aided in recent years with functional imaging (fluorodeoxyglucose-positron emission tomography–computed tomography (FDG PET/CT)). Two metaanalyses have indicated sensitivities of 88.3% to 97% and specificities of 68% to 74.9% in detecting unknown primaries.

INVESTIGATION

Patients presenting with possible head and neck cancer should be referred urgently to a specialist head and neck oncology team. The workup requires confirmation of the histological diagnosis and full examination of the aerodigestive tract for accurate staging and to exclude second primary lesions. Cross-sectional imaging with CT or magnetic resonance imaging (MRI) with contrast enhancement is also essential for staging purposes detailing the anatomical extent of the primary lesion and any nodal involvement. CT provides more limited soft-tissue resolution than MRI and often the two modalities are complementary. Imaging of the chest with chest x-ray or CT is required to exclude pulmonary metastases, especially in those patients with more advanced local disease or a synchronous lung primary. There may be a synchronous primary in 2% to 5% of head and neck cancer patients and these are often tobacco related. The incidence of distant metastases is reported to be between 5% and 30% and the majority is in the lung, although very occasionally bone or liver secondaries are found. The occurrence of metastases correlates with the increasing stage of the primary tumour and the number, size and bilaterality of lymph node involvement at presentation. PET using 18 FDG combined with CT for anatomical data is invaluable now in assisting in identifying potential primary sites in the head and neck territory in patients who present with malignant neck nodes from an otherwise unknown primary. As such, true unknown primaries of the head and neck territory are comparatively rare these days.

All patients with head and neck cancer should be discussed in a multidisciplinary meeting at the time of diagnosis and staging to determine the optimum treatment. The choice is usually between radical surgery with or without postoperative RT (or chemoradiotherapy), or primary radical RT (or concurrent chemoradiation), with possible neck dissection for residual disease. The decision is usually determined by the site of the primary tumour, the size of the primary tumour and consequent functional morbidity, evidence of lymph node involvement and the patient's comorbidity or individual preference. Before embarking on any radical treatment options, there are a number of preparatory steps that need to be assessed.

NUTRITION

Patients with head and neck cancer have many reasons to be malnourished before diagnosis of their malignancy. Many have a background of excessive alcohol intake and the tumour may have resulted in impaired swallowing function or caused oral discomfort. The success of any radical treatment is compromised by inadequate nutrition and morbidity is also increased. It is essential that all patients with head and neck cancer are assessed by a specialist dietician and a speech and language therapist (SALT) before any treatment. They may require enteral feeding before treatment and will certainly need it following reconstructive surgery. Patients receiving radical RT will usually have a course of treatment over many weeks and will develop mucositis and dysphagia in the acute phase. Nasogastric tube or percutaneous gastrostomy should be actively considered in all patients, especially those with large treatment volumes, and is essential for patients being considered for concurrent chemoradiation where the acute toxicity is invariably increased. It is also important for the dietetic and SALT input to continue regularly throughout the treatment course—patients need to be weighed weekly because outcome data show ongoing weight loss to be a negative prognostic factor—and into the recovery phase following treatment, which may last many weeks. Close monitoring with a rehabilitation focus should therefore continue during the follow-up period until tube feeding is no longer required and patients have returned to sufficient oral intake and proven maintained weight.

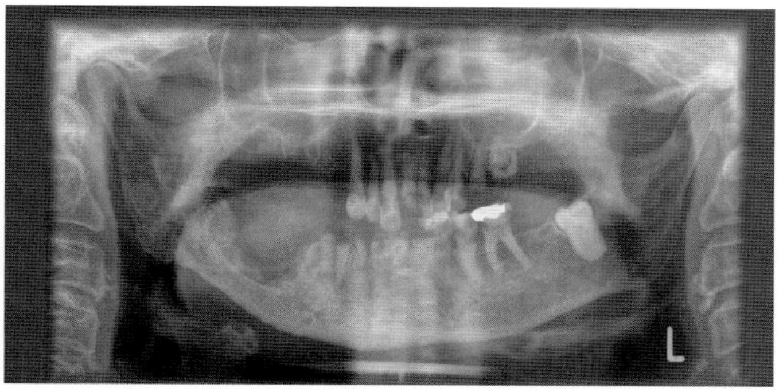

Fig. 22.3 Orthopantomogram of mandible showing osteoradionecrosis on right side.

DENTITION

Patients receiving radical RT for head and neck cancers will often have treatment volumes involving part or all of the mandible and the salivary glands. Following RT, these patients are often left with some xerostomia even with parotid-sparing RT approaches. Saliva has a protective role in neutralising oral acids and reducing dental caries. Tooth decay and dental problems can be increased post RT. Patients need to have a full dental assessment before RT. The ideal is for review by a restorative dentist or maxillofacial team to remove teeth if required. Any problem teeth should be removed and, because this typical patient population has often neglected their oral hygiene, many end up with a dental clearance. Dental extractions should be done a minimum of 2 weeks before commencing RT. Edentulous patients should be reviewed to ensure that dentures are well fitting and will not aggravate their RT reaction by movement.

When taking consent from patients for RT, they must be counselled about the risks of dental problems following the treatment and, in particular, osteoradionecrosis (ORN) of the mandible, which can develop spontaneously but is more likely after dental procedures, particularly extractions (Fig. 22.3). Patients need to be encouraged to use fluoride mouthwash or gel daily and to have regular dental checkups; if dental work is considered necessary, it should be performed by specialist hospital dental teams in view of the high risk of complications.

INDICATIONS FOR RADIOTHERAPY

Definitive Radiotherapy

The chief aim in using RT in head and neck cancer is organ preservation. In early laryngeal cancer, equivalent cure rates are attainable with radical RT and laryngectomy, but the former has the clear advantage of normal voice preservation. In some sites, for example, nasopharyngeal cancer, RT is the only option or the preferred option because of the inaccessible nature of the primary.

Postoperative Radiotherapy

The purpose of postoperative RT is to improve locoregional control. It has recently been estimated that cancer-specific and overall survival at 5 years might be improved by about 10% with postoperative RT.

There are a number of indications for postoperative RT (Table 22.1). In some cases, postoperative RT is mandatory; in other situations the real benefit to the patient is less clear.

Postoperative RT should ideally commence within 6 weeks of surgery as evidence suggests an inferior outcome if started later than this.

Palliative Radiotherapy

As a general rule, RT should be used with curative intent and with standard curative doses. On occasion, however, patients will not be fit to

TABLE 22.1 Indications for Postoperative Radiotherapy

Positive (involved) resection margins
Extracapsular lymph node spread
Close resection margins, that is, <5 mm
Invasion of soft tissues
≥2 nodes involved
> one positive nodal group (i.e. level)
Involved node >3 cm in diameter
Vascular invasion
Perineural invasion
Poor differentiation
Stage III/IV
Multicentric primary
Oral cavity/oropharynx tumours with involved nodes at level IV/V
Carcinoma in situ/dysplasia at resection 'margin/field changes'

Guidelines for cervical nodal irradiation in squamous cell carcinoma of the head and neck.
From Dr M. Henk and the CHART steering committee. A randomised multicentre trial of CHART versus conventional radiotherapy in head and neck cancer. https://doi.org/10.1016/S0167-8140(97)00094-7

undergo any form of radical RT, and RT can provide useful symptom relief using a shorter schedule and limited irradiation volume.

RADIOTHERAPY PLANNING

Once RT has been determined as the treatment modality for patients with head and neck cancer, a number of steps are required before commencing treatment. Patients need to be informed of all possible side effects (see the 'Toxicity of Treatment' section) and need to give consent.

Immobilisation

The next step is to consider immobilisation. Tumours in the head and neck may be relatively small compared with other anatomical sites, and they are also often adjacent to several critical normal structures. It is therefore essential for accurate treatment delivery that patients have good-quality reproducible immobilisation. In general, this involves an individual shell to cover the head, the neck and sometimes the shoulders. These shells are typically thermoplastic devices and are created specifically for the patient during the planning phase. The patient then has subsequent imaging in the mask. Mould room staff or radiographers who make the shell also require information about the patient's position (usually supine) and the orientation of the neck. This is important and is determined by the site one intends to irradiate. It also must consider the primary beam orientation; an extended neck position would be required for treatment of the parotid bed and middle/inner ear to facilitate the exiting dose below the contralateral eye, though with intensity modulated radiotherapy (IMRT) approaches, this may not be required. It is also necessary to consider whether the patient requires a mouth bite or tongue depressor. A mouth bite is used to push the tongue out of the treatment volume in cases of, for example, maxillary antral tumours. A tongue depressor is used to push the tongue into the treatment volume in cases of, for example, oral tongue tumours. Centres vary in their use of these devices because of issues concerning patient comfort and consistency in placement.

The most important issue of any immobilisation device is to know the reproducibility of setup for any particular patient. All centres should know the accuracy of their setup because this is the information required for determining the margin from clinical target volume (CTV) to planning target volume (PTV). In practice, an accuracy of 3 mm can be expected with existing devices, although this can be reduced further with online imaging (see later).

TARGET VOLUMES

Definitive Radiotherapy

When RT (with or without chemotherapy) is the definitive treatment, a gross tumour volume (GTV) will be present and a planning CT scan will allow it to be delineated combined with information from an examination under anaesthesia (EUA), histology and other diagnostic imaging. Help from a specialist radiologist is recommended. The CTV is to account for microscopic spread. Overtly involved nodes should be included in a separate nodal CTV. As will be seen later, this has evolved from a rather 'generous' anatomical approach to a much 'tighter' volumetric approach as long as the GTVs are easily defined. Occult lymph node metastases occur in up to 20% to 30% of N0 neck cases, so prophylactic irradiation is required for many head and neck tumours and is delineated as a separate CTV. Some centres differentiate between high-risk nodes and those at a lower risk and define those by separate nodal CTVs and prescribed doses of irradiation. The site where prophylactic nodal irradiation is not considered is early glottic cancer (T1/T2 disease). The likelihood of nodal involvement has been widely studied and it is clear that the probability increases with site of primary, size of primary and differentiation. Node selection is explored further in Chapter 23 under each head and neck cancer subsite.

The regions of the neck have been divided into levels to allow international consensus on the lymph node anatomy to enable accurate delineation (Fig. 22.4):

- Level I contains the submental and submandibular lymph nodes.
- Level II contains the upper jugular lymph nodes, which are above the hyoid bone.
- Level III contains the midjugular lymph nodes, which are between the hyoid bone and the cricoid cartilage.
- Level IV contains the lower jugular lymph nodes beginning below the cricoid.
- Level V contains the lymph nodes of the posterior triangle.
- Level VI contains the pretracheal lymph nodes.
- Level VII contains the retropharyngeal and retrostyloid nodes.

In unilateral structures (parotid, buccal mucosa, lateral floor of mouth), it is possible to treat the primary site and ipsilateral neck nodes, but in midline structures, bilateral treatment is required because the lymph drainage may be to either side of the neck. Guidelines exist to help with this approach for oropharyngeal cancer. Ipsilateral irradiation has obvious advantages in terms of normal tissue irradiation (and thus toxicity reduction) and complements IMRT (see later).

Postoperative Radiotherapy

The principles discussed in the preceding section on definitive RT are applicable in the postoperative setting, but there are some important additional points to note.

As a general rule, the whole surgical bed where the tumour is located should be included in the postoperative irradiated volume. With CT planning, it often becomes apparent that changes within the subcutaneous tissues will give volumes at risk that are bigger than anticipated. There is less consensus on the CTV in this scenario, but useful guidelines exist..

Unless there is gross residual disease or in cases where RT is planned for the primary site following a neck dissection, a GTV will not be apparent on the planning CT scan. It is often helpful to coregister any diagnostic scans with the planning CT scan in determining more precisely the preoperative GTVs to arrive at a meaningful CTV.

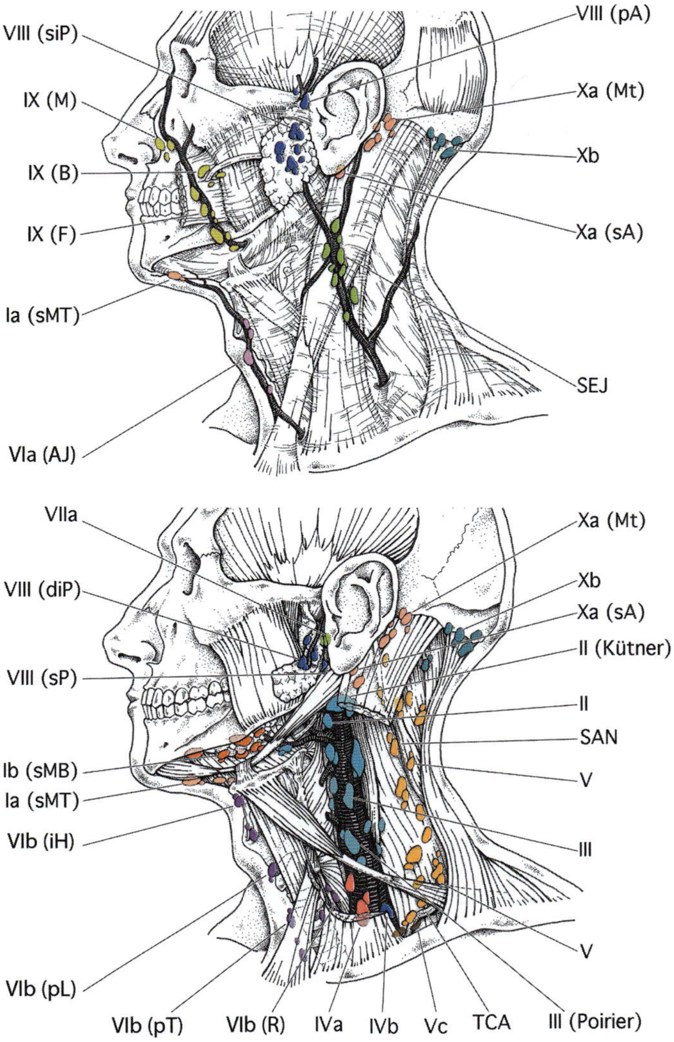

Fig. 22.4 Lymph node levels in the neck. (From Gregoire V, Ang K, Budach W, et al. Delineation of the neck node levels for head and neck tumours: a 2013 update. DAHANCA, EORTC, HKNPCSG, NCIC CTG, NCRI, RTOG, TROG consensus guidelines. *Radiother Oncol.* 2014;110(1):172-181.)

Debate continues on whether to irradiate the neck postoperatively when it is planned to irradiate the primary site and there is no nodal disease identified in the neck dissection specimen. The additional morbidity of irradiating the lower neck to intermediate prophylactic doses is relatively low compared with the rest of the neck, whereas recurrence in those not irradiated is difficult if not impossible to salvage. The decision must rest with the treating clinician, but a factor in that decision-making process will be the adequacy of the neck dissection.

The retropharyngeal nodes (level VIIA) are not routinely sampled in a neck dissection. Depending on the tumour site (and hence the risk of involvement), these should be included if the rest of the neck is to be irradiated postoperatively.

RADIOTHERAPY TECHNIQUE

Conformal Radiotherapy

In the past, conventional planning for head and neck RT has involved orthogonal films taken in the simulator with fields defined directly. With developments in RT planning, it became possible to shape beams to shield normal structures and thereby reduce toxicity. A CT scan with the patient located in the immobilisation device is a prerequisite to the process. The GTV and CTV(s) are defined directly on the CT. Structures to be avoided, including the spinal cord, are outlined separately. The volumes are then used for planning purposes. This approach may still be utilised for small volume irradiation (e.g. early larynx), but most RT in the head and neck territory in the United Kingdom is undertaken now using IMRT.

Intensity Modulated and Image-Guided Radiotherapy in Head and Neck Cancers

Developments in computer and the multileaf collimator (MLC) technology have facilitated the establishment of Intensity-modulated radiotherapy (IMRT) as the standard of care for most if not all head and neck cancer treatment. It has significant advantages in the many subsites within the head and neck territory because of the high degree of conformality that may be achieved and thus normal tissue sparing.

Image-guided radiotherapy (IGRT) is distinct from IMRT. The technique of IGRT is intended to ensure that the target volume as defined at the outset of treatment is treated consistently throughout the course of RT. Organs move and patients move, although immobilisation techniques should ensure that patient movement is less than 3 mm in the head and neck region. IGRT then has as its purpose to correct for motion and setup errors by imaging the treatment area on a daily basis. It has other advantages, as will be seen later.

What Is Intensity Modulated Radiotherapy?

Any radical RT technique aims to treat tumour tissue while minimising the exposure of healthy adjacent normal tissue. In the head and neck region, it is self-evident that there are many normal tissues that potentially need not be treated. The clinical target volume is often complex, with structures nearby which, if damaged, could result in catastrophic sequelae, for example, binocular blindness and myelopathy. Two-dimensional techniques use parallel-opposed fields to minimise these risks by the 'shrinking-field' technique (Fig. 22.5).

CT delineation of target volumes has facilitated the use of three-dimensional conformal RT. By defining a CTV and a margin for setup error to give the PTV, the resultant field with blocks or MLCs will achieve improved conformality and potentially reduced normal tissue dose (Fig. 22.6).

IMRT uses the computer control of the MLC to produce either a finite or an infinite number of subfields within each field to improve

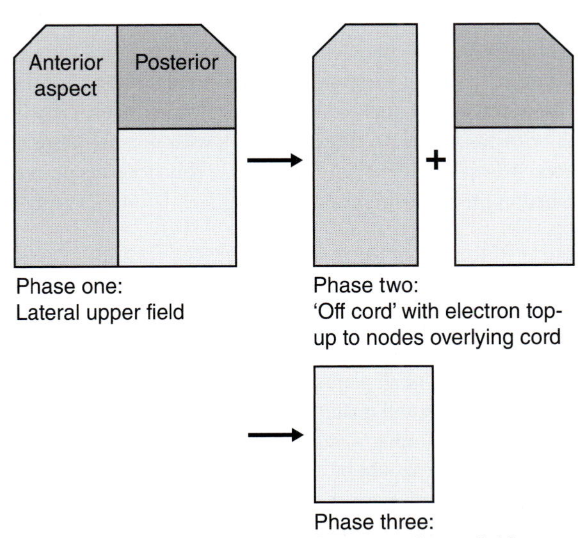

Fig. 22.5 Three-phase shrinking field treatment.

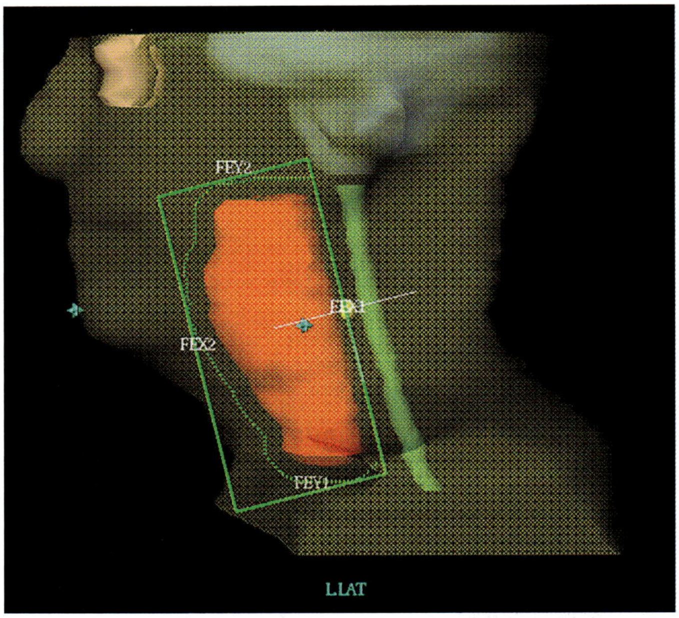

Fig. 22.6 Conformal radiotherapy treatment.

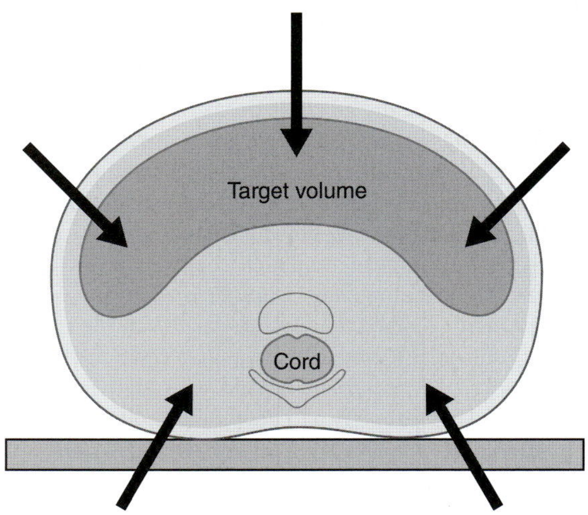

Fig. 22.7 Treating a target volume with normal tissue in the concavity.

target volume coverage. In essence, in a single beam's-eye view, the target volume is seen as a three-dimensional structure and is treated as such. The net effect of such complex beam modulation (Fig. 22.7) is the ability to treat concave target volumes with normal tissues in the concavity. It is self-evident why IMRT has therefore become so well established in the head and neck territory.

Treatment Planning in Intensity Modulated Radiotherapy

It is evident that the process of inverse planning requires absolute clarity of target volume definition (Fig. 22.8). This is not a minor issue, because arriving at definitions, particularly in the head and neck area, is through a process of integration of all planning data. This will include any pretreatment visual inspection and imaging, operative findings, pathology results, postoperative and planning scans and knowledge of patterns of spread. Clearly, this approach should be applied to all RT where accurate target-volume definition is necessary, that is, curative RT, but the ability of IMRT to achieve a high degree of conformality makes this crucial. International updated consensus guidelines from Gregoire et al. (2014) exist for the definition and delineation of the nodes in the cervical chain, which should lead

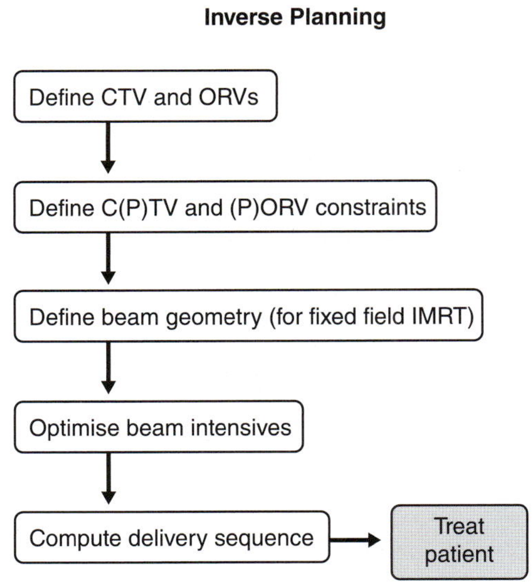

Fig. 22.8 Inverse planning. *C(P)TV*, clinical (Planning) target volumes; *CTV*, clinical target volume; *ORV*, Organ-at-risk volume; *(P)ORV*, (planning) Organ-at-risk volume.

to uniformity between centres and within centres amongst treating teams. More recently, guidelines have been published for the primary tumour and selection of associated CTV (Gregoire et al., 2018) (Fig. 22.9). The fundamental change here is the shift to a volumetric expansion of the defined GTV and two dose levels to reflect the level of risk of microscopic disease. Widespread adoption of these approaches should reduce treatment variation between clinicians and improve clinical outcomes.

The process of inverse planning requires as much clarity on normal tissue volume definition as that of the clinical target volume. In the head and neck region, these organs at risk (OARs) would include the spinal cord, brainstem, brain, optic pathway, cochlea and salivary tissues, depending on the primary site of irradiation. Failure to delineate these accurately could mean that they are irradiated unintentionally beyond conventional tolerance limits, because IMRT achieves its goal of improved conformality, in simple terms, by moving the dose elsewhere. Guidelines now exist that comprehensively describe these normal tissues and should result in consistency. Normal tissues, once delineated, require a specification of dose. These constraints may be specified in terms of maximum doses (e.g. spinal cord) or dose-volume constraints (e.g. parotid glands) and will be determined on the functional unit arrangement (i.e. parallel versus series). The QUANTEC data published by Marks et al. in 2010 detail the dose limits and risks if exceeded and are an invaluable resource.

The Scope of Intensity Modulated Radiotherapy in Head and Neck Tumours

The improvement in conformality in head and neck tumours with IMRT has two important fundamental benefits. First, it facilitates the coverage of complex and especially concave target volumes. Second, it can achieve avoidance of dose-limiting normal tissues.

It is perhaps the avoidance function that is more useful in head and neck tumours. The parallel-opposed technique does, as the name suggests, treat everything in its path. Mucosa and salivary glands that need not necessarily be treated can now be spared by this approach (Fig. 22.10). The net effect is reduced toxicity. This has perhaps been best explored in relation to reducing xerostomia through sparing of one or both parotid glands, as seen in the Nutting et al. (2011). In addition, however, there is the improved tolerability of some of the more intense schedules that have emerged as superior in the management of

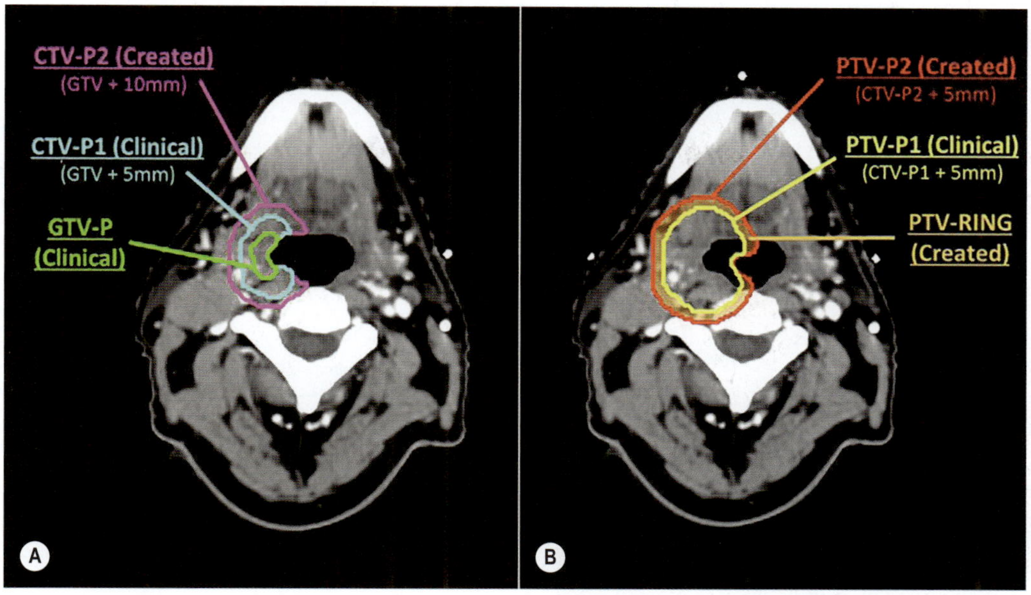

Fig. 22.9 Axial slice from a patient with a T2N1 p16 positive squamous cell carcinoma of the tonsil. (A) The 5 + 5-mm expansion rule, including GTV-P, CTV-P1 and CTV-P2. (B) PTV-P1 *(yellow)* from the clinically delivered plan, as well as the created PTV-P2 and PTV ring structures used for this study. *CTV*, Clinical target volume; *GTV*, gross tumor volume; *P1*, high-dose; *P2*, low-dose; *PTV*, planning target volume. (Reproduced from Corkum MT, Mitchell S, Venkatesan V, Read N, Warner A, Palma DA. Does 5 + 5 equal better radiation treatment plans in head and neck cancers? *Adv Radiat Oncol.* 2019;4(4):683-688. https://doi.org/10.1016/j.adro.2019.06.001)

head and neck tumours, namely, altered fractionation and concurrent chemoradiotherapy.

An improvement in conformality, however, also facilitates comprehensive coverage of the target volume as defined, as well as dose escalation if clinically indicated.

Dose escalation with IMRT needs consideration of radiobiological principles. A single-phase technique is used throughout the whole volume (Fig. 22.11), with different doses specified according to areas of variable risk, for example gross disease, high-risk (e.g. involved nodes postexcision) and low-risk territories (e.g. elective nodes in contralateral neck). Not only is the total dose modified according to perceived risk but so is the dose per fraction. A higher than conventional dose per fraction will have a higher cell kill effect and is important in the area that is dose escalated. This approach is called the *synchronous* or *simultaneous integrated boost (SIB)* technique (Fig. 22.12) and is well established as an approach in IMRT of the head and neck. Care is clearly required in the volume of normal tissue exposed to this, as higher than expected morbidity may result because of the negating effect on normal tissue damage. In areas to receive prophylactic irradiation, the total dose needs to be modified upwards to compensate for the longer elective treatment (e.g. 54 Gray (Gy) in 30 fractions rather than 50 Gy in 25 fractions; see later section) to compensate for repopulation.

It is no wonder that IMRT has become the standard of care for most head and neck cancers.

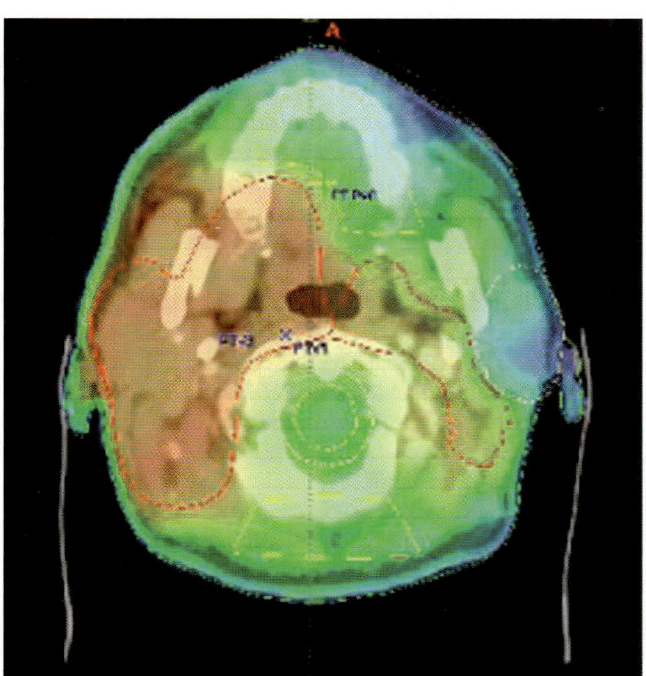

Fig. 22.10 The scope of intensity modulated radiotherapy in sparing the parotid and mucosa.

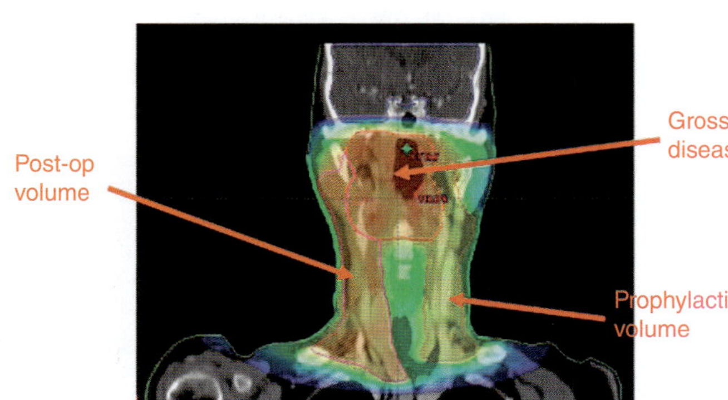

Fig. 22.11 The scope of intensity modulated radiotherapy in sparing the parotid and delivering dose according to risk of disease.

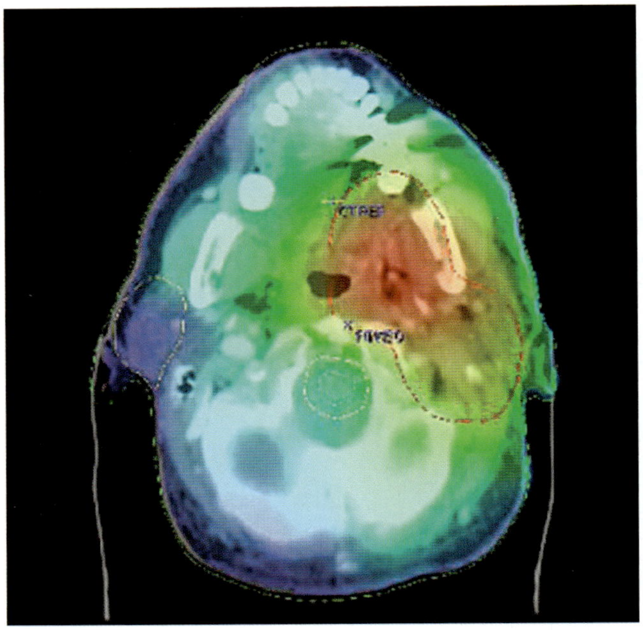

Fig. 22.12 The scope of intensity modulated radiotherapy in treating high-risk areas with the synchronous boost technique.

Image-Guided Radiotherapy

Patients with head and neck tumours need a high degree of reproducibility, and this is generally achieved through good immobilisation techniques. These immobilisation devices cannot achieve complete immobility, and it is for that reason that a CTV–PTV margin exists, even in IMRT (Fig. 22.13). IGRT seeks to reduce this margin, ideally by daily imaging. Put differently, IGRT ensures that the accurately delineated target volume is consistently treated at each fraction. In the case of head and neck cancer when volumetric imaging is used, both bone and soft-tissue landmarks can be identified and the isocenter can then be adjusted on a daily basis. A further advantage of IGRT is in treatment adaptation. For head and neck cancer, by using axial (volumetric) imaging, it is possible to see the impact of treatment on the disease and, where appropriate, to modify the plan so that high-dose target volumes can be reduced if there has been a good response. The complementary approach is where treatment results in a change in body profile, such as, through weight loss, which can impact on received doses and can

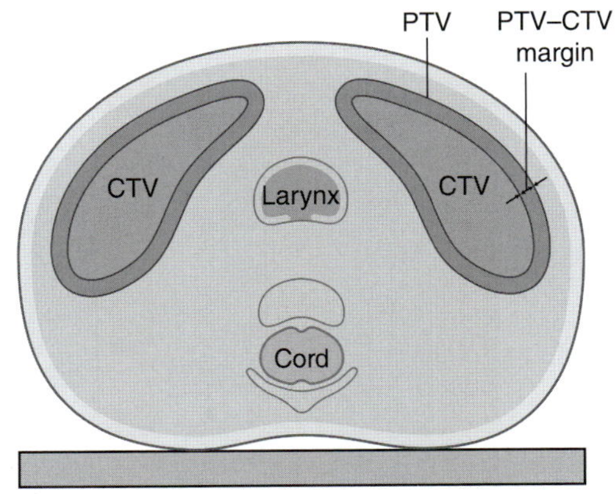

Fig. 22.13 Planning target volume–clinical target volume margins. *CTV*, Clinical target volume; *PTV*, planning target volume.

be clinically significant. Hot spots, if evident, can be addressed through replanning (Fig. 22.14). Technology now exists for this to occur swiftly on the treatment machine, enabling a seamless delivery program of care.

DOSE AND FRACTIONATION

Definitive Radiotherapy

The conventional schedule for RT to head and neck cancer involves the delivery of 70 Gy in 2-Gy fractions over 7 weeks, treating 5 days per week. Shorter schedules remain useful for small-volume treatments: 50 Gy in 16 fractions over 3 weeks or 55 Gy in 20 fractions over 4 weeks.

The Danish Head and Neck Cancer Group (DAHANCA) compared 6 fractions per week with the standard 5 (still using 2 Gy per fraction). In total, 66 to 68 Gy was given in either 6.5 or 5.5 weeks. They showed improved 5-year local control in the moderately accelerated group of 68% versus 56% for standard therapy without chemotherapy. Either the extra treatment was given on Saturday, or the patients were treated twice on Friday (with a ≥6-hour gap).

Another schedule is to use a concomitant boost to the primary site during conventional RT. This provides the first phase of treatment (primary disease plus involved nodes and microscopic spread) in the morning, and then later the same day, a second smaller boost dose is given to the phase 2 volume, involving the gross disease only. The dose is 1.8 Gy daily with a 1.5-Gy boost for the last 12 treatments, resulting

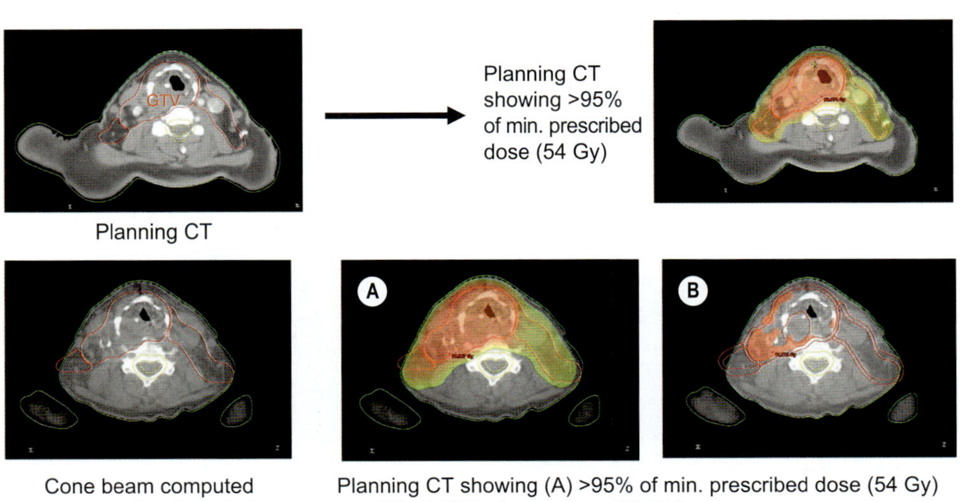

Fig. 22.14 Adaptive radiotherapy.

in a total dose of 72 Gy in 42 fractions given over 6 weeks. This accelerates the overall treatment time.

A recent metaanalysis of fractionation schedules has concluded that there is a survival benefit with altered fractionation. The largest survival benefit (8.2% at 5 years) was evident with hyperfractionation, not dissimilar to the benefits seen with concurrent chemoradiation. Accelerated schedules resulted in a lesser survival gain, although such a schedule would be easier to implement in the clinic than hyperfractionation. To some extent, this debate on fractionation has been superseded by the accelerated hypofractionated schedules (i.e. dose per fraction slightly higher than 2 Gy) used in IMRT, at least in the United Kingdom: 65 to 66 Gy in 30 fractions over 6 weeks would be considered an accepted schedule, with reduced doses (54 Gy typically) to areas of less risk of disease.

Postoperative Radiotherapy

Sites of gross residual disease—that is, the primary and involved nodes—are treated to doses similar to the definitive setting (70 Gy when using 2-Gy fractions or 65 to 66 Gy in 30 fractions). More typically, adjuvant therapy doses of 60 Gy in 30 fractions would be recommended, with the option to boost where there are high-risk pathological findings (extracapsular spread and/or positive/close margins). Lower doses of 50 Gy in 2-Gy fractions (or 54 Gy in 30 fractions) would be given to lower areas of risk of microscopic disease. The DAHANCA group give useful guidance on the approach to volume definition.

CHEMOTHERAPY IN HEAD AND NECK CANCER

There has been much work done looking into chemotherapy agents in head and neck cancer. Many drugs have been shown to have some response in squamous cell cancers of the head and neck, in particular, the platinum compounds, 5-fluorouracil, methotrexate, bleomycin, vinca alkaloids and, more recently, the taxanes. However, the most compelling data are in the use of chemotherapy given concurrently with RT.

Concurrent Chemotherapy and Definitive Radiotherapy

The accepted standard treatment for radical nonsurgical therapy for more advanced head and neck cancer is concurrent cisplatin chemotherapy with radical RT at least in those patients younger than 70 years of age. The evidence for this comes from Pignon's original metaanalysis updated in 2021, which showed a small but significant survival advantage to the combined treatment, but only if the chemotherapy was given concurrently. This benefit was not seen in induction or adjuvant schedules. The overall survival benefit for any chemoradiation schedule was approximately 4% but increased to 8% if cisplatin was the chemotherapy drug chosen. Concomitant chemotherapy is given simultaneously with radiation therapy to improve local and distant control. The mechanisms for action include the elimination of micrometastases and increased sensitivity to the RT.

The standard schedule for concurrent chemoradiotherapy for head and neck cancer involves cisplatin given intravenously on days 1, 22 and 43 of the RT at a dose of 100 mg/m^2. Alternatively (and increasingly in the United Kingdom), the cisplatin is being delivered using the weekly schedule of 40 mg/m^2 for 6 weeks. There is anecdotal evidence that this regimen is better tolerated than the 3-weekly schedule, particularly in the head and neck cancer population, although this is still being debated. Patients require a satisfactory full blood count and adequate renal function throughout. Nutritional support is essential and a feeding tube is advised in all patients undergoing combination treatment. Acute toxicity is usually more severe in these patients and should be looked for and managed aggressively.

Although cisplatin remains the gold standard agent for concurrent chemotherapy, cetuximab, a monoclonal antibody to the epidermal growth factor receptor (EGFR), when given concurrently with RT, has been shown to improve progression-free and overall survival without the added burden of traditional sensitising chemotherapy. It is generally reserved for fit patients in whom all forms of platin-based chemotherapy treatment are contraindicated.

Given the excellent prognosis with HPV-positive head and neck cancers, studies are underway to evaluate the safety of deescalating treatment, especially regarding cisplatin substitution or avoidance of concurrent chemoradiation completely. Mehanna et al. (2019) has, however, cast doubt on the merits of this, and thus platinum-based chemotherapy remains the standard of care.

Concurrent Chemotherapy and Postoperative Radiotherapy

A previous section outlined the range of indications for postoperative RT. Some situations would be considered particularly adverse for locoregional recurrence and, in these cases, consideration should be given to concurrent chemoradiation postoperatively. Two trials by Cooper and Bernier and a consensus view have suggested that such patients would be those with positive primary resection margins, and those with pathologically involved nodes with extracapsular spread.

Induction Chemotherapy

Neoadjuvant or induction chemotherapy has been used to downstage a primary tumour before definitive surgery or RT, and to decrease the incidence of distant metastases. In the Pignon metaanalysis of chemotherapy with RT in head and neck cancer, there was evidence that organ preservation was increased in patients receiving chemotherapy followed by radical RT compared with primary surgery for advanced but resectable laryngeal cancer. Although the original metaanalysis did not show any real survival benefit, a more recent review on updated data has shown that induction schedules may convey a survival advantage of up to 2% to 3%. The majority of these studies used the previous standard induction chemotherapy schedule of cisplatin and 5-fluorouracil (PF). The debate on the role of induction chemotherapy has been ignited with the publication of two key trials using the triplet of docetaxel, cisplatin and 5-fluorouracil, and further ones since reviewed in a metaanalysis that has shown progression-free and overall survival and distant failure rate benefits over PF. To date, however, the only widely accepted setting for which induction chemotherapy has consensus value is in laryngeal preservation in patients with resectable but locally advanced disease, more advanced nasopharyngeal cancer and in some cases of rapidly progressive disease.

SYSTEMIC THERAPY IN THE PALLIATIVE SETTING

Chemotherapy can be used for palliation in patients with recurrent or metastatic head and neck cancer. If patients have not received prior treatment with chemotherapy, cisplatin and 5-fluorouracil could be considered as first-line treatment, or a more outpatient equivalent such as carboplatin and capecitabine could be considered. Monoclonal antibody therapy against EGFR with platinum-based chemotherapy is active and has been shown to improve median overall survival compared with standard chemotherapy alone. More recently, immunotherapy has become established as valuable therapy particularly in those patients whose disease is PDL-1 positive. The option and/or the order of therapy thus will be dependent on the tumour pathology, pace of disease, patient comorbidity and patient and clinician expectations as well as local commissioning approvals.

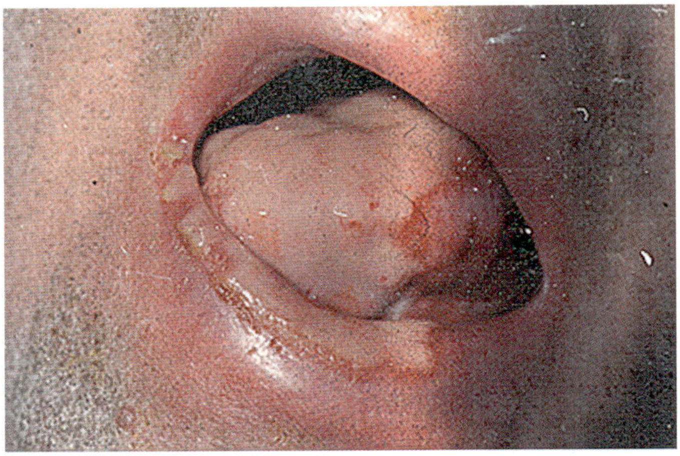

Fig. 22.15 Acute side effects of radiotherapy: Acute mucositis.

TOXICITY OF TREATMENT

RT for head and neck cancer has many side effects that must be effectively communicated to the patient before embarking on treatment. A detailed explanation is essential not only for informed consent but also to improve compliance with the full course of treatment to give the best chance of a successful outcome. As with RT to any part of the body, the side effects (apart from fatigue) relate to structures within the radiation field. They can be divided into acute (early) or late side effects. Reactions will, to some extent, be site specific and are discussed in more detail in Chapter 35. However, it is useful to consider the principles here.

Acute Toxicity

Mucositis will develop in the treatment volume for all patients with head and neck cancer and can be severe and disabling. It may be mild (grade 1/2) but is often severe (grade 3) (Fig. 22.15), especially in those receiving concurrent chemotherapy. Grade 4 mucositis (frank ulceration) rarely occurs in practice. Management includes analgesia using the pain ladder. Opiates may be required at some stage. Topical agents may be used initially and alongside systemic analgesia. Patients must have their weight monitored and nutritional supplements considered. The majority of patients will have a level of discomfort that requires opiate-level analgesia. This can be administered in oral preparations (solutions, syrups etc.) or delivered via feeding tube if present. It can often become difficult for patients to tolerate oral medications, particularly in the latter stages of treatment, but the development of transdermal delivery systems for opiates can be an excellent alternative in patients with head and neck cancer where swallowing is often difficult or uncomfortable and, in the main, transdermal delivery has avoided the need for subcutaneous infusions of an opiate, which were occasionally required in the past for patients with severe symptoms.

Dysphagia secondary to mucositis, loss of taste, loss of appetite and thickened secretions leads to weight loss in patients with head and neck cancer. This should be predicted before treatment and a feeding tube considered in all patients with large treatment volumes, especially those to be treated by chemoradiotherapy. If patients without a tube are struggling and losing weight, a tube may need to be inserted during treatment—this will usually involve a radiologically placed gastrostomy or a temporary nasogastric tube. Prophylactic gastrostomy tube insertion is usually more satisfactory and allows early feeding to be initiated before the patient develops difficulties.

Thickened secretions can be alleviated with carbocysteine, which has a systemic mode of action, or saline nebulisers and acute xerostomia, managed symptomatically.

A skin reaction is seen in any treated area and develops as the treatment progresses. The skin changes from mild redness (Figs. 22.16 and 22.17) to brisk erythema to desquamation; initially, dry changes and peeling progress to moist desquamation (Fig. 22.18). A skincare regimen should include washing with lukewarm water and unperfumed soap, avoiding shaving until treatment is completed and applying regular moisturising cream. Once skin is broken, a barrier product should be used. The optimal regimen is unclear and is often centre specific. Patients should be reviewed regularly posttreatment to monitor the resolution of skin and mucosal reactions.

Fatigue is seen in many patients receiving radical RT. It has been shown that maintaining a level of gentle activity is the best way to overcome the asthenia during therapy. In patients with head and neck cancer, especially those receiving chemoradiotherapy, it is usual to monitor the haemoglobin during RT and to transfuse patients as required to keep the level greater than 12 g/dL. There is evidence that RT is less effective in patients with anaemia, although no good evidence exists that correcting anaemia improves outcomes. Indeed, a review of five key trials using erythropoietin (EPO) found a worse outcome in the treated groups. The conclusion was that EPO should not be administered as an addition to RT outside of the study setting, as myelosuppression can occur and can be life-threatening.

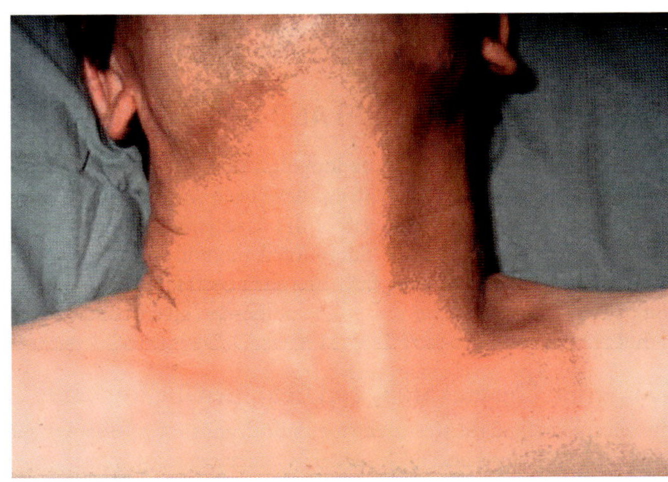

Fig. 22.16 Marked erythema in a patient treated for nasopharynx cancer (neck).

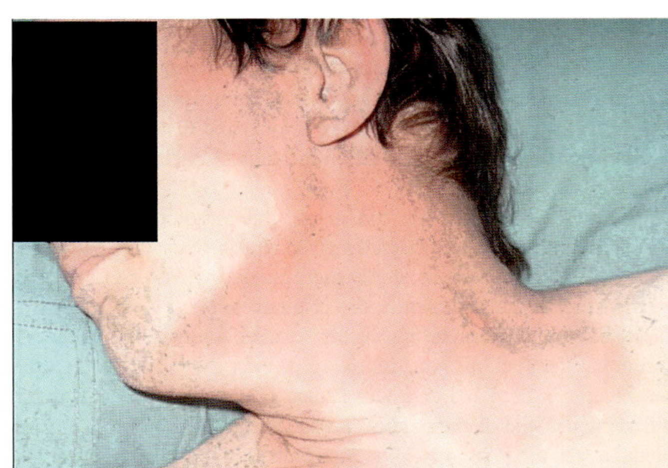

Fig. 22.17 Acute side effects of radiotherapy: Skin erythema with associated dry desquamation.

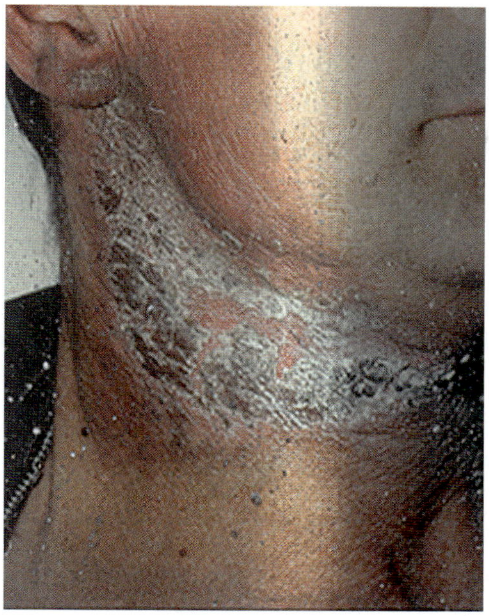

Fig. 22.18 Marked erythema in a patient treated for nasopharynx cancer (face).

Late Toxicity

Skin pigmentation/atrophy can be seen in patients treated with head and neck RT as a result of the doses received by the skin. Skin sparing is achieved where possible as a result of the use of megavoltage RT and modern designs of shells that minimise the bolus effect. Bolus may be used if there is evidence of skin involvement in a tumour, or impending fungation, which will of course enhance the skin dose.

Alopecia can occur and may be outside the primary irradiated area because of the IMRT delivery technique (rotational IMRT). Patients should be warned of the possibility.

Xerostomia is a common late side effect of RT to the head and neck. It most commonly arises because of RT to the parotid gland, although the submandibular gland, sublingual glands and minor salivary glands throughout the mouth can also be included. The risk of xerostomia increases with increasing dose. The initial symptom may become apparent from as early as the first week of therapy, and irreversible damage to the gland will arise with modest doses. It can be a most distressing side effect for patients, and efforts to minimise the dose to one or both salivary glands should be routine during RT planning, given the compelling trial data that first demonstrated the value of IMRT in head and neck cancer. If it develops, patients should be offered artificial saliva preparations. Dental checkups are essential.

ORN is the breakdown of bone in an area treated with RT (see Fig. 22.3). In patients with head and neck cancer, it is most often seen in the mandible and can be triggered by dental extractions. It may mimic local recurrence of a tumour. ORN is difficult to manage as further surgery can exacerbate the problem. The best management is prevention, which means diligent dental assessments, any required treatments before RT and proactive dental hygiene postradiation treatment (e.g. fluoride mouthwashes or gels). The ability of IMRT to conform and the avoidance of high doses to the mandible unless integral to the target volume should also reduce the risk of ORN. Patients must be educated about the risk of dental work after RT and seeking specialist advice for any treatment required. It should be performed under sedation and with antibiotic cover.

Myelitis secondary to RT is a rare but recognised side effect from head and neck RT. There has been considerable debate over what constitutes a safe dose of radiation to the spinal cord. This is complicated because of many variables including volume treated, fraction size and total dose. Different series have described different maximal doses. A safe total dose is 44 to 46 Gy, although consensus is that doses up to 50 Gy in 2 Gy per fraction is acceptable and is clarified in the QUANTEC series. As discussed earlier, IMRT facilitates coverage of volumes with sparing of the spinal cord in the concavity, obviating many of the historical challenges of tumours close to the spinal cord. Some patients may develop Lhermitte's syndrome secondary to early transient myelitis. In Lhermitte's syndrome, patients complain of tingling or electric shocks in the legs. This can be provoked by flexing the neck. These symptoms begin about 6 weeks following the RT and may last a few months. Progression to late damage is rare but is still observed with IMRT.

The RCR consent forms provide a useful summary of the potential short-term (acute) and longer-term or late sequelae and can be accessed online.

FUTURE DEVELOPMENTS

Artificial intelligence (AI) approaches to aid normal tissue and target volume delineation are available and used, and appropriate safety checks in the clinic should streamline the volumising stage. In addition, AI and advanced online imaging will facilitate the change of current practice from radiotherapy planning only at the beginning of treatment, to an adaptive daily planning before each treatment, enabling a more personalised approach to treatment delivery.

Seeking more active systemic agents and embedding immunotherapy into disease management beyond metastatic disease is ongoing.

FURTHER READING

Ang KK, Trotti A, Brown BW, et al. Randomised trial of addressing risk features and time factors of surgery plus radiotherapy in advanced head-and-neck cancer. *Int J Radiat Oncol Biol Phys*. 2001;51(3):571–578.

Bernier J, Cooper JS, Pajak TF, et al. Defining risk levels in locally advanced head and neck cancers: a comparative analysis of concurrent postoperative radiation plus chemotherapy trials of the EORTC (#22931) and RTOG (#9501). *Head Neck*. 2005;27(10):843–850.

Bernier J, Domenge C, Ozsahin M, et al. Postoperative irradiation with or without concomitant chemotherapy for locally advanced head and neck cancer. *N Engl J Med*. 2004;350(19):1945–1952.

Biau J, Lapeyre M, Troussier I, et al. Selection of lymph node target volumes for definitive head and neck radiation therapy: a 2019 update. *Radiother Oncol*. 2019;134:1–9.

Blanchard P, Bourhis J, Lacas B, et al. Taxane-cisplatin-fluorouracil as induction chemotherapy in locally advanced head and neck cancers: an individual patient data meta-analysis of chemotherapy in head and neck cancer group. *J Clin Oncol*. 2013;31(23):2854–2860.

Bonner JA, Harari PM, Giralt J, et al. Radiotherapy plus cetuximab for squamous-cell carcinoma of the head and neck. *N Engl J Med*. 2006;354(6):567–578.

Bourhis J, Overgaard J, Audry H, et al. Hyperfractionated or accelerated radiotherapy in head and neck cancer: a meta-analysis. *Lancet*. 2006;368(9538):844–854.

Brouwer CL, Steenbakkers RJHM, Bourhis J, et al. CT-based delineation of organs at risk in the head and neck region: DAHANCA, EORTC, GORTEC, HKNPCSG, NCIC CTG, NRG oncology and TROG consensus guidelines. *Radiother Oncol*. 2015;117(1):83–90.

Budach W, Hehr T, Budach V, Belka C, Dietz K. A meta-analysis of hyperfractionated and accelerated radiotherapy and combined chemotherapy and radiotherapy regimens in unresectable locally advanced squamous cell carcinoma of the head and neck. *BMC Cancer*. 2006;6:28.

Chatterjee S, Kiyota N, Vaish R, et al. Weekly versus 3-weekly cisplatin along with radiotherapy for locoregionally advanced non-nasopharyngeal head and neck cancers: is the equipoise in literature addressed yet? *Head Neck.* 2023;45(6):1594–1603.

Cooper J, Pajak TF, Forastiere AA, et al. Postoperative concurrent radiotherapy and chemotherapy for high-risk squamous-cell carcinoma of the head and neck. *N Engl J Med.* 2004;350(19):1937–1944.

Evans M, Beasley M. Target delineation for postoperative treatment of head and neck cancer. *Oral Oncol.* 2018;86:288–295.

Fasano M, Corte CMD, Di Liello R, et al. Immunotherapy for head and neck cancer: present and future. *Crit Rev Oncol Hematol.* 2022;174:103679.

Fletcher GH. Elective irradiation of subclinical disease in cancers of the head and neck. *Cancer.* 1972;29:1450–1454.

Fu KK, Pajak TF, Trotti A, et al. A Radiation Therapy Oncology Group (RTOG) phase III randomized study to compare hyperfractionation and two variants of accelerated fractionation to standard fractionation for head and neck squamous cell carcinomas: first report of RTOG 9003. *Int J Radiat Oncol Biol Phys.* 2000;48(1):7–16.

Gregoire V, Ang K, Budach W, et al. Delineation of the neck node levels for head and neck tumours: a 2013 update. DAHANCA, EORTC, HKNPCSG, NCIC CTG, NCRI, RTOG, TROG consensus guidelines. *Radiother Oncol.* 2014;110(1):172–181.

Gregoire V, Coche E, Cosnard G, Hamoir M, Reychler H. Selection and delineation of lymph node target volumes in head and neck conformal radiotherapy. Proposal for standardizing terminology and procedure based on surgical experience. *Radiother Oncol.* 2000;56(2):135–150.

Gregoire V, Eisbruch A, Hamoir M, Levendag P. Proposal for the delineation of the nodal CTV in the node-positive and the post-operative neck. *Radiother Oncol.* 2006;79(1):15–20.

Gregoire V, Evans M, Le Q-T, et al. Delineation of the primary clinical target volumes (CTV-P) in laryngeal, hypopharyngeal, oropharyngeal and oral cavity squamous cell carcinoma: AIRO, CACA, DAHANCA, EORTC, GEORCC, GORTEC, HKNPCSG, HNCIG, IAG-KHT, LPRHHT, NCIC CRG, NCRI, NRG Oncology, PHNS, SBRT, SOMERA, SRO, SSHNO, TROG consensus guidelines. *Radiother Oncol.* 2018;126(1):3–24.

Gregoire V, Levendag P, Ang KK, et al. CT-based delineation of lymph node levels and related CTVs in the node-negative neck: DAHANCA, EORTC, GORTEC, NCIC, RTOG consensus guidelines. *Radiother Oncol.* 2003;69(3):227–236.

IPEM (Institute of Physics and Engineering in Medicine). *Guidance for the clinical implementation of intensity modulated radiation therapy*. York, UK: IPEM; 2008 IPEM Report 96.

Jackson A, Marks LB, Bentzen SM, et al. The lessons of QUANTEC: recommendations for reporting and gathering data on dose-volume dependencies of treatment outcome. *Int J Radiat Oncol Biol Phys.* 2010;76(3 Suppl.):S155–S160.

Jensen K, Friborg J, Hansen CR, et al. The Danish Head and Neck Cancer Group (DAHANCA) 2020 radiotherapy guidelines. *Radiother Oncol.* 2020;151:149–151.

Lacas B, Carmel A, Landais C, et al. Meta-analysis of chemotherapy in head and neck cancer (MACH-NC): an update on 107 randomized trials and 19,805 patients, on behalf of MACH-NC Group. *Radiother Oncol.* 2021;156:281–293.

Lambin P, Ramaekers BLT, van Mastrigt GAPG, et al. Erythropoietin as an adjuvant treatment with (chemo) radiation therapy for head and neck cancer. *Cochrane Database Syst Rev.* 2009(3):CD006158. https://doi.org/10.1002/14651858.CD006158.pub2.

Lemus OML Cao M, Cai B, Cummings M, Zheng D. Adaptive radiotherapy: next generation radiotherapy. *Cancers.* 2024;16(6):1206.

Lengele B, Hamoir M, Scalliet P, Grégoire V. Anatomical bases for the radiological delineation of lymph node areas. Major collecting trunks, head and neck. *Radiother Oncol.* 2007;85(1):146–155.

Marks LB, Yorke ED, Jackson A, et al. Use of normal tissue complication probability models in the clinic. *Int J Radiat Oncol Biol Phys.* 2010;76(3):S10–S19.

Mehanna H, Robinson M, Hartley A, et al. Radiotherapy plus cisplatin or cetuximab in low-risk human papillomavirus-positive oropharyngeal cancer (De-ESCALaTE HPV): an open-label randomised controlled phase 3 trial. *Lancet.* 2019;393(10166):51–60.

Moharti BK, Umapathy H, Bahadur S, Thakar A, Pathy S. Short course palliative radiotherapy of 20Gy in 5 fractions for advanced and incurable head and neck cancer: AIIMS study. *Radiother Oncol.* 2004;71(3):275–280.

Nguyen NT, Doerwald-Munoz L, Zhang H, et al. 0-7-21 Hypofractionated palliative radiotherapy in head and neck cancers. *Br J Radiol.* 2015;88(1049):20140646.

Nutting CM, Morden JP, Harrington KJ, et al. Parotid-sparing intensity modulated versus conventional radiotherapy in head and neck cancer (PARSPORT): a phase 3 multicentre randomized controlled trial. *Lancet Oncol.* 2011;12(2):127–136.

Overgaard J, Hansen HS, Specht L, et al. Five compared with six fractions per week of conventional radiotherapy of squamous-cell carcinoma of head and neck: DAHANCA 6&7 randomised controlled trial. *Lancet.* 2003;362(9388):933–940.

Peters LJ, Goepfert H, Ang KK, et al. Evaluation of the dose for post-operative radiation therapy of head and neck cancer: first report of a prospective randomized trial. *Int J Radiat Oncol Biol Phys.* 1993;26(1):3–11.

Pignon JP, Bourhis J, Domenge C, Designé L. Chemotherapy added to locoregional treatment for head and neck squamous-cell carcinoma: three meta-analyses of updated individual data. *Lancet.* 2000; 355(9208):949–950.

Pignon JP, le Maître A, Bourhis JMACH-NC Collaborative Group. Meta-analyses of chemotherapy in head and neck cancer (MACH-NC): an update. *Int J Radiat Oncol Biol Phys.* 2007;69(2 Suppl): S112–S114.

Pignon JP, le Maître A, Maillard E, Bourhis JMACH-NC Collaborative Group. Meta-analysis of chemotherapy in head and neck cancer (MACH-NC): an update on 93 randomised trials and 17,346 patients. *Radiother Oncol.* 2009;92(1):4–14.

Posner MR, Hershock DM, Blajman CR, et al. Cisplatin and fluorouracil alone or with docetaxel in head and neck cancer. *N Engl J Med.* 2007;357(17):1705–1715.

Royal College of Radiologists. Head and Neck Cancer. In: *Radiotherapy dose fractionation*. 4th ed. RCR; 2024:56–65. https://www.rcr.ac.uk/media/2ahl12m4/07-head-neck-cancer-radiotherapy-dose-fractionation-fourth-edition.pdf.

Royal College of Radiologists. Head and neck consensus statements 2022. Available from: https://www.rcr.ac.uk/our-services/all-our-publications/clinical-oncology-publications/head-and-neck-cancer-rcr-consensus-statements/ (Accessed 23 July 2025).

Royal College of Radiologists National radiotherapy consent forms. National radiotherapy consent forms (rcr.ac.uk)

Szyszko TA, Cook GJR. PET/CT and PET/MRI in head and neck malignancy. *Clin Radiol.* 2018;73(1):60–69.

Vermorken JB, Mesia R, Rivera F, et al. Platinum-based chemotherapy plus cetuximab in head and neck cancer. *N Engl J Med.* 2008;359(11):1116–1127.

Vermorken JB, Remenar E, van Herpen C, et al. Cisplatin, fluorouracil, and docetaxel in unresectable head and neck cancer. *N Engl J Med.* 2007;357(17):1695–1704.

23

Sinonasal, Oral, Larynx and Pharynx Cancers

Christopher D. Scrase

CHAPTER OUTLINE

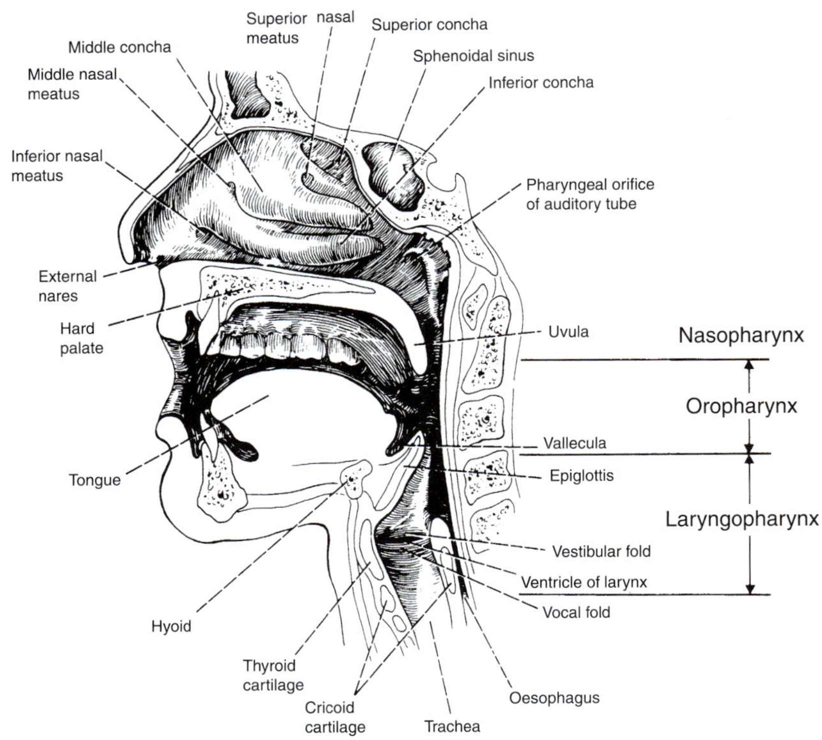

Fig. 23.1 Section of the pharynx, from front to back.

This chapter reviews each anatomical subtype of the head and neck region.

NASOPHARYNX

Anatomy

The nasopharynx is cuboidal in shape and comprises the most superior of the three pharyngeal structures. As such, it has a direct communication with the nasal cavity anteriorly and oropharynx inferiorly (Fig. 23.1).

Anterior Wall

The anterior wall comprises the posterior choanae and nasal cavity.

Posterior Wall

The posterior wall is formed by the tissues of the prevertebral space adjacent to the first and second cervical vertebrae.

Lateral Walls

The pharyngobasilar fascia forms the lateral and posterior walls. Within this is the opening of the eustachian tube and, more posteriorly, a deep recess called the fossa of Rosenmüller (lateral nasopharyngeal recess) (Fig. 23.2).

Superior Wall

Strictly speaking, the roof slopes in an anterior to posterior direction abutting the base of the skull. The sphenoid sinus lies superiorly and the superior component of Waldeyer's ring, the most prominent in childhood, is located here. There is a depression in the mucosa in the midline known as the *pharyngeal bursa* which sometimes extends into the basiocciput.

Inferior Wall

The inferior wall is, in reality, an imaginary horizontal line running from the lower border of the soft palate to the posterior pharyngeal wall.

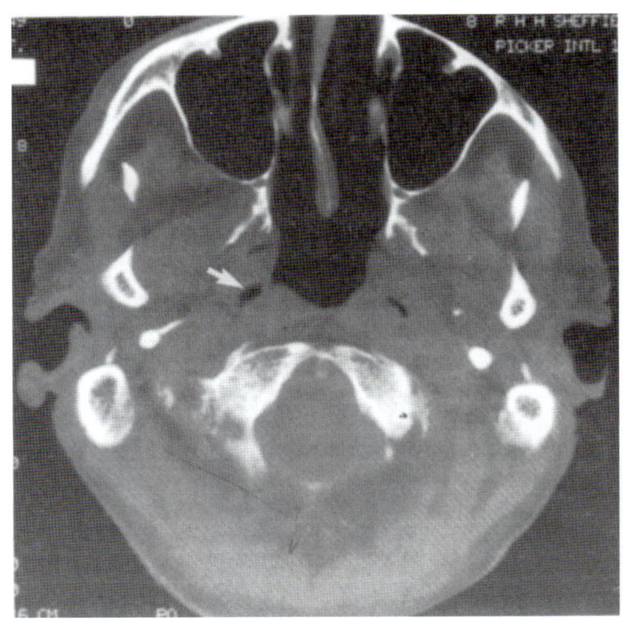

Fig. 23.2 Computed tomography scan showing normal anatomy of the nasopharynx. The fossa of Rosenmüller (pharyngeal recess) is *arrowed*. (Courtesy Dr R. Nakielny, Sheffield, UK.)

Incidence of Nasopharyngeal Tumours

Cancer of nasopharynx (NPC) is rare in the United Kingdom, with an annual incidence rate of 0.39 per 100,000 population. By contrast, NPC is far more common in patients of southern China, North Africa and Alaska origin. The incidence of NPC in the Hong Kong population is between 20 and 30 per 100,000 per year. NPC is also more common in males than females (3:1), with a median age at presentation of 50 years.

Staging System for Nasopharyngeal Tumours

The staging system is based on the International TNM System, updated most recently to version 8:

T1	Tumour confined to the nasopharynx or extends to the oropharynx and/or nasal cavity without parapharyngeal involvement
T2	Tumour with parapharyngeal space extension and/or infiltration of the medial pterygoid, lateral pterygoid and/or prevertebral muscles
T3	Tumour that invades bony structures of the skull base, cervical vertebra, pterygoid structures and/or paranasal sinuses
T4	Tumour with intracranial extension and/or involvement of the cranial nerves, infratemporal fossa, hypopharynx, orbit or masticator space
N1	Unilateral metastases in cervical lymph node(s) and/or unilateral or bilateral metastases in retropharyngeal lymph nodes, ≤6 cm above the caudal border of the cricoid cartilage
N2	Bilateral lymph node(s) ≤6 cm above the caudal border of the cricoid cartilage
N3	Any lymph node >6 cm and/or extension below the caudal border of the cricoid cartilage

Stage Grouping	
Stage 1	T1N0M0
Stage 2	T2N0M0
	T1N1M0
	T2N1M0
Stage 3	T1N2M0
	T2N2M0
	T3N0M0
	T3N1M0
	T3N2M0
Stage 4A	T4N0M0
	T4N1M0
	T4N2M0
	Any T N3M0
Stage 4B	Any T, Any N M1

Aetiology, Pathology and Lymphatic Spread

Squamous cell carcinomas (SCCs) comprise the most common histological type. They may be subdivided into well- to poorly differentiated types, those with a heavy lymphatic infiltrate (lymphoepithelioma), transitional cell tumours and keratinising and nonkeratinising types. The World Health Organization (WHO) usefully classifies nasopharyngeal tumours as follows:

Type 1	Well-differentiated keratinising type SCC (KSCC)
Type 2	Moderately differentiated nonkeratinising type (NKDC)
Type 3	Undifferentiated type typically with an extensive lymphocytic infiltrate (NKUC)

The presence of keratin (i.e. type 1) is associated with local infiltration, whereas type 3 tumours tend to disseminate widely. The WHO III subtype is the most common form of NPC in endemic areas and differs from the squamous type of NPC in its association with the Epstein–Barr virus (EBV) and sensitivity to chemotherapy and radiotherapy (RT).

NPC is thus associated with infection with EBV. EBV DNA is incorporated into the tumour genome. Infection with EBV is common and is the cause of glandular fever. In Hong Kong, almost all children aged 10 years have been infected by the virus. Even in Hong Kong, only a small minority develop NPC. Genetic and dietary factors seem important in tumour development. Genetic alterations include deletion of chromosomal regions at 1p, 14q and 16p and amplification of 4q and 12q. Dietary factors are also important, including eating salt-dried fish (containing carcinogenic nitrosamines) and lack of fresh fruit and vegetables (lack of antioxidants).

Although SCCs form the majority of nasopharyngeal cancers, other pathologies are recognised in this region. These include adenocarcinoma, adenoid cystic carcinoma and lymphoma. Treatment may vary by tumour type according to the propensity for nodal spread and response to radiation, although the principles of technique as described here can still broadly be applied.

It is because of the rich lymphatic supply that these tumours commonly spread and, indeed, present with neck nodes. This spread may be bilateral, but the distribution is dissimilar to other head and neck SCCs and is reflected in the TNM classification outlined earlier. It has been found that 70% to 90% of cases have nodes at some point. Levels 1A/B are rarely involved, whereas levels 2 and 5 (the postcervical chain) can be considered the first-echelon nodes for this tumour site.

Nasopharyngeal cancers have a high propensity for distal haematogenous spread and, as a consequence, distal failure.

Signs and Symptoms

The first presenting symptom is often painless node enlargement confirmed on examination. These are often bilateral in their distribution and, as mentioned earlier, typically involve the posterior cervical chain.

Other common symptoms include nasal obstruction and epistaxis through expansion into the nasal cavity and auditory disturbances, especially unilateral deafness and recurrent otitis media. Examination findings may confirm a mass in the postnasal space and cranial nerve palsies especially of II to VI through direct expansion through bone and via nerve foramina, and IX to XII through compression from Rouvière's node. This node is the most superior of the retropharyngeal node chain and overlies the transverse process of C1.

Patients may report headaches, although other symptoms or signs will usually be readily apparent.

Diagnosis and Staging

The diagnosis may be strongly suspected on clinical grounds alone from the aforementioned findings, especially on nasendoscopic examination, but histological confirmation of any nasopharyngeal mass will be required. Patients should be assessed with rigid and fibre-optic nasendoscopy. Further locoregional staging, best with magnetic resonance imaging (MRI), is mandatory. A computed tomography (CT) scan, although adequate, does not afford the same degree of information, particularly in the base of the skull region.

In the context of neck nodes where a primary is not readily apparent, especially when it lies posteriorly in the upper neck, the finding of EBV genomic material most reliably detected using in situ hybridisation is usually indicative of a clinically inapparent nasopharyngeal primary and treatment should be along the lines of such tumours.

Because nasopharyngeal cancers have a high propensity for systemic spread, a workup for distal disease is essential. As such, haematological and biochemical screens and a CT scan of the chest, abdomen and pelvis should be undertaken. A positron emission tomography–computed tomography (PET/CT) scan may be useful, especially for patients with a suspected occult primary in the nasopharynx.

Treatment

The relative inaccessible nature of the primary tumour and frequent involvement of Rouvière's node dictates that radiation therapy is the main modality for treatment. In addition, and unlike other head and neck SCCs, the presence of substantial neck nodes should not lead to initial surgical excision, as they generally respond well to radiation therapy. Any nodes that have failed to respond adequately or at recurrence can, provided the primary disease is controlled, then be managed by an appropriate neck dissection.

Before radiation therapy, a thorough dental assessment is mandatory with essential treatment performed as necessary.

Small tumours of the nasopharynx (T1-T2N0M0) can be adequately treated with radiation alone. A dose of 70 Gray (Gy) in 33 to 35 fractions or the biological equivalent should be given to the primary site and grossly involved nodes. The majority of nasopharyngeal tumours will, given their advanced staging and comorbidity permitting, be managed with concurrent chemoradiation. The nasopharynx is the one head and neck site where concurrent chemoradiation has been more readily adopted internationally due in part to the Intergroup 0099 Study. This study compared concurrent chemoradiation and adjuvant chemotherapy with RT alone and showed a significant advantage in survival with the combined modality approach. The control arm was particularly inferior, however, when compared with other studies. Further studies and a recent metaanalysis by Blanchard et al. (2021) has, however, supported the concurrent chemoradiation approach and that the addition of induction or adjuvant chemotherapy to concomitant chemotherapy improves further tumour control and survival. The most frequently used concurrent regimen is cisplatin, 100 mg/m^2, on days 1, 22 and 43 of RT and results in an improvement in overall survival of 6% at 5 years compared with RT alone.

Radiation Technique

The technique of Ho formed the basis of the two-dimensional approach to treating nasopharyngeal carcinoma. Treatment fields were vast but adapted according to local staging. Determination of the primary clinical target volume is now very much individualised based on all clinical information, and using intensity modulated radiotherapy (IMRT) facilitates comprehensive coverage while sparing radiosensitive neuronal structures and the salivary glands. The pattern of spread outlined earlier dictates that the whole cervical lymphatic chain should be outlined and treated as routine, although doses prescribed will be determined by whether they are overtly involved and proximal to the primary site or more distal and clinically uninvolved. In other words, even in early cases, at least prophylactic doses of radiation should be given to all nodes. Guidelines with international consensus have recently been published by Lee et al. (2018), which should lead to standardisation and optimisation of volume definitions.

A full head and neck immobilisation device is mandatory, with the shoulders kept well down. A tongue depressor may be used, although sparing of some of the oral cavity, and thus minor salivary glands can be achieved with IMRT. The consensus guidelines suggest tight (5-mm) margins to the primary gross tumour volume (GTV) as the high-dose margin, and lesser doses to the remainder of the nasopharynx. The clinical target volume (CTV) will need to include all areas of potential spread including into the base of the skull and the nerve root foramina. There are many normal tissues to be delineated to optimise sparing including the brainstem, optic nerves and chiasm. The doses recommended are 70 Gy in 33 to 35 fractions given 5 times per week or 65 Gy in 30 fractions, both using 6-MV photons (see Figs. 23.3–23.8).

Complications

The significant volumes of normal tissue ordinarily irradiated can give rise to a range of long-term sequelae. IMRT facilitates salivary

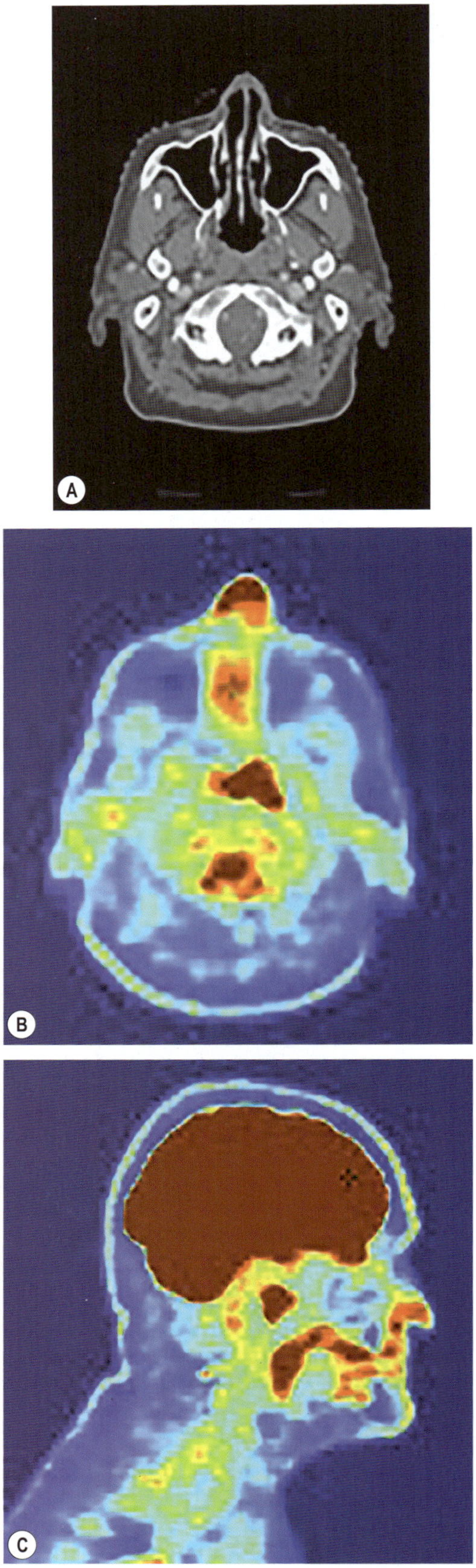

Fig. 23.3 (A) Planning computed tomography scan with complete response to induction chemotherapy. (B) Coregistered diagnostic positron emission tomography–computed tomography (PET/CT) scan prechemotherapy showing a left-sided nasopharyngeal tumour in the axial plane. (C) Coregistered diagnostic PET/CT scan prechemotherapy showing a left-sided nasopharyngeal tumour in the sagittal plane.

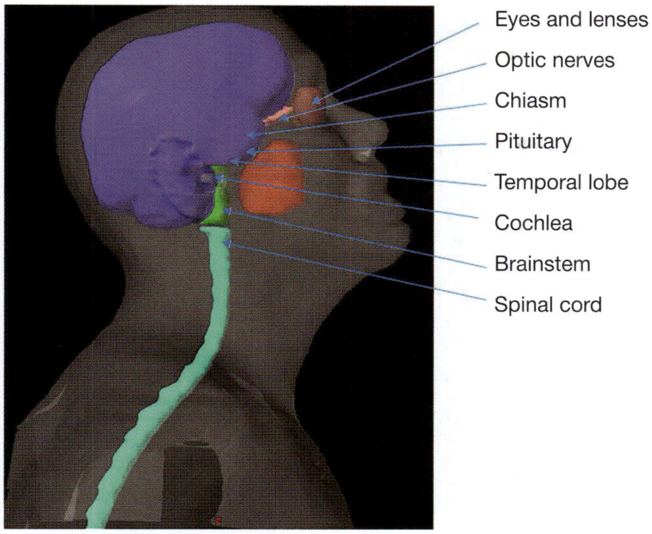

Fig. 23.4 Primary site and proximity to normal tissues.

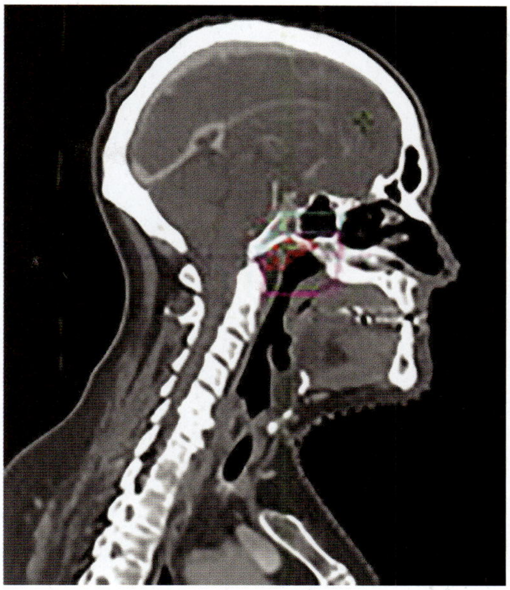

Fig. 23.6 Lower 'prophylactic' dose clinical target volume including part of the sphenoid sinus and clivus in the sagittal plane.

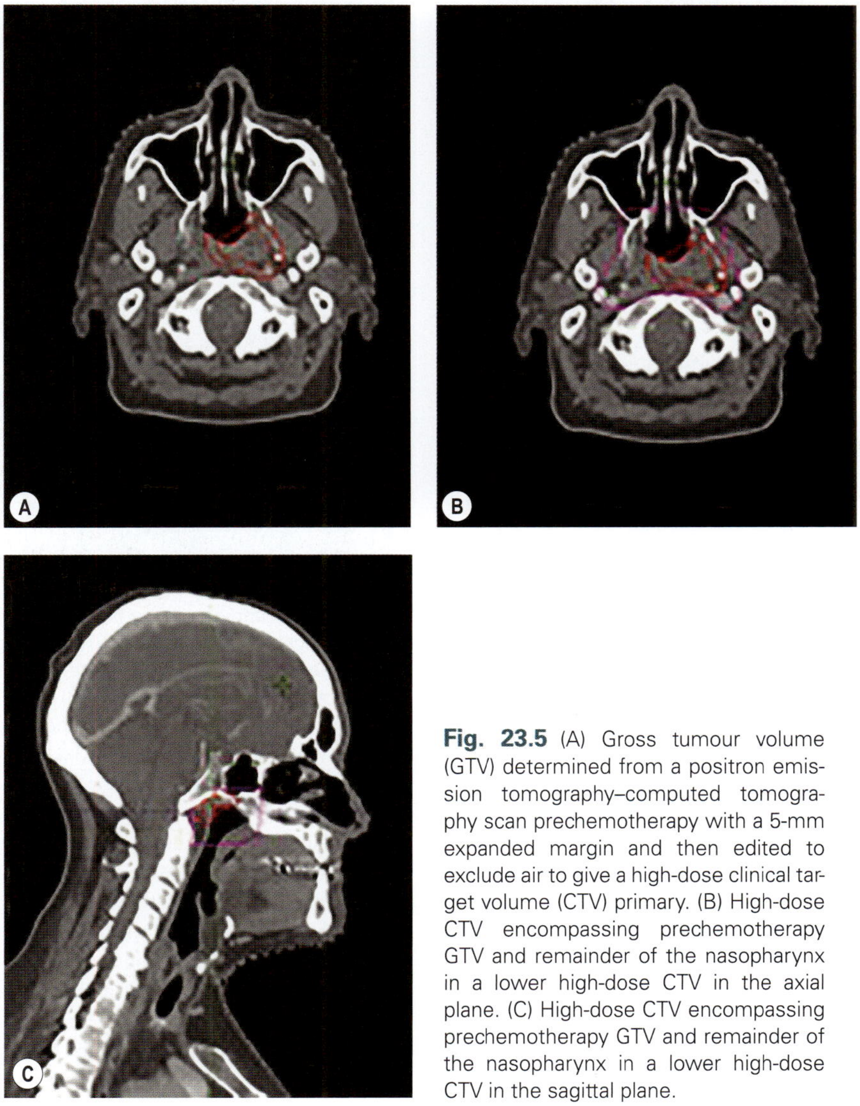

Fig. 23.5 (A) Gross tumour volume (GTV) determined from a positron emission tomography–computed tomography scan prechemotherapy with a 5-mm expanded margin and then edited to exclude air to give a high-dose clinical target volume (CTV) primary. (B) High-dose CTV encompassing prechemotherapy GTV and remainder of the nasopharynx in a lower high-dose CTV in the axial plane. (C) High-dose CTV encompassing prechemotherapy GTV and remainder of the nasopharynx in a lower high-dose CTV in the sagittal plane.

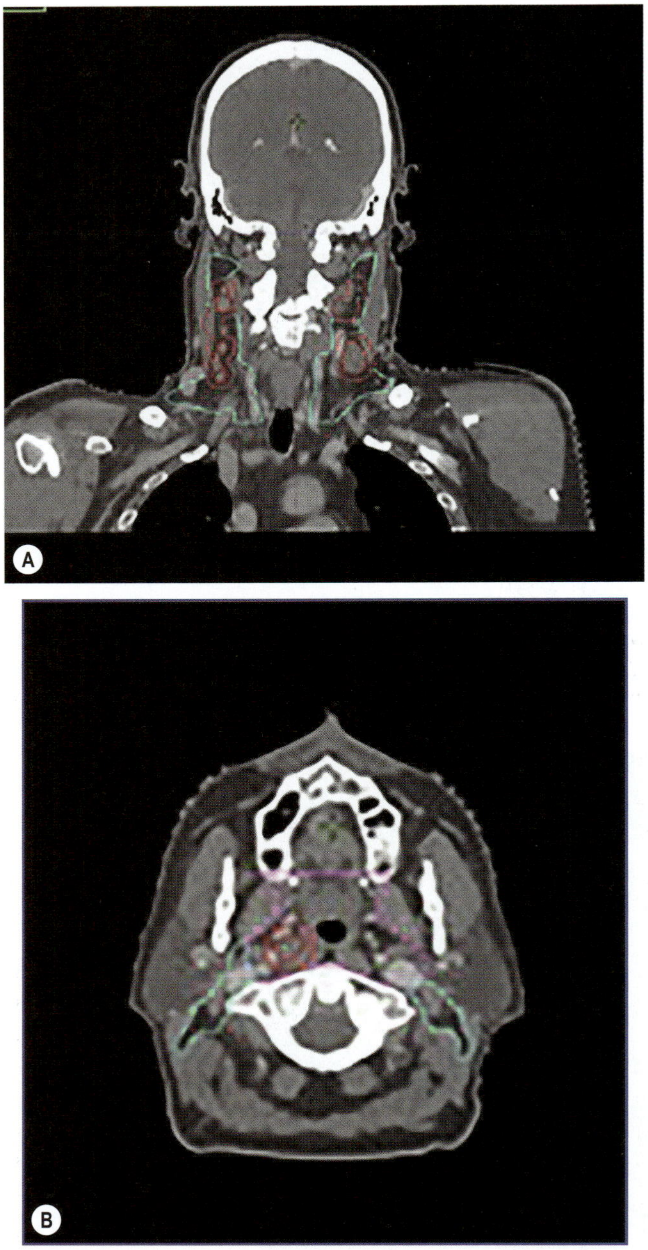

Fig. 23.7 (A) Neck node volumes in the coronal plane with post-chemotherapy nodal volumes in a high-dose clinical target volume (CTV) and remainder of the neck nodes receiving lower prophylactic doses. (B) Neck node volumes in the axial plane with postchemotherapy nodal volumes in a high-dose CTV (right retropharyngeal node) and remainder of the neck nodes receiving lower prophylactic doses.

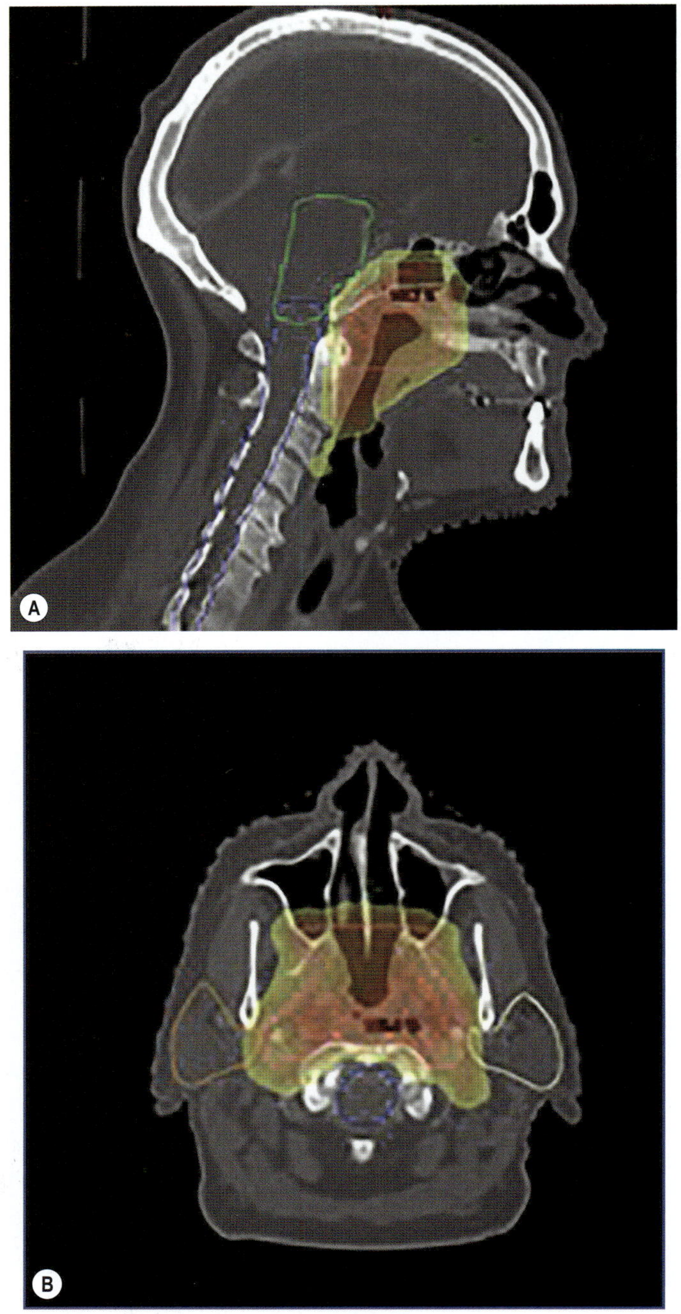

Fig. 23.8 (A) Dose distribution in the sagittal plane encompassing three dose levels spanning prechemotherapy primary gross tumour volume (GTV), clinical target volume (CTV) nasopharynx and prophylactically into the sphenoid sinus and clivus. Note the proximity to the brainstem and spinal cord planning risk volumes. (B) Dose distribution in the axial plane encompassing three dose levels spanning prechemotherapy primary GTV, CTV nasopharynx and prophylactically into the clivus.

gland sparing and while not avoiding chronic xerostomia completely, significantly reduces this without compromising irradiation of adjacent lymph nodes. IMRT also facilitates sparing of other normal tissues, enabling risk reduction of long term sequelae.

High doses of radiation may be delivered to elements of the mandible. As a consequence, there are risks of osteoradionecrosis (ORN) and preventive measures beyond meticulous radiation technique should be adopted. Moreover, the proximity of the pterygoid muscles to the primary target volume will give rise to trismus, and jaw exercises should be encouraged to minimise this.

Endocrine failure as a result of irradiation of the pituitary and thyroid glands, although relatively easy to treat, is a not uncommon outcome in long-term survivors and should be actively sought through routine testing in the follow-up of these patients.

Advanced tumours with extension into the skull base introduce additional tissues exposed to the high doses of radiation that will be necessary to achieve local control. Aspects of the temporal lobes, optic nerves and chiasm and middle and inner ear will be irradiated and, as a consequence, are at risk of late neurological damage. Careful attention to tolerance doses as determined by the QUANTEC data (Chapter 22) should minimise this risk.

Follow-up

Patients should be assessed clinically with endoscopic examination and neck palpation. There is no consensus on the best mode of radiological assessment to determine the completeness of response to treatment. MRI and/or PET/CT scans may have added value.

Results

Effective treatment of early (stage 1–2) tumours of the nasopharynx should give rise to 5-year overall survival rates of 80% to 90%. More advanced tumours, when treated optimally, will result in 5-year survival rates of the order of 50% to 70%.

Late recurrences are recognised, suggesting that follow-up beyond 5 years might be prudent and/or advising patients and primary care practitioners of this so that patients can be referred again without delay. Recurrent disease may, on occasion, be amenable to reirradiation as long as volumes to be treated are relatively small and the patient is prepared to accept the additional risks associated with such an approach. Surgery may be used for small disease in the nasopharynx and for nodal relapses.

NOSE AND NASAL CAVITY

Anatomy

The external nose is like the tip of an iceberg, with a complex array of passageways and air cavities within it that form the nasal cavity and paranasal sinuses. The hair-bearing entrance that forms the vestibule and the mucociliary escalator provides an important initial defence against the inhalation of germs (Fig. 23.9).

The nasal vestibule lies within the aperture of the nostril. It is bounded laterally by cartilage that forms the nasal ala, medially by cartilage that forms the columella and inferiorly by the most anterior portion of the floor of the nose. Importantly, this area is lined by squamous epithelium as an extension from the outside skin.

The nasal cavity or nasal fossa proper lies between the maxillary sinus inferiorly and the eyes and ethmoidal sinus superiorly. It is divided into two by a midline cartilaginous septum.

Superior Wall

The superior wall is composed of the cribriform plate of the ethmoidal sinus. The olfactory apparatus that lies here provides us with our sense of smell.

Inferior Wall

Broader than the superior wall, the inferior wall is formed from the hard palate.

Anterior Wall

The nasal bones and cartilage that form the external nose give rise to the anterior wall.

Posterior Wall

The posterior border of the hard palate and maxillary sinus gives an open passage into the nasopharynx.

Lateral Wall

Three turbinates overlie the lateral wall, which itself is formed from the medial walls of the maxillary sinus inferiorly and the ethmoid sinus superiorly.

Incidence

Many cancer registries combine nasal, paranasal and middle ear tumours together when reporting incidence, as all three types are rare. The incidence of all three types combined is 1:100,000 per year. About two-thirds of all cases arise in the sinuses, giving a true incidence of nasal cancer of about 0.3:100,000. The nasal vestibule is the most common site of origin. Males who have worked in the chromium industry (Glasgow/Teeside, England) or nickel refining (South Wales) are at increased risk of developing this rare cancer. Chromate-induced cancers are often accompanied by a septal perforation.

Staging System

The system used for the nasal cavity is identical to that for ethmoidal sinus tumours in view of the anatomical relationship of these two structures.

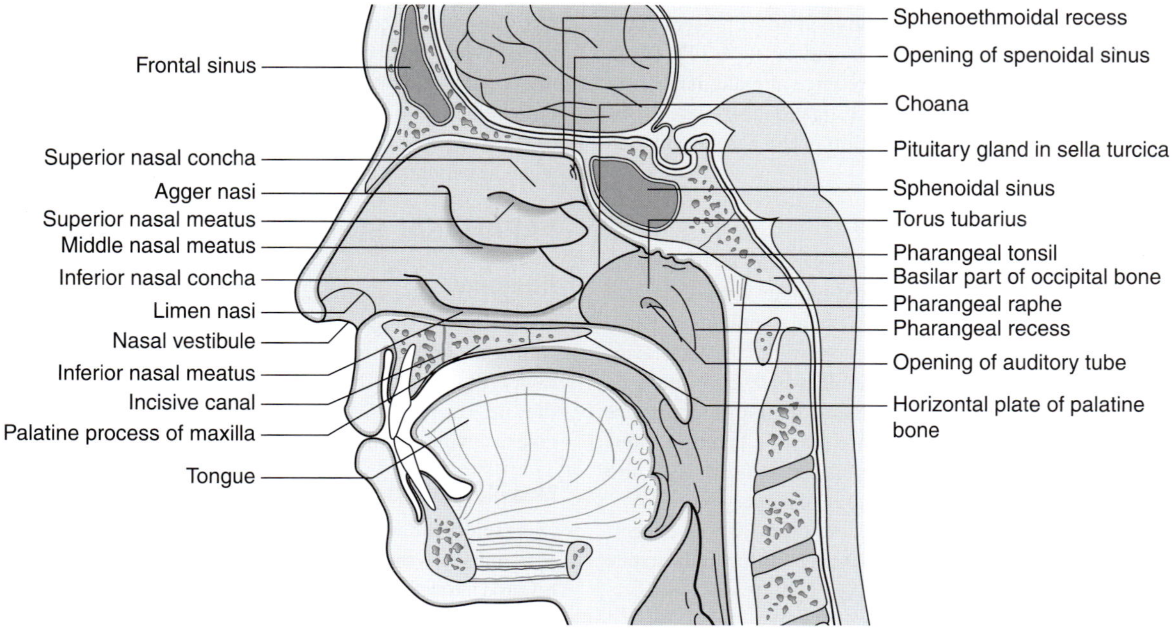

Fig. 23.9 Nose and nasal cavity anatomy.

T1	Tumour restricted to one subsite of the nasal cavity with or without bony invasion
T2	Tumour involves two subsites in a single site or extends to involve an adjacent site within the nasoethmoidal complex, with or without bony invasion
T3	Tumour extends to invade the medial wall or floor of the orbit, maxillary sinus, palate or cribriform plate
T4A	Tumour invades any of the following: anterior orbital contents, skin of nose or cheek, minimal extension to anterior cranial fossa, pterygoid plates, sphenoid or frontal sinuses
T4B	Tumour invades any of the following: orbital apex, dura, brain, middle cranial fossa, cranial nerves other than V2, nasopharynx or clivus

Aetiology, Pathology and Lymphatic Spread

The normal lining of the nasal cavity is pseudostratified columnar ciliated epithelium except for the vestibule, as mentioned earlier, that comprises squamous epithelium with sweat and sebaceous glands.

The aetiology of true nasal cavity tumours is not dissimilar to that of the paranasal sinuses with many environmental factors being implicated. Smoking is associated with the most common histological subtype seen. Such SCCs arise most commonly at the lateral wall.

Other histologies comprise the remaining 20% and include adenocarcinoma, adenoid cystic carcinoma, melanoma, lymphoma, plasmacytoma and sarcoma. Inverted papillomas, themselves rare, can transform or coexist with SCC. Olfactory neuroblastomas (esthesioneuroblastomas) arise from the olfactory tissue at the level of the cribriform plate. Basal cell carcinomas can arise in the vestibule.

The lymphatic drainage of the nasal cavity can be usefully divided into two. The main part of the nasal cavity drains via the nasopharynx to the retropharyngeal nodes and upper deep cervical nodes (levels 2). The lower anterior portion drains additionally to the submandibular (level 1B) and buccofacial nodes (level 9).

Signs and Symptoms

Unlike paranasal sinus tumours, these tumours tend to present comparatively early with obstructive symptoms and epistaxis. However, symptoms of benign disease can blur the presence of malignancy, and SCCs of the lateral wall may, on further investigation, be a late manifestation of maxillary sinus disease. Inspection of the nasal cavity will typically reveal a fleshy outgrowth.

Diagnosis and Staging

Biopsy of the suspected lesion is required. A polypoidal lesion may be snared off and may give rise to an unsuspected tumour when examined pathologically. It may be necessary to perform a lateral rhinotomy to obtain adequate exposure and surgical evaluation of lesions within the nasal cavity.

Except for the small tumour of the vestibule, which can usually be demarcated in the clinic, tumours of the nasal fossa proper require thorough staging with CT and/or MRI. Care must be taken in interpreting benign secretions from malignant infiltration of soft tissue and bone invasion as this may impact on the degree of surgery.

Certain tumour types, for example, adenoid cystic as well as lymphoma, will require exclusion of distal involvement as this may dictate local management.

Treatment

Small tumours of the vestibule can be managed by either surgery or RT. The choice will in part be based on the expected cosmetic outcome.

More advanced tumours of the vestibule or those of the nasal fossa proper will usually require surgical clearance, often followed by RT, especially if it is an SCC in view of the propensity for bone invasion. Lymphomas and plasmacytomas can be managed by primary RT at appropriate doses with or without the addition of chemotherapy.

Inoperable nasal cavity tumours should be managed by combined chemoradiation according to the comorbidity of the patient.

Radiotherapy Technique

Tumours of the vestibule and low anterior nasal fossa tumours may be treated by a direct anterior appositional electron beam or with photons. Given the relatively superficial nature of such tumours, some bolus material is likely to ensure adequate surface dose. Consideration will need to be given to transmission of dose through air spaces.

More advanced tumours and those within the nasal fossa proper frequently require an approach similar to that used for maxillary sinus tumours using IMRT and doses up to 65 Gy in 30 fractions.

CT planning for all but the most superficial tumours facilitates accurate tumour definition and normal tissue avoidance. The true CTV may extend much more posteriorly than initially envisaged and therefore needs to be considered to minimise late relapse as a result of target volume selection.

As with all head and neck tumours, good immobilisation is required. A mouth bite may be used to move the tongue away from the treatment volume (Figs. 23.10–23.12).

Complications

Superficial tumours will inevitably manifest acute skin reactions that usually heal promptly. In the longer term, atrophy of the nasal cartilage may result in some loss of the original nasal profile.

Deeper tumours managed with techniques similar to that used for paranasal sinus tumours may be complicated by damage to the normal tissues in the vicinity. Atrophy of the nasal lining will result in dryness and a tendency towards the development of crusts. Regular use of a saline spray helps to address this. Epiphora will result if there is stenosis of the nasolacrimal duct.

Results

The diversity of pathologies at this site and the relative rarity even of SCC of the nasal cavity give rise to only limited outcome data. Nonetheless, early SCC of the vestibule can be expected to result in cure rates on the order of 80% to 90% at 5 years. More advanced tumours of the vestibule and fossa proper will give rise to cure rates on the order of 40% to 60%. Olfactory neuroblastomas carry a better prognosis, whereas patients with mucosal melanomas generally fare badly.

PARANASAL SINUS TUMOURS

Anatomy

The paranasal sinuses comprise four pairs of linked hollow cavities within the anterior and midportions of the skull that link to the nasal cavity (Fig. 23.13). They are named according to the bone within which they lie. The purpose of the paranasal sinuses is to lighten the bone and give resonance to the voice.

Maxillary Sinuses

Lying under the eyes, these sinuses are pyramidal in shape. The base of the pyramid forms the lateral wall of the nasal cavity, with the apex extending towards the zygomatic process. The superior aspect comprises the floor of the orbit and the ethmoidal sinus, whereas the inferior extent is that of the alveolar process and typically lies just below the floor of the nasal cavity. The infraorbital nerve traverses the roof of the sinus, whereas the first and second molar teeth typically project into the sinus floor. The posterior

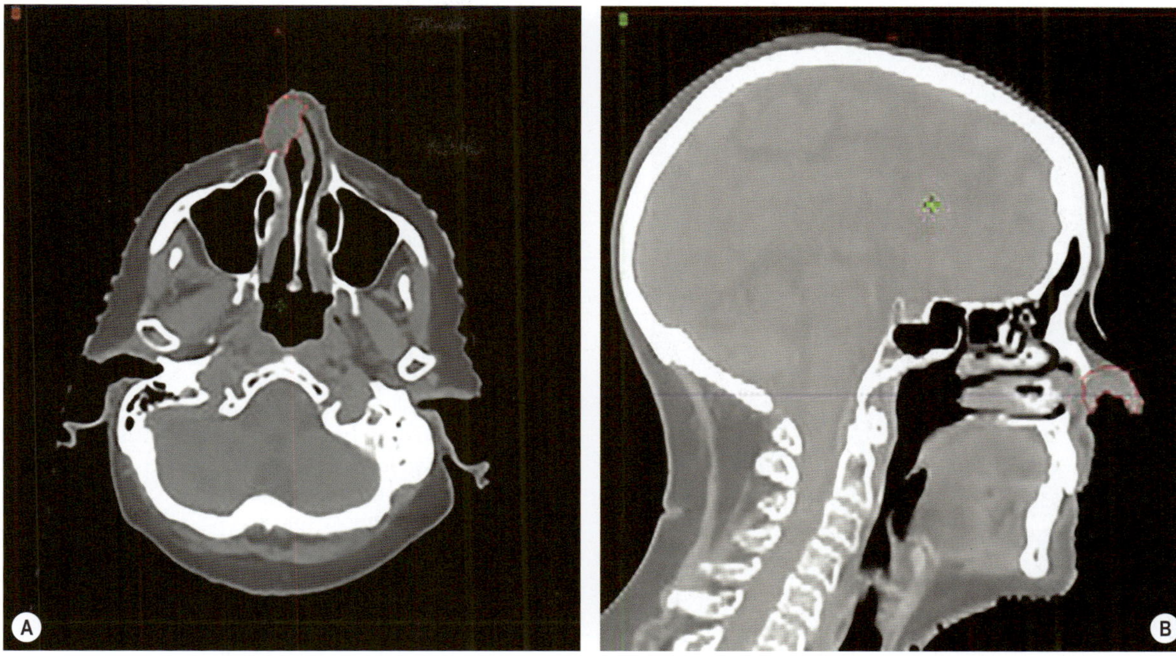

Fig. 23.10 (A) Gross tumour volume (GTV) in the axial plane. (B) GTV in the sagittal plane.

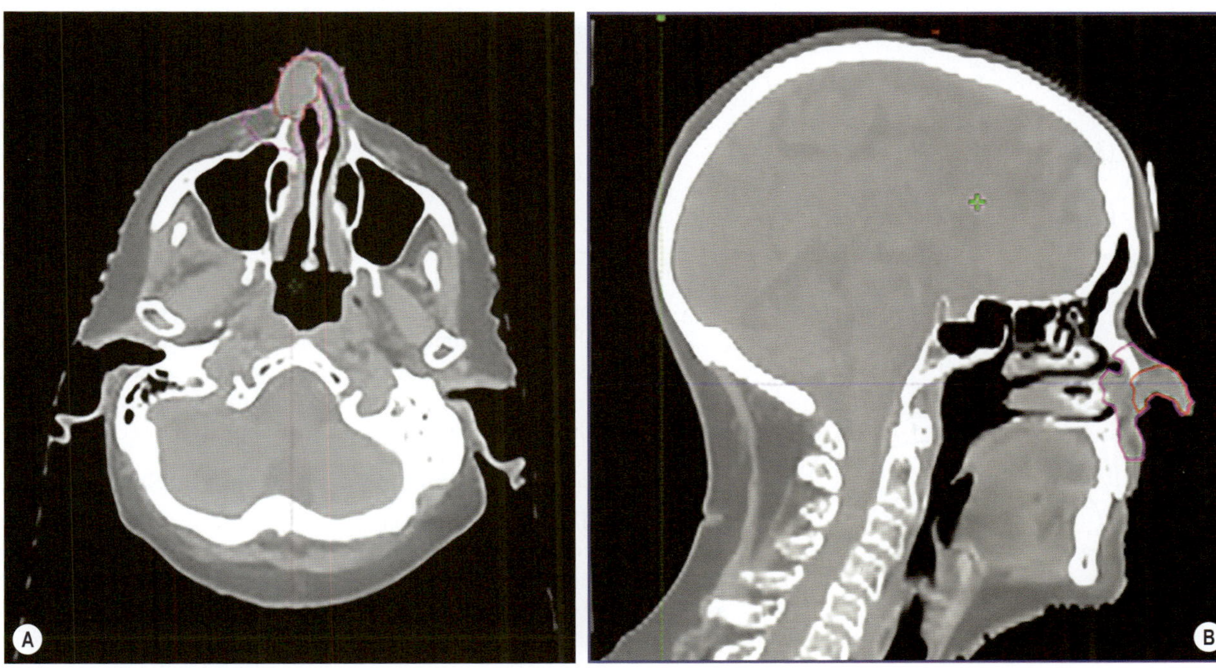

Fig. 23.11 (A) Clinical target volume (CTV) expanded 10 mm in the axial plane. (B) CTV expanded 10 mm in the sagittal plane.

wall abuts the infratemporal and pterygopalatine fossae. The maxillary sinus drains via the ostium maxillare beneath the middle concha.

Frontal Sinus

Lying over the eyes in the frontal bones, these sinuses only reach full size after puberty. They drain into the nasal cavity through the middle meatus beneath the middle concha via the frontonasal duct.

Ethmoid Sinus

Lying on either side of the upper part of the nasal cavity and between the orbits, these sinuses are grouped into three portions: the anterior and middle drain into the nasal cavity via the middle meatus, and the posterior drains via the superior meatus beneath the superior concha. A thin bony lamina (the lamina papyracea) separates the sinus from the orbital and nasal cavities. The optic nerve lies posteriorly to the sinus and the anterior cranial fossa lies superiorly.

Sphenoid Sinus

Lying deep in the skull base beneath the pituitary gland, this sinus, which also develops mainly after puberty, drains into the nasal cavity via the sphenoethmoidal recess above the superior concha of the nasal cavity. The nasopharynx lies inferiorly and the nasal cavity

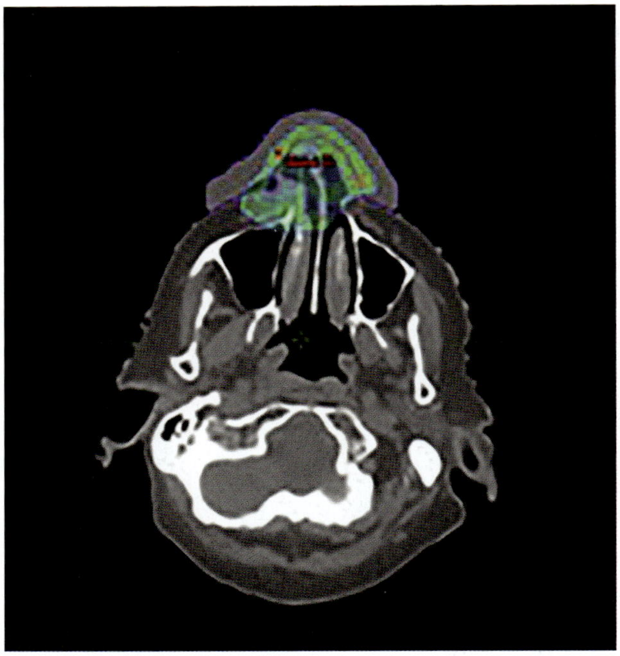

Fig. 23.12 Dose distribution on the axial plane. Note the use of physical bolus to optimise the surface dose.

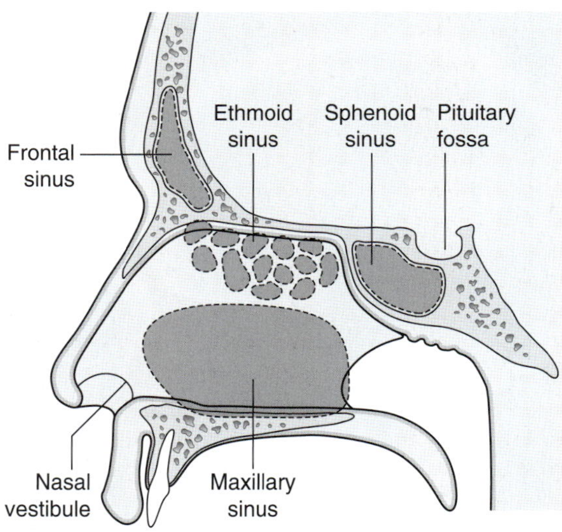

Fig. 23.13 Paranasal sinus anatomy.

anteriorly to the sinus, whereas the optic nerve and cavernous sinuses lie laterally.

Incidence of Paranasal Sinus Tumours

These tumours are rare, with a crude incidence of less than 1/100,000 people per year. Most tumours arise in the maxillary sinus; less commonly, in the ethmoid sinus. Tumours arising de novo in the frontal and sphenoidal sinuses are especially rare. Frequently, multiple sinuses are involved at presentation.

Staging System for Paranasal Sinus Tumours

The TNM system (8th edition) as described here is only applicable to maxillary sinus tumours. The ethmoidal sinuses are classified separately. There is no formal system that applies to tumours of the sphenoidal and frontal sinuses. The N component is as elsewhere for head and neck SCCs.

	Maxillary Sinus	Ethmoidal Sinus
T1	Mucosa only, with no erosion or destruction of bone	One subsite with or without bony invasion
T2	Bone erosion/destruction including extension into the hard palate and/or middle meatus, except extension to the posterior wall of the maxillary sinus and pterygoid plates	Two subsites with or without bony invasion
T3	Bone erosion/destruction of the posterior wall of the maxillary sinus, involvement of the subcutaneous tissues, floor or medial wall of the orbit, pterygoid fossa and ethmoid sinuses	Involvement of the medial wall or floor of the orbit, maxillary sinus, palate or cribriform plate
T4A	Involvement of the anterior orbital contents, skin of the cheek, pterygoid plates, infratemporal fossa, cribriform plate, sphenoidal or frontal sinuses	Involvement of the anterior orbital contents, skin of the cheek, infratemporal fossa, cribriform plate, sphenoidal or frontal sinuses
T4B	Involvement of the orbital apex, dura, brain, middle cranial fossa, cranial nerves (excluding the second division of the Vth cranial nerve), nasopharynx or clivus	Involvement of the orbital apex, dura, brain, middle cranial fossa, cranial nerves (excluding the second division of the Vth cranial nerve), nasopharynx or clivus

Although it does not form part of the TNM staging system, division of maxillary sinus lesions into those arising from the infrastructure—that is, anteroinferiorly—from lesions arising from the suprastructure which lie superoposteriorly, is potentially useful. This division arises from a theoretical line drawn from the medial canthus to the angle of the mandible in a lateral plane (Ohngren's line) (Fig. 23.14).

Aetiology, Pathology and Lymphatic Spread

The healthy sinuses are lined with ciliated columnar epithelium. SCCs comprise the most common histological subtype and, as with other head and neck SCCs, are associated with smoking and, to a lesser extent, excess alcohol. Adenocarcinomas, particularly of the ethmoid sinus, occur and are associated with hardwood furniture manufacturers. Other tumour types include adenoid cystic carcinoma, melanoma and lymphoma.

The lymph system is remarkably sparse and, as such, tumours can be quite advanced without involved nodes. The corollary is that it is rare to present with neck nodes from an unsuspected primary located in the paranasal sinuses. Lymphatic drainage is typically towards the retropharyngeal (Rouvière's node) and upper deep cervical nodes (level II) unless the tumour is particularly anteriorly placed when the buccinator (now referred to as level IX) and level I nodes are at risk as well.

Signs and Symptoms

The complex anatomical relationship with neighboring structures is reflected in the diverse presenting features of these tumours. On the other hand, the air cavities permit substantial expansion and, as such,

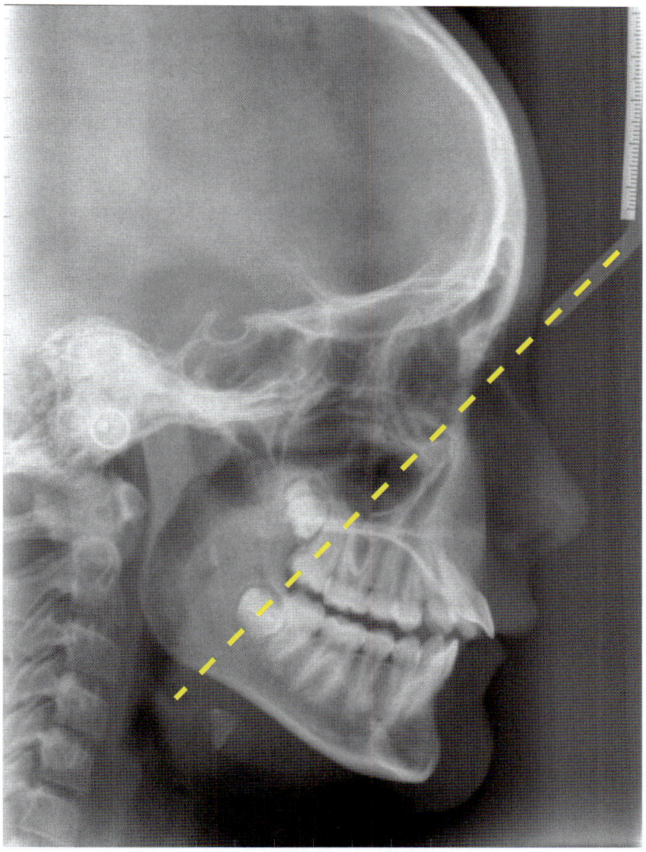

Fig. 23.14 Radiograph illustrating Ohngren's line dividing the suprastructure and infrastructure of the paranasal sinuses.

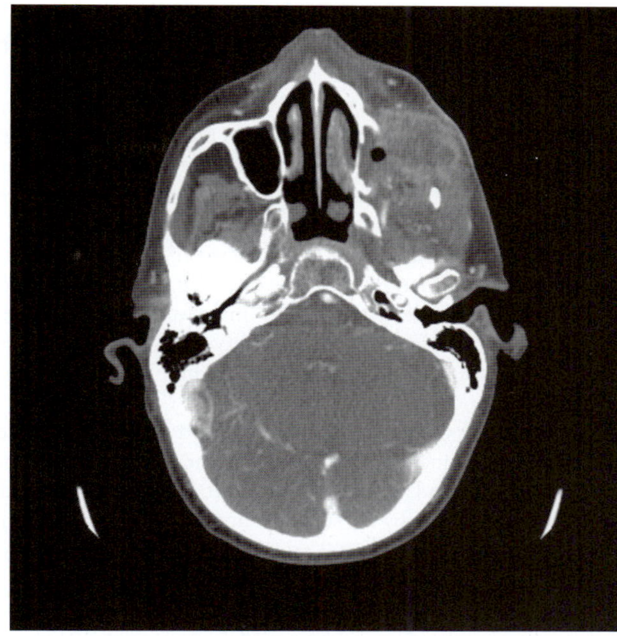

Fig. 23.15 Extensive tumour of the left paranasal sinus territory with extension into subcutaneous tissues and infratemporal fossa.

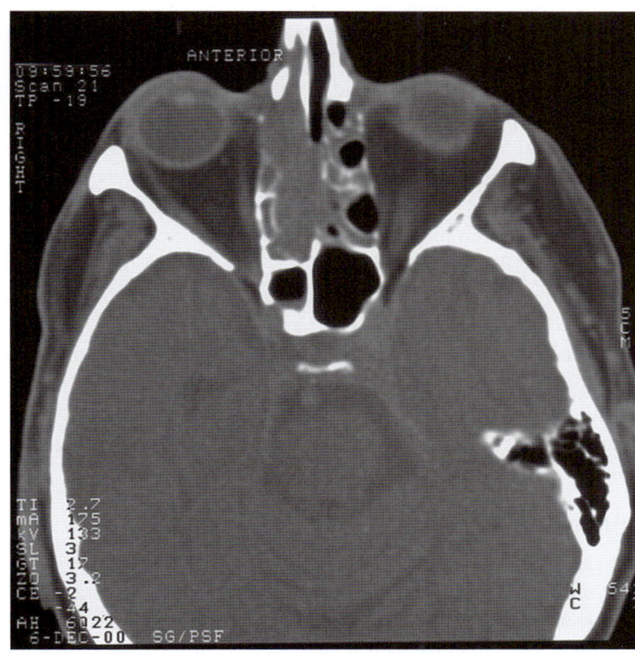

Fig. 23.16 Ethmoid sinus tumour showing close proximity to the optic nerve and chiasma.

these tumours often present late, the early symptoms blurring with benign inflammatory disease.

Maxillary sinus tumours present with symptoms and signs related to the mode of expansion of the tumour: inferiorly, pain related to teeth and ulceration may manifest, whereas inferoposteriorly, there is trismus (Fig. 23.15), superiorly, proptosis and diplopia; medially, there may be nasal stuffiness with discharge, which may not necessarily be bloody; anteriorly and laterally, a soft-tissue mass may emerge in the cheek. If the infraorbital nerve is involved, there will be numbness of the cheek and upper lip.

Ethmoidal sinus tumours frequently present with nasal obstruction. There may, in addition, be a discharge, which again may not be blood stained. Less commonly, there may be bone expansion overlying the superior aspect of the nose (Fig. 23.16). Loss of smell is often overlooked and may indicate tumour.

Bearing in mind the rarity of primary tumours of the sphenoidal sinus, these will typically present with deep-seated pain, often referred to the vertex of the skull, and there may be associated cranial nerve palsies. Frontal sinus tumours may simply present with bony swelling.

Diagnosis and Staging

Initial assessment in the clinic should comprise a thorough examination including the use of a nasal speculum and upper airway endoscopy. The oral cavity must be inspected. A mass may be readily apparent and a sample taken for histological assessment. An examination under anaesthesia will invariably be required.

Plain x-rays may demonstrate bony erosion, but a CT and MRI scan will ultimately both be required to define this more precisely as well as locoregional staging generally. CT scanning gives excellent bony detail whereas MRI scanning gives better distinction of tumour from adjacent soft tissues. Care must be exercised in the interpretation of signal changes on MRI which may reflect inflammatory disease (which often coexists). An orthopantomogram (OPG) will assist in the assessment of tooth preservation.

Treatment

Surgical options include endoscopic resection, craniofacial resection and maxillectomy with or without orbital exenteration or a combination of both. The type of surgery will be determined by the site, tumour type, stage of the tumour and surgical intent. As a general rule, though, surgery and postoperative RT will be indicated for tumours of the maxillary and ethmoidal sinuses except for the rare T1 lesion with complete clearance. Surgery will comprise a partial or total maxillectomy (depending on location and extent), ethmoidectomy and/or sphenoidectomy. Vascularised flap reconstruction is now favoured over obturating the cavity left with a prosthesis, as the quality of life appears improved in such patients and the early concerns of lack of direct viewing of the cavity have been superseded by more advanced imaging in follow-up.

RT may be given as definitive therapy for very advanced disease typically with chemotherapy in fit patients. The role of induction chemotherapy is less clear, but it may improve locoregional disease control and reduce surgical morbidity. On occasion, surgery may follow RT in advanced tumours where there has been a good response.

RT when given postoperatively is delivered to the operative bed comprising the original location of the tumour and known and potential areas of spread. In the definitive setting, the volume irradiated will be determined by all staging information available to the clinician.

Radiotherapy Technique

An immobilisation device should be used. Care should be taken in achieving the optimal head position. In practice, it is often best for the plane of the floor of the orbit to be perpendicular to the treatment couch. A tongue depressor may be used and facilitates movement of the tongue inferiorly *away* from the treatment volume. A full head and neck shell over the shoulders should be used.

Volumes should be delineated on a contrast-enhanced planning CT scan. For postoperative RT, this will include the surgical bed and, given that these tumours are often at an advanced stage, necessitates large volumes of irradiation. Cervical neck nodes should be irradiated to at least prophylactic doses in more advanced cases (i.e. T3/4). Coregistration of images is invaluable in the process of volume delineation. IMRT is the standard of care, given its ability to improve target-volume coverage and sparing of adjacent normal tissues (Figs. 23.17 and 23.18).

The doses used will be determined by treatment intent. Gross disease postoperatively and when used in the definitive setting will demand a higher dose (i.e. 70 Gy in 35 fractions or 65–66 Gy in 30 fractions), with consideration to irradiation of critical normal tissues, even with IMRT techniques.

Complications

The biggest risk with treatment of paranasal sinus tumours is lack of local control, given the generally advanced nature at presentation. On the other hand, those patients who do survive long term or are cured are at risk of treatment-related sequelae.

Late sequelae following surgery relate to fibrosis within the operated bed, potentially exacerbated by RT and issues related to any prosthesis if still used. Some degree of nasal crusting is inevitable and epiphora may occur.

RT with or without surgery will invariably result in some xerostomia as a result of the irradiation of the ipsilateral parotid gland, although some sparing is possible with IMRT. It is for that reason that any teeth remaining following resection should be in healthy condition. Trismus may result and should be actively managed with appropriate jaw exercises. Binocular blindness is a rare but catastrophic complication of maxillary sinus irradiation. Pituitary failure may emerge in long-term survivors.

Given the complex relationship of tumour and normal tissues, particularly the optic chiasm, IMRT is critical to achieve adequate normal tissue sparing.

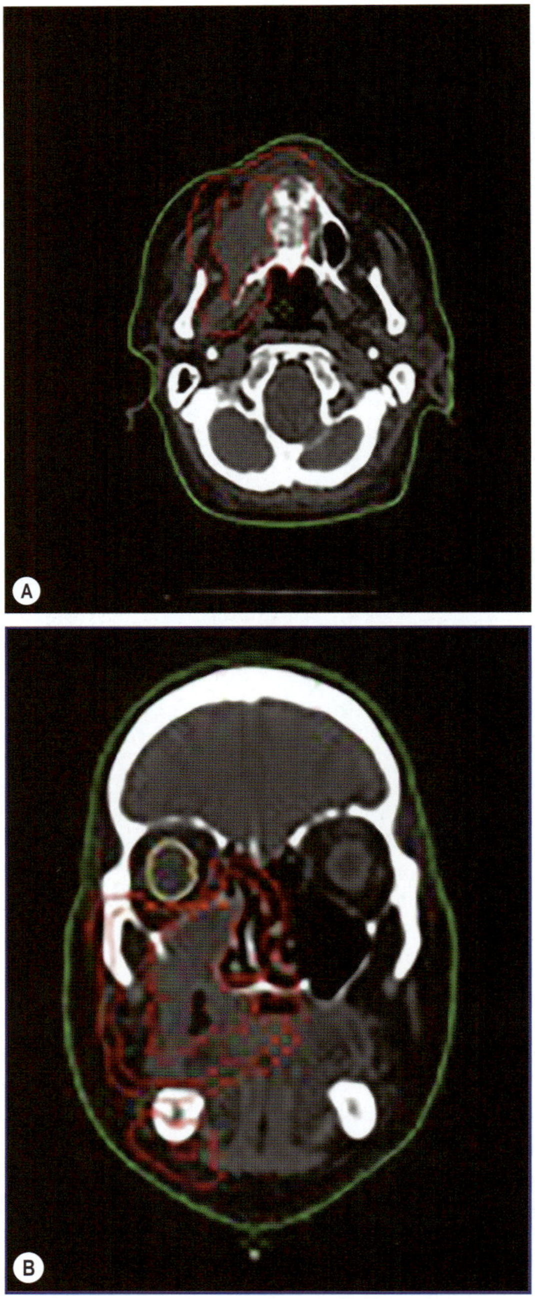

Fig. 23.17 (A) Large right-sided sinus carcinoma in the axial plane with a 10-mm margin adapted to include the whole hard palate to give a high-dose clinical target volume (CTV). (B) The same large right-sided sinus carcinoma in the coronal plane with a 10-mm margin adapted to include the nasal cavity and pterygoid fossa to give a high-dose CTV.

Follow-up

Follow-up is required to monitor for recurrence and manage any long-term sequelae. Cavities should be inspected by endoscope. Imaging with MRI and/or PET/CT has offset early reservations of the reconstructive approach obscuring direct inspection of cavities.

Results

Overall, paranasal sinus tumours lead to a 25% to 30% 5-year survival. Tumours within the infrastructure and where there is good clearance by surgery give rise to more favourable outcomes of the order of 50% 5-year survival.

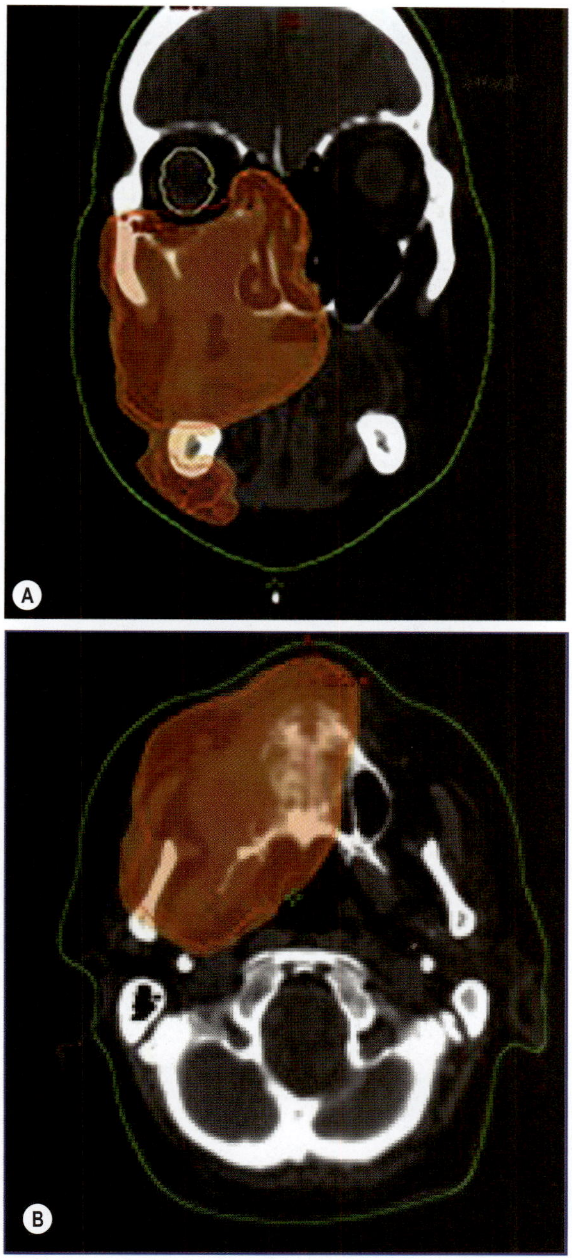

Fig. 23.18 (A) Dose distribution in the coronal plane encompassing the primary site clinical target volume (CTV) and involved upper neck node. (B) Dose distribution in the axial plane encompassing the primary site CTV.

LIP AND ORAL CAVITY CARCINOMA

Anatomy

Cancers of the lip arise from the vermilion (external) border.

The anatomical sites conventionally regarded as constituting the oral cavity are the buccal mucosa, upper and lower alveolus, retromolar trigone, hard palate, tongue (anterior two-thirds: anterior to the circumvallate papillae) and floor of the mouth.

Incidence of Oral Cavity Carcinoma

The oral tongue and then the floor of mouth are the most common subsites. Overall, they are still a rare group of cancers making up 1% to 4% of all malignancies. The incidence of mouth cancer is increasing: from 1992 to 1995, there were 8 cases per 100,000 people. That figure increased to 13 per 100,000 from 2012 to 2014. Although mouth cancer is more common in males, the ratio has fallen to 2:1 with the increasing prevalence of smoking and alcohol use in females.

Staging System for Oral Cavity and Lip Carcinoma (8th Edition)

There are changes from the 7th edition TNM insofar as depth of invasion (DOI) has been shown to be an independent prognostic factor with depths of 4 to 5 mm being an important threshold for the risk of nodal involvement. Clinicians are expected to estimate DOI from palpation. Extrinsic muscle invasion has been removed from T4 status as it has been difficult for histopathologists to define, and it lacked specificity.

T1	Tumour ≤2 cm and DOI ≤5mm
T2	Tumour ≤2 cm and DOI >5 mm but <10 mm or size 2–4 cm and DOI ≤10 mm
T3	Tumour >4 cm and DOI >10 mm
T4a	Tumour invades adjacent structures, for example, through cortical bone of the mandible or maxilla or involving the maxillary sinus or skin of the face
T4b	Tumour invades the masticator space, pterygoid plates or skull base and/or encases the internal carotid artery
N1	Single ipsilateral node ≤3 cm diameter and extranodal extension (ENE)–ve
N2A	Single ipsilateral node >3 cm ≤6 cm and ENE–ve
N2B	Multiple ipsilateral nodes ≤6 cm and ENE–ve
N2C	Bilateral or contralateral nodes ≤6 cm and ENE–ve
N3A	Any node >6 cm and ENE–ve
N3B	Any N and clinically overt ENE+ve

Aetiology, Pathology and Lymphatic Spread

Whereas tumours that occur within the oral cavity share with the majority of other upper aerodigestive tract tumours the etiological factors of exposure to alcohol and tobacco, tumours of the lip tend to be seen in patients with much exposure to sunlight, particularly smokers. Alcohol seems to be less important in the aetiology of cancers of this site. Other risk factors for oral cavity cancers include local trauma (e.g. badly fitted dentures) and leucoplakia. There is an association with betel nut, chewed in many cultures, and also with syphilis, which is still prevalent in some parts of the world.

Cancers of the lip are almost always SCCs, and over 90% of the oral cavity cancers are too. A small proportion of oral cavity tumours are adenocarcinomas or arise from the minor salivary glands of the oral cavity.

Nodal involvement in cancers of the lip occurs rarely (<5% of all cases at presentation), but the incidence is higher with large, poorly differentiated tumours or those at the angle of the mouth (Fig. 23.19). The neck nodes can be a site of potential relapse and therefore must be included in follow-up assessment. Nodal disease can be salvaged surgically but is better anticipated by sentinel node biopsy.

In oral cavity cancers, spread may be local to adjacent structures including the mandible. Nodal involvement is usually primarily to the submental and submandibular glands followed by the upper deep cervical nodes, specifically levels 1A, 1B and 2, although disease can spread directly to levels 3 and 4, so-called *skip* nodes (Fig. 23.20). Midline tumours may develop bilateral nodal spread. Retropharyngeal nodes are rarely involved in this group of cancers.

Signs and Symptoms

Lip cancers present in a similar manner to skin tumours, with visible lesions over the lip. There may be a nonhealing ulcer or persistent

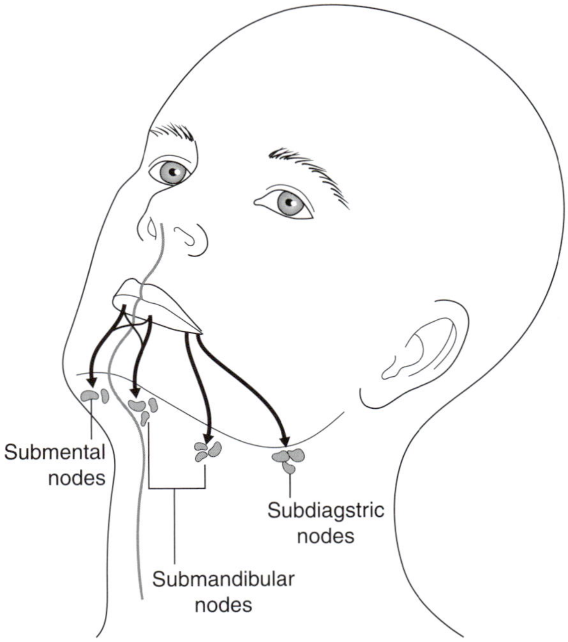

Fig. 23.19 Lymphatic drainage of the lower lip.

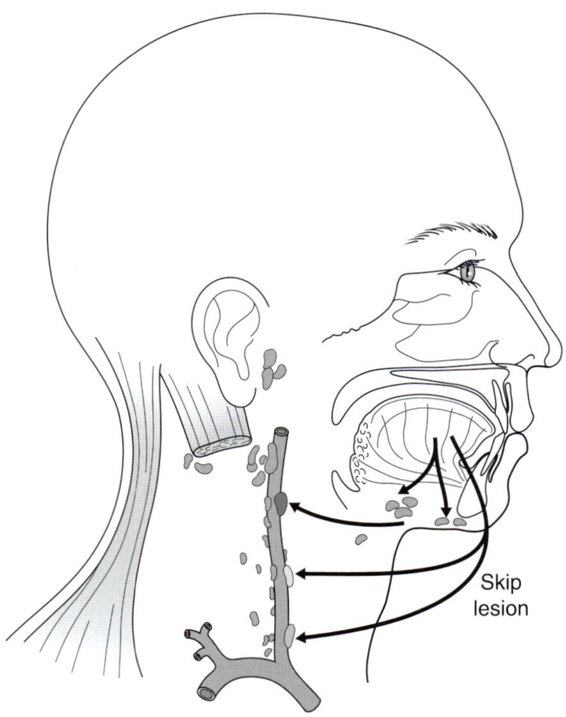

Fig. 23.20 Skip lesion.

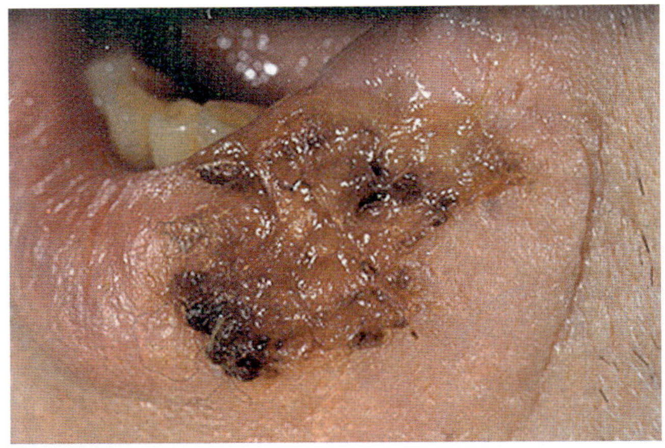

Fig. 23.21 Small-cell carcinoma of the lip.

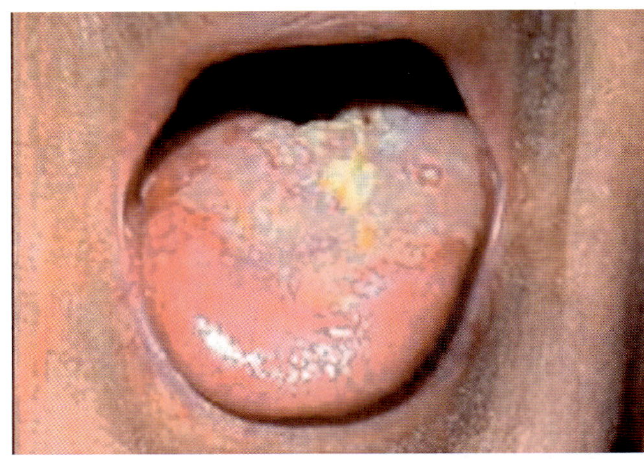

Fig. 23.22 Extensive carcinoma of the dorsum of the tongue.

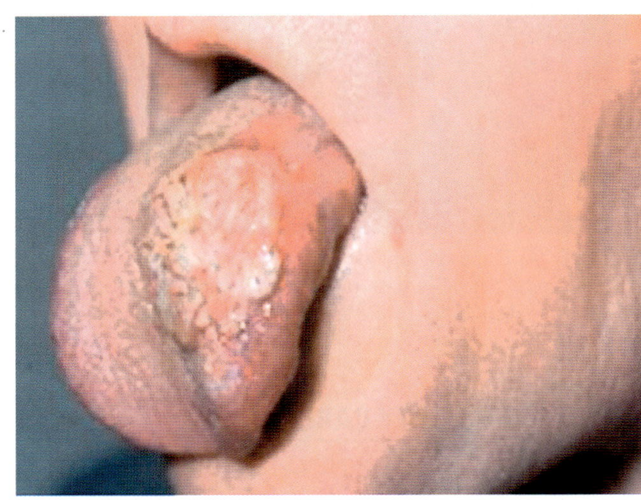

Fig. 23.23 Tumour on the left lateral edge of the tongue.

scabbing. The lesions may be ulcerative or exophytic. There can be discomfort or bleeding associated with the area and occasionally infiltration of adjacent skin or the underlying oral mucosa (Fig. 23.21).

Oral cavity cancers also commonly present with ulcerated lesions. They are often detected at dental checkup and can be associated with leucoplakia or erythroplakia. Local pain can be a symptom and, in more advanced tumours, may radiate to the ear on the involved side (Figs. 23.22 and 23.23).

Diagnosis and Staging

Patients should be referred to a specialist head and neck team for full assessment. Local examination should be performed including full inspection of the oral cavity (Figs. 23.22 and 23.23) and nasendoscopy to examine the rest of the aerodigestive tract. Imaging is required for any tumours in the anterior part of the oral cavity to exclude mandibular involvement (Figs. 23.24 and 23.25). It also assists in the assessment of dentition before any planned RT. For oral cavity tumours, CT

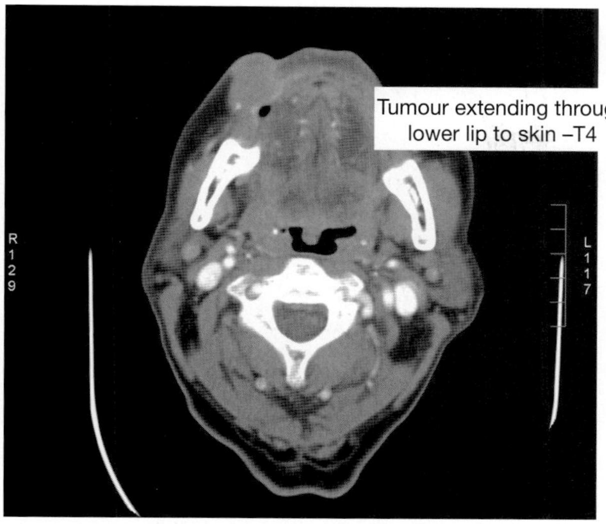

Fig. 23.24 Carcinoma of the buccal mucosa.

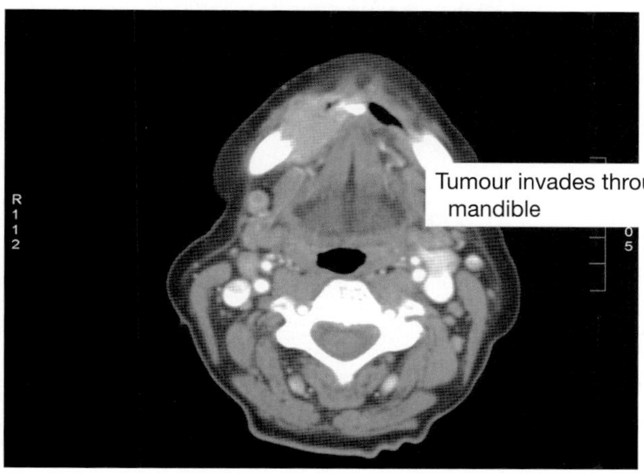

Fig. 23.25 Carcinoma of the lower alveolus.

or preferably MRI of the primary site is required to determine DOI or involvement of adjacent structures (Figs. 23.26–23.29), as with any head and neck cancer, imaging of the neck nodes and chest is required to exclude distant spread.

A biopsy of the lesion is required and can be done in the clinic or as part of an examination under anaesthetic if more detailed information about tumour extent is required.

Sentinel lymph node biopsy can be used for prognostication, staging and identification of occult nodal metastases in tumours where the primary tumour has a DOI more than 2 to 4 mm.

Treatment of Lip Cancers

Most lip cancers occur on the lower lip and, because of their conspicuous position, the majority of these tumours present relatively early and so are regularly curable. Both surgery and RT are treatment options, and the choice between the two often comes down to deciding which will give the better cosmetic/functional result. Very small superficial lesions can be treated by a lip shave, as long as an adequate deep margin is obtained. This will give a very good cosmetic result.

For larger lesions, surgery using a variety of surgical approaches, the choice of which is dependent on the size and location of the lesion and the needs for reconstruction, is preferred, although there is still a place for RT using external beam with/without brachytherapy if available (Fig. 23.30).

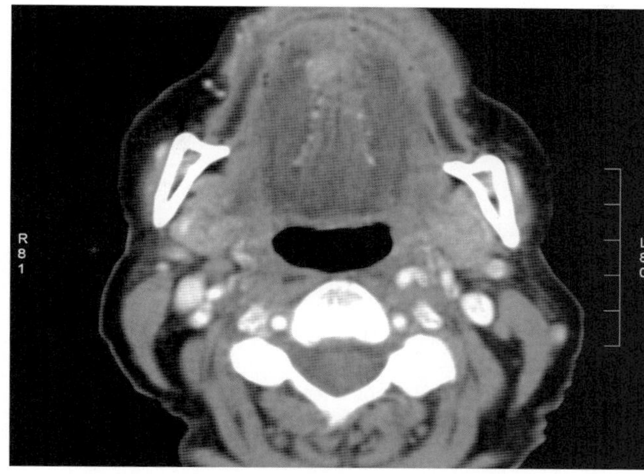

Fig. 23.26 Carcinoma of the anterior floor of the mouth.

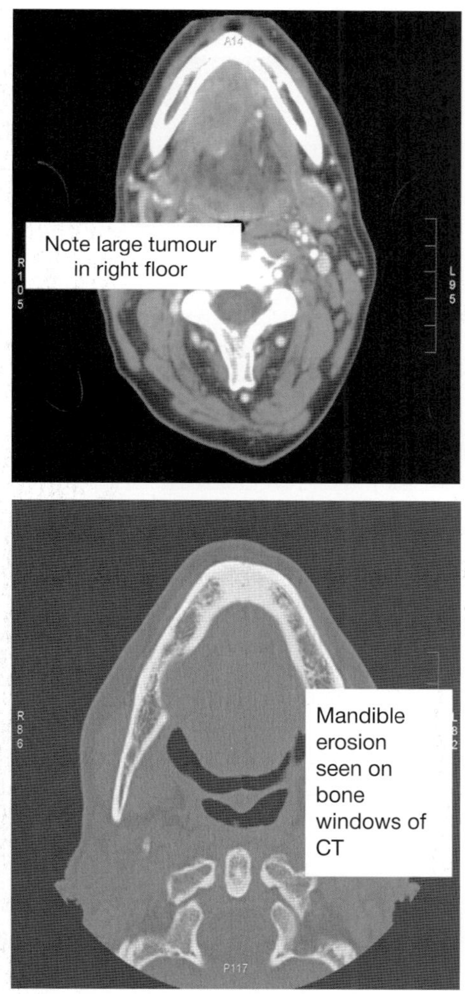

Fig. 23.27 Advanced cancer of the floor of the mouth. *CT*, Computed tomography.

Radiotherapy Technique

For small tumours, the technique will be similar to that used for skin tumours. A margin of at least 1 cm is required around the disease as assessed by inspection and palpation to arrive at a suitable CTV.

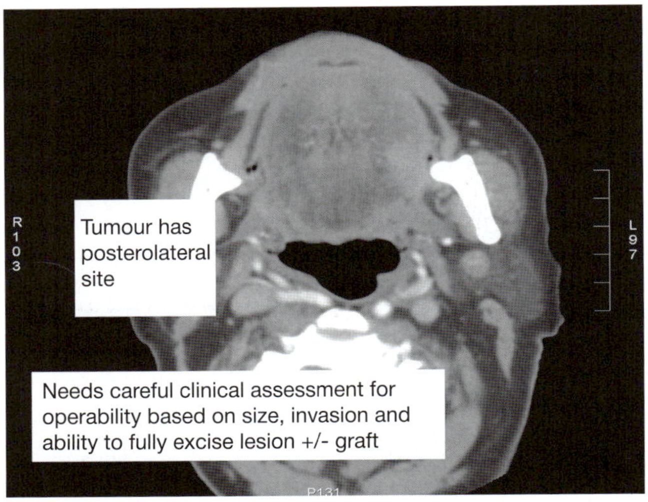

Fig. 23.28 Computed tomography scan showing carcinoma of the left lateral tongue.

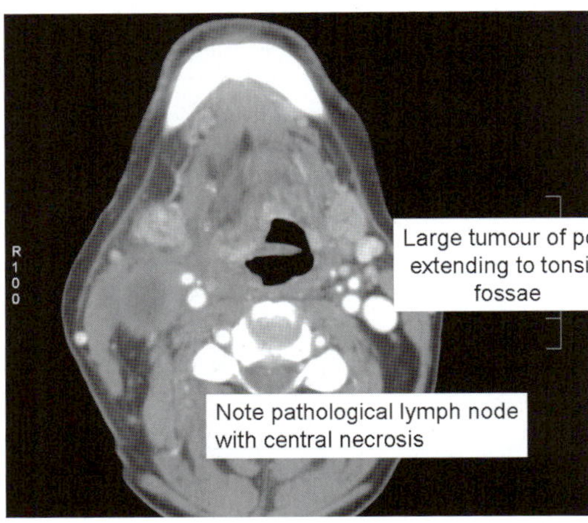

Fig. 23.29 Computed tomography scan showing carcinoma of the base of the tongue.

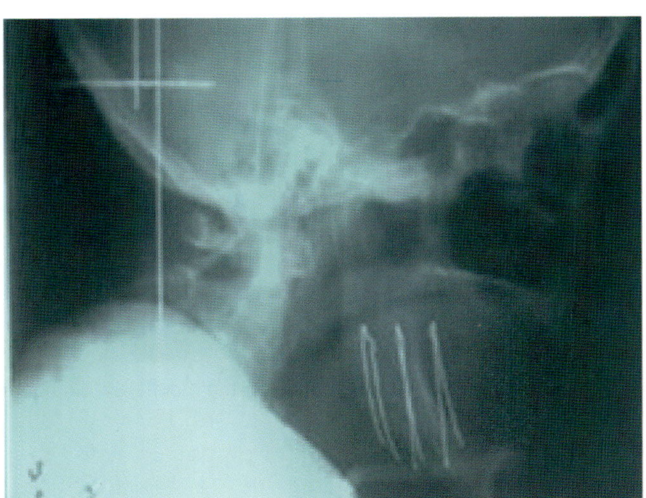

Fig. 23.30 Lateral radiograph showing three iridium hairpin insertions in an early tongue tumour. This effective treatment is rarely used in the United Kingdom today, as both the operator and nurses are irradiated by the iridium sources.

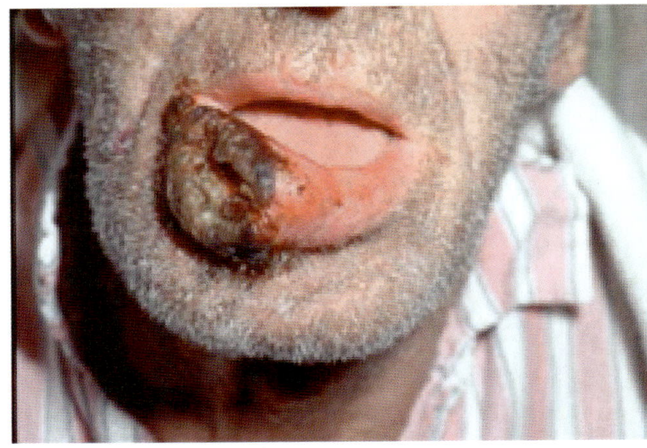

Fig. 23.31 Extensive lip carcinoma.

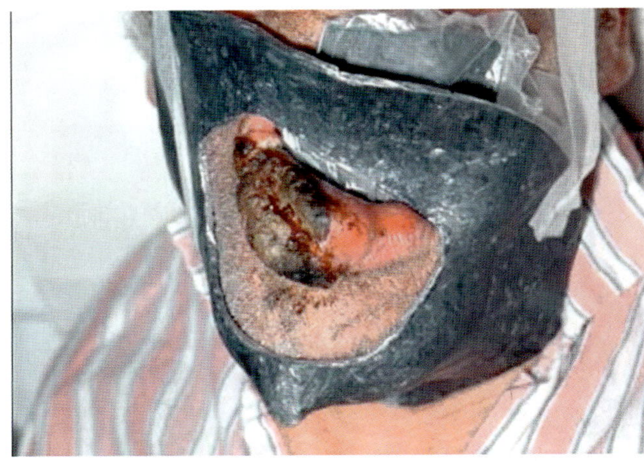

Fig. 23.32 Lead cutout and gum shield for a 300-kV treatment.

An individualised lead cutout and an internal gum shield will usually be used (Figs. 23.31–23.33). This arrangement facilitates appropriate sparing of the adjacent tissues including the unaffected (usually upper) lip and the deeper tissues of the oral cavity. These lesions are usually exophytic, so electrons will often be preferred or orthovoltage if available and, because the energy chosen is likely to be less than 12 MeV, a few millimetres of wax should be placed over the lesion to ensure maximum dose at the tumour surface. The gum shield will require wax on its anterior surface to absorb any backscatter electrons that could potentially enhance the dose to the treated volume. Care will need to be exercised in the degree of underlying bone irradiated that cannot be shielded by the gum shield.

Dose schedules for SCCs of the lip are similar to those for skin cancers and the reader is referred elsewhere. Longer fractionation schedules give better long-term cosmesis than a few large fractions and are preferred. Usual treatment regimens for these tumours range from 50 to 55 Gy in 15 to 20 fractions, treating daily.

Treatment of Cancers of the Oral Cavity

Whereas at many other head and neck sites, primary RT (or, increasingly, chemoradiotherapy) is becoming more usual as first-line treatment, this is not so for oral cavity tumours, where primary surgery retains its place as the preferred management of at least operable disease. High-level evidence to support the use of surgery here is scant, but other evidence does support this approach.

The surgery for oral cavity cancers depends on the extent of the primary. Small T1 and T2 lesions may be suitable for simple excision

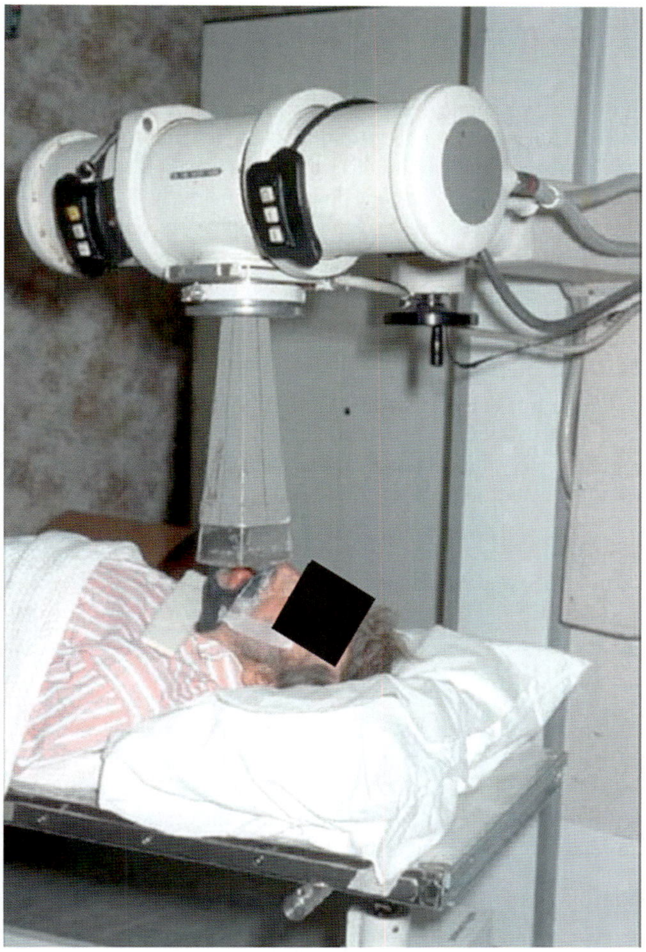

Fig. 23.33 A 300-kV treatment for lip cancer.

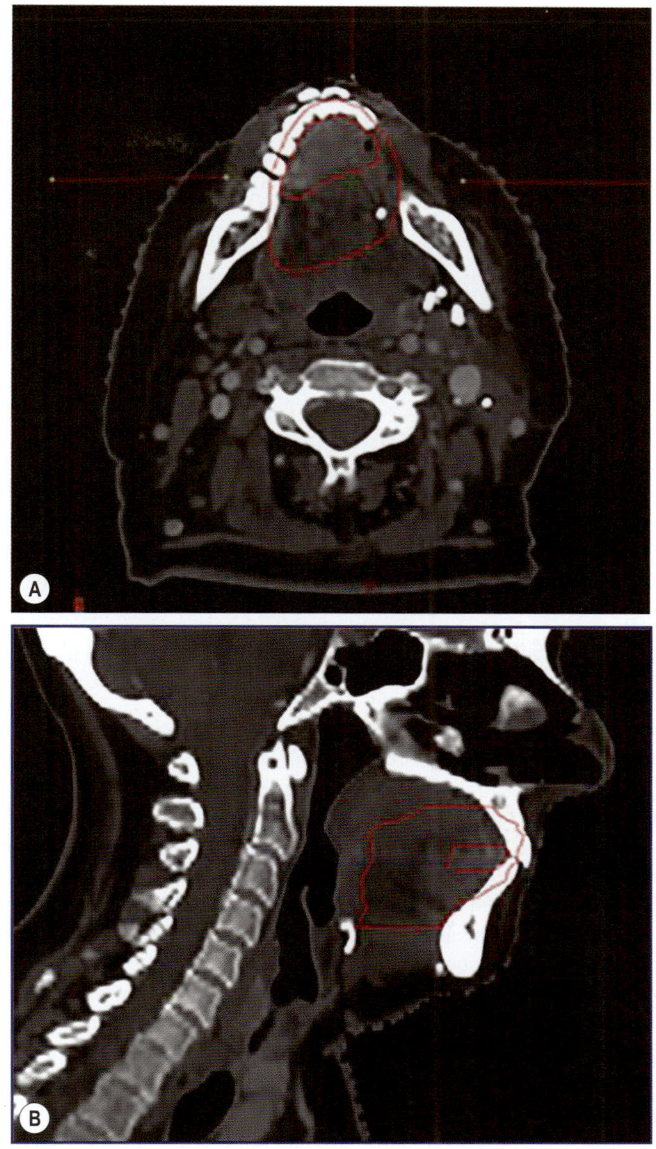

Fig. 23.34 (A) Oral tongue squamous cell carcinoma (SCC) with primary in situ (as deemed inoperable), hence a 10-to-20-mm clinical target volume (CTV) margin as seen in the axial plane. (B) The same oral tongue SCC with primary in situ, with a 10-to-20-mm CTV margin as seen in the sagittal plane.

which may be left to heal or closed with a split-skin graft or free flap. Larger lesions or those with more extensive invasion may require hemimandibulectomy with or without removal of part of the mandible and reconstruction with myocutaneous flaps.

RT remains an integral part of many patients' treatments, as postoperative adjuvant treatment has been established as an important part of the overall management of many of these tumours. In recent years, evidence has accumulated of the value of adding chemotherapy to RT schedules in high-risk patients.

Selection criteria for giving postoperative RT or chemoradiotherapy are widely agreed, even if the evidence level for some of these indications is not high. The reader is referred to Chapter 22 for these criteria.

Radiotherapy Technique

An immobilisation device is used and should include fixation of the shoulders even if it is not intended to irradiate the neck nodes comprehensively. An intraoral device may be used. For tongue tumours, it has as its purpose to move the tongue into the treatment volume and, as a consequence, achieve physical sparing of some of the palate. There is then sparing of some of the minor salivary tissue. For buccal tumours, its intention is different: here, it is helpful to move the tongue *away* from the irradiated mucosa and thereby lessen the toxicity.

Volumes should be defined on a planning CT scan, with coregistration of any imaging undertaken preoperatively. A fundamental decision is whether to treat the neck bilaterally. This decision should be based on the anticipated risk of contralateral spread and will vary according to the tumour site within the oral cavity and the nodal burden assessed at surgery. For well-lateralised tumours, an ipsilateral approach will often suffice, especially if only one lymph node was involved with no extranodal extension (ENE). Relapse in the contralateral neck can potentially be salvaged later. If the neck dissection yields no involved nodes and the nodal count is deemed adequate for a clearance (typically 13–15 nodes), the neck does not need to be irradiated.

There is now consensus on the postoperative primary volume and use of the same principles as those for primary RT described elsewhere in the chapter. Specifically, a preoperative GTV is re-created and expanded 5 mm and combined with the surgical bed (including a flap where indicated) and expanded 5 mm to create a primary site postoperative CTV (Figs. 23.34 and 23.35).

An IMRT approach enables comprehensive coverage of the operated primary site and lymph nodes where irradiated and sparing of clinically significant normal tissues.

The doses of radiation used will be dictated by the surgical findings and follow the principles outlined in Chapter 22. Thus 60 Gy in

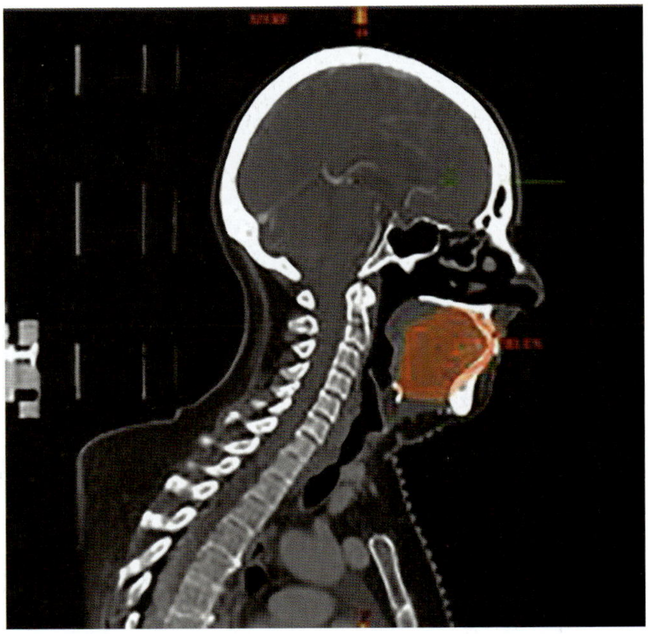

Fig. 23.35 Dose distribution (for high dose) in the sagittal plane.

30 fractions over 6 weeks is typically given with the option of boosting nodes with ENE by another 6 Gy (to 66 Gy).

Complications

Acute reactions with RT to the oral cavity include the usual effects on the skin and mucosa but should be self-limiting. The effect on nutrition can be profound and should be managed aggressively if not proactively.

Late effects will be determined in part by the site of irradiation. Sparing of salivary tissue should be possible and as such, xerostomia should be minimised. Taste and a heightened intraoral sensitivity may result. Fibrosis of the neck may result, although the relative impact of surgery and RT is poorly documented. Mucosal ulceration may occur but usually heals with conservative measures such as antimicrobial mouthwashes. ORN (see Fig. 22.3) can be minimised by meticulous dental hygiene before and following RT. The least amount of mandible should be irradiated while ensuring complete coverage of the volume at risk. Hot spots in the treatment plan should be avoided, particularly overlying the mandible.

Follow-up

Patients should be assessed for recurrence, including in the neck and especially if not treated initially, and for any late effects. Inspection of the primary site is often comparatively straightforward notwithstanding any reconstructive approaches to aid function.

Results of Treatment

Lip Cancer

As mentioned previously, the majority of these tumours present relatively early and if treated with radical RT (or surgery) have an excellent chance of cure. T1 and T2 lesions would be cured in 90% to 100% of patients. Larger or more advanced tumours have a worse prognosis.

Oral Cavity Cancers

The same rules apply for these cancers as others in the head and neck. Small, early cancers have a better prognosis than those with invasion into adjacent structures or nodal involvement. T1 and small T2 lesions of the oral cavity may be cured by surgery alone and the overall survival is 85% to 95%. This can fall to as low as 50% for T4 tumours or those with extensive nodal disease.

OROPHARYNGEAL CARCINOMA

Anatomy

The oropharynx comprises the tonsil, the base of the tongue (otherwise known as the posterior one-third of the tongue) and the undersurface of the soft palate. It is continuous with the nasopharynx superiorly, the hypopharynx inferiorly and the oral cavity anteriorly. The major components of Waldeyer's ring lie within the oropharynx: only the superior component lies within the nasopharynx. The function of the oropharynx is multifactorial: swallowing and respiration, including protection of the airway, phonation, taste and immune surveillance.

Anterior Wall

There is no true anterior wall, as the oropharynx communicates directly with the oral cavity. The anterior tonsillar pillar divides the oral cavity from the oropharynx, whereas the circumvallate papillae (sulcus terminalis) on the surface of the tongue divide the oral tongue from the base of tongue.

Posterior Wall

The posterior wall is formed by the tissues of the prevertebral space adjacent to C2 and C3 and constitutes the posterior pharyngeal wall.

Lateral Wall

The palatoglossal (anterior pillar) and palatopharyngeal (posterior pillar) arches, the faucial tonsil (the tonsil) and a small component of the pharyngeal wall constitute the lateral wall of the oropharynx. The parapharyngeal space lies more lateral still. The internal and external carotid arteries, internal jugular vein, superior cervical ganglion and retropharyngeal nodes lie within this area.

Superior Wall

The superior wall is composed anteriorly of the undersurface of the soft palate. Otherwise, there is a direct opening into the nasopharynx.

Inferior Wall

The hyoid bone constitutes the anatomical boundary between the oropharynx and hypopharynx. The vallecula, which is a trough that lies between the tongue base and the epiglottis, lies within this area. Lingual tonsillar tissue gives the inferior component of Waldeyer's ring.

Incidence of Oropharyngeal Tumours

Cancers of the oropharynx are increasingly common in the developed world. Incidence has tripled in males from 2.0 to 5.8 per 100,000 and doubled in females from 0.8 to 1.7 between 1995 and 2011. While a reduction in the prevalence of smoking in most high-income countries of the past two decades has led to a decline, human papilloma virus (HPV) infection is increasingly driving the net increase.

Of oropharyngeal cancers, the most common are tonsillar (≈60%) (Fig. 23.36), followed by 25% in the base of the tongue and 10% in the soft palate.

Staging System of Oropharyngeal Tumours

Staging has been updated in the latest version of the TNM system (8th edition) to reflect the inherently better prognosis of HPV+ve tumours.

T0	No evidence of primary tumour
T1	Tumour ≤2 cm in greatest dimension
T2	Tumour >2 cm but ≤4 cm in greatest dimension
T3	Tumour >4 cm in greatest dimension or extension to the lingual surface of the epiglottis
T4	Tumour invades the larynx, deep/extrinsic muscle of the tongue, medial pterygoid, hard palate or mandible or beyond

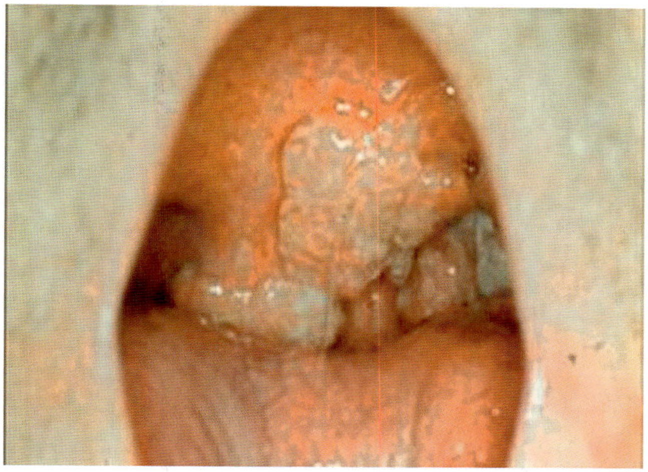

Fig. 23.36 Advanced tonsillar cancer involving the soft palate.

For HPV–ve tumours, the T staging is subdivided into T4A and T4B.

T4A	Tumour invades the larynx, deep/extrinsic muscle of the tongue, medial pterygoid, hard palate or mandible
T4B	Tumour invades the lateral pterygoid muscle, pterygoid plates, lateral nasopharynx or skull base or encases the carotid artery

For nodal status, the differences between HPV+ve and HPV–ve SCC tumours are even more striking.

HPV+ve tumours: clinical staging

cN0	No regional lymph node metastases
cN1	One or more ipsilateral lymph nodes, none larger than 6 cm
cN2	Contralateral or bilateral lymph nodes, none larger than 6 cm
cN3	Lymph nodes >6 cm

HPV+ve pathological staging

pN0	No regional lymph node metastases
pN1	Metastases in 4 or fewer lymph nodes
pN2	Metastases in more than 4 lymph nodes

For HPV-negative tumours, the nodal staging is same as described for oral cavity tumours (see page 367), with extracapsular extension of nodal disease having a significant impact on upstaging.

Aetiology, Pathology and Lymphatic Spread

As with other head and neck cancers, tobacco and alcohol consumption are the most significant risk factors for developing cancers in this region. There are no specific genetic risk factors for this type of tumour. There is a specific group of oropharyngeal carcinomas in younger (often nonsmoker) patients, which are found to be associated with HPV. Although there appears to be distinct histopathological appearances with less differentiation and basaloid-type cells, some argue that such is the positive influence of the HPV status, that the description of the morphological subtype of SCC might be misleading. The presence of HPV can be confirmed by immunochemical staining for the virus-associated protein p16. Moreover, reviews of the outcomes of these specific tumours compared with the typical SCCs indicate an improved prognosis. The intrinsic better prognosis and higher chemoradiosensitivity of HPV-positive tumours is also directing treatment strategies towards treatment deintensification, including omission of concurrent chemotherapy or a reduction in total RT dose, though this is not yet the standard of care.

Histologically, almost all oropharyngeal carcinomas are the squamous cell cancers prevalent in the head and neck region. One variant of SCC of the oropharynx is the lymphoepithelioma. Histologically, it is lymphocyte predominant and may mimic lymphoma. Lymphoepithelioma may arise in the base of the tongue, tonsils or nasopharynx. It is a very radiosensitive variant of SCC. Other cancers in this area include minor salivary gland carcinomas and lymphoma. Mention has already been made of Waldeyer's ring. It is a site of extranodal non-Hodgkin lymphoma, and the tonsil is the most common primary extranodal site of head and neck non-Hodgkin lymphoma.

The oropharynx has a rich lymphatic supply; 60% of oropharyngeal cancers have nodal involvement at presentation. In tonsillar tumours, this is predominantly unilateral spread, unless the primary extends to the midline, and is important when determining volumes to irradiate. Tonsillar cancers drain to the adjacent jugulodigastric or subdigastric node (the so-called *tonsillar node*) within level 2 and then to the remainder of the deep cervical nodes of levels 2 and 3. The remainder of the oropharyngeal cancers are midline structures and therefore can drain to bilateral nodes. Tumours of the soft palate and posterior pharyngeal wall drain to the retropharyngeal nodes and upper deep cervical lymph nodes—that is, level 2. Base of tongue tumours commonly spread to the mid- and upper-cervical nodes—that is, levels 2 and 3.

Signs and Symptoms

Cancers in this region commonly present with sore throat or painful swallowing. Tumours in the tonsillar region or posterior oropharynx may present with earache because of extension into the parapharyngeal space or the sensation of a lump in the throat. Tumour or ulceration in the oropharynx can usually be visualised in the clinic via nasendoscopy. A fine needle aspiration (FNA) or biopsy can often be taken at the time.

As with many head and neck cancers, the presentation may be via a neck mass from secondary lymph nodes. In this case the primary may be identified from tonsillectomy or targeted biopsies guided by PET/CT.

Diagnosis and Staging

Patients with a history of persistent sore throat should be referred urgently to the ear-nose-throat (ENT) clinic. Patients may also be referred urgently for persistent tonsillar swelling or neck lymphadenopathy.

A full history should be undertaken. The importance of comorbidities may determine the preferred treatment modality. This is particularly the case in patients who are heavy smokers or have a history of alcohol intake.

A full ENT examination is performed in the clinic. This allows delineation of the primary. It should include fibre-optic examination to look for synchronous tumours. The neck should be clinically examined for palpable lymph nodes.

Radiological assessment of the primary is essential to complete the staging. This is usually a CT or MRI scan, noting the pros and cons of each approach referenced earlier (Fig. 23.37). This may also reveal pathological lymphadenopathy not identified clinically. Imaging of the chest is also essential for exclusion of metastatic spread or synchronous primary tumours of the lung.

Treatment

Currently, management of primary tumours of the oropharynx is largely nonsurgical and in contrast to most oral cavity tumours. Chemoradiation is the standard of care for younger and healthier patients with more advanced cancers. For early-stage disease, RT alone will suffice.

Management of neck disease, especially in those with more advanced disease, has been strongly debated over the years: Data now favour nonsurgical treatment and follow-up with PET/CT, with surgery

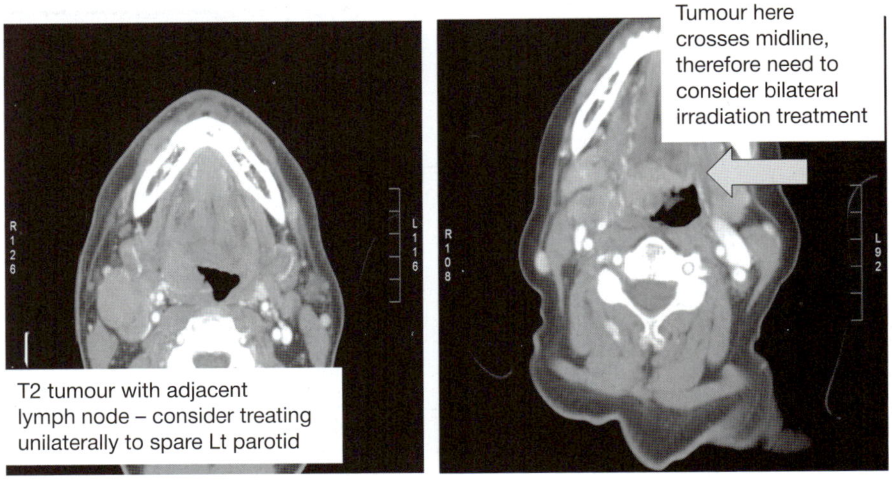

Fig. 23.37 Computed tomography scan showing carcinoma of the tonsil.

reserved for those patients with an incomplete or equivocal response on imaging at 3 to 4 months posttreatment, especially in HPV-positive patients. Neck dissection thus might be preferred in patients with bulky nodes who are HPV–ve.

For early tonsillar cancers, however, there is increasing interest in the role of transoral resection and neck dissection, which in select patients may avoid the need for adjuvant treatments.

Radiation Technique

The patient is treated in an immobilisation device that includes the head and shoulders. The patient is treated supine. The neck will typically be in a 'neutral' or comfortably extended position as this then moves some of the oral cavity out of the primary beam. A tongue depressor is not usually used.

A planning CT scan coregistered with diagnostic scans facilitates precise volume definition. The primary CTV must include reasonable margins to account for microscopic spread. These margins have recently been refined and agreed by consensus. In practice, the GTV is defined on optimal data sets and grown volumetrically with a high-dose margin for the CTV on the order of 5 mm only, and lower-dose larger margins of 10 mm, excluding any air or bone unless affected (Figs. 22.9 and 23.38). This approach means that the older approach of anatomically determined volumes is no longer required and can be expected to reduce the morbidity of treatment. The selection of lymph nodes is based on the known pattern of spread of these tumours. Where a neck dissection has been carried out, this additional information allows for appropriate doses to be specified according to the risk of disease; that is, nodes with extracapsular spread could be irradiated to a high dose.

Larger tumours of the tonsil that approach or cross the midline, which have spread locally to the base of the tongue or are node positive, should be treated with a volume that encompasses the primary and bilateral upper cervical neck nodes.

Other oropharyngeal tumours (i.e. base of tongue, postpharyngeal wall and soft palate) usually require a similar bilateral approach because of the high risk of contralateral lymph node involvement (Figs. 23.39 and 23.40).

Smaller, well-lateralised cancers of the tonsil where the node burden is low (typically fewer than three involved nodes in levels 2/3) can still be treated with unilateral irradiation after discussing the benefit of reduced toxicity versus the possibility of contralateral neck recurrence. Fractionation schedules used in this situation are typically 65 to 66 Gy in 30 fractions over 6 weeks. Concurrent chemotherapy, certainly in younger, fitter patients, forms an important component of this treatment. Indeed, the strongest evidence for concurrent chemoradiotherapy originates from oropharyngeal tumours.

Complications

Acute reactions in the oropharynx are predictable. Mucositis will compromise nutrition and should be managed aggressively. In practice, this often means that these patients have feeding tubes sited before therapy (percutaneous endoscopic gastrostomy (PEG) tube or radiologically inserted gastrostomy (RIG) tube) and opiate analgesia. Acute xerostomia and the often copious mucous production should be managed symptomatically. Skin reactions and reversible alopecia will occur in the irradiated volume.

Chronic xerostomia has been a common side effect of wide-field RT as used here. There is now level one evidence that sparing at least one parotid gland with IMRT techniques results in an improvement in the quality of life of these patients.. Trismus may result from high-dose RT to the pterygoid muscles and should be spared as far as clinically appropriate. Active stretching exercises can also help to alleviate this.

Follow-up

Patients will require follow-up imaging using PET/CT in the vast majority of cases to detect and manage residual disease early, and repeated if there are equivocal lesions which the multidisciplinary team would favour observing.

Results

HPV association has a markedly positive impact on prognosis. Most patients with early-stage disease do well, with 5-year survival rates of 75% to 90%. For more advanced disease, the survival curves diverge such that HPV–ve disease cases plummet to 30% to 60%, whereas HPV+ve cases still fare very well, with 5-year survival rates being maintained even with more advanced disease. It is no wonder that there is ongoing debate about treatment deintensification in HPV+ve patients and treatment intensification in HPV–ve patients.

LARYNX

Anatomy

The larynx is a cartilaginous frame held in position by intrinsic muscles and ligaments. The anterior and lateral parts of this box are formed by the thyroid cartilage. The cricoid cartilage is below the thyroid cartilage, forming a complete ring around the larynx just below the vocal cords.

The larynx is divided into three areas: the supraglottis, glottis and subglottis (Fig. 23.41). The structures of the supraglottis are the epiglottis,

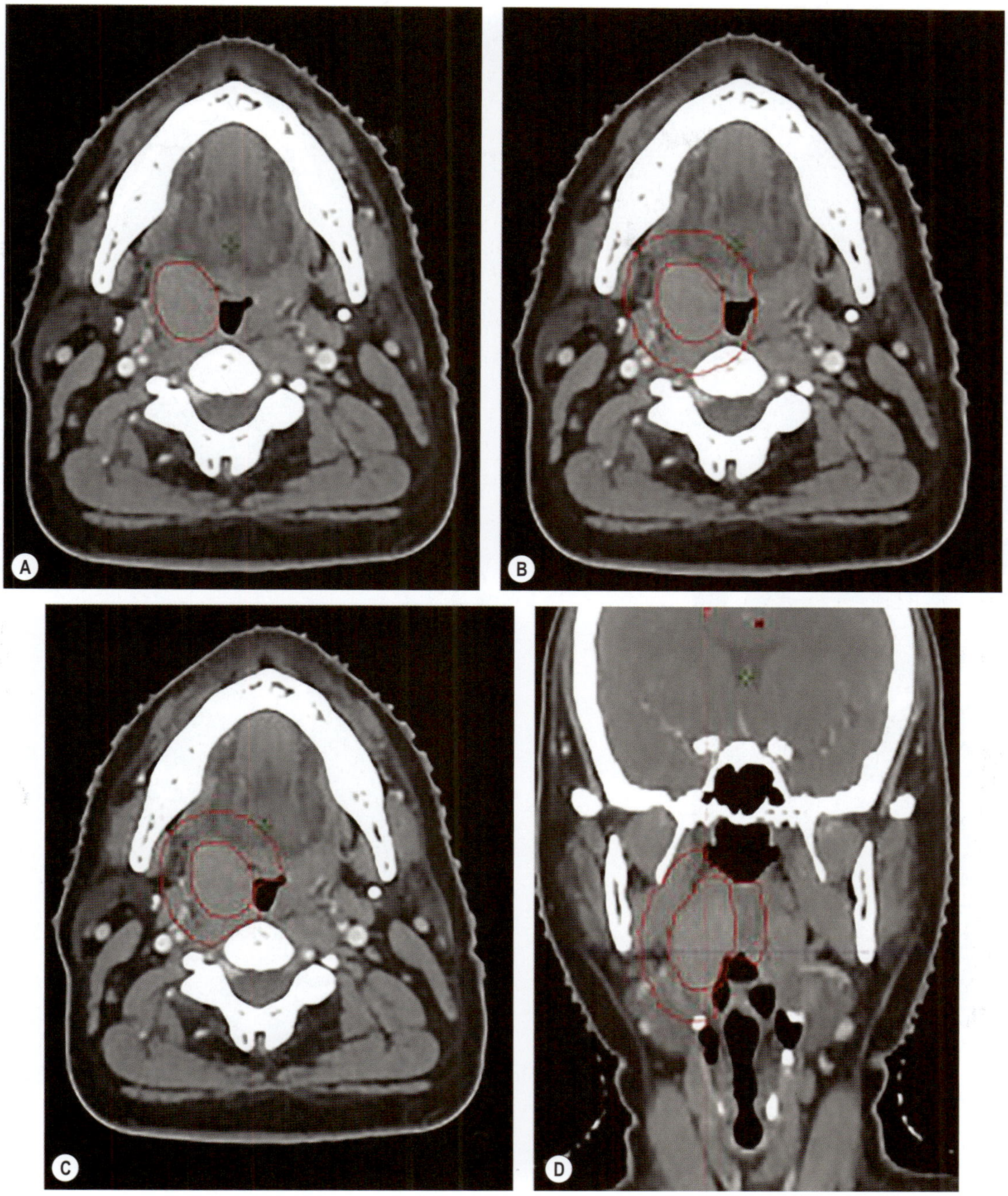

Fig. 23.38 (A) T3 tonsillar squamous cell carcinoma (SCC) in the axial plane on the right side, delineated to give the gross tumour volume (GTV). (B) The same T3 tonsillar SCC in the axial plane on the right side, expanded 10 mm (preferred to 5 mm due to concerns over image quality of the GTV). (C) The same T3 tonsillar SCC in the axial plane on the right side, edited to exclude air and bone to give the high-dose clinical target volume (CTV). (D) The same T3 tonsillar SCC in the coronal plane on the right side, edited to exclude air and bone to give the high-dose CTV.

aryepiglottic folds, arytenoids, ventricular bands (often called the false cords) and ventricular cavities. The true glottis is the area by the vocal cords. The subglottic area is the area beneath the vocal cords and above the trachea.

Incidence of Laryngeal Cancer

There are around 2000 cases of laryngeal cancer in the United Kingdom, which makes the larynx the most common site for head and neck cancer overall, but numbers are falling. The male-to-female ratio is 4.5:1. In some parts of France, Spain and Italy, the incidence of laryngeal cancer can be up to six times more common. Unlike the United Kingdom, where true glottis is the most common site, the supraglottic area is the most common site for laryngeal tumours in southern Europe. Typically, 60% to 70% of tumours begin in the glottis, 25% of cases are supraglottic, 2% only are true subglottic cancer and the remainder are transglottic tumours, in which the precise site of origin cannot be determined.

Staging System for Laryngeal Cancer (8th Edition)

Although the nodal status follows the principle described elsewhere for HPV–ve tumours, the T status is described according to which element of the larynx the tumour is considered to arise from.

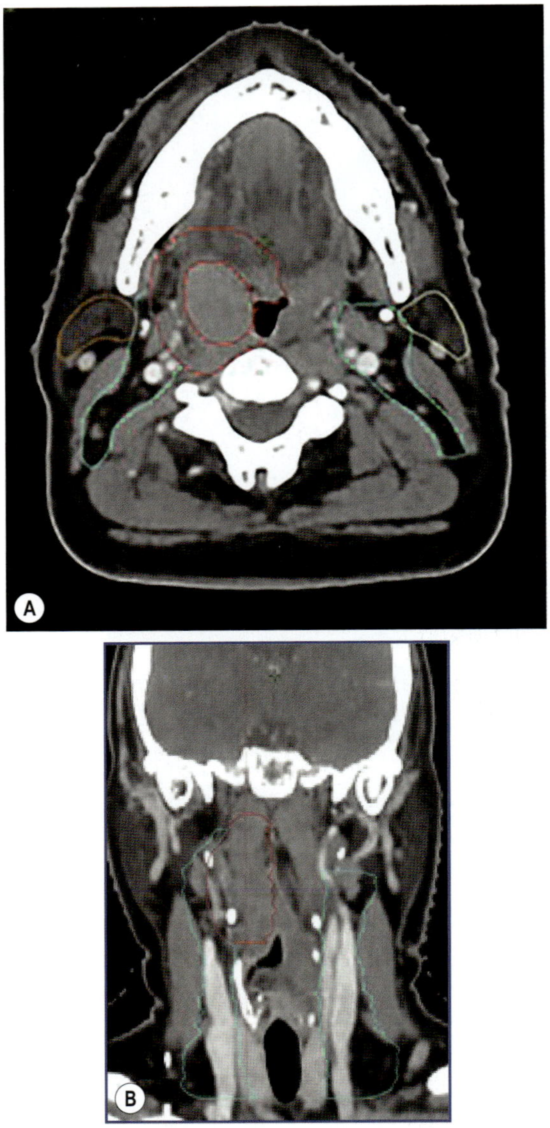

Fig. 23.39 (A) Elective nodal irradiation (bilaterally). (B) Elective nodal irradiation seen in the coronal plane. Note that the contralateral nodal irradiation volume does not extend so far superiorly in line with Royal College of Radiologists consensus statements and affords better contralateral parotid gland sparing.

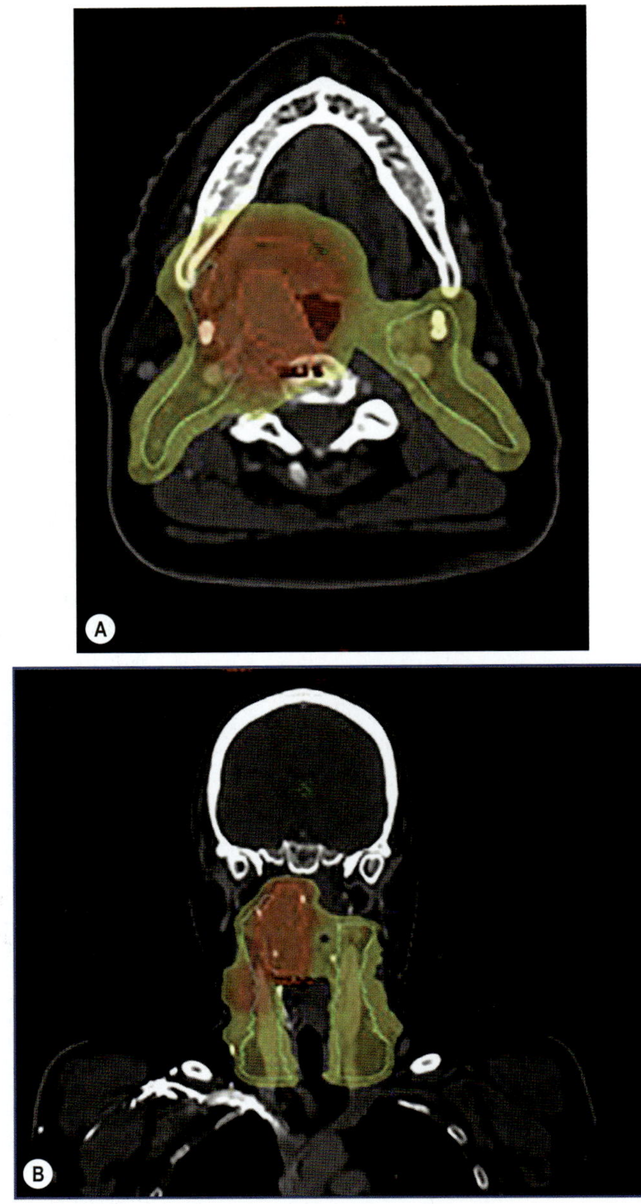

Fig. 23.40 (A) High-dose and elective nodal irradiation seen in the axial plane. (B) High-dose and elective nodal irradiation seen in the coronal plane. Note the high dose given to the right-sided level 3 node.

(1) Supraglottic Larynx

T – Primary Tumour	
T1	Tumour limited to one subsite of the supraglottis, with normal vocal cord mobility
T2	Tumour invades the mucosa of more than one adjacent subsite of the supraglottis or glottis or the region outside the supraglottis (e.g. mucosa of the base of the tongue, vallecula, medial wall of piriform sinus) without fixation of the larynx
T3	Tumour limited to the larynx, with vocal cord fixation and/or invades any of the following: postcricoid area, preepiglottic space, paraglottic space and/or inner cortex of thyroid cartilage
T4A	Tumour invades through the outer cortex of the thyroid cartilage and/or extends beyond the larynx
T4B	Tumour invades the prevertebral space, encases the carotid artery or mediastinal structures

(2) Intrinsic Larynx: Glottis

T – Primary Tumour	
T1	Tumour limited to the vocal cord, with normal mobility A = one vocal cord B = both vocal cords
T2	Tumour extends to the supraglottis and/or subglottis and/or with impaired vocal cord mobility
T3	Tumour limited to the larynx, with vocal cord fixation and/or invasion of the paraglottic space and/or inner cortex of the thyroid cartilage
T4A	Tumour invades through the outer cortex of the thyroid cartilage and/or invades tissues beyond the larynx
T4B	Tumour invades the prevertebral space, encases the carotid artery or invades mediastinal structures

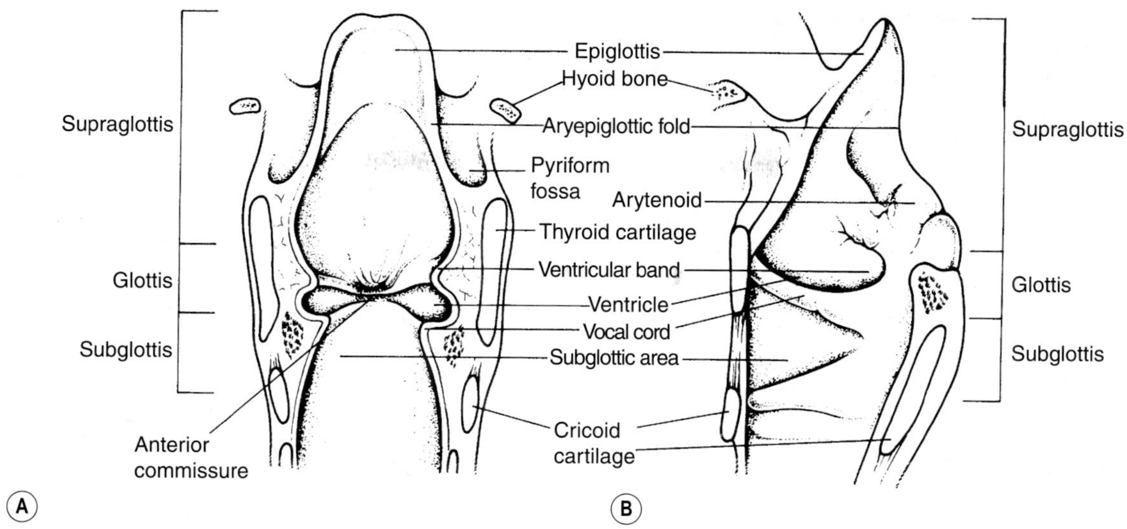

Fig. 23.41 Landmarks of the normal larynx and pharynx from (A) the posterior and (B) the lateral aspect. (Redrawn from Robinson JO. *Surgery*, 7th ed. Longmans, Green and Co.; 1965.)

(3) Subglottis

T – Primary Tumour	
T1	Tumour limited to the subglottis
T2	Tumour extends to the vocal cord(s), with normal or impaired mobility
T3	Tumour limited to the larynx with vocal cord fixation and/or invasion of the paraglottic space and/or inner cortex of the thyroid cartilage
T4A	Tumour invades the cricoid or thyroid cartilage and/or invades tissues beyond the larynx
T4B	Tumour invades the prevertebral space, encases the carotid artery or invades mediastinal structures

Aetiology, Pathology and Lymphatic Spread

As with many head and neck cancers, laryngeal tumours tend to develop in smokers. In contrast with oropharyngeal cancer, HPV infection is not a major cause. The higher incidence of supraglottic cancer in parts of Europe may be caused by the type of alcoholic drink consumed and the use of dark rather than blond tobacco. The true glottis has a poor lymphatic supply and tumours arising from the true vocal cord are relatively slow to metastasise to regional lymph nodes. But supraglottic carcinoma of the larynx spreads far more readily to the lymph nodes within the neck. The incidence of lymph node spread from even T1 and T2 lesions ranges between 27% and 40%, and for T3/T4 lesions the rate of lymph node metastasis is 55% to 65%.

Initially, lymphatic spread is upwards to the jugulodigastric lymph nodes immediately beneath the angle of the jaw (level 2). Tumours also commonly spread to the midjugular lymph nodes (level 3). Over 95% of laryngeal tumours are invasive squamous carcinoma. Although usually well differentiated, some tumours, especially of the supraglottic region, can be poorly differentiated and are more likely to spread to lymph nodes. A common variant of well-differentiated squamous cancer is a verrucous carcinoma. This tumour contains a large amount of keratin and has a heaped-up, warty appearance. Sometimes invasive cancer can be preceded by carcinoma in situ of the epithelium of the vocal cords. However, this usually transforms into invasive cancer within 1 to 2 years of detection.

Signs and Symptoms

The first symptom in more than 90% of patients with true glottic cancer is hoarseness. Comparatively small tumours of the vocal cords can cause marked changes in the voice, and there is National Health Service (NHS) guidance for early referral to exclude cancer. Advanced tumours of the vocal cords may narrow the airway, especially if a vocal cord is paralysed, leading to stridor. This is a whistling noise when the patient breathes and is an oncological emergency. Untreated, the patient will develop progressive dyspnoea and can suffocate. For this reason, patients with stridor should be immediately referred for consideration of an emergency tracheostomy or urgent laser debulking.

Hoarseness is less common as a symptom for early supraglottic cancer. Most patients complain initially of either a sore throat or a foreign body–like sensation in the upper larynx, which they often describe as caused by either a fish bone or a piece of silver paper. Hoarseness only develops when the tumour reaches the vocal cord. More advanced tumours may have pain referred to the ear, and patients may occasionally cough up blood (haemoptysis).

Diagnosis and Staging

Many laryngeal cancers are visible during a flexible fibre-optic examination. As well as visualising the larynx, the neck should be carefully palpated for lymph nodes, especially in the jugulodigastric area.

Patients should then have an examination under anaesthetic when histology is often acquired using rigid fibre-optic endoscopes to inform the staging, which is so critical to subsequent management. The mobility of the vocal cords should be assessed with the patient conscious and anaesthetised. CT and MRI scanning will give further information about the degree of spread, as these imaging modalities may show small, impalpable lymph nodes in the neck or subglottic spread, or disease in the mediastinum, and should be undertaken in all but the earliest cases of laryngeal cancer (Figs. 23.42 and 23.43).

Most patients with laryngeal cancer smoke. Smoking can affect the cardiovascular and respiratory systems. If the patient has chronic obstructive pulmonary disease (COPD) or ischaemic heart disease, this may alter management decisions. Such patients may only be fit for less radical treatments and surgery, or chemoradiotherapy may be contraindicated.

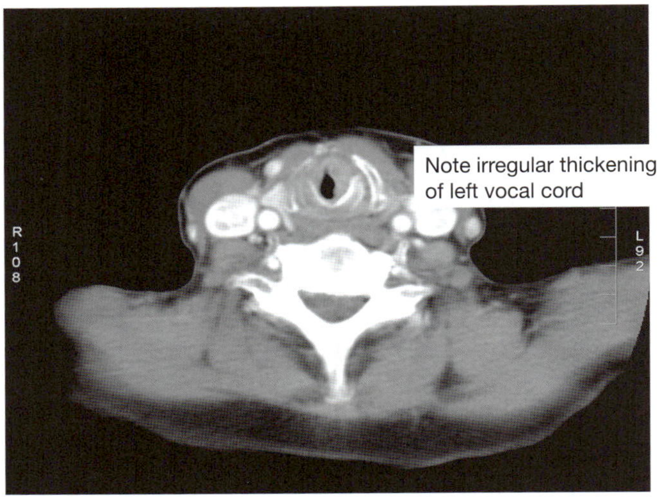

Fig. 23.42 Early carcinoma of the larynx.

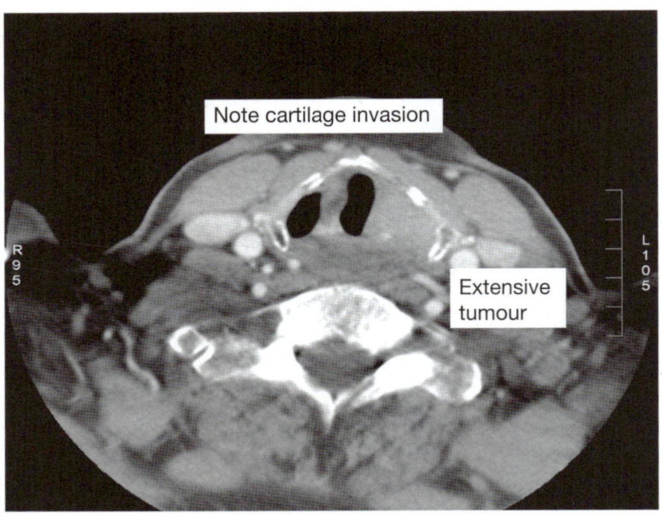

Fig. 23.43 T4 carcinoma of the larynx.

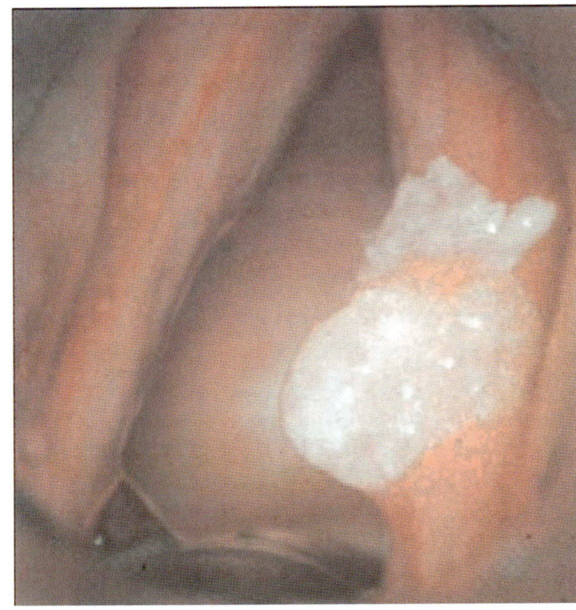

Fig. 23.44 Early (T1) carcinoma of the vocal cord.

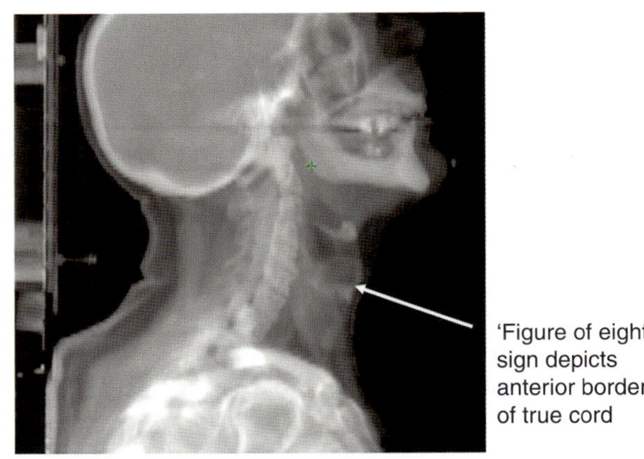

Fig. 23.45 Landmarks for early laryngeal cancer on a digitally reconstructed radiograph.

Treatment of Early Laryngeal Tumours T1 and T2 (Fig. 23.44)

Either RT or transoral laser microsurgery or open partial laryngeal surgery may be employed as initial therapy for early laryngeal tumours. In the United Kingdom, RT with surgical salvage (total laryngectomy) or laser microsurgery and RT as salvage are the most common approaches with comparable efficacy. Treatment selection will, in part, be determined by tumour factors, such as distinctiveness of tumour margin and location on the cord, as well as patient preference.

Radiotherapy Technique for Glottic Cancers (Figs. 23.45 and 23.46)

The larynx is a mobile structure and, although the vocal cord occupies about 1 cm only, the radiation volume should be at least 4 × 4 cm to allow for vocal cord movement during respiration and swallowing, thus encompassing a CTV and internal target volume (ITV). This is determined on a planning CT scan. The vocal cords are easily determined as they sit about 1 cm below the thyroid cartilage promontory. The anterior commissure sits just under the skin and bolus material may be required to ensure adequate dose coverage. Opposed fields or anterior oblique fields with margins to ensure coverage of the planning target volume (PTV) are determined and typically give rise to field sizes of 5 × 5 cm, An IMRT approach, however, enables improved conformality, sparing of the carotid vessels and the '5+5' approach to volume definition (Figs. 23.47–23.50). Dosage schemes in use nationally and internationally range from 50 Gy in 16 fractions over 3 weeks to 63 Gy in 28 fractions over 5.5 weeks using 6-MV photons.

Radiotherapy Technique of Early Supraglottic Carcinomas of Larynx T1, T2 N0

Owing to the fact that supraglottic larynx tumours are more likely to spread to lymph nodes in the neck, most centres advocate prophylactic irradiation of the jugular chain even if there are no palpable lymph nodes or lymph nodes detectable on MRI scanning. Many oncologists incorporate at least the jugulodigastric lymph node within the irradiated volume for part or all of the treatment. Therefore the typical treatment volume for an early supraglottic larynx cancer is slightly longer to enable irradiation, albeit prophylactically, of the level 2 and 3 nodes. Dose fractionation schedules are consistent with large-volume irradiation elsewhere in the head and neck area: that is, 70 Gy in 35 fractions over 7 weeks or 65 to 66 Gy in 30 fractions over 6 weeks.

Complications of Treatment for Early Laryngeal Cancer

Most patients develop a brisk radiation mucositis towards the end of treatment, but this usually resolves within 1 month. A small number

Early intrinsic glottic laryngeal cancer

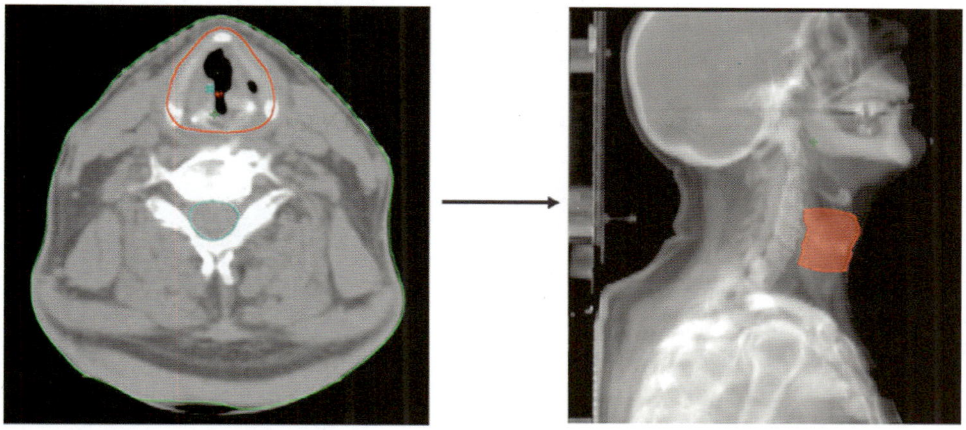

Fig. 23.46 Early vocal cord carcinoma with the clinical target volume seen in the axial and sagittal planes using traditional landmarks.

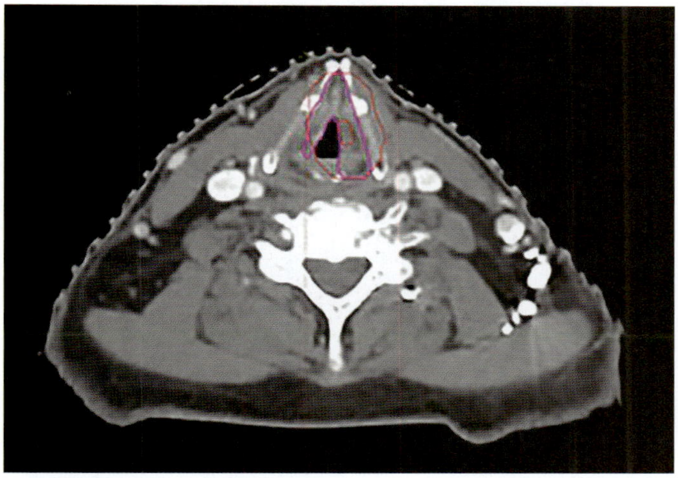

Fig. 23.47 Early vocal cord carcinoma extending towards the anterior commissure, expanded by 10 mm and then edited inside the cartilage to give the clinical target volume.

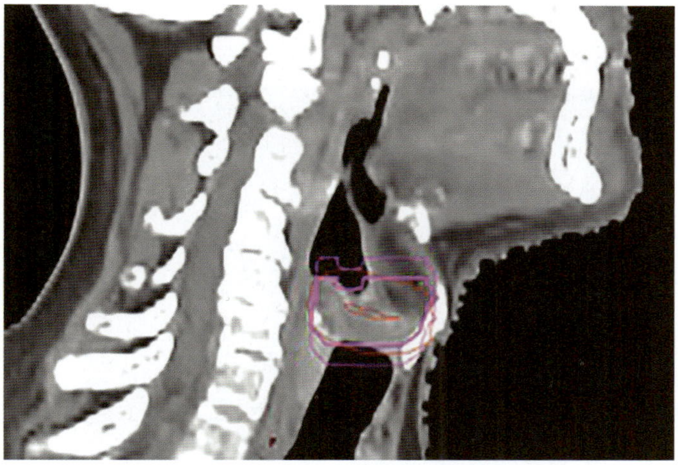

Fig. 23.49 The same vocal cord carcinoma as in Fig. 23.47, seen in the sagittal plane with a 5-mm superior-inferior internal target volume margin.

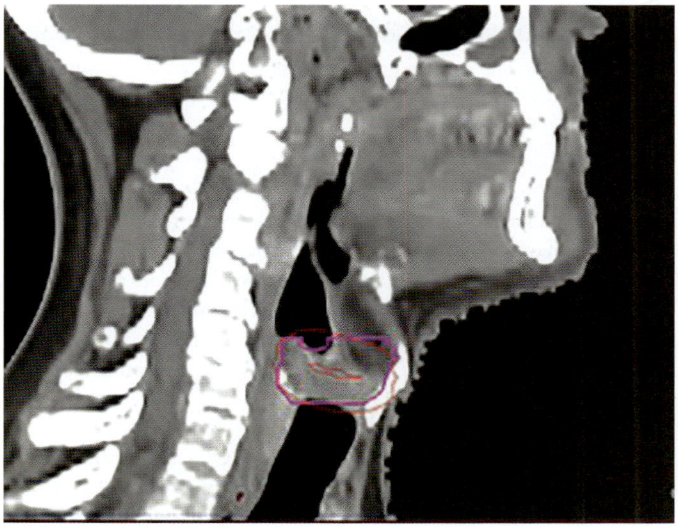

Fig. 23.48 The same vocal cord carcinoma as in Fig. 23.47, seen in the sagittal plane.

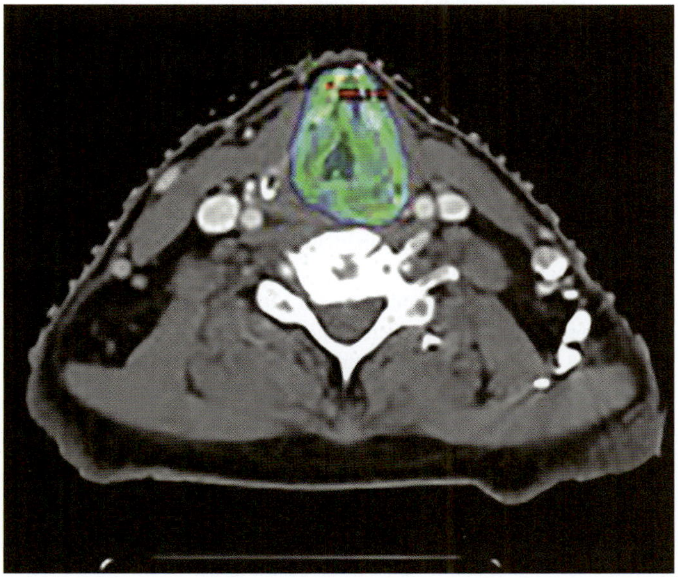

Fig. 23.50 Resultant dose distribution. Note the sparing of the contralateral arytenoid cartilage.

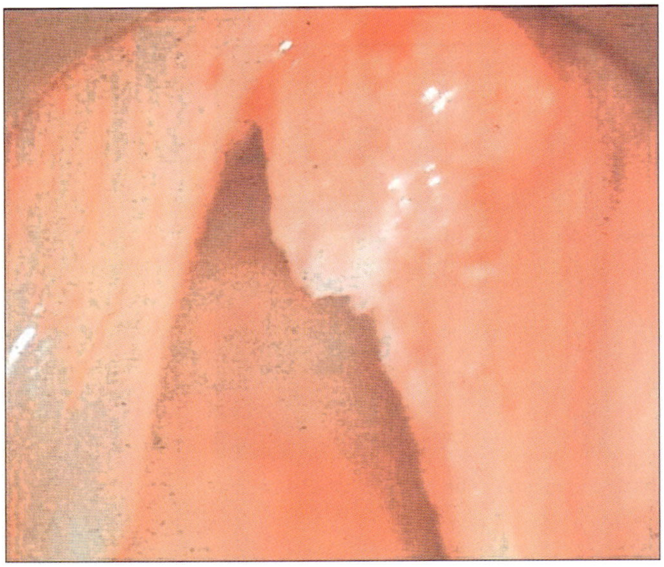

Fig. 23.51 T3 carcinoma of the larynx with a fixed cord.

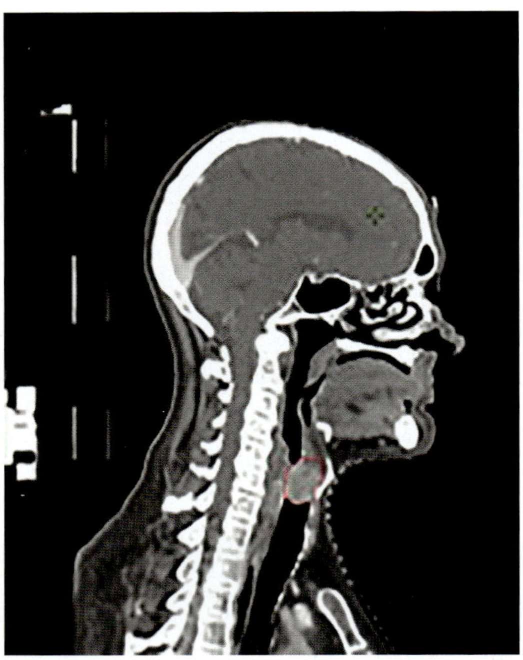

Fig. 23.52 Transglottic T3 carcinoma seen in the sagittal plane.

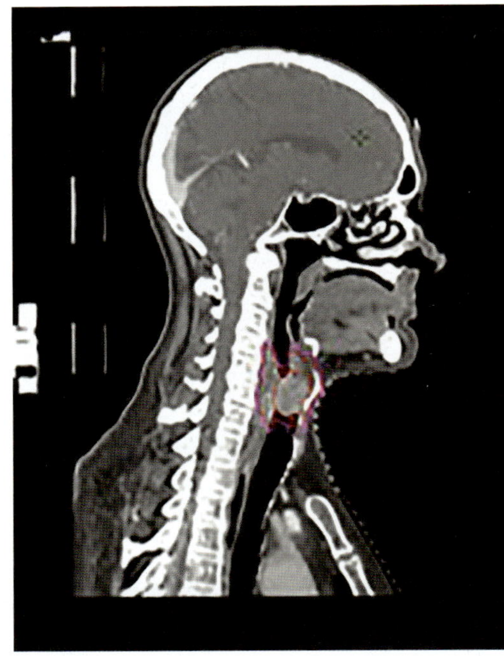

Fig. 23.53 Transglottic carcinoma with a 10-mm margin superior-inferior to generate the clinical target volume.

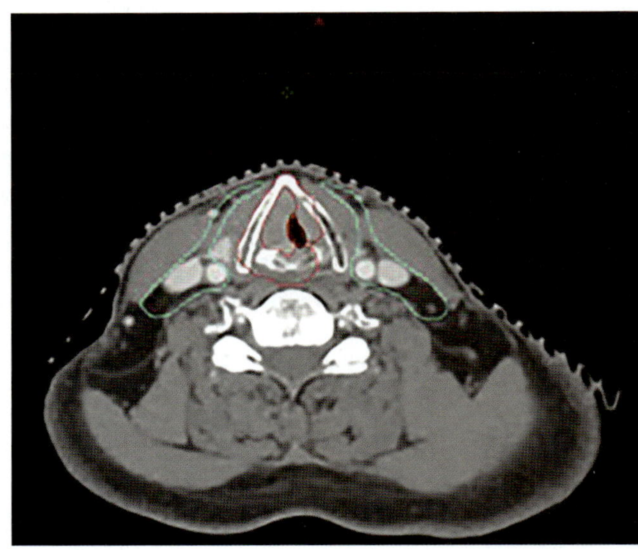

Fig. 23.54 The same transglottic tumour as in Fig. 23.53, with inclusion of the thyroid cartilage on the right due to concerns over early invasion and elective nodal irradiation. As the tumour extended into the subglottis, level 6 nodes were included.

of patients develop persisting laryngeal oedema. This is more common in supraglottic cancers where the incidence can be as high as 25% and more common among heavy smokers. Treatment is by advising cessation of smoking, taking antibiotics if there is evidence of infection and taking corticosteroids. Persistent severe laryngeal oedema may be a reason for tracheostomy. Patients with persisting oedema should be carefully examined for persisting or recurrent tumour. Laryngeal necrosis is rare, with an incidence of less than 1%.

Treatment of Bulky T2 and T3 Glottic and Supraglottic Tumours (Fig. 23.51)

Most of these tumours can be well managed with larynx preservation approaches (Figs. 23.52–23.54). In all cases, nodal irradiation, even if given with prophylactic intent, will be required and is enabled with an IMRT through a synchronous boost technique. In node-negative cases, levels 2 to 4 should be irradiated. If the patient is node positive, the levels 2 to 5 should be treated and level 1B included if level 2 is diseased anteriorly. Concurrent chemotherapy improves outcomes as evidenced in the metaanalysis discussed in Chapter 22. As such, concurrent chemotherapy would be considered the standard of care in fit patients.

Induction chemotherapy followed by RT has had an established role in laryngeal preservation based on the early work of the Veterans Affairs Laryngeal Cancer Study Group, although later work of the Radiation Therapy Oncology Group (RTOG) demonstrated the superiority in terms of laryngeal preservation with concurrent chemoradiotherapy. That said, there is continued interest in the neoadjuvant approach, especially given the superiority of the triplet regimen docetaxel-cisplatin-fluorouracil (TPF), (see Chapter 22).

T4 Laryngeal Cancers

Patients with tumour that extends through the thyroid cartilage or into the base of the tongue do not do well with laryngeal preservation approaches. Similarly, patients with a poorly functioning larynx are better managed with a total laryngectomy if fit enough.

Patients with inoperable disease may be considered for neoadjuvant chemotherapy followed by concurrent chemoradiotherapy, recognising the toxicity of such an approach.

Postoperative Radiotherapy Technique

Incomplete excision of a laryngeal tumour with positive surgical margins is an absolute indication for RT treatment. Laryngeal cancers can spread out of the larynx by infiltration either through the thyroid cartilage or through the thyrocricoid membrane into the soft tissues of the neck—that is, pT4 disease. Such spread, again, is an indication for postoperative therapy, as is extracapsular nodal spread. In cases of involved margins at the primary site and extracapsular spread, concurrent chemotherapy would also be offered in fit patients. The other indications for postoperative RT are considered in Chapter 22.

The tracheostomy opening is a potential site for recurrence, especially if the patient has had an emergency tracheostomy or if there is subglottic tumour. The tracheal stoma should be included in all or part of the treatment. The radiation reaction, though, can be brisk around the tracheostomy, with soreness, desquamation and occasionally bleeding after doses as low as 40 Gy in 20 fractions, and the delivered dose might need some reduction to that delivered elsewhere in the neck.

Results of Treatment

Early Laryngeal Cancers

Local control rates for T1A glottic tumours are around 90% to 93%. For T1B tumours, this drops slightly to 85% to 89% and for T2 tumours, marginally less again.

Local control rates for T1N0 supraglottic tumours range from 77% to 100% whereas for T2N0, this falls slightly to 62% to 83%.

Advanced Laryngeal Cancers

It is possible to get 65% 5-year survival with RT alone in selected T3 glottic cancers. In the past, more advanced transglottic T3 lesions had between 40% and 50% survival if treated by RT alone, rising to about 65% if treated by laryngectomy with postoperative RT if required. The results of RT alone are significantly improved by the administration of concomitant cisplatin chemotherapy, with 4-year survivors with T4 disease exceeding 50%.

HYPOPHARYNGEAL CARCINOMA

Anatomy

The hypopharynx extends posterolaterally in relation to the larynx, at the level of the hyoid bone to about the lower level of the cricoid cartilage (Fig. 23.55). The hypopharynx comprises the piriform fossa, the postcricoid region and the posterior pharyngeal wall, and therefore cancers of these three regions comprise the hypopharyngeal carcinomas. The piriform fossae (or sinuses) are pear-shaped channels that run alongside the larynx and are adjacent to the inner aspect of the thyroid cartilage. The postcricoid region is behind the larynx and runs from the arytenoids to the inferior border of the cricoid cartilage. The posterior pharyngeal wall abuts the prevertebral fascia and extends from the level of the floor of the vallecula to the cricoid cartilage (Fig. 23.56).

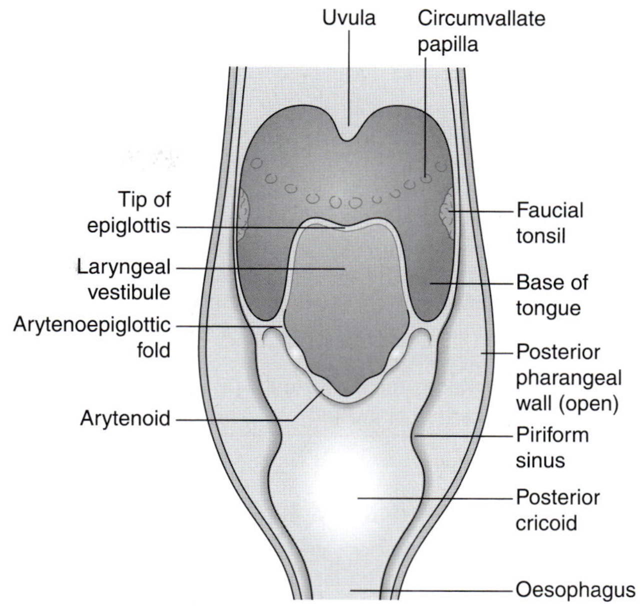

Fig. 23.55 Hypopharyngeal carcinoma anatomy.

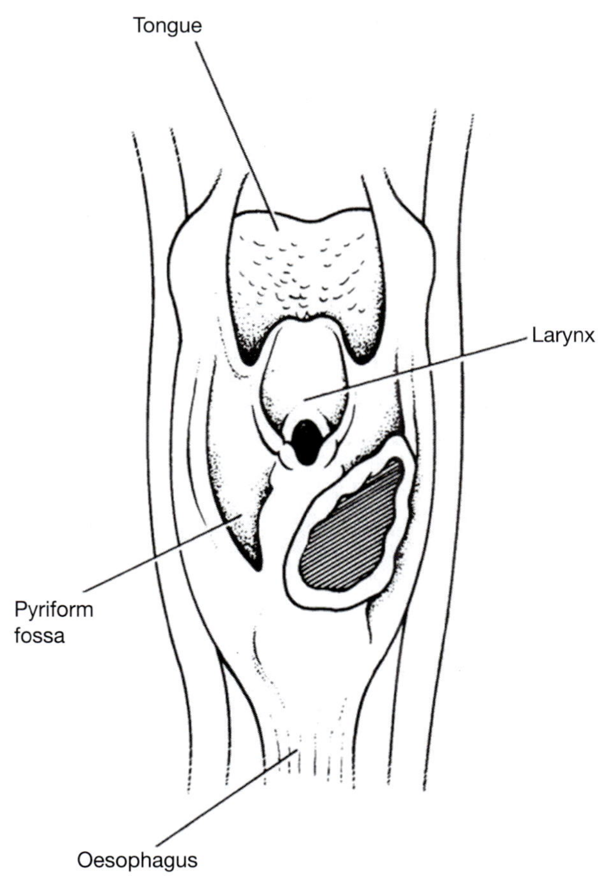

Fig. 23.56 Carcinoma of the hypopharynx (right pyriform fossa). (Reproduced from Macfarlane. *Textbook of surgery*, 7th ed. London: Churchill Livingstone.)

Incidence of Hypopharyngeal Tumours

Cancers of the hypopharynx are uncommon, with an age-standardised incidence rate of 0.63 per 100,000 population. Most arise in the piriform sinuses. These tumours mainly occur in the fifth to seventh decades and are approximately three to four times more common in males than females.

Staging System of Hypopharyngeal Tumours (8th Edition)

T1	Tumour limited to one subsite of the hypopharynx and/or measuring ≤2 cm in greatest dimension
T2	Tumour involves more than one subsite of the hypopharynx or an adjacent site, does not fix the hemilarynx and/or measures >2 cm but not >4 cm in greatest dimension
T3	Tumour measures >4 cm in greatest dimension or fixes the hemilarynx, or extends into oesophageal mucosa
T4a	Tumour invades the thyroid/cricoid cartilage, hyoid bone, thyroid gland, oesophageal muscle or central compartment soft tissue
T4b	Tumour invades the prevertebral fascia, encases the carotid artery or invades mediastinal structures

Regional lymph nodes are staged as per other head and neck sites.

Aetiology, Pathology and Lymphatic Spread

As with other head and neck cancers, tobacco and alcohol consumption are the most significant risk factors for developing cancers in this region. There are no specific genetic risk factors for this type of tumour. Postcricoid cancers may be associated with iron deficiency anaemia as part of Plummer–Vinson syndrome.

Tumours of the hypopharynx are rare in the United Kingdom but are more common in parts of Europe. Piriform fossa tumours are more prevalent in the Mediterranean regions whereas postcricoid tumours are more common in parts of Northern Europe.

Histologically, almost all hypopharyngeal carcinomas are SCCs prevalent in the head and neck region.

The hypopharynx has an extensive lymphatic supply (Fig. 23.57). The majority of piriform fossae cancers have nodal involvement at presentation. There is early spread to the upper and middeep cervical nodes (levels 2 and 3), but the drainage can include all levels including the supraclavicular nodes. Spread can be bilateral. The posterior pharyngeal wall drains to the retropharyngeal nodes (level 7A) and deep cervical lymph nodes. The postcricoid region drains to levels 3 and 4 and the paratracheal nodes (level 6). The extensive nodal drainage generally needs to be considered in RT planning.

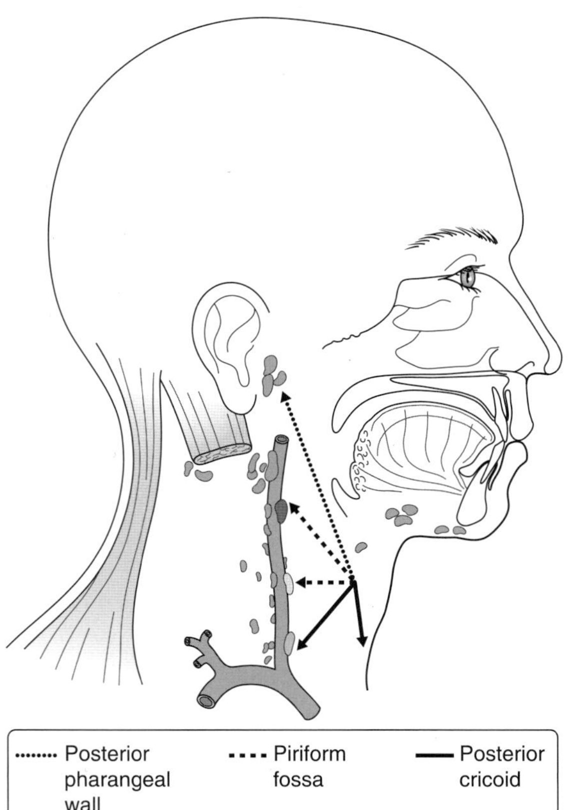

Fig. 23.57 Hypopharynx lymphatic supply.

Signs and Symptoms

Cancers in this region commonly present at an advanced state with sore throat, which may radiate to the ear, or with painful or difficulty swallowing. There may be hoarseness or haemoptysis. Tumour or ulceration in the hypopharynx can usually be visualised in the clinic via nasendoscopy and FNA, or biopsy taken if required.

Many present, however, with a neck mass from secondary lymph nodes.

Diagnosis and Staging

Patients with a history of persistent sore throat should be referred urgently to the ENT clinic. Patients may also be referred urgently for the other symptoms listed earlier or because of the presence of neck lymphadenopathy.

A full ENT examination is performed in the clinic. This allows delineation of the primary and facilitates exclusion of synchronous tumours. Examination should include fibre-optic examination. The neck should be clinically examined for palpable lymph nodes. Patients should have an examination under anaesthesia to assess the extent of the primary and for a biopsy to confirm the tissue diagnosis. Radiological assessment of the primary is essential for full locoregional staging (Fig. 23.58). This may also reveal pathological lymphadenopathy not identified clinically. Ideally, this assessment should be undertaken before biopsy to avoid any artefact that may lead to overstaging, and may be CT or MRI, or both. Imaging of the chest is also essential for exclusion of metastatic spread or synchronous primary tumours of the lung. PET/CT is now recommended in advanced cases and will help to determine the upper and lower extent of disease.

Early consideration of comorbidity factors and performance status should occur to tailor subsequent treatment.

Treatment

Given the advanced nature of most cases, surgery followed by RT (with/without chemotherapy) is the standard of care in fit, motivated patients. Surgery is thus considered the optimal initial treatment for bulky or T4

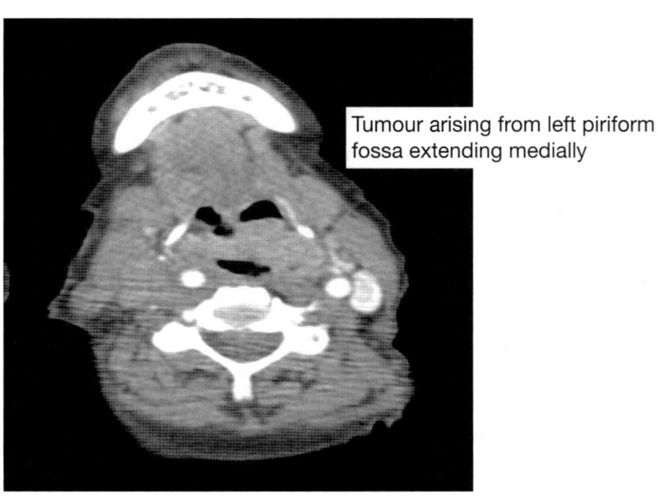

Fig. 23.58 Carcinoma of the piriform fossa.

tumours in this region and usually involves pharyngolaryngectomy. In other instances the aim of organ preservation via treatment with induction chemotherapy followed by RT or concurrent chemoradiotherapy could be considered; that said, many of these patients present malnourished, and a period of nutritional support is often required before embarking on intensive treatment. Even then, up to 25% of patients may not be suitable for any curative treatment. Attempts to improve outcomes nonsurgically with dose escalation have not translated into clinical benefit.

Radiotherapy Technique

Patients are treated in the supine position and immobilised in the usual fashion. The shoulders should be held well down as the primary target volume sits relatively low in the neck and would be clipped by the radiation beam, affecting delivered dose. A planning CT scan facilitates delineation of the primary tumour and nodes. The intimate relationship between areas of the hypopharynx means that primary CTVs are generally quite large themselves. In addition, hypopharyngeal tumours have a high propensity for submucosal spread, and as such, CTV margins need to take that into consideration, specifically superiorly and inferiorly. In practice, this means that the prophylactic CTV could be 15 mm instead of the usual 10 mm. The choice of nodes to include in the irradiation volume—that is, the nodal CTV—is based on the previous discussion, although in practice, all the nodes in the neck are irradiated.

RT prescriptions will follow the principles in Chapter 22. The large volumes characteristic of these tumour sites do not lend themselves to short fractionation schedules as used in early laryngeal disease, and thus 70 Gy in 35 fractions over 7 weeks or 65 to 66 Gy in 30 fractions over 6 weeks would be standard. Concurrent treatment with platinum chemotherapy will generally be an essential component of treatment (Figs. 23.59–23.63).

Complications

Treatment results in a predictable acute reaction of mucositis, which should be managed as discussed earlier. If patients have not undergone a pharyngolaryngectomy (and hence a stoma), they are at risk of aspiration pneumonia, and this should be managed aggressively.

Late complications at this site will include some degree of xerostomia because of the need to extend the volume superiorly, although some sparing will be possible with IMRT. Some patients have permanent dysphagia, either secondary to strictures or late damage to nerves and muscles, leading to uncoordinated swallowing. Sparing of some of the constrictor apparatus may be possible again with IMRT to offset this.

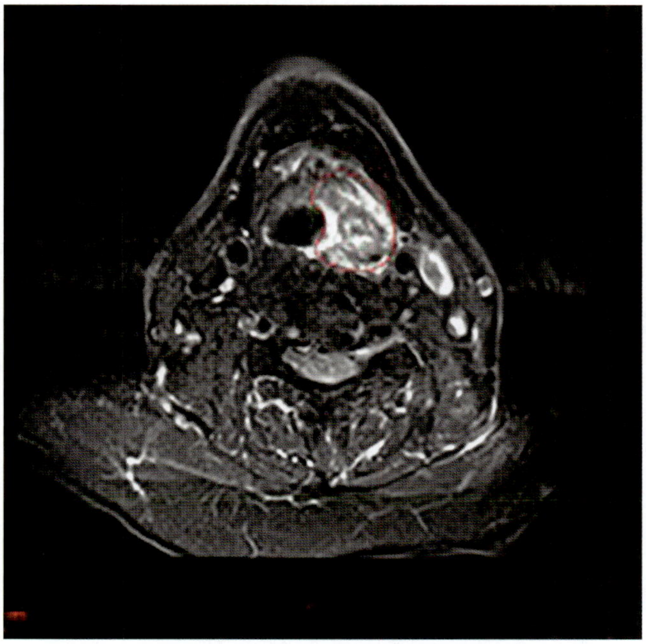

Fig. 23.59 Left-sided hypopharyngeal squamous cell carcinoma delineated on a coregistered diagnostic magnetic resonance imaging scan.

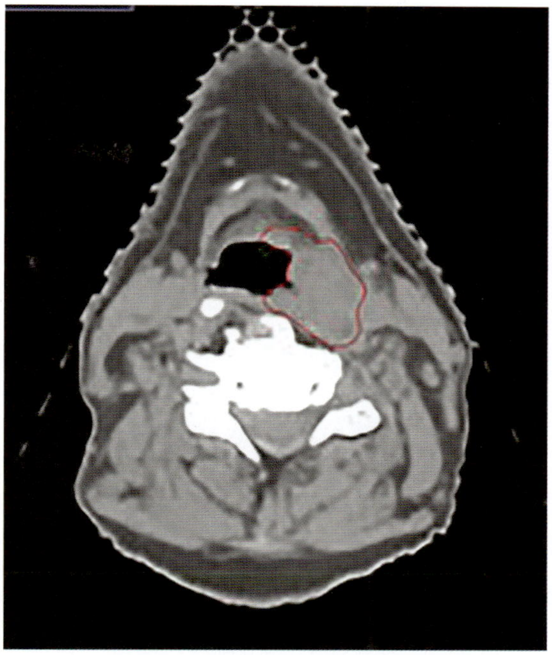

Fig. 23.60 The same tumour as in Fig. 23.59, delineated on a planning computed tomography scan.

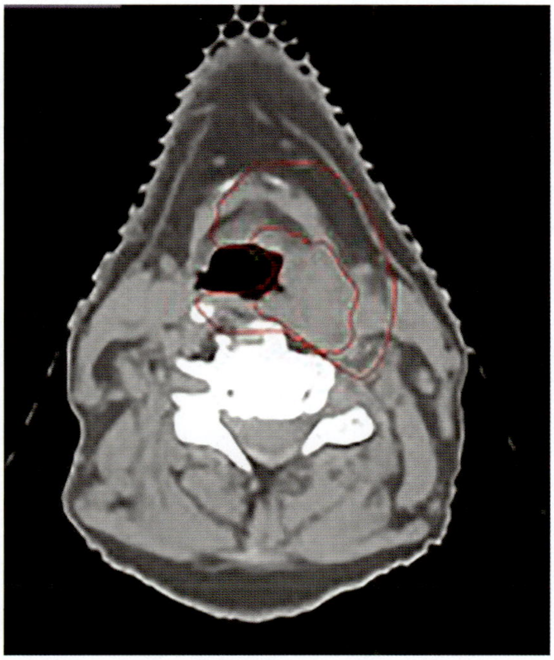

Fig. 23.61 The same tumour as in Fig. 23.59, with a 10-mm margin in the axial plane, taking into account variation between the gross tumour volume seen on a diagnostic magnetic resonance imaging scan and planning computed tomography scan.

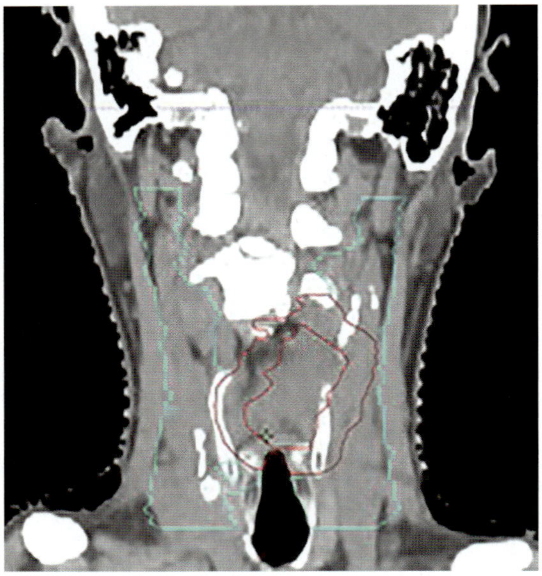

Fig. 23.62 The same tumour as in Fig. 23.59, seen in the coronal plane, with a 10-mm high-dose margin superior-inferior (and a further margin for submucosal extension treated to a lower dose) and the elective nodal volume.

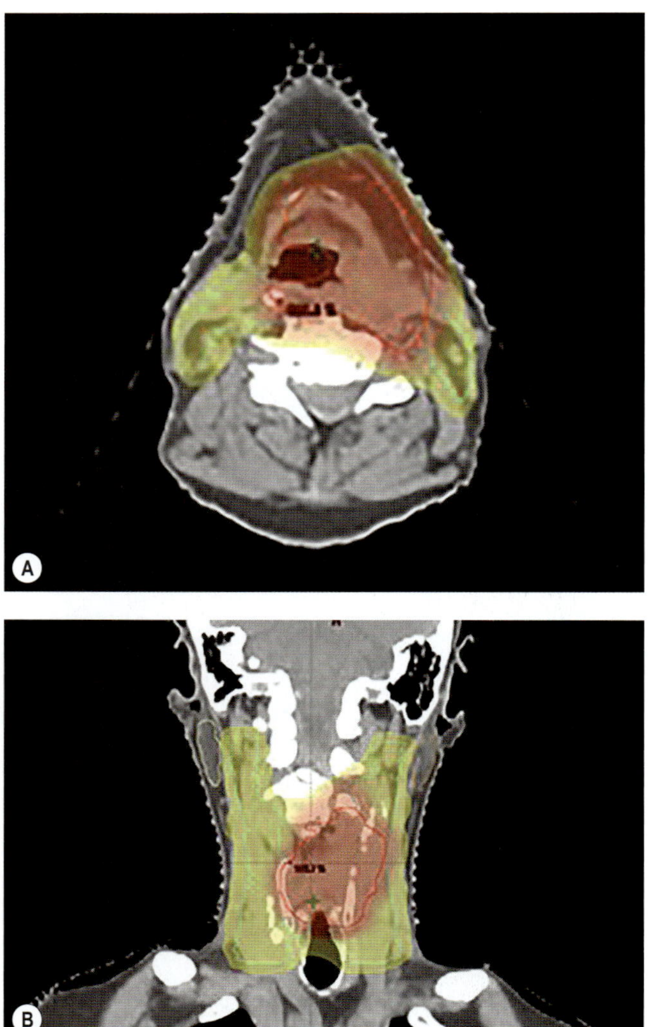

Fig. 23.63 (A) Dose distribution for the same hypopharyngeal tumour as in Fig. 23.59, seen in the axial plane. (B) Dose distribution for the same hypopharyngeal tumour, seen in the coronal plane.

Follow-up

Given that most patients present with advanced disease, a high index of suspicion should remain of residual/recurrent disease. Patients should be supported nutritionally and any late effects managed expectantly. Follow-up imaging will depend on treatment goals.

Results

Overall, the prognosis with hypopharyngeal carcinoma is poor, with an overall 5-year survival rate of 30%, reflecting the late presentation of most cases. Most patients succumb to distal metastases, intercurrent illness or second primaries if locoregional control has been attained. The outcome for tumours diagnosed at an earlier stage is predictably more favourable: treatment of T1 lesions can give rise to local control rates of greater than 85%, but with T2 and T3 lesions, the control falls to less than 60%, translating into 5-year survival rates of about 35%.

For very advanced hypopharyngeal tumours, standard therapy is surgery and postoperative (chemo-) radiation, although the clinician may opt, with the patient, to manage the condition palliatively in the light of an anticipated poor outcome (10% 5-year survival) and the significant morbidity and mortality from treatment.

FURTHER READING

Alpert TE, Morbidini-Gaffney S, Chung CT, et al. Radiotherapy for the clinically negative neck in supraglottic laryngeal cancer. *Cancer J.* 2004;10(6):335–338.

Al-Sarraf M, LeBlanc M, Giri PG, et al. Chemoradiotherapy versus radiotherapy in patients with advanced nasopharyngeal cancer phase III randomized intergroup study 0099. *J Clin Oncol.* 1998; 16(4):1310–1317.

Baujat B, Audry H, Bourhis J, et al. Chemotherapy in locally advanced nasopharyngeal carcinoma: an individual patient data meta-analysis of eight randomized trials and 1753 patients. *Int J Radiat Oncol Biol Phys.* 2006;64(1):47–66.

Bernier J, Domenge C, Ozsahin M, et al. Post-operative irradiation with or without concomitant chemotherapy for locally advanced head and neck cancer. *N Engl J Med.* 2004;350(19):1945–1952.

Blanchard P, Lee AWM, Carmel A, et al. Meta-analysis of chemotherapy in nasopharynx carcinoma 9MAC-NPC): an update on 26 trials and 7800 patients. *Clin Transl Radiat Oncol.* 2021;32:59–68.

Byers RM, Clayman GL, McGill D, et al. Selective neck dissections for squamous cell carcinoma of the upper aerodigestive tract: patterns of regional failure. *Head Neck.* 1999;21(6):499–505.

Candela FC, Kothari K, Shah JP. Patterns of cervical node metastases from squamous carcinoma of the oropharynx and hypopharynx. *Head Neck.* 1990;12(3):197–203.

Chen SW, Tsai M-H, Yang S-N, Liang J-A, Shiau A-C, Lin F-J. Hypopharyngeal cancer treatment based on definitive radiotherapy: who is suitable for laryngeal preservation? *J Laryngol Otol.* 2008;122(5):506–512.

Claus F, De Gersem W, De Wagter C, et al. An implementation strategy for IMRT of ethmoid sinus cancer with bilateral sparing of the optic pathways. *Int J Radiat Oncol Biol Phys.* 2001;51(2):318–331.

Cooper JS, Pajak TF, Forastiere AA, et al. Postoperative concurrent radiotherapy and chemotherapy for high-risk squamous cell carcinoma of the head and neck. *N Engl J Med.* 2004;350(19): 1937–1944.

Department of Veterans Affairs Laryngeal Cancer Study Group. Induction chemotherapy plus radiation compared with surgery plus radiation in patients with advanced laryngeal cancer. *N Engl J Med.* 1991;324:1685–1690.

Dirix P, Vanstraelen B, Jorissen M, Vander Poorten V, Nuyts S. Intensity-modulated radiotherapy for sinonasal cancer: improved

outcome compared to conventional radiotherapy. *Int J Radiat Oncol Biol Phys*. 2010;78(4):998–1004.
Duthoy W, Boterberg T, Claus F, et al. Postoperative intensity-modulated radiotherapy in sinonasal carcinoma. *Cancer*. 2005;104(1):71–82.
Forastiere AA, Goepfert H, Maor M, et al. Concurrent chemotherapy and radiotherapy for organ preservation in advanced laryngeal cancer. *N Engl J Med*. 2003;349(22):2091–2098.
Forastiere AA, Zhang Q, Weber RS, et al. Long-term results of RTOG 91-11: a comparison of three nonsurgical strategies to preserve the larynx in patients with locally advanced larynx cancer. *J Clin Oncol*. 2013;31(7):845–852.
Garden AS, Morrison WH, Clayman GL, Ang KK, Peters LJ. Early squamous cell carcinoma of the hypopharynx: outcomes of treatment with radiation alone to the primary disease. *Head Neck*. 1996;18(4):317–322.
Gowda RV, Henk JM, Mais KL, Sykes AJ, Swindell R, Slevin NJ. Three weeks radiotherapy for T1 glottic cancer: the christie and royal marsden hospital experience. *Radiother Oncol*. 2003;68(2):105–111.
Gregoire V, Ang K, Budach W, et al. Delineation of the neck node levels for head and neck tumours: a 2013 update. DAHANCA, EORTC, HKNPCSG, NCIC CTG, NCRI, RTOG, TROG consensus guidelines. *Radiother Oncol*. 2014;110(1):172–181.
Gregoire V, Evans M, Le Q-T, et al. Delineation of the primary clinical target volumes (CTV-P) in laryngeal, hypopharyngeal, oropharyngeal and oral cavity squamous cell carcinoma: AIRO, CACA, DAHANCA, EORTC, GEORCC, GORTEC, HKNPCSG, HNCIG, IAG-KHT, LPRHHT, NCIC CRG, NCRI, NRG Oncology, PHNS, SBRT, SOMERA, SRO, SSHNO, TROG consensus guidelines. *Radiother Oncol*. 2018;126(1):3–24.
Jackson SM, Hay JH, Flores AD, et al. Cancer of the tonsil: results of ipsilateral radiation treatment. *Radiother Oncol*. 1999;51(2):123–128.
Jang SS, Davis ME, Vera DR, Lai SY, Guo TW. Role of sentinel lymph node biopsy for oral squamous cell carcinoma: current evidence and future strategies. *Head Neck*. 2022;45(1):251–265.
Jones AS, Fish B, Fenton JE, Husband DJ. The treatment of early laryngeal cancers (T1–T2N0): surgery or irradiation? *Head Neck*. 2004;26(2):127–135.
Kam MK, Leung S-L, Zee B, et al. Prospective randomized study of intensity-modulated radiotherapy on salivary gland function in early-stage nasopharyngeal carcinoma patients. *J Clin Oncol*. 2007;25(31):4873–4879.
Lee AW, Ngan RKC, Tung SY, et al. Preliminary results of trial NPC-0501 evaluating the therapeutic gain from concurrent-adjuvant to induction-concurrent chemoradiotherapy, changing from fluorouracil to capecitabine, and changing from accelerated radiotherapy fractionation in patients with locally advanced nasopharyngeal carcinoma. *Cancer*. 2015;121(8):1328–1338.
Lee AW, Ng WT, Pan JJ, et al. International guideline for the delineation of the clinical target volumes (CTV) for nasopharyngeal carcinoma. *Radiother Oncol*. 2018;126(1):25–36.
Lee MS, Ho H-C, Hsiao S-H, Hwang J-H, Lee C-C, Hung S-K. Treatment results and prognostic factors in locally advanced hypopharyngeal cancer. *Acta Otolaryngol*. 2008;128(1):103–109.
Mahenna H, Wong W-L, McConkey CC, et al. PET-CT surveillance versus neck dissection in advanced head and neck cancer. *N Engl J Med*. 2016;374(15):1444–1454.
Melder KL, Geltzeiler M. Induction chemotherapy for locally advanced sinonasal squamous cell carcinoma and sinonasal undifferentiated carcinoma: a comprehensive review. *Cancers*. 2023;15(15):3798.
Ng WT, Chow JCH, Beitler JJ, et al. Current radiotherapy considerations for nasopharyngeal carcinoma. *Cancers*. 2022;14(23):1–15.
Nutting CM, Griffin CL, Sanghera P, et al. Dose-escalated intensity-modulated radiotherapy in patients with locally advanced laryngeal and hypopharyngeal cancers: ART DECO, a phase III randomised controlled trial. *Eur J Cancer*. 2021;153:242–256.
O'Sullivan B, Warde P, Grice B, et al. The benefits and pitfalls of ipsilateral radiotherapy in carcinoma of the tonsillar region. *Int J Radiat Oncol Biol Phys*. 2001;51(2):332–343.
Orus C, León X, Vega M, Quer M. Initial treatment of the early stages (I, II) of supraglottic squamous cell carcinoma: partial laryngectomy versus radiotherapy. *Eur Arch Otorhinologol*. 2000;257(9):512–516.
Parsons TJ, Mendenhall WM, Stringer SP, et al. Squamous cell carcinoma of the oropharynx: surgery, radiation therapy, or both. *Cancer*. 2002;94(11):2967–2980.
Royal College of Radiologists. In: Head and Neck Cancer. *Radiotherapy Dose Fractionation*. 4th ed. London: RCR; 2024, pp. 56–65.
Royal College of Radiologists. *Head and Neck Cancer Consensus Statements*. London: RCR; 2022. Available from: https://www.rcr.ac.uk/our-services/all-our-publications/clinical-oncology-publications/head-and-neck-cancer-rcr-consensus-statements/ (Accessed on 23 July 2025).
Schache AG, Powell NG, Cuschieri KS, et al. HPV-related oropharyngeal cancer in the United Kingdom: an evolution in understanding of disease etiology. *Cancer Res*. 2016;76(22):6598–6606.
Scola B, Fernández-Vega M, Martínez T, Fernández-Vega S, Ramirez C. Management of cancer of the supraglottis. *Otolaryngol Head Neck Surg*. 2001;124(2):195–198.
Shah JP, Candela FC, Poddar AK. The patterns of cervical lymph node metastases from squamous carcinoma of the oral cavity. *Cancer*. 1990;66(1):109–113.
Varghese C, Sankaranarayanan R, Nair B, Nair MK. Predictors of neck node control in radically irradiated squamous cell carcinoma of the oropharynx and laryngopharynx. *Head Neck*. 1993;15(2):105–108.
Wang H-Y, Chang Y-L, To K-F, et al. A new prognostic histopathologic classification of nasopharyngeal carcinoma. *Chin J Cancer*. 2016;35:41.
Wendt CD, Peters LJ, Delclos L, et al. Primary radiotherapy in the treatment of stage I and II tongue cancers: importance of the proportion therapy delivered with interstitial therapy. *Int J Radiat Oncol Biol Phys*. 1990;18(6):1529–1530.
Westra WH. The pathology of HPV-related head and neck cancer: implications for the diagnostic pathologist. *Semin Diagn Pathol*. 2015;32(1):42–53.

24

Thyroid Cancer

Jonathan Wadsley

CHAPTER OUTLINE

INTRODUCTION AND EPIDEMIOLOGY

Thyroid cancer comprises a number of different histological subtypes with very variable clinical behaviour. These include differentiated thyroid cancer (papillary and follicular), medullary thyroid cancer and anaplastic thyroid cancer. The presence of a micropapillary carcinoma of the thyroid is likely to have no impact on life expectancy, whereas anaplastic thyroid cancer is almost always lethal. Although thyroid cancer is uncommon, representing only about 1% of all cancers, it is the most frequently occurring endocrine malignancy and incidence of papillary thyroid cancer is increasing. This rise is largely as a result of the increased use of medical imaging, which detects incidental thyroid lesions that may otherwise never have been discovered. Most of the increase is because of the diagnosis of lower-risk cancers. In spite of the increase in incidence, there has been no increase in mortality. In the United Kingdom, the incidence of thyroid cancer has increased by more than two and a half times since the early 1990s. In 2018, there were around 3900 new cases but only 410 deaths because of thyroid cancer. Differentiated thyroid cancer is highly curable (5-year survival around 95%). It can also affect children and young adults. While the majority of patients with differentiated thyroid cancer will be cured, around 10% to 15% will develop advanced refractory disease, which cannot be cured.

All suspected and confirmed thyroid cancers should be discussed at a thyroid cancer multidisciplinary team meeting. Comprehensive updated international guidelines are available. They include 'Guidelines for the Management of Thyroid Cancer', 2014, by the British Thyroid Association and the Royal College of Physicians and the soon to be updated 'Revised American Thyroid Association Guidelines', 2016 published by the American Thyroid Association. The UK National Institute for Health and Care Excellence (NICE) issued guidance on the assessment and management of thyroid cancer in December 2022 (NG230).

ANATOMY

The thyroid gland is situated in the anterior part of the neck, just above the clavicle and sternum (Figs. 24.1A and B). The gland consists of a right and left lobe joined by an isthmus that crosses the trachea at the second and third cartilaginous rings. The average weight of the thyroid gland is 20 g. The parathyroid glands lie on the posterior surface of both thyroid lobs, and the recurrent laryngeal nerves are in a cleft between the trachea and the oesophagus. Lymphatic drainage from the thyroid can be to nodes superior to the thyroid gland and lateral to the gland and the paratracheal region.

AETIOLOGICAL FACTORS

Differentiated thyroid cancer can affect all age groups, including, rarely, children. In the United Kingdom, currently the highest incidence rates are in the 65-to-69-year age group. Eleven percent of cases are diagnosed in patients 75 years of age or over. The condition is approximately three times more common in females than in males.

Exposure to ionising radiation in childhood, either therapeutic, such as radiotherapy (RT) as a part of acute leukaemia treatment protocols, or associated with environmental exposure, increases the risk of developing thyroid cancer. Following exposure to fallout (particularly radioiodine (RAI)) from the Chernobyl nuclear reactor fire in 1986, there has been a marked increase in well-differentiated thyroid cancer in Russia, Ukraine and Belarus in children and young people, with over 5000 new cases reported. The mortality from the accident has been low, with fewer than 50 deaths and a projected 30-year mortality of 1%. There is, however, no proven relationship between the development of thyroid cancer and administration of iodine-131 for the treatment of benign thyroid disorders such as hyperthyroidism.

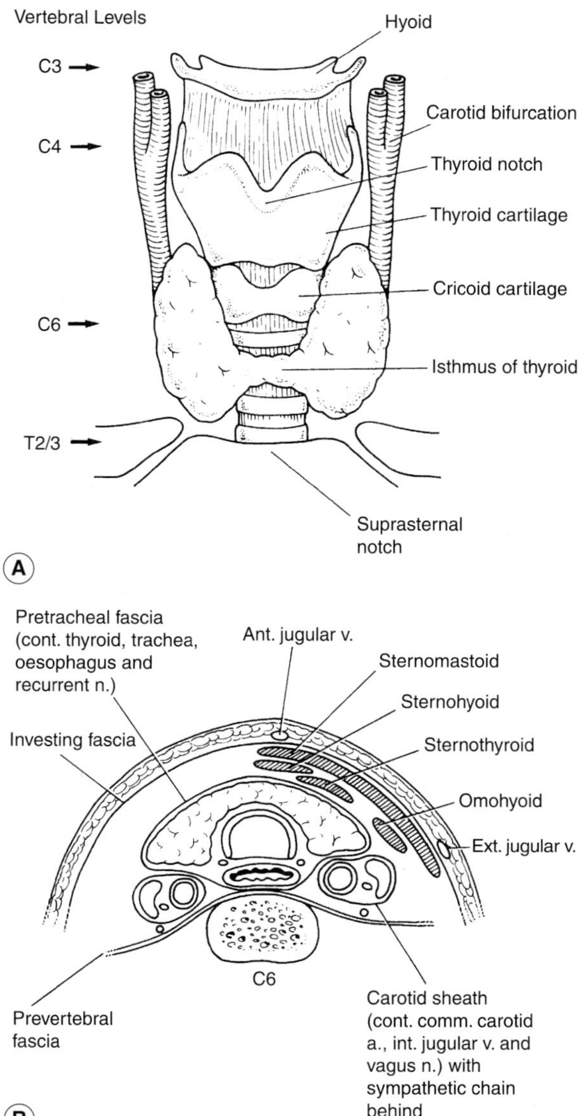

Fig. 24.1 (A) Structures palpable on the anterior aspect of the neck, together with corresponding vertebral levels. (B) Transverse section of the neck through C6 showing the relations of the thyroid gland. (Reproduced from Ellis H. *Clinical anatomy*, 5th ed. Oxford: Wiley-Blackwell; 1975.)

Other medical conditions that affect the thyroid have also been linked to an increased risk of developing thyroid cancer, namely, endemic goitre, which occurs in areas where there is low natural iodine; Hashimoto thyroiditis; a past history of thyroid adenoma; or a family history of thyroid adenoma or cancer.

Some genetic conditions that increase the risk of differentiated thyroid cancer include Gardner syndrome, Cowden syndrome and familial adenomatous polyposis.

Around 25% of cases of medullary thyroid cancer arise as a result of germline mutations in the RET gene and may be associated with multiple endocrine neoplasia syndromes. The remaining sporadic cases of medullary thyroid cancer are frequently found to carry somatic RET mutations.

Differentiated thyroid cancer initiation and progression results from the accumulation of genetic and epigenetic events. These include point mutations of BRAF (predominantly papillary) and RAS (N,H,K-Ras predominantly follicular) genes and chromosomal rearrangements, RET/PTC (papillary, particularly radiation induced) and PAX8/PPARγ (follicular); abnormal miRNA (microRNA) with gene methylation problems also plays a part. These events are described in the 2014 Thyroid Cancer Genome Atlas. P53 and TERT promoter mutations are thought to be later events in the progression to more poorly differentiated thyroid cancer.

Increased knowledge about the molecular alterations underlying the development of thyroid cancer has led to the development of targeted therapies, particularly tyrosine kinase inhibitors active against relevant signalling pathways and, most recently, specific RET inhibitors licensed for the treatment of thyroid cancers with RET fusions or mutations.

PRESENTATION, DIAGNOSIS AND PATIENT PATHWAY

The most common presenting feature of thyroid cancer is a painless lower neck lump. In more advanced cases, patients may complain of a lump on the side of the neck because of the spread to lymph nodes; hoarseness or change in voice, suggesting recurrent laryngeal nerve involvement; stridor; or, rarely, dysphagia. Patients presenting with a thyroid nodule are more likely to have malignancy if the nodule is fixed, there are palpable lymph nodes, vocal cord palsy is present or there is a past history of Hashimoto thyroiditis, previous neck irradiation or a family history of thyroid cancer. Malignancy within a thyroid nodule is also more common if a patient is under 20 years of age or over 60 years of age.

A rapid enlargement of the mass or a rapid development of symptoms, suggesting compression of other structures, may be because of a more rapidly growing anaplastic carcinoma or lymphoma.

In the first instance, the patient should be referred to a neck lump clinic, typically managed by endocrinology, endocrine surgery or ear-nose-throat (ENT) surgery. A history of the development of the mass and any relevant personal past history (including of radiation exposure) or family history of thyroid problems or other endocrine tumours are important. Examination is undertaken to define whether the mass is solitary or multiple, whether it is tender, which might suggest a benign cause, and whether the mass is fixed to the skin or to underlying structures in the neck. Any enlarged lymph nodes within the neck are noted. Development of stridor is a medical emergency demanding urgent hospital admission for management of airway compromise.

Ultrasound and fine needle aspiration cytology (FNAC) are essential investigations for neck masses suspected of being a thyroid cancer. Ultrasound guidance may help in obtaining the aspiration cytology and can help distinguish solid from cystic masses in the neck. It can differentiate between solitary and multiple nodules, help detect involved lymph nodes (if needed by guided FNAC) and provide sonographic features suggesting probable malignancy in some cases. An established system for grading ultrasound appearance should be used, such as the British Thyroid Association 2014 guidelines for ultrasound scoring of thyroid nodules (BTA-U score) (Table 24.1). This can help establish the risk of malignancy and determine whether FNAC is required. FNAC should be reported according to the Royal College of Pathologists Thy classification system (Table 24.2).

While a definite (Thy5) diagnosis can be reached for papillary carcinoma on FNAC, follicular cancers cannot be differentiated from adenomas on FNAC alone, as architectural evidence of either capsular or vascular invasion is required. Lobectomy is therefore usually necessary to reach a diagnosis when Thy3F cytology is reported.

There are no indications for an incisional biopsy of the thyroid, which might compromise future therapeutic interventions, but if thyroid lymphoma or anaplastic thyroid cancer is suspected, an ultrasound-guided core biopsy may be more helpful than FNAC.

TABLE 24.1 British Thyroid Association 2014 Ultrasound U Classification for Thyroid Nodules

U1 (Normal)	No Nodules
U2 (benign)	Hyperechoic or isoechoic with a halo Cystic change with ring-down artefact (colloid) Microcystic or spongiform appearance Peripheral eggshell calcification Peripheral vascularity
U3 (indeterminate)	Solid homogenous markedly hyperechoic nodule with halo (follicular lesions) Hypoechoic with equivocal echogenic foci or cystic change Mixed or central vascularity
U4 (suspicious)	Solid hypoechoic (compared with thyroid) Solid very hypoechoic (compared with strap muscles) Hypoechoic with disrupted peripheral calcification Lobulated outline
U5 (malignant)	Solid hypoechoic with lobulated or irregular outline and microcalcification Papillary carcinoma Solid hypoechoic with lobulated or irregular outline and globular calcification Medullary carcinoma Intranodular vascularity Taller than wide axially (AP > ML) Characteristic associated lymphadenopathy

TABLE 24.2 Royal College of Pathologists 2009 Thy Classification System

Thy1	Nondiagnostic; FNAC needs repeating
Thy2	Nonneoplastic; two diagnostic tests with benign results 3–6 months apart are needed to exclude malignancy
Thy3 F	Follicular lesion; lobectomy required with completion thyroidectomy if malignant histology
Thy3 A	Atypia present; repeat ultrasound and FNAC; consider diagnostic hemithyroidectomy
Thy4	Abnormal, suspicious but not diagnostic of any histological form of thyroid cancer; treatment required depending on histology
Thy5	Diagnostic of thyroid malignancy; surgery required for differentiated thyroid cancer; other management may be more appropriate if other forms of malignancy

FNAC, Fine-needle aspiration cytology.

Radioactive iodine scans can rarely help differentiate nonfunctioning 'cold' nodules within the thyroid, which may represent a malignancy, from 'hot' nodules, which rarely contain a cancer. Usually these scans are not helpful with diagnosis and are much more useful in the postoperative period for diagnosing residual disease or early recurrence.

Cross-sectional imaging with either computed tomography (CT) or magnetic resonance imaging (MRI) scans is not routinely required for early-stage (T1 and T2) lesions, but it can be helpful in planning the extent of surgery in patients with more advanced (T3, T4 or N1) disease.

Thyroid function tests are usually normal in patients with thyroid cancer; calcium, phosphate and thyroglobulin can be sampled for baseline measurement, but thyroglobulin level is not useful in the preoperative phase. If there is any suspicion that the thyroid tumour may be a medullary cancer, the serum calcitonin level is checked.

TABLE 24.3 TNM Staging System from American Joint Committee on Cancer, 8th Edition (2018)

Thyroid Cancer: TNM Classification	
T	Primary tumour, including papillary, follicular, poorly differentiated, Hurthle cell and anaplastic carcinomas
TX	Primary tumour cannot be assessed
T0	No evidence of primary tumour
T1	Tumour 2 cm or less in greatest dimension, limited to the thyroid
T1a	Tumour 1 cm or less in greatest dimension, limited to the thyroid
T1b	Tumour more than 1 cm but not more than 2 cm in greatest dimension, limited to the thyroid
T2	Tumour more than 2 cm but not more than 4 cm in greatest dimension, limited to the thyroid
T3a	Tumour more than 4 cm in greatest dimension, limited to the thyroid
T3b	Tumour of any size with gross extrathyroidal extension invading strap muscles (sternohyoid, sternothyroid or omohyoid muscles)
T4a	Tumour extends beyond the thyroid capsule and invades any of the following: subcutaneous soft tissues, larynx, trachea, oesophagus, recurrent laryngeal nerve
T4b	Tumour invades prevertebral fascia, mediastinal vessels or encases carotid artery
N: Regional Lymph Nodes	
NX	Regional lymph nodes cannot be assessed
N0	No regional lymph node metastasis
N1	Regional lymph node metastasis
N1a	Metastasis in Level VI: pretracheal, paratracheal and prelaryngeal/Delphian lymph nodes; or upper/superior mediastinum
N1b	Metastasis in other unilateral, bilateral or contralateral cervical (Levels I, II, III, IV or V) or retropharyngeal
M: Distant Metastasis	
M0	No distant metastasis
M1	Distant metastasis

Staging performed using the TNM system, 8th edition, American Joint Committee on Cancer (AJCC) is summarised in Tables 24.3 and 24.4. All anaplastic carcinomas are considered T4 tumours. At the latest revision, the AJCC increased the cutoff for age as an adverse prognostic factor from 45 to 55 years.

One major disadvantage of the TNM system is that the presence of positive nodes does not necessarily predict poorer survival, consequently making this staging system less useful in the practical setting than at other cancer sites.

DIFFERENTIATED THYROID CANCER

These tumours are divided into papillary and follicular thyroid cancers and are distinguished by their behaviour, as they are sensitive to thyroid stimulating hormone (TSH), take up iodine and can produce thyroglobulin. All three of these factors are used in their management. It should be remembered that, in general, differentiated thyroid cancer carries a very good prognosis, with 20-year survival of over 85% in those patients who do not develop distant metastasis.

Papillary thyroid cancer is the most common type of thyroid cancer, accounting for almost 80% of all cases, and its incidence is increasing worldwide. These tumours are also derived from the follicular cells of the thyroid and may show psammoma bodies, small flecks of

TABLE 24.4 Thyroid Cancer Stage Groupings from American Joint Committee on Cancer, 8th Edition (2018)

Separate stage groupings are recommended for papillary or follicular (differentiated), medullary and anaplastic (undifferentiated) carcinoma.
Papillary or follicular (differentiated); <55 years of age
Stage I Any T, Any N M0
Stage II Any T, Any N M1
Papillary or follicular (differentiated); ≥55 years of age
Stage I T1a, T1b, T2 N0 M0
Stage II T3 N0 M0; T1, T2, T3 N1 M0
Stage III T4a Any N M0
Stage IVA T4b Any N M0
Stage IVB Any T, Any N M1
Medullary
Stage I T1a, T1b N0 M0
Stage II T2, T3 N0 M0
Stage III T1, T2, T3 N1a M0
Stage IVA T1, T2, T3 N1b M0; T4a Any N M0
Stage IVB T4b Any N M0
Stage IVC Any T, Any N M1
Anaplastic
Stage IVA T1, T2, T3a N0 M0
Stage IVB T1, T2, T3a N1 M0; T3b, T4a, T4b N0, N1 M0
Stage IVC Any T, Any N M1

calcification, on microscopy. The distinctive feature of these tumours is that they have characteristic nuclei (Orphan Annie appearance) and may grow in branching stalks (the so-called papillae). These tumours are often multifocal and may involve the cervical lymph nodes, with less tendency to haematogenous spread when compared with follicular cancers. Papillary carcinoma is three times more common in females than males, with a peak incidence in the third to fourth decade of life.

Follicular thyroid cancer makes up about 10% of thyroid malignancies. It generally affects a slightly older age group than papillary cancer and does not typically involve local lymph nodes. Follicular carcinomas are often solitary within the thyroid gland and may invade the vascular channels and spread via the bloodstream to distant sites.

Management of Differentiated Thyroid Cancer

The aims of treatment are to remove all thyroid cancer tissue and to reduce the risk of recurrent disease as far as possible. This will almost always include the use of surgery, sometimes followed by RAI treatment and TSH suppression. With increasing understanding of risk stratification and the excellent prognosis of many early thyroid cancers, there is a trend towards treatment deescalation and a more individualised approach.

Surgery

Surgery is required for most thyroid cancers, although evidence is accumulating that small cancers (<10 mm) may be managed conservatively with active surveillance. Total thyroidectomy should be offered to patients with T3 or T4 tumours, regional lymph node involvement, adverse histological features or metastatic disease. A thyroid lobectomy alone may be sufficient for patients with T1a(m) to T2N0M0 disease, although high-quality evidence to support this is currently lacking. The UK 'hemi or total thyroidectomy in low risk thyroid cancer' (HoT) trial is addressing this question in a randomised controlled trial.

There is not thought to be a role for prophylactic central or lateral neck dissection, but if structural nodal disease is present, a compartment-orientated neck dissection should be undertaken. 'Cherry picking' of individual involved nodes is not recommended.

Thyroid surgery carries risks of recurrent laryngeal nerve palsy and postoperative hypoparathyroidism due to damage to the parathyroid glands. In expert hands the risks of these complications should be low, but they may require ongoing management when they occur. Patients who have had total thyroidectomy will inevitably require lifelong thyroid hormone replacement. The target range for TSH is discussed later in this chapter.

Up to 20% of patients may develop locoregional recurrence, usually signalled by a rising thyroglobulin or clinically recurrent disease detectable on ultrasound (or rarely other cross-sectional imaging) or palpable in the neck. These patients may remain curable, with appropriate intervention. If operable, surgery should be considered as the first salvage procedure offered.

Radioiodine Treatment

RAI in the form of the isotope iodine-131 has been used in the management of differentiated thyroid cancer for more than 80 years. It exploits the almost exclusive presence of the sodium iodide symporter (NIS), an active transporter of iodine, in the thyroid follicular cell membrane. This allows the delivery of high doses of radiation specifically to thyroid and thyroid cancer cells while causing very little toxicity in other tissues. While RAI is in general a very safe and well-tolerated treatment, increasing recognition of potential late effects, in particular, second malignancy risk, and the excellent prognosis of most thyroid cancers even without this treatment are leading to more careful patient selection.

Iodine uptake into thyroid cells is dependent on TSH levels, and effective RAI treatment requires an elevated TSH. Historically, this has been achieved by withdrawing thyroid hormone replacement therapy, resulting in pituitary production of TSH. More recently, a recombinant human TSH (rhTSH) has been developed. This has been shown to be as effective as thyroid hormone withdrawal in facilitating successful RAI ablation while significantly improving quality of life and is now used routinely. It is also desirable for patients to be in a low iodine state when receiving RAI to maximise uptake. Iodinated contrast for CT scanning should be avoided for at least 8 weeks, iodine containing medications such as amiodarone should be avoided and patients are asked to observe a low-iodine diet for 1 to 2 weeks before treatment.

There are a number of different scenarios in which RAI may be a useful treatment, with differing goals.

Thyroid Remnant Ablation

The aim of RAI ablation is to destroy any residual normal thyroid remnant tissue following total thyroidectomy. This potentially renders thyroglobulin, a highly specific biomarker for residual thyroid or thyroid cancer tissue, a more useful tumour marker, facilitating follow-up.

Adjuvant Treatment

The goal of treatment here is to destroy any remaining microscopic foci of residual thyroid cancer cells. Patient selection for such therapy is based on postoperative risk stratification for recurrence (Table 24.5). Recent randomised trials have demonstrated that adjuvant RAI does not impact recurrence rates for lower-risk differentiated thyroid cancer, which are very low even without RAI. This is reflected in recent guidance such as the UK NICE guideline 2022 (NG230) and is leading to more selective application of this treatment.

Typically, a fixed empirical activity of iodine-131 is administered for ablation or adjuvant therapy. The HiLo and ESTIMABL trials demonstrated that 1.1 GBq is as effective as the more traditional 3.7 GBq both in terms of ablation success rate and in preventing recurrence for

TABLE 24.5 Postoperative Risk of Structural Disease Recurrence, ATA 2015

Risk Group	Clinicopathological Features	Recurrence Risk
Low risk (1%–5%)	Unifocal PTmC	1%–2%
	Intrathyroidal encapsulated FV-PTC	1%–2%
	Intrathyroidal unifocal PTmC, BRAF mut	1%–2%
	Intrathyroidal, <4 cm, BRAF wt	1%–2%
	Minimally invasive FTC	2%–3%
	pN1 without extranodal extension, ≤3 LN involved	2%
	Multifocal PTmC	4%–6%
	Intrathyroidal PTC 2–4 cm	5%
	pN1 ≤5 lymph nodes involved	5%
	pN1, all LN <0.2 cm	5%
Intermediate risk (10%–30%)	pT3, minimal ETE	3%–8%
	Intrathyroidal PTC <4 cm BRAF mut	10%
	pN1, >5 LN involved	20%
	Clinical N1	20%
	PTC, vascular invasion	15%–30%
	PTC, extrathyroidal, BRAF mut	10%–40%
High risk (>30%)	pN1, any LN >3 cm	30%
	PTC >1 cm TERT mut +/– BRAF mut	>40%
	pN1 with extranodal extension, >3 LN involved	40%
	pT4a, gross ETE	30%–40%
	FTC, extensive vascular invasion	30%–55%

patients with T1-3 tumours without other adverse pathological features. The 3.7-GBq dose is still used for patients with high-risk disease.

Therapy

This refers to the treatment of gross residual or metastatic disease with RAI. Typically, higher activities such as 5.5-GBq iodine-131 are used, and there is interest in personalising treatment using dosimetry to deliver a defined absorbed dose to the target, although evidence to justify this approach is as yet limited and further research is required. Repeated therapy may be given, typically at 6-month intervals. RAI therapy can be curative, especially, for example, in younger patients with lung metastases. Even if not completely curative, it can lead to effective disease control for numbers of years.

Radiation Protection Precautions

Because iodine-131 is a γ emitter, precautions need to be taken to avoid unnecessary radiation exposure to others following treatment. Ideally, residual dose rates should be monitored in each patient following treatment, and tailored advice should be provided regarding necessary precautions depending on the rate of fall of activity levels and a careful risk assessment of the patient's circumstances, for example, whether they are responsible for caring for young children. Low activities such as 1.1 GBq can be safely delivered on a day case outpatient basis, but use of higher activities will generally require a short inpatient stay in appropriately designed facilities while radiation levels fall. (See Chapter 8 for more information about radionuclide administration and radiation protection.) Pregnancy must be excluded prior to treatment with RAI. It is recommended that females avoid pregnancy for at least 6 months following RAI. It is reported that there can be an increased risk of spontaneous abortion up to 12 months after RAI. Males are advised to take careful contraceptive precautions for 6 months following RAI.

Toxcity of Radioiodine

Iodine-131 therapy can cause some discomfort and swelling in the neck. Sialoadenitis (inflammation of the salivary glands) can occur because of the preferential iodine uptake by these glands. Radiation cystitis from excretion of RAI is also possible, but both of these are uncommon, especially with the lower activities of RAI used for ablation or adjuvant therapy. Nausea can occur with higher activities.

There is a small risk of hyponatraemia following treatment; risk factors include old age; female gender; presence of hypertension; presence of diabetes; use of thiazide diuretics, angiotensin receptor blockers or angiotensin converting enzyme inhibitors; lung metastasis; and low estimated glomerular filtration rate prior to therapy. Symptoms of this complication include generalised weakness, nausea and vomiting.

There is a small risk of later development of second malignancy following RAI. The risk appears to be dose dependent and is highest for haematological malignancies, but increased risk of other solid tumours has been reported. While the risks are low given the generally excellent prognosis of most patients with differentiated thyroid cancer who will therefore be long-term survivors, this needs to be taken into account, and this is at least in part responsible for the trend to fewer patients being given RAI.

Dynamic Risk Stratification

It is now recognised that a patient's risk of recurrence can be reassessed following completion of treatment and these data used to determine (1) risk of subsequent recurrence, (2) whether ongoing TSH suppression is required and (3) a follow-up strategy. It is recommended that 6 to 9 months following RAI a neck ultrasound scan is undertaken and serum thyroglobulin and thyroglobulin antibody levels measured. Patients can then be allocated to categories of excellent response, indeterminate response and incomplete response (Table 24.6).

Thyroid Stimulating Hormone Levels

All patients who have had a total thyroidectomy require thyroid hormone replacement, typically with levothyroxine (T4). This is required to replace the natural hormone produced by the gland. In some cases it is also desirable to suppress the levels of TSH produced by the pituitary, which can stimulate residual thyroid cancer cells.

In patients with low-risk disease not felt to require RAI, it is recommended that TSH levels are kept towards the lower end of the normal

TABLE 24.6 Dynamic Risk Stratification Following Surgery and Radioiodine, ATA 2015

Category	Imaging and Biochemical Features	Long-Term Structural Recurrence Risk
Excellent response	Negative imaging and suppressed Tg <0.2 ng/mL or stimulated Tg <1 ng/mL with negative TgAb	1%–4%
Indeterminate response	Nonspecific imaging findings, suppressed Tg detectable but <1 ng/mL, stimulated Tg <10 ng/mL, TgAb stable or declining	15%–20%
Biochemical incomplete response	Negative imaging but suppressed Tg ≥1 ng/mL or stimulated Tg ≥10 ng/mL or TgAb rising	20%
Structural incomplete response	Structural or functional evidence of disease regardless of Tg or TgAb levels	50%–85%

range (0.3–2.0). For patients requiring RAI, it is recommended that TSH is suppressed to <0.1 for the first 6 to 9 months following treatment, at which stage dynamic risk stratification should be undertaken to determine whether or not TSH suppression can be relaxed. Patients considered to be at high risk of recurrence or with residual disease should be considered for continued TSH suppression.

Iodine Refractory Differentiated Thyroid Cancer

While patients with advanced disease may respond well to RAI, and a proportion are cured, many will eventually become refractory to RAI and develop progressive disease. This is known as *iodine refractory differentiated thyroid cancer (IRDTC)* and carries a poor prognosis, with median survival of only 3 to 5 years if untreated.

IRDTC responds poorly to conventional cytotoxic chemotherapy. Multikinase inhibitors such as sorafenib and lenvatinib have been shown to significantly improve progression-free survival in this group of patients and are now used routinely. These agents are, however, associated with significant toxicity, and it is recommended that treatment is only started in patients with evidence of disease progression that is at risk of causing significant symptoms. This treatment is palliative, and tumours will inevitably ultimately become resistant.

Recent evidence has demonstrated the benefit of another multikinase inhibitor, cabozantinib, in further extending progression-free survival in patients who have experienced disease progression on a first-line multikinase inhibitor.

A proportion of patients with IRDTC are found to have specific targetable genetic alterations such as RET and NTRK fusions. It is recommended that such alterations are tested for in this group of patients because specific inhibitors are now available and have shown benefits in the second-line setting, on failure of multikinase inhibitors, in these selected patients.

Another development in the treatment of IRDTC is the concept of redifferentiation therapy. The goal of such treatments is to re-establsh expression of NIS in thyroid cancer cell membranes, the loss of which is responsible for cells becoming iodine refractory. This may in turn render the cancer sensitive to RAI. Alterations in the MAP kinase signalling pathway have been found to be responsible for loss of NIS expression, and treatment with BRAF inhibitors (such as dabrafenib) and MEK inhibitors (such as selumtinib and trametinib) that block this aberrant signalling has been shown to reestablish RAI uptake in a proportion of patients. The precise clinical benefit of this approach when compared with the use of multikinase inhibitors remains to be established and continues to be an area of active research interest.

MEDULLARY THYROID CANCER

Diagnosis and Initial Management

Derived from parafollicular C cells, which produce calcitonin, these cancers are part of a familial endocrine cancer syndrome in 25% of the patients who develop medullary thyroid cancer (MTC). MTC is sporadic, without a familial component in 75% of cases. Not all patients with the inherited form give a positive family history, as the condition can skip generations. These familial syndromes can be broadly divided into three types.

Familial MTC can occur by itself, is inherited in an autosomal dominant pattern and is associated with a mutation in the RET protooncogene. If this mutation is present, almost 100% of patients will develop MTC. If it occurs by itself without other endocrine neoplasia, the thyroid cancer may behave in a more indolent manner than when it appears as part of the multiple endocrine neoplasia (MEN) syndromes. MTC is also a component of the familial syndromes MEN 2A (also known as Sipple syndrome) and MEN 2B. Patients may develop phaeochromocytoma in both MEN 2A and 2B, hyperparathyroidism in MEN 2A and ganglioneuromatosis in MEN 2B. MTC may occur relatively early in MEN 2B and be more aggressive.

Patients with any of these syndromes should be offered prophylactic thyroidectomy while still young, before MTC develops. Guidance is available regarding the optimal timing of prophylactic surgery, which varies according to the location of the RET mutation in an individual family.

As this condition is potentially inheritable and is associated with other endocrine tumours, all patients diagnosed with MTC should be offered RET mutation genetic testing with the local clinical genetics service after appropriate counselling, detailing the implications of positive or negative test results for them and their relatives.

Diagnosis in this type of thyroid cancer can be made with FNAC. An elevated serum calcitonin helps confirm the diagnosis. Patients presenting with these tumours require screening for the other potential components of these familial syndromes, in particular for phaeochromocytoma, because this has implications for the safety of any planned surgery. This is generally undertaken by measuring urine or serum catecholamines.

These cases, because of their rarity, should be treated by specialist teams including a surgeon, endocrinologist, geneticist and oncologist.

Because lymph node involvement is common, at a minimum most patients will require total thyroidectomy and prophylactic central compartment node dissection. In patients with clinical or radiological evidence of involvement of lateral neck nodes, lateral neck node dissection will also be required.

RAI does not have a role in the treatment of MTC.

Adjuvant external beam radiotherapy (EBRT) may be considered following surgery in patients with very locally advanced disease, especially when there is concern about the possibility of residual disease.

Serum calcitonin is a specific tumour marker for MTC and is used to monitor patients following completion of primary treatment. A persistently elevated or rising calcitonin requires investigation for residual or recurrent disease. If locoregional recurrence is identified, further surgery should be considered.

Advanced Medullary Thyroid Cancer

Advanced MTC can have a very variable clinical course. Some patients have extremely indolent disease and remain well without treatment for many years, while others experience much more rapidly progressive and symptomatic disease. Patients may experience diarrhoea, thought to be caused by high levels of circulating calcitonin, and in rare cases the tumour may be ACTH secreting, leading to Cushing syndrome.

As with differentiated thyroid cancer (DTC), conventional cytotoxic chemotherapy has little to offer these patients. In recent years the multikinase inhibitors vandetanib and cabozantinib have been shown to extend progression-free survival in patients with progressive MTC and are now used routinely.

The most recent advance has been the development of the specific RET inhibitors selpercatinib and pralsetinib, which have demonstrated significant responses and improved progression-free survival in patients with either germline or somatic RET mutations, and routine testing for these mutations is now recommended to allow access to these treatments when relevant mutations are identified.

ANAPLASTIC THYROID CANCER

Anaplastic thyroid cancer (ATC) is rare, making up fewer than 5% of thyroid malignancies, but is in general aggressive and carries a much worse prognosis than differentiated thyroid cancer, with median survival less than 6 months in many published series. It typically presents in older patients (mean age at diagnosis is 65 years).

ATC develops from the follicular cells, and in some cases, it may develop as a result of dedifferentiation of an existing DTC. In other cases, ATC may develop de novo. Patients typically present with a rapidly growing mass in the neck. The trachea and oesophagus are frequently involved at an early stage, leading to dysphagia, dyspnoea and, later, stridor. The voice may be hoarse because of infiltration of the laryngeal nerves and subsequent vocal cord palsies. Neck node involvement and metastatic spread, usually to the lung, are relatively common, with metastases being present at initial presentation in up to 50% of patients.

Diagnosis generally requires core biopsy, the important differential diagnosis being thyroid lymphoma. Cross-sectional imaging of the neck with either CT or MRI is helpful to assess the local extent of disease and to identify the rare patient who may have operable disease. CT of the chest and abdomen should also be considered in view of the high risk of metastatic disease.

From 30% to 50% of ATC cases will carry a BRAF mutation. Now that specific systemic therapy is available targeting this mutation, it is recommended that BRAF mutation testing is undertaken urgently on diagnosis.

In a small minority, surgery with total thyroidectomy and radical neck dissection may be possible. This may be followed by adjuvant EBRT.

In the majority, surgery is either impossible or inappropriate. Patients with BRAF mutant ATC can now access treatment with dabrafenib and trametinib. Significant and durable responses have been observed in this treatment, and there are reports of successful surgery being undertaken in patients who are sufficiently downstaged.

Patients with BRAF wild type tumours have much more limited treatment options, and management is with EBRT with or without concurrent chemotherapy. Anaplastic thyroid cancers, however, can show a variable radiosensitivity, with some tumours continuing to enlarge, even while undergoing RT.

Palliative chemotherapy, typically carboplatin and paclitaxel, may be considered in selected fitter patients, but results are generally disappointing. Given the relatively high tumour mutational burden in ATC there is growing interest in the role of immunotherapy for this condition.

THYROID LYMPHOMA

Thyroid lymphomas are non-Hodgkin B-cell lymphomas of varying grade and can be associated with Hashimoto thyroiditis. They usually present as an enlarging thyroid mass. Core biopsy is often required in addition to FNAC to determine the grade and type of lymphoma. The majority are high-grade diffuse large B-cell lymphomas, although low-grade tumours do occur. Once a diagnosis of lymphoma has been made, staging is as for other extranodal sites for lymphoma, with CT scan covering all the potential nodal and extranodal lymphoma sites and marrow examination. Treatment is usually with systemic therapy but may be followed with RT.

EXTERNAL BEAM RADIOTHERAPY FOR THYROID CANCER

EBRT, although not used frequently, does have a role in all histological types of thyroid cancer.

Indications for Treatment

Adjuvant Treatment

DTC. Adjuvant radiotherapy is not routinely indicated, but should be considered when there is gross evidence of local tumour invasion at surgery with significant macroscopic residual disease or when there is residual or recurrent tumour that fails to concentrate radioiodine, that is, loco-regional disease where further surgery or radioiodine is ineffective or impractical. In these situations, typically 60 Gy in 30 daily fractions would be prescribed.

MTC. EBRT should be considered only once optimal surgery has been performed and if there is significant risk of local recurrence. This may be where there is macroscopic residual disease or microscopic residual disease on the background of a large volume disease. EBRT should not be used to consolidate inadequate surgery. Again, typically 60 Gy in 30 daily fractions would be prescribed.

Palliation

EBRT may be considered to palliate symptoms in a number of situations for patients with advanced disease, including:

- Spinal cord compression
- Stridor
- Superior vena cava obstruction
- Cerebral metastases with or without surgery
- Solitary or a limited number of bone metastases
- Dysphagia
- Bleeding tumour

Typically, short fractionation regimes such as 30 Gy/10 fractions, or 20 Gy/5 fractions or 8 Gy/1 fraction are used, depending on the clinical situation, frailty and prognosis of the patient.

Anaplastic Thyroid Cancer

Postoperative. Occasional patients have operable disease. In view of the high risk of recurrence, depending on the patient's fitness adjuvant radiotherapy may be considered following surgery. There is some evidence that such a multimodality treatment improves outcomes. Typically, 60 Gy in 30 daily fractions would be prescribed.

Radical. A minority of patients suffering from inoperable but localized anaplastic cancers with good performance status (0–1), no distant metastases may be treated with 60 to 66 Gy in 30 to 33 daily fractions, with or without concurrent chemotherapy as a radical treatment.

In patients with BRAF mutations, it is becoming a more common practice to initiate treatment with a BRAF and MEK inhibitor combination which may lead to downstaging and reconsideration of surgery.

Palliative. A majority of patients are treated by simpler palliative techniques, due to either disease extent or frailty. Parallel-opposed anterior and posterior fields are used with doses of 20 Gy in 5 daily fractions or 30 Gy in 10 daily fractions.

Technique

For radical or adjuvant treatment, especially for DTC and MTC, patients should now be treated with intensity-modulated radiotherapy (IMRT) techniques. This allows more accurate dose distribution and the reduction of dose to organs at risk. It also allows for much greater dose homogeneity superiorly and inferiorly, where the treatment volume may markedly change shape, improving dose distributions for thyroid cancer (Fig. 24.2). It is now standard in centres in the United Kingdom and elsewhere for high-dose radical or adjuvant therapy for DTC, MTC and some good performance status ATC.

IMRT can achieve steep dose gradients between high-dose planning target volume (PTV) and nearby normal tissues. This allows improved protection of organs at risk (OARs) such as spinal cord and parotids, pharyngeal constrictors while achieving dose escalation to tumour-bearing target volumes. The planning process is called inverse planning. Here, the primary high-dose volume (e.g. CTV1 [first clinical target volume] intended dose 60–66 Gy), prophylactic dose volumes (e.g. CTV2 [second smaller clinical target volume],

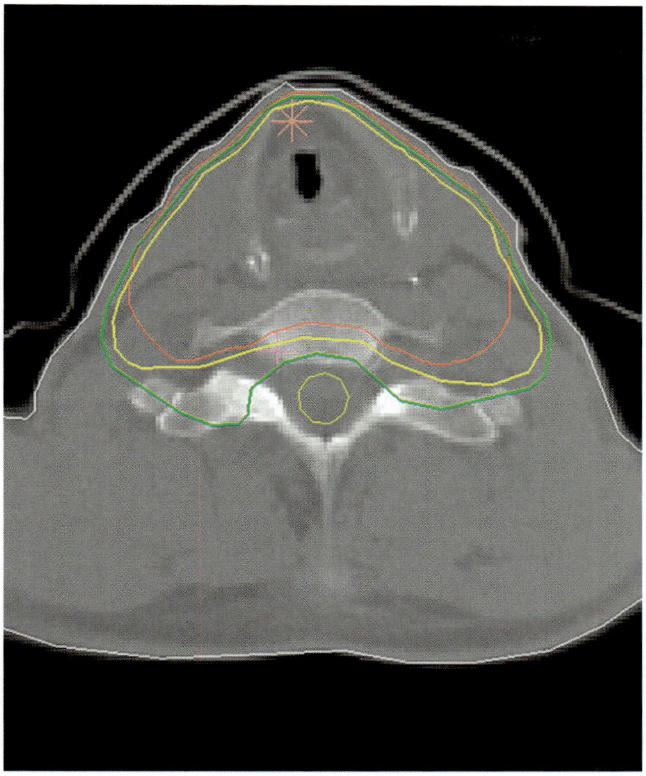

Fig. 24.2 Intensity modulated radiotherapy five-field inverse plan.

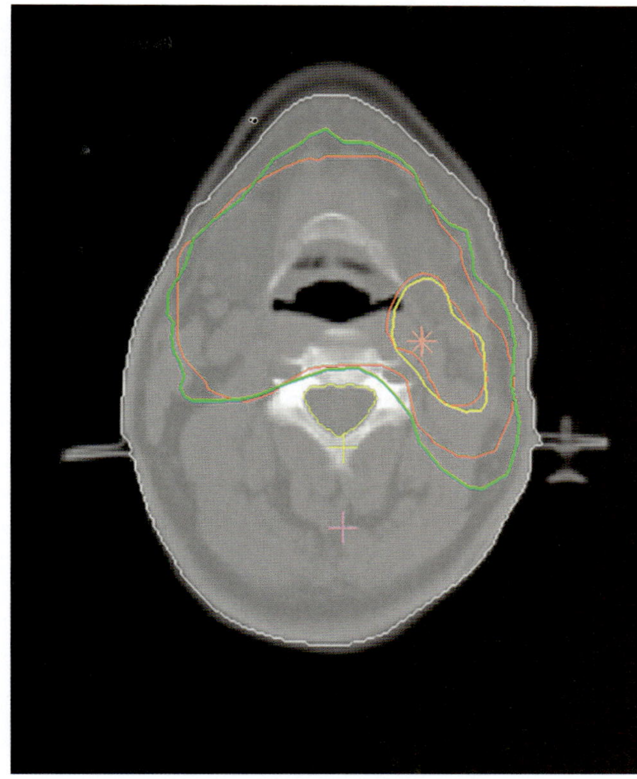

Fig. 24.3 Intensity modulated radiotherapy boost to nodal disease.

delineating microscopic lymph node areas according to published consensus guidelines; intended dose 54 Gy) and OARs (spinal cord dose constraint 46 Gy, parotid median <24 Gy, etc.) are outlined. The planning system, then by several iterations, finds out the best acceptable plan to meet these constraints. This produces superior and more optimal dose distribution and fewer early and late side effects and better quality of life because of improved OAR sparing, confirmed by published trials. Ongoing studies are looking at potentially better local control and survival because of dose escalation.

IMRT can also be used to create plans delivering a concomitant boost to specific areas for dose escalation without extending treatment time (Figs. 24.3 and 24.4).

A minority of patients suffering from anaplastic cancers with good performance status (0–1), no distant metastases and a higher life expectancy may be treated with 60 to 66 Gy using techniques described previously, with or without concurrent chemotherapy, as definitive or neoadjuvant and adjuvant treatments along with surgery. However, the majority are treated with simpler palliative techniques. Parallel-opposed anterior and posterior fields are used with doses of 20 Gy in 5 fractions or 30 Gy in 10 fractions, but if a large irregular volume is to be treated, an IMRT plan is preferred, which gives better dose distribution and allows OAR blocks to be used, even in the palliative situation. The apices of the lungs are usually shielded by multileaf collimators (MLCs) or lead blocks. For palliation of symptoms for metastatic or recurrent cancers, 30 Gy/10 fractions, 20 Gy/5 fractions or 8 Gy/1 fraction can be used, depending on the clinical situation, frailty and prognosis for the patient.

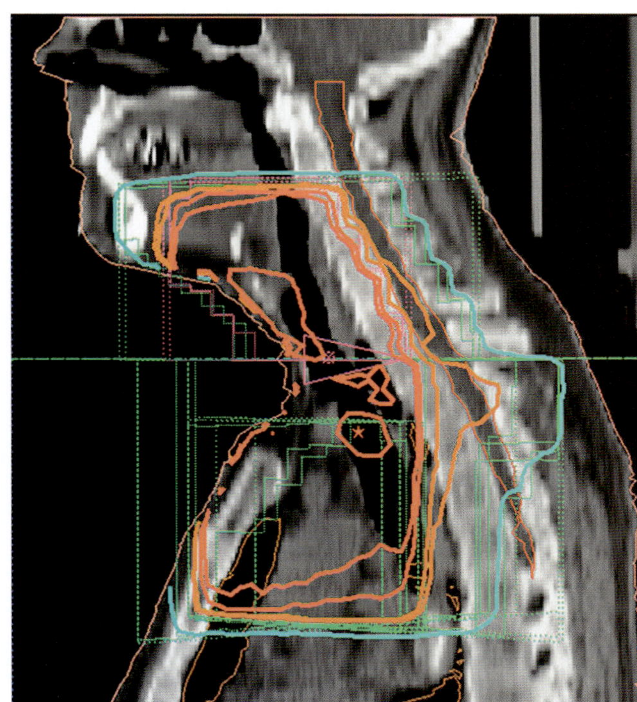

Fig. 24.4 Lateral isodose maps showing dose distribution of intensity modulated radiotherapy boost to nodal disease. *Red*, 100%; *orange*, 50%; *blue*, 20%.

Radiotherapy for Thyroid Lymphoma

RT is usually given after four cycles of chemotherapy, using, for example, the rituximab-cyclophosphamide, doxorubicin, vincristine and prednisone (R-CHOP) chemotherapy regimen. The anatomical PTV is as for other thyroid tumours, but nowadays only the volume on presentation with a margin (involved field) is usually preferred. The dose is usually about 30 to 40 Gy in 15 to 20 fractions for diffuse high-grade lymphomas after chemotherapy. The lower dose is preferred for complete responders. A planned IMRT setup is optimal, with 24 to 30 Gy used in daily 2 Gy/fraction doses; without any chemotherapy, 35 Gy in 20 fractions are used. The maximum acceptable spinal cord dose is no more than 40 Gy, and IMRT will allow doses well below this.

FURTHER READING

Cancer Genome Atlas Research Network. Integrated genomic characterization of papillary thyroid carcinoma. *Cell.* 2014;159: 676–690.

Haugen BR, Alexander EK, Bible KC, et al. 2015 American Thyroid Association management guidelines for adult patients with thyroid nodules and differentiated thyroid cancer: the American Thyroid Association guidelines task force on thyroid nodules and differentiated thyroid cancer. *Thyroid.* 2016;26(1):1–133.

James BC, Mitchell JM, Jeon HD, Vasilottos N, Grogan RH, Aschebrook-Kilfoy B. An update in international trends in incidence rates of thyroid cancer 1973–2007. *Cancer Causes Control.* 2018; 29(4–5):465–473.

Leboulleux S, Bournaud C, Chougnet CN, et al. Thyroidectomy without radioiodine in patients with low-risk thyroid cancer. *N Engl J Med.* 2022;386(10):923–932. https://doi.org/10.1056/NEJMoa2111953

Mallick U, Harmer C, Yap B, et al. Ablation with low-dose radioiodine and thyrotropin alfa in thyroid cancer. *N Engl J Med.* 2012;366(18): 1674–1685.

NICE (National Institute for Health and Care Excellence). *Thyroid cancer: assessment and management.* NICE; 2022. NICE guideline NG230. https://www.nice.org.uk/guidance/ng230

Perros P, Boelaert K, Colley S, et al. Guidelines for the management of thyroid cancer. *Clin Endocrinol.* 2014;81(Suppl. 1):1–122.

Wadsley J, Armstrong N, Bassett-Smith V, et al. Patient preparation and radiation protection guidance for adult patients undergoing radioiodine treatment for thyroid cancer in the UK. *Clin Oncol (R Coll Radiol).* 2023;35(1):42–56. https://doi.org/10.1016/j.clon.2022.07.002

Wadsley J, Beasley M, Garcez K, Hoy S, Newbold K, Boelaert K. Guidelines on the use of systemic therapy in patients with advanced thyroid cancer. *Clin Oncol (R Coll Radiol).* 2023;35(1):57–64. https://doi.org/10.1016/j.clon.2022.10.009

25

Gastrointestinal Cancer

Somnath Mukherjee, Maria Hawkins, Douglas Brand and Emilia Bruton

CHAPTER OUTLINE

CANCER OF THE OESOPHAGUS

Epidemiology

Oesophageal cancer is the seventh most common cancer worldwide (600,000 in 2020) and the sixth most common cause of death (544,000 in 2020). Cancer of the oesophagus has high mortality and marked geographic variation. Globally, the incidence is highest in Eastern Asia for both genders, followed by Southern Africa, Eastern Africa, Northern Europe and South-Central Asia. Squamous cell carcinomas (SCCs) are the most common type globally and are most common in Southeastern and Central Asia (79% of the total global SCC cases); the highest burden of adenocarcinoma (AC) was found in Northern and Western Europe, North America and Oceania (46% of the total global AC cases). Incidence in males is substantially higher than in females, especially in the case of AC (male-to-female ratio AC: 4.4; SCC: 2.7).

Within the western population, an increasing incidence of ACs of the oesophagus and cardia has been observed. Variation in incidence and mortality between countries may reflect diversity of aetiological factors, use of screening and access to healthcare.

In the United Kingdom, an excess of 9200 new cases are diagnosed per year with an annual death rate of around 8000. The peak age of diagnosis is 85 to 89 years. The incidence in males has increased by 11% since the early 1990s (between 1993 and 1995 and between 2016 and 2018), whereas the incidence in females has decreased by 16% in the same period.

Aetiology and Pathology

The most common histological subtypes are SCC and AC, accounting for more than 90% of tumours. More recently, based on whole genome sequencing, mutational signatures have defined aetiologically distinct subgroups of oesophageal AC: the DNA damage repair (DDR) impaired (18%), the mutagenic (53%) and the G;C >A/T dominant (29%).[1] The DDR impaired and mutagenic subgroups have potentially actionable mutations, as can be targeted with DNA-damaging therapy (e.g. poly ADP ribose polymerase (PARP) inhibitors, radiotherapy (RT)) and immunotherapy, respectively.

Risk Factors for Squamous Cell Carcinomas

Alcohol and tobacco make up the largest risk factors for oesophageal SCC in the western world. The relative risk is reported as 6.2 for smokers who do not consume alcohol. Smokers who have significant intakes of alcohol have a 10-to-25-fold increased risk of SCC. Equally, chewing tobacco and betel leaves, as practised in Southern Asia, contributes to the excess risk seen in these regions. Nitrosamines, N-nitroso compounds, aromatic amines and polycyclic hydrocarbons found in alcohol and tobacco, alone or in combination, contribute to the carcinogenic effect.

Patients with iron deficiency anaemia and a diet low in riboflavin (Plummer-Vinson, also called Paterson-Brown Kelly syndrome) are at a higher risk of upper digestive tract SCCs. Tylosis, a hereditary condition characterised by hyperkeratosis of the palms and soles and papilloma of the oesophagus, is associated with a one in three chance of developing oesophageal cancer below the age of 50 years. Long-standing achalasia cardia is associated with a 5% risk of oesophageal squamous carcinoma. Patients with a history of previous cancer of the aerodigestive tract have a 2% to 4% incidence of oesophageal cancer. A higher incidence of SCCs was observed in individuals exposed to ionising radiation.

Risk Factors for Adenocarcinoma

Gastrooesophageal Reflux Disease

Gastrooesophageal reflux disease is commonly referred to as *GORD* or *GERD*. Acid and bile reflux result in intestinal metaplasia of the oesophageal squamous epithelium. The area of metaplastic change looks red on endoscopy, whereas the normal oesophagus has a pearly appearance. This change is called Barrett oesophagus. Obesity and smoking contribute to these changes. The probable morphological sequence is metaplasia → dysplasia → carcinoma, accompanied by a series of genetic events resulting in invasive cancer. The incidence of AC developing in Barrett oesophagus is 0.5% to 1% per year. Chemoprevention, using a combination of high-dose esomeprazole and aspirin, has been shown to reduce the incidence of oesophageal cancer in patients with Barrett oesophagus.[2]

Obesity

Risk of AC of the oesophagus increases with increasing body mass index, with up to threefold increases reported in very obese cohorts.

Alcohol and Tobacco

The association between alcohol and tobacco and oesophageal AC is less robust than for squamous cancer, but several large studies show that there is a moderate increased risk of AC of the oesophagus and the cardia of the stomach.

Anatomy

The oesophagus is a flattened muscular tube of 18 to 26 cm in length with diameters varying from 1.6 to 2.5 cm. The oesophagus starts at the pharyngooesophageal junction at the level of the C5–6 vertebral interspace and ends at the oesophagogastric junction at the level of the T11 vertebra. It is traditionally divided into three segments: cervical, thoracic and abdominal. The cervical segment is about 4 to 5 cm long and extends from the pharyngooesophageal junction (vertebral level C7, distance on endoscopy at about 15 cm) to the thoracic inlet (vertebral level T3, endoscopically at about 18 cm). The thoracic oesophagus extends from the thoracic inlet to the diaphragmatic opening, also called the *hiatus* (vertebral level T9–10, endoscopically at about 37 cm), and is about 20 cm long. The thoracic oesophagus is divided into three segments (upper to T5/carina/24 cm on endoscopy; mid to 32 cm; lower to diaphragmatic opening). The abdominal segment is short, varying from 1 to 2.5 cm, extending from the hiatus to the oesophagogastric junction. The oesophagus moves with respiration and during swallowing, and movement is more prominent in the region of the gastrooesophageal junction (GOJ); this has implications for RT planning.

Lymphatic drainage is of importance to the surgeon and the oncologist. A dense lymphatic network is found in the submucosa, which travels a variable distance longitudinally before penetrating the muscle layer and draining into the periooesophageal lymph nodes. This may explain the extensive intramural spread of the cancer beneath an intact mucosa, and tumour-free margins may not necessarily mean complete tumour resection. The lymphatic drainage of the proximal oesophagus is towards the deep cervical chain and thoracic duct. The distal oesophagus drains into the lower mediastinal, left gastric and coeliac axis nodes.

The oesophageal wall is composed of four layers: the innermost mucosa (nonkeratinised squamous epithelium); submucosal connective tissue; muscularis propria (with inner circular and outer longitudinal layers); and adventitial layer. The myenteric or Auerbach plexus of nerves responsible for coordinating swallowing is located between the inner circular and outer longitudinal layers. The oesophagus has no mesentery or serosal lining, which may explain the relatively easy spread of oesophageal cancer into the surrounding tissues.

Oesophagogastric Junctional Tumours

ACs of the oesophagogastric junction have been divided into three subtypes as proposed by Siewert and Stein.[3] Type 1 junctional tumours primarily arise from the distal oesophagus and involve the junction; type 2 junctional tumours straddle the junction; and type 3 tumours are predominantly in the cardia of the stomach, involving the junction. Type 1 and 2 junctional AC is treated using oesophagus protocols. Type 3 junctional tumours are thought to behave like gastric AC and therefore are treated using gastric protocols.

Clinical Manifestations

Dysphagia and weight loss are the most common initial symptoms in over 90% of patients. Odynophagia (pain during swallowing) is seen in about 50% of patients. Epigastric pains, haematemesis, regurgitation of undigested food and aspiration pneumonia are less common but recognised symptoms. Cough from a tracheobronchial fistula, hoarse voice, superior vena caval obstruction and haemoptysis are less frequent. Pleural effusions and ascites as well as bone pain secondary to metastases can occur. Anorexia and right upper quadrant discomfort/pain may suggest liver metastases. Clinical examination should be directed at any presence of obvious metastatic disease, such as neck or supraclavicular lymph nodes, hepatomegaly, pleural effusions and ascites.

A thorough nutritional assessment by a specialist oncology dietician at baseline and at regular intervals while on treatment is mandatory.

Diagnostic Evaluation

Any patient who presents with recent onset dysphagia and weight loss should be investigated for a possible oesophageal cancer. Many major centres have a fast-track dysphagia endoscopy service available to minimise delay in the diagnosis of the cancer. Oesophageal tumours are staged using the 8th edition of the UICC/AJCC staging system.

In the majority of cases, upper gastrointestinal (GI) endoscopy visualises the tumour and its distance from the incisor teeth. The endoscopist should also define the lower extent of the tumour (if the lumen is traversable) and evaluate the oesophagogastric junction. Multiple biopsies should be taken to maximise the yield. Any associated Barrett segment, its length and its relation to the invasive cancer should be noted.

In patients who are fit for curative treatment, the first step is a multislice computed tomography (CT) scan of the chest and abdomen to exclude obvious metastatic disease. CT has poor sensitivity in predicting the T or N stage. The sensitivity and specificity of CT for T4 disease are 25% and 94%, respectively, and for coeliac node involvement are 30% and 90%, respectively.

In patients with localised disease, further evaluation with fluorodeoxyglucose-positron emission tomography-computed tomography (FDG PET/CT) and endoscopic ultrasound (EUS) is recommended. EUS is useful in evaluating the local T and N stage and has improved the preoperative staging of oesophageal cancer. FDG PET is primarily undertaken to rule out metastatic disease, and based on a metaanalysis, sensitivity and specificity for detection of distant disease are 71% and 93%, respectively.

In patients with hoarseness of voice or haemoptysis/unexplained cough, bronchoscopy is recommended to rule out recurrent laryngeal nerve involvement or tracheobronchial fistula. Endobronchial ultrasound (EBUS) may be required in selective cases to rule out involvement of the respiratory tract.

Patients should have assessment of programmed death-ligand 1 (PD-L1), HER2 and MMR status. PD-L1 expression can be determined using the tumour proportion score and combined positive score. Other markers are likely to become increasingly used in the future, for example, claudin 18.2.

Therapy

General Principles

Dietary assessment and nutritional support are essential components of management. Many patients are symptomatic at diagnosis, and life expectancy is limited in patients with advanced disease; specialist nurses and the palliative care team play a vital role in patient management and should be involved early. For patients undergoing chemotherapy, monitoring of blood count and liver and renal function is mandatory.

For patients suitable for radical surgery, prehabilitation should be considered to optimise physical status.

Surgery

Surgery is the backbone of treatment for resectable tumours of both histological subtypes and is used in combination with either chemoradiotherapy (CRT) or perioperative chemotherapy for all but T1N0 disease. For SCCs, definitive chemoradiation is also a recommended option that should be discussed (see later section).

The surgery involves resection of the primary tumour with an adequate margin along with regional lymph nodes. Two standard surgical techniques have been described for surgical resection of oesophageal cancers: transthoracic (Ivor Lewis technique) and transhiatal. The aim is complete resection. The margin status and the extent of nodal burden are powerful prognostic indicators for relapse-free survival.

For select T1N0M0 tumours, endoscopic resection (using either endoscopic mucosal resection or endoscopic submucosal dissection) may be the treatment of choice and can be considered definitive treatment unless there is an involved margin or risk factors for nodal involvement (e.g. depth of invasion, lymphovascular invasion, poorly differentiated tumour, ulceration, large tumour size).[4]

Perioperative Chemotherapy

Several large, randomised controlled trials have established the role of perioperative chemotherapy in the treatment of patients with locally advanced AC of the oesophagus and GOJ in the United Kingdom.

Updated results from the MRC OE-2 trial of preoperative chemotherapy in patients undergoing curative surgery showed 5-year OS rates of 23% in the combined modality arm compared with 17% in the surgery alone arm.

The MRC OE-05 study compared four cycles of epirubicin, cisplatin and capecitabine (ECX) chemotherapy with two cycles of cisplatin and 5-fluorouracil (5-FU), and failed to show OS advantage for the more intensive regimen.[5]

The FLOT4/AIO study demonstrated the benefit of perioperative FLOT for ACs of the oesophagogastric junction and stomach, and established the new standard of care for these tumours (see gastric section). The recent ESOPEC trial (published in abstract form only) provides further evidence for use of the regimen in oesophageal ACs in addition to those of the oesophagogastric junction.

Neoadjuvant Chemoradiation

Neoadjuvant CRT (CROSS regimen) is considered the standard of care for the treatment of oesophageal SCC and is an option for ACs of the oesophagus and GOJ.

The use of neoadjuvant CRT is based on the results of the randomised phase III CROSS trial,[6] which showed a significant survival advantage for neoadjuvant CRT over surgery alone (49.4 months versus 24 months, hazard ratio (HR) 0.657, $P = .003$), with no increase in postoperative mortality. A long-term follow-up paper demonstrated that the benefit was particularly pronounced for participants with SCC (median OS 81.6 months versus 21.1 months, HR 0.48, $P = .008$).

Typical treatment regimen:

Five weekly cycles of carboplatin AUC2 and paclitaxel 50 mg/m^2

Concomitant RT: 41.4 Gy in 23 fractions or 45 Gy in 25 fractions

Choice of Therapy

For oesophageal and GOJ ACs, both neoadjuvant chemoradiation and perioperative chemotherapy are considered standard-of-care treatments. The choice between the two continues to be debated. The Neo-AEGIS trial compared the CROSS regimen (trimodality therapy) with optimum perioperative chemotherapy (ECX/ECF or FLOT). The trial closed early and was underpowered to detect noninferiority, but no statistically significant difference was observed in 3-year survival between the two groups.[7]

Results from the randomised phase III ESOPEC trial were recently reported (abstract only). This trial compared the CROSS regimen with FLOT4 (docetaxel, oxaliplatin, 5-FU, leucovorin) in patients with oesophageal AC. It demonstrated a significant overall survival benefit with perioperative FLOT (median OS 66 months versus 37 months). These results are likely to result in perioperative chemotherapy being used as the preferred treatment option for ACs.

Adjuvant Immunotherapy

The Checkmate 577 trial[8] evaluated the addition of one year of adjuvant nivolumab in patients with oesophageal/oesophagogastric junction cancer treated with neoadjuvant CRT and surgery and with evidence of residual disease in the resection specimen. It demonstrated a greater median disease-free survival of 22.4 months for patients receiving nivolumab compared with 11.0 months in the placebo arm. PD-L1 testing is not required for this indication.

Radical Radiotherapy

External beam radiation alone or as part of combined modality treatment has been evaluated in both SCC and AC of the oesophagus. Radical radiation treatment alone for treatment of clinically localised oesophageal cancer is not generally recommended in the curative setting. Both local and distant failure rates remain high despite higher doses of radiation, and 5-year survival is reported to be less than 5%. It is therefore infrequently used.

Definitive Chemoradiation

This is an option for all patients with SCC and in patients with AC who are not considered candidates for surgery. Chemoradiation protocols typically use cisplatin and 5-FU (or its oral derivative, capecitabine) with fractionated external beam radiation to a dose of 50 to 60 Gray (Gy). In two phase III trials in SCCs, definitive chemoradiation gave comparable median survival figures of around 15 to 19 months with a 25% to 40% 2-year survival. In the United Kingdom, the CRT with or without cetuximab in patients with oesophageal cancer (SCOPE 1) trial[9] randomised a conventional dCRT regimen (4 cycles of cisplatin and capecitabine, with cycles 3 and 4 being concurrent with radiation, 50 Gy in 25 fractions) to the same regimen with the addition of the epidermal growth factor receptor (EGFR) antagonist cetuximab. Nearly three-quarters of the patients had SCC. Although the trial failed to show benefit of adding cetuximab, it demonstrated unprecedented survival in patients treated with dCRT (median overall survival (OS) of 34.5 months; 95% confidence interval (CI) 24.7–42.3 months), with a 3-year OS of 47.2% (95% CI 38.2–55.7). Treatment failure at 24 weeks was highly predictive of OS (median OS 8.3 versus 42.3 months). The SCOPE regimen became the standard of care in the United Kingdom.

The use of weekly carboplatin/paclitaxel as the chemotherapy component of dCRT is gaining popularity and has been reported in some retrospective series to demonstrate similar efficacy with less toxicity than the conventional cisplatin fluoropyrimidine-based dCRT regimen. FOLFOX has also been studied as an alternative regimen.[10] It did not demonstrate improved outcomes.

Dose escalation has been examined in the ARTDECO and PRODIGE 26/CONCORDE studies. ARTDECO randomised patients between standard dose (50.4 Gy in 28 fractions) RT or high-dose RT, where a simultaneous integrated boost was delivered to the primary tumour to a total dose of 61.6 Gy. No significant difference in local control (LC) or survival was observed between the two regimens.[11] The PRODIGE 26/CONCORDE study assessed dose escalation to 66 Gy in 33 fractions. No increase in toxicity was detected, but there was no improvement in progression-free survival.[9] The SCOPE 2 trial is also looking at dose escalation, comparing 50 Gy in 25 fractions with 60 Gy in 25 fractions, and results are awaited.

Typical treatment prescription:

Radiotherapy: 50 Gy in 25 fractions, concomitant with one of the following concurrent chemotherapy regimens:

- Four cycles of cisplatin 60 mg/m^2 day 1 and capecitabine 625 mg/m^2 twice daily, days 1 to 21 (radiation to commence with C3 and C4)
- Five weekly cycles of carboplatin AUC2 and paclitaxel 50 mg/m^2
- Six cycles of oxaliplatin 85 mg/m^2, leucovorin 200 mg/m^2, bolus fluorouracil 400 mg/m^2 and infusional fluorouracil 1600 mg/m^2

Patients receiving definitive chemoradiation may be considered for salvage oesophagectomy if local recurrence occurs.

Adjuvant Radiation or Chemoradiation

There are no prospective randomised trial data to support the routine use of adjuvant chemoradiation in resected oesophageal cancer. Single-institute series have shown some improvement in LC rates and progression-free survival, but this could be caused by the inherent bias in the studies that the patients were fit enough to receive the adjuvant treatment.

Palliative Radiotherapy

Palliative RT is recommended for local pain, bleeding, dysphagia or LC. Brachytherapy is rarely used. Dose options for palliative RT include single-fraction (8–10 Gy) or fractionated RT (typically 20 Gy/5 fractions; 30 Gy/10 fractions; 36 Gy/12 fractions) using 6-to-15-MV photons.

External Beam Radiation Technique

Radical treatment: RT is delivered preferably using intensity modulated radiotherapy (IMRT), typically using 6-MV photons. Four-dimensional CT (4DCT) planning is recommended for tumours of the lower oesophagus and GOJ because of tumour motion (Figs. 25.1 and 25.2). The tumour and involved nodes are outlined based on the information from the staging CT scan, PET/CT scan and EUS. EUS can detect submucosal spread and gives a more accurate extent of the disease. Clinical target volume (CTV) is derived using a margin of 2 cm in the superior-inferior direction along the course of the oesophagus and 1 cm in the circumferential direction, editing out uninvolved organs at risk (OARs) (heart, lung, large vessels, bone). Planning target volume (PTV) includes a margin of 1 cm in the superior-inferior direction and 0.5 cm circumferentially. Where 4DCT is used, an internal target volume (ITV) is generated taking into account tumour motion during respiratory cycle, and a smaller margin (about 0.5 cm, depending on institutional setup errors) is applied to generate PTV.

Palliative treatment: Gross tumour with a 1.5-to-2-cm margin is identified as PTV. Parallel-opposed fields (anterior/posterior) can be used for palliative RT. Beam energy: 6-to-15-MV photons.

Management of Advanced/Metastatic Disease

Systemic treatment is constantly evolving, and biomarker-driven treatment is being increasingly used in the clinic.

Palliative chemotherapy for oesophageal and GOJ AC is similar to gastric cancer and is discussed together subsequently.

Standard first-line palliative chemotherapy for oesophageal SCCs is a platinum-fluoropyrimidine doublet, but recent trials have supported the addition of immunotherapy, particularly for patients with elevated PD-L1 expression.

KEYNOTE-590[12] investigated the addition of pembrolizumab to chemotherapy and included patients with both SCC and AC (the majority had SCC). The greatest benefit was seen in patients with SCC, with a PD-L1 combined positive score ≥10 (median overall survival 13.9 months versus 8.8 months), although benefit was also seen in other groups.

Checkmate 648[13] investigated the addition of nivolumab to chemotherapy in SCC. Overall, survival was significantly longer with nivolumab, with the greatest increase seen in patients with a PD-L1 tumour proportion score ≥1% (15.4 versus 9.1 months).

Nivolumab is also an option for second-line treatment (in patients not receiving immunotherapy first line) based on the results of the ATTRACTION-3 trial,[14] which demonstrated improved overall survival compared with taxane-based chemotherapy. In this setting, outcomes are not affected by PD-L1 expression.

Other Treatments

Palliative treatment options are tailored to the individual patient and are best discussed in a multidisciplinary setting along with the palliative care team. Oesophageal stenting provides palliation of dysphagia. Endoscopic laser treatment may be suitable for bulky endoluminal squamous tumours.

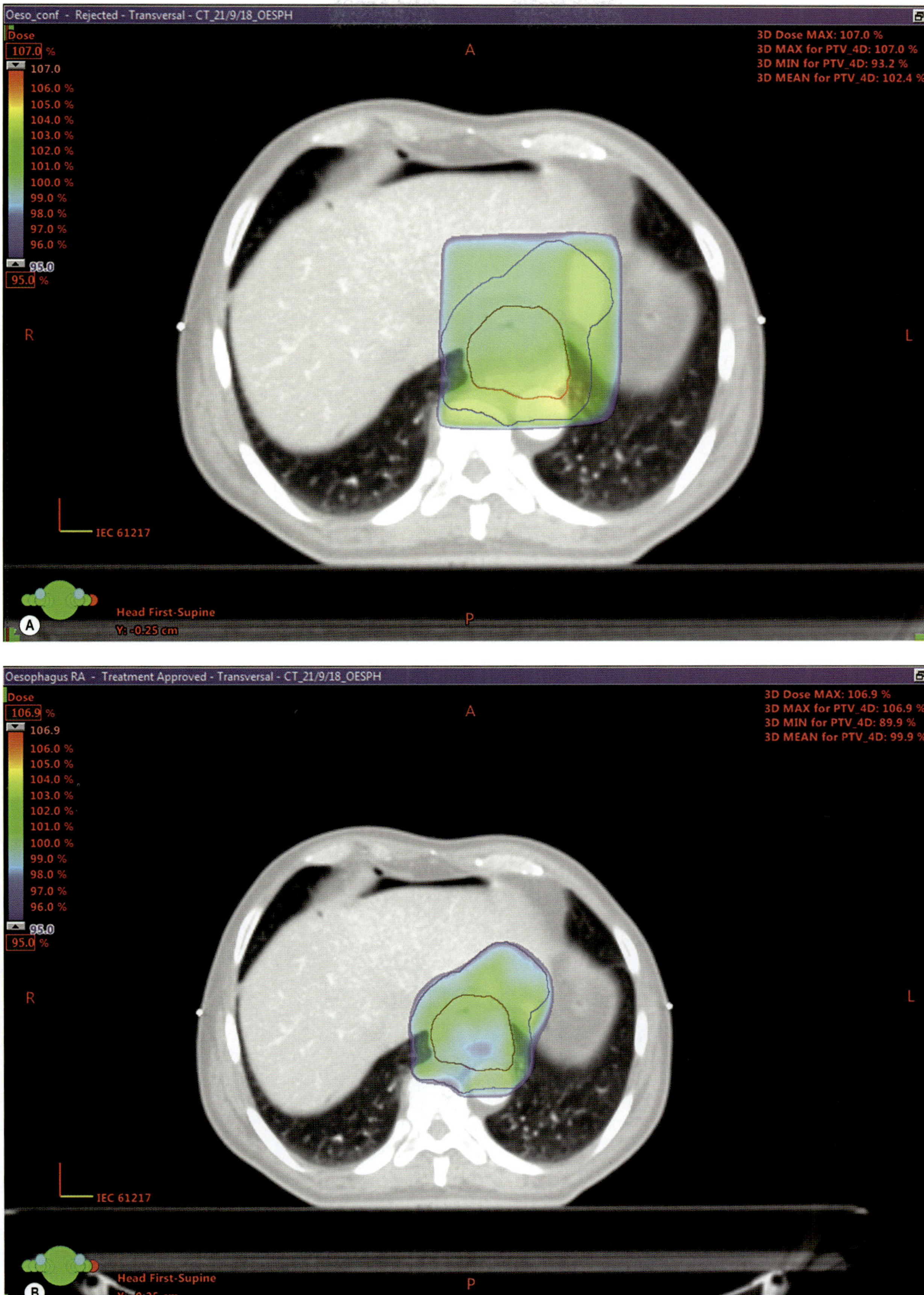

Fig. 25.1 (A) Conformal radiotherapy plan for lower oesophageal cancer. (B) Intensity modulated plan (IMRT/ Rapid Arc) for lower oesophageal cancer.

(continued)

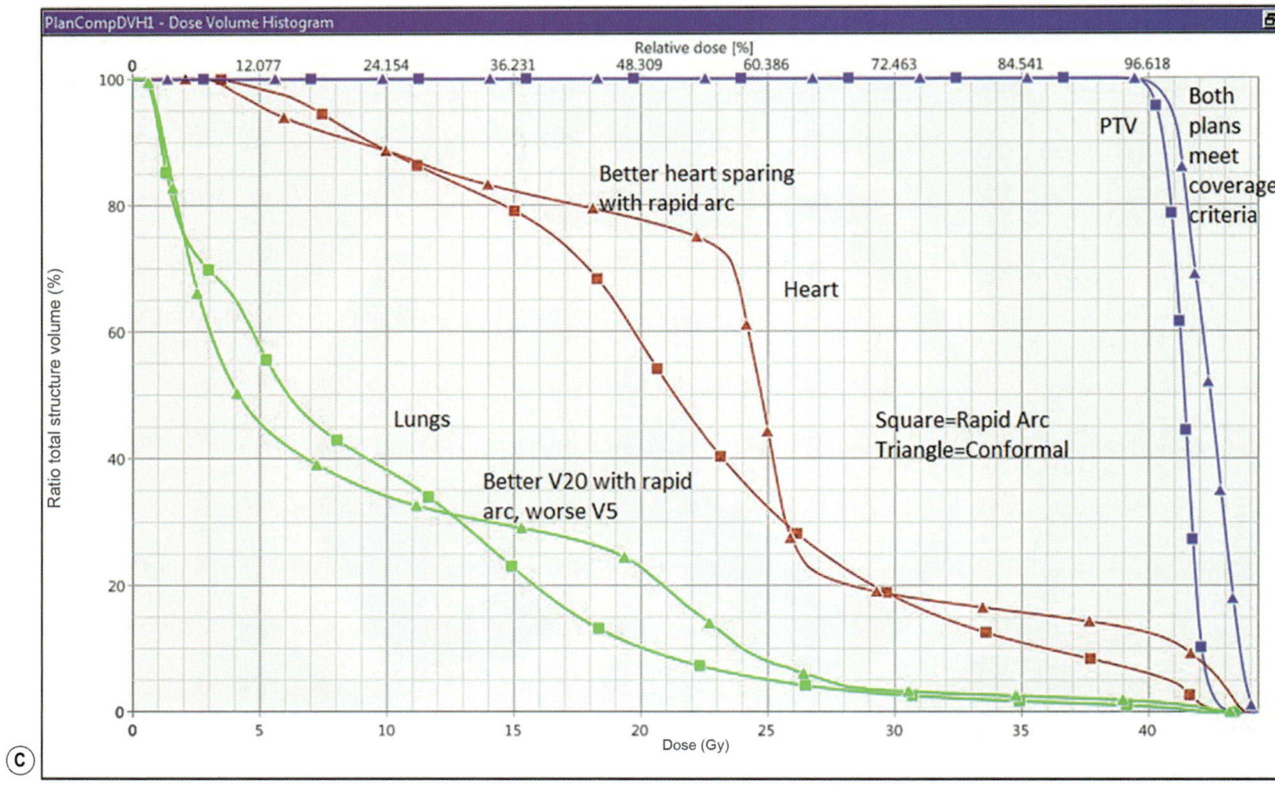

Fig. 25.1—cont'd (C) Dose-volume histogram showing comparative planning target volume coverage, lung and heart doses. (From Aitken KL, Hawkins MA. The role of radiotherapy and chemoradiation in the management of primary liver tumours. *Clin Oncol (R Coll Radiol)*. 2014;26(9):569–580.)

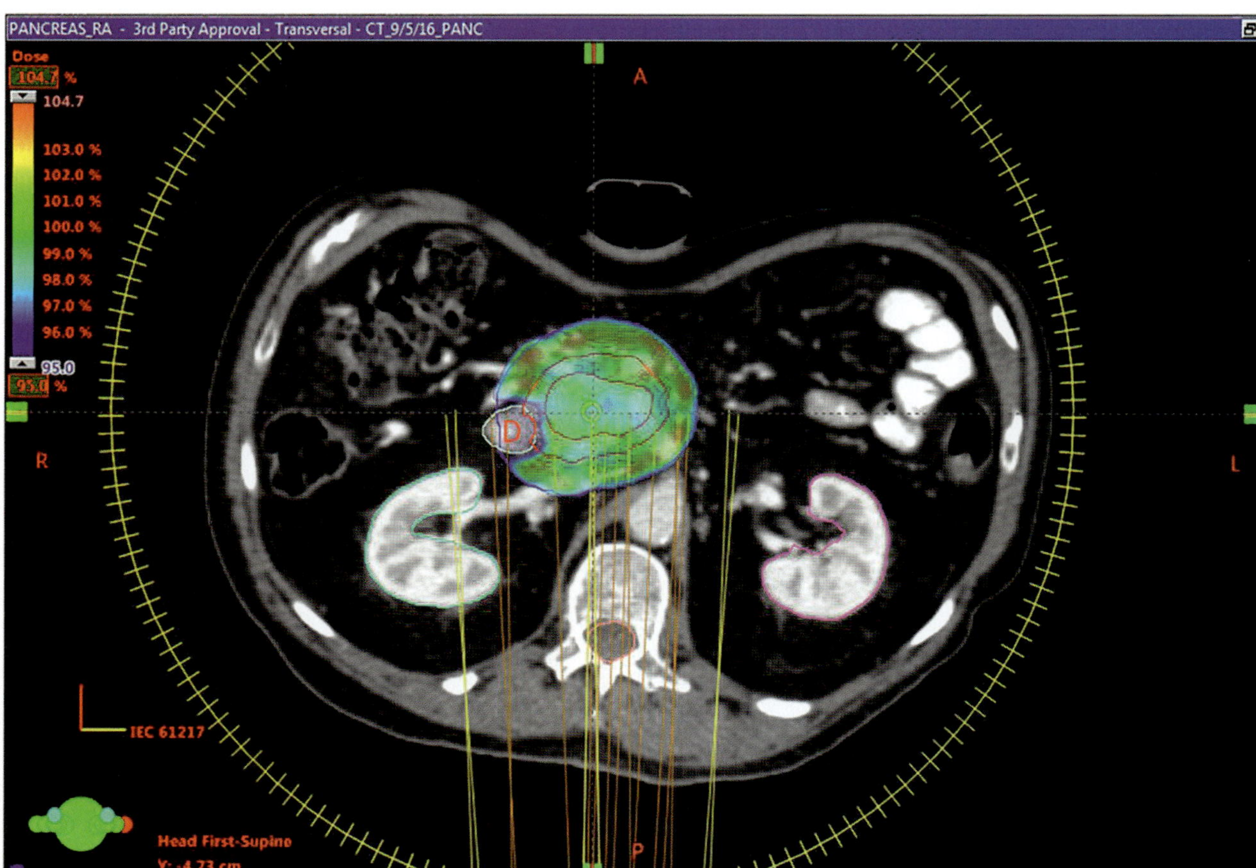

Fig. 25.2 Intensity modulated radiotherapy plan for cancer head of pancreas showing duodenal sparing.

Summary

Management of oesophageal cancer has evolved over the past few decades. Treatment decisions should be made within a multidisciplinary team setting. Careful staging and selection of patients for curative treatments are vital, and surgery should be performed in high-volume specialist centres for best outcome. Combined modality treatments remain the standard of care in the curative setting for all patients with oesophageal cancer except those with very early tumours.

CANCER OF THE STOMACH

Anatomy

The stomach begins at the oesophagogastric junction and ends at the pylorus. It is divided into three parts: cardia (fundus), body and pyloric antrum. The blood supply of the stomach is derived from the branches of the coeliac axis. The regional lymphatics drain into the coeliac axis nodes, splenic hilar, porta hepatis and gastroduodenal and suprapancreatic nodal groups. Venous drainage is primarily through the portal venous system into the liver.

Epidemiology

There is considerable variation in the worldwide incidence of gastric cancer. The highest incidence is seen in Eastern Asia, South America and Eastern Europe (http://globocan.iarc.fr/old/FactSheets/cancers/stomach-new.asp). The incidence in Western Europe is in decline. However, the incidence of tumours of the cardia and oesophagogastric junction has increased. The incidence of stomach cancer has been declining in the United Kingdom since 1930 and has halved since the 1990s. Cancer Research United Kingdom (CRUK) reported 6740 new cases in the United Kingdom in 2015, making this the 17th most common cancer. The incidence is projected to fall further by 17% between the years 2014 and 2035 and to 11 cases per 100,000 people by 2035.

Aetiology

Environmental and genetic factors play a role in the pathogenesis of gastric cancer. Carcinogens implicated in the aetiology include nitrates and nitrites in food, a diet that is high in processed meat and salt and low in fruits and vegetables, smoking and industrial dust exposure. The role of alcohol remains uncertain. Increased risk has been reported with a specific strain of *Helicobacter pylori* (CAG + ve), especially in noncardia lesions, and infection with *H. pylori* has been implicated in around one in three stomach cancers. Pernicious anaemia and previous subtotal gastrectomy for benign conditions, and villous adenomas are thought to be associated with increased risk of gastric cancer after a long period of latency.

Genetic factors include mutations in specific genes, CDH1 and p53. CDH1 encodes for E-cadherin and mutations in this gene are associated with hereditary diffuse gastric cancer. Another familial gastric cancer syndrome is associated with p53 mutations. Gastric cancer is also a component of Li-Fraumeni syndrome, hereditary nonpolyposis colorectal cancer (HNPCC), Peutz-Jeghers polyposis, BRCA-2 mutations and juvenile polyposis.

Pathology

AC constitutes 95% of the gastric cancers. They are classified into intestinal and diffuse types (Lauren classification system). The intestinal type is more common in older patients, high-risk groups and males. The diffuse type is more commonly seen in females and younger patients and carries a poorer prognosis. Other histological types of gastric malignancies include carcinoids, lymphomas and gastrointestinal stromal tumours (GISTs). GISTs are the most common mesenchymal tumours of the GI tract.

More recently, comprehensive molecular characterisation has classified gastric AC into four different subtypes according to The Cancer Genome Atlas (TCGA) research network: (1) Epstein-Barr virus positive (characterised by recurrent *PIK3CA* mutations, extreme DNA hypermethylation and amplification of *JAK2, PD-L1* and *PD-L2*); (2) microsatellite unstable tumours characterised by high mutation rates; (3) genomically stable tumours that are enriched for the diffuse histological variant; and (4) tumours with chromosomal instability (CIN), which show marked aneuploidy and focal amplification of receptor tyrosine kinases. These molecular subtypes provide rationale for targeted therapy for distinct populations of patients with gastric cancer.

Clinical Features

The most common presenting symptoms are anaemia, weight loss, anorexia, haematemesis, melena, upper abdominal pain/discomfort and nausea/vomiting. Occult bleeding is more common than overt haematemesis. Possible clinical findings include anaemia, abdominal mass, left supraclavicular lymphadenopathy and ascites.

Staging

The initial investigations often include an endoscopy. Gastroscopy and biopsy will confirm the diagnosis in the majority of patients. Multiple biopsies increase the sensitivity and yield. The TNM staging system is used for staging gastric cancer. EUS is of value in proximal cardia and junctional tumours to assess operability. Cross-sectional imaging with a spiral CT is the first step to exclude overt metastatic disease. CT is not a sensitive tool for detecting peritoneal spread, and therefore laparoscopy is mandatory before surgery to detect any occult peritoneal spread. Laparoscopy may also help in identifying tumours in the lesser sac, on the surface of the liver and nodal disease. FDG PET imaging may identify metastases not clearly seen on CT, but 25% to 30% of primary gastric cancers are not FDG avid (especially the diffuse type).

PD-L1 and human EGFR 2 (HER2) status should be determined in patients.

Management

The optimal management of gastric cancer should take place within a multidisciplinary setting. Radical treatment in Europe consists of surgery with perioperative chemotherapy, but in other parts of the world different approaches have been used. For example, in the Far East postoperative chemotherapy is the standard of care, and in America postoperative CRT is more commonly used than in Europe. Each of these approaches are discussed in the following sections.

For advanced disease, palliative chemotherapy may be offered for survival benefit and radiation for symptomatic benefit where appropriate. As with oesophageal cancer, involvement of a dietician and palliative care is very important in this disease.

Surgery

The goal of surgery is complete resection. However, only 25% to 30% of patients with gastric cancer may be suitable for potentially curative surgery. Distal tumours can be treated with partial gastrectomy if suitable margins can be obtained; however, proximal tumours usually require a total gastrectomy. The extent of lymphadenectomy—D1 (perigastric nodes) versus more extensive D2 lymphadenectomy (D2 or D3)—is a matter of debate; however, in the United Kingdom, a D2 lymphadenectomy is recommended (NICE guidance). More extensive radical lymphadenectomy has not shown to be of survival benefit but increases morbidity.

Surgery may be the only treatment needed for early lesions (T1N0M0), and endoscopic therapy may be used for very early lesions confined to the mucosa. However, in the majority of patients treated with a curative intent, a combined modality approach is necessary.[15]

The common sites of relapse following a curative resection are locoregional (lymph nodes, gastric bed and anastomosis) and metastatic (liver and peritoneal seeding).

Palliative gastrectomy or gastric bypass procedure can be offered for patients with obstructive symptoms, bleeding or intractable pain.

Perioperative (Neoadjuvant and Adjuvant) Chemotherapy

The relapse rate is high for patients who have had gastrectomy for stages T2 and beyond. This is thought to be mainly because of the locoregional failure (LRF) and micrometastatic disease present at diagnosis. Various adjuvant treatments have been explored to improve survival. Perioperative chemotherapy with epirubicin/cisplatin/5-FU has been shown to improve the disease-free and OS in patients with resectable gastric cancer. The UK Medical Research Council (MRC) MAGIC trial randomised over 500 patients to either surgery alone or three cycles of preoperative ECF (epirubicin 50 mg/m^2, cisplatin 60 mg/m^2, day 1 and infused 5-FU 200 mg/m^2 for 21 days) followed by surgery and then three more cycles of postoperative ECF. Both progression-free and OS were superior in the combined modality arm. Five-year survival rates were 23% in the surgery alone arm and 36% in the perioperative chemotherapy arm.[16] In the United Kingdom, following the publication of this trial, perioperative chemotherapy has become the standard of care for patients with curable and resectable gastric cancers. The addition of bevacizumab to chemotherapy failed to show additional benefit (NCRI ST03).

More recently, a randomised phase III study compared perioperative ECX (epirubicin, cisplatin and capecitabine) with perioperative FLOT4 (docetaxel, oxaliplatin, 5-FU, leucovorin) in AC of the GOJ and stomach. It reported a significant increase in overall survival in the FLOT4 group (median overall survival 50 months versus 35 months with ECX), and FLOT4 has since become the new standard of care for operable cancers of the GOJ and stomach.[17]

The role of immunotherapy is currently evolving for gastric cancer. The recently published KEYNOTE-585 study demonstrated that the addition of perioperative pembrolizumab to chemotherapy improved the pathological complete response rate (12.9% versus 2.0%) but did not demonstrate a significant improvement in event-free survival.[18] The MATTERHORN study is assessing the role of adding durvalumab to preoperative FLOT chemotherapy. Interim results have shown an improvement in pathological complete response rate (19% versus 7%), and the results are awaited for event-free survival outcomes.[19]

Adjuvant Chemotherapy

Compared with the prominent use of perioperative chemotherapy in Europe, adjuvant chemotherapy is widely used in East Asia, including Japan and Korea. The ACTS-GC study (Japan) has confirmed the benefit of adjuvant single-agent S1 chemotherapy for 1 year over surgery alone in a randomised phase III trial involving over 1000 patients (OS 71.7% versus 61.1%; HR 0.67, 95% CI (0.54, 0.83)). The CLASSIC trial (South Korea, Taiwan, China) recruited a similar number of patients and showed a survival benefit for 6 cycles of adjuvant oxaliplatin and capecitabine over surgery alone (5-year overall survival 78% versus 69%; HR 0.66, $P = .0015$). Adjuvant chemotherapy therefore remains the standard of care in East Asia.

Microsatellite Instability: High Tumours

Patients with microsatellite instability-high (MSI-high) gastric cancers have a better prognosis compared to those with non-MSI-high tumours, and there is no added benefit of adjuvant chemotherapy.

Adjuvant Chemoradiation

In North America, adjuvant chemoradiation has been offered for patients with resected gastric cancer based on the results of the Intergroup 0116 randomised trial comparing surgery alone with surgery followed by postoperative chemoradiation with 5-FU and folinic acid (FA). The adjuvant chemoradiation improved the median progression-free survival (19 versus 30 months $P < .0001$) and OS (26 versus 35 months $P < .006$). It is felt that a significant proportion of patients may have had suboptimal lymph node dissection, and the postoperative chemoradiation may have compensated for the inadequate surgery. More recently, the benefit from this approach has been called into question. The Korean ARTIST trial ($n = 458$) compared the addition of CRT with platinum-fluoropyrimidine adjuvant therapy alone. There was no OS benefit, although in a subgroup analysis, 3-year disease-free survival was improved in node-positive patients who received chemoradiation (77.5% versus 72.3%, $P = .04$). The Dutch CRITICS trial compared perioperative ECX chemotherapy versus preoperative ECX and postoperative CRT in patients with cancer of the stomach and GOJ treated with D1/D2 gastrectomy. The trial failed to show any advantage for postoperative CRT (40.8% versus 40.9%, $P = .99$).

The ARTIST 2 trial compared 2 adjuvant chemotherapy regimens with adjuvant chemoradiation. It demonstrated that there was no additional benefit from chemoradiation in patients achieving an R0 resection after D2 gastrectomy.[20]

Neoadjuvant Chemoradiation

At present, there are no phase III data to support the use of neoadjuvant CRT, but the ongoing TOPGEAR and CRITICS II studies are investigating this approach.

The Australian TOPGEAR trial (NCT01924819) is comparing perioperative ECF/ECX chemotherapy with/without preoperative chemoradiation for resectable gastric cancer.

Radiation Techniques

The postoperative radiation target volumes are generated based on the tumour site in the stomach and the known pattern of LRF and need to be tailored to the individual patient's T stage and type of surgery. The CTV includes the gastric/tumour bed; gastric remnant; anastomosis; duodenal stump (where present); nodal stations along the lesser and greater curvature of the stomach, gastroduodenal, coeliac axis, suprapancreatic and retropancreatic nodes; porta hepatis; and splenic groups. Additional nodal groups are included based on the site of the tumour. A margin of 1 cm in all directions (except posteriorly, where a 0.5-cm margin is used) generates PTV. IMRT is recommended. Typical recommended dose constraints for OARs are as follows: kidneys—at least three-quarters of one kidney should receive less than 20 Gy; heart—no more than 30% to receive more than 40 Gy; spinal cord—maximum dose 45 Gy; liver—mean liver dose less than 30 Gy. The standard dose fractionation is 45 Gy in 25 fractions over 5 weeks. The concomitant chemotherapy options include single-agent capecitabine (825 mg/m^2 2 times daily (bd), on days of RT only, as in the ARTIST trial) or cisplatin/capecitabine combination (weekly cisplatin 20 mg/m^2 with capecitabine 575 mg/m^2 bd on days of RT only, as in the CRITICS trial). The patient needs to be monitored carefully with weekly full blood counts, biochemistry, dietetic assessment including weight and adequate measures for GI toxicity (nausea, vomiting and diarrhoea).

Palliative Treatments in Advanced/Metastatic Gastric Cancer

Palliative Chemotherapy

First-line treatment for patients with gastric and GOJ AC has a chemotherapy backbone (typically a platinum and fluoropyrimidine). Additional therapy is determined by HER2 status and PD-L1 expression.

In patients with HER2 + ve gastric cancer, addition of trastuzumab to cisplatin + fluoropyrimidine chemotherapy has been shown to improve both overall and progression-free survival.[21] In the ToGA trial, the subgroup of patients with HER2-positive (FISH + ve or IHC 3 + ve) gastric cancers had 4.2 months' improvement in OS with the addition of trastuzumab to chemotherapy (16 months versus 11.8 months, HR 0.65, 95% CI 0.51–0.83).

Patients with HER2-negative, PD-L1-positive gastric cancer can be offered immunotherapy in combination with chemotherapy. For those with a combined positive score ≥10, either nivolumab or pembrolizumab can be added. For patients with a combined positive score of 5 to **<10, nivolumab can be added.**

This approach improved overall survival in the CheckMate 649 and KEYNOTE-859 trials.

The KEYNOTE-811 trial is assessing the addition of pembrolizumab to trastuzumab-chemotherapy in patients with HER2 + ve gastric cancer. Interim analysis has shown that the addition of pembrolizumab significantly improved progression-free survival (10 months versus 8.1 months).[22]

In patients with tumours that are HER2 negative and have low PD-L1 expression, or in those with contraindications to the above options, chemotherapy alone is offered. Doublet chemotherapy with a platinum and fluoropyrimidine is the standard first-line treatment. Triplet chemotherapy (with either anthracycline or docetaxel) does not improve OS and is more toxic. Cisplatin with 5-FU (or capecitabine) (CF/CX) with/without epirubicin (ECF/ECX) or docetaxel (DCF) are regimens with response rates of 35% to 45% and a median OS of around 9 to 12 months. The REAL-2 study comparing cisplatin versus oxaliplatin and intravenous (IV) 5-FU versus oral capecitabine showed that the four regimens are of similar efficacy.[23] A docetaxel-based regimen, DCF (docetaxel, cisplatin and 5-FU) and irinotecan with cisplatin, produces similar median survival figures of around 9 months.

In an unselected population, the addition of targeted therapy with EGFR inhibitors (panitumumab in the REAL3 trial) or vascular endothelial growth factor (VEGF) inhibitors (bevacizumab in the AVAGAST trial) have failed to show survival benefit over conventional chemotherapy alone in first-line trials.

Second- and subsequent-line chemotherapy options include rechallenge of platinum-fluroropyrimidine, docetaxel, paclitaxel and irinotecan. In addition, MMR-deficient/MSI-high gastric cancers may be offered pembrolizumab monotherapy.

The RAINBOW trial, a double-blind, phase III, randomised trial, demonstrated that the addition of the monoclonal antibody ramucirumab (VEGFR-2 inhibitor) to paclitaxel resulted in a significant survival advantage compared with single-agent paclitaxel, with a median OS of 9.6 months ((95% CI: 8.5–10.8) versus 7.4 months (95% CI: 6.3–8.4), HR = 0.807 (95% CI: 0.678–0.962), $P = .017$). In the phase III REGARD trial, ramucirumab monotherapy significantly improved survival compared with placebo (HR = 0.776, 95% CI: 0.603–0.998, $P = .047$).

Palliative Radiotherapy

In selected patients, palliative RT (8–10 Gy in a single fraction or 20 Gy in 5 fractions, parallel opposed fields, using 4-to-15-MV photons) may help palliate pain, bleeding and obstructive symptoms.

Summary

Management of gastric cancer has improved over the past decade. Most patients with resectable gastric AC are likely to need a combined modality approach for best results. Those with metastatic disease benefit from treatment targeting HER2 and from immunotherapy.

PANCREATIC CANCER

Anatomy

The pancreas lies in the retroperitoneal space transversely along its long axis in the upper abdomen at the level of the first two lumbar vertebrae. It is divided into a head, body and tail. The pancreas is closely related to the surrounding structures including the stomach, duodenum and jejunum, lesser sac, kidneys, transverse colon, liver, spleen and vascular structures including the coeliac axis, superior mesenteric vessels and splenic and portal vein. Pancreatic cancer often locally infiltrates these structures. The pancreatic duct joins the bile duct to form the common bile duct, which opens into the second part of the duodenum through the major papilla. Pancreatic tumours originating from the head can compress the common bile duct, resulting in obstructive jaundice. The pancreas has a complex and extensive lymphatic drainage into the superior and inferior pancreaticoduodenal, coeliac axis, superior mesenteric and porta hepatis nodes. The tumour cells can also spread along the perineural pathways.

Incidence and Epidemiology

CRUK reports an average of 10,452 new cases were diagnosed annually in the United Kingdom between 2016 and 2018. The incidence of pancreatic cancer has been steadily rising in the United Kingdom through the decades, with a 9% rise in the past decade; it is projected to rise by 5% between 2025 and 2040, with a projected incidence of 16,000 per year in 2035. Pancreatic cancer is the 10th most common cancer in the United Kingdom. The mortality rate mirrors the incidence because of the poor prognosis. The causes of this cancer are largely unknown. The strongest association is with smoking, although the association is much less than seen with lung cancer. There is a doubling of incidence of this cancer in cigarette smokers. Exposure to organic chemicals, obesity and alcohol consumption are also thought to increase the risk. Hereditary pancreatic cancer syndromes account for less than 10% of the cancers and include hereditary pancreatitis, familial melanoma, BRCA-2, familial adenomatous polyposis (FAP), HNPCC, Peutz-Jegher and ataxia telangiectasia syndromes. There is an association between diabetes mellitus and pancreatic cancer.

Pathology

Some 90% of tumours in the pancreas are AC; 65% arise from the head of the pancreas. Neuroendocrine tumours, cystadenomas and cystadenocarcinomas are uncommon and have a better prognosis. The tumour spread is through local invasion into adjacent organs, in particular, perineural invasion through splanchnic nerves causing back pain. Lymphatic spread is common into regional and paraaortic lymph nodes. Tumours often metastasise to the liver and peritoneum. More than 80% of patients with pancreatic cancer present with either locally advanced or metastatic cancer that is not amenable for curative treatments.

More recently, based on molecular (mutational, transcriptomic) signatures, several subtypes of pancreatic cancer have been proposed. RNA expression analysis defined four subtypes: (1) squamous; (2) pancreatic progenitor; (3) immunogenic; and (4) aberrantly differentiated endocrine exocrine (ADEX) that correlate with histopathological characteristics.[24] These various subtypes identify opportunities for therapeutic intervention.

Clinical Features

The majority of the early symptoms are nonspecific. Therefore, most patients present with advanced disease. The common presenting symptoms are obstructive jaundice, weight loss, anorexia, back pain and fatigue. Back pain caused by deep perineural invasion may be present in more than 50% of patients. Classically, this pain is referred between the shoulder blades and is partially relieved by sitting up and leaning forwards. Back pain is usually considered to be a sign of inoperability. Less commonly, patients can present with new onset diabetes as a result of pancreatic insufficiency. Rarely, the cancer may be found following a bout of acute pancreatitis.

Clinical examination may reveal jaundice, evidence of weight loss, palpable supraclavicular nodes (Virchow's node) and umbilical nodule (Sister Mary Joseph's nodule). Superficial thrombophlebitis is a paraneoplastic feature. The liver may be enlarged, and there may be epigastric fullness/mass on palpation. Venous thromboembolism is a common association of pancreatic cancer (associated with >10% of cases).

Diagnostic Evaluation and Imaging

A full blood count may reveal anaemia, and biochemical tests confirm obstructive jaundice. CA19.9, a serum tumour marker, is raised in 60% to 90% of patients with pancreatic cancer.

Endoscopic retrograde cholangiopancreatography (ERCP) is an extremely useful investigation for evaluating the ampulla, obtaining cytological specimens and also for biliary drainage. Multislice contrast enhanced dual-phase CT with three-dimensional reconstruction is extremely useful to define the relationship of the tumour to the vessels and surrounding structures, and for detection of metastatic disease. EUS by an experienced endoscopist will help in detecting small lesions, any nodal involvement and, more importantly, venous involvement. Endoscopic ultrasound-guided fine needle aspiration (EUS FNA) may increase the diagnostic sensitivity to near 100% and has been shown to be reliable for presurgical workup.

Laparoscopy is helpful in detecting unsuspected peritoneal disease because up to 30% of patients with locally advanced pancreatic cancer (LAPC) have occult microscopic peritoneal disease.

FDG PET is an important imaging modality in nonmetastatic pancreatic cancer, particularly in those due to undergo resection. The PET-PANC study assessed the benefit of PET/CT in 589 patients with suspected pancreatic cancer. Patients underwent a multidetector CT scan as the standard of care and then a subsequent PET/CT as the experimental investigation.[25] Sensitivity (92.7% versus 88.5%) and specificity (75.8% versus 70.6%) for the diagnosis of pancreatic cancer was superior with PET/CT. PET/CT significantly improved diagnostic accuracy in all scenarios (P <.0002). PET/CT influenced management in 45% of patients and stopped resection in 20% of patients who were due to have surgery. However, the benefit of PET/CT was limited in patients with chronic pancreatitis or pancreatic tumours other than AC. PET/CT should be considered as the standard of care for apparently localised pancreatic cancer, particularly where resection is planned.

In selected patients, magnetic resonance imaging/magnetic resonance cholangiopancreaticogram (MRI/MRCP) may offer a better definition of local and vascular anatomy before surgery.

Therapy

Surgery

Less than 20% of patients have potentially surgically resectable lesions. Standard surgical treatment is pancreaticoduodenectomy pioneered by Whipple and his team in 1935. The distal body and tail of the pancreas tumours may require en bloc resection of the spleen along with the pancreas. The overall 5-year survival following surgical resection is 5% to 20%. For best results, surgery should be performed in high-volume centres with specialist experience. In the absence of distant metastases, features that make a tumour unresectable are based on (1) arterial involvement: tumour involvement/encasement of the superior mesenteric artery (SMA) or coeliac axis greater than 180 degrees or involvement of the first jejunal branch of the SMA; (2) venous involvement: unreconstructable portal vein (PV)/superior mesenteric vein (SMV) or tumour contact with the proximal jejunal branch of the SMV; or (3) invasion of adjacent organs (kidney, adrenal and colon). Tumours are considered to be borderline resectable based on (1) arterial involvement: SMA contact of 180 degrees (or less) or contact with the common hepatic artery without extension to the coeliac axis or hepatic artery bifurcation; or (2) venous involvement: contact with the SMV or PV of more than 180 degrees but suitable vessel proximal and distal to the site of involvement allowing for safe and complete resection and vein reconstruction. Patterns of failure after surgical resection without any adjuvant therapy are well described; 50% to 85% of patients have local relapse, 25% to 35% have peritoneal recurrences and 25% to 90% have liver metastases. Tumour stage, grade and resection margin status are the best predictors for survival after potentially curative surgery.

Adjuvant Therapy

Adjuvant (postoperative) chemotherapy to reduce the risk of cancer recurrence is considered the standard of care in Europe. The ESPAC-1 trial was the first study that confirmed the benefits of adjuvant chemotherapy (5-FU/FA), reporting a survival of 20.1 months (versus 15.5 months in patients not receiving chemotherapy, $P = .0009$). The study also found adjuvant CRT to be detrimental (15.9 months versus 17.9 months, $P = .05$). The CONKO-001 study demonstrated benefits of adjuvant gemcitabine (OS 22.8 months versus 20.2 months, $P = .01$). The ESPAC-3 trial showed that both 5-FU/FA and gemcitabine in the adjuvant setting have similar outcomes; however, gemcitabine was less toxic. The ESPAC-4 trial demonstrated OS benefit for the combination of gemcitabine and capecitabine over gemcitabine alone (28 months versus 25.5 months, $P = .032$).[26] However, subgroup analysis shows that significant benefit is largely confined to patients who have R0 resection. More recently, a randomised phase III trial demonstrated the benefit of modified oxaliplatin, leucovorin, irinotecan and fluorouracil (mFOLFIRINOX) over single-agent gemcitabine. In the Unicancer GI PRODIGE 24/CCTG PA.6 trial, 493 participants were included, and with a median follow-up of 69.7 months, the median OS was 53.5 months in the mFOLFIRINOX arm versus 35.5 months in the gemcitabine arm (HR 0.68, 95% CI 0.54–0.85). The randomised phase III APACT study evaluated the role of nab-paclitaxel in combination with gemcitabine in the adjuvant setting. Although it did not meet the primary endpoint of independently assessed disease-free survival, a small improvement in median overall survival was seen (41.8 versus 37.7 months) with the addition of nab-paclitaxel to adjuvant gemcitabine chemotherapy.

In Europe, mFOLFIRINOX is now the standard adjuvant therapy for patients who are fit enough, with gemcitabine-capecitabine (as in ESPAC-4) or gemcitabine alone as options for less fit patients.

Neoadjuvant Therapy

OS in resectable pancreatic cancer remains poor, and 40% to 60% of patients have a positive resection margin, with a correspondingly poor outcome. There has been a growing interest in the use of neoadjuvant treatment in pancreatic cancer with a view to treating micrometastatic disease, sparing surgery in patients with bad tumour biology and reducing the risk of positive margins.

Several metaanalyses suggest that preoperative treatment may downstage locally advanced and borderline resectable tumours and improve resectability and overall survival; however, downstaging a truly unresectable tumour is rare.[27] The benefit of the neoadjuvant approach is most likely to be in the borderline resectable patients, and this approach is being investigated as part of well-designed randomised clinical trials.

The PREOPANC trial compared neoadjuvant CRT to up-front surgery in both resectable and borderline resectable pancreatic cancer. Although the difference in median survival was only 1.4 months (favouring neoadjuvant CRT), the 5-year overall survival rate was 20.5% with neoadjuvant CRT versus 6.5% with up-front surgery, and this was consistent across the pre-specified subgroups. In addition, an R0 resection rate of 72% was achieved in the neoadjuvant CRT group compared with 43% in the up-front surgery group.

ESPAC-5 is a recently published randomised study that compared immediate surgery with neoadjuvant therapy (either gemcitabine plus capecitabine, FOLFIRINOX or capecitabine-based chemoradiation) in patients with borderline resectable pancreatic cancer. Although there was no significant difference in resection rates, there were increased 1-year overall survival rates in the neoadjuvant treatment groups when compared with immediate surgery.

The Alliance A021501 trial compared the use of preoperative mFOLFIRINOX with or without hypofractionated RT in the neoadjuvant setting for patients with borderline resectable pancreatic cancer.[28] This demonstrated favourable results for the mFOLFIRINOX arm, with an 18-month OS of 66.7%, and 47.3% in the arm receiving hypofractionated RT in addition to mFOLFIRINOX.

Management of Locally Advanced Pancreatic Cancer

Chemotherapy (see the 'Palliative Chemotherapy' section, later) is considered the standard of care for LAPC. Trials of up-front CRT versus chemotherapy alone have shown conflicting results. One large randomised trial of chemotherapy alone versus induction chemotherapy followed by consolidation CRT (the LAP07 study) failed to show benefit for addition of CRT, median OS being 16.5 months and 15.2 months, respectively ($P = .83$).[29] However, CRT was associated with a decrease in local progression (32% versus 46%, $P = .03$) and no increase in grades 3–4 toxicity, except for nausea. Outside clinical trials, CRT is currently considered for patients with prominent local symptoms, or as consolidation following 4 to 6 months of chemotherapy.[30] Where CRT is being considered, capecitabine is the preferred radiosensitiser based on the SCALOP trial which compared radiosensitisation with capecitabine to gemcitabine.[31] Capecitabine is given at a dose of 830 mg/m^2 twice daily on the days of treatment. IMRT and IGRT including 4DCT techniques help optimise tumour dose distribution while minimising radiation dose to the normal tissue.

The SCALOP2 trial examined dose escalation from 50.4 Gy in 28 fractions to 60 Gy in 30 fractions as well as the addition of nelfinavir to capecitabine-based CRT in patients who had received 3 cycles of induction chemotherapy (gemcitabine/nab-paclitaxel). Neither improved overall survival in LAPC, but dose escalation to 60 Gy was well tolerated and 1-year local progression was reduced.[32]

Stereotactic body radiotherapy (SBRT) is being increasingly used as the preferred treatment over CRT. Whereas previous studies using 1-to-3-fraction treatments had reported high incidences of grades 3–4 GI toxicity, a more recent study using 5-fraction regimens has reported early and late grade 3 + toxicity of 2% and 11%.[33] A systemic review of 19 prospective and retrospective SBRT studies has shown 1-year survival of 51.6% and a 1-year LC of 72.3%.[34] A more recent systematic review and metaanalysis compared SABR with conventionally fractionated RT and suggested that SABR may result in an improvement in 2-year OS (26.9% versus 13.7%) but found comparable 1-year overall survival (53.7% versus 49.3%). SABR was associated with lower rates of acute G3/4 toxicity (5.6% versus 37.7%), but there was no significant difference in late toxicity.[35]

External Beam Radiation Techniques

In patients with LAPC, the target volumes are defined using the information from the imaging studies available (EUS, CT, PET/CT, MRI) (Fig. 25.2). IGRT (4DCT) is preferable. Gross tumour volume (GTV) is defined as tumour and any lymph nodes >1 cm in short axis diameter (or smaller nodes that are metabolically active on PET/CT). Prophylactic nodal irradiation of noninvolved nodes is not advocated. Where 4DCT is available, a composite GTV is created to account for tumour motion during multiple phases of respiration. For CRT, CTV is created by a 5-mm expansion of the GTV/composite GTV, and the CTV is then edited off the GI tract. For PTV, 4DCT is the preferred option and when available, a 5-mm expansion around CTV defines PTV. When 4DCT is not available, it is defined as CTV with a 10-mm expansion for the anterior-posterior and lateral margin and a 15-mm expansion for the superior-inferior margin. IMRT is preferred, typically using 6-MV photons, to deliver 50.4 to 54 Gy in 1.8-Gy fractions.

For SBRT, 4DCT, organ compression and/or other motion management strategies including active breathing control/fiducial placement are essential for treatment delivery. PTV is generated by direct expansion of the GTV/composite GTV by 3 to 5 mm. A typical dose-fractionation scheme is 33 to 40 Gy in 5 fractions, typically using 6-MV photons. Dose volume histograms for each of the OARs (liver, kidneys, GI tract, spinal cord) should be critically evaluated before accepting the final plan; in particular, the dose to the GI tract is often critical.

Stereotactic MR-Guided Adaptive Radiation Therapy

Recently SMART has been of interest as a technique that could allow safe dose escalation for tumours in anatomically challenging locations such as the pancreas.

A recently published single-arm phase II study treated patients with borderline resectable or LAPC with SMART prescribed to 50 Gy in 5 fractions demonstrated promising 2-year overall survival from diagnosis of 53.6% and limited severe toxicity (Chuong, 2024).

Palliative Chemotherapy

Single-agent gemcitabine had long been the standard of care for patients with inoperable or metastatic pancreatic AC, with a median survival of about 6 months. More recently FOLFIRINOX (5-FU, FA, irinotecan, oxaliplatin) has demonstrated superior median survival in metastatic pancreatic AC (11.1 months versus 6.8 months in the gemcitabine group, HR 0.57, $P < .001$).[36] The combination of gemcitabine with nab-paclitaxel has also demonstrated a superior OS (8.5 months versus 6.7 months in the gemcitabine group, HR 0.72, $P < .001$).[37] However, grade 3/4 toxicity was higher with the combination of gemcitabine with nab-paclitaxel.

The NAPOLI 3 trial was a randomised phase III trial that compared the NALIRIFOX regimen with gemcitabine/nab-paclitaxel NALIRIFOX and was associated with improved overall survival (11.1 months versus 9.2 months), and both regimens had significant rates of grade 3 toxicity.[38]

Second-line chemotherapy:

Not many patients are suitable for second-line chemotherapy. Survival benefit from second-line chemotherapy is 1 to 2 months and must be carefully weighed against toxicity and quality of life.

Patients receiving FOLFIRINOX as first-line treatment can be considered for gemcitabine treatment. In patients who have received the gemcitabine/gemcitabine combination, an oxaliplatin-based regimen may be appropriate. Alternatively, a combination of liposomal irinotecan with 5-FU may be used. The NAPOLI-1 trial provided evidence for this regimen, showing survival of 6.1 months compared with 4.2 months in the group receiving 5-FU alone.[39]

Supportive Care for Symptom Palliation

Endoscopic biliary stenting of a resectable pancreatic tumour for the release of jaundice is as good as surgical bypass to relieve jaundice. The duodenal obstruction can be relieved by expandable stents. Pain relief is important for the palliation of pancreatic cancer. Severe pain can be caused by infiltration of the coeliac plexus, and this can be relieved by destruction of the plexus by an injection of alcohol, which can be carried out under either x-ray control or CT guidance.

HEPATOCELLULAR CARCINOMA

Epidemiology

Hepatocellular carcinoma (HCC) is a global problem; in males it is the second greatest cause of cancer deaths worldwide, with 80% occurring in poorly developed countries.[40] An estimated 782,500 new liver cancer cases and 745,500 deaths occurred worldwide in 2012, with China alone accounting for half of the cases. The prognosis for liver cancer is very poor (with an overall ratio of mortality to incidence of 0.95). Therefore, the geographical patterns in incidence and mortality are analogous. HCC has a strong male preponderance with a ratio of male to female being 4:1, and its occurrence increases with age, reaching a peak at age 70 years.[20] A risk factor can be identified in 90% of HCC cases, with the most frequent factors being chronic viral hepatitis (types B and C), cirrhosis caused by alcohol intake and aflatoxin exposure. A global epidemiological shift is occurring in the predominant aetiologies, from viral to nonviral causes.[41] All etiologic forms of cirrhosis are associated with increased tumour risk factors, with one-third of cirrhotic patients developing HCC during their lifetime.[42]

Symptomatology

Because most cases occur in patients who already have chronic liver disease, often there are no specific symptoms or worsening of symptoms as a result of underlying disease. Decompensation of disease because of the presence of HCC may occur, manifesting with encephalopathy, variceal bleeding or ascites. There could be jaundice, ascites and bruising right upper quadrant pain, or other GI symptoms such as loss of appetite, nausea, vomiting, diarrhoea, unintentional weight loss and tiredness. Metastatic disease can also cause symptoms: bone pain, for example, because of bone metastases. The physical findings usually reflect the underlying liver disease. Laboratory examination is usually nonspecific and reflects the degree of underlying cirrhosis.

Diagnostics and Classification

Noninvasive diagnosis criteria[43] for HCC are based on a combination of imaging and laboratory findings, which are hallmarks for HCC (arterial hypervascularity and venous/late-phase washout) and depend on the nodule size. A biopsy is only required if the radiological hallmarks of HCC are not seen or systemic treatment is considered. A triphasic CT scan and/or MRI are often the initial diagnosis manoeuvre. The serum alpha-fetoprotein is often elevated in patients with HCC but does not correlate with other clinical features such as stage, size or prognosis.

Clinical staging drives treatment options for HCC and ultimately influences OS and consists of the following factors: liver function and performance status, the ability to deliver optimal liver-directed therapy; and cancer biology.

The liver function is key for deriving prognosis, with Child-Pugh classification[44] being the most commonly used. The Child-Pugh score combines clinical findings (encephalopathy and ascites) with laboratory findings (bilirubin, albumin and prothrombin time) to classify patients in three categories, with grade A having the more favourable outcome and considered suitable for surgery or more aggressive therapies.[44]

Classically, the disease has been classified using tumour numbers, size and overall disease volume as a surrogate for biology. Combining these criteria with the underlying liver function has been used to provide clinical guidance to aid treatment selection. The Barcelona Clinic Liver Cancer (BCLC) staging system is commonly used in this context (Mauro et al., 2022).

General Management Principles

The mainstay of therapy is surgical resection; however, the majority of patients are not eligible for surgery, because HCC is diagnosed late in its course. Options of treatment are determined by both extent of tumour and severity of the underlying liver disease. The approaches of treatment in HCC are constantly evolving, with new treatment and indications being adopted rapidly; however, therapeutic approaches often vary depending on the available expertise. For inoperable patients, locoregional treatments should be considered.

Surgical Therapy

Potentially curative partial hepatectomy is the preferred treatment for HCC in patients with adequate liver functional reserve. The ideal candidate for resection has a solitary HCC (≤5 cm) that is confined to the liver and shows no imaging evidence of invasion of the hepatic vasculature, no evidence of portal hypertension and well-preserved hepatic function (normal bilirubin and platelet count >100,000). Long-term relapse-free survival rates average 40%, and 5-year survival rates as high as 90% are reported in selected candidates. A large number of patients are considered unresectable because of poor liver function rather than tumour size; these patients will be considered for liver transplantation. Invasion of the major portal vein, hepatic vein or adjacent organs (gallbladder) is not suitable for resection.

Liver Transplantation

Orthotopic liver transplantation (OLT) is a suitable option for patients with liver disease (usually cirrhosis) who would not tolerate liver resection and who have a solitary HCC 5 cm (or smaller) in diameter, or up to three separate lesions, none of which is larger than 3 cm, no evidence of gross vascular invasion, and no regional nodal or distant metastases. These criteria (known as the Milan Criteria) help define an ideal candidate, although centres may adopt broader criteria in their practice.[45] When these selection criteria are strictly applied, excellent overall 3-to-4-year actuarial (75%–85%) and recurrence-free survival rates (83%–92%) can be achieved, although these series represent highly selected cases.

The waiting time for transplant means that locoregional treatments may be offered while awaiting transplant. Practice varies, but typically an expected 3-to-6-month wait may prompt bridging therapy consideration. Options include transarterial chemoembolisation (TACE), transarterial radioembolisation (TARE), microwave/radiofrequency ablation and SBRT. Efforts to randomise patients between TACE and SBRT have met issues with recruitment; see the TRENDY trial.[46]

Locoregional Treatments

Although the mainstay of therapy is surgical resection, the majority of patients are not eligible, because of tumour extent or underlying liver dysfunction.

Several other treatment modalities are available, including:

1. Ablative methods: Radiofrequency ablation (RFA), microwave ablation (MWA), cryo or ethanol ablation, radiation therapy and stereotactic RT.
2. Local ablation with radiofrequency or percutaneous ethanol injections (PEIs) are considered the standard of care for patients with BCLC-0 (≤2 cm) and an option for BCLC-A tumours not suitable for surgery. PEI delivered with a 'single-session' multipronged needle has resulted in a complete response of 80% to 90% in tumours smaller than 4 cm. Thermal ablation (MWA or RFA) is the most widely used alternative to PEI. Several randomised controlled studies have shown that RFA has a better LC than PEI (2-year local recurrence rate 2%–18% versus 11%–45%, respectively), mainly in Asian studies. The EASL guidelines (European Association for Study of, European Organisation for, and Treatment of, 2018) recommend that RFA should be used in tumours smaller than 5 cm, with PEI to be used when RFA is not technically possible. For lesions less than 3 cm, away from blood vessels and ducts

and BCLC0, the complete response for both RFA and PEI is greater than 90% and they are considered competitive approaches to resection. Recent metaanalysis has suggested a higher complete response rate with MWA than RFA,[47] transarterial chemoembolisation (TACE) and transarterial radioembolisation (TARE).

3. Arterially directed therapies involve the infusion of particles via a catheter into the arterial branch of the hepatic artery, feeding the portion of the liver where the tumour is located. This is made possible by the dual blood supply to the liver and the hypervascular nature of HCC. The following arterial-directed therapies are currently in use: transarterial bland embolisation (TAE), TA chemoembolisation (TACE), TACE with drug-eluting beads (DEB-TACE) and TA radioembolisation with yttrium-90 microspheres (TARE). The principles of these therapies are to cause ischaemia by eliminating or minimising the blood flow to the tumour, ultimately causing tumour necrosis. TACE has shown survival benefit, and more than 50% of patients achieve an objective response.

Systemic Therapy and Molecularly Targeted Agents

The results with systemic therapy in HCC are poor. The knowledge of molecular events has permitted development of targeted therapies. In 2008, sorafenib was the first agent to have been proven to improve median survival versus placebo in Western patients, 10.7 versus 7.9 months and Eastern populations, 6.5 versus 4.2 months. More recently, the combination of immunotherapy checkpoint inhibitor Atezolizumab plus anti-VEGF Bevacizumab has shown improved overall survival and progression-free survival over sorafenib in the first-line setting and is now an accepted first-line treatment of choice.[48] More recently, phase III data have also supported the use of combination immunotherapy, durvalumab and tremelimumab in the first-line setting.[49] Second-line options include tyrosine kinase inhibitors such as regorafenib and cabozantinib.

Radiation Therapy

Liver-directed external beam radiation was historically limited by the lack of precise tumour imaging to target or on treatment, older RT techniques and the inability to quantify and assess the dose received by a given volume of tissue. The entire liver was often treated with radiation. Therefore, low doses of RT were used, which resulted in a low likelihood of tumour cure or control. Consequently, RT was primarily limited to the palliative setting.

The development of improved treatment planning and dose delivery methods, such as three-dimensional conformal radiation therapy and IMRT, volumetric imaging on treatment and motion management techniques, provided a mechanism not only to target hepatic lesions while sparing uninvolved hepatic parenchyma but also to precisely measure the radiation dose delivered to both the tumour volume and the surrounding normal tissue. RT is not limited by the location of the lesion and can be safely delivered to lesions in a variety of locations. This is attractive where invasive ablative treatments may be difficult, such as close to major vasculature or the dome of the liver.

The use of liver-directed RT significantly increased with the development of SBRT. SBRT uses multiple conformal beams (or volumetric arc therapy) to deliver high doses of RT with rapid-dose falloff beyond the target volume (see Fig. 25.3). Although the complete mechanism

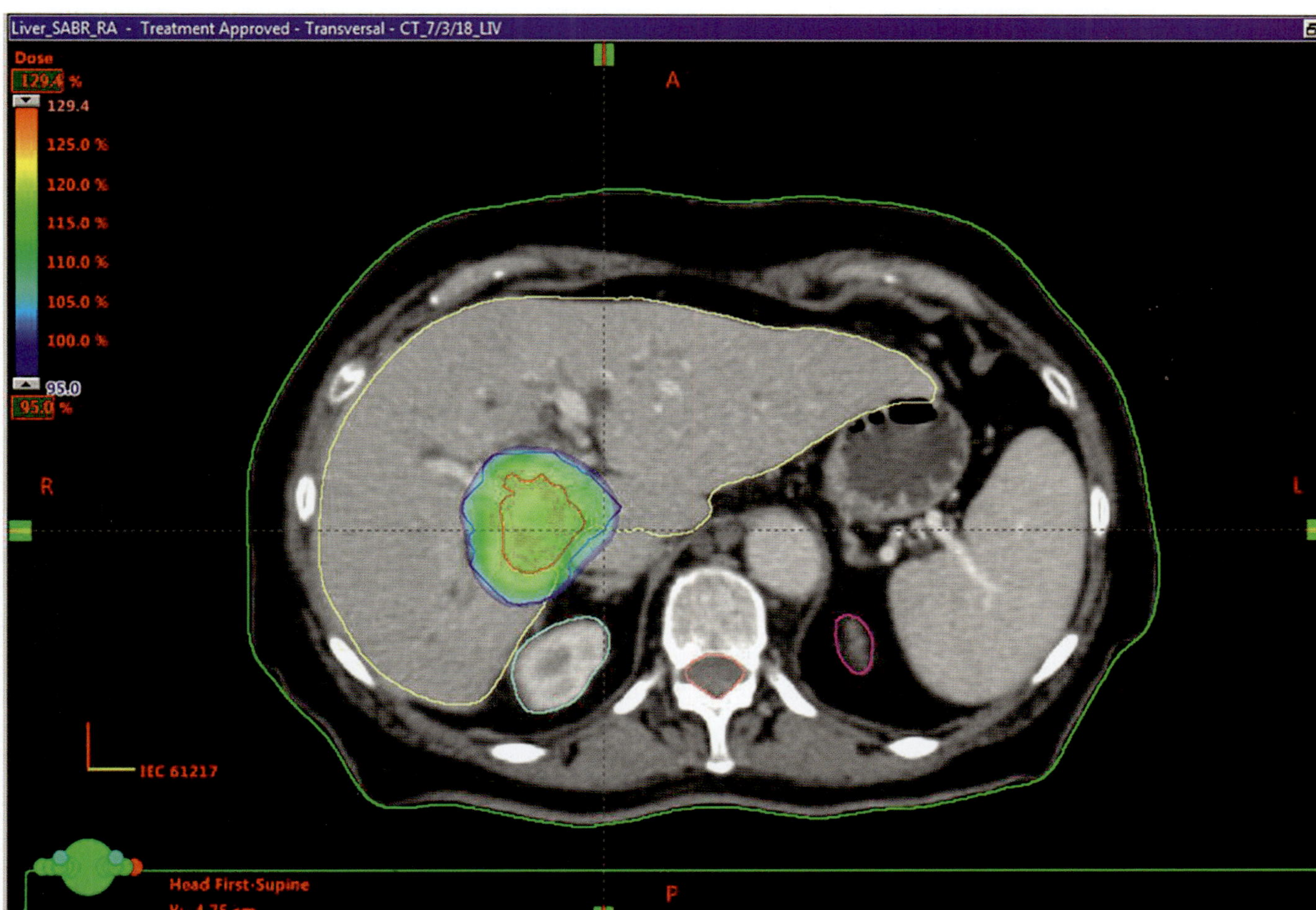

Fig. 25.3 Stereotactic ablative radiotherapy of liver tumour.

underlying SBRT-induced cell death is still a topic of research, the high radiation doses in SBRT are thought to result in an ablative effect on the tumour through vascular injury and immunomodulatory effects,[50] in addition to the DNA damage and cell death seen in conventionally fractionated RT. Given the highly conformal nature of SBRT, precise tumour definition and dose delivery are imperative. In addition to sophisticated treatment-planning software systems, SBRT also depends on accurate target identification, precise and reproducible patient immobilisation and assessment of target and organ motion. LC was reviewed in five studies that treated a total of 394 patients. The median follow-up was 18 months (IQ range 11–29 months). The 1-, 2- and 3-year actuarial LC rates were 93%, 89% and 86%, respectively. A single randomised study has investigated the addition of SBRT to standard-of-care first-line sorafenib for unresectable HCC not suitable for TACE or ablation.[51] Overall survival was significantly improved (HR = 0.72, 95% CI 0.52–0.99). However, interpretation of this study is challenging given the evolving first-line treatment paradigm, specifically the introduction of immunotherapy.

Charged particle therapies have also been employed in the treatment of hepatic tumours. Unlike photon-based RT, which has an exponential dose falloff, particle-based therapy (such as proton therapy) has an extremely rapid dose falloff at the end of its range. Consequently, tumours can be treated more effectively with less toxicity by charged particles than by photons, even in the cirrhotic liver with limited hepatic functional reserve. Hong et al.[52] reported on 92 patients with unresectable HCC or intrahepatic cholangiocarcinoma (IHCC) treated with moderately hypofractionated proton therapy with larger tumours. The median tumour size was approximately 6 cm with a dose prescribed of 58 GyE in 15 fractions. After a median follow-up of 19.5 months, the 1-year LC of 97% was reported; this translated into a 22.5-month median OS. A systematic review of charged particles versus protons[53] included 73 cohorts from 70 noncomparative observational studies. Pooled OS was significantly higher at 1, 3 and 5 years for protons than for conventional RT (relative risk (RR) 1.68, 95% CI 1.22–2.31, $P < .001$; RR 3.46, 95% CI: 1.72–3.51, $P < .001$; RR 25.9, 95% CI: 1.64–408.5, $P = .02$, respectively). LC was also significantly higher for patients treated with protons than for CRT ($P = .013$ and $P < .001$, respectively).

A small randomised study has compared proton beam therapy versus RFA for small recurrent HCCs (mostly after RFA).[54] It showed non-inferior outcomes for proton beam therapy; however, the utility of such data may be limited given the costs of protons. Carbon ion therapy has been utilised, with excellent LC rates seen in a small phase I study[55]).

Principles of Radiation Delivery

A. Immobilisation and motion management

In general for conformal RT and conventional fractionation, a larger margin for internal target coverage is accepted and the setup errors are usually larger to account for uncertainties in tumour localisation (Fig. 25.4). These are accepted, as over large number of fractions, the errors will tend to average out.

SBRT relies on the delivery of accurate high doses to the target, and errors in localisation could result in increased normal tissue toxicity and/or geometric tumour miss. Therefore, the use of techniques or devices to localise the radiation to the tumour,

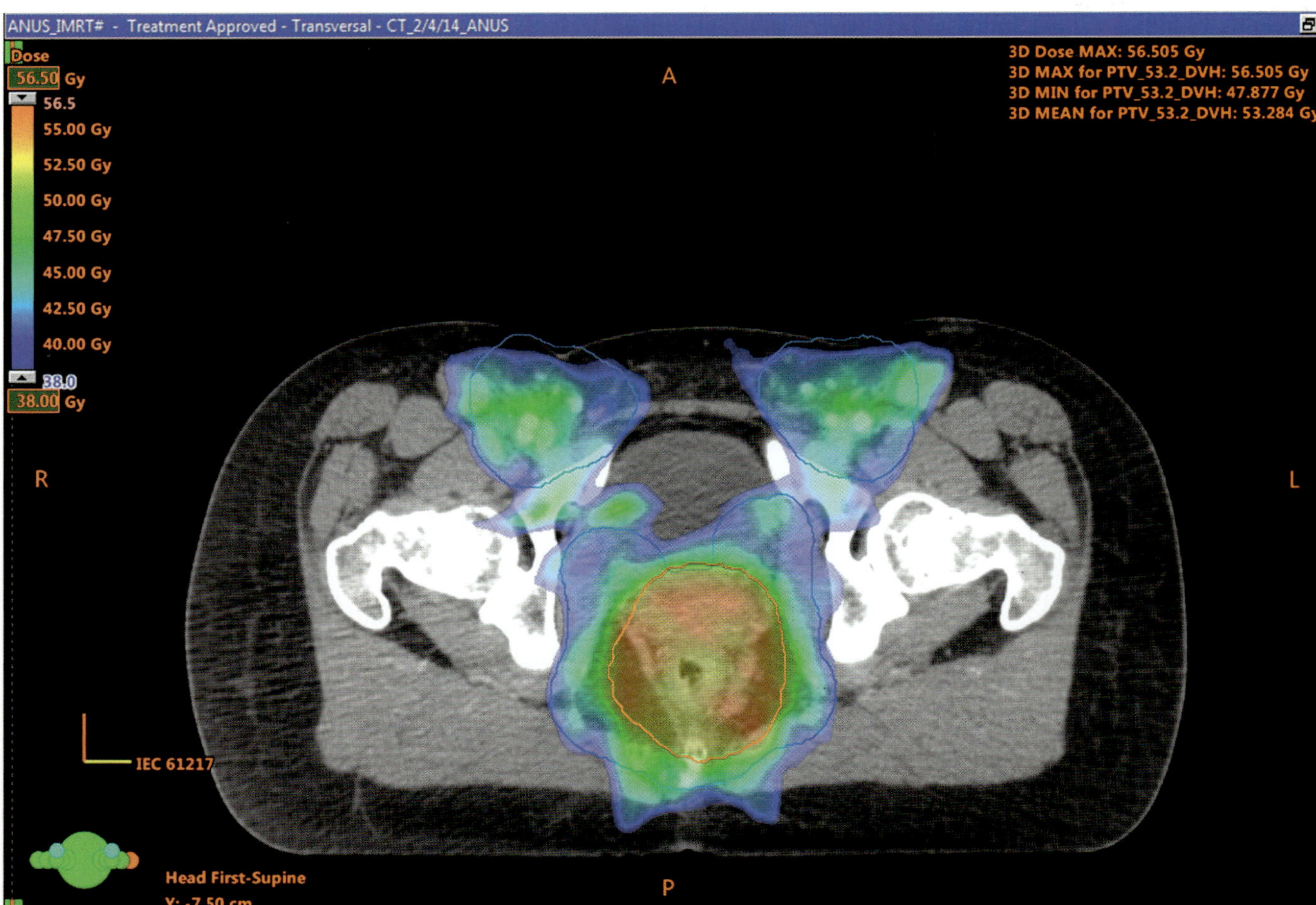

Fig. 25.4 Intensity modulated radiotherapy plan for locally advanced anal cancer showing dose-painted primary tumour and regional nodes.

minimise margins and optimise on-treatment quality assurance is very important. Immobilisation devices are needed to ensure that patients remain in a consistent, reproducible position throughout treatment. There is no universal agreed standard for liver SBRT, but recommendations from groups with experience in SBRT are available. The primary motion with liver RT is respiratory motion, which can be controlled with fixed immobilisation including abdominal compression, breath hold and/or tracking. For immobilisation, vacuum bag systems or fixed body immobilisers can be used. The AAPM suggests a cutoff of 5 mm, after which respiratory management is recommended. The options can be categorised into three types: (1) nongated ITV reduction strategies; (2) active or passive breath-hold techniques; and/or (3) surrogate markers (e.g. fiducial markers or radioopaque lipiodol). A simple margin expansion to account for ITV is then applied based on a 4DCT scan, fluoroscopy and/or cine MRI to capture the full range of motion. These are categorised as ITV methods or motion encompassing methods. An additional margin for setup motion is added for PTV with recommendations ranging between 2 and 5 mm.

B. Localisation

At simulation, IV contrast is considered standard in HCC. Information from the diagnostic triphasic dynamic contrast enhanced CT is particularly useful for tumour visualisation. MRI is integral to localisation, especially in cirrhotic patients or those who are unable to tolerate IV contrast. This may be a dedicated planning position MRI or fusion of diagnostic MRI imaging. The addition of oral contrast is useful to identify GI structures in the vicinity of the tumour.

C. Dose selection and toxicity

HCCs are radiosensitive, and radiation yields excellent local tumour control rates.

Schedules of 33 to 60 Gy in 3 to 5 fractions, biologically effective dose (BED) 60 to 180 Gy_{10} have been used. Actuarial local rates at 1, 2 and 3 years for lesions treated with BED of 100 Gy or less were 94%, 89% and 86%, respectively. Similar LC rates (92%, 89%, and 86%) were seen in lesions treated with BED greater than 100 Gy_{10} (log-rank $P = .972$) (Fig. 25.3) (Ohri et al., 2018). These suggest that there might not be a dose-response relationship within the range of reported doses. It would be reasonable to use 40 to 50 Gy in 5 fractions to achieve an LC of greater than 90% at 2 years. The normal tissue dose constraints are becoming better described as experience with SBRT is increasing.

Radiation-induced liver disease (RILD), which can present in both classic and nonclassic forms, is perhaps the most feared complication of liver irradiation; however, severe toxicity after SBRT is reported in less than 10% of Child-Pugh A patients. The risks are higher in patients with underlying cirrhosis. Predictors of toxicity to RT include baseline Child-Pugh scores, and higher normal liver doses (e.g. mean dose, effective liver dose, doses to 700–900 cc) are associated with liver function decline 3 months post-SBRT. Lower baseline platelet count and portal vein thrombus were also associated with an increased risk. It has been suggested that use of protons may reduce the risk of RILD and improve survival through better liver dosimetry.[56]

Normal tissue complication probability models are now able to predict the risk of classic RILD associated with a given radiation treatment plan. Recently, MRI techniques to map RILD have shown contribution from direct-dose effects and secondary inflammatory effects in the aetiology of RILD.[57]

D. Treatment delivery

Daily online treatment verification is crucial for accurate delivery of RT. The verification should be appropriate to the type of RT delivered and equipment used. Volumetric imaging (such as onboard cone beam CT) or tracking of fiducial markers can be used. Alignment solely on bony anatomy should not be applied, as it may lead to errors in setup. Attention should be given to the organ function of the patient with assessment of status during RT.

Future Perspectives

The treatment of HCC has evolved considerably in the past decade. A multidisciplinary approach and liver function optimisation in every patient have made it possible to offer an option for treatment and disease control and survival extension at any stage of presentation. Prevention is still key in this disease. Therefore, promotion of a healthy lifestyle, including decreasing alcohol and prevention of metabolic syndrome, is important. Sequencing and combination of locoregional treatments need to be investigated systematically in prospective trials, and combinations of locally ablative treatments with systemic treatments are being tested (e.g. TACE3 ISRCTN12053408). Effective adjuvant therapies are needed after curative local treatment. The incorporation of RT in the standard of care with high-level evidence is urgently needed.

BILIARY TRACT CANCERS

Biliary tract cancers (BTCs) are uncommon cancers comprising cholangiocarcinoma (divided into three disease subtypes: intrahepatic, perihilar and extrahepatic), gallbladder and ampullary cancers. They account for around 3% of all GI cancers globally. The overall incidence of cholangiocarcinoma has increased progressively worldwide over the past four decades, and increased mortality was seen in the United States and Europe, representing an area of unmet need.

The incidence of cholangiocarcinoma in the United Kingdom is rising: age-standardised incidence rates of 2.9 in 2001 to 2003 have risen to 4.6 in 2016 to 2018 for BTCs.[58] During that time, 3-year net survival for BTCs increased from 9.2% in 2001 to 12.6% in 2016 to 2018; a modest gain and indicative of the difficulties in treating these cancers.

Cholangiocarcinomas are aggressive tumours. Most patients have advanced-stage disease at presentation, and management requires a multidisciplinary approach. Surgery is the only potentially curative treatment modality for cholangiocarcinoma, but only a minority of patients (<35%) have disease that is amenable to surgical resection with curative intent. Achieving clear resection margins is critical to a better outcome, with median disease-free survival durations of 12 to 36 months reported. Adjuvant capecitabine is now generally offered following results of the randomised BILCAP study.[59] An even smaller subset of patients, typically with hilar cholangiocarcinoma, are candidates for liver transplantation following neoadjuvant chemoradiation.

The historical standard of care for patients with advanced disease was established by the ABC-02 trial, a combination chemotherapy with cisplatin and gemcitabine (CisGem).[60] This has recently been superseded in the first-line setting by gemcitabine/cisplatin/durvalumab, following positive survival data (durvalumab 24.9% versus placebo 12.4%, 2-year survival from the TOPAZ-1 trial).[61]

A large focus of interest is the development of targeted therapies for the treatment of specific mutational subset BTCs:

1. Fibroblast growth factor receptor fusion/rearrangement targeting, for example, pemigatinib[62] and futibatinib[63]
2. Isocitrate dehydrogenase 1 (IDH1) mutations, for example, ivosidenib[64]
3. BRAF V600E mutation, for example, dabrafenib/trametinib[65]
4. HER2 amplification, for example, zanidatamab[66]

In addition, the necessary broad testing may occasionally identify mutational states suitable for basket-type approvals:

1. MSI-high phenotype, for example, pembrolizumab
2. NTRK fusion rearrangements, for example, entrectinib, larotrectinib

Such systemic therapies will form the backbone of treatment for all patients with unresectable BTCs. Efforts are being made to bring the molecularly targeted agents into the first-line setting (e.g. the FIGHT-302 and SAFIR-ABC-10 trials).

RT does not have a clearly defined role in the management of BTCs. Published reports describing RT response are generally of non-randomised, single-institution experiences that are subject to selection bias. Patients with better performance status may receive higher radiation doses. Reports of patients receiving EBRT for bile duct carcinoma have suggested that doses of 40 to 45 Gy result in improved survival outcomes compared with lower doses. These data have been superseded, and now doses of more than 80 Gy are recommended. Tao et al.[67] reported a retrospective analysis of 79 patients with inoperable, locally advanced intrahepatic cholangiocarcinoma and the impact of radiation dose on outcomes. Patients treated to a biologically equivalent dose of 80.5 Gy achieved remarkable levels of long-term LC, OS and progression-free survival (78%, 58% and 39%, respectively, at 3 years). Most (89%) patients had received previous systemic treatment. The median OS time after diagnosis was 30 months; the 3-year OS rate was 44%. Radiation dose was the single most important prognostic factor; higher doses correlated with an improved LC rate and OS. Additionally, a single-arm phase II hypofractionated proton beam study also demonstrated high LC rates in cholangiocarcinoma (2-year LC and OS rates were 94.1% and 46.5%, respectively), with minimal toxicity (7.7% grade 3). The most important data come from the randomised phase II ABC-07 trial, which randomised patients with non-metastatic, unresectable BTCs after 4 cycles of gemcitabine/cisplatin to receive either 4 more cycles of gemcitabine/cisplatin (per ABC-02) or 2 cycles of gemcitabine/cisplatin and then SBRT to the disease.[68] Dose/fractionation was either 50 Gy in 5 fractions (<6 cm) or 67.5 Gy in 15 fractions (≥6 cm), with dose reductions being possible to meet liver constraints. The study did not meet its primary endpoint of PFS, suggesting our selection of patients for SBRT may need further refinement.

The principles of primary SBRT delivery follow HCC principles (see previously).

In the postoperative setting, nodal positive and R1 tumours might benefit from adjuvant CRT. SWOG S0809, a phase II intergroup trial of adjuvant capecitabine and gemcitabine followed by RT and concurrent capecitabine in extrahepatic cholangiocarcinoma and gallbladder carcinoma,[69] was a phase II multicentre study that met the primary objectives. A total of 79 eligible patients were treated (86% completed). For all patients, 2-year survival was 65% (95% CI, 53%–74%); it was 67% and 60% in R0.

Principles of Adjuvant Radiotherapy

Delineation of the CTV should be based on review of the preoperative scans, postoperative scans, clips or markers placed by the surgeon, and surgery summary notes. Review and discussion of the targets with the surgeon are strongly recommended. CTV will include the tumour bed and retropancreatic, coeliac and portal vein nodes with a possible boost to any areas of positive margins (best estimate). Radiation doses of 45 Gy in 25 fractions and 55 Gy in 25 fractions are delivered as a simultaneous integrated boost with concurrent capecitabine.

CANCER OF THE COLON AND RECTUM

Epidemiology

Malignancies of the colon and rectum constitute the fourth most common form of cancer in the United Kingdom, with an annual incidence of 42,900 new cases in 2016 to 2018 (http://www.cancerresearchuk.org/health-professional/cancer-statistics/statistics-by-cancer-type/bowel-cancer#heading-Zero). One in 17 males and 1 in 20 females will be diagnosed with bowel cancer during their lifetime. Incidence rates for bowel cancer are projected to fall by 8% in the United Kingdom between 2023 and 2040, with an estimated 47,000 new cases annually by 2040. In Europe, approximately 538,000 new cases of bowel cancer were estimated to have been diagnosed in 2022. The UK incidence rate is the 22nd highest in Europe for males and the 10th highest for females (https://gco.iarc.who.int/today/en/fact-sheets-cancers). The age-specific incidence rises markedly over the age of 60 years, whereas less than 1% of all cases occur in patients under the age of 40 years.

Aetiology

The majority of rectal cancers develop via the CIN pathways. About 13% are caused by deficient mismatch repair (dMMR).

1. Familial clustering

   Approximately 20% of cases of colorectal cancer are associated with a familial history, and first-degree relatives of patients with invasive colorectal cancer or colorectal adenomas are at increased risk of colorectal cancer. There are well-defined inherited syndromes such as Lynch syndrome (also known as HNPCC) and FAP. It is therefore recommended that all patients with colorectal cancer have a family history investigated and a risk assessment undertaken. A screening colonoscopy every 6 years is recommended for most individuals without a personal history of colorectal cancer and with one first-degree relative with colorectal cancer diagnosed before the age of 50 years, or two first-degree relatives with colorectal cancer diagnosed at any age.[70]

2. Environmental factors

   It is likely that rectal cancer has a different aetiology than colon cancer (https://www.wcrf.org/int/research-we-fund/continuous-update-project-findings-reports/colorectal-bowel-cancer), with high body mass index, body or abdominal fatness, low levels of physical activity, metabolic syndrome and type II diabetes being seen as risk factors. Some data suggest that these are also associated with a poor prognosis. Risk is also increased by excessive consumption of meat (red or processed) and alcohol (moderate/high intake), long-standing ulcerative colitis or Crohn affecting the rectum.

Histopathology and Clinical Features

The vast majority of colorectal cancers are ACs. Macroscopically, they present as an endoluminal mass that protrudes into the lumen and originates from mucosa. The mass could be exophytic or polypoid, and bleeding may be seen in ulcerated, friable or necrotic lesions. They typically show glandular differentiation and mucin formation and stain positively for carcinoembryonic antigen (CEA). Small cell carcinomas, lymphomas, melanomas and adenosquamous carcinomas have been reported.

More recently, a consensus molecular subtype classification based on gene expression data has been described (Consensus Molecular Subtypes, CMS 1–4).[71]

Usually, patients will present with symptoms of rectal bleeding, altered bowel habits or weight loss and are diagnosed by colonoscopy. Asymptomatic patients are diagnosed during routine screening colonoscopy or an imaging performed for other reasons. Rarely, bulky lesions may present with overt bowel obstruction.

Total mesorectal excision (TME) is the procedure used in the treatment of colorectal cancer in which a significant length of the bowel around the tumour is removed. The procedure is mainly used in mid and lower rectal tumours where it is essential to remove the rectum along with the mesorectum up to the level of the levators.

For mesorectal resections, histopathological examination should include a photographic record of the surgical specimen; assessment is a strong quality-control measure. The classification has three grades based on the completeness of the removal of the mesorectum and/or plane of surgical excision and the grade impacts on both local recurrence and survival. The status of the circumferential resection margin (CRM) (i.e. ≤1 mm) and TME quality are surrogates for good oncological outcomes. At least 12 lymph nodes should be examined. The RCP minimum data set for a colorectal surgery histopathology report should be used (https://www.rcpath.org/asset/E94CE4A2-D722-44A7-84B9D68294134CFC).

Pretreatment Staging Evaluations

The aim of pretreatment evaluation is to assess the presence or absence of distant metastatic disease (with CT chest, abdomen and pelvis, and PET/CT and/or MRI (liver) as appropriate), to determine the tumour location and its local extent. An accurate assessment is necessary for rectal cancer with pelvic MRI and/or endorectal USS is required. High-quality pelvic MRI is the most accurate investigation to define locoregional clinical staging of rectal tumours. By detecting extramural vascular invasion (EMVI) and determining the T substage and distance to the CRM, MRI can also predict the risks of local recurrence and should be carried out in select patients for respective preoperative management and to define the extent of surgery. A specialist and dedicated multidisciplinary team comprising surgeons and a medical oncologist, radiation oncologist, gastroenterologist, radiologist and pathologist should discuss all relevant cases of colorectal cancer.

Staging Systems

Colon and rectal cancers are staged using the tumour, node and metastasis (TNM) staging system from the American Joint Committee on Cancer (AJCC)/Union for International Cancer Control (UICC); the current (8th edition, implemented in 2018). The prefixes *p* and *yp* used in the TNM staging system denote pathological staging and pathological staging following neoadjuvant therapy, respectively.

KRAS, BRAF and mismatch repair (MMR) status should be assessed.

Colon Cancer: Treatment Principles

Surgery

Surgery is still the main treatment modality. The aim of surgery is excision of the primary tumour with wide excision margins. The tumour spreads to the lymph nodes located in the mesentery close to the vascular supply for that portion of colon. This portion of node-bearing mesentery is excised along with the bowel. Continuity of the bowel is usually reestablished by a direct anastomosis, between either excised segments of colon or the colon and the terminal ileum.

For select early-stage tumours, endoscopic resection followed by surveillance may be an option. Tumours suitable for endoscopic resection are pT1 ACs confined to the head, neck and stalk of a pedunculated polyp, without any histological features associated with an adverse outcome (lymphatic or venous invasion, grade 3 differentiation, significant tumour budding).

Adjuvant Chemotherapy

Adjuvant chemotherapy is of proven benefit for patients with stage III (node-positive) colon cancer. Six months of 5-FU and FA chemotherapy given to such patients is estimated to reduce the risk of death by 30%, which translates into a 10% to 13% absolute improvement in survival. Two randomised controlled trials have confirmed that the addition of oxaliplatin to 5-FU and FA improves 3-year survival by an additional 7%.

Patients with stage II tumours have derived less benefit from adjuvant chemotherapy. Trials, such as the British QUASAR trial, have shown only a 3.6% increase in 5-year survival in this group of patients. However, stage II includes a heterogeneous group of patients, and multivariate analysis of patterns of relapse have shown major and minor prognostic paramaters that should be taken into account to refine the risk assessment. Major prognostic parameters include pT4 stage, tumour perforation and <12 lymph nodes sampled. Minor prognostic parameters include high-grade tumours, lymphovascular invasion, perineural invasion, presentation with obstruction and high preoperative CEA levels. MSI/MMR status should also be taken into account; patients with MMR-deficient tumours have a better prognosis and do not benefit from adjuvant chemotherapy in the same way as patients with MMR-proficient tumours.

The Xeloda in Adjuvant Colon Cancer Therapy (X-ACT) trial has shown that oral capecitabine is at least as effective as 5-FU and FA. Orally administered capecitabine is an alternative treatment for patients who may not be able to tolerate oxaliplatin-based regimens. Currently, irinotecan-based regimens have not been shown to give an advantage in an adjuvant setting and therefore are not currently recommended.

A shorter course of chemotherapy (3 months) may be selected as a treatment for some patients with colon cancer. The International Duration Evaluation of Adjuvant therapy (IDEA) pooled analysis compared 3 with 6 months of adjuvant chemotherapy for stage III colon cancer. The overarching goal was to reduce chemotherapy-related toxicity, mainly oxaliplatin-induced neuropathy. Patients were classified into low-risk and high-risk groups, suggesting that low-risk patients may be offered only 3 months of treatment.[72]

Neoadjuvant Chemotherapy

The role of neoadjuvant chemotherapy for locally advanced colon cancer was assessed in the FOxTROT trial. This showed that 6 weeks of neoadjuvant FOLFOX can be delivered without increasing perioperative morbidity. The group receiving neoadjuvant treatment had fewer incomplete resections and less recurrent disease within 2 years. No benefit was seen from the neoadjuvant use of panitumumab, and no benefit was seen in MMR-deficient tumours.[73]

Management of Advanced Colorectal Cancer

The median survival for patients with metastatic colorectal cancer has improved vastly over the past few decades. Combination chemotherapy with targeted therapy has improved the median survival beyond 2 years.

Oligometastatic Disease. Patients with resectable liver metastases have an overall 5-year survival of 25% to 30% following hepatic resection and perioperative chemotherapy. Other techniques such as thermal ablation or SBRT may be used in combination with, or as an alternative to, surgery in patients where frailty or anatomical location of the metastasis makes the tumours inoperable.

Resection of lung metastases can achieve 5-year survival of 25% to 35% in carefully selected patients and may be combined with resection of liver metastases.

The addition of cetuximab to chemotherapy was associated with worse overall survival compared with the use of chemotherapy alone (55.4 vs 81 months).[74]

The ORCHESTRA trial[75] examined the role of tumour debulking in addition to standard palliative chemotherapy in patients with multiorgan metastatic colorectal cancer. The trial did not demonstrate an improvement in overall survival. Further study is needed into the role of local therapies in metastatic colorectal cancer.

Chemotherapy for Advanced Disease. Oxaliplatin or irinotecan in combination with fluoropyrimidines (5-FU or the oral prodrug, capecitabine) is the backbone of treatment for advanced/metastatic colorectal cancer. Given as a single agent, fluoropyrimidines have a response rate on the order of 20%. The DNA topoisomerase 1 inhibitor, irinotecan, used in combination with 5-FU and FA (FOLFIRI) yields a response rate of 39%; oxaliplatin with 5-FU and FA (FOLFOX4) has a response rate of 51%, used in first-line therapy. The consecutive use of both regimens (used in either sequence) extends OS to 18 months. One Italian phase III study has shown the chemotherapy triplet (FOLFOXIRI) to be superior to FOLFIRI in the first-line setting (22.6 months versus 16.7 months, HR 0.7, *P* = .03).[76] The chemotherapy triplet is recommended for BRAF mutant patients (who have a particularly poor prognosis).[77] In clinical practice, chemotherapy is frequently combined with targeted agents, both in the first- and second-line settings.

Targeted (Biological) Therapies. Anti-EGFR therapy: Cetuximab and panitumumab are active in combination with irinotecan-5-FU or oxaliplatin-5-FU chemotherapy in the first-line setting in patients who do not harbour *RAS* mutations (exons 3 and 4 of *KRAS*, and exons 2, 3 and 4 of *NRAS*). In *RAS* wild-type populations, an OS of 23 months has been demonstrated with a cetuximab and FOLFIRI combination[78] and an updated analysis of the PRIME study has shown a survival benefit of combining panitumumab with FOLFOX4 (median OS 23.9 months).[79]

Biological agents are indicated for most patients in the first-line setting unless contraindicated. An anti-EGFR therapy may be preferred in the first line (over anti-VEGF therapy) in *KRAS* wild-type patients based on the FIRE3 study that demonstrated an OS benefit for the former combination (FOLFIRI plus cetuximab, 28.7 months versus FOLFIRI plus bevacizumab, 25 months, HR 0.77, *P* = .017).[80]

Anti-VEGF therapy: Bevacizumab, which binds circulating VEGF-A, has demonstrated improved efficacy (OS, PFS, response) in combination with a single-agent 5-FU as well as a 5-FU-irinotecan combination[81] in combination with 5-FU-oxaliplatin; the benefit was seen in terms of PFS only.[82]

Biological agent combinations in second-line setting:

Where bevacizumab has not been used in first-line treatment (typically *KRAS* wild-type patients treated with FOLFIRI-cetuximab as first-line combination), it can be used in combination with FOLFOX4 in the second-line setting because it has demonstrated OS benefit over FOLFOX4 alone (12.9 months versus 10.8 months, HR 0.75, *P* = .001).[83] Where bevacizumab has been used in first line treatment (typically in combination with FOLFOX4 for *KRAS* mutant patients), aflibercept[84] or ramucirumab[85] may be used in combination with FOLFIRI.

Immunotherapy. Immunotherapy has a role in treatment of patients with dMMR/MSI-high tumours. Pembrolizumab has been shown to have activity in the first-line setting and significantly improved progression-free survival in the phase III KEYNOTE-177 trial. There was significant crossover from the chemotherapy arm, but after a median follow-up of 44.5 months, the median overall survival was not reached in the pembrolizumab arm and was 36.7 months in the chemotherapy arm. Median progression-free survival was 16.5 months with pembrolizumab and 8.2 months with chemotherapy[86]).

In the United Kingdom, second-line nivolumab with ipilimumab (after previous chemotherapy treatment) is recommended by NICE based on the results of the CheckMate 142 study, which included 119 patients with metastatic colorectal cancer.[87]

BRAF V600E Mutated Colorectal Cancer. The presence of BRAF mutations is associated with a poor prognosis, with standard-of-care treatment being less effective for these patients. Targeting the BRAF signalling pathway has been shown to be beneficial in the phase III BEACON study[88] and led to the approval of the combination of encorafenib and cetuximab for pretreated BRAF V600E-mutated colorectal cancer. The study demonstrated improved survival (9.3 months) compared to chemotherapy (5.9 months).

Third-Line Options. Both regorafenib and trifluridine/tipiracil are available for fit patients who have progressed on fluoropyrimidines, oxaliplatin, irinotecan, bevacizumab and in case of KRAS WT, anti-EGFR antibodies.

The recently published SUNLIGHT trial[89] showed that the addition of bevacizumab to trifluridine/tipiracil resulted in improved overall survival (10.8 months versus 7.5 months).

Radiotherapy and Colon Cancer

There are very few studies that investigated the role of CRT in colon cancer. One phase III randomised controlled study evaluating adjuvant radiation therapy in patients with locally advanced colon cancers (T3N1, T3N2 and T4anyN) showed similar OS in patients receiving chemotherapy and radiation compared with those treated with chemotherapy alone, but with higher toxicity in patients receiving radiation therapy. Unfortunately, this study was closed because of poor accrual. There are some institutional retrospective reports suggesting a R0 resection rate of 92% to 100%, increased downstaging and a possible reduction in locoregional recurrence following preoperative CRT. The RT doses range between 45 and 50.4 Gy in 25 to 28 fractions with concurrent fluoropyrimidines. The RT fields reflect the tumour location (e.g. sigmoid, descending/ascending colon and proximity to other normal structures). IMRT/VMAT are preferred, and daily volumetric imaging is recommended to aid localisation during treatment delivery. In the palliative setting, either a single fraction of 8 Gy or up to 30 Gy in 10 fractions may be used as a palliative procedure in colon cancer to stop bleeding and reduce pain; however, this depends on the clinical setting.

Follow-up

Follow-up protocols for patients with colonic cancer vary across institutions but, in all cases, the patient will undergo endoscopic examination to rule out any local recurrence or new primary lesions. Patients should also have CT imaging as part of their follow-up protocol as per NICE guidance.

Rectal Cancer: Treatment Principles

The determination of an optimal treatment plan for an individual patient with rectal cancer involves a multidisciplinary approach and incorporates patient preferences. Once the intent of the treatment has been decided (radical or palliative), the consideration of the likelihood of maintaining bowel function and preservation of genitourinary functions needs to be made.

The sequencing of multimodality therapy needs to be carefully considered, especially in patients who present with synchronous metastatic disease and who entertain a curative intent.

A risk-adapted approach is recommended for rectal cancer.[90]

The quality of primary surgery for rectal cancer is of key importance in reducing local recurrence rates. Historically, 5-year local recurrence rates of 20% were common, which led to an interest in offering neoadjuvant RT to reduce the risk of local recurrence.

Specialist colorectal surgeons have been trained in the technique of total mesorectal excision. This technique involves removal of the entire rectum and associated mesorectal fat and reduces the risk of local recurrence at 5 years from 20% to 6%. It has also been shown that the single most important factor for predicting disease recurrence is the circumferential resection margin. The circumferential resection margin is said to be clear if there is no evidence of tumour from either the primary site, or in an associated lymph node that extends to within 1 mm of the inked resection margin around the circumference of the excision specimen. Patients at high risk of local recurrence are typically offered long-course postoperative RT, typically a dose of 45 Gy in 25 fractions over 5 weeks.

Because TME surgery is now the gold standard for surgical excision and recurrence rates have fallen to 5% to 6%, the role of preoperative RT has been brought into question. A recent study from the Netherlands reported after a median follow-up of just over 2 years that the local recurrence rate was 2.4% for patients who received preoperative RT before TME surgery, compared with an 8.2% recurrence rate in patients receiving no preoperative RT. The MRC CR07 study was a large prospective study in which patients with operable rectal cancers were randomised to receive either short-course preoperative RT or primary surgery followed by long-course postoperative RT if the circumferential resection margin was positive. Local recurrence after short-course RT (SCRT) was 4.4% at 3 years compared with 10.6% (P <.0001) for postoperative CRT.

Advances in pelvic imaging, specifically EUS and MRI of the pelvis, can provide excellent soft-tissue definition in perirectal tissues and visualise tumour penetration through the mesorectal fascia. Such patients may then be correctly selected for long-course preoperative RT, to downstage the tumour before surgery.

Patients who are offered long-course RT receive concomitant chemotherapy with either infusional 5-FU at 200 mg/m^2/day continuous schedule OR oral capecitabine, 825 mg/m^2 BD for the duration of RT.

Total Neoadjuvant Therapy

For patients with more locally advanced tumours, neoadjuvant chemotherapy in addition to either CRT or short-course RT can be considered a total neoadjuvant therapy (TNT) approach.

In the RAPIDO trial,[91] patients with high-risk locally advanced rectal cancer were assigned to receive either SCRT followed by chemotherapy or standard-of-care long-course chemoradiotherapy (LCCRT). After 5 years of follow-up, the probability of distant metastatic disease was lower in the experimental arm (23% versus 30.4%). However, rates of locoregional recurrence were higher in the experimental arm (10% versus 6%).

The PRODIGE 23 trial[92] randomised patients to either neoadjuvant FOLFIRINOX followed by LCCRT or just neoadjuvant LCCRT. This group receiving neoadjuvant chemotherapy had higher 3-year disease-free survival rates (76% versus 69%).

Organ Preservation

There is interest in nonsurgical treatment options for rectal cancers as multimodality treatment including surgery can cause significant morbidity, and patients with distal rectal cancers are left with a permanent stoma.

A complete clinical response can be achieved in 10% to 40% of patients after neoadjuvant LCCRT/SCRT. Good outcomes have been reported with a watch and wait policy, although these patients are typically subject to more intensive surveillance protocols to ensure that if local recurrence occurs, surgical salvage is timely. The GRECAR2 study[93] demonstrated no evidence of a difference in oncological outcomes for patients treated with local excision rather than TME after a good response to CRT (residual tumour <2 cm).

The phase II STAR-TREC trial achieved organ preservation in 60% at 12 months. The ongoing STAR-TREC phase III trial is evaluating the optimum therapeutic strategy for achieving organ preservation in early-stage rectal cancers.[94]

In early rectal cancer, the OPERA trial assessed the use of a contact x-ray brachytherapy boost versus an external beam boost in combination with CRT. The group receiving the brachytherapy boost had significantly improved the 3-year organ preservation rate (81% versus 59%).

For more advanced tumours, the OPRA trial provides prospective evidence to suggest that organ preservation is achievable in up to half of patients receiving total neoadjuvant therapy, without a negative impact on survival compared with historical controls.[95]

Early-phase trials have shown promising results for the use of PD-1 blockade for the small proportion of locally advanced rectal cancers that are MMR deficient (5%–10%). After 6 months of follow-up, 100% of the 12 patients had achieved CCR with no evidence of progression or recurrence reported.[96]

Radiotherapy Boost. Delivering a higher dose of radiation to areas of macroscopic disease correlates with an improved response rate and so can be considered for disease lying outside the resection margin or for an organ preservation approach (including patients too frail for surgery but fit for CRT).

Palliative Radiotherapy

Palliative RT can be very helpful in patients with advanced rectal tumours with symptoms of bleeding or intractable pelvic pain. A short course of treatment (20–30 Gy in 5–10 fractions) is often used for such patients.

Radiotherapy Technique

Patient setup: The patient is immobilised supine with feet and popliteal fossa support (e.g. Combifix). Ideally, the bladder should be comfortably full at the time of simulation (>150 mL) and the same instructions for bladder filling should be used during treatment as used for simulation. An anal marker can be placed at the anal verge. IV contrast for visualisation of the pelvic vessels is recommended. Oral contrast does aid delineation of the small bowel and can be used (e.g. gastrografin 10–20 mL in 1L of water taken 40–60 minutes before planning CT). CT slices should not be more than 3 mm thick, and the true pelvis should be imaged (approximately lumbar vertebrae 5 to at least 4 cm below the anal verge/or anal marker).

The diagnostic MRI should be fused with the planning CT to aid in defining the extent of the primary tumour and any nodal spread.

Scan from L5 to 4 cm below the anal marker; recommended slice thickness is 2.5 mm or greater.

Organs at Risk

The following OARs must be delineated (the RTOG normal pelvic atlas for male and female provides pictorial guidance and these atlases are available to download from https://www.nrgoncology.org/About-Us/Center-for-Innovation-in-Radiation-Oncology after completing an access form): small bowel, bladder and right and left femoral heads. Small bowel contouring should include all individual small bowel loops to at least 20 mm above the superior extent of the PTV. It may be helpful to initially delineate the large bowel ± endometrium to exclude these from subsequent delineation of the small bowel.

Technique and Dose

The benefit of IMRT in locally advanced rectal cancer is because of its highly conformal dose distribution to the PTV, allowing dose reduction to the small bowel and other OARs, which is of particular importance when dose escalation is considered. In a metaanalysis of six studies including a total of 859 patients, of which 98.7% received neoadjuvant CRT, IMRT reduced grade 2 or higher acute overall GI toxicity, diarrhoea and proctitis with ORs of 0.38, 0.32 and 0.60, respectively (all P <.05), compared with three-dimensional CRT. IMRT also reduced acute grade 3 (or higher) proctitis compared with three-dimensional CRT (OR, 0.24; P = .03). The use of IMRT or VMAT is now considered the standard of care for rectal RT.

Dose. Short-course preoperative RT: 25 Gy in 5 fractions over 1 week, 45 Gy in 25 × 1.8-Gy fractions, 5 times per week with concurrent fluoropyrimidines.

Long-course postoperative RT: 45 Gy in 25 fractions over 5 weeks with concurrent IV infusional 5-FU or oral capecitabine chemotherapy.

An optional boost to the GTV may be used for disease lying outside the resection margin or for an organ preservation approach. The boost may be delivered consecutively as 5.4 Gy in 3 fractions or as a simultaneous integrated boost (50 Gy in 25 fractions).

Palliative RT: 20 to 30 Gy in 5 to 10 fractions.

Daily volumetric imaging is recommended if IMRT is used.

Treatment Toxicity. During treatment, patients may experience cystitis, proctitis and lethargy. The dose-limiting structure for long-term toxicity is the small bowel, with the associated risk of fibrosis, stricturing and obstruction. The risk of small bowel toxicity is directly related to the volume of irradiated small bowel. With careful planning, the risk of significant small bowel toxicity can be reduced to around 5%. Other long-term toxicities that need to be considered are impotence in male patients, loss of fertility and insufficiency fractures.

Follow-up

Patients with rectal cancer require regular endoscopic follow-up to look for local recurrence and the development of new tumours. In most protocols, regular pelvic MRI combined with CT chest, abdomen and pelvis are undertaken at intervals of 3 to 6 months.

ANAL CANCER

Epidemiology and Aetiology

Anal cancer constitutes 1% of all malignancies of the bowel, with 1400 new cases being diagnosed each year in the United Kingdom. Anal cancer is associated with human papilloma virus (HPV) infection, a history of receptive anal intercourse or sexually transmitted disease. Immunosuppression after organ transplantation of HIV, haematologic malignancies and previous cervix malignancies are also associated with increased risk of developing the cancer; smoking also plays a role. The association with HPV type 16 and 18 (HPV-16, HPV-18) infections is especially strong.

High-grade anal intraepithelial neoplasia (AIN) is associated with HPV infections and is thought to be a precursor for invasive carcinomas; the treatment of high-grade AIN might prevent the development of anal cancer. HPV immunisation is now commonplace, and the future incidence of anal cancer is expected to decrease.

Anatomy

The anus is defined as extending from the rectum to the skin of the perianal region. The superior margin is the palpable upper border of the anal sphincter and puborectalis muscle. Inferiorly, it extends to skin within a 5-cm radius of the anal verge.

There is a transition in the histological type of epithelium lining the anus. Perianal skin is squamous epithelium, which turns to a transitional-type epithelium at the dentate line, and then into the glandular mucosal lining of the rectum.

The anus has a dense lymphatic supply via three main routes. The upper canal drains to perirectal and superior hemorrhoidal nodes. The area round the dentate line drains to hypogastric and obturator nodes. The anal verge and perianal skin drains to superficial inguinal nodes.

Histopathology

Approximately 80% of anal tumours are SCCs (Fig. 25.3). The recognised subtypes are keratinising large cell, nonkeratinising (transitional cell) and basaloid. ACs occur in 10% of cases and tend to arise from the glandular mucosa of the upper anal canal. Other tumour types include lymphomas, melanomas, small cell carcinomas and sarcomas.

Clinical Features

The symptoms often are nonspecific and common symptoms include anal pain and bleeding, pruritus, a mass in the anal region or discharge. Occasionally, tumours may affect the sphincter mechanism and cause incontinence. On examination, patients may present with ulcerated or exophytic lesions, and inguinal lymphadenopathy may be present. Associated features, such as anal warts or leucoplakia, may be present. Inguinal lymph node metastases are noted in 15% of patients, and surgical series show that pelvic nodal spread is present in about 30% of patients at presentation. Systemic metastatic spread is observed in less than 5% of patients at the time of initial diagnosis. Increasing tumour size and depth of penetration into the anal wall increases the risk of nodal metastases.

Diagnostic Workup and Staging

Patients are staged using the UICC/AJCC staging scheme. A full history digital rectal and physical examination including risk factor assessment is followed by an examination under anaesthetic to assess the extent of the tumour and to obtain a biopsy for histological confirmation of the diagnosis. One-third of patients present with enlarged inguinal lymph nodes. These should always be biopsied, as 50% of enlarged lymph nodes are reactive, usually caused by infection associated with the primary tumour. MRI of the pelvis provides improved soft-tissue definition of the primary tumour and pelvic lymph nodes. A CT scan of the chest, abdomen and pelvis completes the staging. PET scanning has been reported to be useful in the evaluation of pelvic lymph nodes, even in patients who have normal lymph nodes on CT imaging. A metaanalysis of 17 clinical studies calculated the pooled specificity and sensitivity for detection of lymph node involvement by PET/CT at 93% and 76%, respectively. The use of PET/CT can either downstage or upstage the patients and has produced treatment plan modifications between 12% and 59% of patients by changes in either radiation dose or fields. However, the PET/CT is not considered a replacement for pelvic MRI and CT. Gynaecologic examination including colposcopy is suggested for female patients because of the association of the anal cancer and HPV. PD-L1 testing may be undertaken in patients with advanced disease where immunotherapy is being considered.[97] HIV testing on patients should be undertaken if the status is unknown, as patients with undiagnosed HIV and low CD4 counts tend to tolerate chemoradiation poorly.

Treatment

Definitive Chemoradiation

Three trials performed between 1987 and 1994 determined concurrent mitomycin C (MMC), 5-FU and RT (MF-CRT) as the standard of care. ACT1 was performed in the United Kingdom and randomised 585 patients to RT alone or MF-CRT, and significantly reduced LRF from 59% to 36%. This benefit was maintained after a median follow-up of 13 years, with a significant reduction in the risk of relapse or death.

A parallel European Organisation for Research and Treatment of Cancer (EORTC) trial of 110 patients with locally advanced disease also showed a significant reduction in the risk of LRF. An RTOG trial (n = 310) demonstrated a significant reduction in LRF colostomy-free survival with MF-CRT compared with 5-FU and RT (F-CRT). All trials used crude RT schedules and a significant treatment gap between the first phase of RT and a subsequent boost.

Three further phase III trials were performed between 1998 and 2008. The RTOG 9811 trial[98,99] of 641 patients found that neoadjuvant and concomitant cisplatin 5-FU resulted in inferior LRF, colostomy-free survival (CFS) and OS when compared with MF-CRT. In the United Kingdom, the largest trial, ACT2,[100] enrolled 940 patients and used a two-phase RT schedule. There was no evidence of a difference in the complete response rate for concurrent cisplatin compared with mitomycin C and no improvement in PFS with the addition of two cycles of maintenance 5-FU cisplatin. Subset analysis did not show any benefit in subsets based on established prognostic factors. However, the cancer outcomes were improved compared with ACT1, and the continuous RT schedule may have contributed to this finding. The ACCORD 03 trial enrolled 307 patients and showed no benefit from the addition of neoadjuvant cisplatin 5-FU chemotherapy. It also compared two doses of boost (15 versus 20–25 Gy) after whole pelvic irradiation. A nonsignificant 5% improvement in LC was seen, although one-third of patients had early-stage disease. These three trials did not demonstrate any benefit from the use of cisplatin concurrently, neoadjuvantly or as adjuvant therapy.

Future data will come from the three embedded trials within the UK PLATO umbrella trial. ACT 3 is a nonrandomised study for patients with resected T1 anal margin tumours. Those with margin >1 mm are observed, while those with margin <1 mm receive CRT 41.4 Gy in 23 fractions. Randomised phase II ACT 4 for patients with T1-2 (<4 cm) N0 tumours randomised 1:2 to receive standard 50.4 Gy in 28 fractions versus deescalated 41.4 Gy in 23 fractions; here, early data have suggested less toxicity with dose escalation (Gilbert et al., 2023). ACT 5 is a randomised phase III trial comparing two dose-escalation arms against the standard 53.2 Gy in 28 fractions for patients with T3/4 or N+ cancers.

Radiotherapy Treatment Principles (Fig. 25.4)

The RT techniques used in previous phase III trials were relatively simple and resulted in substantial irradiation of the surrounding normal tissues (Fig. 25.4). ACT2 used a shrinking field technique, treating the whole pelvis with 30.6 Gy, followed by a reduced treatment volume to all sites of macroscopic disease, giving 19.8 Gy using a generous margin and without a planned gap in treatment. Significant improvement in RT treatment can be achieved with the use of IMRT. This also allows the use of altered doses to the GTV and sparing of normal tissues. The use of IMRT in future trials is supported by the RTOG 0529 single arm phase II trial led by Kachnic et al.[101] In the United Kingdom, we have developed guidance for the multicentre introduction of IMRT,[102] and most UK centres have now implemented IMRT in routine clinical practice. Although long-term effects are not yet fully characterised, IMRT has been increasingly adopted by the radiation oncology community and should no longer be considered investigational for the treatment of anal cancer.

Target Volume: External Beam Radiotherapy. The CTV includes the primary tumour, first station nodes (pararectal, hypogastric and obturator nodes) and presacral and internal iliac nodes. In patients with positive inguinal nodes, the inguinal nodal areas must also be included in the treatment field.

Patient Simulation and Immobilisation. Patients are positioned supine with immobilisation for popliteal fossa or feet and a comfortably full bladder, and the use of IV contrast to aid delineation of pelvic vessels is indicated.

Before pretreatment scan, the clinician will assess the diagnostic imaging and ascertain whether the primary tumour is adequately bolused by the surrounding buttocks, that is, 5 mm of tissue surrounding the main tumour, and consideration of tailored wax or sheet bolus should be given. The distal point of macroscopic disease or anal verge should be delineated with a radioopaque marker before imaging, whichever is more inferior. All patients must be scanned with a comfortably full bladder using a local bladder-filling protocol.

Target Definition. The primary tumour should be visualised with the aid of the diagnostic MRI, CT and PET imaging. A 10-to-15-mm margin to the gross tumour should be considered depending on the stage.

The elective nodes (Table 25.1) should include inguinal, mesorectum, internal and external iliacs and presacral space. If the tumour stage is early and there are no mesorectal nodes, only the lower 50 mm of the mesorectum should be irradiated.

For OARs, see guidance for rectal cancer; in addition, consider defining the external genitalia. For male genitalia, it should include the penis and scrotum out laterally to the inguinal creases. In females, it should include the clitoris, labia majora and minora, out to the inguinal creases. The superior border in both genders should lie midway through the symphysis pubis.

Online volumetric imaging should be performed on days 1 to 5 and weekly thereafter, at a minimum.

The optimal dose and schedule for anal cancer is still under evaluation. The dose recommended for the elective nodes is 40 Gy in 28 fractions over 5.5 weeks; however, a minimum dose of 30.6 Gy in 1.8-Gy per fraction to 36 Gy for negative nodes is acceptable, with tumour and involved nodes receiving doses between 50.4 and 53.2 Gy in 28 fractions over 5.5 weeks.

Systemic chemotherapy should be prescribed concurrently in all patients who are considered fit for standard treatment.

Accepted regimens are:

- Mitomycin, 12 mg/m^2 on day 1 (+/– 42) with 5-FU 1000 mg/m^2 on days 1 to 4 and 29 to 32
- Mitomycin, 12 mg/m^2 on day 1 (+/– 42) with capecitabine 825 mg/m^2 bd on days of RT

Dose reductions in chemotherapy should be considered if patients are elderly or the renal function is impaired.

Treatment-Related Toxicity

In general, IMRT treatments are well tolerated, with patients rarely needing admission for symptom control or skin toxicity. Female patients should be considered for vaginal dilators and counselled about vaginal stenosis and infertility risk.

Follow-up

Assessing the response to primary CRT: A clinical assessment of response by physical examination is typically performed from 6 to 8 weeks following the completion of therapy. There is considerable controversy regarding the optimal time to assess response posttreatment. Initial imaging could be performed around 3 months after treatment, for example, with MRI for local response and CT or PET for distant disease assessment. SCCs regress slowly and continue to decrease in size for up to 26 weeks following therapy. For patients with a clinical complete response, reevaluation every 3 to 6 months with DRE, anoscopy and inguinal node palpation is recommended for 5 years. Based upon the results from the ACT II trial, patients with persistent disease can be watched for up to 6 months following completion of treatment as long as there is no progressive disease during this period of follow-up.

Role of Surgery

Surgical therapy is reserved for patients with recurrent or persistent disease after CRT. Although prognosis is poor overall, an APR offers the potential for long-term survival.

Recurrent disease: Post-CRT, local recurrences can be successfully salvaged with surgery, but locally recurrent anal SCC can be a difficult clinical problem that is associated with profound morbidity and long-term disease control in about 25% to 40% of cases.

Palliative Treatment

Metastatic disease after locoregional treatment may develop in 10% to 20% of patients. The most common site for spread is the liver; however, lung, bone, lymph nodes and skin metastases have been reported. The first-line treatment for advanced anal SCC is carboplatin and paclitaxel, as established by the randomised phase II InterAACT.[103] Median overall survival was 12.3 months for cisplatin/5-FU versus 20 months for

TABLE 25.1 Anatomical Boundaries for Pelvic Lymph Nodes

	Superior	Inferior	Lateral	Medial	Anterior	Posterior
Internal iliac nodes	20 mm above the inferior aspect of sacroiliac joint or 15 mm above the most anterior site of gross tumour, whichever is most superior	The point of levator ani insertion into the obturator fascia and obturator internus	In the upper pelvis, the iliopsoas muscle In the lower pelvis, the obturator internus muscle	In the upper pelvis, 7 mm medial to internal iliac vessels In the lower pelvis, the mesorectum and presacral space	In the upper pelvis, 7 mm anterior to the internal iliac vessels In the lower pelvis, the obturator internus muscle or bone	The bony pelvis
External iliac nodes	See superior border of internal iliac	The inguinal lymph nodes	The iliopsoas muscle	In the upper pelvis, 7 mm medial to the external iliac vessels In the lower pelvis, 10 mm inside the bladder or small bowel	7 mm anterior to the external iliac vessels encompassing all visible benign lymph nodes	The internal iliac lymph node group
Inguinal nodes	The external iliac nodal group	At the inferior slice demonstrating the lesser trochanter	The medial edge of sartorius or iliopsoas	To include all visible lymph nodes or lymphoceles. The spermatic cord in males. The medial third to half of the pectineus or adductor longus muscle in females.	Approximately 5 mm in from the skin surface	The pectineus, adductor longus and iliopsoas
Mesorectal nodes	The level of the rectosigmoid junction, best identified where the superior rectal artery turns anteriorly	The anorectal junction approximately where the levator ani inserts into the sphincter complex	The medial edges of the mesorectal fascia and levator ani		10 mm anterior to the mesorectum into the anterior organs (penile bulb/prostate and seminal vesicles/bladder in males; bladder/vagina/cervix and uterus in females)	The sacrum or coccyx
Presacral nodes	See superior border of internal iliac	The edge of the coccyx	Sacroiliac joints		10 mm anterior to the anterior sacral border encompassing any lymph nodes or presacral vessels	The sacrum
Obturator nodes	Superiorly 3–5 mm above the obturator canal where the obturator artery is sometimes visible	The obturator canal where the obturator artery has exited the pelvis	The obturator internus muscle	Medial: 10 mm into the bladder	The anterior extent of the obturator internus muscle	The internal iliac lymph node group

carboplatin plus paclitaxel (HR 2.0, $P = 0.014$). Second-line treatment with platinum/fluoropyrimidine can be considered. Another recent option is immunotherapy, as it has shown to be effective for a subset of patients in early-phase trials. An objective response with pembrolizumab was seen in 15% of PD-L1-positive patients in KEYNOTE-158. Palliative RT can be offered for patients with symptomatic nodal, bone or skin metastases.

Prognosis

Male gender and positive lymph nodes are independent prognostic factors for higher LRF, anal cancer death and lower survival in both United Kingdom and United States multivariate analysis. P16 positivity and/or HPV negativity are independent prognostic factors for OS.

Gastrointestinal Stromal Tumours

GISTS are the most common mesenchymal tumours of the GI tract. However, they are rare tumours and account for less than 3% of all GI tumours and 5% of all soft-tissue sarcomas. GISTS are defined as c-KIT–positive mesenchymal tumours arising from anywhere in the GI tract or abdomen. The median age at presentation is around 60 years. GISTS are uncommon before the age of 40 years and extremely rare in children. They occur equally in both males and females. The most common site is the stomach (60%–70%), followed by the small bowel (20%–30%). GISTS are thought to arise from the precursors of the interstitial cells of Cajal (ICC), the pacemaker cells that initiate and control peristalsis. Mutations within the KIT and PDGFRA genes are common and have prognostic and predictive value.

GISTS can present as incidental masses in the abdomen. The common presenting complaints include GI bleeding (50%), abdominal pain (20%–50%) and feeling of a mass. The most frequent sites of metastases are the liver (65%) and omentum (often without ascites) (21%). Risk stratification for relapse is assessed using tumour site, size and mitotic index.

In view of the rarity of GISTS, they should be managed by an experienced multidisciplinary team within a specialist cancer centre. Surgery remains the primary treatment for operable tumours. The response rates to chemotherapy are very low. The systemic treatment has been revolutionised by the discovery of the KIT tyrosine kinase inhibitor imatinib, which is effective in 85% of patients with metastatic GISTS. Sunitnib, another multitargeted tyrosine kinase inhibitor, is licenced for second-line use in patients who have progressed or are intolerant to imatinib. Regorafenib is licenced in third line. A small proportion are driven by platelet-derived growth factor receptor instead (or in addition) to KIT. Avapritinib is licenced in certain countries for the treatment of PDGFRA mutated patients, based on strong data from early-phase trials. In the adjuvant setting, imatinib has been shown to improve both the progression-free survival and OS in resected high-risk GISTS.

REFERENCES

1. Secrier ML, De Silva N, Eldridge MD, et al. Mutational signatures in esophageal adenocarcinoma define etiologically distinct subgroups with therapeutic relevance on behalf of the Oesophageal Cancer Clinical and Molecular Stratification (OCCAMS) Consortium 13 Europe PMC Funders Group. *Nat Genet.* 2016;48(10):1131–1141.
2. Jankowski JAZ, de Caestecker J, Love SB, et al. Esomeprazole and aspirin in Barrett's oesophagus (AspECT): a randomised factorial trial [published correction appears in *Lancet.* 2018 Dec 15;392(10164):2552. doi: 10.1016/S0140-6736(18)32970-2.]. *Lancet.* 2018;392(10145):400–408. doi: 10.1016/S0140-6736(18)31388-6.
3. Siewert JR, Stein HJ. Classification of adenocarcinoma of the oesophagogastric junction. *Br J Surg.* 1998 Nov;85(11):1457–1459. doi:10.1046/j.1365-2168.1998.00940.x PMID: 9823902.
4. Pimentel-Nunes P, Libânio D, Bastiaansen BAJ, et al. Endoscopic submucosal dissection for superficial gastrointestinal lesions: European Society of Gastrointestinal Endoscopy (ESGE) guideline—update 2022. *Endoscopy.* 2022;54(6):591–622.
5. Alderson D, Cunningham D, Nankivell M, et al. Neoadjuvant cisplatin and fluorouracil versus epirubicin, cisplatin, and capecitabine followed by resection in patients with oesophageal adenocarcinoma (UK MRC OE05): an open-label, randomised phase 3 trial. *Lancet Oncol.* 2017;18(9):1249–1260.
6. van Hagen P, Hulshof MCCM, van Lanschot JJB, et al. Preoperative chemoradiotherapy for esophageal or junctional cancer. *N Engl J Med.* 2012;366(22):2074–2084.
7. Reynolds JV, Preston SR, O'Neill B, et al. Trimodality therapy versus perioperative chemotherapy in the management of locally advanced adenocarcinoma of the oesophagus and oesophagogastric junction (Neo-AEGIS): an open-label, randomised, phase 3 trial. *Lancet Gastroenterol Hepatol.* 2023;8(11):1015–1027.
8. Kelly RJ, Ajani JA, Kuzdzal J, et al. Adjuvant nivolumab in resected esophageal or gastroesophageal junction cancer [published correction appears in *N Engl J Med.* 2023;388(7):672. https://doi.org/10.1056/NEJMx220014]. *N Engl J Med.* 2021;384(13):1191–1203.
9. Crehange G, M'vondo C, Bertaut A, et al. Exclusive Chemoradiotherapy With or Without Radiation Dose Escalation in Esophageal Cancer: Multicenter Phase 2/3 Randomized Trial CONCORDE (PRODIGE-26. *Int J Radiat Oncol Biol Phys.* 2021;111(3):S5. doi:10.1016/j.ijrobp.2021.07.045.
10. Conroy T, Galais MP, Raoul JL, et al. Definitive chemoradiotherapy with FOLFOX versus fluorouracil and cisplatin in patients with oesophageal cancer (PRODIGE5/ACCORD17): final results of a randomised, phase 2/3 trial. *Lancet Oncol.* 2014;15(3):305–314.
11. Hulshof MCCM, Geijsen ED, Rozema T, et al. Randomized study on dose escalation in definitive chemoradiation for patients with locally advanced esophageal cancer (ARTDECO Study). *J Clin Oncol.* 2021;39(25):2816–2824.
12. Kato K, Cho BC, Takahashi M, et al. Nivolumab versus chemotherapy in patients with advanced oesophageal squamous cell carcinoma refractory or intolerant to previous chemotherapy (ATTRACTION-3): a multicentre, randomised, open-label, phase 3 trial. *Lancet Oncol.* 2019;20(11):1506–1517.
13. Doki Y, Ajani JA, Kato K, et al. Nivolumab combination therapy in advanced esophageal squamous-cell carcinoma. *N Engl J Med.* 2022;386(5):449–462.
14. Kato K, Shah MA, Enzinger P, et al. Keynote-590: phase III study of first-line chemotherapy with or without pembrolizumab for advanced esophageal cancer. *Future Oncol.* 2019;15(10):1057–1066.
15. Lordick F, Carneiro F, Cascinu S, et al. Gastric cancer: ESMO clinical practice guideline for diagnosis, treatment and follow-up. *Ann Oncol.* 2022;33(10):1005–1020.
16. Cunningham D, Allum WH, Stenning SP, et al. Perioperative chemotherapy versus surgery alone for resectable gastroesophageal cancer. *N Engl J Med.* 2006;355(1):11–20.
17. Al-Batran SE, Homann N, Pauligk C, et al. Perioperative chemotherapy with fluorouracil plus leucovorin, oxaliplatin, and docetaxel versus fluorouracil or capecitabine plus cisplatin and epirubicin for locally advanced, resectable gastric or gastro-oesophageal junction adenocarcinoma (FLOT4): A randomised, phase 2/3 trial. *Lancet.* 2019;393(10184):1948–1957.
18. Shitara K, Rha SY, Wyrwicz LS, et al. Neoadjuvant and adjuvant pembrolizumab plus chemotherapy in locally advanced gastric or gastro-oesophageal cancer (KEYNOTE-585): an interim analysis of the multicentre, double-blind, randomised phase 3 study. *Lancet Oncol.* 2024;25(2):212–224.
19. Janjigian YY, Al-Batran S-E, Wainberg ZA, et al. LBA73 pathological complete response (pCR) to durvalumab plus 5-fluorouracil, leucovorin, Oxaliplatin and Docetaxel (FLOT) in resectable gastric and gastroesophageal junction cancer (GC/GEJC): interim results of the global, phase III Matterhorn study. *Ann Oncol.* 2023;34(suppl2):S1315–S1316.
20. Park SH, Lim DH, Sohn TS, et al. A randomized phase III trial comparing adjuvant single-agent S1, S-1 with oxaliplatin, and postoperative chemoradiation with S-1 and oxaliplatin in patients with node-positive gastric cancer after D2 resection: the artist 2 trial. *Ann Oncol.* 2021;32(3):368–374.
21. Bang Y-J, Van Cutsem E, Feyereislova A, et al. Trastuzumab in combination with chemotherapy versus chemotherapy alone for treatment of HER2-positive advanced gastric or gastro-oesophageal junction cancer (ToGA): a phase 3, open-label, randomised controlled trial. *Lancet.* 2010;376(9742):687–697.
22. Janjigian YY, Kawazoe A, Bai Y, et al. Pembrolizumab plus trastuzumab and chemotherapy for HER2-positive gastric or gastro-oesophageal junction adenocarcinoma: Interim analyses from the phase 3 KEYNOTE-811 randomised placebo-controlled trial. *Lancet.* 2023;402(10418):2197–2208.
23. Cunningham D, Starling N, Rao S, et al. Capecitabine and oxaliplatin for advanced esophagogastric cancer. *N Engl J Med.* 2008;358(1):36–46.
24. Bailey P, Chang DK, Nones K, et al. Genomic analyses identify molecular subtypes of pancreatic cancer. *Nature.* 2016;531(7592):47–52.

25. Ghaneh P, Hanson R, Titman A, et al. PET-PANC: multicentre prospective diagnostic accuracy and health economic analysis study of the impact of combined modality 18fluorine-2-fluoro-2-deoxy-d- glucose positron emission tomography with computed tomography scanning in the diagnosis and management of pancreatic cancer. *Health Technol Assess.* 2018;22(7):1–114.
26. Neoptolemos JP, Palmer DH, Ghaneh P, et al. Comparison of adjuvant gemcitabine and capecitabine with gemcitabine monotherapy in patients with resected pancreatic cancer (ESPAC-4): a multicentre, open-label, randomised, phase 3 trial. *Lancet.* 2017; 389(10073):1011–1024.
27. Zhan HX, Xu JW, Wu D, et al. Neoadjuvant therapy in pancreatic cancer: a systematic review and meta-analysis of prospective studies. *Cancer Med.* 2017;6(6):1201–1219.
28. Katz MHG, Shi Q, Meyers J, et al. Efficacy of preoperative mFOLFIRINOX vs mFOLFIRINOX plus hypofractionated radiotherapy for borderline resectable adenocarcinoma of the pancreas: the A021501 phase 2 randomized clinical trial. *JAMA Oncol.* 2022;8(9):1263–1270.
29. Hammel P, Huguet F, Van Laethem JL, et al. Effect of chemoradiotherapy vs chemotherapy on survival in patients with locally advanced pancreatic cancer controlled after 4 months of gemcitabine with or without erlotinib: the LAP07 randomized clinical trial. *JAMA.* 2016;315(17):1844–1853.
30. Balaban EP, Mangu PB, Khorana AA, et al. Locally advanced, unresectable pancreatic cancer: American Society of Clinical Oncology clinical practice guideline. *J Clin Oncol.* 2016;34(22): 2654–2668.
31. Mukherjee S, Hurt CN, Bridgewater J, et al. Gemcitabine-based or capecitabine-based chemoradiotherapy for locally advanced pancreatic cancer (SCALOP): a multicentre, randomised, phase 2 trial. *Lancet Oncol.* 2013;14(4):317–326.
32. Mukherjee S, Virdee P, Shaw R, et al. Scalop-2: a multi-centre randomised trial of induction chemotherapy followed by Capecitabine +/−nelfinavir with high or standard dose radiotherapy for locally advanced pancreatic cancer (LAPC): results of stage 1—the non-randomised dose-finding component. *Ann Oncol.* 2018;29:viii243.
33. Herman JM, Chang DT, Goodman KA, et al. Phase 2 multi-institutional trial evaluating gemcitabine and stereotactic body radiotherapy for patients with locally advanced unresectable pancreatic adenocarcinoma. *Cancer.* 2015;121(7):1128–1137.
34. Petrelli F, Comito T, Ghidini A, Torri V, Scorsetti M, Barni S. Stereotactic body radiation therapy for locally advanced pancreatic cancer: a systematic review and pooled analysis of 19 trials. *Int J Radiat Oncol Biol Phys.* 2017;97(2):313–322.
35. Tchelebi LT, Lehrer EJ, Trifiletti DM, et al. Conventionally fractionated radiation therapy versus stereotactic body radiation therapy for locally advanced pancreatic cancer (CRiSP): an international systematic review and meta-analysis. *Cancer.* 2020;126(10):2120–2131.
36. Conroy T, Ychou M, Bouché O, et al. FOLFIRINOX versus gemcitabine for metastatic pancreatic cancer. *N Engl J Med.* 2011;364(19):1817–1825.
37. Von Hoff DD, Ervin T, Arena FP, et al. Increased survival in pancreatic cancer with nab-paclitaxel plus gemcitabine. *N Engl J Med.* 2013;369(18):1691–1703.
38. Wainberg ZA, Melisi D, Macarulla T, et al. NALIRIFOX versus nab-paclitaxel and gemcitabine in treatment-naive patients with metastatic pancreatic ductal adenocarcinoma (NAPOLI 3): a randomised, open-label, phase 3 trial. *Lancet.* 2023;402(10409):1272–1281.
39. Wang-Gillam A, Hubner RA, Siveke JT, et al. NAPOLI-1 phase 3 study of liposomal irinotecan in metastatic pancreatic cancer: final overall survival analysis and characteristics of long-term survivors. *Eur J Cancer.* 2019;108:78–87.
40. Kew MC. Hepatocellular carcinoma in developing countries: prevention, diagnosis and treatment. *World J Hepatol.* 2012; 4(3):99–104. https://doi.org/10.4254/wjh.v4.i3.99.
41. Singal AG, Kanwal F, Llovet JM. Global trends in hepatocellular carcinoma epidemiology: implications for screening, prevention and therapy. *Nat Rev Clin Oncol.* 2023;20(12):864–884.
42. Pineda JA, Aguilar-Guisado M, Rivero A, et al. Infecciosas Grupo para el Estudio de las Hepatitis Viricas de la Sociedad Andaluza de Enfermedades. Natural history of compensated hepatitis C virus-related cirrhosis in HIV-infected patients. *Clin Infect Dis.* 2009;49:1274–1282.
43. Bruix J, Sherman M, Llovet M, et al. Clinical management of hepatocellular carcinoma. Conclusions of the Barcelona-2000 EASL conference. European Association for the Study of the Liver. *J Hepatol.* 2001;35:421–430.
44. Child CG, Turcotte JG. Surgery and portal hypertension. *Major Probl Clin Surg.* 1964;1:1–85.
45. Lingiah VA, Niazi M, Olivo R, Paterno F, Guarrera JV, Pyrsopoulos NT. Liver transplantation beyond Milan criteria. *J Clin Transl Hepatol.* 2020;8(1):69–75.
46. Méndez Romero A, van der Holt B, Willemssen FEJA, et al. Transarterial chemoembolization with drug-eluting beads versus stereotactic body radiation therapy for hepatocellular carcinoma: outcomes from a multicenter, randomized, phase 2 trial (The TRENDY Trial). *Int J Radiat Oncol Biol Phys.* 2023;117(1): 45–52.
47. Dou Z, Lu F, Ren L, Song X, Li B, Li X. Efficacy and safety of microwave ablation and radiofrequency ablation in the treatment of hepatocellular carcinoma: a systematic review and meta-analysis. *Medicine (Baltimore).* 2022;101(30):e29321.
48. Finn RS, Qin S, Ikeda M, et al. Atezolizumab plus bevacizumab in unresectable hepatocellular carcinoma. *N Engl J Med.* 2020; 382(20):1894–1905.
49. Abou-Alfa GK, Lau G, Kudo M, et al. Tremelimumab plus durvalumab in unresectable hepatocellular carcinoma. *NEJM Evid.* 2022;1(8):EVIDoa2100070.
50. Marciscano AE, Haimovitz-Friedman A, Lee P, et al. Immunomodulatory effects of stereotactic body radiation therapy: preclinical insights and clinical opportunities. *Int J Radiat Oncol Biol Phys.* 2021;110(1):35–52.
51. Dawson LA, Winter KA, Knox JJ, et al. NRG/RTOG 1112: randomized phase III study of sorafenib vs. stereotactic body radiation therapy (SBRT) followed by sorafenib in hepatocellular carcinoma (HCC). *J Clin Oncol.* 2023;41:489.
52. Hong TS, Wo JY, Yeap BY, et al. Multi-institutional phase II study of high-dose hypofractionated proton beam therapy in patients with localized, unresectable hepatocellular carcinoma and intrahepatic cholangiocarcinoma. *J Clin Oncol.* 2016;34(5): 460–468.
53. Qi WX, Fu S, Zhang Q, Guo XM. Charged particle therapy versus photon therapy for patients with hepatocellular carcinoma: a systematic review and meta-analysis. *Radiother Oncol.* 2015; 114:289–295.
54. Kim TH, Koh YH, Kim BH, et al. Proton beam radiotherapy vs. radiofrequency ablation for recurrent hepatocellular carcinoma: a randomized phase III trial. *J Hepatol.* 2021;74(3):603–612.
55. Hoegen-Saßmannshausen P, Naumann P, Hoffmeister-Wittmann P, et al. Carbon ion radiotherapy of hepatocellular carcinoma provides

excellent local control: the prospective phase I PROMETHEUS trial. *JHEP Rep.* 2024;6(6):101063.
56. Sanford NN, Pursley J, Noe B, et al. Protons versus photons for unresectable hepatocellular carcinoma: liver decompensation and overall survival. *Int J Radiat Oncol Biol Phys.* 2019;105(1):64–72.
57. Wei L, Simeth J, Aryal MP, et al. The effect of stereotactic body radiation therapy for hepatocellular cancer on regional hepatic liver function. *Int J Radiat Oncol Biol Phys.* 2023;115(3):794–802.
58. Tataru D, Khan SA, Hill R, et al. Cholangiocarcinoma across England: temporal changes in incidence, survival and routes to diagnosis by region and level of socioeconomic deprivation. *JHEP Rep.* 2023;6(3):100983.
59. Primrose JN, Fox RP, Palmer DH, et al. Capecitabine compared with observation in resected biliary tract cancer (BILCAP): a randomised, controlled, multicentre, phase 3 study. *Lancet Oncol.* 2019;20(5):663–673.
60. Valle J, Wasan H, Palmer DH, et al. Cisplatin plus gemcitabine versus gemcitabine for biliary tract cancer. *N Engl J Med.* 2010; 362:1273–1281.
61. Oh DY, Ruth He A, Qin S, et al. Durvalumab plus gemcitabine and cisplatin in advanced biliary tract cancer. *NEJM Evid.* 2022;1(8): EVIDoa2200015. https://doi.org/10.1056/EVIDoa2200015.
62. Abou-Alfa GK, Sahai V, Hollebecque A, et al. Pemigatinib for previously treated, locally advanced or metastatic cholangiocarcinoma: a multicentre, open-label, phase 2 study. *Lancet Oncol.* 2020;21(5): 671–684. https://doi.org/10.1016/S1470-2045(20)30109-1.
63. Goyal L, Meric-Bernstam F, Hollebecque A, et al. Futibatinib for *FGFR2*-rearranged intrahepatic cholangiocarcinoma. *N Engl J Med.* 2023;388(3):228–239.
64. Zhu AX, Macarulla T, Javle MM, et al. Final overall survival efficacy results of ivosidenib for patients with advanced cholangiocarcinoma with IDH1 mutation: the phase 3 randomized clinical ClarIDHy trial. *JAMA Oncol.* 2021;7(11):1669–1677.
65. Subbiah V, Lassen U, Élez E, et al. Dabrafenib plus trametinib in patients with $BRAF^{V600E}$-mutated biliary tract cancer (ROAR): a phase 2, open-label, single-arm, multicentre basket trial. *Lancet Oncol.* 2020;21(9):1234–1243.
66. Harding JJ, Fan J, Oh DY, et al. Zanidatamab for HER2-amplified, unresectable, locally advanced or metastatic biliary tract cancer (HERIZON-BTC-01): a multicentre, single-arm, phase 2b study. *Lancet Oncol.* 2023;24(7):772–782.
67. Tao R, Krishnan S, Bhosale PR, et al. Ablative radiotherapy doses lead to a substantial prolongation of survival in patients with inoperable intrahepatic cholangiocarcinoma: a retrospective dose response analysis. *J Clin Oncol.* 2016;34:219–226.
68. Hawkins MA, Valle JW, Wasan HS, et al. Addition of stereotactic body radiotherapy (SBRT) to systemic chemotherapy in locally advanced cholangiocarcinoma (CC) (ABC-07): results from a randomized phase II trial. *J Clin Oncol.* 2024;42:4006.
69. Ben-Josef E, Guthrie KA, El-Khoueiry AB, et al. SWOG S0809: a phase II intergroup trial of adjuvant capecitabine and gemcitabine followed by radiotherapy and concurrent capecitabine in extrahepatic cholangiocarcinoma and gallbladder carcinoma. *J Clin Oncol.* 2015;33:2617–2622.
70. Galiatsatos P, Foulkes WD. Familial adenomatous polyposis. *Am J Gastroenterol.* 2006;101:385–398.
71. Guinney J, Dienstmann R, Wang X, et al. The consensus molecular subtypes of colorectal cancer. *Nat Med.* 2015;21(11):1350–1356. doi:10.1038/nm.3967.
72. André T, Meyerhardt J, Iveson T, et al. Effect of duration of adjuvant chemotherapy for patients with stage III colon cancer (IDEA collaboration): final results from a prospective, pooled analysis of six randomised, phase 3 trials. *Lancet Oncol.* 2020;21(12):1620–1629. doi:10.1016/S1470-2045(20)30527-1.
73. Morton D, Seymour M, Magill L, et al. Preoperative chemotherapy for operable colon cancer: mature results of an international randomized controlled trial. *J Clin Oncol.* 2023;41(8): 1541–1552.
74. Bridgewater JA, Pugh SA, Maishman T, et al. Systemic chemotherapy with or without cetuximab in patients with resectable colorectal liver metastasis (New EPOC): long-term results of a multicentre, randomised, controlled, phase 3 trial. *Lancet Oncol.* 2020;21(3):398–411.
75. Gootjes EC, Adhin AA, Bakkerus L, et al. Primary outcome analysis of the ORCHESTRA trial: a randomized phase III trial of additional tumor debulking to first-line palliative systemic therapy for patients with multiorgan metastatic colorectal cancer. *J Clin Oncol.* 2024;42(17_suppl):LBA3502. doi:10.1200/JCO.2024.42.17_suppl.LBA3502
76. Falcone A, Ricci S, Brunetti I, et al. Phase III trial of infusional fluorouracil, leucovorin, oxaliplatin, and irinotecan (FOLFOXIRI) compared with infusional fluorouracil, leucovorin, and irinotecan (FOLFIRI) as first-line treatment for metastatic colorectal cancer: the Gruppo Oncologico Nord Ovest. *J Clin Oncol.* 2007;25(13): 1670–1676. doi:10.1200/JCO.2006.09.0928
77. Cervantes A, Adam R, Roselló S, et al. Metastatic colorectal cancer: ESMO Clinical Practice Guideline for diagnosis, treatment and follow-up. *Ann Oncol.* 2023;34(1):10–32. doi:10.1016/j.annonc.2022.10.003.
78. Van Cutsem E, Köhne CH, Láng I, et al. Cetuximab plus irinotecan, fluorouracil, and leucovorin as first-line treatment for metastatic colorectal cancer: updated analysis of overall survival according to tumor KRAS and BRAF mutation status. *J Clin Oncol.* 2011;29(15):2011–2019. doi:10.1200/JCO.2010.33.5091.
79. Douillard JY, Siena S, Cassidy J, et al. Final results from PRIME: randomized phase III study of panitumumab with FOLFOX4 for first-line treatment of metastatic colorectal cancer. *Ann Oncol.* 2014;25(7):1346–1355. doi:10.1093/annonc/mdu141.
80. Heinemann V, von Weikersthal LF, Decker T, et al. FOLFIRI plus cetuximab versus FOLFIRI plus bevacizumab as first-line treatment for patients with metastatic colorectal cancer (FIRE-3): a randomised, open-label, phase 3 trial. *Lancet Oncol.* 2014;15(10):1065–1075. doi:10.1016/S1470-2045(14)70330-4.
81. Kabbinavar F, Irl C, Zurlo A, Hurwitz H. Bevacizumab improves the overall and progression-free survival of patients with metastatic colorectal cancer treated with 5-fluorouracil-based regimens irrespective of baseline risk. *Oncology.* 2008;75(3-4):215–223. doi:10.1159/000163850.
82. Saltz LB, Clarke S, Díaz-Rubio E, et al. Bevacizumab in combination with oxaliplatin-based chemotherapy as first-line therapy in metastatic colorectal cancer: a randomized phase III study [published correction appears in J Clin Oncol. 2008 Jun;26(18):3110] [published correction appears in J Clin Oncol. 2009 Feb 1;27(4):653]. *J Clin Oncol.* 2008;26(12):2013–2019. doi:10.1200/JCO.2007.14.9930.
83. Giantonio BJ, Catalano PJ, Meropol NJ, et al. Bevacizumab in combination with oxaliplatin, fluorouracil, and leucovorin (FOLFOX4) for previously treated metastatic colorectal cancer: results from the Eastern Cooperative Oncology Group Study E3200. *J Clin Oncol.* 2007;25(12):1539–1544. doi:10.1200/JCO.2006.09.6305.
84. Van Cutsem E, Tabernero J, Lakomy R, et al. Addition of aflibercept to fluorouracil, leucovorin, and irinotecan improves survival in a phase III randomized trial in patients with metastatic colorectal cancer previously treated with an oxaliplatin-based

regimen. *J Clin Oncol.* 2012;30(28):3499–3506. doi:10.1200/JCO.2012.42.8201.

85. Tabernero J, Yoshino T, Cohn AL, et al. Ramucirumab versus placebo in combination with second-line FOLFIRI in patients with metastatic colorectal carcinoma that progressed during or after first-line therapy with bevacizumab, oxaliplatin, and a fluoropyrimidine (RAISE): a randomised, double-blind, multicentre, phase 3 study [published correction appears in Lancet Oncol. 2015 Jun;16(6):e262. doi: 10.1016/S1470-2045(15)70273-1.]. *Lancet Oncol.* 2015;16(5):499–508. doi:10.1016/S1470-2045(15)70127-0.
86. Diaz Jr LA, Shiu KK, Kim TW, et al. Pembrolizumab versus chemotherapy for microsatellite instability-high or mismatch repair-deficient metastatic colorectal cancer (KEYNOTE-177): final analysis of a randomised, open-label, phase 3 study. *Lancet Oncol.* 2022;23(5):659–670.
87. Lenz HJ, Van Cutsem E, Limon ML, et al. First-line nivolumab plus low-dose ipilimumab for microsatellite instability-high/mismatch repair-deficient metastatic colorectal cancer: the phase II CheckMate 142 study. *J Clin Oncol.* 2022;40(2):161–170.
88. Tabernero J, Grothey A, Van Cutsem E, et al. Encorafenib plus cetuximab as a new standard of care for previously treated *BRAF* V600E-mutant metastatic colorectal cancer: updated survival results and subgroup analyses from the Beacon study. *J Clin Oncol.* 2021;39(4):273–284.
89. Prager GW, Taieb J, Fakih M, et al. Trifluridine-tipiracil and bevacizumab in refractory metastatic colorectal cancer. *N Engl J Med.* 2023;388(18):1657–1667.
90. Glynne-Jones R, Wyrwicz L, Tiret E, et al. Rectal cancer: ESMO clinical practice guidelines for diagnosis, treatment and follow-up. *Ann Oncol.* 2017;28(suppl_4):iv22–iv40.
91. Bahadoer RR, Dijkstra EA, van Etten B, et al. Short-course radiotherapy followed by chemotherapy before total mesorectal excision (TME) versus preoperative chemoradiotherapy, TME, and optional adjuvant chemotherapy in locally advanced rectal cancer (RAPIDO): a randomised, open-label, phase 3 trial. *Lancet Oncol.* 2021;22(1):29–42.
92. Conroy T, Bosset JF, Etienne PL, et al. Neoadjuvant chemotherapy with FOLFIRINOX and preoperative chemoradiotherapy for patients with locally advanced rectal cancer (UNICANCER-PRODIGE 23): a multicentre, randomised, open-label, phase 3 trial. *Lancet Oncol.* 2021;22(5):702–715.
93. Rullier E, Rouanet P, Tuech JJ, et al. Organ preservation for rectal cancer (GRECCAR 2): a prospective, randomised, open-label, multicentre, phase 3 trial. *Lancet.* 2017;390(10093):469–479.
94. Bach SP, de Wilt JH, Peters F, et al. STAR-TREC phase II: Can we save the rectum by watchful waiting or transanal surgery following (chemo)radiotherapy versus total mesorectal excision for early rectal cancer? *J Clin Oncol.* 2022;40(16_suppl):3502.
95. Garcia-Aguilar J, Patil S, Gollub MJ, et al. Organ preservation in patients with rectal adenocarcinoma treated with total neoadjuvant therapy. *J Clin Oncol.* 2022;40(23):2546–2556.
96. Cercek A, Lumish M, Sinopoli J, et al. PD-1 blockade in mismatch repair-deficient, locally advanced rectal cancer. *N Engl J Med.* 2022;386(25):2363–2376.
97. Marabelle A, Cassier PA, Fakih M, et al. Pembrolizumab for previously treated advanced anal squamous cell carcinoma: results from the non-randomised, multicohort, multicentre, phase 2 KEYNOTE-158 study. *Lancet Gastroenterol Hepatol.* 2022;7(5):446–454.
98. Ajani JA, Winter KA, Gunderson LL, et al. Fluorouracil, mitomycin, and radiotherapy vs fluorouracil, cisplatin, and radiotherapy for carcinoma of the anal canal: a randomized controlled trial. *JAMA.* 2008;299:1914–1921.
99. Gunderson LL, Moughan J, Ajani JA, et al. Anal carcinoma: impact of TN category of disease on survival, disease relapse, and colostomy failure in US Gastrointestinal Intergroup RTOG 98-11 phase 3 trial. *Int J Radiat Oncol Biol Phys.* 2013;87(4):638–645.
100. James RD, Glynne-Jones R, Meadows HM, et al. Mitomycin or cisplatin chemoradiation with or without maintenance chemotherapy for treatment of squamous-cell carcinoma of the anus (ACT II): a randomised, phase 3, open-label, 2 × 2 factorial trial. *Lancet Oncol.* 2013;14:516–524.
101. Kachnic LA, Winter K, Myerson RJ, et al. RTOG 0529: a phase 2 evaluation of dose-painted intensity modulated radiation therapy in combination with 5-fluorouracil and mitomycin-C for the reduction of acute morbidity in carcinoma of the anal canal. *Int J Radiat Oncol Biol Phys.* 2013;86:27–33.
102. Muirhead R, Adams RA, Gilbert DC, et al. Anal cancer: developing an intensity-modulated radiotherapy solution for ACT2 fractionation. *Clin Oncol (R Coll Radiol).* 2014;26(11):720–721.
103. Rao S, Sclafani F, Eng C, et al. International rare cancers initiative multicenter randomized phase II trial of cisplatin and fluorouracil versus carboplatin and paclitaxel in advanced anal cancer: InterAAct. *J Clin Oncol.* 2020;38(22):2510–2518. https://doi.org/10.1200/JCO.19.03266.
104. Crosby T, Hurt CN, Falk S, et al. Chemoradiotherapy with or without cetuximab in patients with oesophageal cancer (SCOPE1): a multicentre, phase 2/3 randomised trial. *Lancet Oncol.* 2013;14(7):627–637.
105. Ford HER, Marshall A, Bridgewater JA, et al. Docetaxel versus active symptom control for refractory oesophagogastric adenocarcinoma (COUGAR-02): an open-label, phase 3 randomised controlled trial. *Lancet Oncol.* 2014;15(1):78–86.
106. Liu CQ, Ma YL, Qin Q, et al. Epidemiology of esophageal cancer in 2020 and projections to 2030 and 2040. *Thorac Cancer.* 2023;14(1):3–11.
107. Obermannová R, Alsina M, Cervantes A, et al. Oesophageal cancer: ESMO clinical practice guideline for diagnosis, treatment and follow-up. *Ann Oncol.* 2022;33(10):992–1004.
108. Sung H, Ferlay J, Siegel RL, et al. Global cancer statistics 2020: GLOBOCAN estimates of incidence and mortality worldwide for 36 cancers in 185 countries. *CA Cancer J Clin.* 2021;71(3):209–249.
109. Chuong MD, Lee P, Low DA, et al. Stereotactic MR-guided on-table adaptive radiation therapy (SMART) for borderline resectable and locally advanced pancreatic cancer: a multi-center, open-label phase 2 study. *Radiother Oncol.* 2024;191:110064.
110. Aitken KL, Hawkins MA. The role of radiotherapy and chemoradiation in the management of primary liver tumours. *Clin Oncol (R Coll Radiol).* 2014;26(9):569–580.
111. European Association for the Study of the Liver. EASL clinical practice guidelines: management of hepatocellular carcinoma. *J Hepatol.* 2018;69(1):182–236.
112. Mauro E, Forner A. Barcelona Clinic Liver Cancer 2022 update: linking prognosis prediction and evidence-based treatment recommendation with multidisciplinary clinical decision-making. *Liver Int.* 2022;42(3):488–491. https://doi.org/10.1111/liv.15180.
113. Ohri N, Tomé WA, Mendez Romero A, et al. Local control after stereotactic body radiation therapy for liver tumors. *Int J Radiat Oncol Biol Phys.* 2021;110(1):188–195.
114. Park JW, Chen M, Colombo M, et al. Global patterns of hepatocellular carcinoma management from diagnosis to death: the BRIDGE study. *Liver Int.* 2015;35(9):2155–2166.
115. Argilés G, Tabernero J, Labianca R, et al. Localised colon cancer: ESMO clinical practice guidelines for diagnosis, treatment and follow-up. *Ann Oncol.* 2020;31(10):1291–1305.

116. Garant A, Vasilevsky CA, Boutros M, et al. Morpheus phase II–III study: a pre-planned interim safety analysis and preliminary results. *Cancers (Basel).* 2022;14(15):3665.
117. Gerard JP, Barbet N, Schiappa R, et al. Neoadjuvant chemoradiotherapy with radiation dose escalation with contact x-ray brachytherapy boost or external beam radiotherapy boost for organ preservation in early cT2-cT3 rectal adenocarcinoma (OPERA): a phase 3, randomised controlled trial. *Lancet Gastroenterol Hepatol.* 2023;8(4):356–367. https://doi.org/10.1016/S2468-1253(22)00392-2.
118. Alexandra Gilbert, Joanne Webster, Sarah Brown, Joanna Copeland, Sharon Ruddock, Duncan Gilbert et al. ESTRO Congress 2023 https://www.estro.org/Congresses/ESTRO-2023/1438/highlightsofprofferedpapers-latestclinicaltrials/13339/standardvsdosereducedchemoradiotherapyinanalcancer
119. Singal AG, Kanwal F, Llovet JM. Global trends in hepatocellular carcinoma epidemiology: implications for screening, prevention and therapy. *Nat Rev Clin Oncol.* 2023 Dec;20(12):864–884. doi:10.1038/s41571-023-00825-3 Epub 2023 Oct 26. PMID: 37884736.

26

Tumours of the Thorax

Kamalram Thippu Jayaprakash, Cathryn Crockett and Gerard G. Hanna

CHAPTER OUTLINE

LUNG CANCER

Lung cancer is the second most common cancer in the United Kingdom and, because of the high mortality rate, is the most common cause of death from cancer, with 35,895 deaths in 2014 (Cancer Research UK). Most of these deaths are preventable, because smoking causes around 85% of cases, but lung cancer in never-smokers is being increasingly recognised as our understanding of these tumours rapidly evolves.

As a result of the long induction period from exposure to tobacco and other carcinogens until the development of cancer, the incidence of lung cancer today reflects smoking habits of the population in previous decades. The incidence of lung cancer in males in Britain has been falling since 1990 but is rising in females because they took up smoking later than males. Similarly, the incidence of cancer in developing countries continues to rise in parallel with the increasing prevalence of smoking. Other proven causes of lung cancer include ionising irradiation and asbestos. Exposure to diesel fumes and a diet low in fruit and vegetables are probable causes of lung cancer.

However, only 10% to 15% of smokers eventually develop lung cancer. There is probably an interplay between genetic susceptibility of the disease and exposure to carcinogens.

Pathology

Histologically, lung cancer is grouped into the more common *non-small cell lung cancer (NSCLC)*, which consists of adenocarcinoma, squamous cell carcinoma and not otherwise specified, and *small cell lung cancer (SCLC)*, with the percentage of cases in the United States in the years 2010 to 2014 shown in parentheses: small cell (13%), adenocarcinoma (47%) and squamous carcinoma (23%). There are other uncommon lung cancer types, such as large cell carcinoma (1.6%) and adenoid cystic carcinoma (National Cancer Institute). The incidence of squamous and small cell carcinomas is falling and that of adenocarcinoma is rising.

However, with the development of new non-cytotoxic cancer treatments directed against specific molecular targets, the genotype of cancer and whether it expresses the programmed death ligand are becoming much more important than the morphology of lung cancer. There are various well-established laboratory techniques and assays to test for genetic alterations where a biological agent is available, and science and technology in this area is fast expanding. An example is ctDNA, in which DNA sequencing produces much faster turnaround time compared to tissue-based molecular profiling.

Mesothelioma, a cancer of the pleura, which is almost always caused by exposure to asbestos, is increasing in incidence, again reflecting the induction period from exposure to the development of disease.

Symptoms

Primary

Lung cancer often presents in the advanced stage by the time patients develop symptoms predominantly because of spread to the mediastinum, causing central chest pain, dysphagia and hoarseness (attributed to compression of the oesophagus and recurrent laryngeal nerve, respectively) or because of growth into a main or lobar bronchus, causing cough, haemoptysis, breathlessness and infection. A pleural or pericardial effusion may also cause dyspnoea. Direct extension into the chest wall causes pain. If the tumour is in the apex of the lung and infiltrates into the brachial plexus, Pancoast syndrome develops. This results in pain or sensory loss of the C7/8 T1 dermatomes and wasting of the small muscles of the hand.

Recent studies have demonstrated benefits of lung cancer screening, which is being increasingly adopted in various countries, including the United Kingdom. This shift in focus to early detection will result in more early-stage disease being diagnosed, which improves survival outcomes in lung cancer.

Metastases

Unfortunately, up to 25% of patients present with symptoms of metastatic disease beyond the thorax. Common sites of metastases are bone (producing pain), brain (producing seizures, headaches and hemiparesis), liver and adrenals.

Paraneoplastic Syndromes

Tumours may produce proteins that have hormonal activity producing various biochemical abnormalities. Recognised syndromes include hyponatraemia secondary to antidiuretic hormone secretion (almost always produced by small cell carcinoma), hypercalcaemia because of parathyroid hormone-like protein (almost always produced by squamous cell carcinoma) and Cushing syndrome because of adrenocorticotropic hormone (ACTH). Antigens expressed by the tumour may lead to cross-tissue reactivity and syndromes suggestive of autoimmune disease.

Diagnosis and Staging

Patients presenting with the preceding symptoms require a clinical examination, particularly focusing on the chest, including palpation of the supraclavicular fossa, which is a common site for lymph node metastases. Investigation then proceeds with a full blood count and biochemical tests of renal and liver functions and bone chemistry. Thereafter, radiology includes a chest x-ray and a computed tomography (CT) scan of the chest and upper abdomen with intravenous contrast administration. If the disease can be treated with curative intent, fluorodeoxyglucose-positron emission tomography (FDG PET) scan is performed. These examinations provide the stage and will, in most cases, demonstrate the site, which can most easily be biopsied to confirm the diagnosis.

The basis of PET scanning is the increased metabolic activity of cancer, which avidly takes up glucose. Following administration of 18-fluorodeoxy-D-glucose (18F-FDG), there is emission of positrons from tumour-bearing areas. The PET scan is usually combined with a CT scan taken on a hybrid machine, a PET/CT scanner, so that the areas of high uptake can be coregistered with the anatomy provided by the CT. Lesions that have PET activity equal to or less than the mediastinal blood pool are deemed negative and those with higher activity, positive. PET scanning will demonstrate metastases that were not previously identified in up to 20% of cases of confirmed lung cancer. In a patient with a small peripheral lesion, PET can help characterise the lesion; malignant lesions tend to be positive, and benign negative. Algorithms have been developed to estimate the probability of malignancy based on patient demographics, growth and PET and CT characteristics. The use of PET/CT imaging and information is essential when undertaking radiotherapy (RT) target volume delineation.[1]

The PET scan is also useful for demonstrating spread to local lymph nodes in the hilum and mediastinum. However, such PET abnormalities should usually be confirmed, if possible, by ultrasound-guided biopsy, by either a bronchoscope or an oesophagoscope, as benign conditions such as sarcoidosis and infection can produce significant 18F-FDG uptake in lymph nodes. Mediastinal histological staging aids with RT planning.[2] If diagnostic material is not obtained by endoscopy, the mediastinal lymph nodes can be surgically sampled by mediastinoscopy. In this procedure a small incision is made above the suprasternal notch. Then, the mediastinoscope is carefully inserted by dissection in front of the trachea, and lymph nodes are removed for pathological examination.

If the tumour is seen to involve a lobar bronchus, bronchoscopy may be required. If metastases are identified, it is often advisable to biopsy one of the affected organs to confirm both the diagnosis and stage of the cancer. If the only site of disease is the periphery of the lung, a CT-guided biopsy is required for pathological diagnosis. However, this test is associated with a small risk of pneumothorax and haemoptysis, which rarely can be fatal. Therefore, if the patient has poor pulmonary function, assessed by a battery of lung function tests such that performing a biopsy poses an unacceptable risk to the patient or the lesion is inaccessible to biopsy, a clinical diagnosis based on imaging is acceptable, particularly for early-stage disease. There are CT- and FDG PET-based prediction models[3,4] that would further improve the confidence of diagnosis. Magnetic resonance imaging (MRI) can be used in specific situations such as Pancoast tumours to determine the extent of invasion of adjacent structures such as vertebrae or the neurovascular bundle that would determine the extent of surgery. MRI with contrast is the best test for demonstrating brain metastases and should be performed for all patients with stage III NSCLC, and CT brain with contrast should be done for patients with stage II NSCLC who are planned for curative-intent treatment. Brain imaging should be performed in patients with symptoms suggestive of brain metastases irrespective of the stage of disease and in SCLC where MRI is preferred if prophylactic cranial RT is not considered.

The diagnostic pathway for lung cancer is complex and often prolonged, which may result in delay in initiating treatments. Diagnostic bundles such as the one developed by the UK National Optimal Lung Cancer Pathway may help streamline and expedite investigations.[5]

Staging

The NSCLC staging system is based on the TNM (tumour, node, metastases) scheme and divides patients into prognostic groups for treatment. The eighth edition of this classification is shown in Table 26.1.[6] The ninth edition is due to be published soon.

Screening

Because of the poor prognosis of lung cancer, mainly as a result of the advanced stage at presentation, screening has been proposed to reduce the mortality of the disease. Using a chest x-ray to detect lung cancer before it produces symptoms has proved unsuccessful. However, a large North American trial involving over 50,000 subjects aged 55 to 74 years, with a significant smoking history, showed that screening with CT reduced both mortality from lung cancer and overall mortality. This latter finding is extremely important and is unique in cancer screening where studies of other sites have only shown a reduction in cancer-specific mortality. A reduction in overall mortality is the gold standard for the evaluation of a screening program as it excludes a significant detriment from overdiagnosis. That is, detecting cancers that would never produce illness during the patient's lifetime and diagnosing these asymptomatic cancers would merely expose the subject to the hazards of treatment such as surgery, RT and chemotherapy, without any improvement in survival. Despite the incontrovertible evidence of benefit, at the time of this writing, screening for lung cancer has not been introduced universally across the United Kingdom.

TABLE 26.1 TNM Staging Classification (8th Edition): T, N and M Descriptors for the 8th Edition of TNM Classification for Lung Cancer

Category	Description
T: Primary Tumour	
Tx	Primary tumour cannot be assessed or tumour proven by presence of malignant cells in sputum or bronchial washings but not visualised by imaging or bronchoscopy
T0	No evidence of primary tumour
T1s	Carcinoma in situ
T1	Tumour ≤3 cm in greatest dimension surrounded by lung or visceral pleura without bronchoscopic evidence of invasion more proximal than the lobar bronchus (i.e. not in the main bronchus)[a]
T1a (mi)	Minimally invasive adenocarcinoma[b]
T1a	Tumour ≤1 cm in greatest dimension[a]
T1b	Tumour >1 cm but ≤2 cm in greatest dimension[a]
T1c	Tumour >2 cm but ≤3 cm or in greatest dimension[a]
T2	Tumour >3 cm but ≤5 cm or tumour with any of the following features[c]: – Involves main bronchus regardless of distance from the carina but without involvement of the carina – Invades visceral pleura Associated with atelectasis or obstructive pneumonitis that extends to the hilar region, involving part or all of the lung
T2a	Tumour >3 cm but ≤4 cm in greatest dimension
T2b	Tumour >4 cm but ≤5 cm in greatest dimension
T3	Tumour >5 cm but ≤7 cm in greatest dimension or associated with separate tumour nodule(s) in the same lobe as the primary tumour or directly invades any of the following structures: chest wall (including the parietal pleura and superior sulcus tumours), phrenic nerve, parietal pericardium
T4	Tumour >7 cm in greatest dimension or associated with separate tumour nodule(s) in a different ipsilateral lobe than that of the primary tumour or invades any of the following structures: diaphragm, mediastinum, heart, great vessels, trachea, recurrent laryngeal nerve, oesophagus, vertebral body, carina
N: Regional Lymph Node Involvement	
Nx	Regional lymph nodes cannot be assessed
N0	No regional lymph node metastasis
N1	Metastasis in ipsilateral peribronchial and/or ipsilateral hilar lymph nodes and intrapulmonary nodes, including involvement by direct extension
N2	Metastasis in ipsilateral mediastinal and/or subcarinal lymph node(s)
N3	Metastasis in contralateral mediastinal, contralateral hilar, ipsilateral or contralateral scalene or supraclavicular lymph node(s)
M: Distant Metastasis	
M0	No distant metastasis
M1	Distant metastasis present
M1a	Separate tumour nodule(s) in a contralateral lobe; tumour with pleural or pericardial nodule(s) or malignant pleural or pericardial effusion[d]
M1b	Single extrathoracic metastasis[e]
M1c	Multiple extrathoracic metastases in one or more organs

[a]The uncommon superficial spreading tumour of any size with its invasive component limited to the bronchial wall, which may extend proximal to the main bronchus, is also classified as T1a.

[b]Solitary adenocarcinoma ≤3 cm with a predominantly lepidic pattern and ≤5-mm invasion in any one focus.

[c]T2 tumours with these features are classified as T2a if ≤4 cm in greatest dimension or if size cannot be determined and T2b if >4 cm but ≤5 cm in greatest dimension.

[d]Most pleural (pericardial) effusions with lung cancer are as a result of tumour. In a few patients, however, multiple microscopic examinations of pleural (pericardial) fluid are negative for tumour and the fluid is nonbloody and not an exudate. When these elements and clinical judgment dictate that the effusion is not related to the tumour, the effusion should be excluded as a staging descriptor.

[e]This includes involvement of a single distant (nonregional) lymph node.

(From Goldstraw P, Chansky K, Crowley J, Rami-Porta R, Asamura H, Eberhardt WEE, Nicholson AG, Groome P, Mitchell A, Bolejack V; International Association for the Study of Lung Cancer Staging and Prognostic Factors Committee, Advisory Boards, and Participating Institutions. The IASLC Lung Cancer Staging Project: Proposals for revision of the TNM stage groupings in the forthcoming (eighth) edition of the TNM Classification for Lung Cancer. *J Thorac Oncol.* 2016;11(1):39–51.)

MANAGEMENT OF NONSMALL CELL LUNG CANCER

EARLY-STAGE NSCLC

Surgery

In patients with early-stage NSCLC who are fit, surgery is the standard treatment. The standard surgical procedure involves lobectomy and lymph node dissection. However, this is associated with significant risks to the patient, with an overall 90-day mortality of 3% and, depending on pulmonary reserve and the extent of surgery, a long-term risk of dyspnoea. Mortality and morbidity increase sharply in patients with impaired cardiopulmonary reserve. Therefore, before surgery, the patient requires careful assessment with cardiopulmonary function (e.g. spirometry, measurement of transfer factor, echocardiography), and if these tests are significantly below normal (typically <40% predicted), a cardiopulmonary exercise test is advised before proceeding with thoracotomy.

The surgical technique has evolved over the years from open thoracotomy to laparoscopic thoracotomy, and robotic-assisted thoracotomy is now routinely offered in many centres. The role of pneumonectomy is questionable because of the high mortality (≤8%) and risk of disabling breathlessness following surgery. However, advances in RT techniques allow management of these patients with RT.

Sublobar resection such as segmentectomy or wedge resection are being increasingly used. Recently, two large, randomised studies[7,8] for small tumours (≤2 cm) showed that sublobar resection offers similar disease-free survival and overall survival compared to conventional lobar resection. Sublobar resection can now be considered in patients with small tumours who have poor pulmonary function, but given excellent outcomes with RT in this group, a balanced discussion of treatment options with patients is vital.

Radical Radiotherapy

Radical RT is an alternative curative treatment option where surgery is contraindicated and/or the patient is not fit for surgery because of comorbidity and/or if the patient declines surgery.

Thoracic RT is particularly challenging because the tumour is a moving target within a region surrounded by critical and radiosensitive structures, such as the lung parenchyma, heart and spinal cord. In addition, because of the low electron density of the lung, the planning system must be able to accurately model photon absorption both within the lung and at air tissue interfaces to ensure that the tumour is not underdosed or that surrounding critical normal organs are not overdosed. Lung RT techniques have transformed in the past decade, which is helping to expand the utility of this treatment modality even to operable early-stage NSCLC. Ongoing studies are comparing radical RT with surgery, and results of these studies are expected in the coming years.

RT Techniques and Fractionation Schedules

Radical RT is delivered by three techniques: continuous hyperfractionated accelerated radiotherapy (CHART), stereotactic ablative body radiotherapy (SABR) and conventional RT, which may be delivered using either standard or hypofractionated dose fractionations.

Continuous Hyperfractionated Accelerated Radiotherapy. CHART for early-stage NSCLC is an efficacious RT schedule. In this regimen, 36 fractions of 1.5 Gy are given 3 times daily, to give a total dose of 54 Gy in only 12 consecutive days. This schedule exploits two of the five radiobiological principles where delivering a radical course of RT in 12 days addresses accelerated repopulation of tumour cells, and small fraction size aims to minimise late normal tissue toxicities. CHART demonstrated an absolute 2-year overall survival improvement of 9% when compared to RT delivered to a dose of 60 Gy using a 2-Gy fraction size.[9] Despite this significant survival benefit, CHART has not been widely adopted due to the requirement that RT be delivered over the weekend, and therefore it has more recently been superseded by SBRT.

Stereotactic Body Radiotherapy/Stereotactic Ablative Body Radiotherapy. SBRT or SABR refers to the delivery of highly conformal, ablative doses in a small number of fractions. RT planning principles involve delivery of inhomogeneous dose within the target, with rapid dose fall-off outside the target volume. SBRT has transformed the treatment landscape for early-stage NSCLC where cases previously deemed inoperable are now able to undergo curative-intent RT, making significant improvement to patients' lives. Because this technique was adopted for peripherally located tumours, its use has now expanded to more central tumours.

In deciding suitability for SBRT, location of the tumour plays a key role, which in turn helps determine the right RT dose fractionation.[10] For a peripherally located tumour (Fig. 26.1), commonly used SBRT doses are 54 Gy/3 fractions and 55 Gy/5 fractions when tumour is closer to the chest wall. There are various descriptions used to define central and ultracentral zones. A commonly accepted definition for *central zone* is by the International Association for the Study of Lung Cancer (IASLC), which defines it as a tumour within 2 cm of any mediastinal critical structures, including the bronchial tree, oesophagus, heart,

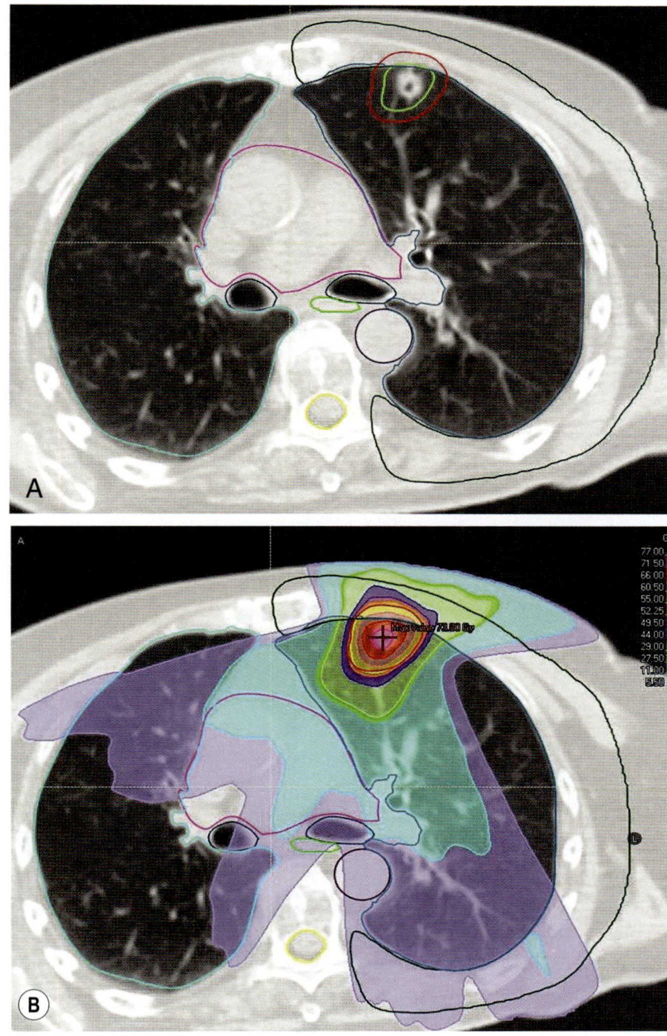

Fig. 26.1 An example of a peripheral zone tumour treated with stereotactic body radiotherapy (SBRT) to a dose of 55 Gy/5 fractions. (A) A cavitating tumour in the lung, close to the chest wall. Contouring of tumour and organs at risk are shown (*light green*, four-dimensional gross tumour volume; *red*, planning target volume; *yellow*, spinal canal; *turquoise*, lungs; *purple*, great vessels; *pink*, heart; *blue*, proximal bronchial tree; *green*, oesophagus; *dark green*, left chest wall). (B) SBRT radiation dose colour wash.

major vessels, spinal cord, brachial plexus and phrenic and recurrent laryngeal nerves (Fig. 26.2). However, there are other definitions for central zone. Two have been used in RTOG trials: in RTOG 0236 it is a tumour within 2 cm of the proximal bronchial tree (PBT), described as the distal 2 cm of the trachea, carina, main bronchi and major lobar bronchi up to their first bifurcation; and in RTOG 0813 it is a tumour within 2 cm of the PBT or touching the mediastinal pleura. Various SBRT fractionations are used for central zone tumour, with 60 Gy/8 fractions (Fig. 26.3) being the most common, and other fractionations in use calling for 5-fraction schedules to a total dose of 50 to 60 Gy.

Definitions for *ultracentral zone* are also inconsistent. Delivery of SBRT to an ultracentral zone target should be carefully considered and ideally be done within a clinical trial due to concerns of treatment-related mortality due to the delivery of ablative doses to radiosensitive airways and the oesophagus, great vessels and spinal cord. Until recently either conventionally fractionated, hypofractionated or hypofractionated-accelerated RT schedules, such as 60 Gy/15 fractions, has been the standard RT fractionation. The SUNSET trial,[11] which

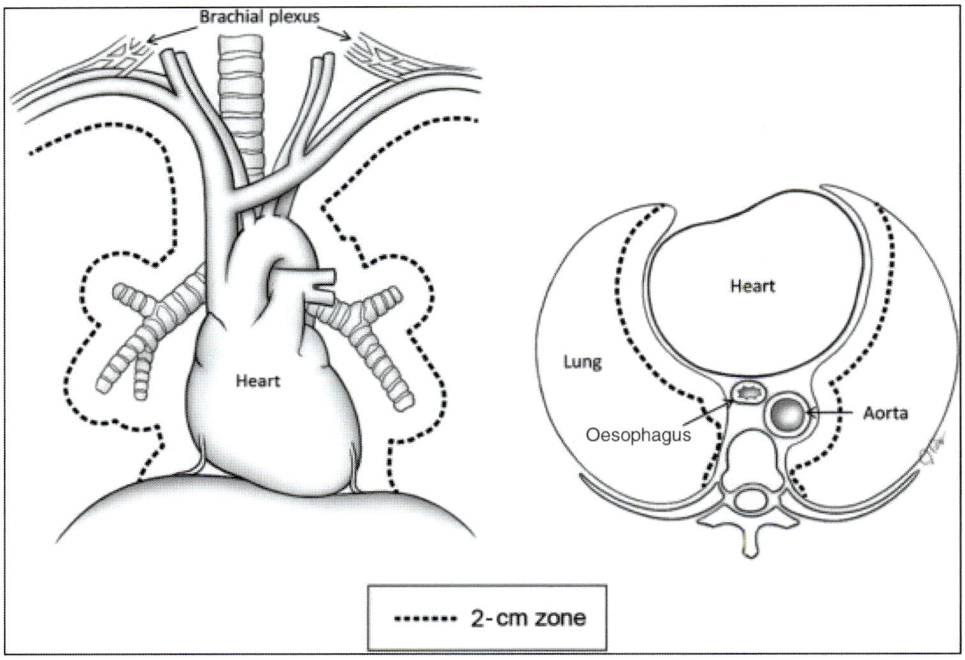

Fig. 26.2 International Association for the Study of Lung Cancer definition of central zone: a tumour within 2 cm in all directions of any mediastinal critical structures, including the bronchial tree, oesophagus, heart, brachial plexus, major vessels, spinal cord, phrenic nerve and recurrent laryngeal nerve.

evaluated 60 Gy/8 fractions, demonstrated the safety of SBRT for ultracentral zone tumours defined by a planning target volume (PTV) that abuts or overlaps with the central bronchial tree, oesophagus or pulmonary vessels, and this option could be considered for carefully selected patients with primary lung tumours where there is no airway invasion and not on anticoagulants, with appropriate SBRT planning parameters as used in the trial. However, recruitment to clinical trials, if available, is encouraged for tumours in the ultracentral zone.

Single-fraction SABR schedules for early-stage NSCLC are becoming popular. A single dose of 30 to 34 Gy is recommended.[12]

Conventional and Hypofractionated-Accelerated Radiotherapy. Radical RT using the conventional fraction size of 2 Gy to a total dose of 60 to 66 Gy is a standard fractionation for NSCLC and is commonly used in early-stage NSCLC where SBRT is not possible and CHART is not available. Radiation dose escalation trials increasing radiation dose beyond 60 to 66 Gy have not been shown to improve outcomes thus far. However, biologically guided RT dose escalation may be beneficial, and more advanced RT techniques such as MRI-guided adaptive RT that might provide opportunity to reduce margins and proton beam therapy could potentially allow further radiation dose escalation trials.

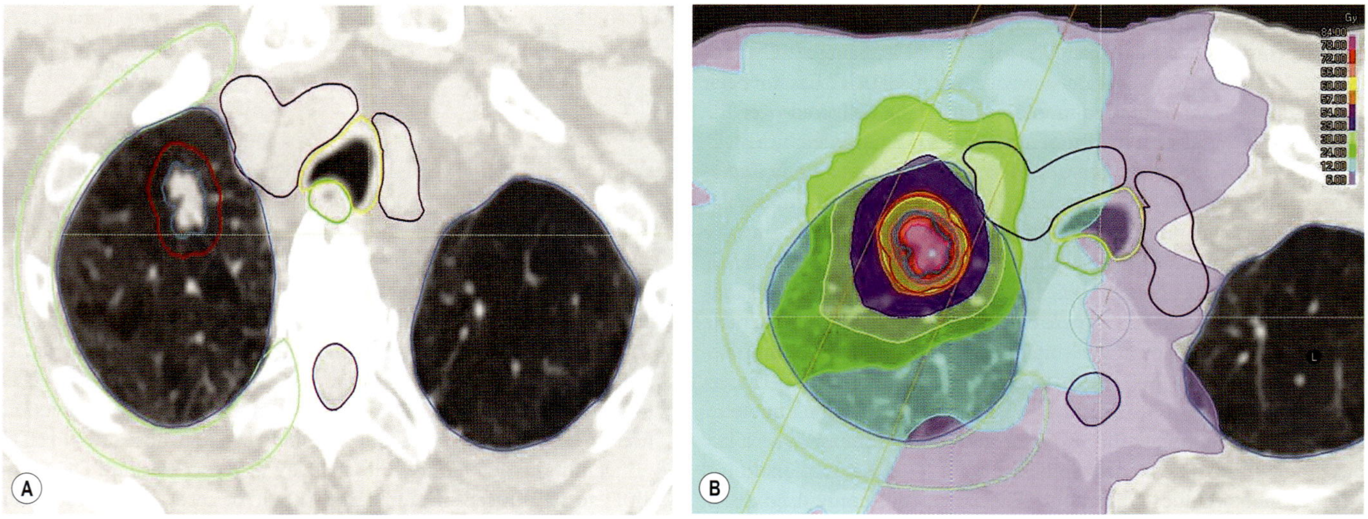

Fig. 26.3 An example of an International Association for the Study of Lung Cancer (IASLC) central zone tumour treated with stereotactic body radiotherapy (SBRT) to a dose of 60 Gy/8 fractions. (A) A solid tumour in the IASLC central zone in the right lung. Contouring of tumour and organs at risk are shown (*light blue*, four-dimensional gross tumour volume; *red*, planning target volume; *dark blue*, spinal canal; *blue*, lungs; *purple*, great vessels; *yellow*, trachea; *green*, oesophagus; *light green*, right chest wall). (B) SBRT radiation dose colour wash.

Hypofractionated-accelerated RT schedules are attractive as they address accelerated repopulation and are delivered in small fraction numbers compared to conventional fractionation. One commonly used schedule is 55 Gy/20 fractions. This schedule was evaluated in the SOCCAR trial[13] in stage III patients and demonstrated safety when used with chemotherapy either concurrently or sequentially, with a promising 2-year survival outcome, and this trial forms the base for using this fractionation in early-stage NSCLC.

Another hypofractionated-accelerated RT schedule, 60 Gy/15 fractions, was initially introduced and used in Canada and is becoming increasingly popular.[14] This schedule provides a higher biologically effective dose (BED) compared to other non-SABR fractionations and is recommended for ultracentral zone tumours (Fig. 26.4). This fractionation has also been used for locally advanced NSCLC.

Immobilisation and Preplanning Image Acquisition

Patients should be planned with the aid of CT. Patients should lie supine, with arms abducted and elbows flexed, in an immobilisation device that incorporates hand bars for the patient to grip. To ensure consistency of position and patient comfort, a vac bag is used in most centres, combined with lateral and sagittal lasers aligned with tattoos to ensure a consistent position between planning and treatment and to minimise movement in all planes as well as rotation between fractions. If the patient is unable to abduct their arms, or in the case of an apical (Pancoast) tumour, consistency of position is achieved with the aid of an Orfit shell. The patient is usually instructed to breathe normally. Contrast is used for central tumours to accurately contour lymph nodes and normal structures such as the heart and blood vessels. If there is collapse or consolidation of the whole or part of the lung, contrast can help delineate tumour from uninflated lung.

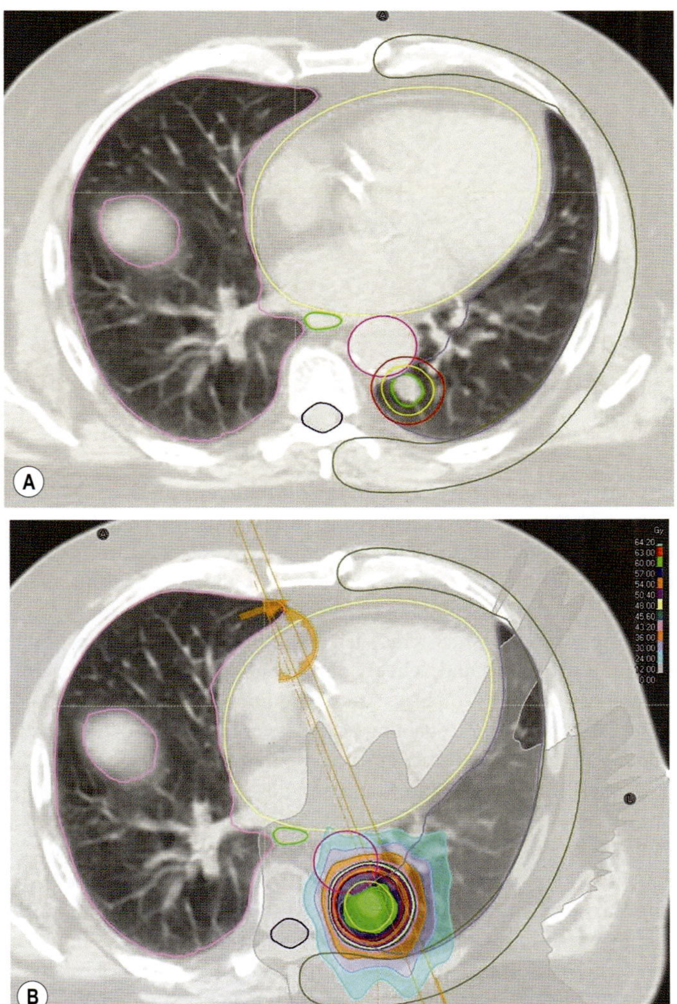

Fig. 26.4 An example of an ultracentral zone tumour treated with hypofractionated-accelerated radiotherapy to a dose of 60 Gy/15 fractions. (A) A solid tumour in the left lung, lower lobe, abutting the great vessels (aorta). Contouring of tumour and organs at risk are shown (*light green*, four-dimensional gross tumour volume; *yellow*, clinical target volume; *red*, planning target volume; *dark blue*, spinal canal; *purple and pink*, lungs; *pink*, great vessels; *yellow*, heart; *green*, oesophagus; *olive green*, left chest wall). (B) Stereotactic body radiotherapy radiation dose colour wash.

Respiratory Motion Mitigation

One of the challenges in RT planning for lung cancer is to address respiratory motion as otherwise it would lead to either the tumour being inadequately covered or organs at risk (OARs) receiving unnecessary radiation dose. In the past, to be certain that the target volume was covered, a larger than necessary margin was used, which would result in excessive OARs being irradiated.

Advances in technology allow us to integrate respiratory motion during the preplanning image acquisition process and thereby mitigate respiratory motion specific to patients. There are various methods of motion management available that are broadly classified into passive and active strategies.[15] Four-dimensional computed tomography (4DCT) is central when considering a passive motion management strategy in which tumour motion is captured in various phases of a respiratory cycle and the patient-specific margin is generated using the internal target volume (ITV) or mid-V or mid-P approach. In an active motion management strategy, the patient is treated during a particular phase of the respiratory cycle, with a deep inspiratory breath-hold technique being commonly used. Respiratory gating and tracking is another active motion mitigation technique, in which tumour motion is tracked using an external surrogate marker, and the patient is only treated in a particular preplanned phase of a respiratory cycle.

Further advances in technology include dynamic tumour tracking where the tumour is tracked with an implanted fiducial or fluoroscopic-based noninvasive technique. These newer technologies allow further refining of RT technique to deliver RT more precisely.

Target Volume Delineation

The gross tumour volume (GTV) encompassing the primary tumour is delineated. A margin, usually 5 mm, is added to the GTV to create a clinical target volume (CTV) to account for microscopic extension of the tumour, but this margin is not required for SBRT treatments. The CTV is then expanded by an appropriate margin depending on the individual centre's protocol for managing day-to-day movement of patients (typically, this is 5 mm in all directions) to produce a PTV. If motion mitigation has not been applied, an extra margin for respiratory motion will need to be added.

Organs-at-Risk Tolerances

In addition to the issue of respiratory motion, lung cancer is surrounded by many radiosensitive OARs, and they need to be carefully contoured, which is particularly important when SBRT is used. The following OARs are required to be contoured on a three-dimensional CT scan depending on the tumour location: spinal cord, lungs, oesophagus, heart, trachea, PBT, chest wall, brachial plexus for upper lobe tumours and spleen, liver, stomach, and bowel for lower lobe tumour depending on their location. OAR dose metrics for SBRT are given in Table 26.2.[16] There is growing evidence for variation in radiosensitivity of cardiac substructures, and therefore cardiac substructure segmenting is likely to become an integral part of lung RT contouring.

TABLE 26.2 Planning Dose Constraints for Stereotactic Body Radiotherapy

		1 FRACTION		3 FRACTIONS		5 FRACTIONS		8 FRACTIONS		
Structure	**Metric**	**Optimal**	**Mandatory**	**Optimal**	**Mandatory**	**Optimal**	**Mandatory**	**Optimal**	**Mandatory**	**End Point**
BrachialPlex	$D_{0.1cc}$		15 Gy		24 Gy	30.5 Gy	32 Gy	35 Gy	39 Gy	Grade 3+ neuropathy
Bronchus_Prox	$D_{0.1cc}$		20.2 Gy		30 Gy	35 Gy	38 Gy		40 Gy	Grade 3+ stenosis/ fistula
Chestwall	$D_{0.1cc}$	30 Gy		36.9 Gy		43 Gy				Grade 3+ fracture/pain
	D_{30cc}			30 Gy						
Oesophagus	$D_{0.1cc}$		15.4 Gy		25.2 Gy		35 Gy		40 Gy	Grade 3+ stenosis/ fistula
GreatVes	$D_{0.1cc}$		30 Gy		45 Gy		53 Gy	60 Gy	65 Gy	Grade 3+ aneurysm
Heart+A_Pulm	$D_{0.1cc}$		22 Gy	26 Gy	30 Gy	29 Gy	38 Gy	40 Gy	46 Gy[a]	Grade 3+ pericarditis
Lungs (nonlung lesions) and lungs—internal target volume (lung lesions)	V_{20Gy}	10%	15%	10%	15%	10%	15%	10%	15%	Grade 3+ pneumonitis
	D_{mean}	8 Gy		8 Gy		8 Gy		8 Gy		
Skin	$D_{0.1cc}$		26 Gy	33 Gy		39.5 Gy		48 Gy		Grade 3+ ulceration
	D_{10cc}		23 Gy	30 Gy		36.5 Gy		44 Gy		
Trachea	$D_{0.1cc}$		20.2 Gy		30 Gy	35 Gy	38 Gy		40 Gy	Grade 3+ stenosis/ fistula

[a]If not achievable, drop prescription dose to 50 Gy.

(From Diez P, Hanna GG, Aitken KL, et al. UK 2022 consensus on normal tissue dose-volume constraints for oligometastatic, primary lung and hepatocellular carcinoma stereotactic ablative radiotherapy. *Clin Oncol.* 2022;34(5):288–300.)

Image segmentation of OARs can be a lengthy process, and this task can be performed by other RT professionals such as radiographers and dosimetrists with appropriate training. There are a growing number of vendors that offer automated contouring tools that could also greatly aid in this process.

RT Planning and Delivery

The best dose distribution, that is, good coverage of the tumour with the lowest dose to critical normal organs, is obtained by employing intensity modulated radiotherapy (IMRT). Studies have demonstrated that IMRT improves dosimetry[17] and possibly survival of patients.[18] This requires careful contouring of OARs and complex planning software that can both accurately model electron transfer and optimise the dose distribution to ensure that the PTV is not underdosed and that the OAR is not overdosed. However, in the specialised situation of SBRT, significant inhomogeneity is allowed within the PTV, with hot spots up to 140% being acceptable, although OAR tolerances must not be exceeded; otherwise, serious or even fatal side effects can result. Various techniques of IMRT are used, including step and shoot, or more commonly, arc therapy, where the output and shape of the beam are continually modulated as the treatment head rotates around the patient. The beam energy is usually 6 MV or less to reduce the effect of secondary buildup at the lung tumour interface.

Modern linear accelerators are equipped with on-board cone beam CT including 4DCT so that the tumour can be accurately imaged with the patient in the treatment position, and if necessary, adjustments made before each fraction is delivered. Anatomical changes due to response to tumour may result in the resolution of preexisting atelectasis and benign pleural effusion, and treatment may lead to the development of new collapse and reactive pleural effusion. These changes need to be carefully analysed, ideally with online review, and rescan and replan may be required in some cases.

More advanced RT systems such as MRI Linac allow the possibility of online adaptation and delivery of precision RT delivery with gating capabilities. Newer CT Linacs are now quipped with artificial intelligence (AI)-based tools, enabling us to deliver adaptive RT. These additional technological advances may help improve the therapeutic radio of thoracic RT and even allow radiation dose escalation.

Special Situations

Patients with lung cancer may also have interstitial lung disease (ILD) (Fig. 26.5), which can increase the risk of severe radiation pneumonitis that may lead to treatment-related morbidity and mortality. There are several types of ILD, with varying prognoses and risks of developing radiation pneumonitis. The GAP analysis would help predict prognosis from an ILD perspective for idiopathic pulmonary fibrosis patients,[19] but advice from an ILD specialist is recommended before RT is considered for these patients. A recent trial, ASPIRE, has demonstrated the safety of SBRT, and therefore radical RT in this setting should be considered in consultation with ILD teams.

Patients with lung cancer may present with more than one tumour and are at high risk of developing subsequent new lung cancer. Therefore, there will be a need to treat more than one tumour either

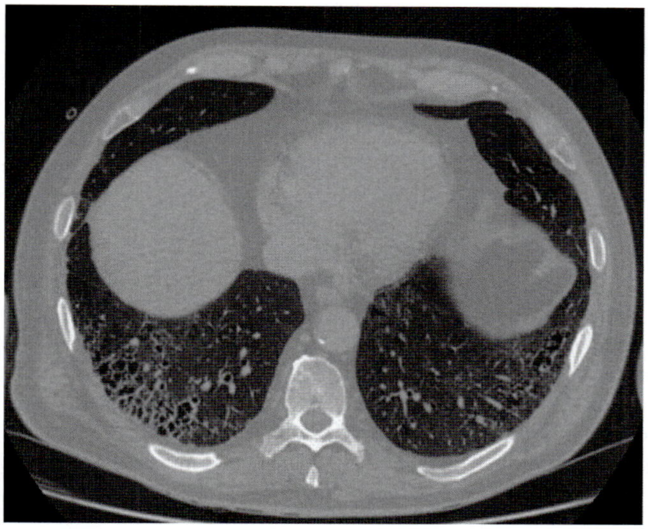

Fig. 26.5 Computed tomography appearances showing background lung parenchymal chances typically seen in idiopathic pulmonary fibrosis.

simultaneously or sequentially. In these circumstances, a close discussion with the RT physics team would help choose the ideal fractionation schedule, and if there is any overlap with the previous course of radiation, a reirradiation pathway should be followed whereby image registration, previous dose deposition, dose recovery and cumulative OAR dose constraints should be considered (Fig. 26.6).

Follow-up

The main objectives for follow-up are to detect recurrences early, identify new lung cancer that may be amenable to curative-intent treatment, identify cases of palliative-intent treatments and identify any potential treatment-related complications.

There is no consensus on follow-up protocols following radical-intent treatment for early-stage NSCLC. It is widely accepted to perform 6 monthly CT scans for up to 5 years if the patient is fit and suitable for further surgical and oncological treatments. The role of routine imaging in patients who are unfit for further active treatment is questionable and, in these circumstances, it is preferable to direct imaging guided by their symptoms.

Differentiating post-RT changes from tumour recurrence can be challenging, particularly for post-SBRT patients. Radiological features of infiltration into adjacent structures, bulging margins, sustained growth, mass-like growth, spherical growth, craniocaudal growth and loss of air bronchograms would suggest local recurrence rather than post-RT changes.[20]

LOCALLY ADVANCED NSCLC

Locally advanced NSCLC (stage III) is a heterogeneous disease. It includes large tumours and/or those with spread to lymph nodes or other central structures such as the mediastinum or great blood vessels. Management generally involves either a surgical approach or chemoradiation.

Operable Disease

Patients with low-volume stage III disease, and of an appropriate fitness level, may be candidates for surgery within a multimodality approach. Traditionally, this would include surgery followed by adjuvant chemotherapy. However, the recently published CheckMate 816 trial has demonstrated an event-free survival benefit of neoadjuvant chemoimmunotherapy in patients with up-front resectable, driver mutation negative disease.[21] Two other trials (NADIM and KEYNOTE-671) have reported promising results in relation to the use of perioperative immunotherapy with or without chemotherapy.[22,23]

Adjuvant Therapy

In cases where the resected tumour is found on postoperative histology to have spread to the lymph nodes, adjuvant platinum-based chemotherapy is offered with the aim of sterilising occult metastatic disease. However, the overall benefit is relatively small, with an improvement in 5-year survival of less than 5%, and side effects are significant. There

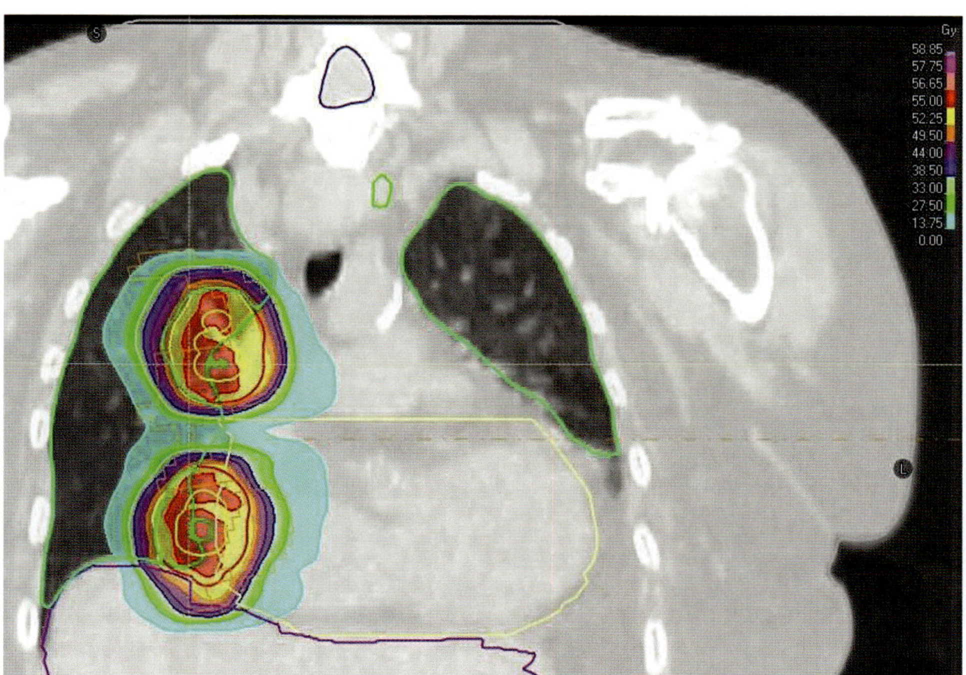

Fig. 26.6 Radiotherapy plan of two synchronous lung primaries treated with 55 Gy/20 fractions; radiation dose colour wash shown.

is currently no clinical trial evidence directly comparing neoadjuvant systemic therapy strategies to those delivered adjuvantly.

For patients with a sensitising epidermal growth factor receptor (EGFR) mutation, the FLAURA study has shown that the use of adjuvant therapy with osimertinib for 3 years is associated with a significant survival benefit[24] and is therefore recommended.

Postoperative RT (PORT) is considered if the tumour is thought to be incompletely resected (R1 or R2) by either the surgeon or the pathologist. The evidence of benefit for PORT is limited, and it should never be used without careful selection, as a metaanalysis of clinical trials (albeit using obsolete techniques and in unselected patients) showed an excess mortality of up to 20% for PORT. Furthermore, the LungART study in patients with completely resected N2 NSCLC did not show any benefit with the use of PORT as compared to no adjuvant RT. Therefore, PORT requires careful planning to ensure that the dose to the remaining lung is kept to a minimum. The placement of clips by the surgeon at sites where the cancer is seen invading structures beyond the limit of resection can help define the CTV.

Inoperable Disease

Combined Modality Treatment

Chemoradiotherapy

In cases of locally advanced disease where surgery is not an option, combining chemotherapy concurrently with the delivery of radiation (Fig. 26.7) produces superior survival results compared with giving treatments sequentially. However, concurrent chemoradiation produces significant morbidity and an overall mortality rate of 3%, and therefore should only be used in patients of good performance status (0 or 1) and adequate organ (particularly heart and lung) function. The drugs used are usually cisplatin and etoposide, as these drugs can be given at full doses with radical (60 Gy or more) radiation. Carboplatin can be used either as a single agent or combined with paclitaxel (in NSCLC) as a less toxic alternative to cisplatin, but the evidence of benefit is not as convincing as for cisplatin.

The use of consolidation immunotherapy following concurrent chemoradiation has emerged as a new standard of care following the results of the landmark PACIFIC randomised trial that reported a statistically significant improvement in both progression-free survival and overall survival.[25]

Surgery, Radiotherapy and Chemotherapy

For selected cases, there is some evidence that a combined approach of surgery, RT and chemotherapy (trimodality therapy) is best. This can be given electively when RT, usually with concurrent chemotherapy, is delivered before surgery in cases of locally advanced lung cancer with spread to either the mediastinal lymph nodes or to adjacent soft tissue as in Pancoast tumours. This approach is associated with significant postoperative mortality and requires close cooperation with the operative and oncology teams to ensure that only suitable patients are treated and that the treatment program is delivered without unplanned gaps. In this regimen, two cycles of chemotherapy are combined with a course of RT at a subradical dose of 45 Gy in 25 fractions, and surgery performed within 3 to 5 weeks of completion of radiation.

Organs-at-Risk Tolerances

In the thorax, the radiation oncologist is confronted with minimising dose to several critical organs that can be affected by radiation with serious, sometimes fatal, consequences including the lungs, heart, oesophagus, spinal cord and brachial plexus against the need to treat a cancer with a radical dose. Specific tolerances have been developed by empirical study over many years, and in particular, the heart is now considered a critical structure where excess radiation has been associated with early death following thoracic RT. The tolerances for the various organs, with the commonly used RT doses used for curative treatment, are given in Table 26.3. These planning doses are a guide, and it is important to remember that patients with pulmonary disease, especially interstitial lung disease,[26] will have reduced tolerance. However, consistent information regarding the interplay of patient factors, that is, preexisting cardiopulmonary function with radiation, is somewhat sparse and inconsistent. Patients with impaired performance status (2 or worse) should generally not be given concurrent chemoradiation and those with impaired pulmonary function indices (spirometry and transfer factor) of less than 40% of normal, corrected for age and gender, and particularly those with pulmonary fibrosis, should only be treated after careful consideration. Full information about the possible consequences (particularly breathlessness and death) of

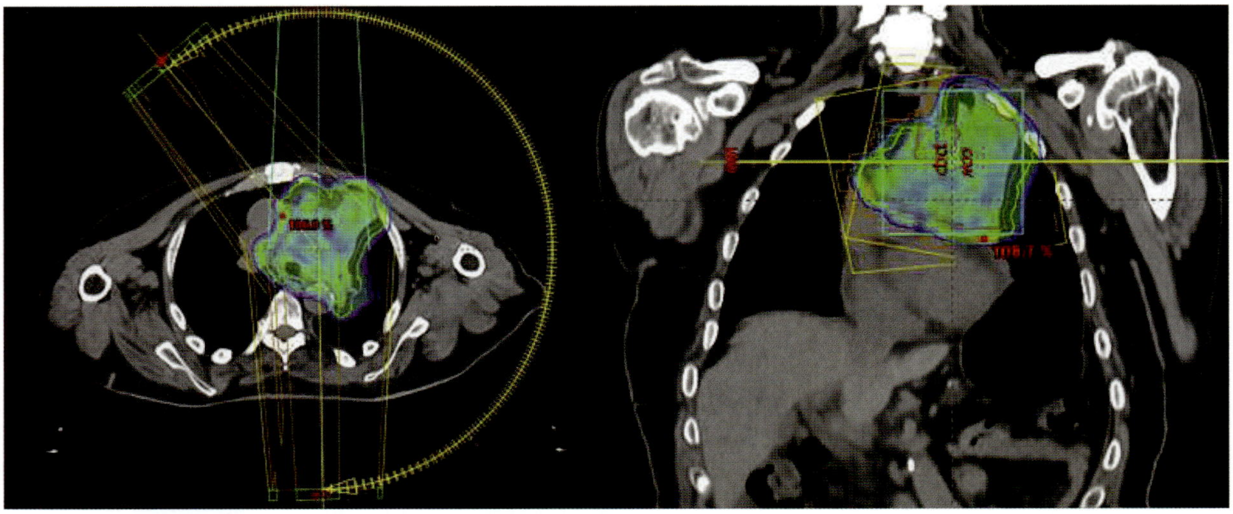

Fig. 26.7 An axial and coronal slice of the radiotherapy (RT) plan of a patient with T4N3M0 left-sided nonsmall cell lung cancer who was treated with concurrent chemoradiotherapy. The RT dose delivered was 60 Gy/30 fractions. Contours: Gross tumour volume *(red)*, internal target volume *(orange)* and planning target volume *(blue)*. A 95% dose colour wash is visible showing the excellent conformity of the plan.

TABLE 26.3 Planning Dose Constraints for Radical Radiotherapy, Total Dose 60–66 Gy in 30–33 Fractions or 55 Gy in 20 Fractions

Lung

These constraints are a guide, and important clinical considerations should be taken into account such as pulmonary function and alternative forms of treatment.

Mean Lung Dose

>20 Gy (considered unacceptable), 18–20 Gy high risk of pneumonitis, 15–18 Gy moderate risk, <15 Gy low risk

DV 20 Gy (% volume of lung minus planning target volume receiving 20 Gy)

>40% very high risk of pneumonitis only acceptable with specific consent, 35%–40% very high risk, 30%–35% high risk, 20%–30% moderate risk, <20% low risk

Oesophagus

No more than 12 cm should receive total dose.

Spinal Cord

60–66 Gy @ 2 Gy per fraction: 50 Gy @ 2 Gy per fraction up to 54 Gy is deemed acceptable if the tumour is close to the cord and the patient is at risk of spinal cord compression if treatment fails.

55 Gy @ 2.75 Gy per fraction: 42 Gy, 50 Gy is deemed acceptable if the tumour is close to the cord and the patient is at risk of spinal cord compression if treatment fails.

Brachial Plexus

No more than 0.5 cc, should receive 60 Gy for 60–66 Gy in 30–33 fractions or 53 Gy for 55 Gy in 20 fractions.

Heart

No more than one-third should receive total dose.

radiation should be provided. Patients will usually opt for treatment, despite the risks, as the outlook for even early-stage untreated lung cancer is very poor.

Radiotherapy Fractionation Schedules

There is no good evidence that for conventionally fractionated radiation, a dose in excess of 60 Gy (or equivalent) given as a sole modality or combined with chemotherapy is beneficial to patients with locally advanced NSCLC. This does not mean that most lung cancers are controlled with 60 Gy but simply that controlled trials of doses greater than 60 Gy have either shown no benefit or in some cases, have shown actual inferior results, probably due to the higher experimental dose producing greater normal tissue toxicity.

However, the studies that evaluated 60 Gy often employed dose prescriptions that did not correct for the reduced electron density within the lung or used what now would be considered obsolete planning systems. Therefore, the dose actually delivered may well have been considerably greater than 60 Gy, and so many centres will prescribe 64 to 66 Gy in 32 to 33 fractions to allow for this factor. In the United Kingdom, a commonly used dose for radical treatment of the lung is 55 Gy in 20 fractions.

Acute Radiotherapy Effects

General fatigue and oesophagitis are common. Oesophagitis is managed with antacids (sometimes combined with a local anaesthetic) and analgesics; soluble paracetamol is used initially, but there should be a low tolerance for administering opiates to maintain hydration and nutrition. Patients should be advised to adopt a bland diet avoiding extremes of temperature. In severe cases, meals may have to be liquidised and oral nutritional supplements prescribed; in such cases dietetic input is important. With conventionally fractionated RT, significant skin reactions are rare. However, palliative RT and some SBRT plans will give an appreciable dose to the skin, resulting in erythema and indeed in some cases moist desquamations. The radiation plan should be reviewed before treatment and patients warned about the possibility of radiation dermatitis and instructed on appropriate skin care.

Late Radiotherapy Effects

Some degree of pneumonitis and fibrosis is an inevitable consequence of radical RT, and it is important that other specialists are aware of this complication because it can be radiologically misdiagnosed as local recurrence. The severity of this side effect depends on radiation and patient factors as mentioned earlier. It is important that patients and their medical attendants are also aware that this complication can develop in the months following RT to ensure that early and aggressive treatment is given. Patients typically present with dry cough, fever and shortness of breath. A chest x-ray may show a hazy appearance in the irradiated area. Therapy is supportive, including oxygen and high-dose steroids. Although there is no evidence of benefit, antibiotics are also often coprescribed to exclude an infective aetiology. There is growing evidence that the lymphopenia associated with RT to locally advanced NSCLC increases the risk of opportunistic infections such as *Pneumocystis jirovecii*, and this is an important differential diagnosis to consider in patients with dyspnoea, cough and patchy consolidation on chest x-ray.

There is no satisfactory treatment for neurological complications of RT, and every effort should be made (even in the case of palliative RT) to avoid exceeding the radiation tolerance of the spinal cord and brachial plexus. Oesophageal stricture and pericardial effusion are seen in the longer term, but with modern RT planning these problems should occur in less than 5% of patients. Long-term cardiac morbidity and mortality is the subject of active research. Some studies have reported on specific key cardiac structures that can be outlined and actively avoided during the RT planning process in an effort to reduce the risk of long-term cardiac toxicity.[27,28] There is also work looking at how best to optimise a patient's cardiac status prior to starting RT. It is now clear that radiation-induced cardiac dysfunction can be misdiagnosed as pneumonitis and may be responsible for excess mortality in the year following radical RT. Treatment is again supportive with the prescription of medication for cardiac failure.

OLIGOMETASTATIC NSCLC

The oligometastatic state was first postulated by Hellman and Weichselbaum in 1995 as a disease state consisting of a low volume of metastatic lesions that may be treated aggressively with curative potential, with either surgery or ablative RT. It is thought to be an 'intermediate state' somewhere between localised and polymetastatic disease. A strict definition of oligometastatic disease still does not exist, although the presence of up to five metastatic lesions in three different organs seems acceptable to most clinicians and definitions by international associations. The lesions may be synchronously diagnosed alongside the primary tumour or develop metachronously. Several prospective phase II trials, including the SABR COMET study, investigating the potential additional benefit of local ablative therapy to systemic therapy in the synchronous oligometastatic setting, have reported promising survival results in favour of combination treatment.[29–31] The results of the confirmatory phase II SARON trial[32] in this setting are still awaited.

POLYMETASTATIC NSCLC

Systemic Treatment

Over the past number of years, the systemic therapy landscape available to patients of good performance status with advanced (stage III and IV) NSCLC has changed dramatically.[33] The types of systemic treatment available include chemotherapy, immunotherapy or targeted drugs. The decision regarding which type of treatment a patient receives is dependent upon both disease and patient factors. Disease factors include the histological subtype, programmed death ligand 1 (PD-L1) expression, the presence of gene mutations and the general behaviour of the disease, for example, aggressive/rapidly progressing. Patient factors include performance status and the presence of comorbidities.

Chemotherapy

It was previously established that the quality and quantity of life of patients with metastatic NSCLC may be improved by the judicious use of a platinum agent combined with one other drug: gemcitabine, paclitaxel, docetaxel or vinorelbine (doublets). A metaanalysis has shown a modest increase in survival of 3 months with platinum doublets compared with best supportive care. Clinical trials have shown that overall, for all types of NSCLC combined, no particular doublet was superior, with response rates of around 25%, a similar median survival of 8 to 10 months and 1-year survival of 30% to 40%. A metaanalysis showed cisplatin doublets produced a statistically significant better response rate and marginally better survival when compared with carboplatin-based combinations for all indications. However, in the palliative setting, this difference was almost imperceptible, and given the palliative nature of this type of chemotherapy, the toxicity, particularly nausea and vomiting, and hearing loss caused by cisplatin, most clinicians prefer a carboplatin combination for the palliative treatment of NSCLC. The addition of a third drug did not increase response rates or survival. However, a large trial compared cisplatin platinum combined with either gemcitabine or the antifolate drug pemetrexed. The trial was designed to compare the results by histological type. The results showed a clear advantage for the pemetrexed combination for adenocarcinoma, whereas gemcitabine was superior for squamous carcinoma. A further trial has shown that in cases of adenocarcinoma, continuing the pemetrexed as a single agent following the combination therapy (providing the tumour does not progress on doublet therapy) improves survival. More recently, trials have demonstrated an additive survival benefit with immunotherapy delivered alongside platinum-based chemotherapy[34,35] in patients with tumours with PD-L1 expression of <50% in the first-line setting. If PD-L1 expression is 50%, patients may be eligible for single-agent immunotherapy first line, which will be discussed in more detail in the next section.

In the second-line setting, docetaxel as a single agent for squamous carcinoma or combined with nintedanib, a drug that inhibits the development of blood vessels in adenocarcinoma, has shown to produce a survival benefit. However, docetaxel produces significant toxicity and is now being replaced with immunotherapy, if not received first line.

Immunotherapy

For cancer to progress, it needs to overcome the immune response of the host (patient).

Some of the mechanisms by which a cancer achieves this have recently been identified. In particular, lung cancer cells have shown to express a ligand that suppresses the activities of killer T cells that would normally kill cancer cells, a process known as *programmed death.*

Therapies have been developed that block this action of the cancer cell by binding with the ligand or receptor and thus effectively reactivating the body's own immunity against the cancer. These drugs are particularly effective where a high percentage of tumour cells express the ligand (PD-L1 ≥50%). In such cases, drugs such as pembrolizumab have been proven to be superior to chemotherapy in the first-line setting.[36]

In patients with a relatively low expression of PD-L1 (<50%), chemotherapy with or without immunotherapy is used first. However, pembrolizumab and similar drugs such as nivolumab are superior to second-line chemotherapy following initial cytotoxic treatment. Occasionally, even in patients with widespread metastases, a sustained response to immunotherapy is seen. The dramatic effect of these drugs in advanced disease has led to trials being devised to test the value of immune therapy in the early disease setting, particularly combining immunotherapy with RT.

Targeted Therapy

A large number of mutations can be detected in lung cancer cells. Specific therapies have been developed to target some of these mutations. Multiple mutations have now been identified for which established (licenced) therapies have been developed. These mutations are uncommon, but two of the most common amongst them are EGFR and anaplastic lymphoma kinase (ALK), found in about 10% and 5%, respectively, of patients with NSCLC. These mutations are almost exclusively found in adenocarcinoma and are more prevalent in nonsmokers and Asian patients. The drugs targeted at EGFR include osimertinib,[37] dacomitinib, afatinib, erlotinib and gefitinib. These drugs are superior to chemotherapy both in efficacy (response rate) and side effects. This is a fast-developing field. Drugs targeting the ALK gene[38] include crizotinib, ceritinib, alectinib and brigantinib in the first-line setting and lorlatinib in the second line. Other, less common targetable mutations include ROS-1, BRAF V600 and METex14 skipping alteration with drugs available in the first-line setting, RET fusion and KRAS G12C with drugs available in the second-line setting and NTRK fusion with a drug available in the third-line setting.

SBRT/SABR

More recently, newer clinical concepts have been developed that are distinct from oligometastatic disease.[39] These states largely arise from the polymetastatic setting in patients initially treated with systemic therapy and include oligoresistance (mixed response to systemic therapy with some lesions responding but others progressing), oligopersistance (good response generally but some persistent lesions still present) and oligoprogression (good response generally but some progressive lesions seen). The use of ablative RT in these scenarios has been postulated as a way of targeting resistant clones. The recently reported NRG-LU002 trial,[40] which included patients with oligopersistant disease randomised to receive consolidation RT in addition to systemic therapy or systemic therapy alone, unfortunately failed to show a survival benefit, however. The results of further ongoing research in this area from studies such as the HALT study are eagerly awaited.

Palliative Radiotherapy

Patients who are not candidates for radical treatment by virtue of advanced stage of disease or poor performance status can benefit from palliative RT. The extent of the tumour and symptoms determine the treatment volume. Generally, large fields are used for palliation to encompass the tumour and adjacent areas of likely spread/subclinical extension to avoid marginal recurrence or the need for retreatment during the patient's lifetime. However, it is acceptable to treat part of the gross tumour to avoid significant toxicity (particularly oesophagitis), especially in a patient with poor performance status. Thus, in a patient with a peripheral primary and mediastinal disease, radiation is usually directed solely at the latter site.

The patient is simulated and treated supine, usually hands by the side; however, in cases where the tumour extends to the chest wall, one or both arms need to be abducted out of the fields. Simple parallel field arrangements are used, but the tolerance of the spinal cord must not be exceeded, as some patients can survive long enough to be at risk of radiation myelitis. Therefore, oblique fields and/or shielding may be required, which can also be employed to reduce the dose to the oesophagus and lung parenchyma. It is often helpful to delineate a GTV, expand this by 1.5 cm in all directions, and then utilise isocentric fields to encompass this volume, and where possible, shield normal tissue. Field sizes of up to 15 × 10 cm are typically used, but no more than 10 cm of the oesophagus should receive the prescribed dose to avoid inducing severe and prolonged dysphagia.

The doses used for palliative treatment were established by a series of British Medical Research Council (MRC) trials published between 1991 and 1996 that also produced evidence of the effectiveness of palliative RT for the common symptoms of lung cancer: haemoptysis will be relieved in most (up to 90%) patients, and cough and pain will improve in over half of patients treated. The doses employed are 10 Gy in 1 fraction (for patients of poor performance status), 17 Gy in 2 fractions 1 week apart, 20 Gy in 5 fractions or 36 to 39 Gy in 12 or 13 fractions, depending on the extent of both intra- and extrathoracic disease. For fit patients, even those with advanced disease, a higher dose improves survival at the cost of increased side effects, particularly oesophagitis.

Other than a single fraction of 10 Gy and 20 Gy fractionated, all these doses exceed cord tolerance. In the modern era, it is unacceptable to subject patients to the risk of developing radiation myelitis, so every department should have in place protocols to limit the dose to the cord. This may require formal CT planning, particularly if doses in excess of 30 Gy are employed. Retreatment is challenging as usually the spinal cord will have previously received a dose close to tolerance. However, if oblique fields can be employed to avoid the spinal cord, palliative doses up to 30 Gy can be delivered. A review of seven studies involving a total of 159 patients suggests similar levels of palliation as reported in first-line studies can be achieved.

Bone Metastases

Bone pain and pathological fracture are common complications of lung cancer. An 8-Gy single fraction delivered in a parallel pair or direct field can improve pain.

Brain Metastases

Brain metastases are common in lung cancer, with up to half of patients with advanced disease developing intracerebral disease, and as a consequence, suffering from the disabling symptoms of headache, ataxia, hemiparesis and fits. Dexamethasone is used to reduce cerebral oedema, and improvement in symptoms is often seen within a few days. The landmark QUARTZ trial reported that the addition of palliative whole brain irradiation to steroid therapy is of no benefit.

However, patients of good performance status, with disease controlled elsewhere and limited volume of disease, can be treated with ablative therapy, which has been shown, in contradistinction to whole brain radiation, to improve quality of life. Surgery or radiosurgery (using the Gamma Knife or a specially adapted LINAC) can be used to ablate brain metastases. Generally, up to three metastases can be treated in one session with low morbidity, and because of the noninvasive nature and day case administration, this form of RT is increasingly being preferred over surgery.

The value of adjuvant whole brain RT (30 Gy in 10 fractions) following ablative treatment to treat microscopic disease is being increasingly questioned as to whether this prophylactic therapy reduces the rate of intracranial relapse, because no overall survival benefit is found and radiation-induced lethargy, alopecia and cognitive impairment are significant side effects. Therefore, the practice of many centres is to monitor patients following ablative therapy with 3 monthly MRI scans and offer further ablative therapy to new metastases as they arise.

There has been some research into the use of hippocampal avoidance[41] or concurrent memantine administration with whole brain RT to try to reduce neurocognitive toxicity. However, a definite conclusion regarding their benefit has yet to be drawn.

SMALL CELL LUNG CANCER

Natural History

There is a tendency for this cancer disease to disseminate widely and rapidly, with 80% of patients presenting with metastatic disease and often with a short history of symptoms of a few weeks before diagnosis. Spread is local, via the lymphatics and haematogenous systems, and SCLC is often associated with a high prevalence of paraneoplastic phenomena.

Staging and Diagnosis

The investigation and staging for SCLC are generally the same as for NSCLC, with the aim of establishing the diagnosis and determining if the patient has disease limited to the chest that can be irradiated without exceeding normal tissue tolerance. The TNM system is now used for SCLC. However, it is still useful to classify patients using the 'Veteran's Classification' as having limited-stage disease (LS-SCLC). LS-SCLC is disease confined to one hemithorax and adjacent supraclavicular lymph nodes, which are encompassed in a 'tolerable RT portal' (field). Extensive stage disease (ES-SCLC) is where disease has spread beyond the chest and regional lymph nodes and cannot be encompassed in a tolerable RT field. Patients with LS-SCLC are usually assessed with further staging tests that may include PET scanning with a view to curative treatment with chemotherapy and RT. ES-SCLC disease is usually managed with palliative systemic anticancer therapy up front, and prognostic factors include performance status, age and abnormal biochemistry.

Management

Limited-Stage SCLC

The standard of care in limited-stage SCLC is concurrent chemoradiotherapy, with four cycles of etoposide with platinum (either cisplatin or carboplatin) and with RT delivered either at cycle 1 or as early as possible in the treatment course. In patients with bulky tumours, it may be preferrable to deliver RT at the third cycle or at the completion of chemotherapy to reduce the size of the RT treatment field. Following the completion of chemotherapy and thoracic RT, if the patient has a response to treatment, prophylactic cranial irradiation may be considered. Also, given the results of the Adriatic study, adjuvant immunotherapy with durvalumab should be considered.[42]

Extensive-Stage SCLC

Chemotherapy

Combination chemotherapy produces a response in over 60% of patients with extensive disease. Responders experience improvement in quality of life and survival. However, a significant proportion of patients present in very poor clinical condition with advanced organ failure, and only supportive care is appropriate in this situation. In those patients who receive chemotherapy, the duration of response is short and the overall median survival is around 8 months. Several chemotherapy regimens exist and most are equivalent in terms of response; therefore, in the palliative situation, a combination of etoposide and carboplatin (EC) is the standard therapy as this regimen is generally well tolerated. Single-agent therapy has been tried, but because of lower response rates leading to uncontrolled symptoms, palliation and survival were inferior to combination chemotherapy. Normally four cycles of chemotherapy are delivered. More prolonged, alternating regimens or dose-intensive chemotherapy have been found to be of no benefit.

Recently a number of studies have shown that the addition of immunotherapy with PD-L1 inhibitors such as atezolizumab and durvalumab along with EC chemotherapy improves survival. After the four initial cycles of chemoimmunotherapy, the immunotherapy agent is continued as a maintenance therapy until progression.

For patients with a response to chemotherapy, prophylactic cranial irradiation (PCI) and thoracic consolidation irradiation (TCI) may be considered. However, the use of PCI reduced significantly with the use of immunotherapy in ES-SCLC, with uncertainty about the safety of the combination and how best to time the delivery.

Retreatment with chemotherapy on relapse can be considered if the patient remains in good performance status, particularly if several months have elapsed since initial treatment. The regimens used for retreatment are the combination of cyclophosphamide, adriamycin and vincristine (CAV) or topotecan as a single agent. If the disease-free interval is greater than 6 months, retreatment with EC can be of benefit. Responses, however, are of short duration. Patients who do not respond to first-line therapy and those who have relapse within 3 months of treatment are unlikely to respond to further chemotherapy.

Radiotherapy

RT to the thorax, given sequentially or concurrently, has been shown to improve the survival of patients with LS-SCLC.[43] The best results are obtained if the RT is given concurrently with chemotherapy as early as possible in the treatment course; using this approach, 5-year survival of 20% can be obtained. However, patients need to be in good performance status and the disease of such a volume that it can be treated to an adequate dose without risking severe toxicity. If concurrent chemoradiation is not feasible, sequential RT can be used, providing the patient responds to initial chemotherapy. A recent trial showed similar results using either 66 Gy in 33 daily fractions or 45 Gy in 30 fractions bidaily when combined concurrently with cisplatin and etoposide. Radiation doses of similar biological potency are used for sequential treatment. The RT technique is the same as that employed for NSCLC.

Prophylactic Cranial Irradiation

Brain metastases are a common problem in SCLC and without prophylactic irradiation develop in approximately 20% and 50% of patients with LS-SCLC and ES-SCLC, respectively. PCI reduces the incidence of brain metastases and improves the survival of patients with limited SCLC who have successfully undergone chemotherapy and thoracic RT. No benefit has been found for giving a dose higher than 25 Gy in 10 fractions. PCI is given after chemotherapy to avoid radiosensitisation by cytotoxic chemotherapy and to limit its use to those patients who have responded to chemotherapy and therefore are most likely to benefit from this treatment.

The patient's head is immobilised with an Orfit mask in the supine position and a planning CT performed. A parallel pair technique is used comprising two opposed lateral fields. The orbits, most of the parotid glands and the oral cavity can be shielded with multileaf collimators (MLCs). This approach is better than using head rotation to conform to the traditional anatomical line drawn from the outer margin of the orbit, outer canthus and through the lower tragus used to set up the fields, as this arrangement often underdoses the middle cranial fossa and provides inadequate shielding of the parotid glands. Both fields are irradiated daily. The dose is prescribed to the midpoint intersection of both beams.

However, a dose of this order is known to cause significant side effects in NSCLC and there is some evidence that patients with SCLC suffer long- and short-term central nervous system (CNS) sequelae from cranial irradiation. Therefore, RT techniques that reduce the dose to the hippocampus have been developed to potentially reduce these serious side effects. Clinical trial evidence suggests that hippocampal sparing does reduce neurotoxicity but at the risk of increased failures in the avoidance area. At present, hippocampal sparing may be considered but is not widely practised.

Although PCI also reduces the incidence of brain metastases in patients with ES-SCLC who respond to chemotherapy, the effect on overall survival is small and somewhat uncertain, and because of side effects and the generally poor survival, patients with ES-SCLC must be carefully counselled before considering treatment with PCI.

Common acute side effects are headache, tiredness, nausea and reversible alopecia. These can be treated with steroids or other antiemetics. In the 12 weeks following PCI post irradiation, somnolence, cognitive impairment and lethargy are common complaints. These are self-limiting, however, and do not predict late neurotoxicity. Patients with SCLC have a limited life span, so the true incidence of late neurological damage is not known.

Thoracic Consolidation Irradiation

TCI may be considered in patients with ES-SCLC who respond well to chemotherapy and who have thoracic dominant disease. However, the role of TCI in this setting is uncertain. A number of studies have shown improved local control and a trend to improved overall survival in the preimmunotherapy era.[44] However, as studies of immunotherapy in ES-SCLC did not permit TCI, the use of TCI has significantly diminished. Where TCI is offered, a dose of 30 Gy in 10 fractions is appropriate.

The Role of Surgery and SBRT in Early-Stage SCLC

Less than 10% of patients have stage I (T1, T2) disease and, occasionally, these patients have surgical resection to remove an undiagnosed pulmonary nodule. Small retrospective studies suggest that these patients may do well with standard chemotherapy and RT. There is no evidence that patients with more advanced disease, T3 or N2 benefit from surgical treatment. A number of papers have reported the successful use of SBRT in the treatment of stage I LS-SCLC.[45] Where used in this manner, it is preferable to deliver SBRT before any planned systemic therapy.

NEUROENDOCRINE TUMOURS

Pulmonary carcinoid tumours are rare, accounting for only 1% of all lung tumours, but the lung is the primary site of 25% of all carcinoid tumours.[46] The biological aggressiveness of carcinoid tumours is variable, but most are well differentiated and rarely metastasise. These tumours are found in main, lobar or segmented bronchi and present with cough, haemoptysis or local obstructive symptoms.

Surgery is the treatment of choice. Unlike bronchial carcinoma, carcinoid tumours do not exhibit extensive submucosal spread and therefore surgical techniques such as sleeve resection that enable significant volumes of lung to be preserved can be performed without compromising local control and are particularly useful for tumours originating in main bronchi. Five-year survival rates in excess of 90% have been reported following resection.

By contrast, patients with histologically atypical carcinoids (poorly differentiated, pleomorphic cells, increased mitosis and necrotic areas) have a much higher risk of metastases to organs such as the liver, bones, adrenals and CNS and therefore a poorer survival. However, the disease often runs an indolent course, with patients surviving for many years with metastatic disease: the median survival from diagnosis is around 10 years.

As well as conventional imaging, such as CT scanning, radiolabelled octreotide (octreoscans) can be useful in establishing the extent of disease. Carcinoids may produce excess catecholamines and kinins leading to the carcinoid syndrome, which is characterised by facial flushing (often provoked by stress or alcohol), diarrhoea and, in the long term, fibrosis and incompetence of the right-sided heart valves. Such patients have raised levels of catecholamine metabolites in urine such as 3-methoxy-4-hydroxy mandelic acid (UMA) and hydroxyindoleacetic acid (HIAA).

Treatment of patients with locally advanced disease or metastatic disease is palliative. Somatostatin analogues such as octreotide and lanreotide block the release of catecholamines and can improve the symptoms of carcinoid syndrome in 80% of cases. Radionuclide treatment can help if the tumour takes up compounds such as radiolabelled octreotide. RT is used for palliation for chest symptoms as well as metastatic disease.

No chemotherapy combination has clearly been shown to be beneficial in this disease. The cytotoxic combinations used are those prescribed for small cell carcinoma, that is, cisplatin or carboplatin combined with etoposide, although response rates are low, generally less than 20%. However, everolimus (an immunosuppressant originally developed to prevent rejection following organ transplantation) has been found to improve survival in patients with advanced neuroendocrine tumours and is now the systemic treatment of choice.

MESOTHELIOMA

Mesothelioma is a malignant tumour of the pleura, and the majority of cases are caused by exposure to asbestos. There are two main types of asbestos fibres: serpentiles (white asbestos) and amphiboles (blue asbestos). White asbestos fibres are pliable, curly and easily broken down in the lung, releasing magnesium, iron and silica. About 90% of industry used this type and, fortunately, it is rarely associated with mesothelioma. Blue asbestos fibres, however, are rigid and nonpliable. Lung phagocytes repeatedly attempt to break down these fibres and eliminate them. It is thought that this chronic inflammatory response leads to eventual mesothelial cell proliferation, mutation and malignancy. This may explain the long latency period of 20 to 40 years from first exposure to asbestos and development of this tumour. Asbestos was commonly used for insulation in buildings and homes, ships and car parts. It is estimated that the risk of development of this disease is greatest in males born around 1945 to 1950, of whom it is anticipated that 1 in 150 will die of mesothelioma.[47]

In Turkey, there is a high incidence of mesothelioma. At first this was thought to be a result of asbestos-like mineral fibres in the soil. However, these nonasbestos-related tumours are hereditary in nature and have been found to be associated with carriage of an autosomal dominant gene.

Natural History

The majority of patients will progress rapidly and succumb to their illness within 12 months, although occasionally patients may remain stable for some time with or without treatment.[48]

Most patients present with a pleural effusion, but in the later stages of the illness, the tumour encases and constricts the lung and invades the chest and mediastinum, causing pain, dyspnoea and sometimes dysphagia. Night sweats are seen in advanced disease. Although metastases are commonly found at postmortem, disease beyond the thorax rarely causes symptoms during the patient's lifetime.

Prognostic groups are based on the following factors: patient age, gender, weight loss and performance status, tumour histology and clinical stage, values of haemoglobin, leucocyte ($>8.3 \times 10^9$/L) and platelet count ($>400 \times 10^9$/L) at presentation. There are several different staging systems, but they are mostly based on surgical staging and therefore are of no value for the majority of patients.

Initial Assessment and Treatment

A CT scan is used to establish a provisional diagnosis, and there should be a low threshold for performing this imaging in cases of persistent pleural effusion, particularly in patients who have been exposed to asbestos. The next step is to establish a diagnosis and provide optimum control of any pleural effusion. Although the diagnosis can be suggested by cytology, confirmation by histology is usually required. This is usually done with a thoracoscopy, where the scope is introduced into the pleural space and abnormal tissue is biopsied and the effusion drained. Control of the effusion is by the introduction of talc into the pleural space, which causes inflammation of the pleural surfaces, which then fuse together, preventing reaccumulation of fluid. If the lung does not reexpand, the placement of a permanent drain provides drainage. This procedure can be performed under general anaesthetic or in a conscious patient with sedation.

Surgery

Apart from thoracoscopy, there is no established role for surgery in mesothelioma. A trial of debulking surgery showed a small improvement in the time to recurrence of pleural effusion but no improvement in survival. Radical surgery involving removal of the lung and pleura (radical pleuropneumonectomy) has high mortality, approaching 10%, and has largely been abandoned in the United Kingdom following the results of the Mesothelioma and Radical Surgery (MARS) 1 and 2 trials, which showed no benefit of trimodality therapy (chemotherapy, surgery and RT) compared with the standard approach of systemic therapy.[49]

Radiotherapy

RT has a limited role in mesothelioma.[50] Although in the past, irradiation was used prophylactically to prevent disease developing in scars from surgical intervention, recent randomised trials of PORT have shown no benefit. The frequency of surgical scar recurrence in these trials was much lower than that historically observed, probably because minimally invasive techniques are used and possibly because of the increasing use of chemotherapy. RT can produce palliation of pain, particularly where the disease infiltrates the chest wall, but unfortunately, although initial benefit is seen, recurrence of pain is common. Administering RT to the hemithorax following pneumonectomy or pleurectomy to delay local progression is extremely difficult to achieve without exceeding lung tolerance, and deaths as a result of radiation pneumonitis have been reported following pneumonectomy and RT. Therefore, this form of wide-field RT for mesothelioma is not recommended outside a clinical trial.

Systemic Therapy

Systemic therapy with either cytotoxic chemotherapy or immunotherapy is the only treatment modality for mesothelioma that has shown proven benefit in terms of quality of life or survival benefit.[51] The evidence is indirect in that the trials that have established the value of chemotherapy randomised patients between single-agent cisplatin and a combination with an antifolate drug, either pemetrexed or raltitrexed. Both trials showed an improvement in survival for the combination, implying that chemotherapy is superior to supportive care. A UK trial compared chemotherapy with supportive care and showed no significant benefit. However, the drugs used in this study (vinorelbine or the combination of mitomycin, vinblastine and cisplatin) were probably suboptimal, and most clinicians would offer fit patients with mesothelioma the option of palliative chemotherapy. There is no standard second-line option for mesothelioma.

The CheckMate 743 trial showed that the combination of nivolumab plus ipilimumab improved overall survival as compared to chemotherapy in the first-line treatment of mesothelioma.[52] This immunotherapy doublet is now the treatment of choice for patients fit enough to receive systemic therapy.

THYMOMA AND THYMIC MALIGNANCIES

Thymic malignancies represent a spectrum of diseases ranging from benign thymoma to malignant thymic cancer. Thymomas and thymic cancers typically present as a mediastinal mass.[53] However, they are well-known for associated paraneoplastic syndromes such as myasthenia gravis and red cell aplasia. These syndromes can persist following complete resection of the tumour. Thymoma has an unpredictable clinical behaviour that does not correlate with the pathological findings and may recur after many years.

Symptoms

Thymoma can present as an incidental finding on x-rays or symptoms of a paraneoplastic syndrome. Spread occurs via the lymphatics or by the haematogenous route.

Diagnosis

Investigations should concentrate on identifying the extent of disease in the anterior mediastinal and possible areas of spread followed by biopsy.[54]

Pathology and Natural History

Thymomas can be classified as epithelial or lymphocytic. Mixed and spindle forms also exist. The tumour can behave unpredictably regardless of the pathological appearance. Differentiation between benign and malignant disease is determined by the presence of gross invasion of adjacent structures, metastasis or microscopic evidence of capsular invasion.

Management

Surgical resection is the treatment of choice. Locally invasive, large or unresectable tumours should be treated with multimodality therapy. The tumour is chemosensitive, and over half of patients will respond to cisplatin-based regimens. Chemotherapy can be used for locally advanced disease, followed by, if feasible, surgery and PORT (50 Gy in 25 fractions), or if the tumour is not resectable, by RT alone. PORT is used in the treatment of both thymoma and thymic carcinoma. Evidence for the use of PORT for patients with an R0 resection is largely informed by two large database analyses and an updated metaanalysis.[55]

In completed resected thymoma or thymic carcinoma (R0), with no capsular invasion and Masaoka-Koga stage I disease, PORT is not recommended. In completed resected thymoma or thymic carcinoma (R0) with capsular invasion and Masaoka-Koga stages II–IV disease, PORT[42] may be considered to a dose of 45 to 50 Gy in 1.8 to 2.0 Gy per fraction. In patients with thymoma or thymic carcinoma with a R1 resection, PORT is recommended to a dose of 54 Gy in 1.8 to 2.0 Gy per fraction. In patients with thymoma or thymic carcinoma with gross positive margin disease (R2) resection, PORT should be offered to a dose of 60 to 70 Gy in 1.8 to 2.0 Gy per fraction.

Local recurrence may occur late, often 5 or more years after initial surgery, and is frequently associated with more undifferentiated histology. The treatment is similar to initial presentation. In view of the propensity for late recurrence, 10-year survival figures are considered more reliable. Thymomas are also usually radiosensitive. In patients who have localised isolated recurrences, RT alone can be used as local treatment.

CONCLUSION

Tumours of the thorax and, in particular, lung cancer, remain a common cause of disability and death. Although the outcome is generally poor, there has been progress in the past two decades through the judicious use of newer RT techniques where both early-stage and locally advanced disease tumours that can be treated aggressively with SABR and IMRT/VMAT techniques, respectively. Minimally invasive surgery has also contributed to the improvement in clinical outcomes over recent years. Systemic therapy in the treatment of lung cancer has undergone a revolution in the past decade with the now widespread use of immunotherapy and targeted inhibitors of oncogene-derived molecular targets. Key to systemic management is molecular and immune profiling, and these agents are now being used as neoadjuvant and adjuvant therapies. RT remains an effective and key modality of therapy in thoracic cancers.

REFERENCES

1. Konert T, Vogel W, MacManus MP, Nestle U, Belderbos J, Grégoire V, Thorwarth D, Fidarova E, Paez D, Chiti A, Hanna GG. PET/CT imaging for target volume delineation in curative intent radiotherapy of non-small cell lung cancer: IAEA consensus report 2014. *Radiother Oncol.* 2015;116(1):27–34.
2. Steinfort DP, Kothari G, Wallace N, Hardcastle N, Rangamuwa K, Dieleman EMT, Lee P, Li P, Simpson JA, Yo S, Bashirdazeh F, Nguyen P, Jennings BR, Fielding D, Crombag L, Irving LB, Yasufuku K, Annema JT, Ost DE, et al. Systematic endoscopic staging of mediastinum to guide radiotherapy planning in patients with locally advanced non-small-cell lung cancer (SEISMIC): an international, multicentre, single-arm, clinical trial. *Lancet Respir Med.* 2024;12(6):467–475.
3. McWilliams A, Tammemagi MC, Mayo JR, Roberts H, Liu G, Soghrati K, Yasufuku K, Martel S, Laberge F, Gingras M, Atkar-Khattra S, Berg CD, Evans K, Finley R, Yee J, English J, Nasute P, Goffin J, Puksa S, et al. Probability of cancer in pulmonary nodules detected on first screening CT. *N Eng J Med.* 2013; 369(10):910–919.
4. Herder GJ, van Tinteren H, Golding RP, Kostense PJ, Comans EF, Smit EF, Hoekstra OS. Clinical prediction model to characterize pulmonary nodules: validation and added value of 18 F-fluorodeoxyglucose positron emission tomography. *Chest.* 2005;128(4): 2490–2496.
5. Lung Clinical Expert Group. National Optimal Lung Cancer Pathway. August 2017. https://www.roycastle.org/app/uploads/2019/07/National_Optimal_LUNG_Pathway_Aug_2017.pdf
6. Goldstraw P, Chansky K, Crowley J, Rami-Porta R, Asamura H, Eberhardt WEE, Nicholson AG, Groome P, Mitchell A, Bolejack V; International Association for the Study of Lung Cancer Staging and Prognostic Factors Committee, Advisory Boards, and Participating Institutions. The IASLC Lung Cancer Staging Project: proposals for revision of the TNM stage groupings in the forthcoming (eighth) edition of the TNM Classification for Lung Cancer. *J Thorac Oncol.* 2016;11(1):39–51.
7. Saji H, Okada M, Tsuboi M, Nakajima R, Suzuki K, Aokage K, Aoki T, Okami J, Yoshino I, Ito H, Okumura N, Yamaguchi M, Ikeda N, Wakabayashi M, Nakamura K, Fukuda H, Nakamura S, Mitsudomi T, Watanabe S-I, et al. Segmentectomy versus lobectomy in small-sized peripheral non-small-cell lung cancer (JCOG0802/WJOG4607L): a multicentre, open-label, phase 3, randomised, controlled, non-inferiority trial. *Lancet.* 2022;399(10335): 1607–1617.

8. Altorki N, Wang X, Kozono D, Watt C, Landrenau R, Wigle D, Port J, Jones DR, Conti M, Ashrafi AS, Liberman M, Yasufuku K, Yang S, Mitchell JD, Pass H, Keenan R, Bauer T, Miller D, Kohman LJ, et al. Lobar or sublobar resection for peripheral stage IA non-small-cell lung cancer. *N Engl J Med.* 2023;388(6):489–498.
9. Saunders M, Dische S, Barrett A, Harvey A, Gibson D, Parmar M. Continuous hyperfractionated accelerated radiotherapy (CHART) versus conventional radiotherapy in non-small-cell lung cancer: A randomised multicentre trial. *Lancet.* 1997;350(9072):161–165.
10. SABR UK Cosortium. Stereotactic Ablative Body Radiation Therapy (SABR): A Resource. Version 6.1, January 2019. https://www.sabr.org.uk/wp-content/uploads/2019/04/SABRconsortium-guidelines-2019-v6.1.0.pdf
11. Giuliani ME, Filion EJ, Faria S, Kundapur V, Vu TTT, Lok BH, Raman S, Bahig H, Laba JM, Lang P, Louie AV, Hope A, Rodrigues GB, Bezjak A, Campeau M-P, Duclos M, Bratman S, Swaminath A, Salunkhe R, et al. Stereotactic radiation for ultra-central non-small cell lung cancer: a safety and efficacy trial (SUNSET). *Int J Radiat Oncol Biol Phys.* 2024;120(3):669–677.
12. Greenwood H, Hassan J, Fife K, Ajithkumar TV. Thippu Jayaprakash K. Single-fraction stereotactic ablative body radiotherapy for primary and extracranial oligometastatic cancers. *Clin Oncol (R Coll Radiol).* 2023;35(12):773–786.
13. Maguire J, Khan I, McMenemin R, O'Rourke N, McNee S, Kelly V, Peedell C, Snee M. SOCCAR: A randomised phase II trial comparing sequential versus concurrent chemotherapy and radical hypofractionated radiotherapy in patients with inoperable stage III non-small cell lung cancer and good performance status. *Eur J Cancer.* 2014;50(17):2939–2949.
14. Zeng KL, Poon I, Ung Y, Tsao M, Zhang L, Cumal A, Louie AV, Cheung P. Accelerated hypofractionated radiotherapy for centrally located lung tumours not suitable for stereotactic body radiotherapy or chemoradiotherapy. *Clin Oncol.* 2023;35(2):e173–e181.
15. Crockett C, Salem A, Thippu Jayaprakash K. Shooting the star: mitigating respiratory motion in lung cancer radiotherapy. *Clin Oncol (R Coll of Radiol).* 2022;34(3):160–163.
16. Diez P, Hanna GG, Aitken KL, van As N, Carver A, Colaco RJ, Conibear J, Dunne EM, Eaton DJ, Franks KN, Good JS, Harrow S, Hatfield P, Hawkins MA, Jain S, McDonald F, Patel R, Rackley T, Sanghera P, et al. UK 2022 consensus on normal tissue dose-volume constraints for oligometastatic, primary lung and hepatocellular carcinoma stereotactic ablative radiotherapy. *Clin Oncol.* 2022; 34(5):288–300.
17. Gleeson I, Jayaprakash KT. A dosimetric comparison of radical radiotherapy techniques in non-small cell lung cancer. *Lung Cancer.* 2020;139:S37–S38.
18. Fornacon-Wood I, Chan C, Bayman N, Banfill K, Coote J, Garbett A, Harris M, Hudson A, Kennedy J, Pemberton L, Salem A, Sheikh H, Whitehurst P, Woolf D, Price G. Faivre-Finn C. Impact of introducing intensity modulated radiotherapy on curative intent radiotherapy and survival for lung cancer. *Front Oncol.* 2022;12:835844.
19. Ley B, Ryerson CJ, Vittinghoff E, Ryu JH, Tomassetti S, Lee JS, Poletti V, Buccioli M, Elicker BM, Jones KD, King TE Jr, Collard HR. A multidimensional index and staging system for idiopathic pulmonary fibrosis. *Ann Intern Med.* 2012;156(10):684–691.
20. Ronden MI, Palma D, Slotman BJ, Senan S. Brief report on radiological changes following stereotactic ablative radiotherapy (SABR) for early-stage lung tumors: a pictorial essay. *J Thorac Oncol.* 2018;13(6):855–862.
21. Forde PM, Spicer J, Lu S, Provencio M, Mitsudomi T, Awad MM, Felip E, Broderick SR, Brahmer JR, Swanson SJ, Kerr K, Wang C, Ciuleanu T-E, Saylors GB, Tanaka F, Ito H, Chen K-N, Liberman M, Vokes EE, et al. Neoadjuvant nivolumab plus chemotherapy in resectable lung cancer. *N Engl J Med.* 2022;386(21): 1973–1985.
22. Wakelee H, Liberman M, Kato T, Tsuboi M, Lee S-H, Gao S, Chen K-N, Dooms C, Majem M, Eigendorff E, Martinengo GL, Bylicki O, Rodríguez-Abreu D, Chaft JE, Novello S, Yang J, Keller SM, Samkari A; KEYNOTE-671 Investigators. Perioperative pembrolizumab for early-stage non-small-cell lung cancer. *N Engl J Med.* 2023;389(6):491–503.
23. Provencio M, Nadal E, González-Larriba JL, Martínez-Martí A, Bernabé R, Bosch-Barrera J, Casal-Rubio J, Calvo V, Insa A, Ponce S, Reguart N, de Castro J, Mosquera J, Cobo M, Aguilar A, Vivanco GL, Camps C, López-Castro R, Morán T, et al. Perioperative nivolumab and chemotherapy in stage III non-small-cell lung cancer. *N Engl J Med.* 2023;389(6):504–513.
24. Wu Y-L, Tsuboi M, He J, John T, Grohe C, Majem M, Goldman JW, Laktionov K, Kim S-W, Kato T, Vu H-V, Lu S, Lee K-Y, Akewanlop C, Yu C-J, de Marinis F, Bonanno L, Domine M; ADAURA Investigators. Osimertinib in resected EGFR-mutated non-small-cell lung cancer. *N Engl J Med.* 2020;383(18):1711–1723.
25. Antonia SJ, Villegas A, Daniel D, Vicente D, Murakami S, Hui R, Yokoi T, Chiappori A, Lee KH, de Wit M, Cho BC, Bourhaba M, Quantin X, Tokito T, Mekhail T, Planchard D, Kim Y-C, Karapetis CS, PACIFIC Investigators. Durvalumab after chemoradiotherapy in stage III non-small-cell lung cancer. *N Engl J Med.* 2017;377(20):1919–1929.
26. Goodman CD, Nijman SFM, Senan S, Nossent EJ, Ryerson CJ, Dhaliwal I, Qu XM, Laba J, Rodrigues GB, Palma DA; International Association for the Study of Lung Cancer Advanced Radiation Technology Committee. A primer on interstitial lung disease and thoracic radiation. *J Thorac Oncol.* 2020;15(6):902–913.
27. Banfill K, Giuliani M, Aznar M, Franks K, McWilliam A, Schmitt M, Sun F, Vozenin MC, Finn CF; IASLC Advanced Radiation Technology committee. Cardiac toxicity of thoracic radiotherapy: existing evidence and future directions. *J Thorac Oncol.* 2021;16(2): 216–227.
28. Walls GM, O'Connor J, Harbinson M, Duane F, McCann C, McKavanagh P, Johnston DI, Giacometti V, McAleese J, Hounsell AR, Cole AJ, Butterworth KT, McGarry CK, Hanna GG, Jain S. The association of incidental radiation dose to the heart base with overall survival and cardiac events after curative-intent radiotherapy for non-small cell lung cancer: results from the NI-HEART Study. *Clin Oncol (R Coll Radiol).* 2024;36(2):119–127.
29. Palma DA, Olson R, Harrow S, Gaede S, Louie AV, Haasbeek C, Mulroy L, Lock M, Rodrigues GB, Yaremko BP, Schellenberg D, Ahmad B, Senthi S, Swaminath A, Kopek N, Liu M, Moore K, Currie S, Schlijper R, et al. Stereotactic ablative radiotherapy for the comprehensive treatment of oligometastatic cancers: long-term results of the SABR-COMET phase II randomized trial. *J Clin Oncol.* 2020;38(25):2830–2838.
30. Iyengar P, Wardak Z, Gerber DE, Tumati V, Ahn C, Hughes RS, Dowell JE, Cheedella N, Nedzi L, Westover KD, Pulipparacharuvil S, Choy H, Timmerman RD. Consolidative radiotherapy for limited metastatic non-small-cell lung cancer: a phase 2 randomized clinical trial. *JAMA Oncol.* 2018;4(1):e173501.
31. Gomez DR, Tang C, Zhang J, Blumenschein GR Jr, Hernandez M, Lee JJ, Ye R, Palma DA, Louie AV, Camidge DR, Doebele RC, Skoulidis F, Gaspar LE, Welsh JW, Gibbons DL, Karam JA, Kavanagh BD, Tsao AS, Sepesi B, et al. Local consolidative therapy vs. maintenance therapy or observation for patients with oligometastatic non-small-cell lung cancer: Long-term results of

a multi-institutional, phase II, randomized study. *J Clin Oncol.* 2019;37(18):1558–1565.
32. Conibear J, Chia B, Ngai Y, Bates AT, Counsell N, Patel R, Eaton D, Faivre-Finn C, Fenwick J, Forster M, Hanna GG, Harden S, Mayles P, Moinuddin S, Landau D. Study protocol for the SARON trial: A multicentre, randomised controlled phase III trial comparing the addition of stereotactic ablative radiotherapy and radical radiotherapy with standard chemotherapy alone for oligometastatic non-small cell lung cancer. *BMJ Open.* 2018 Apr 17;8(4):e020690.
33. NICE (National Institute for Health and Care Excellence). Lung cancer: Diagnosis and management. NICE guideline (NG122). Published 28 March 2019. Last updated 8 March 2024. https://www.nice.org.uk/guidance/ng122/chapter/Treatment#systemic-anti-cancer-therapy-sact-for-advanced-non-small-cell-lung-cancer
34. Gandhi L, Rodríguez-Abreu D, Gadgeel S, Esteban E, Felip E, Angelis FD, Domine M, Clingan P, Hochmair MJ, Powell SF, Cheng S Y-S, Bischoff HG, Peled N, Grossi F, Jennens RR, Reck M, Hui R, Garon EB; KEYNOTE-189 Investigators. Pembrolizumab plus chemotherapy in metastatic non-small-cell lung cancer. *N Engl J Med.* 2018;378(22):2078–2092.
35. Paz-Ares L, Luft A, Vicente D, Tafreshi A, Gümüş M, Mazières J, Hermes B, Şenler FC, Csőszi T, Fülöp A, Rodríguez-Cid J, Wilson J, Sugawara S, Kato T, Lee KH, Cheng Y, Novello S, Halmos B; KEYNOTE-407 Investigators. Pembrolizumab plus chemotherapy for squamous non-small-cell lung cancer. *N Engl J Med.* 2018;379(21):2040–2051.
36. Reck M, Rodríguez-Abreu D, Robinson AG, Hui R, Csőszi T, Fülöp A, Gottfried M, Peled N, Tafreshi A, Cuffe S, O'Brien M, Rao S, Hotta K, Leiby MA, Lubiniecki GM, Shentu Y, Rangwala R, Brahmer JR; KEYNOTE-024 Investigators. Pembrolizumab versus chemotherapy for PD-L1-positive non-small-cell lung cancer. *N Engl J Med.* 2016;375(19):1823–1833.
37. Ramalingam SS, Vansteenkiste J, Planchard D, Cho BC, Gray JE, Ohe Y, Zhou C, Reungwetwattana T, Cheng Y, Chewaskulyong B, Shah R, Cobo M, Lee KH, Cheema P, Tiseo M, John T, Lin M-C, Imamura F; FLAURA Investigators. Overall survival with osimertinib in untreated, EGFR-mutated advanced NSCLC. *N Engl J Med.* 2020;382(1):41–50.
38. Shaw AT, Bauer TM, de Marinis F, Felip E, Goto Y, Liu G, Mazieres J, Kim D-W, Mok T, Polli A, Thurm H, Calella AM, Peltz G, Solomon BJ; CROWN Trial Investigators. First-line lorlatinib or crizotinib in advanced ALK-positive lung cancer. *N Engl J Med.* 2020;383(21):2018–2029.
39. Patel PH, Palma D, McDonald F, Tree AC. The dandelion dilemma revisited for oligoprogression: treat the whole lawn or weed selectively? *Clin Oncol.* 2019;31(12):824–833.
40. Iyengar P, Hu C, Gomez DR, Timmerman RD, Simone CB II, Robinson CG, et al. NRG-LU002: Randomized phase II/III trial of maintenance systemic therapy versus local consolidative therapy (LCT) plus maintenance systemic therapy for limited metastatic non-small cell lung cancer (NSCLC). *J Clin Oncol.* 2024;42:(16_suppl): 8506.
41. Brown PD, Gondi V, Pugh S, Tome WA, Wefel JS, Armstrong TS, Bovi JA, Robinson C, Konski A, Khuntia D, Grosshans D, Benzinger TLS, Bruner D, Gilbert MR, Roberge D, Kundapur V, Devisetty K, Shah S, Usuki K, et al. Hippocampal avoidance during whole-brain radiotherapy plus memantine for patients with brain metastases: Phase III trial NRG Oncology CC001. *J Clin Oncol.* 2020;38(10):1019–1029.
42. Cheng Y, Spigel DR, Cho BC, Laktionov KK, Fang J, Chen Y, Zenke Y, Lee KH, Wang Q, Navarro A, Bernabe R, Buchmeier EL, Chang J W-C, Shiraishi Y, Goksu SS, Badzio A, Shi A, Daniel DB; ADRIATIC Investigators. Durvalumab after chemoradiotherapy in limited-stage small-cell lung cancer. *N Engl J Med.* 2024;391(14):1313–1327.
43. Simone CB II, Bogart JA, Cabrera AR, Daly ME, DeNunzio NJ, Detterbeck F, Faivre-Finn C, Gatschet N, Gore E, Jabbour SK, Kruser TJ, Schneider BJ, Slotman B, Turrisi A, Wu AJ, Zeng J, Rosenzweig KE. Radiation therapy for small cell lung cancer: an ASTRO clinical practice guideline. *Pract Radiat Oncol.* 2020;10(3):158–173.
44. Slotman BJ, van Tinteren H, Praag JO, Knegjens JL, El Sharouni SY, Hatton M, Keijser A, Faivre-Finn C, Senan S. Use of thoracic radiotherapy for extensive stage small-cell lung cancer: a phase 3 randomised controlled trial. *Lancet.* 2015;385(9962):36–42.
45. Safavi AH, Mak DY, Boldt RG, Chen H, Louie AV. Stereotactic ablative radiotherapy in T1-2N0M0 small cell lung cancer: a systematic review and meta-analysis. *Lung Cancer.* 2021;160: 179–186.
46. Jurkiewicz K, Miciak M, Kaliszewski K. Review of the literature and current state of knowledge on the management of lung neuroendocrine neoplasms. *Clin Cancer Invest J.* 2023;12(6):1–5.
47. Liu B, van Gerwen M, Bonassi S, Taioli E. Epidemiology of environmental exposure and malignant mesothelioma. *J Thorac Oncol.* 2017;12(7):1031–1045.
48. Brims F. Epidemiology and clinical aspects of malignant pleural mesothelioma. *Cancers (Basel).* 2021;13(16):4194.
49. Lim E, Waller D, Lau K, Steele J, Pope A, Ali C, Bilancia R, Keni M, Popat S, O'Brien M, Tokaca N, Maskell N, Stadon L, Fennell D, Nelson L, Edwards J, Tenconi S, Socci L; MARS 2 Investigators. Extended pleurectomy decortication and chemotherapy versus chemotherapy alone for pleural mesothelioma (MARS 2): a phase 3 randomised controlled trial. *Lancet Respir Med.* 2024;12(6):457–466.
50. Hanna GG, John T, Ball DL. Controversies in the role of radiotherapy in pleural mesothelioma. *Transl Lung Cancer Res.* 2021;10(4):2079–2087.
51. Tanvetyanon T, Simon GR. Systemic therapy options for peritoneal mesothelioma. *J Natl Compr Canc Netw.* 2024;22(8):e247031.
52. Baas P, Scherpereel A, Nowak AK, Fujimoto N, Peters S, Tsao AS, Mansfield AS, Popat S, Jahan T, Antonia S, Oulkhouir Y, Bautista Y, Cornelissen R, Greillier L, Grossi F, Kowalski D, Rodríguez-Cid J, Aanur P, Oukessou A, et al. First-line nivolumab plus ipilimumab in unresectable malignant pleural mesothelioma (CheckMate 743): a multicentre, randomised, open-label, phase 3 trial. *Lancet.* 2021;397(10272):375–386.
53. Minervini F, Kocher GJ. When to suspect a thymoma: Clinical point of view. *J Thorac Dis.* 2020;12(12):7613–7618.
54. Markowiak T, Hofmann H-S, Ried M. Classification and staging of thymoma. *J Thorac Dis.* 2020;12(12):7607–7612.
55. Tateishi Y, Horita N, Namkoong H, Enomoto T, Takeda A, Kaneko T. Postoperative radiotherapy for completely resected Masaoka/Masaoka-Koga stage II/III thymoma improves overall survival: an updated meta-analysis of 4746 patients. *J Thoriac Oncol.* 2021;16(4):677–685.

27

Breast Cancer

Ian Kunkler

CHAPTER OUTLINE

ANATOMY

Most of the breast tissue extends from the edge of the sternum to the anterior axillary line and from the second or third to the sixth or seventh costal edge. It overlies the second to the sixth ribs. Breast tissue can be found beyond these areas as high as the clavicle and laterally to the edge of the latissimus dorsi muscle.

The mammary glands are composed of approximately 12 lobes separated by fibrous tissue and surrounded by fat. Each lobe consists of multiple ductulolobular units lined by two layers of cells. The luminal layer is made up of epithelial cells and the outer layer of contractile myoepithelial cells.

Lymphatic Drainage

The principal lymphatic drainage of the breast (Fig. 27.1) is to the axillary nodes lying between the second and third intercostal spaces. Additional drainage occurs to the supraclavicular nodes through the pectoralis major and to the internal mammary chain adjacent to the sternum.

PATHOLOGY

Epidemiology

Worldwide, breast cancer is the most common form of malignancy in females and accounts for 30% of female cancers. The International Agency for Research on Cancer estimates that the incidence in 2020 was 2.6 million cases per year with nearly 685,000 deaths worldwide. This accounts for 36% of all cancers. The highest incidence is in industrialised countries. The highest incidence is in Belgium and the lowest in countries of Southeast Asia and Africa. In the United Kingdom, breast cancer is the most common cancer, accounting for 15% of all new cancers. From 2016 to 2018 in the United Kingdom there were on average 55,920 new cases of breast cancer and 11,499 deaths over the same period (cancerresearchuk.org). In 2018 there were 234,087 new cases of breast cancer. One in eight females in the United Kingdom will develop breast cancer during their lifetime. Nearly half (48%) of breast cancer is diagnosed in females age 65 years or older. The incidence is highest in the United Kingdom in females age 90 years or older. About one-quarter (24%) of new breast cancers occur in females age 75 years or over. Since the early 1990s, the incidence of breast cancer has risen by about one-fifth (19%). It has risen in females and is stable in males. The incidence in the United Kingdom is estimated to rise between 2014 and 2035 to 210 cases per 100,000 females. Unfortunately, mortality from breast cancer in less developed regions is continuing to rise, in part because of lack of access to modern diagnostic facilities and treatment.

Female breast cancer is rare below the age of 30 years. The incidence rises rapidly during the reproductive years. It is lower in younger females (<45 years), but rates are rising. After the age of 50 years, the incidence rises at a lower rate. Male breast cancer is rare in the United Kingdom (370 cases per year from 2016 to 2018), accounting for only 1% of breast cancer cases.

Encouragingly, the mortality of breast cancer is declining in the European Union and the United States, mostly attributed to earlier detection and better systemic treatment. In England and Wales, 78% of females diagnosed with breast cancer survive for 10 years or more and about two-thirds (65%) survive for 20 years or more. Nearly half a million females (491,300) were living with breast cancer in the United Kingdom at the end of 2010. In the United Kingdom, there were about 8838 new cases per year (2016–2018) of ductal carcinoma

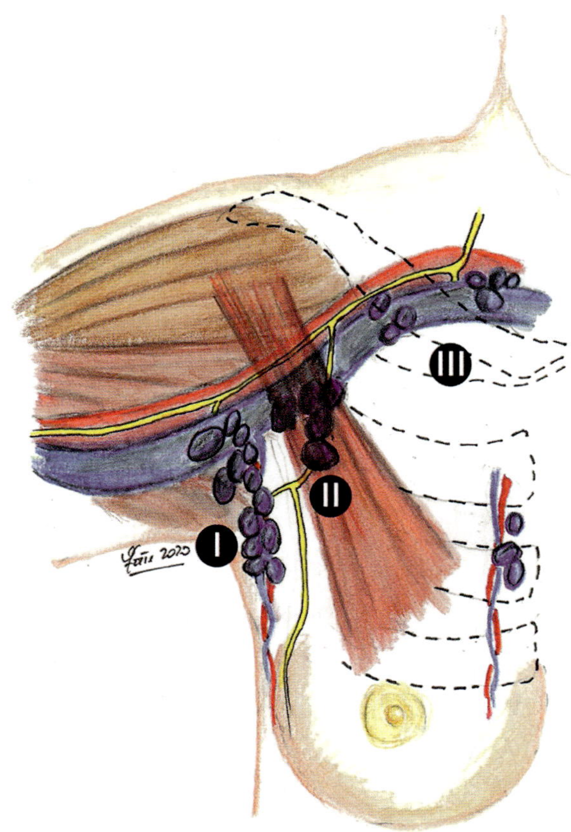

Fig. 27.1 Diagram of lymphatic drainage of the breast showing the position of levels I to III axillary lymph nodes. (Reproduced with permission from Cirocchi R, Amabile MI, De Luca A, et al. New classification of axillary lymph nodes and their anatomical-clinical correlations in breast surgery. *World J Surg Oncol.* 2021;19(1):93.)

TABLE 27.1 Risk Factors for Breast Cancer

Hormonal and reproductive	Early age of the first menstruation Late age of the last menstruation The first reported pregnancy at a late age (after 30 years of age) No pregnancies Postmenopausal condition Use of oral contraception Use of hormone replacement therapy
Related to physiological factors and health status	Older age (increased risk from 35 years of age) Family history of breast cancer Breast, ovarian and endometrial cancer in the past Occurrence of benign changes in the breasts, proceeding with the presence of atypical hyperplasia Ionising radiation, used in connection with, for example, Hodgkin lymphoma therapy Rapid growth in adolescence and high growth in adulthood Infection with an oncogenic virus (e.g. Epstein-Barr)
Nutritional	Western-type diet Excessive consumption of fats, especially animal fats High consumption of red and fried meat High iron intake Development of overweight/obesity after menopause Low consumption of fresh vegetables and fruits Low intake of phytoestrogens (isoflavones, lignans)
Other lifestyle-related	Regular moderate/high alcohol consumption Lack of regular physical activity Night work

From Smolarz B, Nowak AZ, Romanowicz H. Breast cancer-epidemiology, classification, pathogenesis and treatment (review of literature). *Cancers (Basel)* 2022;14(10):2569.

in situ (DCIS), a preinvasive form of breast cancer. The peak rate of DCIS was in females age 65 to 69 years. There has been a 200% rise in the incidence of DCIS since the early 1990s in the United Kingdom, in part because of the development of breast screening programs. Metastatic disease remains a major challenge, with a prevalent population of 57,515 for the period 2020 to 2021 in England, and is almost always fatal within 5 to 10 years. The outcome of metastatic breast cancer has not changed much over the past 20 to 30 years.

Aetiology

The aetiology of breast cancer is not fully understood but involves a complex interaction between a variety of modifiable and nonmodifiable factors and is determined by genetic, environmental, nutritional and hormonal elements. These factors are listed in Table 27.1. More than 90% of breast cancers are the result of sporadic somatic mutations.

Genetic Factors

High-Risk Mutations. It is estimated that 5% to 10% of breast cancers have a genetic basis. Mutations in high-penetrance genes (BRCA1/2) and other genes explain the concentration of cases in high-risk families. Abnormal amplification and mutations of both oncogenes and antioncogenes are involved in the pathogenesis and progression of breast cancer. Nearly 25% of breast cancer cases are related to family history. The sisters and daughters of a female with breast cancer have a threefold increased risk of developing the disease. The risk of breast cancer for a female whose sister is affected is doubled. Females who have a first-degree relative with breast cancer have a 1.75 times higher risk. In females with two or more first-degree relatives with breast cancer, there is a 2.5-fold increased risk of breast cancer. Females with premenopausal or bilateral breast cancer are at a particularly high risk. Multiple germline mutations predispose a female to breast cancer. These include mutations in BRCA1 and BRCA2 (both located on chromosome 17), p53, PTEN, CDH1, CHEK2, PALB2 and ATM. BRCA1 and BRCA2 mutations confer the highest level of risk of breast cancer and also predispose to ovarian cancer. The BRCA1 gene is a suppressor gene that encodes nuclear protein that maintains genomic stability. Its mutations are mainly associated with triple-negative breast cancer (absent oestrogen receptor (ER), progesterone receptor (PgR) and human epidermal growth factor receptor 2 (HER2) expression). Approximately 5% to 10% of all breast cancers and 20% to 25% of all hereditary breast cancers are caused by BRCA1/2 mutations. BRCA1 and BRCA2 genes are inherited in an autosomal-dominant manner. BRCA2 mutations are associated with oestrogen receptor (ER)-positive tumours but have a lower risk of ovarian cancer than BRCA1 mutations. Germline mutations in p53 give rise to the Li-Fraumeni syndrome (childhood sarcomas, brain tumours and early onset breast cancer), and mutations in PTEN give rise to Cowden disease.

The mode of inheritance is usually autosomal dominant with incomplete penetrance. Note that the genetic susceptibility can be passed on by both males and females. Most cases of breast cancer with a genetic basis will have occurred by the age of 65 years. Those at substantial risk include females with:

- Three first- or second-degree relatives with breast or ovarian cancer
- One first-degree relative with bilateral breast cancer
- Two first- or second-degree relatives with breast cancer diagnosed before the age of 60 years or ovarian cancer at any age on the same side of the family

First-degree relatives are mother, sister or daughter. Second-degree relatives are grandmother, granddaughter, aunt or niece. Other features in the family history that increase the risk of breast cancer include male breast cancer and paternal history of breast cancer (two or more relatives on the father's side of the family). The Manchester score should be used to determine referral for genetic testing. The new guidance takes account of cancer subtype. Genetic testing should also be considered for patients with male breast cancer, triple-negative breast cancer before the age of 60, a personal history of ovarian cancer or patients with high-risk ethnic backgrounds such as those of Ashkenazi Jewish heritage. HER2-positive breast cancers carry less risk of BRCA1/2 mutations. Testing is subject to change and its use increasing.

Low-Penetrance Breast Cancer Susceptibility Genes. In sporadic cases, there may be many low-penetrance 'modifier' genes associated with breast cancer. Single-nucleotide polymorphisms (SNPs) explain a large proportion of the risk in females with a strong family history. SNPs also contribute to the development of nonfamilial breast cancer in females, accounting for about 16% of genetic risk. Genome-wide association studies have identified more than 70 variants. Each variant may be associated with a small increased risk for breast cancer in an individual. Modifier genes are found in a number of pathways including steroid metabolism, DNA damage response, immunomodulation and detoxification of environmental carcinogens.

Acquired Factors

Benign Breast Disease. A few benign conditions, specifically atypical ductal hyperplasia or atypical lobular hyperplasia in the breast, increase the risk of breast cancer by four to five times compared to the general population. In females with atypical hyperplasia with a first-degree relative diagnosed with breast cancer, the risk of developing breast cancer is approximately nine times higher.

Risk Factors for Breast Cancer

Menstruation. The epithelium of the breast proliferates during ovulatory cycles. This may be because of the stimulus of either progesterone or oestrogen. This proliferation causes temporary growth of the milk-secreting glandular tissue in preparation for possible pregnancy. If the menarche starts at or after the age of 15 years, there is about a 30% reduction in risk of breast cancer compared to its onset before the age of 12 years. If menstruation continues after the age of 55 years, the risk of breast cancer is doubled compared with a normal menopause at age 45 years. Early menarche and late menopause almost certainly confer an increased risk of breast cancer by prolonging the period in which both breasts are exposed to high levels of oestradiol (and possibly progesterone). Each 1-year delay in menopause increases the risk of breast cancer by 3%.

Oral Contraceptive Pill and Hormone Replacement Therapy. Prolonged use of hormonal contraception increases the relative risk (RR) of breast cancer. The risk is 1.2 to 1.4, with a higher risk the longer the individual took hormonal contraception (1.09 if taken for less than 1 year versus 1.38 if taken for more than 10 years). The RR of breast cancer persisted for at least 5 years in females who took oral contraception for 5 or more years but was not increased if taken for less than 5 years. Oral contraceptives suppress the production of oestradiol and progesterone. Reductions in oestrogen levels may protect against breast cancer. Oral oestrogens, either as the contraceptive pill or as hormone replacement therapy (HRT), may accelerate the development of breast cancer. The absolute risk of developing breast cancer on oral contraceptives is small and is not associated with an increase in mortality. The use of HRT for even a limited period (1–4 years) confers an increased risk of breast cancer. The RR of breast cancer for HRT is 1.66 for current users compared with those who have never used it. Combined therapy for periods of 5 years or more confers a higher risk. The risk of breast cancer falls substantially after 2 years of stopping HRT. Combined HRT both increases the risk of developing breast cancer and increases the chances the cancer will be discovered at a more advanced stage. This is due to its influence in reducing the effectiveness of mammography by creating denser breast tissue. The Women's Health Initiative study concluded that those who take oestrogen only had no increased risk of breast cancer. Taking HRT for more than 10 years more than doubles the risk of breast cancer. There is an excess of invasive lobular cancers in females who develop breast cancer while taking combined HRT.

Pregnancy. The risk of breast cancer in a female rises with her age at first pregnancy. It is three times higher in females who have their first baby over the age of 30 years, compared with those under the age of 18 years.

A first full pregnancy at a young age (e.g. in one's 20s) and later increasing the number of births reduces the risk of breast cancer.

Lactation. Females who have breast-fed their children are slightly less prone to breast cancer. A longer duration of lactation reduces the risk of ER-positive and PgR-positive and –negative breast cancer.

Mammographic Density. Greater density of the breast on mammography is a strong factor in determining breast cancer risk and is seen in both premenopausal and postmenopausal females. Breast density is influenced by both genetic and nongenetic factors.

Diet and Lifestyle. Risk factors for breast cancer at critical times of exposure interact with and impact the normal transformation of the breast, either directly or by modulating the hormonal regulatory environment.

Nutrition and lifestyle may be principally responsible for large variations in breast cancer between countries and marked changes in these rates between migrating populations. Asian females, for example, experience much higher rates of breast cancer after moving to the United States.

Dietary fat, whose effects are mediated by oestrogens, is thought to be a key risk factor for breast cancer. Obesity is particularly associated with breast cancer in postmenopausal females who tend to develop ER-positive breast cancer. In addition, irrespective of menopausal status, obese females have poor clinical outcomes. An increased intake of calories, sugar, alcohol and saturated fats increases the risk of developing breast cancer. Consumption of alcohol increases the incidence of breast cancer in both pre- and postmenopausal females. An intake of 35 to 44 grams of alcohol per day can increase the risk of breast cancer by 32%. The association between smoking and breast cancer is controversial, but the risk of breast cancer is increased (RR 1.54) for females who drink and smoke. There is accumulating evidence that females who start smoking at an early age are at increased risk of breast cancer. Active smoking before a first full-time pregnancy is especially harmful.

Physical Exercise. Physical exercise also appears to have a protective effect against breast cancer in postmenopausal females. The protective effects of physical activity, although the mechanism is unknown, are likely to be through changes in sex hormone levels, immune function, adiposity and insulin-related hormones. Being physically active can change the levels of some hormones, including oestrogen and insulin. Physical activity can lower levels of oestrogen and insulin. High levels of insulin stimulate the production of insulin-like growth factors, which increase breast cancer risk by stimulating cell turnover. Females who are most active have a 12% lower risk of developing breast cancer compared with females who are least active. The more active a female is, the less their risk of breast cancer. The risk of breast cancer falls by 5% for every 2 hours per week a female spends doing moderate to vigorous activity. Even moderate exercise has a protective effect. Benefits are seen in females with and without a family history of breast cancer.

Ionising Radiation. The breast is one of the tissues most sensitive to the induction of malignancy by ionising radiation. Exposure to ionising radiation increases the risk of breast cancer. This is true of females who historically underwent low-dose breast irradiation for benign mastitis. There was a higher risk of breast cancer in females who received radiotherapy (RT) in the past as part of cancer therapy or who underwent control chest radiography for pneumonia or tuberculosis. The risk of breast cancer was highest in females exposed to ionising radiation at a young age.

There is a linear relationship between dose and incidence of breast cancer with doses up to 4 Gray (Gy). Beyond this, the incidence plateaus. It has been calculated that one extra breast cancer per year after 10 years may be caused by radiation from a single mammogram among 2 million females over the age of 50 years. The risk of breast cancer is well validated for females irradiated before the age of 40 years, with an RR of 1.1 to 2.7 at 1 Gy.

Females irradiated in their teenage years by mantle RT for Hodgkin disease, where the mediastinal fields commonly treat the medial part of both breasts, have an increased risk of breast cancer by a factor of 1 in 7 if they were age 20 to 29 years when treated by mantle RT. The risk rises to 50% at the age of 50 years for females treated before age 20 years.

Children irradiated by the atomic bombs dropped on Nagasaki and Hiroshima during World War 2 showed an increased risk of breast cancer with dose.

Ductal Carcinoma In Situ and Lobular Carcinoma In Situ

Breast cancer arises in the terminal duct lobular unit. Premalignant in situ carcinoma can be divided into two types, lobular carcinoma in situ (LCIS) and DCIS, without evidence of penetration on light microscopy of the basement membrane. This classification was based on the belief that LCIS arose from lobules and DCIS from ducts, but this is now known to be incorrect and both arise from the terminal duct lobular unit. DCIS occurs in 25% of breast cancers. There are over 8300 new cases of DCIS per year in the United Kingdom. With the advent of breast screening, the diagnosis of DCIS has increased three to four times and now accounts for 20% of screen-detected cancers. Some 90% of DCIS cases are confined to one segment of the breast. DCIS is a heterogeneous disease based on histology, genetic alterations and clinical course, and controversy exists over which lesions require treatment (Van Seijen et al., 2019). Whether it is preinvasive or noninvasive, DCIS is often included in the definition (stage 0) of breast cancer. It is characterised as a proliferation of neoplastic luminal cells limited to the ductolobular system of the breast. DCIS has the potential to progress to invasive cancer, with DCIS cells invading the basement membrane and the parenchyma. A number of different mechanisms have been suggested. In the independent lineage model, in situ and invasive populations originate from different lineages. In the convergent phenotype model, different genotypes of DCIS may lead to the same phenotype of invasive cancer. In the evolutionary bottleneck model, it is proposed that only a subpopulation of cells with particular genetic features are able to overcome an evolutionary bottleneck and invade the parenchyma. In the multiclonal invasion model, many clones of DCIS have the capacity to escape through the ducts and become invasive. It is possible therefore that DCIS might become invasive by one or more of these mechanisms.

Mutations in the TP53, PIK3CA and GATA3 genes have been linked to aggressive forms of DCIS. TP53 mutations are specifically associated with high-grade DCIS. Most of the genetic alterations seen in DCIS are also seen in invasive cancer, which often accompanies DCIS. DCIS differs from invasive cancer in the higher prevalence of HER amplification (34% versus 10%–15%). The pathway of development of low- and intermediate-grade DCIS is thought to differ from that of high-grade disease. Low-grade DCIS shows a loss in the 17q chromosome, whereas high-grade DCIS often shows a 17q gain. The immune environment plays an important role in determining the risk of progression of DCIS. A strongly active immune signature is associated with lesions at the highest risk.

DCIS is categorised as low grade, intermediate grade or high grade based on combinations of architecture, cell morphology and the presence of necrosis. Untreated high-grade DCIS has the highest progression to invasive breast cancer.

There are two principal histological types: comedo and noncomedo. The most common noncomedo types are solid, cribriform, papillary and micropapillary. More than 90% of cases of DCIS present asymptomatically, with malignant calcifications at screening mammography. Only 75% of all DCIS lesions contain calcification, so mammography commonly underestimates the extent of the disease. Magnetic resonance imaging (MRI) is more effective at detecting multifocality and detecting cancers that are mammographically occult. Other presentations are Paget disease of the nipple, nipple discharge or a lump. Core biopsy is able to establish a diagnosis in 90% of screen-detected cases. DCIS is associated with a substantial risk of progression to invasive carcinoma, with a mean delay of about 7 years. It is estimated that 14% to 53% of DCIS cancers progress to invasive cancer. However, progression is not inevitable, is not orderly and does not occur within a predictable timescale.

Lobular Carcinoma In Situ

LCIS is associated with an increased risk of invasive cancer in both breasts, particularly infiltrating ductal carcinoma of no special type at a rate of 1% to 2% per year. Initial treatment for LCIS is active surveillance to monitor for progression of LCIS to invasive disease.

Invasive Breast Cancer

Malignant tumours mainly arise from the glandular epithelium (adenocarcinomas). Breast cancers are classified as 'of no special type' or 'of special type'. The majority (80%) are of no special type. The histological types of breast cancer are listed in Table 27.2.

TABLE 27.2 Classification of Invasive Breast Cancer

1. No special type
2. Special type
   a. Tubular
   b. Mucoid
   c. Cribriform
   d. Papillary
   e. Medullary
   f. Classic lobular

Invasive cancers have traditionally been classified by their microscopic appearance and by histological grade. Grading is based on nuclear pleomorphism, degree of glandular formation and frequency of mitoses. The Bloom-Richardson system of grades 1, 2 and 3 from least to most malignant is widely adopted (Fig. 27.2). Grading yields useful prognostic information. Both disease-free survival and overall survival are shorter for high-grade cancers.

If an excess of 25% of the main tumour mass contains noninvasive (in situ) disease, and if in situ disease is present in the adjacent breast tissue, the tumour is described as having an *extensive in situ component*. Such patients were previously thought to be at risk of developing invasive cancer elsewhere in the breast and were formerly not suitable for breast conservation. This is no longer true, and such patients can be treated by breast-conserving surgery.

Lymphatic or vascular invasion within the tumour confers an increased risk of local and distant recurrence.

Inflammatory carcinomas are typified by an oedematous and erythematous breast and are often associated with an ill-defined underlying mass. Histologically, there is often tumour infiltration of the subdermal lymphatics, and the prognosis is poor. In contrast, medullary carcinoma is slow growing and has a much better prognosis.

Lobular invasive carcinomas were formerly thought to have a higher incidence of bilaterality and of multicentricity. Studies have shown that most invasive lobular cancers are clonal and not more commonly truly multicentric nor more often bilateral. Paget disease of the nipple is commonly associated with an underlying ductal adenocarcinoma.

MOLECULAR CLASSIFICATION OF BREAST CANCER

Breast cancer is a very heterogeneous disease. There are at least four different molecular subtypes of breast cancer: luminal A and B, HER2 enriched and basal-like. These subtypes can be determined on formalin-fixed paraffin-embedded samples either using a multigene assay or indirectly reconstructed with immunochemically measured steroid receptors: ER, PgR and HER2 status in addition to proliferation status assessed by Ki67. Although there is significant overlap between the intrinsic subtypes and immunohistochemistry, there are some that differ. For example, not all basal types are triple negative and not all luminal-A tumours are ER and PR positive. Luminal breast cancers are generally ER positive and constitute about 70% of all cases of breast cancer in western populations. The luminal-A subtype is usually ER or PgR positive or both and HER2 negative and with low Ki67. The luminal B-like subtype is ER positive and/or PgR positive and HER2 negative and usually has a higher histological grade and a worse prognosis than luminal-A tumours. The HER2 subtype is HER2 positive and ER and PgR negative and makes up 15% to 20% of breast cancers. A more recent classification is HER2 low. HER2-low tumours account for 50% to 60% of all breast cancers. HER2-low tumours have immunohistochemistry scores of 1 to 2, an HER2-positive sore of 3 or more and an HER2 negative score of 0. The basal-like subtype is HER2 negative and

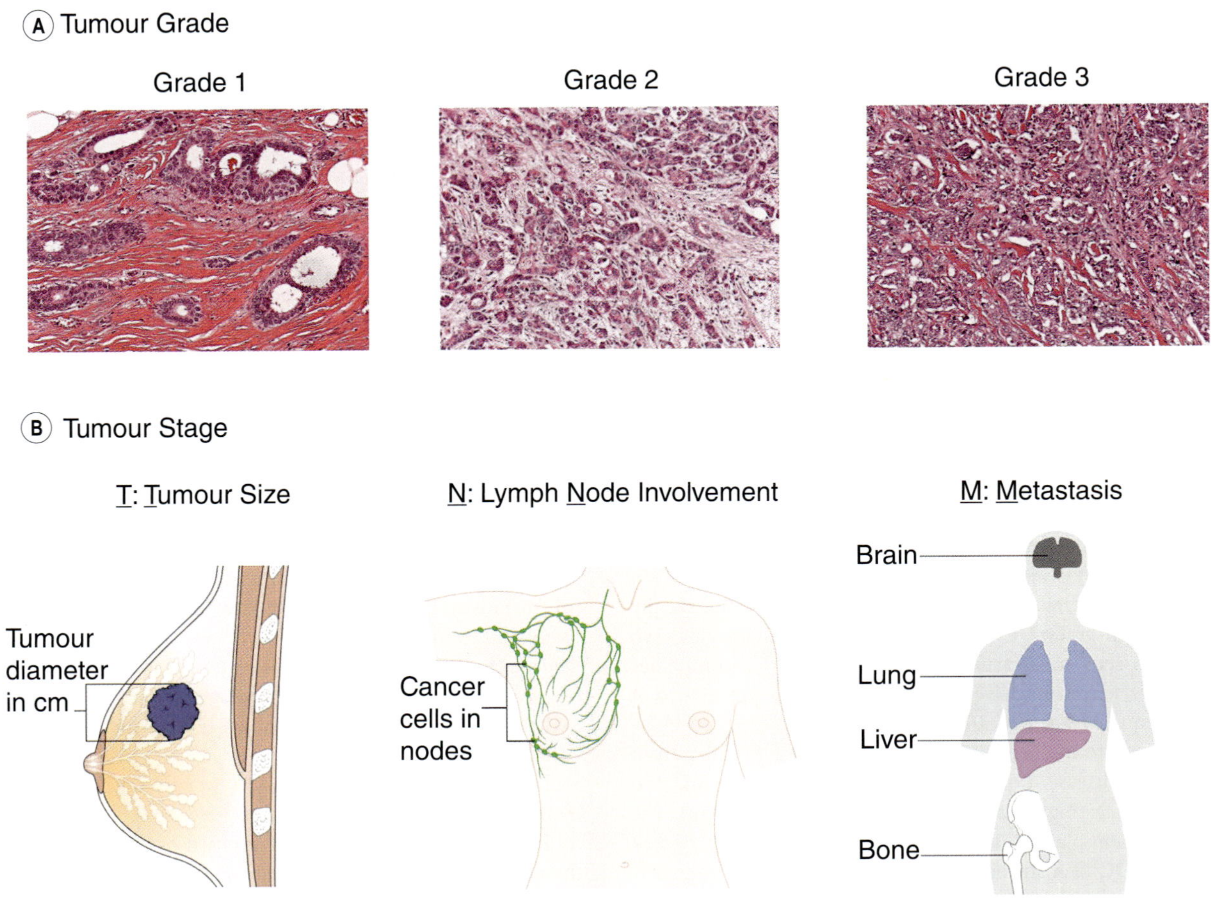

Fig. 27.2 Conceptual overview of tumour grading and staging. (From Lal S, McCart Reed AE, de Luca XM, Simpson PT. Molecular signatures in breast cancer. *Methods*. 2017;131:135–146.)

ER and PgR negative (triple negative) and represents 15% to 20% of breast cancers. The characteristics of the molecular subtypes are shown in Fig. 27.3.

The 50-gene signature PAM50 can reliably classify breast cancer into the main intrinsic subtypes with 93% accuracy and is the basis of the Prosigna test. The latter combines the PAM50 assay with clinical information to assess the risk of distant relapse in postmenopausal females with hormone receptor (HR)-positive, node-negative or node-positive early breast cancer and the need for adjuvant chemotherapy.

MULTIDISCIPLINARY MANAGEMENT OF BREAST CANCER

Patients with suspected breast cancer or recurrent disease should be referred to a specialist breast unit for assessment and treatment. The requirements of a specialist breast centre are summarised in the European Society of Breast Cancer Specialists guidelines (2020) (Biganzoli et al., 2020). The management plan (sequence and timing of staging investigations, pathology, imaging and selection of therapy) should be formulated within a multidisciplinary team (surgeons, medical and clinical oncologists, radiologists, pathologists and specialist nurses). The multidisciplinary team should meet weekly to discuss preoperative and postoperative cases with recurrent or metastatic disease. Comorbidities, quality of life and the patient's wishes should be taken into account. Practice should be evidence based and recorded in national/local written protocols and standards against which compliance should be regularly audited. Decision aids and support of patients by patient advocates and specialist nurses may facilitate shared decision-making.

DIAGNOSIS

The patient may notice a lump on their breast on routine or casual self-examination. Sometimes it is detected as part of a clinical examination for other reasons or as a result of routine examination in hospital or detected on mammographic screening.

Breast Screening

Results from eight randomised trials have shown that breast screening mammography reduces breast cancer mortality by at least 20%. Standard screening mammography will detect two to eight cancers per 1000 mammograms. Digital breast tomosynthesis increases this yield by 1.6 cancers per 1000 mammograms. Screening by ultrasound, especially in females with dense breasts, detects a further 4.4 cancers per 1000 screening examinations. However, the positive predictive value of ultrasound is only 3% to 8%. Screening by MRI has a high sensitivity of 90% to 93% compared to 48% to 63% for mammography and ultrasound combined in trials of asymptomatic females at high risk of breast cancer.

The National Health Service (NHS) breast screening program by mammography (Fig. 27.4) in the United Kingdom started in 1988. All eligible females age 50 to 70 years are invited for screening every 3 years. From 2021 to 2022, 62.3% of females age 50 to 71 years took up their invitation to breast screening. This was below the standard of 70%. Uptake was adversely affected by the COVID-19 pandemic. Detection rates were highest for small invasive cancers (3.4 per 1000 females) and lowest for noninvasive or microinvasive cancers (1.9 per 1000 females). Detection rates were lowest for females age 45 to 49 years (5.6 per 1000) and highest for females age 71 years or over (16.8 per 1000). Small

Molecular subtype	Luminal A	Luminal B	HER2	TNBC
ER/PR	+		–	
HER2	–	+		–
Frequency[a]	50%–60%	30%	10%	10%–20%
Grade[b]	Low		High	
Prognosis[c]	Good		Poor	
5-y survival rate[d]	94.3%	90.5%	84.0%	76.9%
Treatment	Endocrine therapy			
		Anti-HER2 therapy		
	Chemotherapy			

Fig. 27.3 Characteristics of breast cancer molecular subtypes. *ER*, Estrogen receptor; *HER2*, human epidermal growth factor receptor 2; *PR*, progesterone receptor; *TNBC*, triple-negative breast cancer. *a*, Frequency derived from Al-thoubaity FK. Molecular classification of breast cancer: a retrospective cohort study. *Ann Med Surg (Lond)* 2019;49:44–48; Hergueta-Redondo M, Palacios J, Cano A, Moreno-Bueno G. "New" molecular taxonomy in breast cancer. *Clin Transl Oncol.* 2008;10(12):777–785. *b*, Grade derived from Engstrøm MJ, Opdahl S, Hagen AI, et al. Molecular subtypes, histopathological grade and survival in a historic cohort of breast cancer patients. *Breast Cancer Res Treat.* 2013;140(3):463–473. *c*, Prognosis derived from Hennigs A, Riedel F, Gondos A, et al. Prognosis of breast cancer molecular subtypes in routine clinical care: A large prospective cohort study. *BMC Cancer.* 2016;16(1):734; Fragomeni SM, Sciallis A, Jeruss JS. Molecular subtypes and local-regional control. *Surg Oncol Clin N Am.* 2018;27(1):95–120. *d*, Five-year survival rate derived from latest survival statistics of SEER Cancer Stat Facts: Female Breast Cancer Subtypes (https://seer.cancer.gov/statfacts/html/breast-subtypes.html). (Reproduced with permission from Burguin A, Diorio C, Durocher F. Breast cancer treatments: updates and new challenges. *J Pers Med.* 2021;11(8):808.)

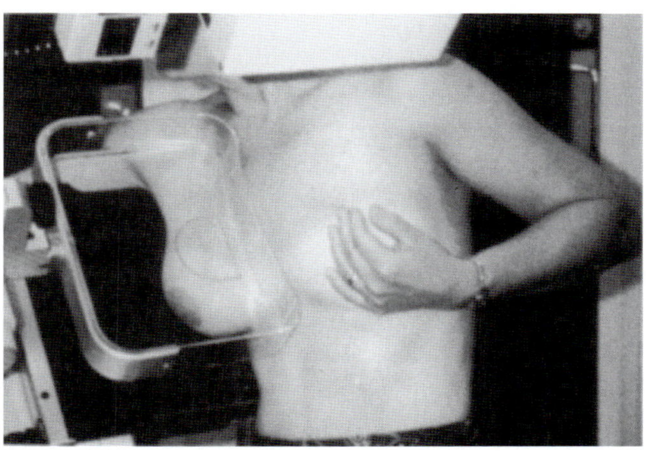

Fig. 27.4 Patient undergoing mammography. (Courtesy Rotherham Breast Screening Service.)

cancers (less than 15 mm in diameter) accounted for 47.8% of those with invasive cancer. It is estimated that, assuming the reduction in mortality continued for 10 years after breast screening ended, for every 235 females invited for screening, one breast cancer death would be prevented (i.e. 43 breast cancer deaths per 10,000 females invited for screening). Overdiagnosis is difficult to estimate (i.e. where females have their cancer treated by surgery, RT and systemic therapy, but it is unknown whether or not the cancer would have become clinically overt during their lifetime). The best estimate of overdiagnosis in the screened population is about 11% (defined as excess incidence in the screened population as a proportion of the long-term suspected incidence).

In addition, some females experience pain on mammography. About 4% of females screened are recalled for further mammography and sometimes biopsy. A clear explanation is required for patients about the risks and benefits of breast screening.

The vast majority (99%) of patients with screen-detected breast cancer will have surgery: 70% postoperative RT, 70% endocrine therapy and 25% chemotherapy. Each treatment has its attendant morbidities, including adverse psychological effects.

Features suggestive of malignancy on mammography are small microcalcifications, stellate opacities with strands extending into the surrounding tissues (Fig. 27.5) or distortion of architecture. The sensitivity of mammography is reduced in dense breasts seen in younger females. Mammography may also show enlarged nodes in the axilla. About 15% of cancers are mammographically occult, and nearly 4% are neither palpable nor visible on mammography.

The benefits of breast screening in reducing breast cancer deaths have to be balanced against the harms of false-positive recall. Overdiagnosis, that is, detection of screen-detected cancers that would not have been detected clinically over a female's lifetime, is the most serious harm because it would probably lead to overtreatment.

Clinical Assessment

Triple assessment is required (history and examination; breast imaging (usually mammography and ultrasound) and core biopsy of suspicious lesions). A full history is required, including details of breast-related symptoms, particularly breast pain, nipple discharge, changes noted in the skin (erythema, dimpling) or shape of the breast, indrawing or distortion of the nipple, axillary lumps and systemic symptoms of weight loss, anorexia, nausea, vomiting, bone pain, breathlessness, headache or motor or sensory disturbance. A full menstrual history should be taken including onset of menarche, menopause, parity, age of first pregnancy, breast-/bottle-feeding and use of the contraceptive pill and HRT. Family history of breast and ovarian cancer should be collected

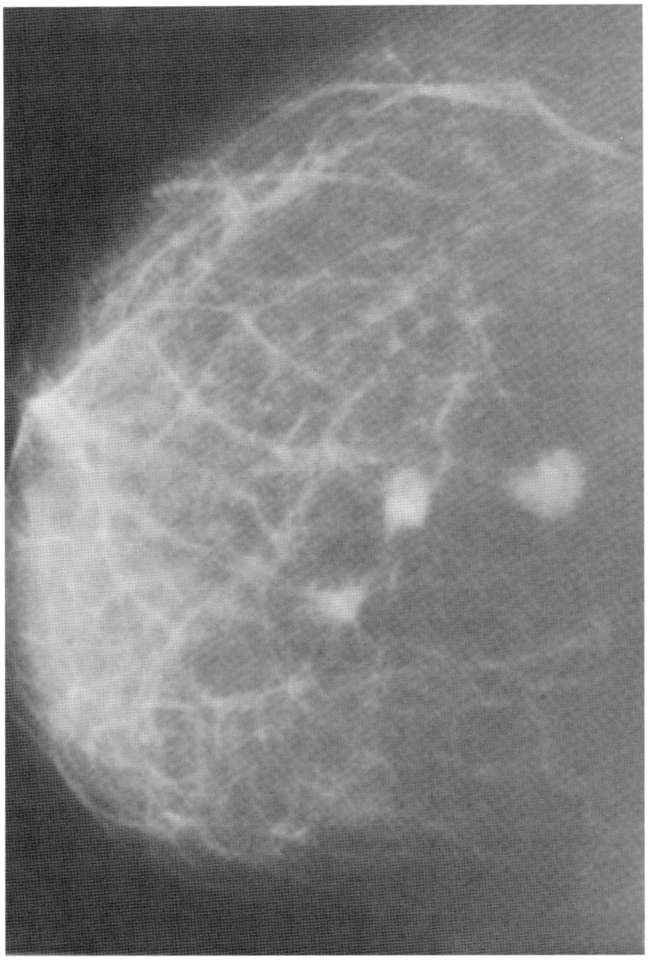

Fig. 27.5 Mammogram showing three spiculated tumours in the breast. (Courtesy Dr R. Peck, Sheffield, UK.)

and recorded, and in families with multiple members on either the paternal or maternal side of the family, consideration should be given to calculating a Manchester score.

Breast Ultrasound

Ultrasound of the breast has an important role in helping to distinguish benign from malignant lesions, particularly when mammography is normal or equivocal. Malignant tumours tend to show an irregular echo-poor pattern (Fig. 27.6A) compared with the smooth outline of a benign fibroadenoma (Fig. 27.6B). Colour Doppler ultrasound may show changes caused by increased tumour vasculature both in primary tumours and lymph nodes. Both the breast and the regional nodes should be imaged.

Magnetic Resonance Imaging

MRI should be available in the preoperative assessment of biopsy-proven invasive breast cancer. It is recommended when there is a discrepancy between the extent of local disease based on clinical examination, mammography and ultrasound (e.g. in invasive lobular breast cancer). It may have an important role in the assessment of (1) the local extent of the primary tumour; (2) multifocality in younger females where the density of the breast is often a limiting factor to the resolution of mammography; (3) familial cases of breast cancer with BRCA mutations; and (4) breast implants. MRI may show 10% to 30% additional invasive cancer in patients presenting with a unifocal lesion. However, MRI may lead to an overestimation of the size of lesions, potentially resulting in unnecessary mastectomies. MRI results

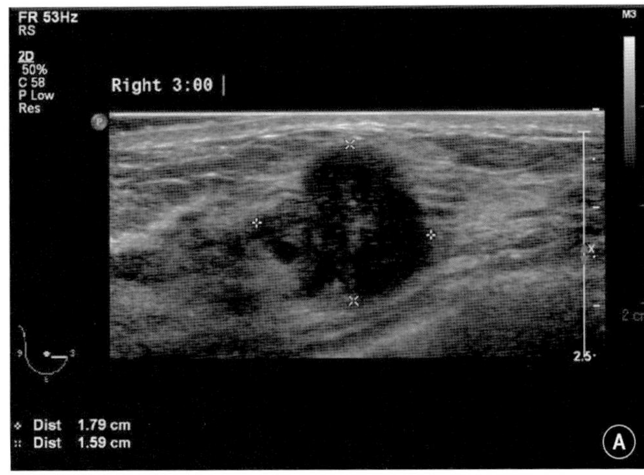

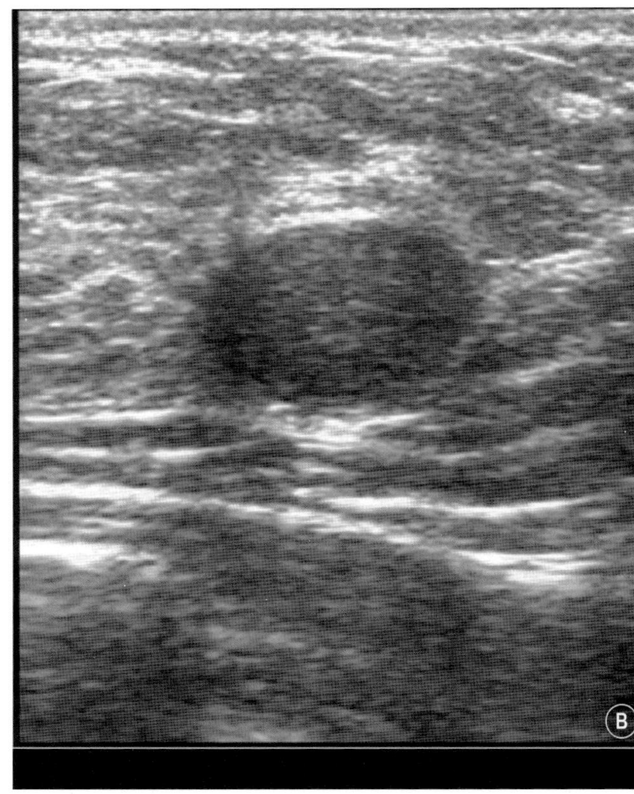

Fig. 27.6 Ultrasound of the breast showing an irregular mass lesion characteristic of a cancer (A) compared with well-defined margins of benign fibroadenoma (B). (Reproduced with permission from Dixon JM (Ed.), *ABC of Breast Diseases* (4th ed.). Chichester. Wiley Blackwell; 2012.)

in false-positive findings in 10% to 15% of patients. Biopsy should be considered where a lesion appears on MRI alone. MRI may also show recurrent cancer in the breast (Fig. 27.7).

Positron Emission Tomography

Positron emission tomography (PET) has a role in excluding metastases. Positron emission tomography-computed tomography (PET/CT) scanning is based on the uptake of fluorine-18. Its resolution is only 5 to 6 mm, so it cannot identify very small lesions. PET may generate false positives with metabolic uptake in inflammatory or other non-malignant conditions. Its advantages are that it may show responses to neoadjuvant systemic therapy earlier than computed tomography (CT) or MRI and may show regional or distant metastases (e.g. bone metastases) not detected on other imaging in patients at high risk of

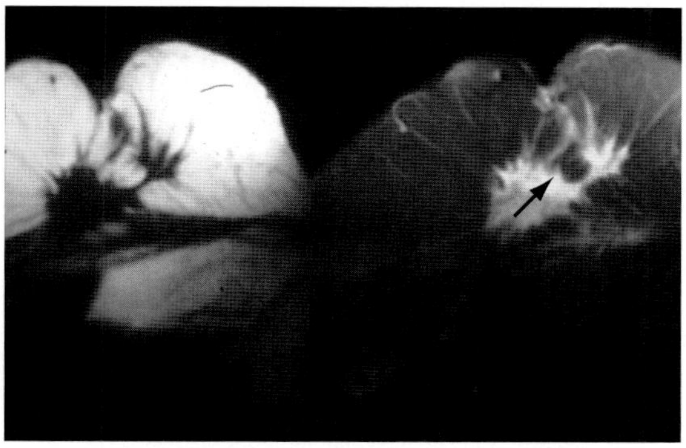

Fig. 27.7 Magnetic resonance imaging scan showing recurrent cancer in the breast. (Courtesy Prof J.M. Dixon, Edinburgh Breast Unit.)

recurrence, as well as locally advanced and inflammatory breast cancer. In addition, it may provide clarity where other imaging is equivocal.

Obtaining a Histological Diagnosis

It is important to obtain a histological diagnosis of breast cancer to confirm suspicious clinical or radiological features. If the tumour is palpable (usually ≥1 cm), core biopsy under local anaesthetic is recommended; stereotactic image-guided core biopsy is recommended for impalpable lesions. Tumour from core biopsy should be stained for ER, PgR and HER2 status and graded. Core needle biopsy is essential if preoperative systemic therapy is planned and a clip inserted to ensure accurate removal of the original tumour-bearing area. Fine needle aspiration cytology (FNAC) does not make a reliable distinction between invasive and in situ disease but is helpful in the diagnosis and treatment of breast cysts. Suspicious axillary lymph nodes should be examined histologically or cytologically.

STAGING

Staging is important to assess the local, regional and metastatic spread of breast cancer because management may differ significantly depending on the extent of the disease. Staging involves clinical, radiological and sometimes laboratory assessment. The simplest clinical staging system that is still in use is shown in Table 27.3. However, the TNM classification of the International Union Against Cancer (Table 27.4) has gained widespread acceptance.

TABLE 27.3 Clinical Staging of Breast Cancer

Stage	Clinical Findings
1	Freely movable (on underlying muscle); no suspicious nodes
2	As stage 1 but mobile axillary node(s) on the same side
3	Primary more extensive than stage 1, e.g. skin invaded wide of the primary mass or fixation to muscle. Axillary nodes, if present, are fixed; or supraclavicular nodes involved.
4	Extension beyond the ipsilateral chest wall area, e.g. opposite breast or axilla; or distant metastases.

Staging Investigations

For patients with T1–2, N0, M0 disease, a full blood count, liver biochemistry and chest radiograph are usually recommended. For patients with (1) T3 or T4 tumours, (2) N1–3 or MI or (3) T0–2, N0 disease with symptoms that could be caused by metastatic disease (e.g. unexplained bone pain or weight loss), a CT scan of the chest and abdomen and a bone scan are recommended.

All patients with locally recurrent disease following mastectomy (Figs. 27.8 and 27.9) or breast-conserving therapy or those with regional or metastatic recurrence require a CT scan of the chest, abdomen and pelvis.

MANAGEMENT OF DUCTAL CARCINOMA IN SITU

Given the uncertainties about which DCIS lesions will progress to invasive cancer, there is a risk that some patients whose DCIS lesions may never progress are being overtreated (Van Seijen et al., 2019). Complete surgical excision remains the core treatment. Surgical options are breast-conserving surgery or mastectomy. Controversy therefore remains on

TABLE 27.4 TNM Classification of Breast Cancer (8th Edition)

Stage T Primary Tumour	Clinical Findings
TX	Primary tumour cannot be assessed.
T0	No evidence of primary tumour
TiS	Carcinoma in situ
TiS (DCIS)	Ductal carcinoma in situ (DCIS)
TiS (LCIS)	Lobular carcinoma in situ (LCIS)
TiS (Paget)	Paget disease of the nipple not associated with invasive carcinoma and/or (Paget) carcinoma in situ (DCIS and/or LCIS) in the underlying breast parenchyma. Carcinomas in the breast parenchyma associated with Paget disease are categorised based on the size and characteristics of the parenchymal disease, although the presence of Paget disease should still be noted.
T1	Tumour ≤2 cm in greatest dimension
T1mi	Microinvasion ≤0.1 cm in greatest dimension
T1a	>0.1 cm but <0.5 cm in greatest dimension
T1b	>0.5 cm but <1 cm in greatest dimension
T1c	>1 cm but <2 cm in greatest dimension
T2	>2 cm but <5 cm in greatest dimension
T3	>5 cm in greatest dimension
T4	Tumour of any size with direct extension to chest wall and/or to skin (ulceration or skin nodules)
T4a	Extension to chest wall (does not include pectoralis muscle invasion only)
T4b	Ulceration, ipsilateral satellite skin nodules or skin oedema (including peau d'orange)
T4c	Inflammatory carcinoma

(continued)

TABLE 27.4 TNM Classification of Breast Cancer (8th Edition)—cont'd

Stage T Primary Tumour	Clinical Findings
Regional Lymph Nodes	
NX	Regional lymph nodes cannot be assessed (e.g. previously removed)
N0	No regional lymph node metastases
N1	Metastases in ipsilateral level I, II axillary lymph nodes
N2	Metastases in ipsilateral level I, II axillary lymph node(s) that are clinically fixed or matted; or in clinically detected[a] ipsilateral internal mammary lymph node(s) in the absence of clinically evident axillary lymph node metastasis
N2a	
N2b	
N3	Metastasis in axillary lymph node(s) fixed to one another (matted) or to other structures
N3a	Metastasis only in clinically detected[a] internal mammary lymph node(s) and in the absence of clinically detected axillary lymph node metastasis
N3b	
N3c	Metastasis in ipsilateral infraclavicular (level III axillary) lymph node(s) with or without level I, II axillary lymph node involvement; or metastasis in ipsilateral supraclavicular lymph node(s) with or without axillary or internal mammary lymph node involvement
	Metastasis in infraclavicular lymph node(s)
	Metastasis in internal mammary and axillary lymph nodes
	Metastasis in supraclavicular lymph node(s)
M Distant Metastasis	
M0	No distant metastases
M1	Distant metastases
pTNM Pathological Classification	
pT: Primary Tumour The pathological classification requires the examination of the primary carcinoma with no gross tumour at the margins of resection. A case can be classified pT if there is only a microscopic tumour in a margin. The pT categories correspond to the T categories.	Note: When classifying pT, the tumour size is a measurement of the invasive component. If there is a large in situ component (e.g. 4 cm) and a small invasive component (e.g. .5 cm), the tumour is coded pT1a.
pN: Regional Lymph Nodes The pathological classification requires the resection and examination of at least the low axillary lymph nodes (level I). Such a resection will ordinarily include six or more lymph nodes. If the lymph nodes are negative, but the number ordinarily examined is not met, classify as pN0.	
pNX	Regional lymph nodes cannot be assessed (e.g. previously removed, or not removed for pathological study)
pN0	pN0 No regional lymph node metastasis[b]
pN1 larger than 2.0 mm	No regional lymph node metastasis[b]
pN1mi	Micrometastases; or metastases in one to three axillary ipsilateral lymph nodes; and/or in internal mammary nodes with metastases detected by sentinel lymph node biopsy but not clinically detected[b]
pN1a	
pN1b	Micrometastases (0.2 mm–2 mm and/or >200 cells)
pN1c	Metastasis in one to three axillary lymph node(s), including at least one larger than 2 mm in greatest dimension
	Internal mammary lymph nodes
	Metastasis in one to three axillary lymph nodes and internal mammary lymph nodes
pN2 pN2a Metastasis in four to nine axillary lymph nodes, including at least one that is larger than 2 mm	Metastasis in four to nine ipsilateral axillary lymph nodes, or in clinically detected[b] ipsilateral internal mammary lymph node(s) in the absence of axillary lymph node metastasis Metastasis in clinically detected internal mammary lymph node(s), in the absence of axillary lymph node metastasis
pN2b pN3	
pN3a	Metastasis in 10 or more ipsilateral axillary lymph nodes (at least one larger than 2 mm) or metastasis in infra-clavicular lymph nodes
pN3b	
pN3c	Metastasis in clinically detected[b] internal ipsilateral mammary lymph node(s) in the presence of positive axillary lymph node(s); or metastasis in more than three axillary lymph nodes and in internal mammary lymph nodes with microscopic or macroscopic metastasis detected by sentinel lymph node biopsy but not clinically detected
	Metastasis in ipsilateral supraclavicular lymph node(s)

(continued)

TABLE 27.4 TNM Classification of Breast Cancer (8th Edition)—cont'd

Stage T Primary Tumour	Clinical Findings
Posttreatment ypN:	
Posttreatment yp 'N' should be evaluated as for clinical (pretreatment) 'N' methods (see 'Regional Lymph Nodes' section). The modifier 'sn' is used only if a sentinel node evaluation was performed after treatment. If no subscript is attached, it is assumed that the axillary nodal evaluation was by axillary node dissection.	
The X classification will be used (ypNX) if no yp posttreatment sn or axillary dissection was performed.	
N categories are the same as those used for pN.	

[a]Clinically detected is defined as detected by clinical examination or by imaging studies (excluding lymphoscintigraphy) and having characteristics highly suspicious for malignancy or a presumed pathological macrometastasis based on fine needle aspiration biopsy with cytological examination. Confirmation of clinically detected metastatic disease by fine needle aspiration without excision biopsy is designated with an (f) suffix, e.g. cN3a(f).

[b]Isolated tumour cell clusters (ITCs) are single tumour cells or small clusters of cells not more than 0.2 mm in greatest extent that can be detected by routine H and E stains or immunohistochemistry. An additional criterion has been proposed to include a cluster of fewer than 200 cells in a single histological cross section. Nodes containing only ITCs are excluded from the total positive node count for purposes of N classification and should be included in the total number of nodes evaluated.

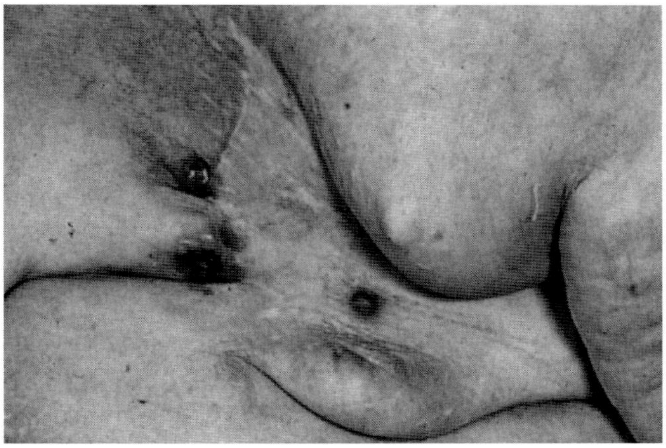

Fig. 27.8 Nodular local recurrence on the skin flaps of a mastectomy scar.

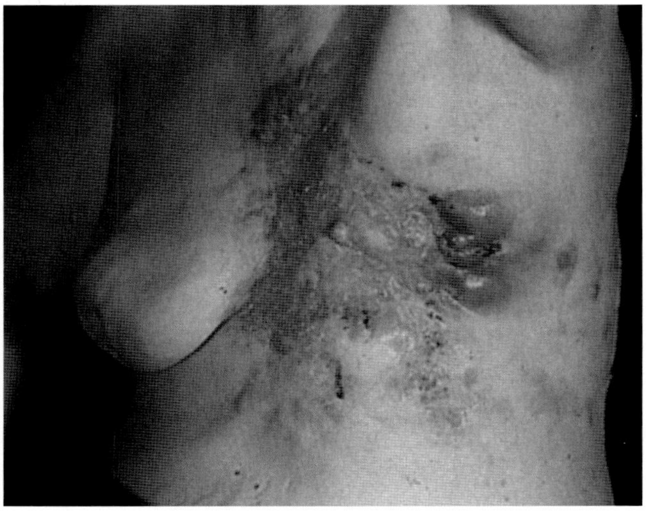

Fig. 27.9 Widespread nodular recurrence over left chest wall following mastectomy, extending to the other breast.

which patients can be kept under surveillance alone after breast-conserving surgery and which need adjuvant RT or endocrine therapy.

With adequate therapy, 99% of patients will survive following treatment. Where the prognosis is good, the morbidities associated with particular treatments (particularly from RT) need to be carefully weighed against the benefits of treatment. A palpable mass should undergo core biopsy. Impalpable malignant calcifications should be biopsied by stereotactic wire localisation. Paget disease of the nipple should undergo punch biopsy. Microdochectomy or total ductal excision should follow a smear of nipple discharge for malignant cells.

The rationale for mastectomy or whole breast irradiation as treatment for DCIS is related to the potential for multicentric disease and/or the presence of occult invasive cancer. Multifocal disease in the same quadrant is not unusual in patients with DCIS. Following wide excision and negative margins, 24% to 43% of patients will have residual DCIS in the same quadrant. Mastectomy remains the treatment of choice for multicentric DCIS and for large unicentric lesions too extensive for breast-conserving surgery. Recurrence rates (invasive and DCIS) after mastectomy are usually less than 1%, with a 5-year median follow-up. Regular mammography of the contralateral breast should be carried out because there is an increased rate of contralateral breast cancer of 2% to 11% over a lifetime. If the extent of the lesion is not more than 3 to 4 cm, an attempt at conservative surgery may be made, aiming to achieve complete excision.

ROLE OF POSTOPERATIVE RADIOTHERAPY FOR DUCTAL CARCINOMA IN SITU

The risk of recurrence (both DCIS and invasive) is reduced by about one-half with postoperative RT (for which the standard dose fractionation is 40 Gy in 15 fractions over 3 weeks or 26 Gy in 5 fractions over 1 week to the whole breast) for all grades of DCIS. However, the absolute benefits in low-grade disease are very small. Four randomised trials have assessed the impact of postoperative RT after breast-conserving surgery for DCIS (NSABP B-17, European Organisation for Research and Treatment of Cancer (EORTC) 10853, UK/ANZ and SweDCIS) (Table 27.5). All employed 50 Gy in 25 daily fractions over 5 weeks without a boost dose to the site of excision. All showed a reduction in DCIS and invasive recurrence. Pooled data from these trials in a Cochrane review showed that RT halved the risk of recurrence

TABLE 27.5 Summary of Four Reported Prospective Randomised Trials that Have Evaluated the Benefit of Adding Radiation Treatment after Lumpectomy for Ductal Carcinoma In Situ[a]

				IPSILATERAL LOCAL RECURRENCE, %			
Study	**No. of Patients**	**Follow-up**	**Outcome**	**Lumpectomy without RT**	**Lumpectomy with RT**	**Decrease with RT**	***P***
NSABP B-17 Wapnir et al. (1)	813	>12 y median	Cumulative incidence at 12 y	32.9	15.8	52	<.05
EORTC 10853 Bijker et al. (2)	1010	10.5 y median	Actuarial at 10 y	26	15	42	<.0001
Swedish Trial Holmberg et al. (3)	1046	8 y mean	Cumulative incidence at 12 y	32[b]	16[b]	50	<.05
UK/ANZ Trial[c] Houghton et al. (4)	1030	4.4 y median	Crude incidence	13.6	5.6	59	<.0001

[a]EORTC = European Organisation for Research and Treatment of Cancer; NSABP = National Surgical Adjuvant Breast and Bowel Project; RT = radiation treatment; UK/ANZ = United Kingdom, Australia, and New Zealand.

[b]Estimated from curves.

[c]The UK/ANZ trial used a 2 × 2 factorial design evaluating excision (lumpectomy) ± radiation ± tamoxifen. The data given in table are limited to the analysis of radiation treatment.

From Solin LJ. The impact of adding radiation after breast conserving surgery for ductal carcinoma in situ. *J Nat Cancer Inst.* 2010;41:187–192.

References
1. Wapnir I, Dignam J, Julian TB, et al. Longterm outcomes after invasive breast tumor recurrenve (IBTR) in women with DCIS in NSABP B-17 and B-24 (abstract 520). *J Clin Oncol.* 2007;25 (suppl):7s.
2. Bijker N, Peterse JL, Duchateau L, et al. Risk factors for recurrence and metastasis after breast-conserving therapy for ductal carcinoma-in-situ: ten-year results of European Organisation for Research and Treatment of Cancer randomized phase III trial 10853. *J Clin Oncol.* 2006;24:3381–3387.
3. Holmberg L, Garmo H, Grandstrand B, et al. Absolute risk reductions for local recurrence and metastasis after post-operative radiotherapy after sector resection for ductal carcinoma in situ of the breast. *J Clin Oncol.* 2008;26:1247–1252.
4. Houghton J, George WD, Cuzick J, et al. Radiotherapy and tamoxifen in women with completely excised ductal carcinoma in situ of the breast in the UK, Australia, and New Zealand: randomised controlled trials. *Lancet.* 2003;362:95–102.

after breast-conserving surgery at 10 years. About half the recurrences were DCIS and half invasive. In the Cochrane review, older patients (>50 years) derived more benefit from RT than younger patients. The addition of RT to breast-conserving surgery did not affect overall or breast cancer-specific survival. None of the trials, however, were prospectively designed for subgroup analysis. International practice varies with all grades of DCIS following breast-conserving surgery and clear margins being treated by postoperative RT in some Western countries. In the United Kingdom, practice tends to be more selective, with postoperative RT confined to higher-grade tumours. The definition of a truly low-risk group that could be safely treated by breast-conserving surgery alone has proven difficult to determine. Studies suggest that even in apparently low-risk patients, the overall risks of invasive recurrence may be up to 10% to 20% at 15 years. In a population-based cohort of 10,090 females from the Netherlands between 1989 and 2004, 15 years after DCIS diagnosis the cumulative incidence of invasive breast cancer was 1.9% after mastectomy, 8.8% after breast-conserving surgery and RT and 15.4% after breast-conserving surgery alone (Elshof et al., 2016). A biological signature in combination with clinical data (DCISionRT) may identify patients with DCIS who benefit from RT, but its clinical utility is uncertain.

The role of a boost dose (16 Gy in 8 fractions) after breast-conserving surgery and whole breast irradiation has been studied in the BIG 3.07 DCIS boost trial. This trial also compared standard dose fractionation (50 Gy in 25 daily fractions over 5 weeks) to hypofractionation (42.5 Gy in 16 daily fractions over 3.5 weeks) in nonlow-risk DCIS. Eligibility criteria were at least one of the following risk factors: age younger than 50 years, symptomatic presentation, palpable tumour, microscopic tumour size 15 mm or larger, multifocal disease, intermediate or high nuclear grade, central necrosis, comedo histology or radial margin smaller than 10 mm or a combination. There was an absolute gain in local control from a tumour bed boost of 4.4% at 5 years (92.7% in the no-boost group and 97.1% in the boost group). The boost group had a rate of grade 2 or higher breast pain and induration. Hypofractionated RT was shown to be as safe and effective as conventionally fractionated radiation. A tumour boost is recommended for nonlow-risk DCIS after breast-conserving surgery and clear margins of at least 1 mm.

There is no indication for axillary dissection or irradiation of the peripheral lymphatics in DCIS, because the risk of positive axillary nodes is 4% or less.

Endocrine Therapy for DCIS

There are wide international variations in the use of adjuvant endocrine therapy for ER-positive DCIS. Some would argue this is overtreatment for a localised disease with an excellent prognosis. The role of adjuvant tamoxifen following breast-conserving surgery has been studied in two placebo randomised controlled trials (NSABP and UK/ANZ). In the NSABP trial, tamoxifen reduced invasive recurrence. In the UK/ANZ trial, only recurrent DCIS was reduced. Tamoxifen had no impact on overall survival in either trial. Despite these trial results, in the United Kingdom, tamoxifen is rarely given for DCIS (in contrast to the United States, where nearly half of patients with ER-positive DCIS receive tamoxifen), because it is associated with deep vein thrombosis, menopausal symptoms and endometrial cancer. Anastrozole, an alternative to tamoxifen, can cause arthralgia, vaginal dryness, hypercholesterolaemia and menopausal symptoms.

Prognosis of DCIS

The overall prognosis of DCIS is excellent, with more than 97% of patients alive and disease free 10 or more years following diagnosis. The 20-year mortality rate from DCIS is about 3.3%. Patients with low-grade DCIS have a superior breast cancer-specific survival rate compared to intermediate and high-grade lesions.

PROGNOSTIC AND PREDICTIVE FACTORS FOR INVASIVE BREAST CANCER

The prognosis for breast cancer in the United Kingdom has substantially improved over the past 3 decades. Five-year survival is now 85%

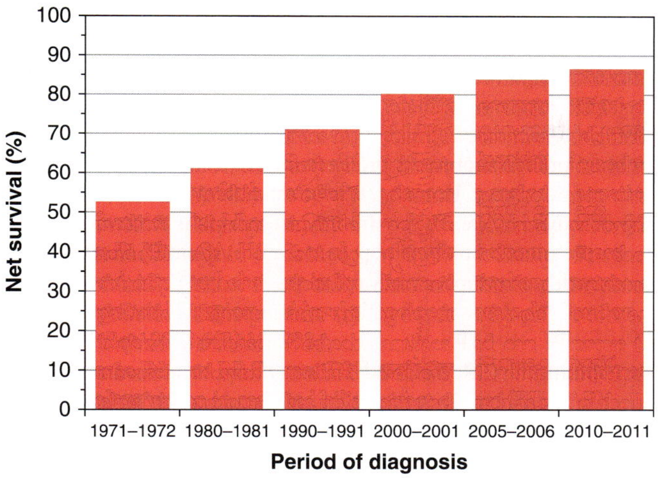

Fig. 27.10 Breast cancer: Age-standardised 5 year net survival, women aged 15–99, in England and Wales. (Reproduced with permission from Cancer Research UK, cancerresearchuk.org)

compared with about 50% in the 1970s (Fig. 27.10), and 75.9% of patients survive 10 years or more. The following are the main prognostic factors.

Stage

Prognosis is excellent for stage 1 disease at diagnosis, with 98% 5-year survival, falling progressively to 15% for stage 4. The St. Gallen Breast Cancer Consensus has established three well-accepted categories of risk (Table 27.6). These are defined by age, axillary node status, histological and/or nuclear grade, presence or absence of lymphovascular invasion and HER2 status.

TABLE 27.6 St. Gallen Breast Cancer Consensus Risk Categories

Low risk	Node negative AND all of the following features: Primary tumour (pT) ≤2 cm, AND Grade 1 AND Absence of extensive peritumoral vascular invasionΔ, AND HER2/neu gene neither overexpressed nor amplified◊, AND Age ≥35
Intermediate risk	Node negative AND at least one of the following features: Primary tumour (pT) >2 cm, OR Grade 2–3, OR Presence of extensive peritumoural vascular invasionΔ, OR Oestrogen receptor (ER) and progesterone receptor (PR) absent HER2/neu gene overexpressed or amplified, OR Age <35 years Node positive (1–3 involved nodes) AND ER and/or PR expressed AND HER2/neu gene neither overexpressed nor amplified
High risk	Node positive (1–3 involved nodes) AND ER and PR absent or HER2/neu gene overexpressed or amplified Node positive (4 or more involved nodes)

Δ, Extensive peritumoral vascular invasion (i.e. neoplastic emboli seen in two or more blocks of the tumour) was a recognised discriminating feature of increased risk; its presence defined intermediate-risk for node-negative disease but did not influence risk category for node positive.

◊, HER2/neu overexpression or amplification must be determined by quality-controlled assays using immunohistochemistry or FISH analysis.

Age

Age is an independent prognostic factor. Females age 35 years or younger have a higher risk of locoregional recurrence and distant relapse. Tumours in females younger than age 35 years are more likely to be high grade, ER and PgR negative and HER2 positive. These females are more prone to local recurrence, being diagnosed at an advanced stage and having a lower 5-year survival compared with older premenopausal patients. Encouragingly, the rates of local recurrence in young females with breast cancer are falling. Adjuvant systemic therapy and a radiation boost to the tumour bed after whole breast irradiation reduce the risk of recurrence by 50%. A study from the Netherlands of 1000 females with nonmetastatic breast cancer younger than age 35 years showed that the 5-year risk of local breast recurrence was 3.2%, and 3.8% for chest wall recurrence after mastectomy.

Tumour Size

Tumour size is a strong independent prognostic factor for overall and recurrence-free survival. A positive correlation has been found between tumour size and the number of involved axillary lymph nodes. The St. Gallen Breast Cancer Consensus Panel classifies tumours larger than 2 cm as intermediate or high risk, even where there are no other adverse prognostic factors.

Axillary Node Status

Nodal status is the strongest independent prognostic factor in breast cancer. If the axillary nodes are not involved, the 5-year survival rate is 98%. If the nodes are involved, the 5-year survival rate falls to 84%. There is a direct correlation between the number of involved nodes and survival. Nodal micrometastases or isolated tumour cells in lymph nodes should not influence risk allocation.

Tumour Grade

Tumour grade remains an important prognostic factor, with significantly better survival for grade 1 compared with grades 2 and 3. The Gene Expression Grade Index is able to classify grade 2 lesions into two groups at high and low risk of recurrence. There is uncertainty as to the role of grade 2 in defining intermediate-risk prognosis. Unfortunately, 50% of patients fall into the grade 2 category.

HER2/Neu Status

HER2 status is both a prognostic and predictive factor in breast cancer. The HER2 gene regulates a protein on the surface of cells that promotes their growth (see the 'HER2-Positive Breast Cancer' section). In patients with HER2-positive breast cancer, the cancer cells make too many copies of, or overexpress, the HER2 gene. HER2 protein overexpression or gene amplification is an adverse prognostic factor. HER2 expression is seen in 15% to 20% of breast cancers and is associated with a higher risk of recurrence and shorter survival.

HER2-Low Breast Cancer

HER2-low breast cancer is a recently defined subset of HER2-negative breast cancers that has an HER2 immunohistochemical (IHC) score of 1+, a score of 2+, or an in situ hybridisation (ISH)-negative phenotype. HER2 low is considered to represent 45% to 55% of breast cancers. It is more common in HR-positive breast cancer (43%–67%). In advanced breast cancer, its incidence ranges from 35% to 63%. The biology of HER2-low breast cancer is poorly understood and seems to represent a subset of breast cancers with considerable heterogeneity. Most HER2-low tumours are of the luminal molecular subtype, have a low Ki67 proliferation index and are less responsive to neoadjuvant chemotherapy, with a pathological complete response (pCR) rate between 9% and 36%. It is unclear whether HER2-low breast cancer is a distinct biological/clinical subgroup or what prognostic significance it has. HER2-low expression has been shown to be highly unstable during disease progression.

Lymphovascular Invasion

Lymphovascular invasion is an adverse prognostic factor in axillary node-negative disease. There are conflicting results as to whether or not it is a poor prognostic factor in axillary node-positive disease.

Tumour Infiltrating Lymphocytes

Tumour infiltrating lymphocytes (TILs) in the tumour and in the stroma carry a good prognosis and are predictive of response to chemotherapy.

PIK3CA Mutations

PIK3CA mutations have been shown to predict response to PI3kinase inhibitors in ER-positive, HER2-negative metastatic breast cancer.

Prognostic Indices

PREDICT (http://www.predict.nhs.uk/) is an online tool for patients with early-stage breast cancer to predict prognosis and benefits from adjuvant chemotherapy, endocrine therapy and trastuzumab. Based on a breast cancer patient's clinical features, PREDICT provides standardised 5- and 10-year survival estimates displayed in easy-to-follow charts.

Hormone Receptor Status

HR status is both a prognostic and predictive factor in breast cancer. About 70% to 75% of invasive breast cancers are ER positive. At least 1% of ER-positive cancer is required for hormonal therapy. ER is the only established predictive marker for response to endocrine therapy. PgR is expressed in more than 50% of ER-positive tumours but rarely in ER-negative tumours. ER status is moderately prognostic and highly predictive of response to hormonal therapy. PgR status is strongly prognostic but weakly predictive of response. ER and PgR status have been validated with level I evidence.

Ki67

The Ki67 protein represents proliferation status and predicts sensitivity to chemotherapy. However, it is not standardised and is not widely used in standard care. The commonly used cutoff is 20%. Ki67 is moderately prognostic but weakly predictive of response, and there is no level I evidence to support its validation.

Molecular Subtype

IHC staining for ER, PgR and HER2 is used to approximate breast cancer molecular subtype (Fig. 27.3). Molecular subtype is prognostic of overall survival, with the best outcomes for luminal A and the worst for basal subtype. Luminal-B tumours have an intermediate prognosis.

MOLECULAR PROFILING IN BREAST CANCER MANAGEMENT

Multigene assays (Fig. 27.11) are used to individualise chemoendocrine therapy in ER-positive, HER2-negative early breast cancer (Lal et al., 2017). The available 21-gene assay (Oncotype DX) and the 70-gene assay (MammaPrint) quantify products of a reverse transcriptase chain reaction for key genes involved in the development of breast cancer. They are incorporated into an algorithm that estimated likely benefit from systemic chemotherapy. Data from the TAILORx and RxPONDER trials demonstrate that most patients with zero to three involved axillary nodes derive no advantage from systemic chemotherapy. Patients with ER-positive, HER2-negative, node-negative early breast cancer with a low genomic score can avoid neoadjuvant

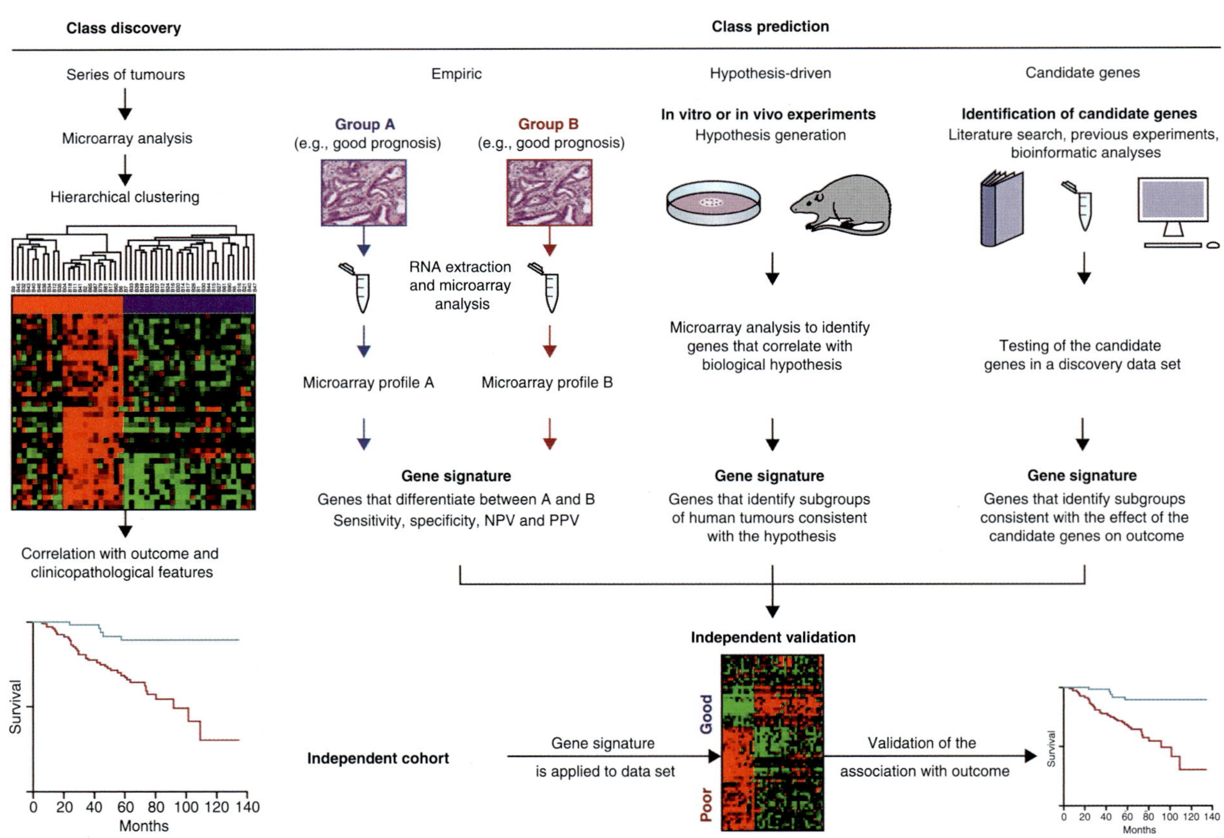

Fig. 27.11 Class discovery and class prediction analysis of microarray-based gene expressing profiling data. (Reproduced with permission from Reis-Filho JS, Pusztai L. Gene expression profiling in breast cancer: classification, prognostication and prediction. *Lancet.* 2011;378(9805):1812–1823.)

or adjuvant chemotherapy. The role of Oncotype DX and MammaPrint in patients with one to three positive nodes remains controversial.

Using the 70-gene signature in the MINDACT trial, patients judged to have low genomic risk and high clinical risk had similar distant metastasis-free survival regardless of application of chemotherapy.

Prosigna and EndoPredict gene expression signatures provide prognostic information on patients with ER-positive, HER2-negative disease treated with endocrine therapy. These assays provide information on risk of late as well as early relapse and so are useful in selection of patients for extended adjuvant endocrine therapy. Finally, gene expression signatures have no role in decision-making for very low-risk disease (e.g. pT1a-b, pN0, grade 1 or strongly ER positive) or if all clinicopathological factors imply low risk or high risk, respectively.

Progress in identification of molecular signatures to predict benefit from adjuvant RT is much less advanced, and none are sufficiently validated for clinical application.

ENDOCRINE THERAPY

Endocrine therapy is based on blocking the effects of oestrogen, which stimulates tumour growth or inhibits its production. Oestrogen passes through the cell membrane and binds ER alpha, one of the two species of ER, to ligand, leading to phosphorylation and transcription. Most of the oestrogen is sited in the nucleus, but some probably exists in the cell membrane where it may interact with growth factors. Activation of membrane ER by either oestrogen or tamoxifen and the ensuing activation of growth factor signalling may be a cause of tamoxifen resistance in certain patients who overexpress HER2. It is possible that a combination of ER-targeted therapy and growth factor receptor-targeted therapy might reverse tamoxifen resistance. Cross talk between growth factor receptor pathways and ER might elucidate the relationship between PgR expression and response to a variety of hormone therapies. As a result of an active growth factor kinase cascade, the transcription of the PgR gene may be inhibited. Hence, in some tumours, PgR negativity may be a surrogate for active growth factor signalling. This would suggest that ER-positive, PgR-negative tumours would respond better to aromatase inhibition than to selective oestrogen receptor modulators (SERMs), as in HER2-positive tumours. Indeed, the ATAC trial showed better outcomes in PgR-negative tumours with anastrozole than tamoxifen. There are accumulating data that ER-positive, PgR-negative tumours are a discrete subset, with a tendency to higher growth factor receptor activity, relative resistance to SERMs and greater sensitivity to aromatase inhibitors such as anastrozole and letrozole.

ER status is predictive for disease-free and overall survival. Irrespective of stage, ER positivity predicts for longer disease-free and overall survival. Higher recurrence and lower survival rates are found in ER-negative patients. The PgR status may also help. Oestrogen stimulates PgR production in normal reproductive tissue and in human breast cancer cell lines. The highest response and disease-free survival rate is seen in ER-positive, PgR-positive tumours. Very few tumours are ER negative and PgR positive, consistent with the production of PgRs being dependent on oestrogen synthesis. The lowest response and disease-free survival rates are seen in ER-negative, PgR-negative tumours.

MASTECTOMY OR BREAST CONSERVATION FOR INVASIVE BREAST CANCER

Historical Background

Radical mastectomy and postoperative RT was the standard local treatment for early breast cancer up to the 1970s based on the Halstedian hypothesis in 1907 that breast cancer spread in an orderly way from the primary site to the regional nodes. The Halsted mastectomy involved removal of the breast and as much of the peripheral lymphatics as possible. Lymphatic spread was considered of critical import and spread via bloodstream largely unappreciated. The Halsted radical mastectomy carried substantial physical and psychological morbidity. The Halstedian hypothesis was challenged by the Fisher hypothesis in the 1970s that dissemination of breast cancer was a systemic disease at the time of diagnosis, even when there was only evidence of locoregional disease. This paradigm was modified by the Spectrum hypothesis of Hellman in 1994 (Hellman, 1994), which stated that breast cancer was a heterogeneous disease varying from one that remained locoregional throughout its course to systemic when first detectable. The concept of breast-conserving surgery was proposed by Sir Geoffrey Keynes, a surgeon working at St. Bartholomew's Hospital. In a small series of 250 patients using interstitial radium needles, he showed in 1937 that clinical outcomes were no different to the standard surgical approach. However, his approach was ignored until tested by studies of breast-conserving surgery and postoperative whole breast irradiation in France by Calle at the Institut Curie in Paris in the 1960s. Subsequent trials confirmed that breast-conserving surgery could achieve similar clinical outcomes to mastectomy with less morbidity without compromising overall survival.

CURRENT SURGICAL PRACTICE FOR EARLY BREAST CANCER

Breast-conserving surgery remains the standard of care for most cases of early breast cancer. When considering the possibility of breast-conserving surgery, the ratio between the tumour size and the breast volume, mammographic appearance or histology from excision or core biopsy is important. Tumours in excess of 3 cm have previously been considered unsuitable for breast-conserving therapy unless the breast size is sufficiently large to allow adequate excision. Greater flexibility in offering breast conservation is now possible with the availability of newer oncoplastic surgical techniques to reshape the breast or fill the tissue defect from local excision by a fat graft or a perforator flap. Preoperative systemic therapy with chemotherapy or hormonal therapy, as appropriate, can also allow sufficient tumour shrinkage for breast-conserving surgery rather than mastectomy. Patients who have clinical or radiological evidence of multifocal disease or have an extensive intraduct component (EIC) are now also candidates for breast conservation. Involved margins after breast-conserving surgery should be reexcised. Mastectomy may be required if it is not possible to clear the margins. Patients should be fully involved in the decision-making process.

There is evidence that local recurrence rates following breast-conserving surgery are higher in younger females. Females under age 35 years have a higher risk of local recurrence after breast-conserving surgery and RT. This may in part be because of the difficulty of identifying cancers by mammography in younger females who tend to have more radiodense breasts or the more aggressive biology of the disease in younger females.

Invasive Lobular Cancer

Lobular cancer is commonly classified as multifocal, although most are clonal so are likely to be unifocal. They are poorly visualised by mammography and often have higher reexcision rates. Breast-conserving surgery is usually possible, but mastectomy is often required as many invasive lobular cancers are large at diagnosis. It is also associated with a classical pattern of metastatic spread that differs from other breast cancer subtypes, with a higher rate of metastatic disease involving the pleura, the peritoneum and the gynaecological and gastrointestinal (GI) tracts.

Prophylactic Surgery for Hereditary Breast Cancer

Whether females with BRCA1 and BRCA2 mutations can be treated by mastectomy or breast-conserving surgery remains controversial. The cumulative risk of contralateral breast cancer 20 years after a breast cancer diagnosis in a cohort of 3886 patients was 40% for BRCAI mutation carriers and 26% for BRCA2 carriers. Local recurrence is more common in the first 5 to 7 years after primary therapy, particularly in triple-negative breast cancer, which commonly occurs in BRCA1 mutation carriers. There are no prospective randomised trials comparing mastectomy and breast-conserving therapy in BRCA carriers. Overall, the evidence suggests no increase in the risk of true local recurrence in BRCA mutation carriers. However, there is an increased risk of new cancers in the conserved breast. While contralateral mastectomy reduces the risk of development of breast cancer, its impact on survival is unclear. While it is the case that there is an increased risk of a second primary cancer in the ipsilateral breast and contralateral breast in BRCA mutation carriers, bilateral mastectomy, while frequently advised and carried out, is not mandatory. The risks for the patient should be individualised, taking into account the type of BRCA mutation, age of the patient, risk of death from the index cancer and effect of therapy employed for the treatment of the index case on the risk of a subsequent cancer. BRCA mutation status should be known prior to surgery. In patients with triple-negative breast cancer, neoadjuvant chemotherapy can be started while awaiting genetic testing and counselling. Most patients with known BRCA mutations opt for bilateral mastectomy.

When considering contralateral prophylactic mastectomy in BRCA mutation carriers, one should take into consideration that there is also a significantly increased risk of ovarian cancer (Morrow, 2022).

Reconstruction After Mastectomy

Mastectomy is a mutilating operation, but much can be achieved in remodelling the breast by use of autologous tissue or implants. Most patients should be offered the possibility of immediate breast construction, if locally available.

Conservation Therapy (Limited Surgery and Postoperative Radiotherapy)

In patients with T1 and small T2 tumours (≤5 cm), some form of local surgery should be considered. The most popular choice is a wide local excision to obtain clear histological margins (typically at least 1–2 mm). If the margins are found to be involved, a reexcision to clear the margins by at least 1 mm is recommended. If reexcision of the margins still shows the tumour at the margin, further reexcision or mastectomy should be considered.

A variety of oncoplastic techniques are available to allow larger resections while maintaining the natural shape of the breast. Reduction mammoplasty is possible in small- and medium-sized breasts. Criteria for breast conservation are summarised in Table 27.7.

TABLE 27.7 Criteria for Breast-Conserving Therapy

1. Tumours ≥3 cm
2. Satisfactory cosmetic result anticipated
3. Postoperative whole breast radiotherapy technically feasible
4. Medically fit for surgery
5. Clear histological margins at primary excision or reexcision
6. Able to attend regular clinical and mammographic follow-ups

Local Recurrence After Breast-Conserving Therapy

The treatment of choice for local recurrence after breast-conserving surgery and postoperative RT is a mastectomy. A second breast-conserving procedure is not often commonly offered to females who have recurrences or who develop second cancers in the treated breast many years after the index cancer. A recent metaanalysis showed no detriment to overall survival by a second breast-conserving procedure.

POSTOPERATIVE RADIOTHERAPY

Dosage and Fractionation

Whole Breast and Postmastectomy. The development of shortened (hypofractionated) dose fractionation schedules (Table 27.8) has been

TABLE 27.8 Patient and Treatment Characteristics in Four Randomised Trials Testing Hypofractionated Radiotherapy After Surgery for Early Breast Cancer

	START P[1]	START A[2]	START B[3]	Ontario[4]
Years accrual	1986–1998	1998–2002	1999–2001	1993–1996
Total number of patients	1410	2236	2215	1234
Standard arm (Gy/fr/weeks)	50/25/5	50/25/5	50/25/5	50/25/5
Test arm A (Gy/fr/weeks)	42.9/13/5	41.6/13/5	40.0/15/5	42.5/16/3.1
Test arm B (Gy/fr/weeks)	39/13/5	39/13/5	NA	NA
Mean age (years)	54.5	57.2	57.4	Not reported
Node+ (%)	32.7	28.8	22.8	0
Mastectomy (%)	0	15	8	0
Tumour size (%)	42.5[a]	48.6[b]	35.9[b]	20.0[b]
Boost (%)	74.5	60.6	42.6	0
Chemotherapy (%)	13.9	35.5	22.2	11
Regional radiotherapy (%)	20.6	14.2	7.3	0

[a]Clinical T-stage.

[b]Pathological stage.

Reproduced with permission from Yarnold J. Pushing the frontiers of radiobiology: a special feature in memory of Sir Oliver Scott and Professor Jack Fowler. Changes in radiotherapy fractionation-breast cancer. *Br J Radiol.* 2019;92:20170849.

References
1. Yarnold J, Ashton A, Bliss JM, et al. Fractionation sensitivity and dose response of late adverse effects in the breast after radiotherapy for early breast cancer: long-term results of a randomised trial. *Radiother Oncol.* 2005;75:9–17.
2. Bentzen SM, Agrawal RK, Aird EG, et al. The UK standardisation of breast radiotherapy (START) trial A of radiotherapy hypofractionation for treatment of early breast cancer: a randomised trial. *Lancet Oncol.* 2008;9:331–341.
3. Bentzen SM, Agrawal RK, Aird EG, et al. The UK standardisation of breast radiotherapy (START) trial B of radiotherapy hypofractionation for treatment of early breast cancer: a randomised trial. *Lancet.* 2008;371:1098–1107.
4. Whelan T, Mackenzie R, Julian J, et al. Randomized trial of breast irradiation schedules after lumpectomy for women with lymph node-negative breast cancer. *J Natl Cancer Inst.* 2002;94:1143–1150.

TABLE 27.9 Rates of Local Tumour Relapse in Four Randomised Trials Testing Hypofractionated Radiotherapy After Surgery for Early Breast Cancer

Trial	Randomisation (Gy/fraction)	% 5-Year Local Relapse (95% CI)	% 10-Year Local Relapse (95% CI)
START P[1,2]	50.0/25	7.9 (5.4–10.4)	12.1 (8.8–15.5)
	42.9/13	7.1 (5.4–10.4	9.6 (6.7–12.6
	39.0/13	9.1 (6.4–11.7)	14.8 (11.2–9.2)
START A[2,3]	50.0/25	3.4 (2.3–5.1)	6.7 (4.9–9.2)
	41.6/13	3.1 (2.0–4.7)	5.6 (4.1–7.8)
	39.0/13	4.4 (3.1–6.2)	8.1 (6.1–10.7)
START B[2,4]	50.0/25	3.3 (2.4–4.6)	5.2 (2.7–5.2)
	40.0/15	1.9 (1.2–3.0)	3.8 (2.7–5.2)
Ontario[5]	50.0/25	3.2[a]	6.7[b]
	42.5/16	2.8[a]	6.2[b]

[a]Absolute difference 0.4% (95% CI (–1.5 to +2.4%))

[b]Absolute difference 0.5% (95% CI (–2.5 to +3.5%))

CI, Confidence interval.

Reproduced with permission from Yarnold J. Pushing the frontiers of radiobiology: a special feature in memory of Sir Oliver Scott and Professor Jack Fowler. Changes in radiotherapy fractionation-breast cancer. *Br J Radiol.* 2019;92:20170849.

References

1. Owen JR, Ashton A, Bliss J, et al. Fractionation sensitivity and dose response of late adverse effects in the breast after radiotherapy for early breast cancer: long-term results of a randomised trial. *Radiother Oncol.* 2005;75:9–17.
2. Haviland JS, Owen JR, Dewar JA, et al. The UK stardardisation of breast radiotherapy (START) trials of radiotherapy hypofractionation for treatment of early breast cancer: 10-year follow up results of two randomised trials. *Lancet Oncol.* 2013;14:1086–1094.
3. Bentzen SM, Agrawal RK, Aird EG, et al. The UK standardisation of breast radiotherapy (START) trial A of radiotherapy hypofractionation for treatment of early breast cancer: a randomised trial. *Lancet Oncol.* 2008;9:331–341.
4. Bentzen SM, Agrawal RK, Aird EG, et al. The UK standardisation of breast radiotherapy (START) trial B of radiotherapy hypofractionation for treatment of early breast cancer: a randomised trial. *Lancet.* 2008;371:1098–1107.
5. Whelan TJ, Pignol JP, Levine MN, et al. Long-term results of hypofractionated radiation therapy for breast cancer. *N Engl J Med.* 2010;362:513–520.

a major trend in the deescalation of adjuvant RT for breast cancer supported by level I evidence from clinical trials. The European Society for Radiotherapy and the Oncology Advisory Committee in Radiation Oncology Practice provide useful guidelines on patient selection and dose and fractionation for external beam radiotherapy (Meattini et al., 2022). Historically, the empirical standard dose and fractionation regimen following breast-conserving surgery and mastectomy was 50 Gy in 25 fractions of 2 Gy over 5 weeks.

It was hypothesised that breast cancer may be as sensitive as late-reacting tissues to fraction size. Accordingly, hypofractionation should not be disadvantageous for breast cancer as long as the total dose is appropriately reduced. Indeed, hypofractionation may be advantageous in local control by minimising accelerated tumour repopulation. Total dose has to be reduced to compensate for nonlinear increase in normal tissue and anticancer effects, more particularly, for late-reacting normal tissues than for self-renewal tissues.

TABLE 27.10 Clinically Assessed Moderate or Marked Adverse Effects for Patients Treated by Breast Conservation Surgery in Four Randomised Trials Testing Hypofractionated Radiotherapy

Trial	Randomisation (Gy/Fraction	% Breast Shrinkage at 10 Years (95% CI)	% Excellent or Good Breast Cosmesis at 10 Years (95% CI)
START pilot	50.0/25	63.8	
	42.9/13	74.4	
	30.0/13	58.0	
START A	50.0/25	34.2 (29.9–39.2)	
	41.6/13	31.4 (27.2–36.0)	
	39.0/13	30.0 (25.7–34.8)	
START B	50.0/25	31.2 (27.9–34.9)	
	40.0/15	26.2 (23.1–29.6	
Ontario	50.0/25		71.3[a]
	42.5/16		69.8[a]

[a]Absolute difference 1.5%(95% CI (–6.9 to +9.8))

CI, Confidence interval.

Reproduced with permission from Yarnold J. Pushing the frontiers of radiobiology: a special feature in memory of Sir Oliver Scott and Professor Jack Fowler. Changes in radiotherapy fractionation-breast cancer. *Br J Radiol.* 2019;92:20170849.

There was a statistically significant reduction in normal tissue effects for the schedule of 40 Gy in 15 fractions in the START B trial. The START pilot trial and the START A trial aimed to produce estimates of alpha/beta ratios for local control and normal tissue effects unconfounded by differences in treatment time (each arm was delivered over 5 weeks). The START B and Ontario trials tested the noninferiority of 15 and 16 fractions of 2.7 Gy over 3 and 3.2 weeks, respectively, on local control and normal tissue effects compared to 50 Gy in 25 fractions over 5 weeks. There was a statistically significant reduction in normal tissue effects for the schedule of 40 Gy in 15 fractions in the START B trial. Both trials were shown to be at least as effective as conventionally fractionated RT. Details of the pivotal trials of hypofractionated RT for invasive cancer treated by breast-conserving surgery are summarised in Tables 27.8–27.10. No cases of damage to the brachial plexus were seen in the START B trial, so it is considered safe for regional nodal irradiation. Most of the trial data relate to breast irradiation after breast-conserving surgery. Moderate fractionation after mastectomy is underrepresented. Patients treated with mastectomy were not included in the Ontario trial and represented only 10% of the population in the START B trial. However, there are no biological grounds for that similar efficacy, and toxicity should not apply for chest wall irradiation. However, moderate hypofractionation should be advised for patients undergoing breast construction or nodal irradiation.

More recently, the FAST and FAST-FORWARD trials have tested even shorter ultrahypofractionated dose fractionation schedules. The FAST trial assessed normal tissue effects and local control of 30 Gy in 5 fractions of 6 Gy or 28 Gy in 5 fractions of 5.7 Gy, both given once a week over 5 weeks, compared to conventional 50 Gy in 25 fractions over 5 weeks in 915 females with node-negative breast cancer. There were more adverse effects on breast cosmesis with the regimen of 30 Gy in 5 fractions and 2 Gy in 5 fractions compared to 50 Gy. The critical outcome of adjuvant breast irradiation is local control. The local failure rate was low (1.3% at 10 years), reflecting the inclusion of low-risk patients treated with adjuvant endocrine therapy. However, the FAST trial was underpowered to detect differences in local failure rate (Whelan et al., 2020).

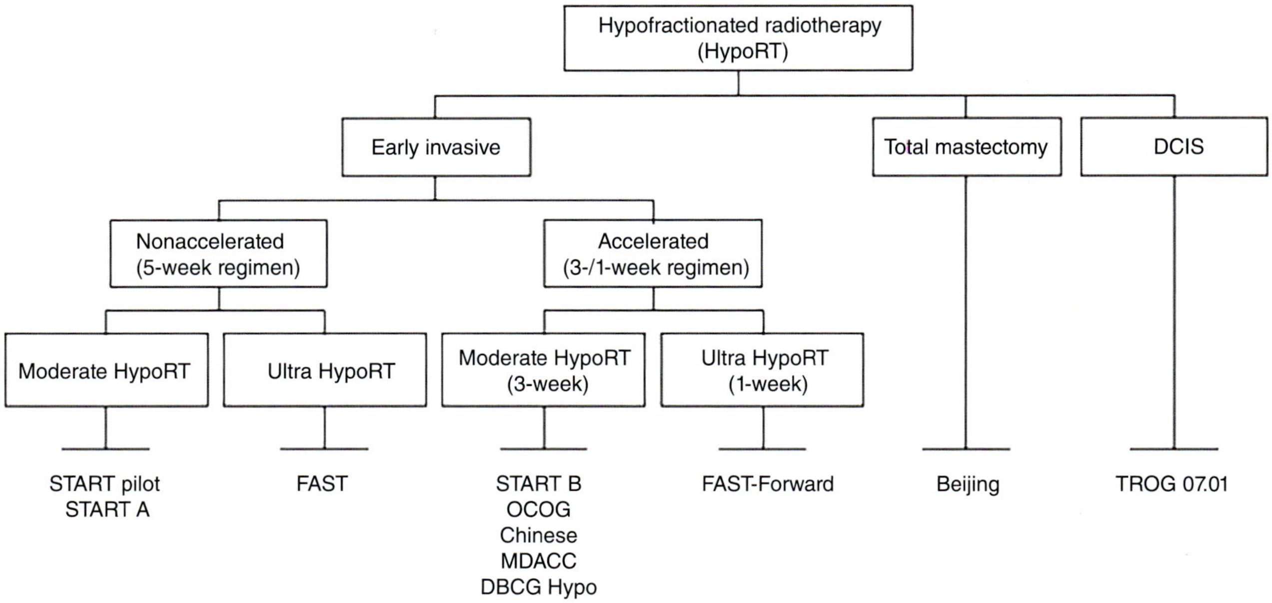

Fig. 27.12 Schema of trials of hypofractionated radiation therapy. *DBCG*, Danish Breast Cancer Group; *DCIS*, ductal carcinoma in situ; *MDACC*, MD Anderson Cancer Center; *OCOG*, Ontario Clinical Oncology Group; *START*, Standardisation of Breast Radiotherapy Trial; *TROG*, Trans-Tasman Radiation Oncology Group. (Reproduced with permission from Kim N, Kim YB. Journey to hypofractionation in radiotherapy for breast cancer: critical reviews for recent updates. *Radiat Oncol J.* 2022;40(4):216–224.)

The FAST-FORWARD trial compared 27 Gy in 6 fractions of 5.4 Gy to 26 Gy in 5 fractions of 5.2 Gy to moderately hypofractionated RT (40 Gy in 15 fractions) in over 4000 patients with pN0 or in pNI patients with early breast cancer treated by breast-conserving surgery or mastectomy. The experimental arms were noninferior in terms of local control, but the 27-Gy arm was associated with more normal tissue events, whereas that was not the case for the 26-Gy arm. In light of the COVID-19 pandemic, many centres have adopted the regimen of 26 Gy in 5 fractions for adjuvant RT to the breast or chest wall, while retaining moderate fractionation (e.g. 40 Gy in 15 fractions) for patients receiving regional nodal irradiation where the evidence of efficacy and safety of ultrahypofractionated RT is still under investigation. Other centres may retain moderately hypofractionated dose schedules for the breast until longer follow-up of the FAST-FORWARD trial is available, because both local recurrence and radiation toxicity may occur late. In addition, breast size was not described in the trial. It is therefore possible that there may be different normal tissue effects in patients with larger breasts (Levy and Rivera, 2020). The Royal College of Radiologists of London consensus statement recommends 26 Gy in 5 fractions for whole breast and chest wall irradiation (Lewis et al., 2021). The TROG 07.01 DCIS boost trial showed the equivalence of moderate hypofractionation (42.5 Gy in 16 fractions) to standard fractionation for nonlow-risk DCIS. Moderate hypofractionation is therefore a reasonable option following breast-conserving surgery for DCIS. Fig. 27.12 shows the schema of trials of hypofractionation after breast-conserving therapy and mastectomy for invasive cancer and for breast-conserving therapy for DCIS.

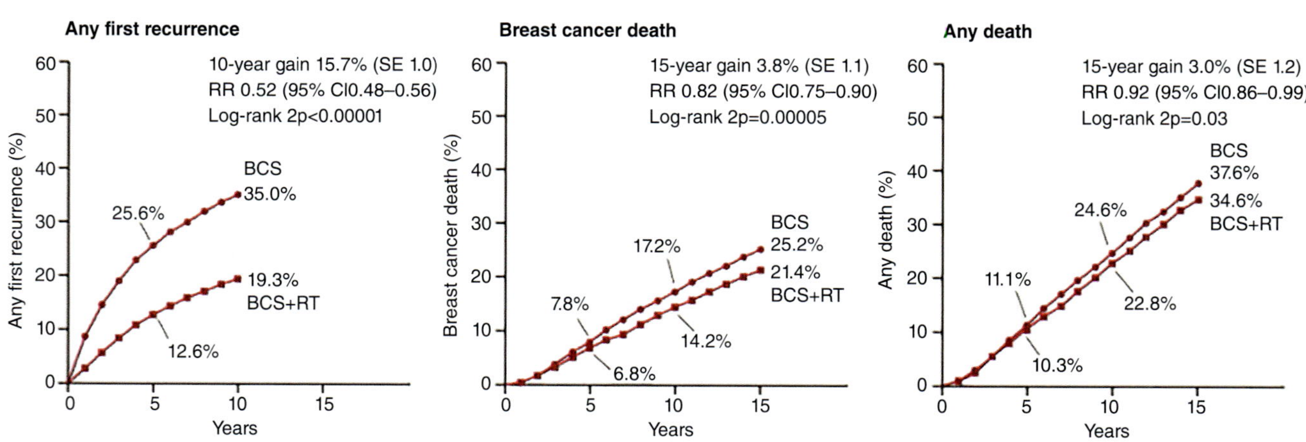

Fig. 27.13 Effect of radiotherapy after breast-conserving surgery on 10-year risk of any (locoregional or distant) first recurrence and on 15-year risks of breast cancer death and death from any cause in 10,801 females (67% with pathologically node-negative disease) in 17 trials. BCS = breast conserving surgery, RT = radiotherapy, RR = risk ratio. (Reproduced with permission from Early Breast Cancer Trialists' Collaborative Group (EBCTCG); Darby S, McGale P, et al. Effect of radiotherapy after breast-conserving surgery on 10-year recurrence and 15-year breast cancer death: meta-analysis of individual patient data for 10,801 women in 17 randomised trials. *Lancet.* 2011;378(9804):1707–1716.)

TABLE 27.11 Trials of Breast-Conserving Surgery With or Without Whole Breast Irradiation After Breast-Conserving for Early Breast Cancer

Study	No. of Patients	Median Follow-up (years)	Age (years)	Tumor Size (cm)	Treatment After Surgery	LR (%)	Statistical Significance for RT/No RT Comparison
Fisher et al., 1995	1009	8	Any age	<1	Tamoxifen RT + tamoxifen RT + placebo	17 3 9	<0.001
Fyles et al., 2004	769	5.6	>50	≤5	Tamoxifen RT + tamoxifen	8 1	0.001
Blamey et al., 2013	1135	13.9	<70	<2	None RT Tamoxifen RT + tamoxifen	1.9% pa 0.7% pa 0.8% pa 0% pa	<0.001
Potter et al., 2007	869	4.5	Postmenopausal (mean, 66)	≤3	Tamoxifen or AI Tamoxifen or AI + RT	6 2	<.001
Forrest et al., 1996	585	5.7	<70	≤4	Tamoxifen RT + tamoxifen	24.5 5.8	<0.001‡
Winzer et al., 2010	361†	10	45–75	≤2	None RT Tamoxifen RT + tamoxifen	34 10 8 9	<0 .001
Hughes et al., 2013	636	10.5	≥70	≤2.0	Tamoxifen RT + tamoxifen	9 2	<0.001
Tinterri et al., 2009	749	5.0	55–75	<2.5	None RT	3 1	0.07
Kunkler et al., 2023	1326	10.0	≥65	≤3	Tamoxifen or AI + RT	9.5 0.9	<0.001

†, 347 analysed.

‡, Calculated by LW from data in the paper.

AI, Aromatase inhibitor; *LR*, local recurrence; *RT*, radiation therapy.

Modified from Kunkler IH, Williams LJ, Jack WJL, Cameron DA, Dixon JM; PRIME II investigators. Breast conserving surgery with or without irradiation in women aged 65 years or older with early breast cancer (PRIME II): a randomised controlled trial. *Lancet Oncol.* 2015;16(3):266–273.

Fisher B, Anderson S, Redmond SK et al. Reanalysis and results after 12 years of follow up in a randomised clinical trial comparing total mastectomy with lumpectomy with or without irradiation in the treatment of breast cancer. *N Eng J Med.* 1995;333:1456–1461; Fyles AW, McCready DR, Manchul LA. Tamoxifen with or without breast irradiation in women 50 years of age or older with early breast cancer. *N Eng J Med.* 2004;351:963–970; Blamey RW, Bates T, Chetty U, et al. Radiotherapy or tamoxifen after conserving surgery for breast cancer of excellent prognosis: British Associaion of Surgical Oncology (BASO) II trial. *Eur J Cancer.* 2013;49:2294–2302; Potter R, Gnant M, Kwasny W, et al. Lumpectomy plus tamoxifen or anastrazole in women with favorable early breast cancer. *Int J Rad Oncol Biol Phys.* 2007;68:334–340; Forrest AP, Stewart HJ, Everington D, et al. Randomised controlled trial of conservation therapy for breast cancer: 6-year analysis of the Scottish trial. *Lancet.* 1996;348;708–713; Winzer KJ, Sauerbrei W, Braun M, et al. Radiation and tamoxifen after breast conserving surgery updated results of a 2 x 2 randomised trial in patients with low risk of recurrence. *Eur J Cancer.* 2010;46:95–101; Hughes KS, Schnaper LA, Berry D, et al. Lumpectomy plus tamoxifen with or without irradiation age 70 years or older with early breast cancer: longterm follow up of the CALGB 9343. *J Clin Oncol.* 2013;31:31:2382–2387; Tinterri C, Gatzemeier W, Zanini V, et al. *Breast.* 2009;18:373–377.

Partial Breast Irradiation. Moderate hypofractionation (e.g. 40 Gy in 15 fractions) and ultrahypofractionated regimens (e.g. 26 Gy in 5 fractions) are recommended. Twice daily fractionation should not be offered.

Postoperative Radiotherapy After Breast-Conserving Surgery. In general, postoperative whole breast irradiation should be delivered following wide local excision as part of breast-conserving therapy. The Early Breast Cancer Trialists' Collaborative Group (EBCTCG) meta-analysis of randomised trials of breast-conserving surgery with or without RT shows a halving of the risk of first recurrence, irrespective of risk category (EBCTCG 2011). The addition of postoperative RT after breast-conserving surgery (Fig. 27.13) reduced first recurrences (most of which were local) by 15.7% at 10 years, and this translated into a modest 3.8% reduction in breast cancer mortality at 15 years. Individual trials of breast-conserving surgery with or without breast irradiation are summarised in Table 27.11.

There are much less randomised data on the role of postoperative RT in older patients, particularly over the age of 65 years, receiving adjuvant endocrine therapy. The most mature data are from the CALGB 9343 trial in which 636 ER-positive patients age 70 years and older with TI, N0 tumours treated with 5 years of adjuvant tamoxifen were randomised to postoperative whole breast irradiation or no RT. At 10 years, 90% of patients in the tamoxifen group (95% CI 85%–93%) compared with 98% in the tamoxifen + RT group (95% CI 96%–99%) were free from locoregional recurrence. In the PRIME II

TABLE 27.12 Ongoing Trials of Omission of Radiotherapy After Breast-Conserving Surgery

Trial ClinicalTrials. gov Identifier, Trial Status	Design, Target, Accrual	Demographics	Pathologic	Hormone Receptors (all require HER2- tumours)	Additional RT Omission Criteria	Primary Outcome	Other
IDEA[1] NCT02400190 Closed to accrual	Prospective single-arm cohort 200 eligible patients enrolled	Female Age 50–69 Postmenopausal	Unifocal pT1 pN0-pN0(i+) Margins ≥2 mm No grade requirement	ER+ and PgR+	Oncotype DX Recurrence Score ≤18	5-year LRR	
LUMINA[2] NCT01791829 Closed to accrual	Prospective single-arm cohort 500 patients In investigational cohort	Female Age ≥55	Unifocal T1 pN0(i+) not specified	ER ≥1% and PgR >20%	Exclude if central Ki67	5-year IBR	Nonlobular histologies only No EIC or LVI
PRECISION[3] NCT02653755 Closed to accrual	Prospective Phase II cohort 345 patients in investigational cohort	Female Age 50–75	Unicentric pT1 pN0–pN0(i+) No tumour on ink Grade 1–2 (cN0 allowed if ≥70)	ER ≥10% or PgR+	Prosigna PAM50 low Risk of Recurrence score (i.e. luminal-A subtype)	5-year LRR	Optional survey component on decision comfort/regret
PRIMETIME[4] ISRCTN: 41579286 Open to accrual	Prospective cohort 1550 patients in RT omission cohort	Female Age ≥60	Unifocal pT1 pN0 (i+) Margins ≥1 mm Grade 2	ER+ (PgR incorporated into IHC4+C score)	IHC4+C risk category very low (<5% distant recurrence rate at 10 years)	5-year IBR	Postmenopausal females <60 with comorbidities placing at significant risk of RT toxicity
EXPERT[5] NCT02889874 Open to accrual	Randomised, noninferiority, phase III 1170 patients randomised	Female Age ≥50	Unifocal pT1 pN0–pN0 (i+) No tumour on ink Grade 1–2	ER ≥10% and PgR ≥10%	Prosigna PAM50 Risk of Recurrence ≤60 and luminal-A subtype	Noninferiority of RT omission to adjuvant RG, followed up to 10 years	PRO, QALY, fear of recurrence assessment
DEBRA[6] NCT04852887 Open to accrual	Randomised, noninferiority, phase III 1670 patients randomised	Female or male Age 50–69	Unicentric pT1 pN0 (i+ not allowed) No tumour on ink No grade requirement	ER ≥1% or PgR ≥1%	Oncotype DX recurrence Score ≤18	Noninferiority of RT omission to adjuvant RT, followed up to 10 years	PRO, QoL, distress of recurrence assessment

All trials are in patients who complete breast-conserving surgery with plan/willingness of 5-year adjuvant endocrine treatment and generally disallowed neoadjuvant systemic treatment or chemotherapeutic or biologic treatment.

EIC, Extensive intraductal component; *ER+*, oestrogen receptor positive; *HER2–*, human epidermal growth factor receptor 2 negative; *IBR*, ipsilateral breast recurrence; *LRR*, locoregional recurrence; *LVI*, lymphovascular invasion; *PgR+*, progesterone receptor positive; *PRO*, patient-reported outcome; *QALY*, quality-adjusted life-year; *QoL*, quality of life; *RT*, radiotherapy.

Reproduced with permission from Allen SG, Speers C, Jagsi R. Tailoring the omission of radiotherapy for early-stage breast cancer based on tumor biology. *Semin Radiat Oncol.* 2022;32(3):198–206.

References

1. The IDEA Study (Individualized Decisions for Endocrine Therapy Alone). https://clinicaltrials.gov/study/NCT02400190

2. A Prospective Cohort Study Evaluating Risk of Local Recurrence Following Breast Conserving Surgery and Endocrine Therapy in Low Risk Luminal A Breast Cancer (LUMINA). https://clinicaltrials.gov/study/NCT01791829

3. The PRECISION Trial (Profiling Early Breast Cancer for Radiotherapy Omission): A Phase II Study of Breast-Conserving Surgery Without Adjuvant Radiotherapy for Favorable-Risk Breast Cancer. https://clinicaltrials.gov/study/NCT02653755

4. Kirwan CC, Coles CE, Bliss J; PRIMETIME Protocol Working Group; PRIMETIME Protocol Working Group. It's PRIMETIME. Postoperative Avoidance of Radiotherapy: Biomarker Selection of Women at Very Low Risk of Local Recurrence. *Clin Oncol (R Coll Radiol).* 2016 Sep;28(9):594–596.

5. EXamining PErsonalised Radiation Therapy for Low-risk Early Breast Cancer (EXPERT). https://clinicaltrials.gov/study/NCT02889874

6. De-Escalation of Breast Radiation Trial for Hormone Sensitive, HER-2 Negative, Oncotype Recurrence Score Less Than or Equal to 18 Breast Cancer (DEBRA) (DEBRA). https://clinicaltrials.gov/study/NCT04852887

trial of 1386 patients with axillary node-negative T1-2 (<3 cm), pN0, M0 HR-positive breast cancer randomised to whole breast irradiation or no RT following breast-conserving surgery with minimum 1-mm clear margins, the local recurrence rate in the irradiated arm at 10 years of follow-up was significantly lower (0.9% (95% CI 0.1–1.7) versus 9.5% (95% CI 6.8–12.3), $P < 0.001$), but the absolute difference was modest (8.6%) (Kunkler et al., 2023). Overall survival at 10 years without RT after breast-conserving surgery is the same with or without RT. Overall survival was not compromised in either trial. The National Institute for Care and Clinical Excellence (NICE, 2018) suggests consideration of omission of RT for invasive cancer in females if margins are clear, there is a low absolute risk of local recurrence (≥65 years, T1, N0, ER positive, grade 1 or 2) and they are willing to take adjuvant endocrine therapy for a minimum of 5 years.

There are ongoing trials (Table 27.12) incorporating molecular assay risk stratification in HR-positive patients to refine the selection of low-risk patients for the omission of RT (PRIMETIME, LUMINA, IDEA, PRECISION, DEBRA, EXPERT).

Timing of Postoperative Radiotherapy. Postoperative RT should normally be started around 1 month after breast-conserving surgery where chemotherapy is not indicated, allowing time for the surgical wound to heal. Local recurrence rates do not increase if RT is delayed until 4 to 5 months after the last breast surgery in most, but not all, studies (Recht, 2021).

Computed Tomography Simulation

Standard adjuvant RT planning is CT based. Radiation planning techniques have expanded to forward-planned field-in-field and intensity modulated radiotherapy (IMRT). This range of techniques with better visualisation of target volume (breast, regional nodes and critical structures, e.g. heart, brachial plexus) has allowed treatment to be individualised and risks of morbidity to be diminished. The adoption of three-dimensional CT planning has enabled a move from field placements based on anatomical landmarks to individualised delineation of target volumes and critical structures and better homogeneity of dose distribution, while minimising dosage to organs at risk (OARs). There is a growing body of evidence that achieving more homogeneous dose distributions across the breast volume gives rise to less acute toxicity (pain, skin erythema and desquamation) and late toxicity (breast fibrosis, impaired cosmesis and telangiectasia).

The evidence that postoperative irradiation after mastectomy and breast-conserving therapy improves survival (by mechanisms which remain unclear) and that older RT techniques compromised survival by cardiac damage underpins efforts to optimise maximal antitumour effect with the lowest risk of morbidity.

Full CT scanning of the breast and/or peripheral lymphatics requires the patient to be planned with the ipsilateral arm abducted behind the head or with both hands holding a bar in front of the patient to fit into the bore of most CT scanners. For treatment of the breast alone, the patient should be scanned in the treatment position from the lung apices to the bottom of the lungs, and the breast and nodal fields from the mastoid to the bottom of the lungs. Some of the level I and II axillary nodes are usually incorporated with the tangential fields to the breast (Fig. 27.14).

Where the internal mammary nodes are to be included as part of regional nodal irradiation, breath-hold techniques with wide tangents or rotational techniques to minimise cardiac irradiation are recommended.

Respiratory Gated Radiotherapy

One of the most important principles of adjuvant RT for breast cancer is the minimisation of dose to the heart. The 2005 EBCTCG trial showed in approximately 40,000 females in 78 randomised trials of adjuvant RT that the beneficial effects of RT were counterbalanced by a 30% increase in cardiac deaths. The deaths were predominantly a result of ischaemic heart disease. Active breathing control is one of the key techniques to reduce cardiac and lung irradiation. It involves computer-controlled temporary suspension of breathing in a reproducible cycle.

Following respiratory training, the patient is positioned in a CT scanner without immobilisation (Figs. 27.15 and 27.16). RT is delivered in maximal deep inspiration when the heart is maximally displaced, posteriorly away from the treatment beams (Fig. 27.16). The lung volume irradiated is also reduced. Patients suitable for deep inspiratory breath-hold technique are summarised in Table 27.13. Some

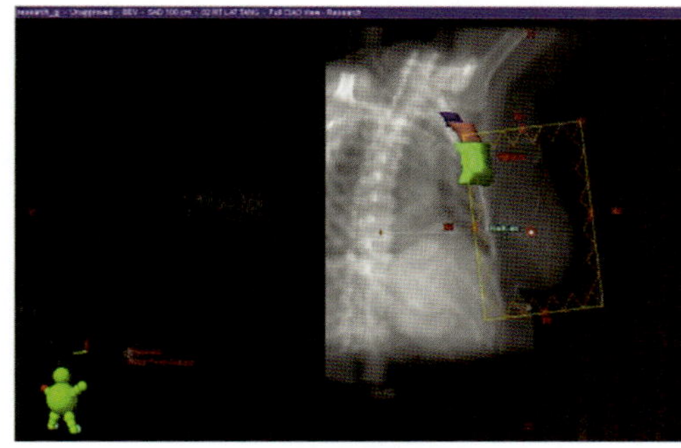

Fig. 27.14 Average nodal coverage of tangential fields, lateral view. (Reproduced with permission from Jacobson G, Bunda-Randall N, Wen S, Miller M. Axillary lymph node coverage with 3-dimensional tangential field irradiation and correlation with heart and lung dose. *Adv Radiat Oncol.* 2017;2(4):630–635.)

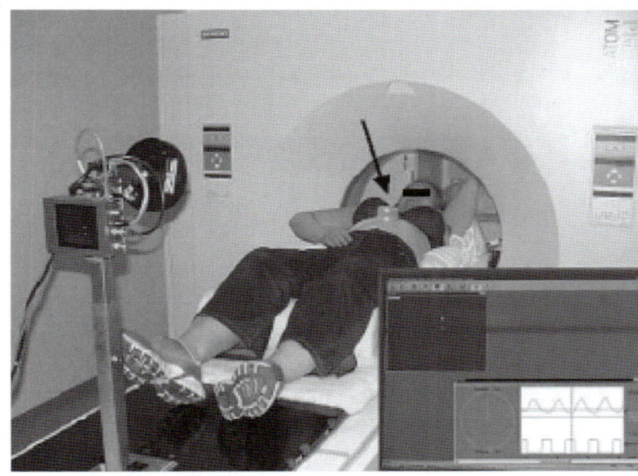

Fig. 27.15 The Varian RPM system displayed in the computed tomography scanner facility. A passive infrared light-reflecting marker *(arrow)* is placed on the patient's chest wall over the xiphoid process. The vertical motion of the marker is tracked by an infrared-sensitive video camera and the input projected onto a computer screen breathing curve. The *insert* shows the gating computer screen with the video camera view and the breathing curve. (Reproduced with permission from Pedersen AN, Korreman S, Nyström H, Specht L. Breathing adapted radiotherapy of breast cancer: reduction of cardiac and pulmonary doses using voluntary inspiration breath-hold. *Radiother Oncol.* 2004;72(1):53–60.)

TABLE 27.13 Criteria for Deep Inspiratory Breath-Hold Techniques to Reduce Cardiac Irradiation

1. Breast conservation where tumour bed is in the lower part of the breast or postmastectomy where cardiac shielding may shield the tumour bed
2. When cardiac doses is likely to exceed guidelines of safety
3. When maximum heart depth is 1 cm on the digital reconstructed radiograph
4. Patients with established cardiac issues or risk factors for cardiac disease

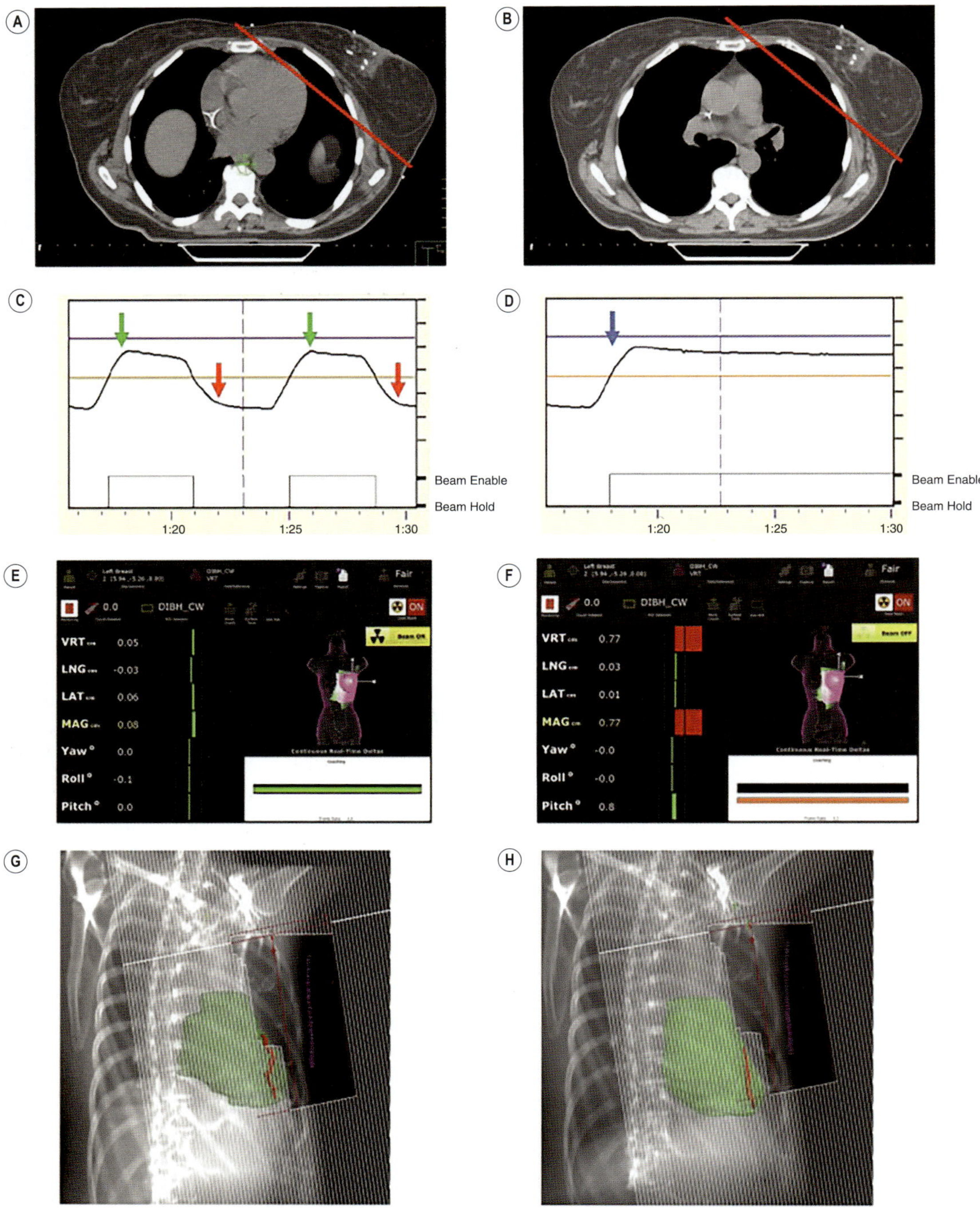

Fig. 27.16 Deep inspiration breath hold (DIBH) techniques and examples of anatomic and dosimetric advantages. (A,B) Axial CT slices from the same level of the breast in free breathing (A) and DIBH (B) CT scans. The red line indicates the tangential radiation field used for whole breast radiation treatment. Note that the heart is easily excluded in the DIBH scan. (C,D) DIBH respiratory tracings and real-time patient monitoring (RPM) using optical tracking at inspiration (green arrow) and expiration (red arrow) during free breathing. (D) RPM tracings confirm appropriate chest excursion during DIBH, with a stable breath hold tracing. After inspiration (blue arrow) with DIBH, the beam would be on during the sustained breath hold. (E) AlignRT screenshot illustrates a reference surface on the chest wall (CW) used for alignment with a region of interest (left breast), which is matched during surface tracking, and with DIBH, when the left breast is within the preset thresholds, as indicated by the dynamic green bars on the side of the panel, the treatment beam is enabled. (F) With expiration or any movements of the left breast outside of tolerance, the green bars turn red and the radiation beam is held. This process continues until the whole radiation dose is delivered daily. (G,H) Digitally reconstructed radiographs from a patient in during free breathing (G) and voluntary DIBH (vDIBH) (H) demonstrating the favorable shift in heart (green) and left anterior descending artery (LAD) (red) positions in relation to CW tangent with vDIBH. (Reproduced with permission from Bergom C, Currey A, Desai N et al. Deep inspiration breath hold: techniques and advantages for cardiac sparing during breast cancer irradiation. *Frontiers in Oncology.* 2018;8:1–10.)

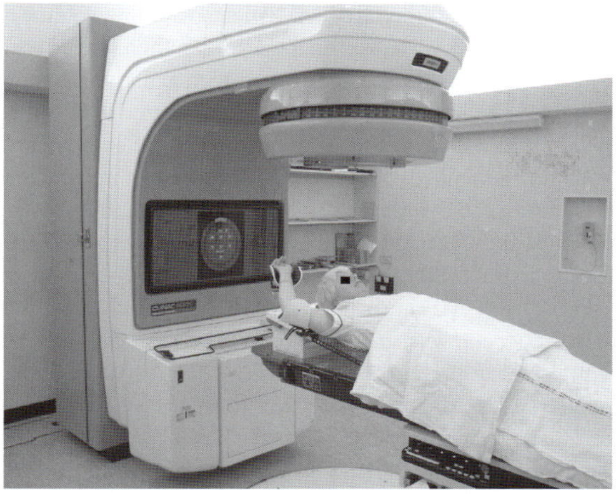

Fig. 27.17 Patient lying on an inclined breast board for chest wall/breast, supraclavicular fossa and internal mammary chain. (Courtesy Mrs J. Cameron, Edinburgh Cancer Centre.)

form of immobilisation is essential to provide a reproducible treatment setup. A variety of devices are in use. These may include a breast board (Fig. 27.17) that fits onto the simulator and treatment couch and a custom-made foam mould from the head to the knees. The patient is treated supine with the arm abducted to 90 degrees. The breast board can be inclined to a range of angles to flatten the chest wall/breast.

This technique simplifies matching and avoids the need for rotating the collimator. The disadvantage is that it increases the volume of lung irradiated in the shoulder field. Alternatively, the patient can lie supine with the arm abducted to 90 degrees. Rotation of the collimator is needed to keep the posterior beam edge parallel to the slope of the contour. The disadvantage is difficulty in matching the chest wall to the shoulder field.

For the large or very mobile breast, some additional form of immobilisation (shell or sling) is needed. The very mobile breast tends to fall laterally, moving the posterior beam edge farther back than the midaxillary point and increasing the volume of lung irradiated. The immobilising device will bring the breast medially and reduce the volume of lung irradiated. Treating the patient prone is an alternative technique for large-breasted patients.

Separate fields are planned to cover (1) the supraclavicular fossa, axilla and, if desired, upper internal mammary chain and (2) the chest wall/breast. Individualised CT planning is needed to ensure adequate coverage while limiting transmitted dosage to the underlying heart and lungs.

The UK HeartSpare randomised trial showed that for large-breasted females with estimated breast volumes greater than 750 cm^3, the supine voluntary breath-hold technique provided better cardiac sparing reproducibility than a free-breathing prone position. Mean heart doses and left anterior descending coronary artery mean doses for supine voluntary breath-hold and prone treatments, respectively, were 0.4 and 0.7 (P <0.001) and 2.9 and 7.8 ($P \leq 0.001$). Fig. 27.18 shows the field edge closer to the left anterior descending coronary artery with supine voluntary breath hold compared to prone treatment in the same patient. The supine position was also more comfortable for patients.

MANAGEMENT OF THE AXILLA

Some form of surgical procedure to obtain nodal histology is advised in virtually all females with operable breast cancer. Given the morbidity of axillance node clearance, particularly the risks of permanent lymphoedema and numbness, nodal assessment has been deescalated. Sentinel node biopsy in which at least one sentinel lymph is identified and removed has become the standard procedure for females with early breast cancer who have clinically and ultrasonically negative nodes. Females with palpable nodes should undergo axillary node dissection if they have not received preoperative systemic therapy. Sentinel node biopsy avoids the morbidity of axillary dissection and has become the standard of care in nodal staging of patients without metastases on axillary ultrasound. The sentinel node is the node most likely to drain the primary tumour. It is identified first by the injection of a radioactive tracer, a vital blue dye or a combination of both. The combination of both techniques is now used less after neoadjuvant chemotherapy. In most patients the sentinel node is in the axilla, but in a few medially placed tumours, it may be in the internal mammary chain. The axilla is normally explored to identify the sentinel node and is identified either by the blue colour of the dye within it or by the high radioactivity scintillation count within the node. If the sentinel node biopsy is positive, the options are no further treatment, complete axillary dissection or axillary irradiation. In specialist centres,

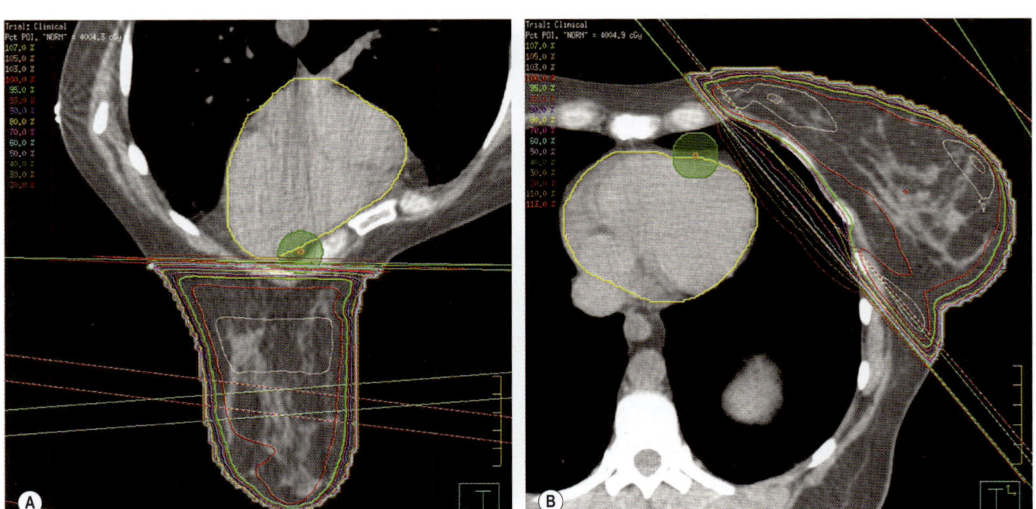

Fig. 27.18 Axial computed tomography slices of (A) prone and (B) supine voluntary breath-hold treatment plan from the same patient, demonstrating the anatomical and dosimetric relationship between breast tissue, heart *(yellow outline)* and left anterior descending coronary artery *(green colour wash with orange bull's-eye)*. (Reproduced with permission from Bartlett FR, Colgan RM, Donovan EM, et al. The UK HeartSpare study (Stage IB): randomised comparison of a voluntary breath-hold technique and prone radiotherapy after breast conserving surgery. *Rad Oncol.* 2015;114(1):66–72.)

TABLE 27.14 UK Guidelines on Axillary Surgery Following Neoadjuvant Chemotherapy

Clinically node-negative axilla (cN0)
1. In many patients, sentinel node biopsy (SNB) may be carried out before or after neoadjuvant chemotherapy (NACT) with equivalent prognostic information.
2. In cN0 patients with unexpected sentinel node metastases, SNB after NACT may be of increased prognostic value compared with up-front SNB.
Clinically node-positive axilla (cN1)
1. Patients can be safely considered for SNB after NACT. Four nodes should be removed with dual mapping.
2. If SNB shows evidence of a complete pathological response within the nodes, offer axillary radiotherapy.
3. If SNB shows isolated tumour cells, micrometastases or macrometastases, offer axillary lymph node dissection.
Patients presenting with extensive axillary node metastases (clinically/radiologically) may, after multidisciplinary team discussion, need to proceed to axillary lymph node dissection or completion of NACT.

Reproduced with permission from Gandhi A, Coles C, Makris A, et al. Axillary surgery following neoadjuvant chemotherapy—multidisciplinary guidance from the Association of Breast Surgery, Faculty of Clinical Oncology of the Royal College of Radiologists, UK Breast Cancer Group, National Coordinating Committee for Breast Pathology and British Society of Breast Radiology. *Clin Oncol.* 2019;31(9):664–668.

sentinel node biopsy has 97% accuracy. In patients with clinically negative axilla (cN0) undergoing neoadjuvant systemic therapy, the guidance from the Association of Breast Surgery, Faculty of Clinical Oncology of the Royal College of Radiologists, UK Breast Cancer Group and National Coordinating Committee for Breast Pathology and British Society of Breast Radiology (Gandhi et al., 2019) recommends that sentinel node biopsy be carried out before or on completion of neoadjuvant chemotherapy carried out after systemic therapy (Table 27.14). Three nodes should be removed by dual mapping. Because there is no definitive evidence to indicate optimal treatment following a complete pathological response in biopsy-proven axillary metastases, axillary irradiation is currently offered. Patients with low-volume residual axillary disease after neoadjuvant chemotherapy on sentinel node biopsy should be treated by a level III axillary clearance because studies show a high rate of residual disease in the axilla if the sentinel node post neoadjuvant chemotherapy is involved.

For patients with clinically involved axillary nodes, a level III axillary clearance up to the level of the medial end of the first rib is recommended. Normally, there should be at least 10 axillary nodes in a level III clearance, and commonly there are 20 to 30. The local control in the axilla from a level III clearance is similar to a selective policy of axillary RT in patients with one or more involved nodes on a four-node lower axillary sample. With either policy, the axillary recurrence rates is similar, 5% at 5 years.

REGIONAL NODAL IRRADIATION

Axillary irradiation is an alternative to axillary node clearance. In the EORTC 10891/22023 AMAROS trial, 4823 patients with T1-T2, N0 breast cancer were randomised if they had one to two positive sentinel nodes to axillary node clearance or axillary irradiation. The 10-year axillary recurrence rates, the primary endpoint (for which the trial was underpowered), was 0.93% (95% CI 0.18–1.68) after axillary clearance, and 1.82% after axillary RT (95% CI 0.74–2.94) were not significantly different refers to the axillary recurrence rates after axillary clearance or axillary RT. Neither disease-free nor overall survival differed. At 5 years, lymphoedema (arm circumference >10% in the ipsilateral upper or lower arm or both) was significantly more frequent after axillary node clearance (24.5%) compared with 11.9% for axillary RT. Patients with low-volume axillary disease (one to three involved sentinel nodes) can therefore be spared the morbidity of axillary clearance and treated with axillary irradiation. For more extensive axillary disease with more than three involved sentinel nodes, it is unclear if axillary irradiation is adequate and axillary clearance is still recommended. The EBCTCG showed that in females treated with or without postmastectomy irradiation including the supraclavicular fossa, axilla and internal mammary chain, there was an 8% reduction in breast cancer mortality at 20 years in the one to three node-positive group (Fig. 27.19). A Danish internal mammary node trial showed a 3.7% survival benefit, with greater gains in N2 disease and in N1 disease with central/medial tumours. The EORTC 22922/10925 internal mammary node trial (Poortmans et al., 2021) showed at median follow-up of 15.7 years that overall survival was 73.1% (95% CI 71.0–75.2) in the internal irradiation arm and 70.9% (95% CI 68.6–72.9) in the control arm, which was not significantly different. There was no difference in cardiovascular deaths, second cancers or contralateral breast cancer between the two arms. However, limiting dosage to the heart may be difficult. For such patients, proton therapy may be an option if there is access to it.

Can we identify particular subgroups that benefit from RNI? The trial populations of the MA.20 and EORTC IMC trials differed. The MA.20 trial studied patients with N1 (85%) and high-risk node-negative (10%) disease. The EORTC trial recruited N0 (44%) and N1 (43%) patients. The larger N0 group in the EORTC trial is likely to have had a lower risk of internal mammary nodes because the latter are associated with axillary node metastases. It is not clear how much benefit is derived from supraclavicular as opposed to internal mammary node irradiation. Given that regional node irradiation only added 3% to 5% improvement in disease-free survival and 1% to 1.6% in overall survival, the absolute benefit from treating any one of these sites is even less. In addition, supraclavicular relapse has a bad prognosis similar to that of de novo supraclavicular node involvement (N3), whereas clinically involved internal mammary nodes have a relatively good prognosis. Both the MA.20 and EORTC trials employed axillary clearance, so it is not clear how the results apply to the current practice of sentinel node biopsy. It is possible that internal mammary node irradiation could be an effective salvage therapy for internal mammary node relapse, but there are no data to support this, and it would be difficult to prove. Where the absolute benefits of internal mammary node irradiation are very small, the decision on whether to irradiate the internal mammary nodes or not must be balanced against the risks of radiation pneumonitis (1% absolute increase and 4% lymphoedema in the MA.20 trial). Although neither the MA.20 nor the EORTC trial reported any increase in cardiac events, the risk of increased cardiac dosage is higher with left-sided compared with right-sided tumours. It may therefore only be reasonable to treat the internal mammary nodes if anatomy is favourable, minimising doses to the heart and lungs. Breath-hold techniques are advised to minimise dose to the heart (Figs. 27.15 and 27.16).

Irradiation of the Supraclavicular Nodes

Recurrences in the supraclavicular region are uncommon in patients with uninvolved or one to three involved axillary nodes. Recurrence in the supraclavicular nodes in patients with four or more involved axillary nodes occurs in around 3% to 5% of patients in recent studies. It is unknown what the impact of supraclavicular recurrence is on clinical outcomes, because it has not been investigated separately from internal mammary nodal irradiation.

Irradiation of the Internal Mammary Nodes

Metastases in the internal mammary nodes are seen in 5% or fewer patients who are pN0 and 20% to 50% of patients who are pN1 on pathological assessment of the axillary nodes. In addition, clinical recurrence occurs

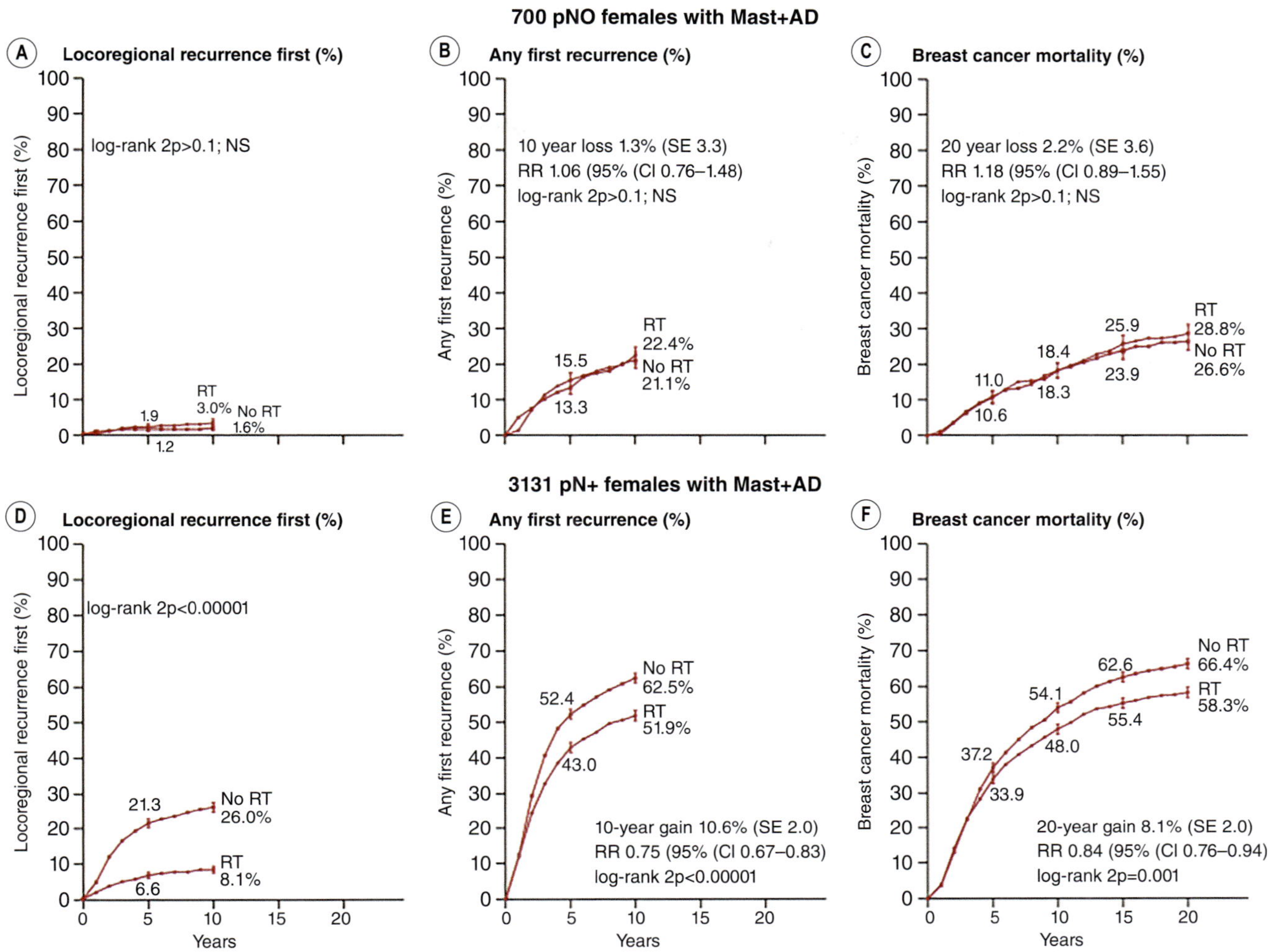

Fig. 27.19 Effect of radiotherapy after mastectomy and axillary dissection *(Mast + AD)* on 10-year risks of locoregional and overall recurrence and on 20-year risk of breast cancer mortality in 1314 females with one to three pathologically positive nodes (pN1–3) and in 1772 females with four or more pathologically positive nodes *(pN4 +)*. (Reproduced with permission from Early Breast Cancer Trialists' Collaborative Group (EBCTCG); McGale P, Taylor C, et al. Effect of radiotherapy after mastectomy and axillary surgery on 10-year recurrence and 20-year breast cancer mortality: meta-analysis of individual patient data for 8135 women in 22 randomised trials. *Lancet.* 2014;383(9935):2127–2135.)

in less than 1% of patients. The proximity of the heart sets a constraint on irradiating the internal mammary nodes in the adjuvant setting.

Indications for internal mammary irradiation:

1. Patients at high risk of locoregional recurrence (i.e. T4 or four or more axillary macrometastases)
2. Patients with one to three positive nodes where regional nodal irradiation is advised, taking into account risk factors (e.g. central/medial location of primary in the breast, laterality and likely dose to the heart and lungs)

Morbidity of Axillary Treatment

Side effects of an axillary clearance include postoperative seroma and numbness in the upper limb. Lymphoedema occurs in 7% to 8% of cases. If axillary RT is added to the dissection, the risk of lymphoedema is substantially higher (30%–40%).

After conventionally fractionated RT (e.g. 45–50 Gy in 20–25 fractions) to the axilla, the risk of lymphoedema is about 3% to 5%, that is, lower than after axillary dissection. However, there is an increased risk of long-term restriction of shoulder movement and a small risk of brachial plexopathy (≤1%). Brachial plexopathy is a rare but serious complication and is usually irreversible. Very careful attention to RT technique with avoidance of overlap between axillary and breast/chest wall fields or moving the patient between the treatment of these fields is essential.

Postmastectomy Radiotherapy

More than half of the locoregional recurrences following mastectomy occur on the chest wall. The mastectomy scar is the most common site of recurrence (Figs. 27.8 and 27.9). Postmastectomy RT is standard in females with four or more involved axillary nodes and for T3 NI tumours. The role of adjuvant RT following mastectomy in patients with one to three involved nodes remains controversial, and both guidelines and practice vary. Before 1997, it was accepted that postmastectomy irradiation improved locoregional control but not survival. However, in 1997 two landmark randomised trials conducted in Denmark and Canada showed a 9% to 10% survival benefit from the addition of locoregional RT following mastectomy to adjuvant CMF (cyclophosphamide, methotrexate and 5-fluorouracil) chemotherapy. The much larger Danish trial of over 3000 high-risk premenopausal patients showed that a significant advantage accrued to patients receiving adjuvant irradiation (10-year survival 54% versus 45%). A trial from the same trial group showed a similar 9% survival (45% versus 36%) benefit in high-risk postmenopausal females receiving locoregional regional irradiation in

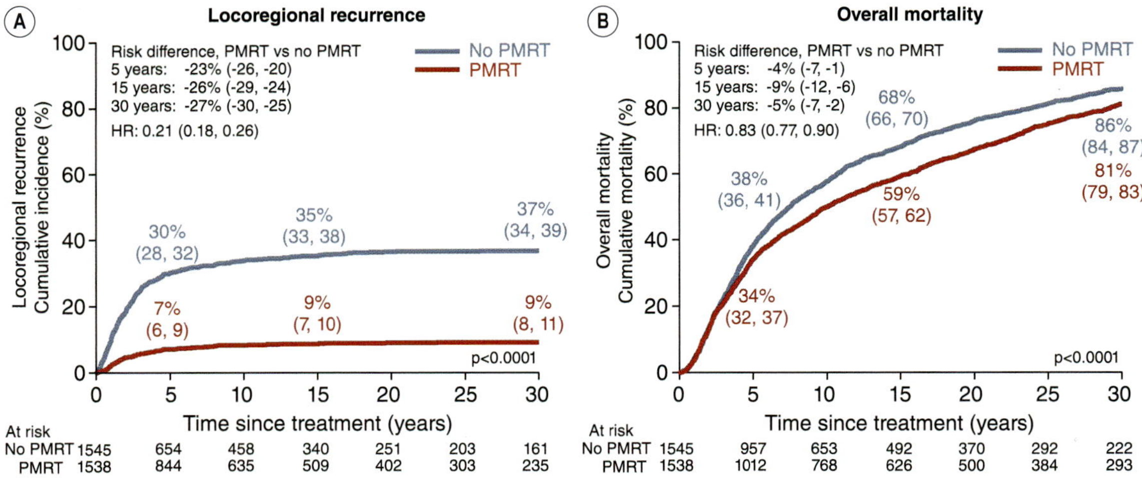

Fig. 27.20 Postmastectomy radiotherapy in high-risk breast cancer patients given adjuvant systemic therapy. (Overgaard M, Nielsen HM, Tramm T, et al. Postmastectomy radiotherapy in high-risk breast cancer patients given adjuvant systemic therapy. A 30-year long-term report from the Danish breast cancer cooperative group DBCG 82bc trial. *Radiother Oncol.* 2022;170:4–13. https://doi.org/10.1016/j.radonc.2022.03.008.)

addition to adjuvant tamoxifen. However, the survival advantage of the benefits of RT only emerged late (i.e. at 10 years). In both the Danish and Canadian trials, all of the peripheral lymphatics (axilla, supraclavicular and internal mammary chain) were irradiated. It is not clear whether irradiation of all of these areas, particularly the internal mammary chain, is essential. The RT technique in the Danish trial differed from the use of a pair of tangential fields in most UK centres to treat the chest wall. A combination of electron beam with limited penetration beyond the chest wall was used to treat the medial part of the chest wall and was matched with a photon field to treat the lateral half of the chest wall. Ten-year follow-up data showed no excess of cardiac morbidity or mortality in the RT plus systemic therapy group compared with those receiving systemic therapy alone. The 30-year results of the DBCG82bc trial showed a cumulative incidence of locoregional recurrence of 9% in the irradiated arm and 37% in the nonirradiated arm in patients who received systemic therapy (HR 0.21 (95% CI 0.18–0.6)). RT reduced breast cancer mortality (56% versus 67% (HR 0.75 (CI 0.69–0.82))) and overall mortality (81% versus 86%) at 30 years (P <0.0001). The 30-year results of the trial are summarised in Fig. 27.20. The results confirm the validity of the Spectrum hypothesis of Hellman (see the 'Mastectomy or Breast Conservation for Invasive Breast Cancer' section). The results of the Danish trial also emphasise the importance of good RT technique in minimising the dose to the heart.

The 2014 Oxford overview of randomised trials of postmastectomy RT (EBCTCG et al., 2014) shows a survival advantage from postmastectomy RT not only in patients with four or more involved nodes but also in those with one to three involved nodes. For 1314 females treated by axillary clearance and one to three positive nodes, RT reduced locoregional recurrence (P <.0001), overall recurrence (RR 0.68, 95% CI 0.57–0.82, P = .00006) and breast cancer mortality (RR 0.80, 95% CI 0.67–0.95, P = .01) (Fig. 27.19). The Oxford overview shows that the higher the baseline risk of recurrence, the higher the survival benefit. This latter observation contrasts with a retrospective analysis of the Danish postmastectomy RT trials, which showed a greater survival benefit for patients with low-risk features and luminal subtype. These contradictory findings might be explained by the complex interaction of local control and better systemic therapy. It is not clear whether more aggressive locoregional therapy should be recommended in more aggressive tumours. On the basis of the results of the Oxford overview, some have argued that postmastectomy RT should be recommended for all patients with one to three positive nodes. However, the locoregional recurrence in unirradiated patients was 16.5% at 5 years and 20.3% at 10 years, higher levels than those seen in the United States and other countries. It is therefore difficult to extrapolate from the EBCTCG analysis to all patients with one to three positive nodes. It remains unclear which subsets benefit.

Consideration also has to be given to the serious side effects of nodal irradiation (lymphoedema, pneumonitis, cardiac damage and second malignancy).

It is known that the risk of local recurrence increases with the cumulative number of risk factors (high tumour grade, nodal involvement and lymphovascular invasion). How these factors should be weighted in the selection of patients for postmastectomy RT is not clear.

Guidelines on postmastectomy RT for patients with one to three involved nodes vary. NICE guidelines recommend adjuvant RT for all patients with axillary macrometastases (NICE 2018).

The 2019 St. Gallen Breast Cancer Consensus Panel (Burnstein et al., 2019) recommended postmastectomy RT to the chest wall and regional lymph nodes in cases of four or more positive nodes, or one to three positive nodes with triple-negative histology. The panel were divided on whether females should receive postmastectomy RT in HER2-positive and/or ER-positive tumours with one to three involved lymph nodes and larger (>5 cm) node-negative tumors. Postmastectomy RT was not advised for T2 N0 cancers. Postmastectomy RT recommendations by the panel were the same for females undergoing immediate reconstruction.

The joint US Association of Clinical Oncology, American Society for Radiation Oncology, and Society of Surgical Oncology guidelines on postmastectomy RT is more nuanced for T1–T2 N1 tumours with one to three positive nodes (Recht et al., 2016) for a heterogeneous population with different risk factors for recurrence. They argue that many of these patients are at lower risk of recurrence and that many North American studies of mastectomy without irradiation have lower 5-to-10-year actuarial rates of locoregional failure, with the most recent rates being lower than 10%. For some subsets of patients, they consider that the risk of locoregional failure may be outweighed by the risks of toxicity. They suggest omitting postmastectomy RT in some women, such as those with limited life expectancy due to old age or comorbidities, or lower tumour burden, or only one node-positive and/or small size tumour, or substantial response to neoadjuvant chemotherapy, or biological characteristics associated with better outcomes and survival and/or greater effectiveness of systemic therapy.

In addition, adjuvant chest wall irradiation is indicated for:

1. Close or involved surgical margins
2. Chest wall recurrence following mastectomy

Currently in the United Kingdom, the MRC/EORTC SUPREMO trial, now in the follow-up phase, is the only prospective trial that is evaluating the role of chest wall irradiation in patients after mastectomy and axillary node clearance with one to three involved nodes or who are node negative with other risk factors (grade 3 and/or lymphovascular invasion receiving contemporary systemic therapy and, where appropriate, anti-HER2 therapy). It has a biological substudy, TRANS SUPREMO, seeking a molecular signature of radiosensitivity. Hopefully, it may provide the basis for selecting patients for postmastectomy RT on the basis of biological and clinicopathological factors. In the absence of more definitive evidence, the pros and cons of postmastectomy RT in females with one to three positive nodes will have to be discussed in multidisciplinary teams on an individual basis.

Local Recurrence After Mastectomy

If local recurrence occurs on the chest wall, spot recurrence should be locally excised if feasible. Of patients treated by local excision alone, 60% to 70% will develop a second local recurrence. For multiple spot recurrences (see Figs. 27.7 and 27.8), this is unlikely to be practical. Radical RT (40 Gy in 15 daily fractions) to the chest wall and the supraclavicular fossa should be considered if not given previously. If irradiation of the supraclavicular fossa is omitted, recurrence rates at this site may be as high as 28%.

For an isolated axillary recurrence, a level III clearance should be considered. Axillary irradiation is only considered if there is macroscopic disease remaining after a clearance or a previous clearance has been undertaken. Most of the available evidence does not support the use of axillary irradiation for patients with extracapsular spread who have undergone a level III axillary clearance.

Target Volumes and Techniques for Locoregional Irradiation

In choosing a technique, guiding principles should be homogeneous irradiation of the target areas, avoidance of overlap of the chest wall/breast with fields to the peripheral lymphatics and minimising dosage to critical structures (lung, heart and the brachial plexus). This is not an easy task, because of the variation in shape and thickness of the chest wall and breast in the craniocaudal and transverse planes. In addition, the sternum slopes when the patient is lying flat. The proximity of the lung and heart to the target volume means that some lung is commonly irradiated. Dose inhomogeneity is exacerbated by lung effects because of scatter and lung transmission.

INTENSITY MODULATED RADIOTHERAPY

IMRT has become available to provide a more even distribution of radiation dose across the breast/chest wall while reducing unwanted irradiation of critical organs such as the lung and heart. IMRT allows the fluence intensity to be varied across the beam. Virtual simulation, which incorporates a laser positioning system and a CT scanner and treatment planning system, has replaced simulation in many centres. Constraints may be put on doses to critical organs and to the breast and chest wall. It has been shown that IMRT can reduce by 3% to 5% the dose to the top and bottom of the breast where hot spots commonly occur with conventional wedged fields using two-dimensional planning (Figs. 27.21A and B). The Cambridge IMRT trial comparing forward-planned IMRT to two-dimensional planning showed that IMRT improved the mean volumes receiving more than 107% and less than 95% of the prescribed dose compared with control. Despite the better target coverage and reduced cardiac dosage from three-dimensional

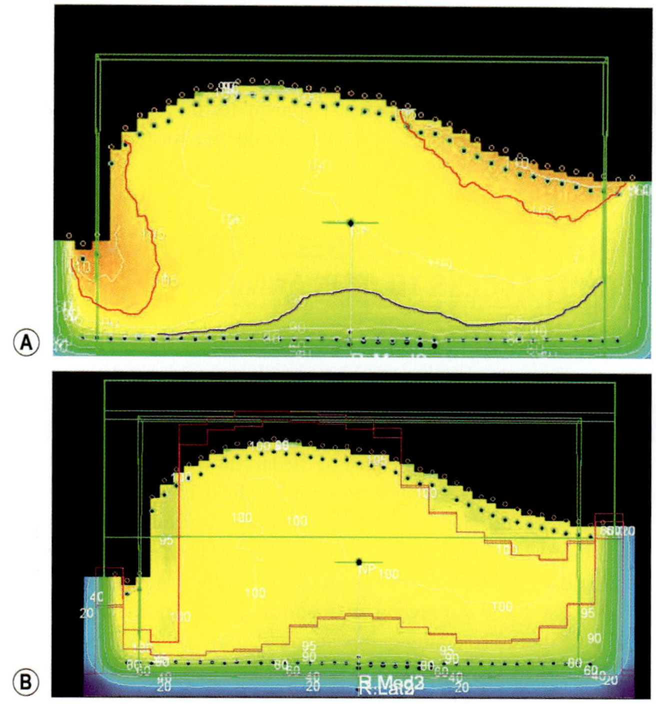

Fig. 27.21 Two beam's-eye view images of the same breast with the isodoses displayed as a colour wash. (A) The dose distribution for a standard two-field plan is shown. The high-dose areas equal to or above 107% of the prescribed dose are shown by the deeper orange colour *(outlined in red)*. The lower-dose areas equal to or below 95% of the prescribed dose are shown by the green colour *(outlined in blue)*. (B) The dose distribution is improved by the addition of two additional multi leafed collimator (MLC) shaped fields, which have the effect of decreasing the regions of higher dose and boosting the regions of lower dose. (Reproduced with permission from Barnett GC, Wilkinson J, Moody AM, et al. A randomised controlled trial of forward-planned radiotherapy (IMRT) for early breast cancer: baseline characteristics and dosimetry results. *Radiother Oncol.* 2009;92(1):34–41.)

planning over two-dimensional planning, the normal tissue complication probability (NTCP) for the lung may increase.

RECOMMENDED DOSE CONSTRAINTS

Based on the RT quality assurance of the Danish HYPO trial testing hypofractionation, suggested guidelines for 40 Gy in 15 daily fraction plans are that the maximum dose to less than 25% of the ipsilateral lung should be 17 Gy (V17 Gy 25%); less than 10% and 5% of the heart should receive 17 Gy and 35 Gy, respectively. If the left anterior descending coronary artery is delineated, the maximum should be 17 Gy. The dose to the contralateral breast should be as low as possible (Thomsen et al., 2021).

Dose Constraints on Cardiac Irradiation

The German breast cancer expert panel (Duma et al., 2019) recommend the following dose constraints: mean heart dose, less than 2.5 Gy; D_{mean}LV (mean dose left ventricle), less than 3 Gy; $V5_{LV}$ (volume of LV receiving ≥5 Gy), less than 17%; $V23_{LV}$ (volume of LV receiving ≥23 Gy), less than 5%; D_{mean}LAD (mean dose left descending coronary artery), less than 10 Gy; $V30_{LAD}$ (volume of LAD receiving ≥30 Gy), less than 2%; $V40_{LAD}$ (volume of LAD receiving ≥40 Gy), less than 1%.

Volumetric Arc Therapy

There is limited experience with volumetric modulated arc therapy (VMAT). It can provide similar or superior target coverage, better sparing of normal tissues with fewer monitor units and shorter delivery times. It has advantages where bilateral breast irradiation is required with a single isocentre and asymmetric arcs. Simultaneous irradiation boost is also possible. However, the German Society of Radiation Oncology guidelines (2019) on heart-sparing techniques conclude that neither VMAT nor tangential IMRT is as effective for heart sparing in patients with standard anatomy (Piroth et al., 2019).

TRADITIONAL FIELD BORDERS (FOR CENTRES WITHOUT ACCESS TO CT PLANNING)

Shoulder Field

A direct anterior megavoltage field covers the supraclavicular fossa and axilla. The upper margin should be at the level of the thyrohyoid groove. The lateral margin should encompass the lateral border of the axilla.

The shoulder joint and the part of the larynx within the field should be shielded. Some centres angle the shoulder field 15 degrees to exclude the spinal cord, although this is not essential as long as the dosage and fractionation are within cord tolerance. The lower border of the shoulder field should be nondivergent to avoid overlap with the tangential fields.

The axillary and supraclavicular nodes are commonly at the same depth, and therefore a single anterior field may suffice. Some centres use a small direct posterior field (posterior axillary boost) to supplement the dose to the axillary nodes. The posterior field is often treated on alternate days unless the midaxillary separation exceeds 20 cm.

Supraclavicular Field

Where the axillary clearance shows four or more nodes to be involved at pathological staging, irradiation of the medial supraclavicular fossa should be given. If the axilla is to be cleared, the surgeon should be asked to place metal clips up to the medial extent of the axillary dissection to ensure that the lateral margin of the supraclavicular field abuts on, but does not overlap, the field of the axillary clearance.

If there are one to three involved nodes and other adverse prognostic factors, for example, grade 3 histology or T3, supraclavicular RT can be considered in fit patients.

NEOADJUVANT THERAPY

In patients who have undergone neoadjuvant therapy with hormonal therapy or chemotherapy and the axillary nodes are positive cytologically and/or clinically or radiologically suspicious, and if the nodal status is YpN− after neoadjuvant therapy, irradiation of the supraclavicular fossa should be considered. If the nodal status is positive after neoadjuvant therapy (ypN+), irradiation of the supraclavicular fossa is recommended.

Chest Wall and Breast

The chest wall or breast is treated isocentrically and can normally be encompassed in a pair of wedged tangential fields (Fig. 27.22), keeping the posterior beam edges parallel to minimise divergence into the lung. This should cover the scar of local excision or of the mastectomy. Before three-dimensional scanning (at 2-to-3-mm intervals), it is helpful to place temporary radiopaque markers at the margins of the breast/chest wall, while acknowledging that these may not represent the true margins of the clinical target volume (CTV)p_Breast.

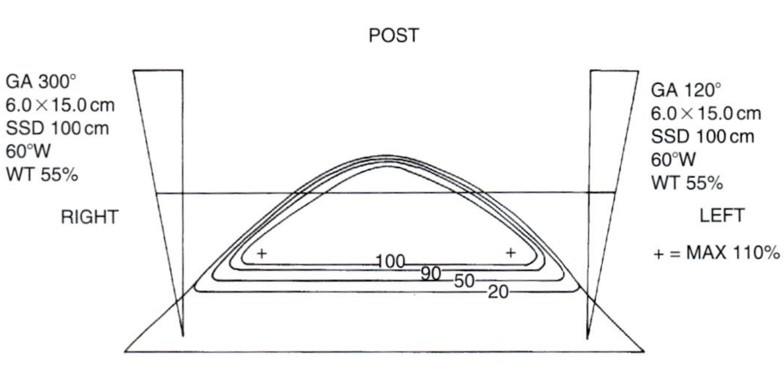

Fig. 27.22 Isodoses of a pair of wedged tangential breast fields.

Delineation of the Target Volume

To date, the target volume has been the weakest link in the planning chain. The European Society for Therapeutic Radiology and Oncology (ESTRO) consensus guidelines on target volume definition for breast/chest wall and regional nodes are recommended for early breast cancer (Offersen et al., 2015). It should be emphasised that they do not apply to locally advanced disease, for which planning should be individualised. The target volumes for the regional nodes are shown in Table 27.15.

THE BREAST AND CHEST WALL AND DELINEATION OF THE TARGET VOLUME

The CTV should be delineated on CT slices sequentially. For the whole breast (CTVp_breast), the CTV includes the soft tissues of the breast down to the fascia. It is often not possible to identify clearly the borders of the breast. The posterior border of the CTVp_breast is the ventral side of the pectoralis major muscle, or in its absence, the exterior side of the ribs and intercostal muscles. The ventral border is 5 mm underneath the skin surface with the exception of T4 cancer where full dosage to the skin is advised. The upper border is the inferior edge of the sternoclavicular joint. The medial border is the ipsilateral edge of the sternum. The lateral thoracic vessels at the lateral border of the breast can be a useful guide to the lateral border of the breast, although it may not be necessary to delineate CTV_breast that far lateral if glandular tissue is clearly visible.

The CTVp_breast should include the primary tumour bed and any margin around it. Virtual simulation of the breast is shown in Fig. 27.23.

Typical dose distributions in the breast and adjacent structures are shown in Fig. 27.24. Field-in-field dose compensation can reduce hotspots (Figs. 27.23A–C).

Radiopaque markers should be placed and the imaginary margins of the breast around along the mastectomy scar. The margins of the CTVp_thoracic wall are similar to the breast. Unless there is invasion of the skin (T4), there is no need to include the pectoral major muscle and ribs in the VCTVp_thoracic wall.

For the planning target volume (PTV), a margin is added to the CTV to take account of patient movement and setup error. The treatment plan should comply with ICRU 50 criteria so that the breast PTV should receive no less than 95% and no more than 107% of the prescribed dose.

Dose Prescription to the Breast

Dose prescription to the breast is 40 Gy TAD in 15 daily fractions over 3 weeks (6-10-MV photons) or 26 Gy in 5 daily fractions over 1 week.

Dose Prescription to the Axilla

The dose should be specified both medially at 3-cm depth from the anterior skin surface (point B) and laterally at half the patient's thickness in the middle of the posterior-anterior beam (point A). The dose should not vary by 5% or more, and maximally by 10% or more across the CTV.

Dose Prescription to the Axilla or Supraclavicular Fossa

Dose prescription to the axilla or supraclavicular fossa is 40 Gy in 15 daily fractions over 3 weeks (6-10-MV photons).

TABLE 27.15 Locoregional Target Volumes

The Axilla
Level 1: CTVn_L1 (Clinical Target Volume, Nodes)
Identification of axillary level I is influenced by surgical scarring from sentinel node biopsy or axillary node clearance. The medial border abuts on the lateral border of CTVn_L2. Superiorly, the axillary vein should be included with a 5-mm margin. The superolateral border of CTVn_L2 should be delineated 1 cm inferior and medial to the humeral head. More inferiorly, the lateral border is limited by an imaginary line between the lateral border of the pectoralis major and the anterolateral edge of the deltoid muscle. The inferior limit in the midaxillary line is around the level of the fourth to fifth ribs. The posterosuperior border of CTVn_L1 is the ventral edge of the subscapular and deltoid muscles, omitting the thoracodorsal artery and vein.
Level 2: CTVn_L2
CTVn_L2 lies posterior to the pectoralis minor muscle. The medial limit is the medial border of pectoralis minor. The superior border includes the axillary artery, which lies above the axillary vein, with an extra slice preferably to take account of partial volume effect. The posterior limit extends to a 5-mm margin posterior to the axillary vein into the surrounding fat, normally corresponding with the chest wall. The lateral border is the lateral border of the pectoralis minor muscle where artefacts may be seen following axillary node dissection. In the latter case, the inferior border may be adjusted to exclude the surgical bed from the level II volume.
CTVn Interpectoralis
The interpectoral lymph nodes (Rotter nodes) lie anterior to pectoralis minor and posterior to pectoralis major. The superior, inferior, lateral and medial limits largely reflect the borders of CTVn_L2.
Level 3: CTVn_L3
CTVn_L3 lies medial to pectoral minor and CTVn_L2 and is known at the infraclavicular volume. The medial border is the clavicle and the junction between the subclavian and internal jugular veins. The superior border includes the subclavian artery with an additional slice for partial volume effect and medially follows the superior border of CTVn_L2 and links to the superior limit of CTVn_L4. The superior border is the clavicle. The inferior border is a 5-mm extension into the fat inferior to the subclavian vein. The posterior limit is the 5-mm posterior to the subclavian vessels.
Level 4: CTVn_L4
This is usually known as the supraclavicular volume. The medial limit is the internal jugular vein (without a margin, i.e. excluding the common carotid artery and the thyroid gland). The superior border is the cranial level of the arch of the subclavian artery (i.e. there is a 5-mm margin superior to the subclavian vein). To account for the partial volume effect and computed tomography scan slice thickness, the superior limit is delineated one slice superior to the subclavian arch. Anterolaterally, the border is the posterior side of the sternocleidomastoid and sternothyroid muscles and the clavicle.
The most lateral part is the connective tissue between the lateral border of the anterior scalene muscle and the clavicle, and links with the medial border of CTVn_L3. The inferior border of CTVn_L4 includes the subclavian vein with a 5-mm margin, so linking to the cranial border of CTVn_IMN. The pleura is the posterior limit.

Internal Mammary Nodes: CTVn_IMN

The superior limit is the inferior limit of CTVn_L4 (Table 27.15), delineated 5 mm around the internal thoracic artery. The inferior limit is normally the superior side of the fourth rib but may be extended with one more intercostal space to the fifth rib. The medial border is 5 mm to the internal thoracic vein or the sternum, whichever is the closest. The lateral border is the internal mammary artery and vein with a 5-mm margin. The posterior border is the pleura. The anterior limit is the anterior limit of the vascular area.

DELINEATION OF THE TARGET VOLUME AND LOCO-REGIONAL DOSE PRESCRIPTION

The heart is a complex structure for contouring. Atlases have been developed to assist with contouring of the left ventricle and coronary arterial segments on RT CT planning. This may assist in research on the relationship between segment doses and cardiac outcomes.

Dose Prescription to the Internal Mammary Nodes

Dose prescription to the internal mammary nodes is 40 Gy TAD in 15 daily fractions over 3 weeks (6-10-MV photons).

Limiting Volume of Lung Irradiated. At the time of simulation, the thickness of lung encompassed in the tangential fields should be measured (the central lung distance perpendicularly from the inner aspect of the chest wall to the posterior beam edge). The central lung distance should not exceed 3 cm. If it exceeds 3 cm, consideration should be given to bringing the medial and/or lateral margins of the fields inwards, as long as this does not involve skimping on the coverage of the wide excision or mastectomy scars. To avoid divergence into the lung, the posterior beam edges should be kept parallel.

Skin Bolus. To overcome the skin-sparing effect of megavoltage, skin bolus (0.5–1 cm depending on the energy of photons) should be applied to the chest wall to ensure full skin dosage in patients where the skin is involved by tumour. Practice varies in the use of bolus for postmastectomy RT when the skin is not involved. Some centres apply bolus to a limited area above and below the scar (where recurrences are most common) or to the whole of the chest wall, either for the whole or part of the course of RT. It is not clear which approach is optimal.

Field Matching. One of the main challenges in breast/chest wall planning is to match the tangential fields to the shoulder field. Immobilisation should minimise movement between the treatment of fields to avoid the risk of overdosage or underdosage at the junction. Fields may be matched using the light beam, and lasers by eye using couch rotation (usually 5–6 degrees) and some collimator rotation. Alternatively, the following can be used:

1. A half beam block to counteract beam divergence, allowing the field edges to be abutted. Asymmetric jaws facilitate this. The match plane can be vertical or angled.
2. A vertical hanging block.
3. A single isocentre with blocks, avoiding the need for couch movement between fields.

Dosimetry. Planning is based on multislice CT scanning of the breast and/or peripheral lymphatics. An adequate dose for most patients is 6-to-10-MV photons. Wedges are needed to compensate for missing tissue. Lung transmission increases the dose to the posterior breast. A correction factor of 10% may be needed. Variations in depth dose across the breast may be around 20%, particularly in larger breasts. Buildup (the distance over which the dose builds up) to 100% is 5 to 10 mm from the skin surface for 6-MV photons.

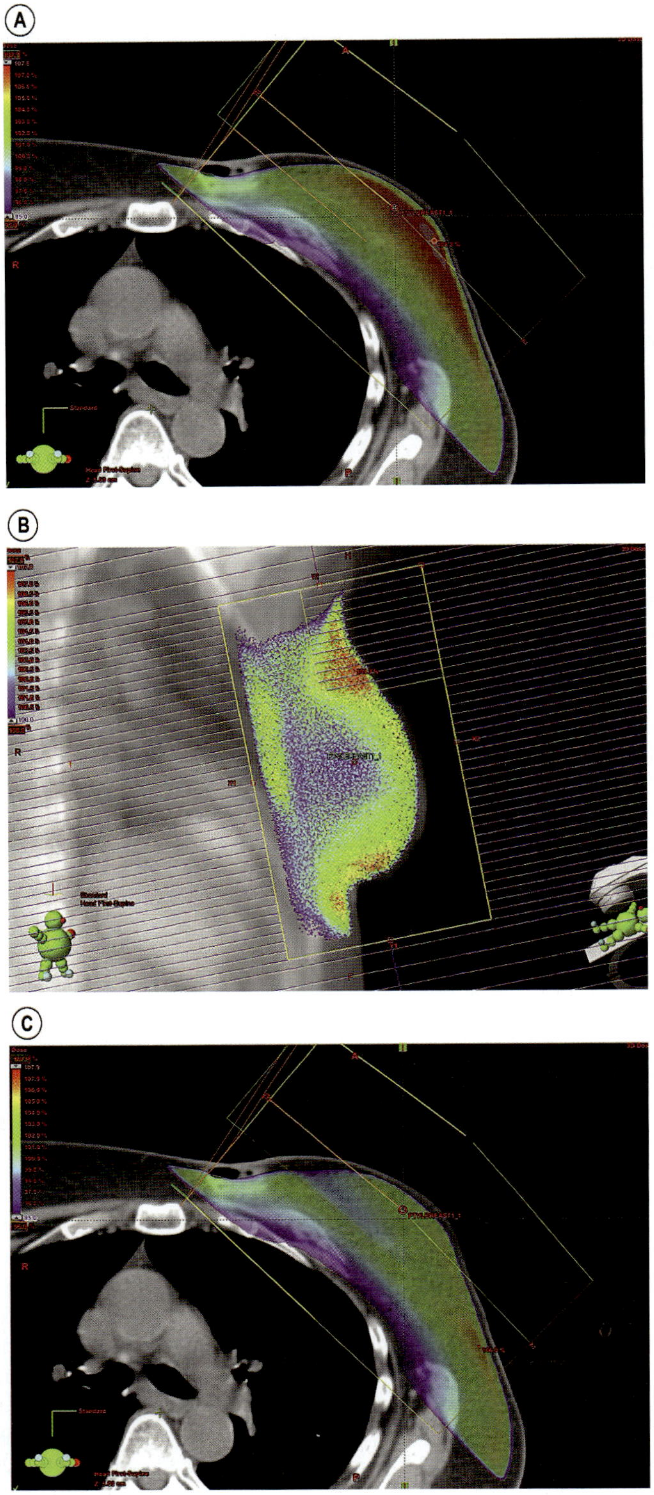

Fig. 27.23 (A) Dose colour wash showing hotspot on a superior slice. (B) Field in field MLc compensation. (C) Dose colour wash showing improved dosimetry due to field in field dose compensation. (Reproduced with permission from Macleod N, Macintyre A, Canney PA. What are the minimum standards of radiotherapy planning and dosimetry for 'hypofractionated' radiotherapy in breast cancer. *The Breast.* 2010;19:172–175.)

Dose, Energy and Fractionation. Megavoltage irradiation (6-MV photons) is used for the tangential field to the chest wall or breast. For patients with larger breasts, higher-energy (10-MV) photons may be needed.

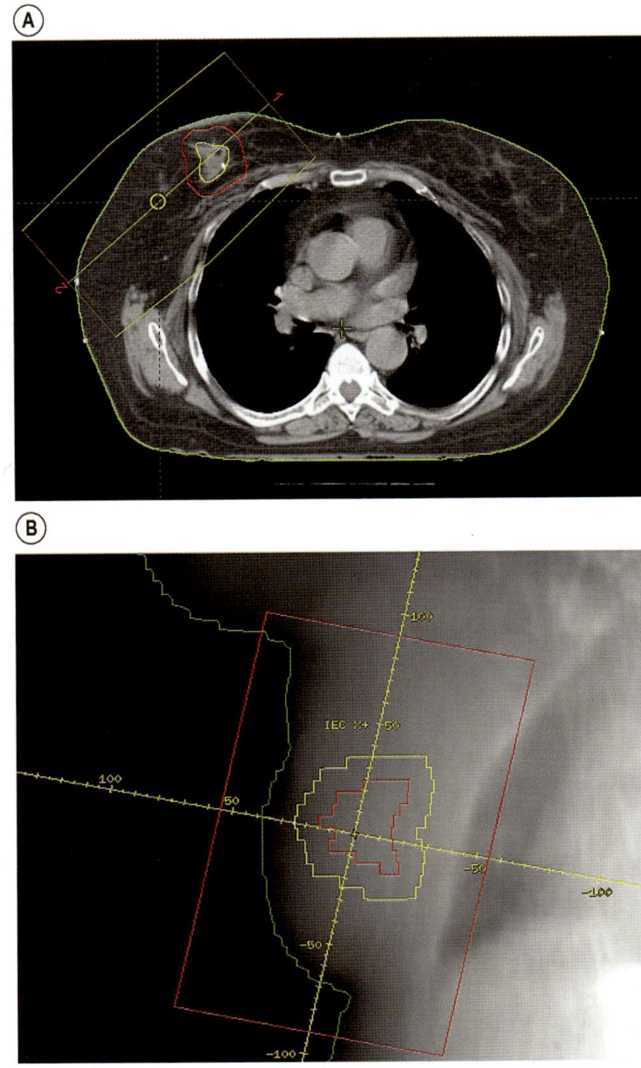

Fig. 27.24 (A) Virtual simulator image of tangential fields placement. Note clips helping to identify tumour bed. (B) Virtual simulator image of beams eye view. (Reproduced with permission from Macleod N, Macintyre A, Canney PA. What are the minimum standards of radiotherapy planning and dosimetry for 'hypofractionated' radiotherapy in breast cancer. *The Breast.* 2010;19:172–175.)

Boost to Primary Tumour Volume After Whole Breast Irradiation. Some form of boost of irradiation to the site of excision of the primary tumour is desirable to bring the tumour dose to 60 Gy in females under the age of 50 years. This is most commonly delivered by electrons. Excellent results can also be achieved by implantation with high dose rate (HDR) or low dose rate (LDR) interstitial implantation. The excellent cosmetic results achievable from postoperative whole breast irradiation are shown in Fig. 27.25. Either form of boost will give comparable local control. However, interstitial implantation requires significant practical expertise, and its use is in decline in the United Kingdom and the United States. Worldwide, LDR afterloading systems, sources and iridium have been withdrawn. HDR brachytherapy with iridium-192 using the MammoSite system is practised in a limited number of centres. The MammoSite HDR system has a catheter comprising a multilumen tube with balloon assembly (Fig. 27.26). The balloon is inflated to fit the size of the excision cavity. An iridium-192 source is inserted into the balloon to deliver the required dose. On completion of therapy, the balloon is deflated and the catheter removed.

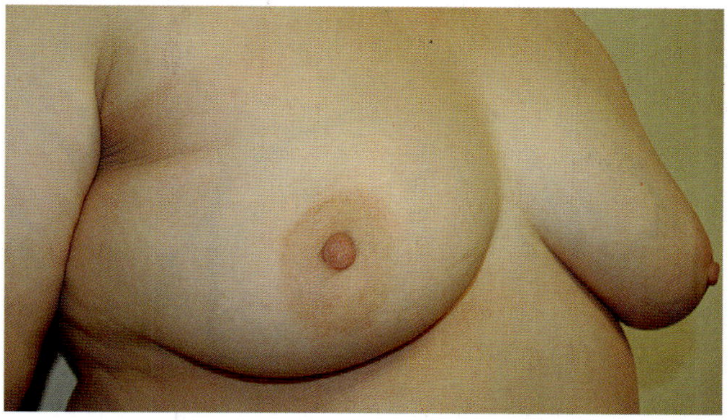

Fig. 27.25 Excellent cosmetic result of postoperative radiotherapy and iridium implant following lumpectomy for early carcinoma of the left breast. (Courtesy Prof. Mike Dixon, Edinburgh, UK.)

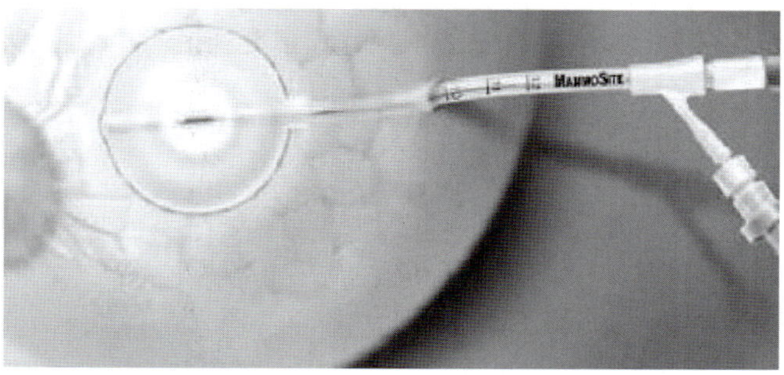

Fig. 27.26 Breast brachytherapy with MammoSite.

A large EORTC trial (Fig. 27.27) of over 5500 patients showed an overall 40% reduction in the risk of local recurrence with the use of the boost. Patients with clear margins after wide local excision were treated with whole breast irradiation (50 Gy in 25 fractions over 5 weeks) and randomised to either a boost (electrons, 10 Gy) or implant. Age was an independent risk factor for recurrence. In females under the age of 40 years, the local recurrence with the boost was 10% compared with 20% without the boost.

The absolute reduction in recurrence was smaller in females over the age of 40 years, but it was still statistically significant up to the age of 50 years. Long-term follow-up of the trial at 20 years showed the cumulative incidence of ipsilateral breast tumour recurrence was 16.4% (99% CI 14.1–18.8) in the no-boost group versus 12.0% (CI 9.8–14.4) in the boost group. The proportional reduction in risk for all risk groups was similar. The absolute reduction in risk was highest in the highest-risk group (i.e. youngest patients). The risk was 36% in the no-boost versus 24.2% in the boost group for females under age 40 years; 19.4% (14.7–24.1) versus 13.5% (9.5–17.5) in females age 41 to 50 years; 13.2% (9.8–16.7) versus 10.3% (6.3–14.3) in females age 51 to 60 years; and 12.7% (7.4–18.0) versus 9.7% (5.0–14.4) for females older than age 60 years. At 20 years, the cumulative incidence of severe fibrosis was 1.8% (99% CI 1.1–2.5) in the no-boost group versus 5.2% (99% CI 3.9–6.4) in the boost group (P <.0001). On this basis, for patients with clear excision margins, a boost is recommended for females up to age 59 years or with an unfavourable biological profile. For older patients the risks of a boost probably outweigh the benefits. In patients for whom reexcision of positive margins is not possible, an electron boost would still be indicated.

Indications for Breast Boost. NICE 2018 guidelines (NICE, 2018) recommend offering an external beam boost to the tumour bed for females with invasive breast cancer and a high risk of local recurrence, following whole breast RT. High-risk factors include age younger than 60 years, high-grade histology, axillary node positive, T3 or T4 tumours and positive or close excision margins (<1 mm).

Breast Boost Technique. The EORTC 22881-10882 trial used an extra 16 Gy as the boost dose. However, increased rates of moderate to severe fibrosis rose significantly by 15% at 10 years (28.1% versus 13.2%, P <.001). Conventionally, planning of the boost had been based on a variety of information (mammogram, operation note and position of the scar) and treated with a single electron field. This clinically based approach was often inaccurate compared with using the position of the surgical ligaclips placed at the margins of the tumour bed (Fig. 27.23A). There is also evidence that electron-based treatment often underdoses the tumour bed compared with photon-based techniques. Advanced RT techniques (IMRT and image-guided radiotherapy (IGRT)) enable a simultaneous integrated boost to be delivered within the breast during daily RT sessions compared with the sequential boost.

IMRT provides better dose homogeneity within the boost volume than a single electron field. This is more convenient to patients and provides cost savings. Studies are in progress to establish whether IMRT and IGRT may have an advantage in reducing boost volumes and the risks of fibrosis. In the United Kingdom, in the IMPORT-HIGH trial of patients with early breast cancer at higher than average risk being treated by breast-conserving surgery, IMRT is being assessed, delivering a simultaneous integrated boost, to test whether RT side effects can be reduced. The control group receive whole breast irradiation (40 Gy in 15 fractions) followed by a sequential photon boost of 16 Gy in 8 fractions with 36 Gy in 15 fractions to the low-risk volume; 40 Gy in 15 fractions to the involved quadrant; and dose escalation to the tumour bed of 48 Gy or 53 Gy in 15 fractions with concomitant boost (Fig. 27.28).

The appropriate electron energy, usually 9 to 12 MeV, is chosen according to the depth of the breast tissue at the site of the tumour-bearing area. This should be accurately measured on the planning CT postoperatively. To avoid transmission of unwanted irradiation to the underlying lung, a Perspex degrader of appropriate thickness can be interposed between the electron applicator and the skin to attenuate the beam. The boosted volume should cover the tumour-bearing area with a margin of 1 to 2 cm (to take account of the inbowing of electron isodoses at depth) judged from clinical, mammographic and perioperative findings. Surgeons place metal clips at the site of the excision, which assist the clinical oncologist in identification of the tumour bed. Alternatively, a field-in-field technique may be used for the breast boost.

Electron Boost Dose. An electron boost dose is 10 Gy in 5 daily fractions over 1 week or 16 Gy in 8 daily fractions, or a radiobiologically equivalent dose, for example, 12 Gy in 4 daily fractions.

PARTIAL BREAST IRRADIATION

Whole breast irradiation has to date been the standard of care following breast-conserving surgery. The case for partial breast irradiation is based on observations that most ipsilateral local recurrences occur close to the original site of excision (the tumour bed). The tumour bed can be identified by titanium surgical clips. The development of advanced RT techniques has allowed dose to be matched to the spatial variation in risk of local recurrence. There are a variety of partial breast irradiation techniques, including external beam, interstitial brachytherapy and intraoperative. There is mature level I evidence for interstitial brachytherapy and for external beam radiotherapy (EBRT). In the GEC ESTRO noninferiority trial, 1328 patients age 40 years or older, pTis or pT1–2a (lesions of ≤3-cm diameter), pN0/pNmi and M0 breast cancer (stages 0, 1 and 2A) were treated with breast-conserving surgery and randomised to whole breast irradiation or to accelerated partial breast irradiation (APBI) with multicatheter brachytherapy. At 10 years of follow-up, the cumulative incidence of local recurrence

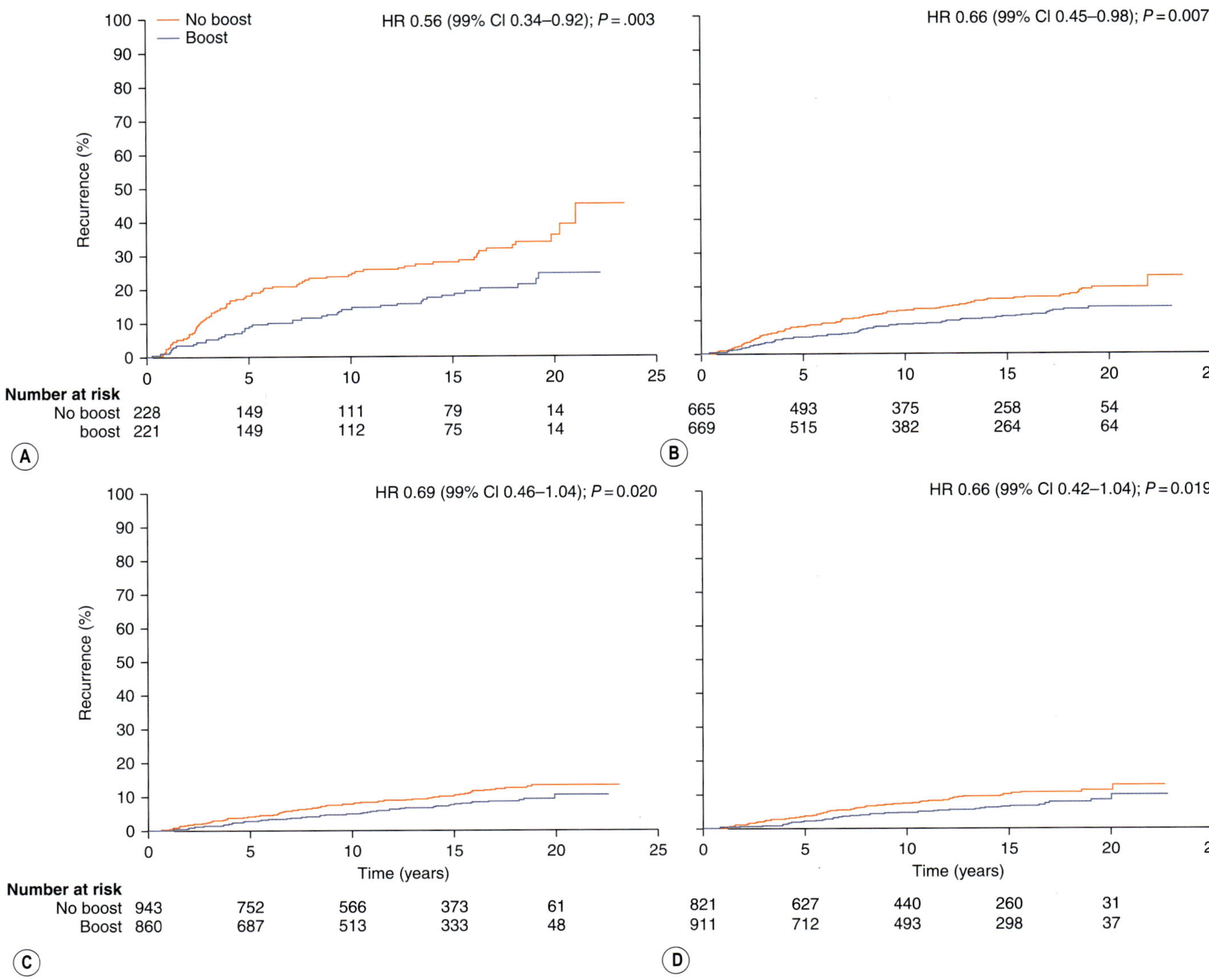

Fig. 27.27 The European Organisation for Research and Treatment of Cancer 22881-10882 Boost vs. No-Boost trial. Cumulative incidence of ipsilateral breast tumour recurrence by age. For patients age 40 years or younger, 71 patients in the no-boost group versus 42 in the boost group had recurrence (A); for patients age 41 to 50 years, 108 versus 74 had recurrence (B); for patients age 51 to 60 years, 100 versus 64 had recurrence (C); and for patients age older than 60 years, 75 versus 57 had recurrence (D). *HR*, Hazard ratio. (Reproduced with permission from Bartelink H, Maingon P, Poortmans P, et al. Whole breast irradiation with or without a boost for patients treated with breast conserving surgery for early breast cancer: 20-year follow-up of a randomised phase 3 trial. *Lancet Oncol.* 2015;16(1):47–56.)

was noninferior for APBI (3.51% (95% CI 1.99–5.03)) with APBI and 1.58% (95% CI 0.37–2.8) with whole breast irradiation. In the larger UK IMPORT-LOW trial of 2018 patients age 50 years or older with unifocal grade 1–3 breast cancer, 3 cm or less with zero to three positive nodes and minimum 2-mm clear margin were randomised to whole breast irradiation (control), 40 Gy to whole breast or 40 Gy to partial breast, and 36 Gy to whole breast or 40 Gy to partial breast only, in 15 daily fractions. At median follow-up of 72 months, the cumulative incidence of local relapse was 1.1% (95% CI 0.5–2.3) in the control group, 2% (95% CI 0.02–1.2) in the reduced group and 0.5% (95% CI 0.2–1.4) in the partial breast group. Both the reduced group and partial breast group were noninferior. Late toxicity to the breast (cosmesis or breast hardness) was similar or significantly less in the partial breast irradiation group compared to whole breast irradiation group. Potential advantages therefore of accelerated partial breast irradiation are patient convenience and reduction in acute and late normal tissue toxicities.

The European Society for Radiotherapy and Oncology Advisory Committee in Radiation Oncology Practice provided consensus guidelines in 2022 on eligibility criteria for partial breast irradiation. These are:

1. Luminal-like subtype
2. Small tumour (≤3 cm)
3. Grade 1 or 2
4. Low- and intermediate-grade DCIS
5. Age 50 or older
6. Unicentric or unifocal

Intraoperative Radiotherapy. The role of intraoperative radiotherapy (IORT) as a method of partial breast irradiation for early breast cancer remains controversial. A number of phase III randomised trials have evaluated IORT. The ELIOT (ELectron InOperative Therapy) trial used a single dose of intraoperative electrons (21 Gy) to the tumour bed following wide local excision. This was an equivalence trial. The

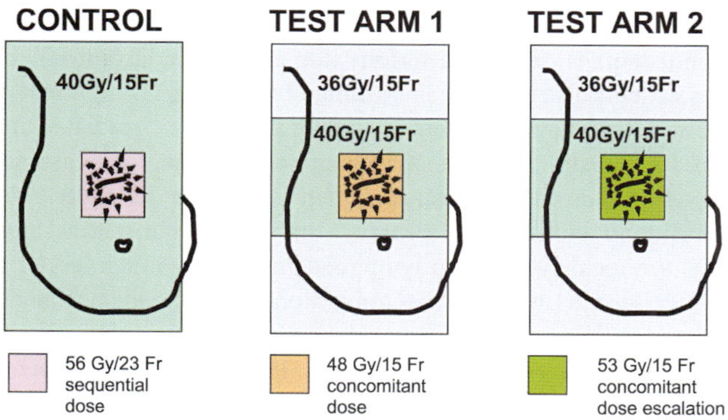

Control: 40Gy in 15 fractions to the whole breast followed by a sequential photon boost of 16Gy in 8 fractions to the tumour bed (Total- 56Gy in 23 fractions sequential dose)

Test Arm 1 and 2: 36Gy in 15 fractions to the low risk volume of the breast, 40Gy in 15 fractions to the index quadrant and dose escalation to the tumour bed with two dose levels of 48Gy and 53Gy in 15 fractions as concomitant boost

Fig. 27.28 Study schema of UK IMPORT HIGH trial. (Reproduced with permission from Coles CE, Brunt AM, Wheatley D, Mukesh MB, Yarnold JR. Breast radiotherapy: less is more? *Clin Oncol.* 2013;25(2):127–134.)

ipsilateral breast tumour recurrence rate at 15 years was significantly higher in the IORT group compared with the whole breast irradiation group (12.6 versus 2.4%).

The TARGIT-A trial evaluated IORT with a 50-kv device with a range of sizes of spherical applicators (Fig. 27.29) delivering a single dose of 20 Gy to the tumour bed over 15 to 20 minutes following wide local excision. This was planned as a noninferiority trial with a margin of 2.5% at 5 years. Additional EBRT was given if there were additional risk factors identified on the pathology excision specimen (15% of the IORT arm). Follow-up of the TARGIT-A trial shows that after a median follow-up of 8.6 years, the 5-year risk of local recurrence in the TARGIT-IORT arm was 2.11% compared to 0.95% in the whole breast irradiation arm. IORT with is not currently recommended outside prospective studies.

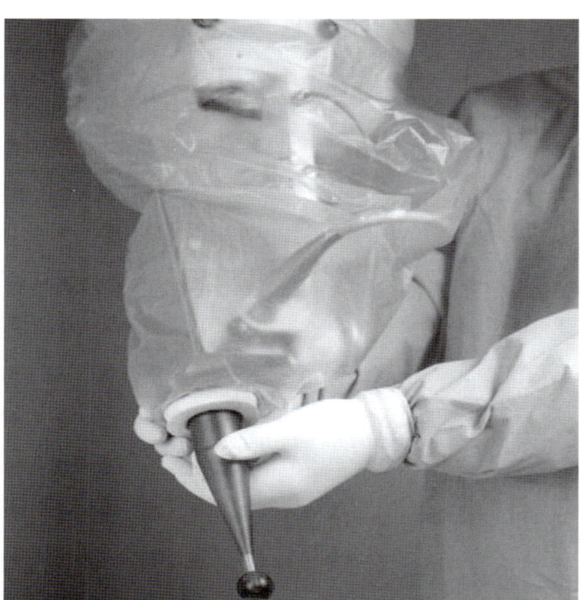

Fig. 27.29 Intrabeam intraoperative radiotherapy.

PROTON BEAM THERAPY

Proton beam therapy utilises high-energy charged particles as opposed to x-rays. It has the advantage of delivering radiation dose to a defined depth optimising target coverage and reducing toxicity to adjacent organs, particularly the heart, lungs and contralateral breast. To date, there are is no level I evidence on the clinical benefits of locoregional RT with protons. Proton beam facilities are currently available in a limited number of centres due to their complexity and high cost. However, there are examples (Fig. 27.30) where it can reduce dose to the heart where patients are intolerant of deep inspiratory breath hold to limit cardiac exposure or in the case of pectus excavatum where the heart lies particularly close to the chest wall. Prospective ongoing trials in the United States (RADCOMP), the Danish Breast Cancer Collaborative Group trial and the UK PARABLE trial are comparing protons with photons with cardiac toxicity +/– patient-reported outcomes as their primary endpoints. As yet, proton beam therapy is not a standard of care in most countries for breast cancer. The German Society of Radiation Oncology (DEGRO) guidelines recommend that protons should be considered in circumstances where presently known cardiac constraints cannot be achieved by alternative approaches and it is anticipated that the patients have a long life expectancy.

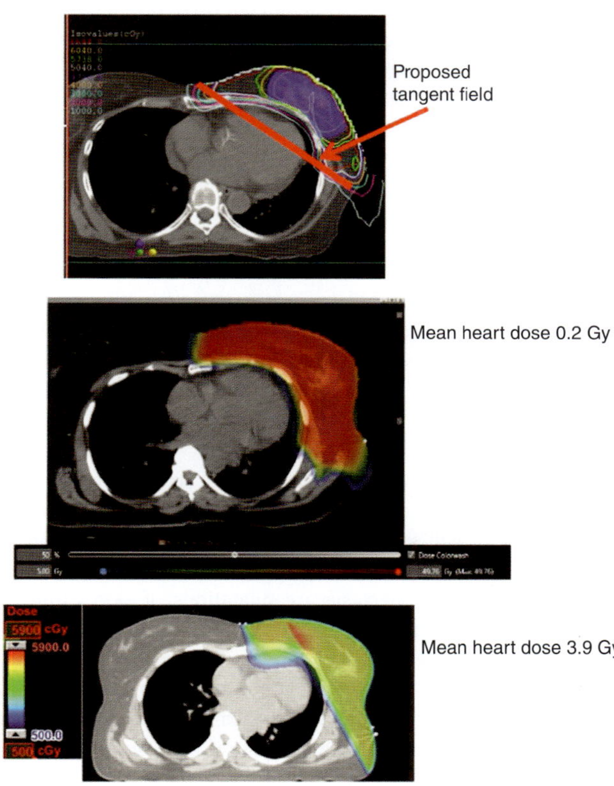

Fig. 27.30 A 53-year-old female with pT1cN0, ER/PR+m HER2-, IDC (invasive ductal carcinoma) of L breast s/p BCS (breast conserving surgery) and Ac_T (adriamycin, cyclophosphamide and taxol [paclitaxel]) chemotherapy, accepted for whole breast radiotherapy but did not tolerate deep inspiration breath-hold. Tangent fields would have resulted in large portions of the left anterior descending coronary artery and left ventricle receiving high doses. Patient was therefore simulated for proton therapy and strong target coverage was achieved with near complete cardiac sparing, with a mean heart dose of 0.3 Gy (colour version of figure is available online). (Reproduced with permission from Braunstein LZ, Cahlon O. Potential morbidity reduction with proton radiation therapy for breast cancer. *Sem Rad Oncol.* 2018;28(2):138–149.)

Morbidity of Radical Radiotherapy

The most common toxicities following breast-conserving surgery and postoperative irradiation to the breast and/or regional nodes are acute dermatitis, arm or breast oedema, myositis, breast fibrosis, rib fractures, lung fibrosis and pneumonitis. Less common complications are cardiac damage (Taylor et al., 2007; Darby et al., 2013), brachial plexopathy and second malignancies (Grantzau et al., 2013).

Acute Dermatitis

Acute radiation dermatitis can occur within 1 day after the start of RT. Acute skin toxicity is a result of impaired repopulation of the epidermis. Features include varying intensities of erythema, itching, hyperpigmentation and discomfort.

Skin Care During Treatment

The following guidance is based on the recommendations of the Society of Radiographers (https://www.sor.org).

Patients are advised to wear loose-fitting natural fibre clothing adjacent to the skin, for example, a cotton T-shirt. The skin should be washed gently with soap and water and gently patted dry. Avoid heat, rubbing and cooling pads/ice, wax for hair removal and all depilatory creams/products and adhesive tape.

To minimise irritation, a moisturising cream that is free of sodium lauryl sulphate is advised. Topical antibiotics should be avoided, unless there is a microbiologically proven infection. Deodorants can continue to be applied, as long as they do not act as an irritant; deodorants should be stopped if the skin is broken. Direct sun exposure should be avoided and high-factor sun block applied to exposed skin.

If the skin is broken, appropriate dressings/products can be applied to minimise further trauma. Nonadhesive non- or low-paraffin/petroleum jelly products are recommended. Gentian violet should not be applied.

Monitoring of skin reactions after completion of treatment should be arranged through community nursing services or a general practitioner.

Breast Swelling

Swelling of the breast occurs in around 30% of patients following breast-conserving surgery and postoperative RT and settles spontaneously in most cases.

Breast Pain

Acute, sharp, electric-shock–like pains or a dull ache within the irradiated breast commonly occurs 0 to 21 days after the start of treatment. Reassurance that it will settle and simple analgesia are often all that is required.

Telangiectasia. Telangiectasia are dilatations of skin capillaries. They have the appearance of spidery red or purple clusters and impair cosmesis. The dilatations develop 2 months to sometimes longer than 6 months progressively after treatment and then stabilise but are permanent. It is important that patients are warned of their development. Telangiectasia are associated with the use of skin bolus or electron breast boosts, particularly using more than 10 MeV compared with low-energy photons or electrons. Forward-planned IMRT has a lower risk of inducing telangiectasia than standard RT. No treatment is normally advised.

Chest Wall Pain/Fibrosis

Chest wall pain, skin fibrosis and contracture occur after breast-conserving surgery and postoperative RT, as well as following postmastectomy irradiation. High-energy electrons (>10 MeV) are associated with an increased risk of breast fibrosis. Maximising dose homogeneity within the breast (avoiding the volume of the breast receiving >107%) is important to minimising breast fibrosis.

Lymphoedema

Lymphoedema is one of the serious side effects of adjuvant RT that causes patients distress and can be difficult to manage. Lymphoedema of the arm is particularly likely to occur if the axilla is irradiated after a level III axillary clearance. Arm lymphoedema may increase progressively and eventually plateau, often years after its onset. With the decline in axillary node clearance and increase in sentinel node biopsy, the incidence of arm lymphoedema is very much less (1%–5%) after sentinel lymphadenectomy alone. Lymphoedema may be associated with sensory and motor deficit (associated with damage to the brachial plexus) and pectoral fibrosis. This combination of locoregional morbidities was associated with older RT techniques and when peripheral lymphatic irradiation was combined with axillary node dissection. In extreme cases of severe lymphoedema, the limb may be flail and useless. Patients with lymphoedema are more prone to cellulitis of the arm, which should be promptly assessed and treated with antibiotics.

Avoidance of trauma to the skin of the arm (e.g. using long-sleeved gloves for gardening), manual lymphatic drainage and compressing bandages or garments are recommended.

Following breast-conserving surgery, the incidence of breast or arm oedema is usually related to axillary node dissection rather than axillary nodal irradiation.

Brachial Plexopathy

Brachial plexopathy is a potential major complication of regional nodal irradiation. Fortunately, it is now rare (<1%), but it was more common in the past with older RT techniques employing higher doses per fraction and when regional nodal irradiation was often combined with level III clearance. The incidence of brachial plexopathy was significantly higher when the total dose to the axilla exceeded 50 Gy. Clinical features include paraesthesia in the affected arm/hand, pain in the shoulder or upper limit, motor weakness and sensory deficit, muscle wasting and loss of tendon reflexes. C7 is particularly affected, with lesser involvement of C6 and C8. The median interval between irradiation and onset of brachial neuropathy is typically 1 to 4 years, although onset can sometimes occur as late as 26 years after radiation therapy and as early as 3 months. Modest hypofractionation (46 Gy in 20 fractions) is not associated with radiation-induced brachial plexopathy. The UK hypofractionation regimen of 40 Gy in 15 daily fractions is considered safe. The important differential diagnosis is malignant infiltration of the brachial plexus. Suspected cases require referral to a neurologist and investigation by MRI and, if appropriate, nerve conduction studies. Clinical symptoms and nerve conduction studies cannot always distinguish between malignant infiltration and radiation-induced brachial plexopathy. Painless upper cervical trunk lesions with lymphoedema usually suggest radiation injury, and painful lower cervical trunk lesions with Horner syndrome usually indicate tumour infiltration. MRI findings characteristic of radiation-induced brachial plexopathy are hyperintensity on T2. A mass is suggestive of malignant brachial infiltration. Metastases show enhancement on gadolinium-enhanced images.

There are no effective treatments for radiation-induced brachial plexopathy. Hyperbaric oxygen was found to be ineffective. Coordinated care among the surgeon, oncologist, neurologist, palliative care specialist, physiotherapist, occupational therapist and general practitioner is needed.

Cardiac Damage

Radiation-induced heart disease encompasses coronary artery disease, pericarditis, myocardial dysfunction and valvular heart disease.

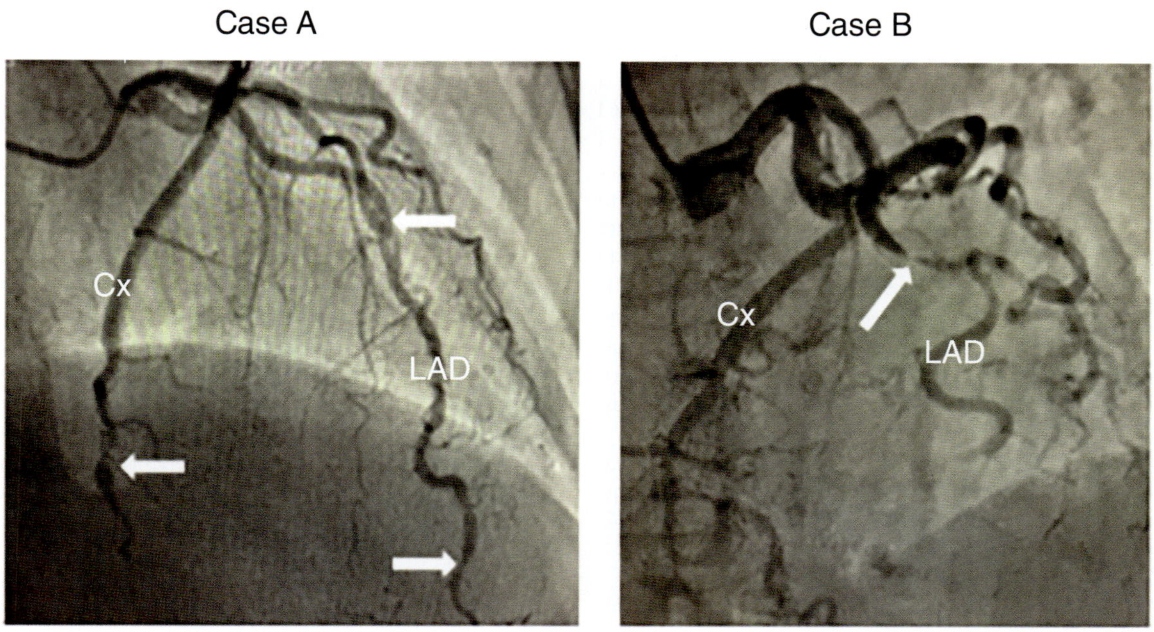

Fig. 27.31 Effects of adjuvant radiotherapy on the coronary arteries. Coronary heart disease in two patients (Case A and B) with previous radiotherapy for left-sided breast cancer. *White arrows* mark areas of diffuse obstructive coronary atheroma in both the left anterior descending coronary artery (LAD) and circumflex coronary artery in Case A and a more discrete severe lesion in the mid-LAD in Case B, causing reduced flow into the distal vessel. *Cx*, Circumflex coronary artery; *LAD*, left anterior descending coronary artery. (Courtesy Dr M. Denvir, University of Edinburgh. Reproduced with permission.)

The pathophysiological effects of irradiation from in vitro and in vivo studies occur at both the microvascular and macrovascular levels and include endothelial damage, inflammation, oxidative effects and cytokine activity, which accelerate the process of atherosclerosis. The coronary arteries are damaged directly, and the pericardium and myocardium become fibrosed. The microvasculature is damaged and valvular stenosis may occur. Doses as low as 2 Gy may cause endothelial inflammation and induce atherosclerosis (Fig. 27.31). The consequences of coronary damage are perfusion defects, ischaemia and fibrosis of the myocardium.

The majority of other radiation-related cardiac abnormalities are late events, occurring 10 to 15 years after RT. In general, radiation-induced cardiotoxicity occurs at an earlier age than the normal population. Cardiac mortality was found to be higher in patients with left-sided compared to right-sided tumours in predominantly older RT trials where the dose to cardiac structures was substantial. With the implementation of three-dimensional planning, mean heart doses have fallen from 13.3 Gy in the 1970s to 4.7 Gy in the 1990s and 2.3 Gy by 2006. These reductions have reduced the risk of radiation-induced cardiac deaths in females without cardiac risk factors. However, even with low mean heart doses, some parts of the heart may receive 40 to 50 Gy. Thus, mean heart dose often does not reflect risks of radiation-induced cardiotoxicity. Angiographic studies of patients who underwent left-side chest wall or breast irradiation showed significant stenosis of the mid and distal left anterior descending artery. The median dose to the damaged and undamaged coronary segments was 30.3 and 26.3 Gy, respectively. Echocardiography can show a significant fall in myocardial deformation.

Cardiac damage can occur with relatively low doses. Data among 963 females who had a major coronary event after RT for breast cancer between 1958 and 2011 in Sweden and Denmark compared with 1205 control females who did not have a major coronary event showed a linear increase in major coronary events with mean dose to the heart by 7.4% per Gy with no apparent threshold (Darby et al., 2013). The increase in acute major coronary events was seen within the first 5 years after RT and persisted into the third decade after irradiation. There are higher risks of radiation-induced cardiac events in patients with established risk factors for coronary heart disease. However, the proportionate risk of major cardiac events was similar in females with or without cardiac risk factors.

Radiation can cause valvular disease, typically affecting the left-sided valves, with aortic regurgitation being the most common. Rarely, it may result in aortic stenosis, mandating surgical intervention. There is limited literature on doses to the cardiac valves from adjuvant RT for breast cancer. Tangential fields in the 1990s delivered less than 2 Gy to the whole heart. Dosage of less than 30 Gy is considered unlikely to cause cardiac damage. However, doses to the internal mammary chain, particularly from direct photon fields, were much higher and did not vary much from the 1970s to 1990s. It is estimated that a dose of approximately 12 Gy to the internal mammary chain in the 2000s would nearly double the risk of ischaemic heart disease and the 30-year absolute risk by a few percentage points. Dose fractionation regimens with 1.8 to 2.0 or 2.5 to 3 Gy per fraction seem to confer similar cardiac risk up to 10 to 15 years. Over 3 Gy per fraction may increase risk.

Myocardial perfusion defects (ischaemic areas of the level ventricle) have been identified in patients irradiated for breast cancer. However, the clinical significance of these abnormalities is not known. The site of these left ventricular perfusion defects is mainly influenced by the borders of the RT fields rather than the distribution of the coronary vessels. This implies that they are caused by damage to the microvasculature of the myocardium rather than coronary artery damage. Damage to the coronary arteries has been demonstrated in breast cancer patients who have undergone adjuvant irradiation and occurs particularly in arterial segments likely to have received high radiation doses (Fig. 27.31).

Radiation-induced pericarditis is a rare acute complication, usually occurring soon after exposure.

Prophylactic supraclavicular irradiation does not appear to increase the risk of stroke.

More data are needed on the combined cardiotoxic effects of anthracycline-based adjuvant chemotherapy. Anti-HER2 therapy with trastuzumab is also cardiotoxic. Chemotherapy-induced toxicity is classified as Type I (anthracyclines) and Type II (trastuzumab). Type I damage is to cardiac myocytes and is judged irreversible. In Type II damage, there is no structural change and damage is reversible. Little is known of these combined cardiotoxic effects or their interaction with other known risk factors (smoking, hypercholesterolaemia, premature menopause). There are wide variations among patients in proneness to radiation-induced toxicity and some evidence of variation in genetic susceptibility. Appropriate imaging-based screening procedures and biomarkers of the risk of cardiac damage are needed because cardiac events may occur 10 to 15 years or more after radiation exposure. Answers to these questions will inform prevention strategies for breast cancer survivors in whom cardiac exposure cannot be avoided.

A significantly higher risk of cardiac death was seen with a linear dose-response relationship in the Japanese survivors of the atomic bomb.

Lung Damage

There are two phases of lung toxicity. The first is a subacute inflammatory phase known as radiation pneumonitis. The second phase is late radiation fibrosis. Radiation pneumonitis is uncommon. It presents acutely with cough, shortness of breath or fever. On auscultation of the chest, there may be crackles or no added sounds. It is thought that cytotoxic damage to the type II pneumocytes and vascular endothelial cells primarily initiates radiation damage. These tissue changes include abnormalities of surfactant-containing lamellar bodies within type II pneumocytes; increases in surfactant production are detected in bronchoalveolar lavage samples within hours of radiation. The immediate phase (within hours or days) is clinically silent. It features an inflammatory response inducing a leucocytic infiltration leading to intraalveolar oedema and vascular congestion. There follows a latent phase (days to weeks) featuring the accumulation of thick secretions from an increase in goblet cells and ciliary malfunction. Subsequently, there is an acute exudative phase (weeks to months) of hyaline membrane formation, type II pneumocyte proliferation, endothelial and epithelial shedding and clinical symptoms of radiation pneumonitis. There follows an intermediate phase (months) mirroring progression of changes noted previously, destruction of hyaline membranes, regeneration of capillaries and fibroblast migration. Finally, there is a fibrotic phase (months to years) of progressive fibrosis with deposition of collagen by fibroblasts distorting alveolar spaces and reducing lung volumes.

The risk of pneumonitis is related to the volume irradiated. The risk of lung toxicity varies with RT technique and the volumes irradiated. Most patients do not experience any limitation of their exercise tolerance. The addition of regional nodal irradiation to breast irradiation significantly increases the risk of pneumonitis.

A number of cytotoxic agents increase the risk of radiation pneumonitis: taxanes, cyclophosphamide, gemcitabine, doxorubicin, mitomycin C, vincristine and bevacizumab. Chest radiograph and CT scan may show pulmonary infiltrates in the irradiated volume. These usually stabilise by a year after RT. Some may resolve or progress over 5 or more years. The risks of pneumonitis are less than 5% if a third axillary field is added to the breast fields if the average lung distance is 3 cm or less. It is unclear whether the risk of pneumonitis is increased by chemotherapy.

Lung function tests may show restrictive ventilatory changes and impaired diffusion capacity that are reversible. Treatment of radiation pneumonitis is with high-dose steroids (prednisone 60 mg per day for 14 days), tailed off by 10 mg per day over 1 to 2 weeks.

Rib Fractures

Rib fractures, as a result of ischaemic osteoradionecrosis with or without soft-tissue necrosis, can develop around 1 year after conventionally fractionated breast RT but are rare (0.1%–5%). Treatment is normally conservative.

Carcinogenesis

Adjuvant locoregional irradiation increases very modestly the risk of cancer in the contralateral breast in females age 45 years or younger. The RR is about 1.2. In a second primary trial undertaken by the Danish Breast Cancer Cooperative Group (Grantzau et al., 2013) in 46,176 females treated between 1982 and 2007 with or without irradiation, RT significantly increased the risk at 10 to 14 years and 15 or more years of lung cancer (HR 1.27; 95% CI 1.04–1.55) and connective tissue (soft-tissue sarcomas (HR 2.96; 95% CI 1.17–6.18)) but did not significantly increase oesophageal cancer (HR 1.17; 95% CI 0.56–2.44). Soft-tissue sarcomas within irradiated fields usually occur 8 to 10 years after treatment but occasionally earlier (1–2 years). Prognosis for angiosarcoma is poor.

ADJUVANT AND NEOADJUVANT SYSTEMIC THERAPY

Patients with early breast cancer and no evidence of metastatic disease should undergo surgery. Most will need some form of systemic therapy. Systemic therapy can be given before surgery (neoadjuvant) in the case of large tumours to downsize them or if evidence of pathological complete response (pCR) provides useful prognostic information (e.g. in HER2-positive disease and triple-negative breast cancer) (Fig. 27.32). Alternatively, systemic therapy can be given after surgery (adjuvant).

ADJUVANT HORMONAL AND CYTOTOXIC THERAPY

Rationale

It is generally accepted that a substantial number of patients with apparently localised breast cancer harbour systemic micrometastases. These micrometastases are currently beyond the detection of conventional staging.

All patients should be considered for some form of adjuvant systemic therapy to try to eradicate micrometastases. Selection of therapy is based on tumour burden and molecular subtype. Factors to be taken into consideration are tumour size, tumour grade, axillary node status, oestrogen/progesterone receptor and HER2 status. The PREDICT tool (see the section titled Prognostic Indices) is often used as a useful adjunct for both clinician decision-making and to help patients understand the concept of the benefits of adjuvant therapy. It is important to understand that the estimates using PREDICT are only a guide, and there are various limitations to the algorithm. The addition of information on tumour biology from intrinsic subtypes (luminal A, luminal B, HER2 enriched and triple negative) may help estimate likely response to systemic therapy. Luminal-A tumours (low grade, high ER and PR expression, low proliferation and low-risk gene expression scores) are usually candidates for endocrine therapy alone (unless they have high-risk features and are treated like luminal-B tumours). Luminal-B tumours express ER but little or no PR, normally have high-risk features (high grade or high proliferation and high risk gene expression scores) and systemic chemotherapy is often indicated.

For patients with ER-positive HER2-negative cancers who are considered to be at higher risk of recurrence, most centres recommend a combination of anthracycline and taxane chemotherapy. Increasing the dose intensity has been shown to improve outcomes with accelerated anthracyclines and has become a standard practice in many centres

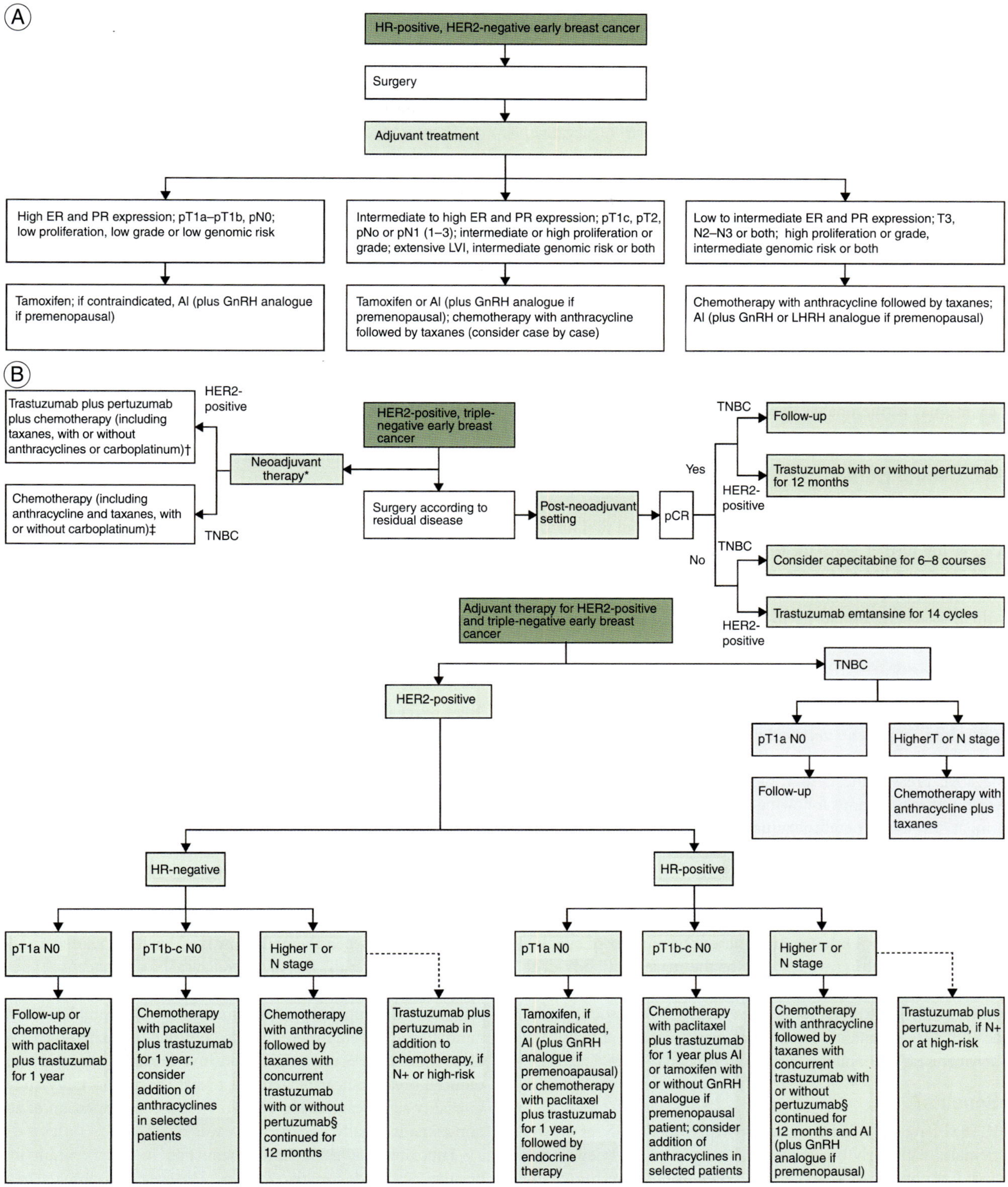

Fig. 27.32 Treatment algorithm for HR-positive and HER2-negative early breast cancer (A) and HER2-positive and triple-negative early breast cancer (B). (Reproduced with permission from Loibl S, Poortmans P, Morrow M, Denkert C, Curigliano G. Breast cancer. *Lancet.* 2021;397(10286):1750–1769.)

(EBCTCG, 2019). For moderate-risk cancers where chemotherapy is indicated, or for patients with prior cardiac disease, shorter-course treatment with TC (docetaxel/cyclophosphamide) may be preferred and, being anthracycline free, has the advantage of less long-term cardiac toxicity and reduced risk of haematological malignancies.

Most patients with HER2-positive cancers will be considered for adjuvant systemic chemotherapy and anti-HER2 therapy, with the exception of those with pT1a N0 disease. Lower-risk HER2-positive cancers may be offered treatment with 12 weeks of paclitaxel together with 1 year of adjuvant trastuzumab, while higher T-stage or node-positive patients are more commonly treated in the neoadjuvant setting with combination chemotherapy with an anthracycline followed by a taxane, trastuzumab and pertuzumab dual anti-HER2 therapy, or docetaxel, carboplatin and dual anti-HER2 therapy.

The neoadjuvant setting offers a number of advantages, most importantly the ability to assess the tumour response to treatment and the option of tailoring the treatment depending on the response. Adjuvant pertuzumab is only used for patients with node-positive disease or in the neoadjuvant setting.

For patients with triple-negative (ER/PR- and HER2-negative) breast cancer, the gold standard is also neoadjuvant chemotherapy, with the exception of patients with small node-negative cancers. The practice-changing KEYNOTE-522 trial demonstrated that the addition of pembrolizumab, a checkpoint inhibitor, significantly improved the pCR rate and event-free survival when added to carboplatin-, paclitaxel- and anthracycline-based neoadjuvant chemotherapy, followed by adjuvant pembrolizumab for 9 further cycles of adjuvant therapy (Schmid et al., 2022). This agent is, however, associated with a number of immune-mediated toxicities, and careful patient counselling is essential. For small node-negative triple-negative breast cancers, less intensive chemotherapy with a combination of some of the aforementioned agents may be reasonable, depending on patient comorbidities, overall treatment benefit and patient wishes.

Residual Cancer Burden

A residual cancer burden (RCB) score is usually calculated by pathologists following neoadjuvant chemotherapy and is a useful tool for risk stratification for further adjuvant therapy after surgery. For patients with HER2-positive breast cancer, there is good evidence from the landmark KATHERINE trial that a switch from postoperative adjuvant trastuzumab +/− pertuzumab to 14 cycles of adjuvant trastuzumab emtansine can significantly reduce the risk of disease recurrence and improves overall survival (von Minckwitz et al., 2019). Six months of adjuvant capecitabine has been shown to reduce recurrence in patients with HER2-negative residual disease after neoadjuvant chemotherapy, but in this study, no patients received neoadjuvant carboplatin, so it is uncertain what the benefit of this approach will be for patients with triple-negative breast cancer. In triple-negative breast cancer, there are now a number of options following surgery, based on the response to treatment. Adjuvant pembrolizumab is continued as part of the KEYNOTE-522 protocol, but some clinicians may also recommend the addition of adjuvant capecitabine for those with residual disease following neoadjuvant therapy. As triple-negative breast cancer with residual disease following neoadjuvant treatment is unfortunately associated with particularly poor outcomes, there are a number of ongoing clinical trials in this setting using some of the newer antibody-drug conjugate drugs, and these may show improved outcomes.

In patients with high-risk HER2-negative breast cancer associated with germline BRCA1/2 mutations, 1 year of adjuvant olaparib, a poly ADP ribose polymerase (PARP) inhibitor, is recommended (Tutt et al., 2021).

Who Benefits?

The EBCTCG have provided a series of 5-yearly metaanalyses of over 75,000 females with early breast cancer. The group's overview shows clearly that both hormonal therapy (tamoxifen or oophorectomy) and cytotoxic therapy (CMF or anthracycline-containing combination chemotherapy) reduce the RR of relapse or death by up to 30% at 10 years. The overall survival benefits are more modest, with a 4% to 12% gain in overall survival. The benefits in overall survival are greater in premenopausal than postmenopausal females. In females over the age of 70 years, there are few data on the benefit of adjuvant chemotherapy and some evidence that the degree of benefit falls with increasing age.

Following polychemotherapy, females age 50 to 59 years gain a 14% reduction in risk of death compared with 8% in females age 60 to 69 years. Life expectancy is likely to be prolonged on average by 4 years for females under the age of 50 years and by 1 to 3 years in females over the age of 50 years. Adjuvant chemotherapy reduces 10-year breast cancer mortality by 27%. For a female who has a 50% chance of dying from breast cancer under the age of 50 years, the approximate reduction in risk of death is 13.5%. For a female with a 10% risk of death at 10 years, the risk of death is about 8%.

There is evidence that anthracycline-containing regimens increase the probability of survival compared with nonanthracycline-containing regimens such as CMF but at the cost of greater toxicity, particularly myelosuppression. For patients at sufficient risk, a combination of a taxane and an anthracycline is recommended.

Adjuvant Endocrine Therapy

British physician George T. Beatson first identified the potential role of oestrogen in breast tissue. He observed that rabbits stopped lactating after oophorectomy. Based on these findings, he undertook an oophorectomy in 1895 on a premenopausal patient with inoperable breast cancer. The patient had a complete remission and lived for a further 4 years. Beatson's work set the foundation of modern hormonal therapy in breast cancer. In current practice, 5 to 10 years of adjuvant endocrine therapy is standard for females with ER-positive breast cancer. Tamoxifen or a steroidal (exemestane) or nonsteroidal (letrozole or anastrozole) aromatase inhibitor is suitable for postmenopausal females. Extending adjuvant endocrine therapy from 5 to 10 years reduces the risk of recurrence further in patients at high risk of recurrence (e.g. node-positive or high genomic score (see the 'Further Reading' section)). Premenopausal patients for whom adjuvant chemotherapy is not indicated because of a low risk of recurrence can be treated by tamoxifen alone.

Adjuvant Tamoxifen

The EBCTCG review of 194 randomised trials showed that 5 years of adjuvant tamoxifen in ER-positive patients reduced breast cancer mortality by 31% and was superior to 1 to 2 years of tamoxifen. In a subsequent EBCTCG metaanalysis, 5 years of adjuvant tamoxifen significantly reduced the risk of recurrence during the first 10 years and the risk of breast cancer mortality by about one-third during the first 15 years (Fig. 27.33) (Davies et al., 2011). Females with ER-rich tumours have 3 to 10 times the benefits of ER-poor patients. Life expectancy is increased by 2 to 3 years in females on tamoxifen for 2 to 3 years. If tamoxifen is added to chemotherapy in ER-rich tumours, additional benefit accrues, as also happens when chemotherapy is added to tamoxifen. In addition, tamoxifen reduces the risk of contralateral breast cancer.

There is an advantage to extending tamoxifen beyond 5 years. The ATLAS trial compared 12,984 females who had completed 5 years of tamoxifen and were randomised to continue tamoxifen for 10 years or discontinue it at 5 years. In ER-positive females, extended tamoxifen reduced breast cancer recurrence, breast cancer mortality and overall mortality significantly (Fig. 27.34). The standard duration of adjuvant tamoxifen is usually 5 years.

Tamoxifen confers a similar reduction in risk of death in node-positive and node-negative females. However, the absolute reduction in risk is greater in node-positive females. The absolute gain in 10-year survival between 5 years of tamoxifen and no tamoxifen is 6% in node-negative and 11% in node-positive females. It confers benefit in both premenopausal and postmenopausal ER-positive females. Adding tamoxifen to chemotherapy in ER-positive patients confers additional benefit. All patients who are ER positive regardless of their menopausal or nodal status should be considered for adjuvant endocrine therapy for 5 years.

Aromatase Inhibitors

In postmenopausal females, the ovary no longer produces oestrogen. Instead, it is mainly synthesised from nonglandular tissue (e.g.

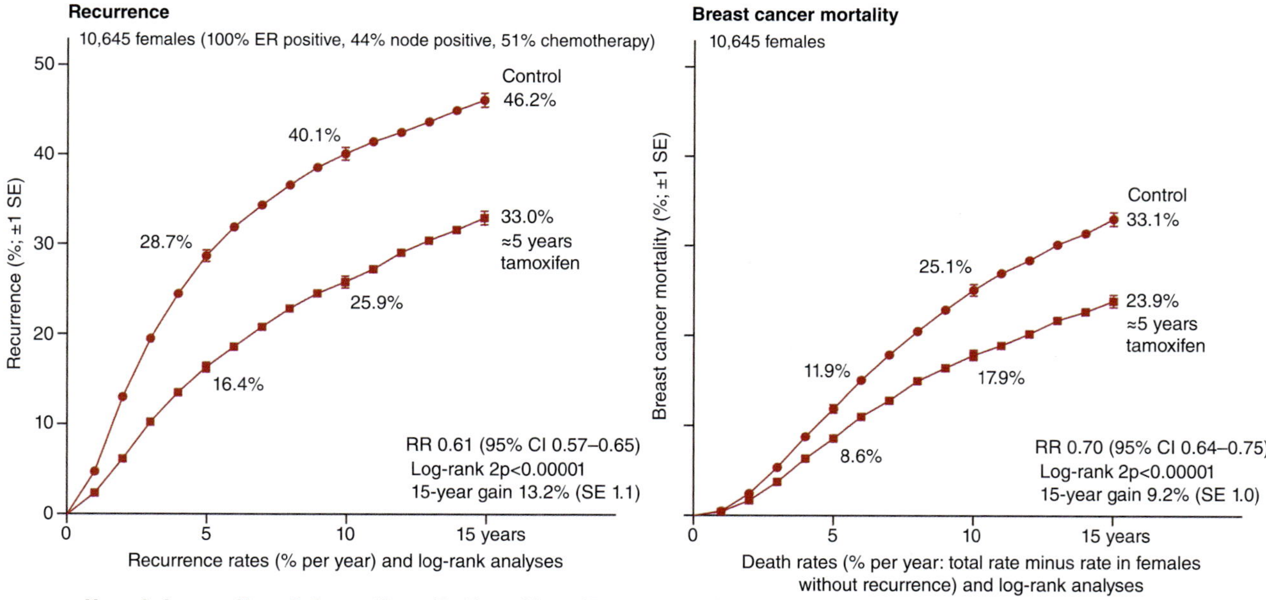

	Years 0–4	Years 5–9	Years 10–14	Years 15+
Tamoxifen	3.74 (891/23819)	2.62 (454/17315)	2.06 (220/10657)	1.75 (88/5034)
control	6.71 (1466/21862)	3.46 (499/14420)	2.11 (182/8620)	1.76 (71/4045)
Rate ratio	0.53 (SE 0.03)	0.68 (SE 0.06)	0.97 (SE 0.10)	0.88 (SE 0.16)
(O–E)/V	−343.3/535.1	−82.5/217.5	−3.3/93.3	−4.4/35.5

Years 0–4	Years 5–9	Years 10–14	Years 15+
1.79 (SE 0.08)	2.25 (SE 0.11)	1.54 (SE 0.11)	1.48 (SE 0.16)
2.46 (SE 0.10)	3.23 (SE 0.13)	2.28 (SE 0.14)	1.89 (SE 0.19)
0.88 (SE 0.05)	0.66 (SE 0.05)	0.68 (SE 0.08)	0.88 (SE 0.14)
−84.4/244.8	−95.8/233.2	−38.6/99.4	−5.7/42.6

Fig. 27.33 Effects of about 5 years of tamoxifen on the 15-year probabilities of recurrence and of breast cancer mortality, for ER-positive disease. Outcome by allocated treatment in trials of about 5 years of adjuvant tamoxifen. Event rate ratio (RR) is from summed log-rank statistics for all time periods. Gain (and its SE) is absolute difference between ends of graphs. ER = oestrogen receptor. O–E = observed minus expected, with variance V. (Reproduced with permission from Early Breast Cancer Trialists' Collaborative Group (EBCTCG); Davies C, Godwin J, Gray R, et al. Relevance of breast cancer hormone receptors and other factors to the efficacy of adjuvant tamoxifen: patient-level meta-analysis of randomised trials. *Lancet.* 2011;378(9793):771–784.)

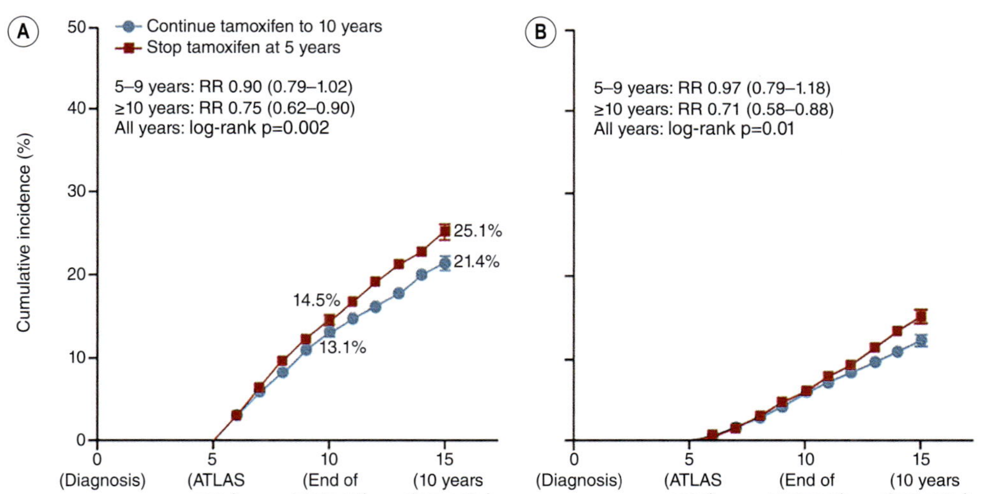

	5–9 years	10–14 years	≥15 years
Continue tamoxifen to 10 years	2.83% (428/15115)	1.96% (165/8439)	2.54% (24/945)
Stop tamoxifen at 5 years	3.16% (471/14889)	2.66% (214/8038)	3.03% (26/859)
Rate ratio, from (O-E)/V	0.90 (SE 0.06)	0.74 (SE 0.09)	0.85 (SE 0.26)
Log-rank O-E and variance V	−24.8/224.7	−29.1/94.7	−2.1/12.5

	5–9 years	10–14 years	≥15 years
Continue tamoxifen to 10 years	1.17% (SE 0.09)	1.38% (SE 0.12)	1.64% (SE 0.39)
Stop tamoxifen at 5 years	1.21% (SE 0.09)	2.01% (SE 0.15)	2.29% (SE 0.47)
Rate ratio, from (O-E)/V	0.97 (SE 0.10)	0.70 (SE 0.10)	0.79 (SE 0.27)
Log-rank O-E and variance V	−3.2/94.0	−27.2/77.5	−2.5/10.6

Fig. 27.34 Adjuvant Tamoxifen: Longer Against Shorter (ATLAS) trial. Recurrence (A) and breast cancer mortality (B) by treatment allocation for 6846 females with ER-positive disease. *Error bars* show SE (Standard Error). Recurrence rates (RR) are percentage per year (events per patient-years of follow-up). Death rates (overall rate: rate in females without recurrence) are percentage per year (SE). (Reproduced with permission from Davies C, Pan H, Godwin J, et al. Long-term effects of continuing adjuvant tamoxifen to 10 years versus stopping at 5 years after diagnosis of oestrogen receptor-positive breast cancer: ATLAS, a randomised trial. *Lancet.* 2013;381(9869):805–816.)

subcutaneous fat, muscle and liver) through the aromatase enzyme. The first two generations of aromatase inhibitors caused significant side effects because they also inhibited other steroid hormones such as aldosterone and cortisol.

Third-generation aromatase inhibitors have much greater specificity and are classified as either steroidal (type 1) or nonsteroidal (type 2). Steroidal aromatase inhibitors inhibit the aromatase enzyme irreversibly. Nonsteroidal aromatase inhibitors are reversible competitive inhibitors. Aromatase inhibitors provide greater reductions in recurrence in more advanced stage 2 to 3, HER2-positive and high-grade disease. The standard duration of an aromatase inhibitor is 5 years, particularly for stage 1 disease. Longer duration up to 10 years can be beneficial for higher-risk patients, although patients still remain at risk of recurrence beyond 10 years. Benefits have to be carefully weighed against toxicity and impact on quality of life.

The role of aromatase inhibitors as an alternative to tamoxifen or in combination with it was explored in the ATAC trial. This trial of over 9000 postmenopausal node-negative and predominantly ER-positive patients at a median follow-up of 68 months showed a significantly longer disease survival in the anastrozole alone group over tamoxifen alone (HR 0.86; 95% CI .78–.97, $P = .01$). In addition, there was a highly significant reduction in risk of contralateral breast cancer in the anastrozole alone group. The incidence of endometrial cancer, vaginal bleeding and discharge, venous thromboembolism and cerebrovascular accidents was also reduced in the anastrozole-treated group. However, musculoskeletal symptoms and bone fractures were more common with anastrozole.

In the BIG 1-98 trial, 8028 postmenopausal patients with endocrine-sensitive breast cancer were randomised to 5 years of tamoxifen (20 mg daily), 5 years of letrozole (25 mg daily), 2 years of tamoxifen followed by 3 years of letrozole or 2 years of letrozole followed by 3 years of tamoxifen. Analysis of the comparison of the tamoxifen (5 years) and letrozole (5 years) with a median follow-up of 25.8 months showed a significant advantage survival of letrozole over tamoxifen (84.0% versus 81.4%, respectively). Patients on tamoxifen had significantly more thromboembolic events. Patients on letrozole had significantly more bone fractures (5.7% versus 4%, respectively, $P = .001$) and deaths from cardiac or cerebrovascular causes.

In the TEAM trial, postmenopausal patients were randomised to up-front tamoxifen versus exemestane, tamoxifen followed by exemestane or exemestane alone. At a median follow-up of 30.6 months, disease-free survival was improved by 4.7% with exemestane compared with tamoxifen alone (95% CI 2.8–6.8). However, there was no difference between exemestane alone or when switched to exemestane from tamoxifen. There were significantly fewer contralateral breast cancers in the exemestane group compared with tamoxifen.

The EBCTCG undertook a metaanalysis of 31,920 patients in randomised trials of aromatase inhibitors versus tamoxifen (EBCTCG, 2015). They compared subgroups (5 years of aromatase inhibitors, 5 years of tamoxifen or 2–3 years of tamoxifen followed by aromatase inhibitors to complete 5 years of treatment and 2–3 years of an aromatase inhibitor followed by tamoxifen). A greater reduction in recurrence was seen in patients taking an aromatase inhibitor during any point of the trial (Fig. 27.35).

Adjuvant Hormonal Therapy After 5 Years of Tamoxifen

From 60% to 70% of breast cancers are ER positive. Despite the efficacy of adjuvant endocrine therapy, 50% of breast cancer recurrences and 66% of deaths occur after the initial 5 years of tamoxifen. This implies that ER-positive breast cancer is a chronic relapsing disease that may remain quiescent for many years. This high rate of late relapse was the basis for investigating extending adjuvant endocrine therapy beyond 5 years. In this extended adjuvant setting, reductions in breast cancer recurrence must be balanced against the cumulative toxicity of longer endocrine therapy.

Extended adjuvant hormonal therapy with more potent aromatase inhibitors, such as letrozole and exemestane, may reduce the risk of recurrent breast cancer in patients treated initially with tamoxifen. In the National Cancer Institute of Canada (NCIC) MA17 trial, 1918 patients who had received 4.5 to 6 years of an adjuvant aromatase inhibitor were randomised to 2.5 mg of letrozole or placebo for a further 5 years. The 5-year disease-free survival in the extended letrozole group was 96% compared with 91% in the placebo group (HR 0.66; $P = .01$). This benefit was independent of nodal status. However, there was no difference in overall survival between the two groups.

Toxicity of Tamoxifen

Postmenopausal symptoms of hot flushes, vaginal dryness and sexual dysfunction are experienced by 20% to 40% of patients. Cognitive deficits also occur (as they do after cytotoxic chemotherapy). These symptoms can significantly interfere with a patient's quality of life. Tamoxifen increases the development of benign endometrial changes, such as hyperplasia. The risk of endometrial cancer is largely confined to postmenopausal females, who should be monitored for symptoms of endometrial hyperplasia or cancer. The risk of endometrial cancer is about 0.02%. Premenopausal females treated with tamoxifen have no known increased risk of uterine cancer and as such require no additional monitoring beyond routine gynaecological care.

Care should be taken to avoid giving tamoxifen concurrently with chemotherapy because it increases the risk of thrombosis. Tamoxifen should therefore only be started once chemotherapy has been completed.

Tamoxifen Plus Chemotherapy

Treatment with both tamoxifen and chemotherapy gives added benefit in both node-positive and node-negative females with ER-positive disease. This also applies to postmenopausal ER-positive patients. However, in ER-negative, node-negative females, the NSABP B-23 trial showed no benefit of the addition of tamoxifen to chemotherapy.

Adjuvant Ovarian Suppression

The Oxford overview showed a highly significant increase in recurrence-free survival (25%) in premenopausal females under the age of 50 years treated by oophorectomy (EBCTCG, 2022).

For node-positive premenopausal females, the gains in recurrence-free and overall survival at 15 years were 10.5% and 13%, respectively. Much smaller but still statistically significant benefits in both these parameters were seen in premenopausal node-negative females. Because tamoxifen and chemotherapy became standard adjuvant therapy, the role of ovarian suppression became unclear. A number of prospective trials and a metaanalysis of ovarian suppression using gonatropin releasing hormone (GnRH) showed no gain from addition of ovarian suppression to tamoxifen or chemotherapy.

The Suppression of Ovarian Function (SOFT) trial compared tamoxifen, tamoxifen plus ovarian suppression and a combination of the aromatase inhibitor exemestane plus ovarian suppression in premenopausal females. Adjuvant therapy was given for 5 years. Options for ovarian suppression were surgical oophorectomy and radiation-induced ovarian suppression or GnRH agonist treatment with triptorelin.

The Tamoxifen and Exemestane Trial (TEXT) compared tamoxifen plus ovarian suppression with the combination of the aromatase inhibitor exemestane and ovarian suppression in 3066 premenopausal patients. At a median follow-up of 67 months, the estimated disease-free survival was 86.6% in the tamoxifen + ovarian suppression group

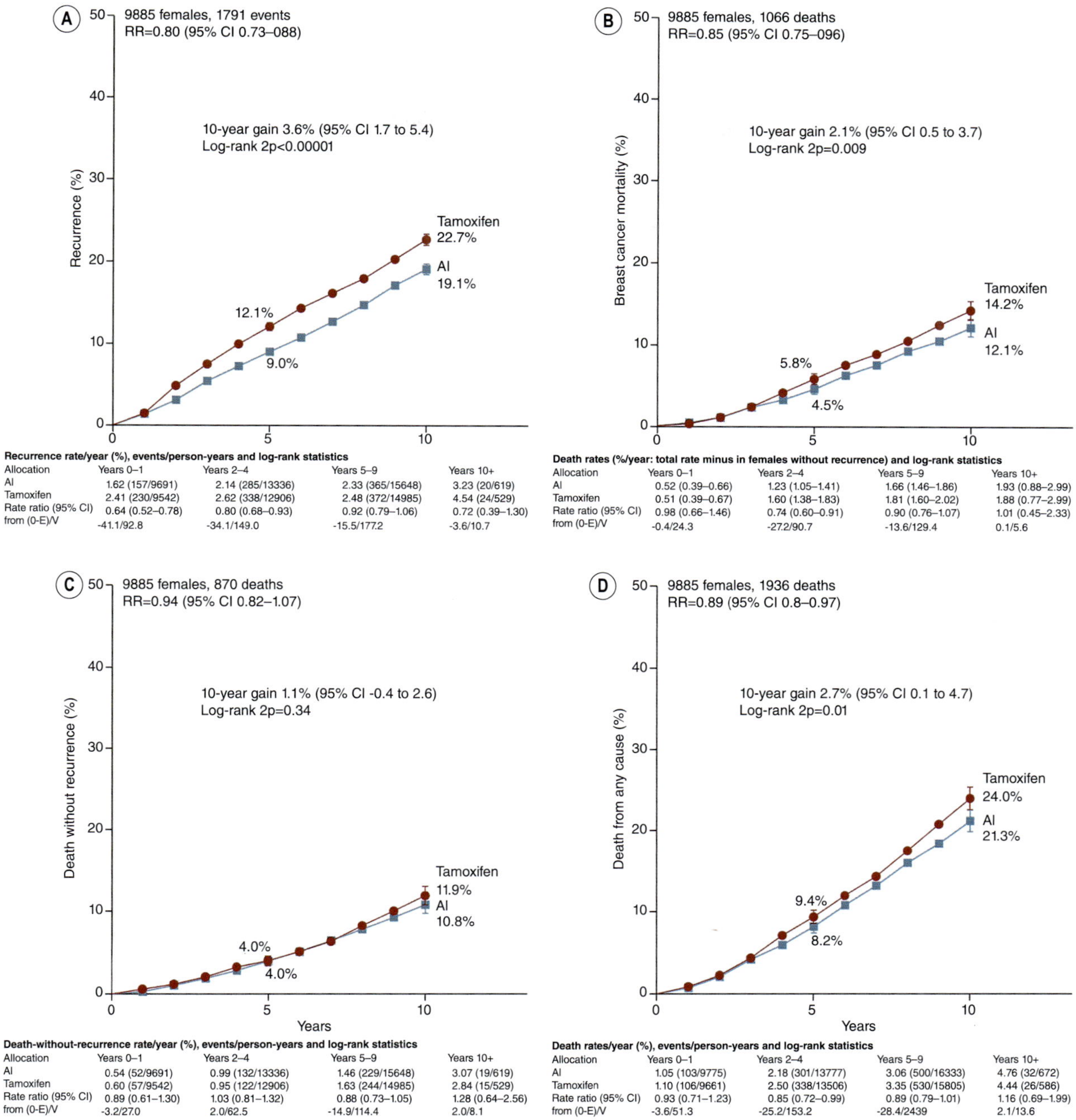

Recurrence rate/year (%), events/person-years and log-rank statistics

Allocation	Years 0–1	Years 2–4	Years 5–9	Years 10+
AI	1.62 (157/9691)	2.14 (285/13336)	2.33 (365/15648)	3.23 (20/619)
Tamoxifen	2.41 (230/9542)	2.62 (338/12906)	2.48 (372/14985)	4.54 (24/529)
Rate ratio (95% CI)	0.64 (0.52–0.78)	0.80 (0.68–0.93)	0.92 (0.79–1.06)	0.72 (0.39–1.30)
from (0-E)/V	-41.1/92.8	-34.1/149.0	-15.5/177.2	-3.6/10.7

Death rates (%/year: total rate minus in females without recurrence) and log-rank statistics

Allocation	Years 0–1	Years 2–4	Years 5–9	Years 10+
AI	0.52 (0.39–0.66)	1.23 (1.05–1.41)	1.66 (1.46–1.86)	1.93 (0.88–2.99)
Tamoxifen	0.51 (0.39–0.67)	1.60 (1.38–1.83)	1.81 (1.60–2.02)	1.88 (0.77–2.99)
Rate ratio (95% CI)	0.98 (0.66–1.46)	0.74 (0.60–0.91)	0.90 (0.76–1.07)	1.01 (0.45–2.33)
from (0-E)/V	-0.4/24.3	-27.2/90.7	-13.6/129.4	0.1/5.6

Death-without-recurrence rate/year (%), events/person-years and log-rank statistics

Allocation	Years 0–1	Years 2–4	Years 5–9	Years 10+
AI	0.54 (52/9691)	0.99 (132/13336)	1.46 (229/15648)	3.07 (19/619)
Tamoxifen	0.60 (57/9542)	0.95 (122/12906)	1.63 (244/14985)	2.84 (15/529)
Rate ratio (95% CI)	0.89 (0.61–1.30)	1.03 (0.81–1.32)	0.88 (0.73–1.05)	1.28 (0.64–2.56)
from (0-E)/V	-3.2/27.0	2.0/62.5	-14.9/114.4	2.0/8.1

Death rates/year (%), events/person-years and log-rank statistics

Allocation	Years 0–1	Years 2–4	Years 5–9	Years 10+
AI	1.05 (103/9775)	2.18 (301/13777)	3.06 (500/16333)	4.76 (32/672)
Tamoxifen	1.10 (106/9661)	2.50 (338/13506)	3.35 (530/15805)	4.44 (26/586)
Rate ratio (95% CI)	0.93 (0.71–1.23)	0.85 (0.72–0.99)	0.89 (0.79–1.01)	1.16 (0.69–1.99)
from (0-E)/V	-3.6/51.3	-25.2/153.2	-28.4/2439	2.1/13.6

Fig. 27.35 Five years of aromatase inhibitors versus 5 years of tamoxifen. (A) Recurrence. (B) Breast cancer mortality. (C) Death without recurrence. (D) Death from any cause. (From Early Breast Cancer Trialists Collaborative Group (EBCTCG). Aromatase inhibitors versus tamoxifen in early breast cancer: patient-level meta-analysis of the randomised trials. *Lancet.* 2015;386(10001):1341–1352.)

and 84.7% in the tamoxifen group (HR 0.83, 95% CI 0.66–1.04, $P = .10$). There was significant benefit from ovarian suppression in the whole study population. However, for patients at sufficient risk to require chemotherapy and who remained premenopausal, the addition of ovarian suppression improved disease outcomes. In a combined analysis of the SOFT and TEXT trials, at a median follow-up of 68 months, disease-free survival was 91.1% in the exemestane-ovarian suppression group and 87.3% in the tamoxifen-ovarian suppression group.

In the SOFT and TEXT trials, the 5-year breast cancer recurrence rates were significantly lower among premenopausal females who received the aromatase inhibitor exemestane plus ovarian suppression compared with those who received tamoxifen plus ovarian suppression. Adding ovarian suppression to tamoxifen did not result in significantly reduced recurrence rates over those treated with tamoxifen alone.

The American Society of Clinical Oncology (2016) recommends that ovarian suppression in addition to adjuvant endocrine therapy should be considered for premenopausal females with ER-positive breast cancer at higher risk of recurrence based on tumour stage, grade, nodal status or other biological features. If the patient has risk factors to warrant adjuvant chemotherapy, this would also justify ovarian suppression. Ovarian suppression was particularly encouraged in females under the age of 35 years where the SOFT trial showed particular benefits. For low-risk premenopausal patients (stage 1 or node-negative with tumour ≤1 cm), ovarian suppression was not recommended.

Ovarian suppression should be started 2 weeks before starting chemotherapy to preserve ovarian function in females age 35 to 40 years, irrespective of the ER status of the tumour.

The additional toxicity of ovarian suppression and aromatase inhibitors in young females needs to be weighed against the benefits. Adding ovarian suppression to tamoxifen increases menopausal symptoms, depression and toxicity with potential long-term health impacts such as hypertension, diabetes and osteoporosis. When exemestane is combined with ovarian suppression, adverse sexual, musculoskeletal and bone-density effects are more common than with tamoxifen plus ovarian suppression.

Adjuvant CDK4/6 Inhibition

The National Institute for Care and Excellence recommends 2 years of abemaciclib as an option for adjuvant treatment of HR-positive, HER2-negative, node-positive early breast cancer in adults whose disease is at high risk of recurrence, defined as pathological tumour involvement in (a) at least four positive axillary lymph nodes, or (b) one to three positive axillary lymph nodes, and at least one of the following criteria: grade 3 disease (defined as at least 8 points on the modified Bloom–Richardson grading system or equivalent) or primary tumour size of at least 5 cm.

Neoadjuvant Chemotherapy and HER2 Positive Breast Cancer

Neoadjuvant chemotherapy (NACT) has been widely adopted to try to induce a tumour response before surgery. NACT has three principal advantages.

First, it provides information on in vivo chemosensitivity. If there is no response to a particular regimen, it can be discontinued and changed. Second, it allows conversion of mastectomy to breast-conserving surgery if there is sufficient tumour shrinkage and may convert inoperable to operable disease. Breast-conserving surgery is considered safe after NACT. It may also allow more time to plan surgery or for genetic testing. Third, it provides prognostic information because a pCR in the primary tumour or nodes is a good prognostic sign. If there is no residual disease after NACT, either invasive or noninvasive, this is described as a pCR. Criteria for patients who have a higher probability of a pCR are age younger than 40 years, smaller tumour size (2.0 cm), grade 3, ductal histology, triple negative, ER/PgR negative, HER2 positive receiving transtuzumab and Ki67 greater than 14%. Criteria for those with a lower probability of pCR are age older than 60 years, grade 1, lobular histology, ER/PgR positive and Ki67 less than 14%. The pCR rates are now anticipated to exceed 50% to 60% for patients with ER-negative HER2-positive or triple-negative breast cancer treated with modern neoadjuvant regimens. The pathological assessment after NACT using the TNM classification is preceded by 'yp'. A complete response in the breast is ypT0/is and in the nodes ypN0. Although the influence of NACT on outcome is clear for invasive disease, the same is not true for DCIS where the significance of residual DCIS is unclear. In terms of disease-free and overall survival, preoperative (neoadjuvant) chemotherapy is as effective as postoperative chemotherapy. It is particularly suitable for HER2-positive and triple-negative breast cancers where there is a good correlation between pCR and survival. A further benefit of NACT is identifying patients after surgery who have no pCR and are candidates for further chemotherapy such as capecitabine for triple-negative breast cancer or Kadcyla (ado-trastuzumab emtansine) for HER2-positive disease.

The 2018 EBCTCG metaanalysis comparing neoadjuvant and adjuvant chemotherapy in 4756 females showed more than two-thirds of patients allocated to NACT achieved a partial or complete response. Patients allocated to NACT were more likely to undergo breast-conserving surgery than patients undergoing adjuvant chemotherapy. There were differences in distant recurrence or breast cancer mortality (EBCTCG, 2018). Patients with ER-negative high-grade tumours were most likely to achieve a pCR. A number of trials have shown pCR rates up to 83% in HER2-positive disease.

TABLE 27.16 Neoadjuvant or Adjuvant Chemotherapy

Epirubicin 90 mg/m^2 IV	Day 1
Cyclophosphamide 600 mg/m^2 IV	Day 1
Repeated every 21 days for 3 cycles	
Docetaxel (Taxotere) 100 mg/m^2 repeated every 21 days for 3 cycles after 3 cycles of EC	Day 1

EC, Epirubicin and cyclophosphamide; *IV*, intravenously.

With NACT, a pCR can be achieved in the axilla in 41% to 75% of patients with triple-negative or HER2-positive breast cancer. The EBCTCG metaanalysis does not provide information on axillary lymph node status before and after NACT. The policies for surgical management have changed with sentinel node biopsy often replacing axillary node dissection. Sentinel node biopsy after NACT in patients who had a positive axilla before NACT is regarded as accurate if at least three sentinel nodes are removed and examined. Whether axillary dissection or RT should be undertaken when there has been a pCR in the axilla is unknown. A US trial (NSABP B-51) is assessing the role of axillary irradiation in patients whose axilla has been converted from node positive to node negative by NACT.

In patients undergoing NACT, the primary and axillary nodes (if involved) should be marked by a metal clip because these may be difficult to locate if there has been a good response to NACT. Similar regimens can be used for neoadjuvant and postoperative adjuvant chemotherapy. For NACT, a sequential regimen of a combination of epirubicin and cyclophosphamide (EC) followed by docetaxel (Taxotere) is suggested (Table 27.16).

The RCB has been shown to correlate with long-term outcomes. The RCB assesses the size of the primary tumour, the cellularity of the invasive component, the dimensions of the largest axillary nodal metastasis and the number of pathologically involved nodes. The risk of distant metastasis increased from 2.4% with RCB-1 to 53.6% for RCB-111.

Anti-HER2 Neoadjuvant Therapy

Clinical outcomes have been transformed by the addition of anti-HER2 targeted therapy combined with standard chemotherapy. The NEOSPHERE study evaluated neoadjuvant transtuzumab plus pertuzumab with docetaxel as NACT in stage 2 and 3 invasive breast cancer compared to anthracycline-based chemotherapy in the adjuvant setting. The highest pCR rate was in the NACT arm with dual targeted therapy (45%) compared to trastuzumab or pertuzumab alone with docetaxel (29% and 24%, respectively).

Postoperative Chemotherapy and HER2 Positive Breast Cancer

Historically, adjuvant chemotherapy has evolved from early regimens with CMF to the incorporation of anthracyclines and more recently the introduction of taxanes. Deescalation of chemotherapy, which is facilitated by better tools to assess risk of recurrence to identify patients who do not need it and thereby avoiding the risks of toxicity, is part of a general pattern has been a major recent advance in management.

Postoperative adjuvant chemotherapy should be initiated within the first few weeks after surgery and precede adjuvant RT (if required). The key clinicopathological parameters for determining the need for adjuvant chemotherapy are locally advanced disease with involved nodes; larger tumour size; low expression of ER, PR or both; high tumour grade or proliferation index; HER2 status; age of the patient; and presence of lymphovascular invasion. A recommended schema for patients with early breast cancer requiring chemotherapy for HR-positive,

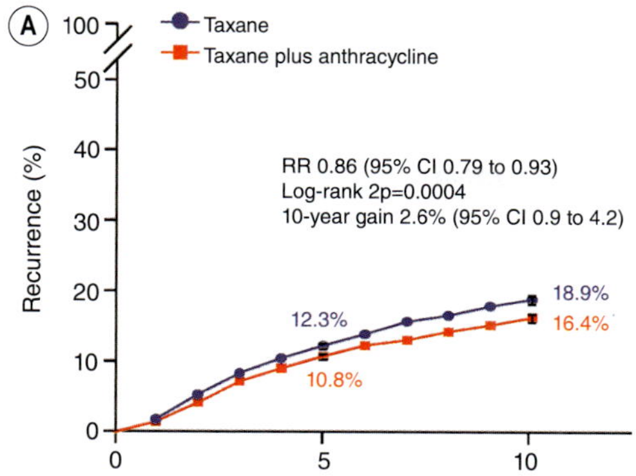

Recurrence rates per year (% [events per person-years]) and log-rank analyses

Allocation	Years 0–4	Years 5–9	Years ≥10
Taxane plus anthracycline	2.34% (900/38514)	1.37% (158/11575)	0.95% (4/420)
Taxane	2.63% (1008/38389)	1.65% (188/11388)	0.76% (3/396)
RR (95% CI)	0.87 (0.79–0.95)	0.80 (0.64–0.99)	1.83 (0.36–9.22)
(0-E)/V	-63.8/443.9	-19.1/83.3	0.9/1.5

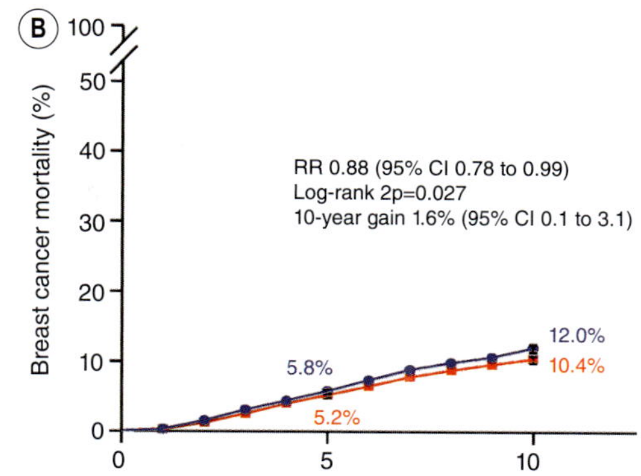

Death rates per year (% [95% CI]: total rate-rate in participants without recurrence) and log-rank analyses

Allocation	Years 0–4	Years 5–9	Years ≥10
Taxane plus anthracycline	1.05% (0.95–1.15)	1.24% (1.04–1.44)	1.10% (0.14–2.06)
Taxane	1.15% (1.04–1.25)	1.42% (1.21–1.63)	1.38% (0.28–2.48)
RR (95% CI)	0.89 (0.78–1.02)	0.85 (0.68–1.06)	0.88 (0.26–2.92)
(0-E)/V	-244/208.8	-13.0/79.0	-0.4/2.7

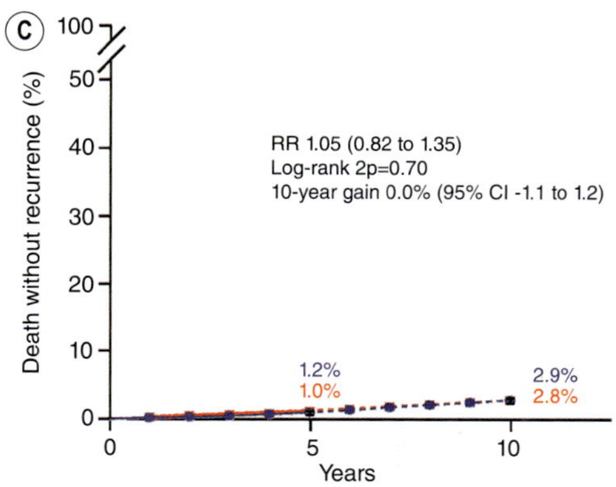

Rates of death without recurrence per year (% [events per person-years]) and log-rank analyses

Allocation	Years 0–4	Years 5–9	Years ≥10
Taxane plus anthracycline	0.24% (91/38514)	0.35% (41/11575)	1.19% (5/420)
Taxane	0.21% (79/38389)	0.36% (41/11388)	1.26% (5/396)
RR (95% CI)	1.15 (0.85–1.56)	0.91 (0.58–1.42)	0.64 (0.16–2.61)
(0–E)/V	5.9/41.4	-1.9/19.2	-0.9/2.0

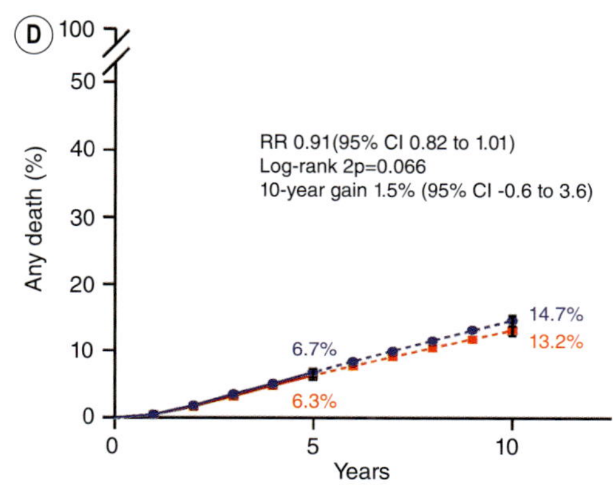

Death rates per year (% [events per person-years]) and log-rank analyses

Allocation	Years 0–4	Years 5–9	Years ≥10
Taxane plus anthracycline	1.28% (510/39707)	1.57% (195/12404)	2.19% (10/456)
Taxane	1.35% (537/39815)	1.76% (217/12345)	2.53% (11/435)
RR (95% CI)	0.93 (0.82–1.05)	0.86 (0.71–1.05)	0.77 (0.31–1.91)
(0–E)/V	-18.5/250.2	-149/98.2	-1.2/4.6

Fig. 27.36 Early Breast Cancer Trialists' Collaborative Group (EBCTCG) patient-level metaanalysis of randomised trials comparing taxane regimens versus without anthracycline. Analyses included 18,103 participants (9076 in taxane plus anthracycline group, 9027 in taxane only group). 10-year cumulative risk of any invasive recurrence (A), breast cancer mortality (B), death without recurrence (C)*, and any death (D)*. Error bars show 95% CI. O–E = observed minus expected. RR = rate ratio. V = variance. 2p = two-sided p value. *Smoothed after 5 years (denoted by dotted line). (Reproduced with permission from Elsevier, Early Breast Cancer Cancer Trialists' Collaborative Group (EBCTCG) patient-level meta-analysis of randomised trials comparing taxane regimens versus without anthracycline. 10 year cumulative risk of outcomes with taxane plus anthracycline versus without anthracycline. *Lancet.* 2023;410:1277–82.)

HER2-negative, HER2-positive and triple-negative breast cancer is shown in Figs. 27.32A and B (Loibl et al., 2021). Multigene assays can also be used, in particular in ER-positive, node-negative, HER2-negative patients, to assess risk more accurately. Anthracycline- and taxane-containing combination chemotherapy would be the standard regimen in most centres and is usually given sequentially over 18 to 24 weeks.

Growth factor support may be required because of the high incidence of neutropenia with some anthracycline-containing regimens (e.g. docetaxel, doxorubicin and cyclophosphamide, TAC) and is essential if aiming to give an accelerated anthracycline regimen.

A metaanalysis in 2023 of 100,000 females in 86 randomised trials of anthracycline-containing and taxane-containing chemotherapy (EBCTCG, 2023) concluded that a combination of taxane- and anthracycline-containing regimens is the most effective at reducing breast cancer recurrence and death (Fig. 27.36). In addition, higher cumulative doses of anthracycline plus taxane deliver the greatest gains. This evidence counters the current trend in guidelines supporting nonanthracycline-based chemotherapy, such as 4 cycles of docetaxel cyclophosphamide.

Physicians should consult local protocols for chemotherapy regimens.

Approximately 15% to 20% of breast cancers are HER2 positive and are associated with aggressive behaviour and a poor prognosis. HER2-positive tumours are classified as those 3+ on IHC or 2+ on IHC with HER2 gene amplification on in situ hybridisation testing. Trastuzumab is a monoclonal antibody against HER2 and can be given either intravenously or subcutaneously. It binds to and prevents activation of the receptor, inhibiting downstream signalling for proliferation

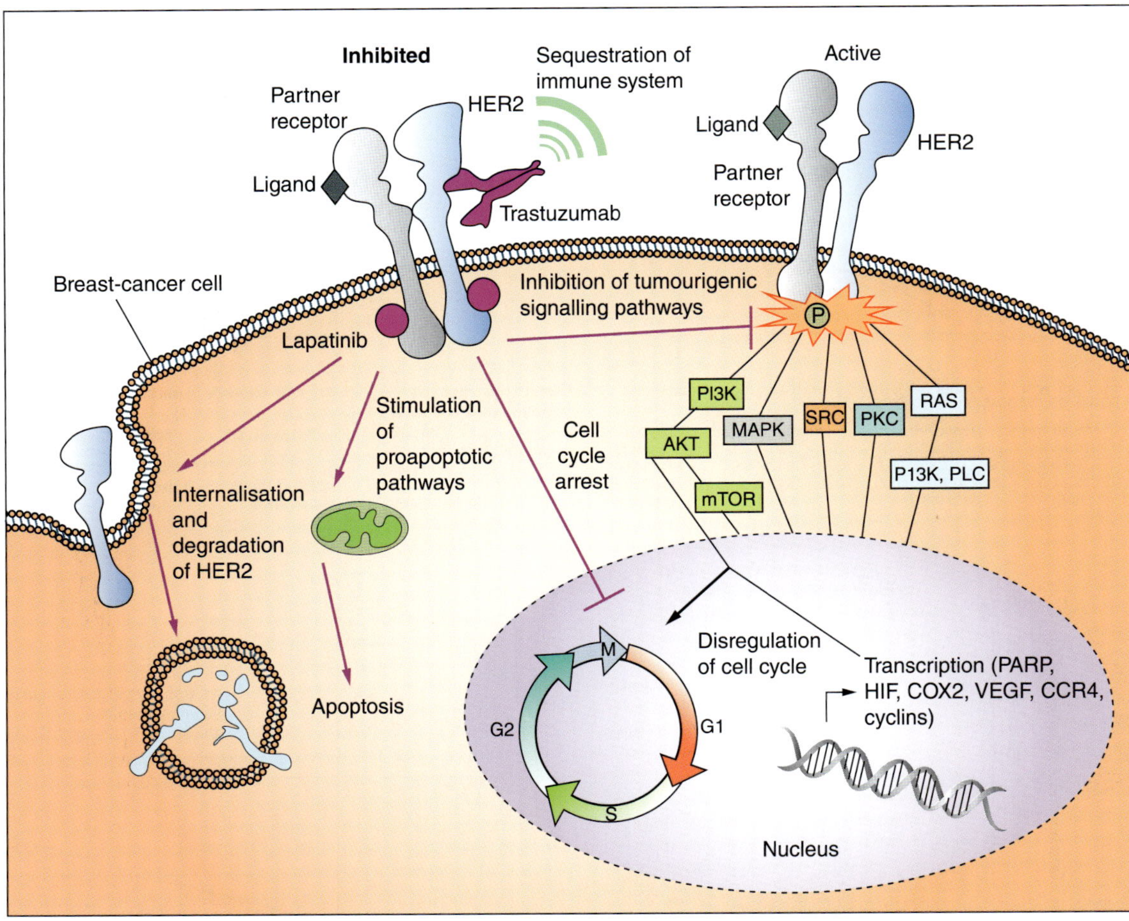

Fig. 27.37 Mechanism of action of current therapies for HER2-expressing breast cancer. Constitutively, active HER2 receptors on the surface of HER2-expressing breast cancer cells dimerise with other HER receptors, activating downstream signalling pathways that mediate tumourigenic cell proliferation, survival and invasion. Trastuzumab prevents constitutive activation of HER2, induces internalisation and degradation of the protein and stimulates the immune system to recognise HER2-overexpressing cells. Lapatinib binds to HER2 and HER1 and inhibits tumourigenic receptor signalling. (Reproduced with permission from Jones KL, Buzdar AU. Evolving novel anti-HER2-strategies. *Lancet Oncol.* 2009;10(12):1179–1187.)

(Fig. 27.37). Pertuzumab, a more recently developed drug, blocks the dimerisation of HER2 (Fig. 27.38) and works synergistically with trastuzumab, increasing the pCR rate in the neoadjuvant setting.

Four major randomised trials (the NSABP B-31, Intergroup N9831, BCIRG 006 and HERA trials) have assessed the role of trastuzumab in the adjuvant setting (Table 27.17). The addition of trastuzumab for 1 year to a sequence of anthracycline-taxane adjuvant chemotherapy in the NSAPB B-31 trial improved overall survival (HR 0.63, 95% CI 0.54–0.73, P <.001). Two years of trastuzumab in the HERA trial was no more effective than 1 year of therapy. Shorter durations of trastuzumab have been evaluated, with conflicting results. The large UK PERSEPHONE study randomised over 2000 patients to either 6 or 12 months of adjuvant trastuzumab and with a median follow-up of over 5 years. This confirmed noninferiority of the shorter duration (HR 1.07 (90% CI 0.93–1.24)), together with less cardiac toxicity. However, the French PHARE trial involving 3384 patients addressing the same question did not demonstrate noninferiority of 6 months of trastuzumab, and clinical practice following publication of both of these studies has generally continued to favour the longer duration of treatment over one year (Table 27.18), with the exception of lower-risk patients.

Cardiac function should be monitored approximately every 3 months in patients on trastuzumab by left ventricular cardiac ejection fraction. If the latter falls, trastuzumab may have to be temporarily or permanently suspended. Rarely, cardiac failure may occur (around 1%) with sequential anthracycline and trastuzumab, but this rises to 4% if given concurrently and is thus contraindicated.

Adjuvant Chemotherapy in Older Patients

Older, fit patients age 70 years or older should be treated with combination chemotherapy because single-agent therapy results in poorer outcomes. Patients' fitness should be carefully assessed, and geriatric assessment is advised. Toxicity should be closely monitored.

Adjuvant Bisphosphonates

Adjuvant bisphosphonates (zoledronic acid or sodium clodronate) are recommended for postmenopausal females with invasive breast cancer at higher risk of recurrence. They also reduce treatment-related bone loss. An EBCTCG metaanalysis demonstrated that adjuvant bisphosphonates reduce breast cancer mortality (Fig. 27.39) and improve disease-free survival and distant disease-free survival, irrespective of tumour biology or type of bisphosphonate used in postmenopausal but not premenopausal females.

Rare side effects of bisphosphonates include osteoradionecrosis of the jaw, atypical femoral fractures and osteonecrosis of the external auditory canal. The optimum duration for bisphosphonate therapy is uncertain, but it can be used for 2 to 5 years.

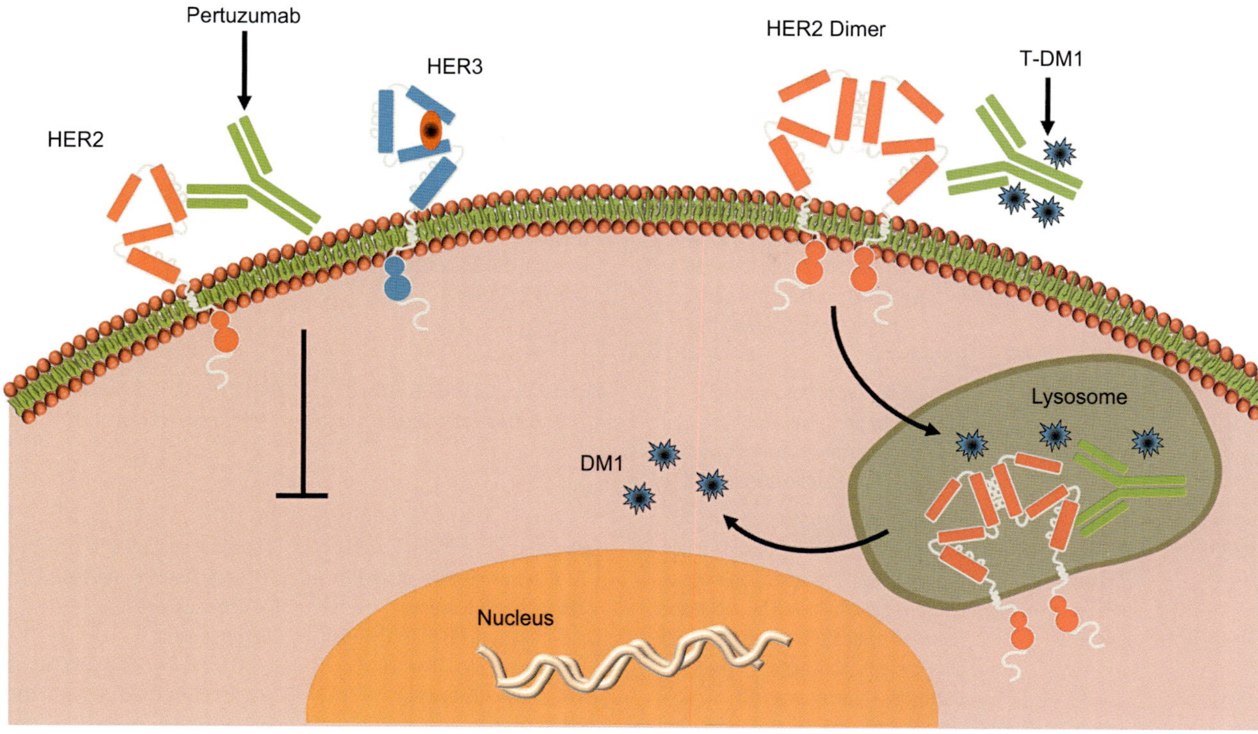

Fig. 27.38 Trastuzumab emtansine and pertuzumab mechanism of action. (Reproduced with permission from Dixon JM (Ed.). *ABC of Breast Diseases* (4th ed.). Chichester. Wiley-Blackwell; 2012.)

MANAGEMENT OF LOCALLY ADVANCED BREAST CANCER

Locally advanced breast cancer (LABC), or stage 3 breast cancer, refers to tumours larger than 5 cm in diameter (T3) or associated with involvement of the skin or chest wall (T4), inflammatory breast cancer (T4d) or with fixed axillary nodes (N2-3) or ipsilateral supraclavicular nodes (M1). LABC still presents a major challenge in management. With breast screening and greater public awareness, its incidence is falling, accounting for about 4% of European patients presenting with breast cancer. A typical example is shown in Fig. 27.40. These are a very heterogeneous group of tumours, with widely differing natural histories. Historically, results with surgery and RT were disappointing, with high levels of locoregional and systemic failure. Substantial improvements have been achieved with the addition of systemic therapy. Much of the published literature is based on case series, with mixed populations of patients, some including patients with inflammatory breast cancer and others not. Often, in studies of systemic therapy, locoregional therapy is not well defined. There are limited internationally agreed guidelines on management (Cardoso et al., 2017).

Clinical Features

The main features of LABC are skin nodules, peau d'orange (T4b), inflammatory changes (T4d), ulceration and fixity to the chest wall (T4a), fixed axillary nodes (N2) or lymphoedema (N3). Local pain, bleeding, ulceration and infection are common symptomatic problems. The natural history of locally advanced disease varies widely. In some patients, distant metastatic disease will rapidly supervene; in others, the disease remains locoregional without metastases.

Diagnosis

Diagnosis should be confirmed by core biopsy of the primary tumour and suspicious nodes.

Mammography may show the extent of malignant calcification but may not be appropriate for patients with gross bleeding or fungating tumours. Ultrasound may show site and extent. MRI is useful for assessing the extent of axillary/internal mammary node spread and invasion of skin and pectoral fascia.

Principles of Management

Neoadjuvant chemotherapy is usually the first step in the multimodal management of LABC. All chemotherapy should, if possible, be given before surgery. Surgery, RT and systemic therapy in different combinations need to be tailored to the clinical features of the patient's cancer to maximise locoregional control and reduce the risk of distant metastases.

For patients with operable disease, the choice is between breast-conserving surgery with oncoplastic procedures or mastectomy, if negative margins can be obtained, followed by adjuvant systemic therapy and RT or NACT followed by surgery and RT. A radiopaque marker should be placed in the tumour under image guidance to assist in identification of the primary in case of pCR. NACT shrinks the tumour in 20% to 40% of cases, allowing breast-conserving surgery in some cases where mastectomy would otherwise have been mandated. For patients with inoperable locally advanced disease, systemic therapy, surgery and RT are indicated.

Choice of Systemic Therapy

Data on the optimum chemotherapy for LABC are similarly sparse (Cardoso et al., 2017). Anthracycline- and taxane-based regimens are the standard NACT regimens. If sufficient tumour debulking has been achieved for surgery, this should be followed by postoperative RT. If there is no response and the tumour remains inoperable, radical RT should follow. The specific choice of neoadjuvant therapy will depend on patient fitness and tumour biology (histological grade, receptor status), and the rate of downstaging would be expected to be similar to the response rates in neoadjuvant therapy, with patients with HER2-positive disease being the most likely to achieve downstaging.

TABLE 27.17 Results From Major Trials Addressing Efficacy of Trastuzumab in Adjuvant Treatment of Breast Cancer

Trial	No. Patients; Years of Observation	Trial Arms	Disease-Free Survival Compared With Experimental Arm	Overall Survival Compared With Experimental Arm
BCIRG006	3222; 5 years	Doxorubicin + cyclophosphamide followed by docetaxel followed by docetaxel + trastuzumab, followed by trastuzumab; docetaxel + carboplatin + trastuzumab followed by trastuzumab	HR .64 (*P*= –.001)[a], HR 0.75 (*P*= .04)[b]; 75% versus 84% versus 81%; 257 versus 185 versus 214 events	HR 0.63 (*P*= .001); HR .77 (*P*= .04); 87% versus 92% versus 91%; 141 versus 94 versus 113 events
NCCTG N9831 & NSABP B-31	4046; 8.4 years	Doxorubicin + cyclophosphamide followed by paclitaxel; doxorubicin + cyclophosphamide, followed by paclitaxel + trastuzumab, followed by trastuzumab	HR 0.60 (*P*= .001); 62% versus 74%; 680 versus 473 events	HR .63 (*P*<.001); 75% versus 84%; 418 versus 286 events
NCCTG N9831	2184; 6 years DFS analysis at 5 years follow-up	Doxorubicin + cyclophosphamide followed by paclitaxel (A); doxorubicin + cyclophosphamide, followed by paclitaxel, followed by trastuzumab (B); doxorubicin + cyclophosphamide, followed by paclitaxel + trastuzumab (C)	Sequential arm: HR .69 (*P*<.001); 72% versus 80% (A versus B); 225 versus 165 events Concurrent arm: HR 0.77 (*P*= .020); 80% versus 84% (B versus C); 174 versus 139 events	Sequential arm: HR 0.88 (*P*= .343); 88% versus 89% (A versus B); 108 versus 96 events Concurrent arm: HR 0.78 (*P*= .102); 90% versus 92% (B versus C) 96 versus 76 events
HERA	5099; 8 years	4 cycles of standard chemotherapy; 4 cycles of standard chemotherapy followed by trastuzumab (1 year); 4 cycles of standard chemotherapy followed by trastuzumab (2 years)	HR 0.99 (*P*= .86); 82% versus 81% (2 years versus 1 year); 367 versus 367 events (2 years versus 1 year); HR .76 (*P*= .001); 71% versus 65% (1 year versus observation); 471 versus 570 events (1 year versus observation)	HR 1.05 (*P*= 0. 63); 86% versus 88% (2 years versus 1 year); 196 versus 186 events; HR 0.76 (*P*≤.001); 83% versus 77% (1 year versus observation) 278 versus 350 events (1 year versus observation)
FNCLCC-PACS04	3010; 3 years	FEC or epirubicin + docetaxel followed by trastuzumab	HR 0.86 (*P*= .41); 78% versus 81%; 70 versus 59 events	HR 1.27 (*P*= NR); 96% versus 95%; 18 versus 22 events
FinHER	232; 5.1 years	Docetaxel or vinorelbine, followed by FEC; docetaxel or vinorelbine + trastuzumab followed by FEC	HR 0.65 (*P*= .12); 73% versus 83%; 31 versus 22 events	HR 0.55 (*P*= .09); 82% versus 91%; 21 versus 22 events
PHARE	3380; 2 years	Trastuzumab (6 months); trastuzumab (12 months)	HR 1.28 (*P*= .29); 94% versus 92%; 175 versus 219 events	NA
ALLTO	8381; 4.5 years	Lapatinib; trastuzumab; trastuzumab followed by lapatinib; lapatinib + trastuzumab	HR 0.84 (*P*= .048); 88% lapatinib + trastuzumab versus 86% trastuzumab	HR .80 (*P*= .78); 95% lapatinib + trastuzumab versus 94% trastuzumab
ExteNET	2840; 2–3 years	Docetaxel (12 months); docetaxel (12 months) followed by neratinib	HR 0.67 (*P*= .009); 92% versus 94%; 109 versus 70 events	NA
TEACH	3147; 4 years	Placebo versus lapatinib	HR 0.83 (*P*= .053); 83% versus 87%; 264 versus 210 events	HR 0.99 (*P*= .96); 94% versus 94%; 97 versus 92 events

[a]HR 0.64 (*P* <.001 for doxorubicin + cyclophosphamide followed by docetaxel versus doxorubicin + cyclophosphamide, followed by docetaxel + trastuzumab, followed by trastuzumab.)

[b]HR 0.75.

FEC, Fluorouracil (5-FU) + epirubicin + cyclophosphamide; *HR*, hazard ratio; *NA*, not applicable. (*P* = .04 for doxorubicin + cyclophosphamide followed by docetaxel versus docetaxel + carboplatin + trastuzumab, followed by trastuzumab.)

Modified and reproduced with permission from Loibl S, Gianni L. HER2-positive breast cancer. *Lancet*. 2017;389(10087):2415–2429.

TABLE 27.18 Treatment Schedule for Adjuvant Trastuzumab

8 mg/kg intravenous loading dose Then 6 mg/kg every 21 days for 1 year

Locoregional Therapy

If erythema or inflammatory changes or peau d'orange resolve with NACT, mastectomy and axillary clearance should follow. Postoperative RT is given to the chest wall and, if there are four or more involved axillary nodes, is given to the medial supraclavicular fossa. There is no good evidence to determine whether or not the internal mammary nodes should be irradiated. Breast-conserving therapy for LABC is not usually feasible. However,

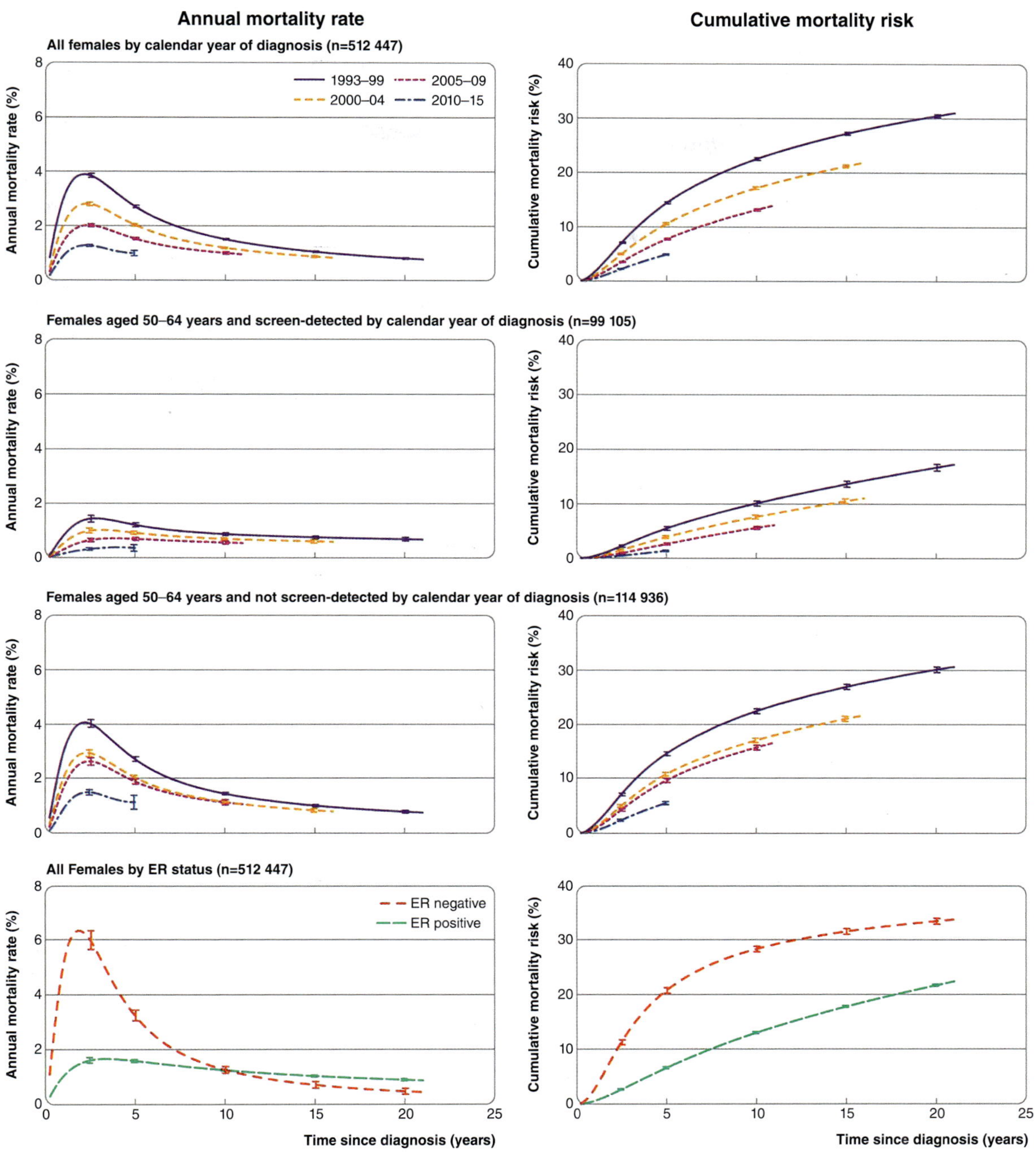

Fig. 27.39 Breast cancer mortality. Crude annual breast cancer mortality rates and cumulative breast cancer mortality risks in 512,447 females with early breast cancer by time since diagnosis according to calendar period of diagnosis: for all females *(top panel)*; for females age 50 to 64 years (who would all have been eligible for screening) according to whether their cancer was screen-detected *(middle panels)* and according to oestrogen receptor status *(bottom panel)*. *Vertical lines* are 95% confidence intervals. *ER*, Oestrogen receptor. (Reproduced with permission from Taylor C, McGale P, Probert J, et al. Breast cancer mortality in 500,000 women with early invasive breast cancer diagnosed in England, 1993–2015: population based observational cohort study. *BMJ*. 2023;381:e074684.)

there are some patients in whom the degree of debulking achieved by chemotherapy does make breast-conserving therapy possible. In addition, there are selected patients suitable for breast-conserving surgery with very small tumours that involve the skin early because of their proximity to the inframammary fold where the amount of breast tissue is small.

Target Volume

The target volume should include the chest wall or breast (in the case of conservative surgery) and, if the axilla has not been cleared, the peripheral lymphatics.

Technique

The principles of radical RT for early breast cancer apply also to locally advanced disease, both for the intact breast or following mastectomy. The only difference is that 0.5 to 1 cm of skin bolus should be applied to the breast or chest wall to ensure that the skin receives a full dose (to overcome the skin-sparing effect of megavoltage RT). Axillary surgery is not normally carried out at staging, and therefore the peripheral lymphatics will normally be irradiated. If mastectomy and a level III axillary clearance have been carried out, the axilla should not be irradiated.

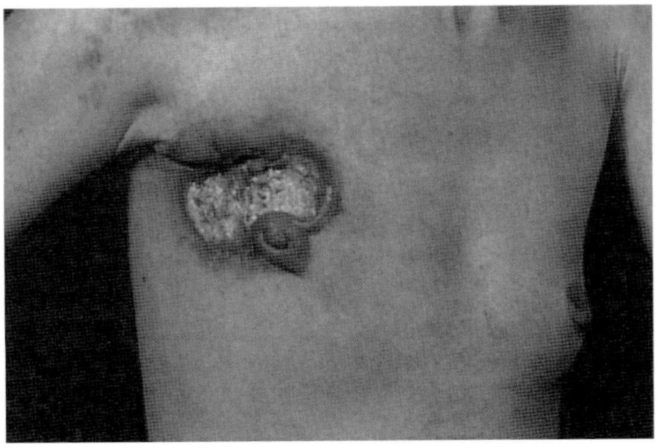

Fig. 27.40 Locally advanced and inoperable carcinoma of the right breast (T4).

Dosage and Fractionation (Radical)

Dosage and fractionation for LABC is 40 Gy in 15 daily fractions over 3 weeks (6-10-MV photons).

A boost of 10 Gy in 5 daily fractions (if the primary tumour is sufficiently small) is to be encompassed within the boost volume.

Locoregional Palliative Radiotherapy

In some patients, radical RT is not advised because of poor medical condition, advanced age or evidence of metastatic disease elsewhere. Locoregional recurrence occurs in approximately 5% to 15% of patients in trials treated by locoregional RT after breast-conserving surgery or mastectomy. Palliative RT can be very effective with minimal toxicity for symptomatic relief of local bleeding, ulceration from localised advanced disease, pain or discharge from skin metastases or flap recurrence after mastectomy, or axillary involvement with or without upper limb lymphoedema. Palliative RT to limited volumes is often possible in areas treated with radical locoregional RT. Responses are usually only partial but may be sufficient for symptomatic relief and may be prolonged. Dry or moist desquamation usually settles within 2 to 3 weeks.

Technique

The technique should be simple, either with parallel-opposed or tangential fields at megavoltage confined to the macroscopic area of tumour with 1-to-2-cm margins with bolus or a single electron field using a Perspex degrader to bring up the skin to full dose.

Dose

The dose is 36 Gy in 6 fractions of 6 Gy given once or twice weekly over 6 weeks, particularly in frail patients.

Inflammatory Breast Cancer

Inflammatory breast cancer (IBC) is rare (2%–4% of breast cancer) but has an aggressive course, accounting for 8% to 10% of breast cancer deaths. It requires a multidisciplinary approach with systemic therapy central to its treatment (Chainitikun et al., 2020). The diagnosis is based on rapid development of skin erythema and oedema or peau d'orange involving at least one-third of breast skin with or without an underlying breast mass. Skin changes may be due to tumour emboli in the dermal lymphatics and are present in around 75% of cases on pathological assessment. IBC has higher rates of HER2 overexpression than non-IBC.

The triple-negative subtype has the worst outcome. Bone is the most common site of metastasis in all subtypes. Liver metastases are common in HER2-positive patients.

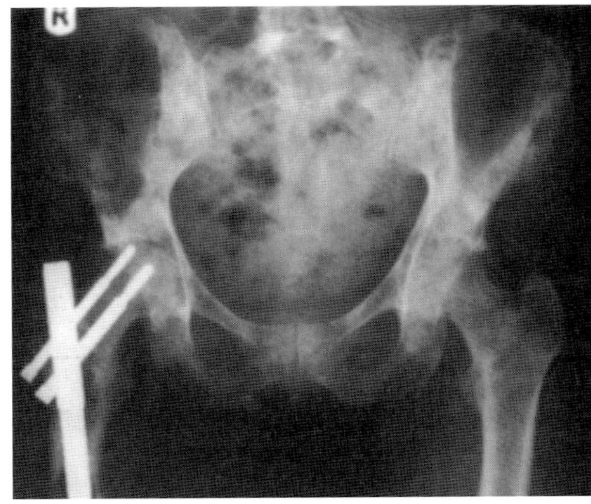

Fig. 27.41 Radiograph of pelvis showing pinning of pathological fracture of right hip as a result of extensive mixed and sclerotic disease from breast cancer.

Treatment

Neoadjuvant chemotherapy is central to treatment, with the aim of achieving a pathologically complete response. Treatment should be based on tumour biology and patient fitness.

The highest pCR rates are achieved in ER-negative subtypes. HER2-positive patients should receive dual HER2 blockade with trastuzumab and pertuzumab.

If the skin changes settle with neoadjuvant chemotherapy, mastectomy and axillary clearance are advised followed by postoperative RT to the chest wall and, if four or more axillary lymph nodes are involved, to the medial supraclavicular fossa with dose fractionation as for non-inflammatory breast cancer. Skin bolus should be applied to the chest wall to ensure full dose to the skin.

Role of Surgery

Surgery used to have a limited role in the management of locally advanced disease. It encompassed (1) initial core biopsy for diagnosis and ER status; (2) mastectomy and axillary clearance in operable patients; (3) mastectomy (ideally with myocutaneous flap reconstruction) for residual masses after chemotherapy and radical RT; (4) palliative debriding of infected and/or necrotic areas to reduce odour; and (5) stabilisation of pathological fractures e.g. of the hip (Fig. 27.41). For inflammatory breast cancer (T4d), only patients with complete clinical resolution of inflammatory changes following chemotherapy should be considered for mastectomy. Mastectomy as a primary procedure or when inflammatory changes persist after neoadjuvant systemic therapy is likely to be followed rapidly by recurrence in the skin flaps. Increasingly, surgery is being offered after neoadjuvant therapy and is followed by RT. Many patients with locally advanced breast cancer are now treated by breast conservation if there is a good response to systemic therapy. There is now considerable evidence that breast conservation is safe in this setting.

Trials of adjuvant chemotherapy in patients with stage 3 disease are rare. The Oxford overview of randomised trials of adjuvant systemic therapy does contain some patients with large operable cancer. The overview showed that all patients gained from adjuvant chemotherapy irrespective of tumour size. On this basis it is reasonable to extrapolate the results of the overview to patients with operable stage 3A disease.

Principles of Management of Advanced and Metastatic Disease

Multidisciplinary management is essential in view of the complexities of advanced disease and must be adapted to the differing requirement

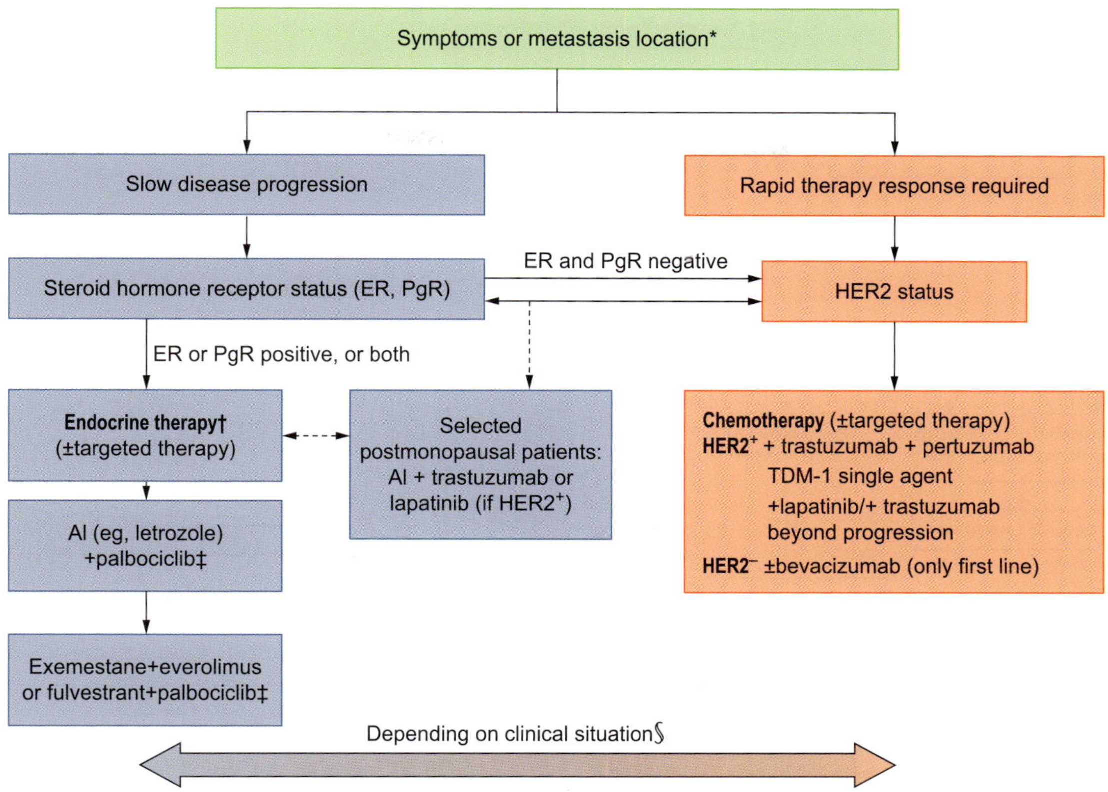

Fig. 27.42 Previous treatments and patients' preferences are key elements in deciding the individual therapeutic steps. (Figure updated after the publication of Bossung V, Harbeck N. Angiogenesis inhibitors in the management of breast cancer. *Curr Opin Obstet Gynecol.* 2010;22:79–86.) Treatment decisions can thus differ for an individual patient. In patients with HR-positive HER2-negative tumours, endocrine therapy should be the first option unless there is life-threatening disease. Chemotherapy is always an additional therapy option depending on the course of disease. ER = oestrogen receptor. PgR = progesterone receptor. AI = aromatase inhibitor. TDM-1 = trastuzumab emtansine. *If bone metastases: + bisphosphonates or denosumab. †Always combine with ovarian suppression or ablation in premenopausal patients. ‡So far, only one line of palbociclib therapy is evidence-based. §Only applicable if ER or PgR positive, or both. (Reproduced with permission from Elsevier, Harbeck N, Gnant M. Breast Cancer. *Lancet.* 2017;389:1134–1150.)

of individual patients. Psychosocial support is needed from the time of diagnosis from specialised oncology nurses. In general, patients should be aware that metastatic breast cancer is incurable but amenable to treatment, often with control of the disease for several to many years. Given that treatment is palliative, a careful and difficult balance has to be struck between tumour response, toxicity and adverse effects on quality of life.

The minimum of staging is history, physical examination, full blood count, liver function tests, CT scan of chest and abdomen and bone scan. The brain should not routinely be imaged in asymptomatic patients.

The choice of treatment must consider the age, general medical condition, comorbidities (including organ dysfunction) and performance status of the patient, menopausal status, ER and HER2 status, additional biomarker status (e.g. PIK3CA, programmed death ligand 1 (PD-L1) expression), response to previous therapies and toxicities, breast cancer susceptibility gene status (e.g. BRCA1, BRCA2, PALB2), number and sites of metastatic involvement, requirement for urgent symptom/disease control, psychological factors, patient preference and the tempo of the disease to date. There are three general forms of systemic therapy: hormonal therapy, chemotherapy and HER2 targeted therapy. Concomitant endocrine and chemotherapy should not be administered outside a trial setting. Chemotherapy may be in combination or by single agent. Candidate palliative chemotherapy schedules are shown in Tables 27.20 to 27.27. Single agent responses rates are shown in Table 27.28.

One of the major recent advances in the treatment of ER-positive, HER2-negative metastatic disease is the addition of CDK4/6 inhibitors in combination with endocrine therapy. For ER-negative disease and for patients with ER-resistant ER-positive disease, aggressive disease or rapidly evolving visceral disease, chemotherapy is the treatment of choice in fit patients. For these patients, or those with triple-negative or low/moderate ER-positive cancers, there are multiple options available and the choice of treatment will depend on patient priorities, fitness and comorbidities, disease-free or progression-free interval, prior responses to therapy and line of therapy. Types and durations of chemotherapy regimens should be individualised and take account of patients' preference, although increasingly, treatments are now given until unacceptable toxicity or progression.

Response to endocrine therapy should be assessed every 2 to 4 months or after 2 to 4 cycles of chemotherapy. To date, there is no multigene technology to support choice of treatment in advanced breast cancer beyond a clinical trial setting. The general schema of systemic therapy for metastatic cancer (Harbeck et al., 2017) is summarised in Fig. 27.42. A recommended treatment algorithm for ER-positive, HER2 negative (Fig. 27.43A), HER2 positive (Fig. 27.43B) and triple negative (Fig. 27.43C) metastatic cancer is shown. The level of the evidence base for most recommendations is low (Cardoso et al., 2017; Sauter and Razaq, 2024), and it should be noted that treatment guidelines and recommendations evolve frequently.

Endocrine therapy is normally the initial treatment of choice for most patients with ER- and/or PgR-positive HER2-negative metastatic breast cancer with disease in the bone, skin or lymph nodes. As long as

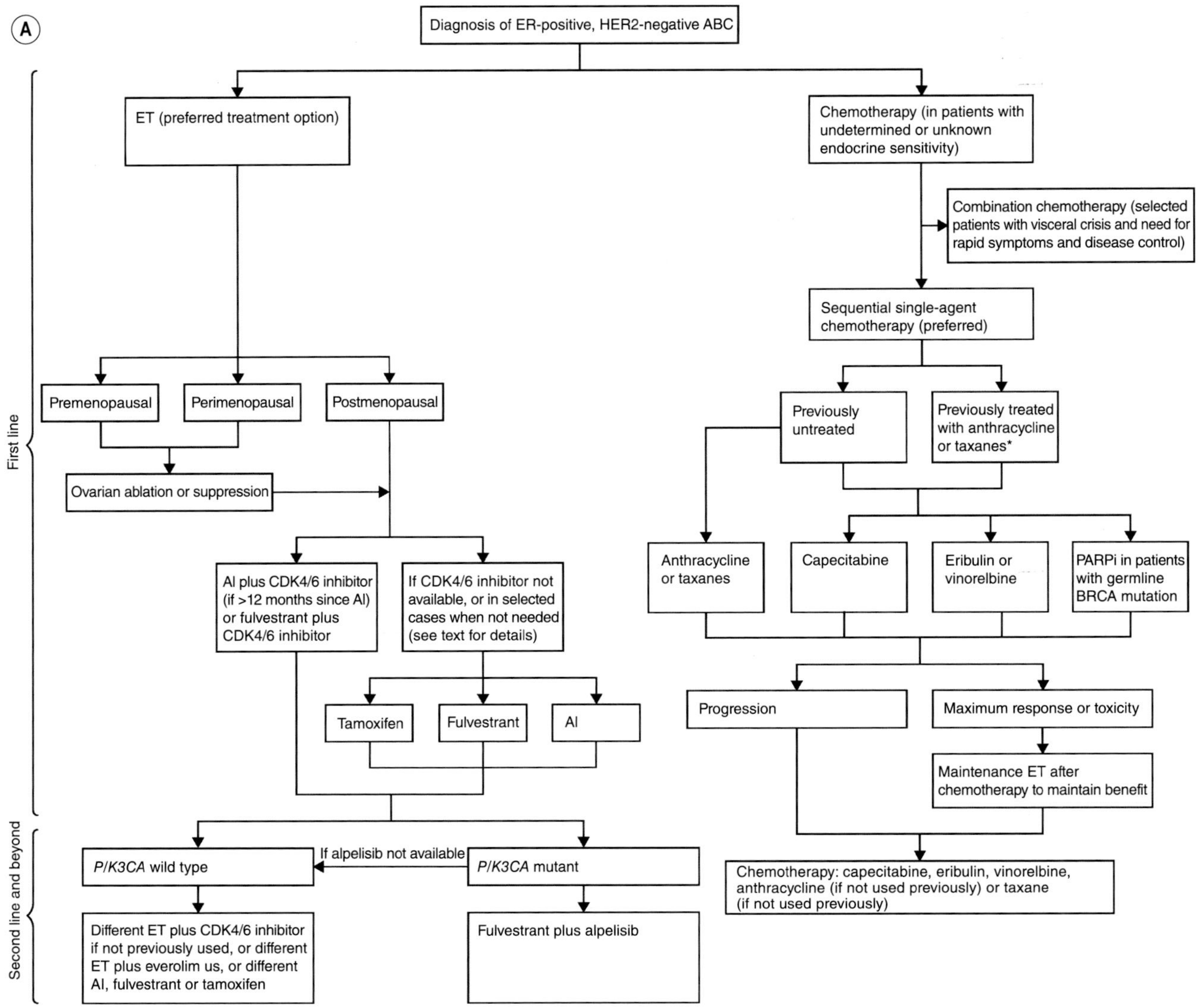

Fig. 27.43 Treatment algorithm for ER-positive and HER-2 negative metastatic breast cancer (A), HER2-positive metastatic breast cancer (B), and triple-negative breast cancer (C). *Rechallenge with taxanes or anthracyclines is possible (if cumulative dose is not reached and DFI ≥12 months). Patients with PD-L1-positive or BRCA-mutated breast cancer should first receive a checkpoint inhibitor with taxane, then PARPi (no data available for checkpoint inhibitors as second-line therapy). *ABC*, Advanced breast cancer; *AI*, aromatase inhibitor; *DFI*, disease-free interval; *ET*, endocrine therapy; *PARPi*, poly(ADP-ribose) polymerase inhibitor. (Reproduced with permission from Loibl S, Poortmans P, Morrow M, Denkert C, Curigliano G. Breast cancer. *Lancet*. 2021;397(10286):1750–1769.)

(continued)

there is not rapid evolution of disease, sequential endocrine therapy is advised. The optimal sequence for HR-positive, HER2-negative disease is uncertain. The choice of endocrine agent will depend on menopausal status, previous endocrine therapy and patient preference.

Treatment of ER Positive, HER2 Negative Breast Cancer

HR-positive, HER2-negative postmenopausal patients with metastatic breast cancer

First-line option is normally a nonsteroidal aromatase inhibitor (letrozole or anastrozole) with or without a cyclin-dependent kinase 4/6 inhibitor such as ribociclib, palbociclib or abemaciclib. Other options are fulvestrant, a selective ER degrader, and tamoxifen. Tamoxifen as first-line therapy is inferior to aromatase inhibitors as first-line therapy in terms of progression-free survival.

Progressive disease on first-line endocrine therapy in postmenopausal patients with HR-positive, HER2-negative metastatic breast cancer

In the event of progression of disease on first-line endocrine therapy, subsequent endocrine options include exemestane +/− everolimus, fulvestrant + a CDK4/6 inhibitor, megestrol (a progestogen), elacestrant (in patients with ESR1 mutations), olaparib or talazoparib (where there is a BRCA1 or 2 mutation), chemotherapy, trastuzumab deruxtecan (for HER-low disease) or abemaciclib alone (in the absence of use of a CDK4/6 inhibitor).

HR-positive, HER2-negative premenopausal patients with metastatic breast cancer

Recommended first-line therapy is tamoxifen and/or ovarian ablation. Ovarian ablation can be by oophorectomy or medical therapy with a gonadotrophin-releasing hormone (e.g. goserelin). Tamoxifen should be continued until disease progression. Once the patient is postmenopausal after oophorectomy, the endocrine therapy options are as for postmenopausal HR-positive, HER2-negative metastatic breast cancer.

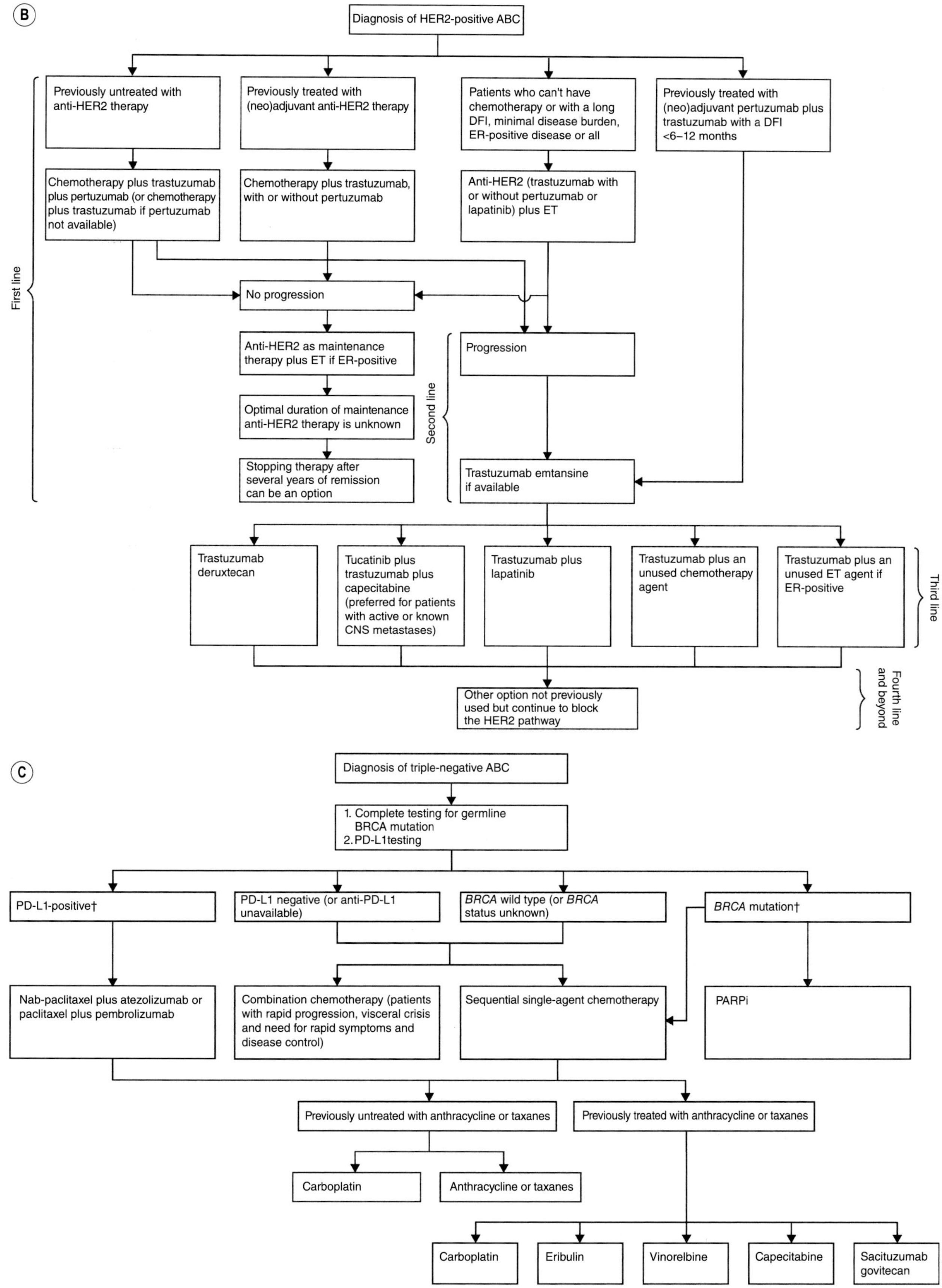

Fig. 27.43—(cont'd)

Biopsy of Metastatic Lesions

The role of repeat biopsy of metastatic lesions has become a more important consideration, as breast cancers can change subtype over time, more commonly by loss (rather than gain) of expression of ER or HER2 receptor. As novel agents are increasingly being tested and thus approved based on a specific tumour subtype, consideration should sometimes be given to repeating a biopsy, as this might facilitate a different treatment option.

The genome of a metastatic clone may be similar to the primary tumour at diagnosis. However, whole genome sequencing has shown that breast cancer metastases may undergo extensive genomic changes, acquiring multiple new somatic mutations and driver mutations by the time they become clinically overt. Many sites of metastases are difficult and invasive to sample, but patients may be willing to undergo biopsy of recurrent lesions for the purpose of molecular profiling. This may help our understanding of clonal evolution and mechanisms of treatment resistance and identify pathways which may be future therapeutic targets (Yates et al., 2017).

CDK4/6 Inhibitors

More recently, a CDK4/6 inhibitor (palbociclib, abemaciclib and ribociclib) has been added to an aromatase inhibitor as first-line therapy for postmenopausal ER-positive, HER2-negative patients with metastatic breast cancer (with the exception of those relapsing less than 1 year from the end of adjuvant aromatase inhibitor). CDK4/6 inhibitors work by inhibiting the transition from the G0/G1 to S phase of the cell cycle, which is mediated by, among other factors, CDK4/6 and cyclin-D, resulting in Rb phosphorylation and subsequently the release of the transcription factor, E2F. The mechanism of action of CDK4/6 inhibitors is shown in Fig. 27.44. The cyclin D/CDK4/6 pathway is commonly overexpressed. All of these agents are given orally and show gains in progression-free survival and overall survival in endocrine-sensitive and endocrine-resistant metastatic breast cancer. The only predictive biomarker for CDK4/6 benefit is ER positivity. The results of randomised trials (PALOMA-2, MONARCH-3, MONALEESA-2 and MONALEESA-7) supporting the use of a CDK4/6 inhibitor in combination with endocrine therapy are shown in Table 27.19. All significantly improved progression-free survival compared to endocrine therapy alone. MONALEESA-7 was confined to premenopausal patients. In postmenopausal patients a combination of palbociclib, ribociclib and abemaciclib reduced progression-free survival events by 42%, 56% and 54%, respectively. A combination of any one of the three agents is approved for first-line therapy for endocrine-sensitive, HER2-negative metastatic breast cancer presenting de novo or when relapse occurs more than 12 months after the completion of adjuvant endocrine therapy. The use of CDK4/6 inhibitors delays the start of chemotherapy by approximately 1 year, and they are the standard of care for first-line therapy of metastatic ER-positive, HER2-negative breast cancer.

All the CDK4/6 inhibitors are in general very well tolerated. Palbociclib and ribociclib cause more haematological toxicity (typically asymptomatic neutropenia), while abemaciclib causes more GI toxicity (diarrhoea) than the other two agents. Ribociclib is associated with prolonged QTc on electrocardiograph (ECG) (with risk of tachycardia) and abnormal liver function tests. However, the overall survival data for ribociclib are the most convincing among the three agents.

Optimal management after first-line CDK4/6 inhibitor therapy is unclear. In general, the principle is to try to use an endocrine therapy-based approach until the disease is considered endocrine therapy resistant, and for those patients who were commenced on single-agent endocrine therapy for metastatic disease before the development of CDK4/6 inhibitors, or chose to have single-agent treatment in the first-line setting, there is evidence for all three CDK4/6 inhibitors that fulvestrant with any of these agents improves progression-free survival over fulvestrant alone in the second-line setting.

Oral Selective Oestrogen Receptor Degraders

Oral SERDs are also in clinical trials at present, and it is unclear at this stage where these agents will fit into treatment algorithms in the future. Oral SERDs are a novel drug class for treatment of ER-positive metastatic breast cancer resistant to other hormonal agents. SERDs that have been evaluated in phase II and III trials include EMERALD (elacestrant), SERENA-2 (camizestrant), AMEERA-3 (amcenestrant) and ACELERA (giredestrant).

Patients who are most likely to benefit from hormonal therapy for relapsed disease have one or more of the following characteristics:

- Disease-free survival over 2 years
- Soft-tissue or bone-predominant disease
- Older postmenopausal patients

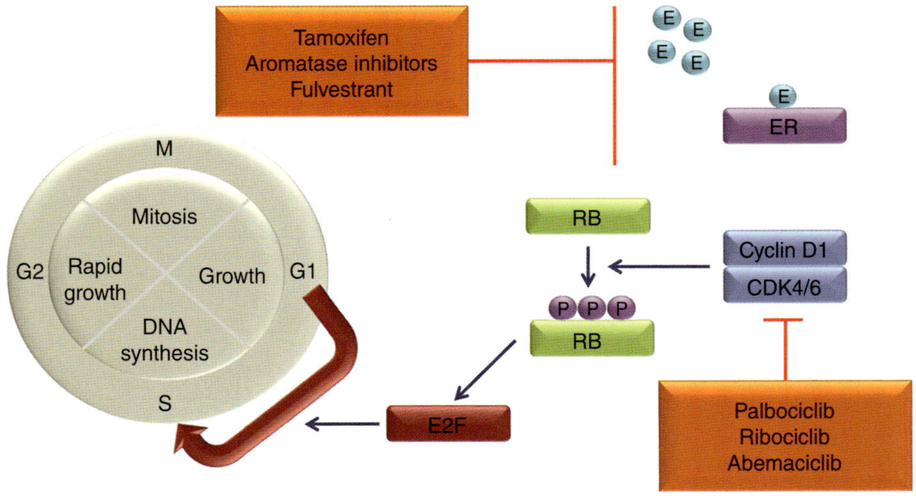

Fig. 27.44 Schematic overview of the mechanism of action of CDK4/6 inhibitors. *CDK*, Cyclin kinase D; *E2F*, transcription factor E2F; *E*, oestrogen receptor; *p*, phosphorylated; *RB*, retinoblastoma tumour suppressor protein. (Reproduced with permission from Loibl S, Furlanetto J. Integrating CDK4/6 inhibitors in the treatment of patients with early breast cancer. *Breast*. 2022;62(Suppl 1):S70–S79.)

TABLE 27.19 **Results From Pivotal Prospective Randomised Controlled Trials Investigating Palbociclib, Ribociclib and Abemaciclib Combined With an Endocrine Partner in the Treatment of First-line Patients With HR + Metastatic Breast Cancer**

Trial Details	PALOMA-2[13,26]	MONALEESA-2[12,15]	MONALEESA-3[20,22,24]	MONALEESA-7[18,25]	MONARCH-3[14,29]
CDK4/6 inhibitor	Palbociclib	Ribociclib	Ribociclib	Ribociclib	Abemaciclib
Endocrine therapy	Letrozole	Letrozole	Fulvestrant	Goserelin plus tamoxifen or NSAI	NSAI
Menopausal status	Postmenopausal	Postmenopausal	Postmenopausal	Pre-/perimenopausal	Postmenopausal
Sample size	666	668	365 (1L therapy)	672	493
Median follow-up (months)	90	80	70.8	53.5	70.2
mPFS combination arm (months)	24.8	25.3	33.6	23.8	28.2
mPFS control arm (months)	14.5	16	19.2	13	14.8
mPFS HR (95% CI)	0.58 (0.46–0.72)	0.57 (0.46–0.7)	0.55 (0.42–0.72)	0.55 (0.44–0.69)	0.54 (0.42–0.69)
mPFS p value	<0.001	<0.001	NA	<0.001	>0.001
mOS combination arm (months)	53.9	63.9	67.6	58.7	67.1
mOS control arm (months)	51.2	51.4	51.8	48	54.5
mOS HR (95% CI)	0.956 (0.777–1.177)	0.76 (0.63–0.93)	0.67 (0.5–0.9)	0.76 (0.61–0.96)	0,754 (0.584–0.974)
mOS p value	0.3378	<0.001	NA	<0.001	0.0301[a]
% ≥1 dose reduction due to AE (combination arm)	36%	50.6%	NA	31%	46.5%
% treatment discontinuation (combination arm)	9.7%	7.5%	NA	4%	16.5%

[a]Results from preplanned interim analysis. The statistical significance threshold for abemaciclib superiority was not met.

1L, First-line; *AE*, adverse events; *mOS*, median overall survival; *mPFS*, median progression-free survival; *NSAI*, nonsteroidal aromatase inhibitor.

Reproduced with permission from Grinshpun A, Tolaney SM, Burstein HJ, Jeselsohn R, Mayer EL. The dilemma of selecting a first line CDK4/6 inhibitor for hormone receptor-positive/HER2-negative metastatic breast cancer. *NPJ Breast Cancer.* 2023;9(1):15.

Sites of Metastases and Impact on Management

The timing and intensity of therapy are influenced by the aggressiveness of the disease and the patient's symptoms. Disease limited to bone and soft tissues tends to take a more indolent course with longer survival. By contrast, in patients with visceral disease the course is usually more aggressive and associated with shorter survival.

For patients in visceral crisis (severe organ dysfunction based on symptoms, signs and/or laboratory investigations and rapid progression of disease), there is an urgent requirement for prompt disease control using combination chemotherapy. Hepatic visceral crisis includes rapidly increasing bilirubin >1.5 times the upper limit of normal in the absence of Gilbert syndrome or obstruction of the biliary tract. Lung visceral crisis includes rapid increase in dyspnoea at rest, not relieved by drainage of a pleural effusion, if present.

Other factors which may point to aggressive disease include:

- A short disease-free interval (<2 years)
- ER- and PgR-negative tumour
- Triple-negative tumour (ER, PgR and HER2 negative)
- HER2-positive disease
- Germline BRCA1 or BRCA2 mutations
- Nonresponse to prior therapy
- CNS involvement
- Multiple sites of disease

For nonvisceral, triple-negative disease, sequential therapy with single-agent chemotherapy may be recommended. The treatment of choice will depend, as previously mentioned, on a variety of both patient and disease factors, and a clinical trial should always be something to consider if the patient is fit enough and keen to consider these.

Physicians should always check evidence-based local protocols for chemotherapy regimens.

Treatment of Metastatic HER2-Positive Disease

For patients with HER2-positive breast cancer, the standard of care for first-line therapy of metastatic disease usually involves a taxane (docetaxel or paclitaxel) in combination with trastuzumab and pertuzumab, with the chemotherapy agent usually being discontinued after 18 to 24 weeks and the dual anti-HER2 therapy continuing until unacceptable toxicity or progressive disease. For patients with ER-positive, HER2-positive breast cancer, endocrine therapy is usually initiated once the cytotoxic drug is withdrawn. The CLEOPATRA trial demonstrated improved overall survival of over 56 months, although with recent advances this figure is likely now to be an underestimate of median overall survival (Swain et al., 2015).

The trials supporting first-, second- and third-line anti-HER2 therapy are summarised in Fig. 27.45, along with their progression-free and overall survival rates. Survival rates have been dramatically prolonged (Miglietta et al., 2022).

First Line

The current standard of care established by the CLEOPATRA trial is dual HER2 blockade with trastuzumab and pertuzumab in combination

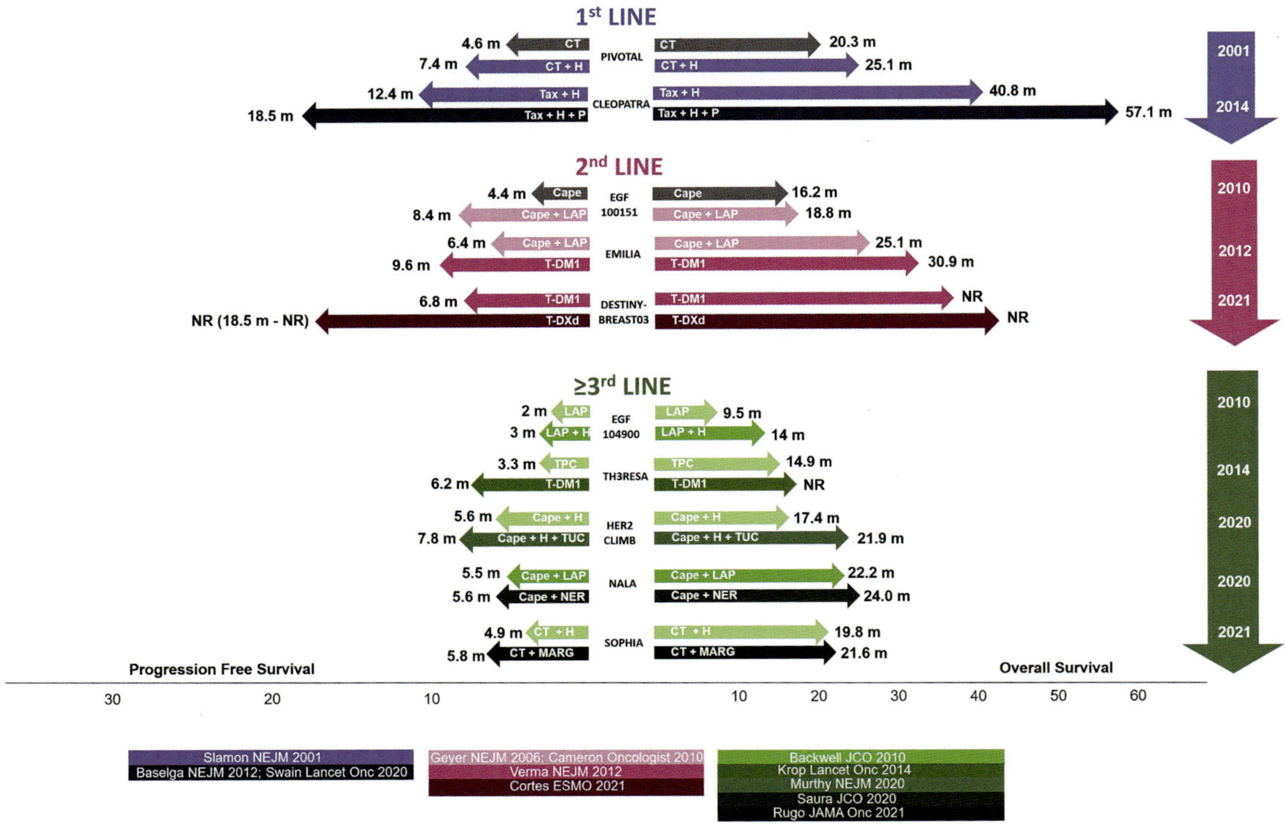

Fig. 27.45 Progression-free survival and overall survival results from major randomised clinical trials testing anti-HER2 strategies according to treatment line. (Reproduced with permission from Miglietta F, Bottosso M, Griguolo G, Dieci MV, Guarneri V. Major advancements in metastatic breast cancer treatment: when expanding options means prolonging survival. *ESMO Open*. 2022;7(2):100409.)

with the taxane docetaxel. Pertuzumab has a complementary mechanism of action (see Fig. 27.38) to that of trastuzumab, binding the extracellular domain 11 of HER2 and inhibiting ligand-dependent dimerisation of HER2-HER3 and diminishing signalling via intracellular pathways (e.g. phosphatidylinositol 3-kinase (PI3K/AKT)). This combination extended median overall survival to 57.1 months compared to 40.8 months with docetaxel and trastuzumab alone.

Second Line

The EMILIA trial had established TDM-1 as the preferred second-line anti-HER2 therapy. Trastuzumab emtansine (TDM-1) is an antibody-drug conjugate made up of trastuzumab, stably linked to a very potent chemotherapy drug (DM-1) derived from maytansine. The mechanism of action of TDM-1 is shown in Fig. 27.38. TDM-1 was approved for patients with metastatic disease progressing on a taxane plus trastuzumab or within 6 months of completing therapy with anti-HER2 therapy. However, recent data on the antibody-drug conjugate deruxtecan (T-DXd) demonstrated impressive superiority of trastuzumab deruxtecan over TDM-1 as preferred second-line therapy. T-DXd is composed of the monoclonal antibody trastuzumab, a cleavable linker and a topoisomerase inhibitor as the payload. The permeability of the payload and the high permeability of the payload contribute to a bystander effect in which the payload can express its anticancer properties on cancer cells close to the one that the antibody conjugate binds to. The DESTINY BREAST-03 trial in patients previously treated with a taxane and trastuzumab showed that T-DXd is more effective than TDM-1 as second-line therapy (Hurvitz et al., 2023; Cortes et al., 2022). The benefit extended to patients irrespective of ER status, previous line of therapy, brain metastasis and visceral disease. The side effects of T-DXd include nausea, neutropenia and, most importantly, interstitial lung disease.

T-DM1, however, may still be appropriate as a second-line agent for use in patients with contraindications to T-DXd, low volume or slowly progressive disease. Increasingly, some high-risk patients may also have had prior exposure to T-DM1 in the adjuvant setting, which may make this not an optimal choice, depending on the relapse-free interval.

Third Line

It is not known whether HER-positive breast cancers will respond to T-DM1 after progression on T-DXd. The HER2CLIMB trial randomised patients to tucatinib, capecitabine and trastuzumab and is widely available as an option after progression on two prior lines of anti-HER2 therapy, which could include treatment in the neo-/adjuvant setting. Tucatinib appears to have particular efficacy for patients with brain metastases, and in a subset analysis of this study, 291 patients with brain metastases were evaluated for response and survival. The median OS was 9.1 months longer in the tucatinib-combination group (21.6 months; 95%, CI 18.1–28.5) versus the placebo-combination group (12.5 months; 95%, CI 11.2–16.9). This was a landmark analysis for breast cancer patients with brain disease as historically, patients with brain metastases have been excluded from many clinical trials to date, even though this is unfortunately one of the most common clinical challenges in HER2-positive breast cancer.

For those patients who have not yet received T-DXd, this is an option in third and subsequent lines of therapy. Combining the tyrosine kinase inhibitor, lapatinib, with capecitabine (Table 27.20) can also offer palliation in heavily pretreated HER2 positive patients.

TABLE 27.20 Palliative Capecitabine and Lapatinib

Capecitabine 1000 mg/m^2 twice daily orally on days 1–14 every 21 days
Lapatinib 1250 mg orally once daily until disease progression

TABLE 27.21 Palliative Schedule of Trastuzumab

Loading dose 4 mg/kg intravenously by infusion over 90 minutes
If loading dose is tolerated, subsequent weekly doses of 2 mg/kg intravenously by infusion over 30 minutes

TABLE 27.22 Palliative Doxorubicin/Epirubicin and Cyclophosphamide

Doxorubicin intravenously 60 mg/m^2 or epirubicin 75 mg/m^2
Cyclophosphamide intravenously 600 mg/m^2 Given every 3 weeks

TABLE 27.23 Palliative Regimen With Docetaxel

Docetaxel 75 or 100 mg/m^2
Repeated every 21 days for up to 6 courses
Dose reduction to 75 mg/m^2 if liver function disturbed or toxicity Prophylaxis with growth colony stimulating factor if using docetaxel 100 m/m^2

TABLE 27.24 Palliative Capecitabine

1250 mg/m^2 twice daily orally days 1–14 every 21 days
Consider starting frailer patients at 1000 mg/m^2

TABLE 27.25 Palliative Eribulin

1.23 mg/m^2 (1.4 mg/m^2 eribulin mesylate) intravenously over 2–5 minutes, day 1 and day 8, every 21 days until disease progression

TABLE 27.26 Palliative Vinorelbine

25–30 mg twice weekly (or days 1 and 8 every 21 days if used in combination schedules)
60 mg/m^2 orally weekly for cycles 1–3, then increasing to 80 mg/m^2 except if neutrophil count falls to <500/mm^3 more than once during first three cycles between 500 and 1000 mm^3

TABLE 27.27 Palliative Gemcitabine and Paclitaxel

Gemcitabine intravenously 1250 mg/m^2 days 1 and 8
Paclitaxel 175 mg/m^2 intravenously day 1 every 21 days

TABLE 27.28 Single-Agent Chemotherapy First-Line Responses Rates in Metastatic Breast Cancer

Paclitaxel/Docetaxel	36%–68%
Doxorubicin and epirubicin	40%
Cyclophosphamide	36%
Mitoxantrone (mitozantrone)	27%
Methotrexate	26%
5-Fluorouracil	28%
Vinorelbine	40%–52%
Gemcitabine	23%–37%
Eribulin	29%

TABLE 27.29 Side Effects of Chemotherapy and Route of Administration

Capecitabine Oral
- Severe nausea or vomiting
- Diarrhoea
- Stomach pains
- Loss of appetite
- Constipation
- Fatigue/weakness
- Back/joint/muscle pain
- Headache
- Hand-Foot syndrome

Carboplatin (Usually Given Intravenously)
- Reduced blood count
- Nausea, vomiting and/or diarrhoea
- Hair loss (reversible)
- Confusion

Cisplatin (Usually Given Intravenously)
- Reduced blood count
- Allergic reactions
- Nausea, vomiting
- Tinnitus and hearing loss
- Renal damage

Cyclophosphamide (Given Intravenously or Orally)
- Reduced blood count
- Nausea, vomiting
- Abdominal pain
- Anorexia
- Hair loss (reversible)
- Impaired fertility
- Bladder damage
- Pulmonary or cardiac toxicity (at high dose)

Docetaxel (Taxotere) (Given Intravenously)
- Reduced blood count
- Allergic reactions
- Fluid retention with weight gain; ankle or abdominal swelling
- Peripheral neuropathy
- Nausea
- Diarrhoea
- Mouth ulcers
- Hair loss
- Fatigue and weakness

(continued)

TABLE 27.29 Side Effects of Chemotherapy and Route of Administration—cont'd

Doxorubicin (Given Intravenously)
• Reduced blood count
• Mouth ulcers
• Nausea, vomiting
• Hair loss (reversible)
• Cardiac damage
Eribulin (Given Intravenously)
• Reduced blood count
• Fatigue/weakness
• Hair loss
• Nausea
• Peripheral neuropathy
Etoposide (Given Intravenously)
• Reduced blood count
• Nausea, vomiting
• Mouth ulcers
• Allergic reactions
• Hypotension (during administration)
• Anorexia
• Diarrhoea and abdominal pain
• Flulike symptoms
• Bronchospasm
5-Fluorouracil (Given Intravenously)
• Reduced blood count
• Mouth ulcers
• Diarrhoea
• Dry skin
• Photosensitivity
Gemcitabine (Given Intravenously)
• Reduced blood count
• Nausea, vomiting
• Fever and flulike symptoms
• Rash
Methotrexate (Given Intravenously, Intrathecally or Orally)
• Reduced blood count
• Mouth ulcers
• Skin rashes and photosensitivity
• Hair loss (reversible)
• Liver damage
• Kidney damage (at high dose)
• Seizures
Paclitaxel (Taxol) (Given Intravenously)
• Reduced blood count
• Allergic reactions
• Mouth ulcers
• Peripheral neuropathy
• Nausea, vomiting
• Diarrhoea
• Anorexia
• Altered taste
• Hair loss
• Joint pains
Vinorelbine (Given Intravenously or Orally)
• Low blood count
• Nausea
• Vomiting
• Fatigue/weakness
• Constipation
• Diarrhoea
• Dizziness

The optimum period of anti-HER2 therapy is uncertain. Nor is it known how long it should be continued in patients who obtain a complete radiological response to anti-HER2 therapy. Stopping it may be an option after several years of durable response, keeping open the possibility of reintroduction if there is recrudescence of disease.

Treatment of Metastatic Triple-Negative Breast Cancer

For metastatic triple-negative breast cancer, a recommended treatment algorithm is shown in Fig. 27.43C.

Triple-negative breast cancer is unfortunately very prone to aggressive metastatic dissemination and is associated with a poor prognosis, with a median overall survival of around 18 months, although the development of novel agents is likely to improve this.

For advanced triple-negative breast cancer, chemotherapy is indicated, and a number of chemotherapy options are available. For those with early relapse or aggressive disease, combination first-line chemotherapy may be the most appropriate option and the choice will depend on prior treatment, timing of relapse, patient fitness and patient wishes. A clinical trial should always be considered, and there are often clinical trials available in the first-line setting for triple-negative breast cancer.

A recent advance for triple-negative breast cancer is immunotherapy, to enhance host immunity against the tumour. Tumour mutational burden is a measure of tumour foreignness and immunogenicity because mutated antigens are identified by T cells to elicit a cytotoxic response. Tumours with a high mutational burden are more likely to respond to immunotherapy. PD-L1 IHC expression is the most commonly used biomarker. Treatment with an immune checkpoint inhibitor, pembrolizumab, can be combined with paclitaxel, nab-paclitaxel or carboplatin and gemcitabine in the case of pembrolizumab, in up to 40% of patients who are PD-L1 positive. The addition of a checkpoint inhibitor can modestly improve progression-free survival compared to placebo. Side effects of immunotherapy from triggering a heightened immune response are unpredictable. They include inflammatory and autoimmune complications, affect any organ. Most often they affect the skin, colon, liver, joints, endocrine organs and lungs. Serious side effects include cardiac, neurological, and renal impairment.' Fatigue is the commonest side effect, usually mild but rarely can be severe. It is important to exclude pituitary, thyroid, diabetes and other endocrine disorders e.g. adrenal insufficiency.

In second-line treatment, various options are also available. Sacituzumab govitecan is a novel antibody-drug conjugate that was shown in the ASCENT trial to be superior to treatment of physician's choice in patients who had already received two lines of chemotherapy, one of which had to be for metastatic disease.

Capecitabine is an oral fluoropyrimidine with a slow release of 5-FU. The usual dose is 1000 mg/m^2 twice daily for 14 days. GI or renal toxicity may be dose limiting.

The TNT study, which compared standard docetaxel to carboplatin in TNBC, demonstrated the superiority of carboplatin in germline BRCA1/2-positive patients alone but similar efficacy for both agents in unselected TNBC patients.

Eribulin, vinorelbine and gemcitabine, or retreatment with an anthracycline, are all valid later-line options based on patient fitness, wishes and prior treatment exposure and response.

For germline BRCA1/2-associated triple-negative breast cancer, platinum-based chemotherapy is recommended.

Around 10% of all triple-negative breast cancers are germline BRCA1/2 associated. Deleterious mutations in BRCA1/2 genes that participate in homologous recombination-guided DNA repair mechanism result in the affected cells being dependent on single strand break-repairing pathways regulated by the enzyme PARP. PARP inhibition is the mainstay of treatment for metastatic tumours with BRCA1/2 mutations, leading to the accumulation of irreparable DNA damage (Miglietta et al., 2022).

There are two approved PARP inhibitors for BRCA-associated metastatic breast cancer: olaparib and talazoparib. In the OLYMPIAD trial, patients with HER2-negative breast cancer with BRCA1/2 mutations, after no more than two prior lines of chemotherapy without progression, were randomised to olaparib or single-agent therapy of the physician's choice (capecitabine, eribulin or vinorelbine). In the EMBRACA trial, patients with BRCA1/2 mutations with no more than three lines of prior therapy for metastatic breast cancer were randomised to talazoparib or a single agent of the physician's choice (capecitabine, vinorelbine or gemcitabine). Both olaparib and talazoparib reduced the risk of progression or death by 42% and 46%, respectively, compared to single-agent chemotherapy, but neither improved overall survival. The main toxicity of both agents is haematological, and they are generally well tolerated but are not universally approved to date.

Morbidity of Chemotherapy (Adjuvant and for Metastatic Disease)

The morbidity of adjuvant cytotoxic therapy may be both physical and psychological. The anthracyclines (doxorubicin and epirubicin) cause complete, although reversible, alopecia. They are also potentially cardiotoxic, and cardiac function, judged clinically and by electrocardiogram and cardiac ejection fraction, should be adequate before use. The risk of symptomatic cardiac dysfunction, for example, using a combination of 5-FU, epirubicin (at a dose of 100 mg/m^2) and cyclophosphamide (FEC-100), is 2% at 8 years. The risk of cardiac death is less than 1% if guidelines on maximum cumulative dose are respected. There appears to be no added risk of cardiotoxicity from combining taxanes with anthracyclines. With cumulative doses of anthracyclines, the long-term risk of inducing leukaemia increases. More recently, cognitive dysfunction has been recognised as a complication of chemotherapy caused by damage to the frontal cortex. The risk factors for this are unknown. The taxanes are associated with fluid retention, peripheral neuropathy and allergic reactions. The common toxicities of a selection of anticancer agents used in treating breast cancer are summarised in Table 27.29. Nausea and vomiting can be reduced by the use of steroids and anti-5HT3 antagonists.

Bone Marrow Involvement

Bone marrow involvement complicates the delivery of cytotoxic therapy because the associated leukopenia and thrombocytopaenia of impaired marrow function may compromise the delivery of full-dose chemotherapy. Doses of chemotherapy have to be reduced to 50% or less of the standard dosage. Weekly low-dose IV epirubicin (20 mg/m^2) is generally well tolerated. If chemotherapy is successful, haemoglobin, white count and platelet levels should eventually rise. Bone marrow involvement is not an absolute indication for cytotoxic therapy, because responses are seen in ER-positive patients. However, rapidly evolving bone marrow infiltration will require chemotherapy.

Growth Factor Support

For patients who are experiencing treatment delays because of febrile leucopenia, treatment with granulocyte colony-stimulating factor (GCSF) is recommended. A single injection of pegylated GCSF is common. Common side effects include pain and redness at the injection site and bone pain.

BONE METASTASES: PREVENTION AND TREATMENT

Approximately 20% to 30% of patients present with bone metastases as the first site of metastatic disease. They are associated with more aggressive tumours, particularly in younger females with large tumours, higher grade or several involved axillary lymph nodes. Bone metastases will develop in 60% to 70% of patients at some stage in the course of their disease. Patients with relatively indolent bone metastases live for many years, and less than 1 year if aggressive visceral metastases develop. Bone metastases cause significant morbidity because of pain, pathological fractures, hypercalcaemia or spinal cord compression. Patients with bony metastases should be considered for long-term bisphosphonate therapy.

Approved agents for patients with bone metastases include denosumab (120 mg subcutaneously every 4 weeks, IV pamidronate 90 mg over ≥2 hours, and zoledronic acid (4 mg given IV over ≥15 minutes every 3–4 weeks)). Dosage must be adjusted according to renal function because bisphosphonates are renally excreted and potentially nephrotoxic.

Oral clodronate (1600 mg daily) is an alternative, but its bioavailability is limited and GI intolerance is common. Patients at risk of pathological fracture should be referred to an orthopaedic surgeon for consideration of mechanical stabilisation (Fig. 27.41) followed by postoperative palliative RT.

Palliative Radiotherapy for Bone Metastases

Palliative RT can achieve response rates in pain relief on the order of 60% and complete pain relief in 10% to 25% of patients. The framework of palliative RT has been altered by better control of metastatic disease with systemic therapy. This has enabled longer-term symptom control and the importance of prevention of bony complications in a chronic disease. The availability of stereotactic body radiotherapy (SBRT) might achieve longer-term symptom control compared to traditional palliative dose-fractionation schedules. Candidates for SBRT are those with predicted longer life expectancy.

Technique

Single or parallel-opposed fields are used in palliative RT. Single fields suffice for the thoracic, lumbar spine and sacroiliac joints. The cervical spine can be treated by a single posterior field, but this will cause a sore throat because of the exit dose through the mouth. Lateral opposed fields reduce the dose to the mouth and resultant mucositis. Traditionally, one vertebral body above and below the symptomatic one is included in the treatment volume.

Dose

Single fractions of 8 Gy are recommended at megavoltage. Approximately 20% of patients will require retreatment after a single fraction of 8 Gy. Following surgical stabilisation, fractionated RT is given: 20 Gy in 5 fractions over 1 week at megavoltage.

BRAIN METASTASES

The incidence of brain metastases in breast cancer is about 5%, and around 14% of patients will develop brain metastases during the course of their disease. HER2-positive and triple-negative breast cancers are more likely to metastasise to the brain.

Neurosurgical resection, stereotactic radiosurgery and whole brain radiotherapy (WBRT) are the cornerstones of palliative treatment. The aim is to relieve the symptoms (nausea, headaches, seizures, hemiparesis and impaired higher function). Neurosurgical resection has a role for large metastases where a combined surgery and radiation approach is needed, relief of mass effect to improve functional status and enabling tapering of corticosteroids. Biopsy may be required of brain lesions in patients with a long disease-free interval. Neurosurgical intervention can also distinguish between progressive brain metastases and radiation-induced necrosis.

With better control of extracranial disease, the importance of preserving cognitive function is recognised while maintaining intracranial tumour control. Techniques such as hippocampal-sparing WBRT and stereotactic radiosurgery are applicable to an increasing number of patients. For limited disease in the brain, the preferred approach for lesions larger than 2.5 cm is stereotactic radiosurgery and surgery. For solitary brain metastases, choice of treatment is influenced by site of metastasis, comorbidities, tumour size, extent of oedema and patient preference.

Stereotactic radiosurgery is well established for patients with one to three brain metastases with good performance status. It has the advantage of delivering higher dose-conformal RT in a single session without causing significant delay in the delivery of systemic chemotherapy or immunotherapy. Stereotactic radiosurgery alone has been shown to be feasible for up to five to 10 metastases. The maximum tolerated doses of radiation vary from 24 Gy for lesions up to 20 mm in size, 18 Gy for lesions 21 to 30 mm and 15 Gy for lesions 31 to 40 mm. WBRT is reserved for those patients in whom stereotactic radiosurgery or stereotactic radiotherapy cannot be performed, for example, for leptomeningeal disease, multiple metastases or medical contraindications.

Technique for WBRT: Parallel opposed fields encompassing the whole skull with the inferior border on a line from the outer canthus to the CI-C2 intervertebral space covering the base of the skull.

Dose: 20 Gy in 5 daily fractions over 1 week (4-6-MV photons)

For systemic therapy of brain metastases (see 'Principles of Management of Advanced and Metastatic Disease' page 488).

Prognosis for brain metastases is poor, with a median overall survival of 9.3 months, ranging from 18 months for HR-positive, HER2-positive breast cancer to 4.4 months for triple-negative breast cancer (Watase et al., 2021).

OLIGOMETASTATIC DISEASE

The concept of oligometastatic disease was introduced by Hellman and Weichselbaum, radiation oncologists at the University of Chicago in 1995. They postulated an intermediate state of metastatic disease involving one or a limited number of metastases (up to five) and that this was associated with less aggressive and biologically diverse tumour biology in which all the stages of metastatic progression have not evolved. About 50% of patients with metastatic breast cancer have one to three metastases at presentation. However, the current definition of oligometastic disease is image rather than biologically based. Oligometastatic disease is a heterogeneous and biological diverse condition whose boundaries are as yet not well defined. Its existence is based on the assumption that it is not simply metastatic disease diagnosed at an earlier stage but is associated with primary tumours with restricted capacity for dissemination (Strauss and Chmura, 2022). For it to be a distinct biological entity, a molecular signature for it has to be identified. That is not yet the case. Because there are no biomarkers, the 2020 ESTRO-ASTRO consensus statement defines the oligometastatic state based on imaging and clinical judgment (Lievens et al., 2020). The evidence base for the efficacy of treatment is evolving but still weak, mostly retrospective or prospective nonrandomised studies with limited level I evidence to underpin best practice.

Oligometastatic disease is subdivided into synchronous and metachronous disease. Synchronous oligometastases are present at the time of diagnosis. Metachronous oligometastases (oligorecurrence) is metastatic disease that appears after the primary management of nonmetastatic cancer. Patients who may derive benefit for treatment of oligometastatic disease are characterised by (1) low tumour burden, (2) long disease-free interval and (3) the ability to ablate all metastatic sites. There is preclinical evidence that oligometastatic lesions may represent resistant tumour subclones leading to intratumoural heterogeneity. By eliminating these tumour subclones, it is postulated that the effectiveness of systemic therapy can be preserved and wider dissemination of disease limited.

Management of Oligometastatic Disease

Ablative highly conformal hypofractionated image-guided radiotherapy (HIGRT) or stereotactic ablative radiotherapy (SABR)/SBRT with steep dose gradients sparing adjacent normal tissue is being evaluated to treat metastatic sites. Many of the studies of SBRT in bone metastases include but are not limited to breast cancer. Typically, SBRT is delivered in 1 to 5 fractions of 8 Gy. In the phase II COMET trial, patients with one to five metastatic sites from multiple histologies including breast cancer were randomised to standard care or HIGRT. The progression-free survival was superior with HIGRT, 11.6 versus 5.4 months, as was overall survival, 50 versus 28 months, at a follow-up of 51 months. The cumulative incidence of new metastases between the arms was not different when adjusted for death as a competing event. In the phase III COMET trial, the reproducibility of the survival benefit is being studied when adjusted by stratification factors (e.g. histology, use of chemotherapy and number of metastases) not undertaken in the phase II trial. SBRT has also been shown to be effective in the long-term control of limited (one to three) oligometastatic bone metastases with single doses of 20 Gy with very limited toxicity. In patients who have been responsive to endocrine therapy, SABR may delay or avoid the need for more toxic systemic therapy. SBRT for spinal oligometastatic disease can achieve durable local progression-free survival of 80% or more with median follow-up of 9 to 24 months, but level I data are needed before it can be considered a standard of care for eligible patients. Integrating SBRT with systemic therapy and immunotherapy is under investigation. The optimal timing of systemic therapy and SBRT is unknown.

BREAST CANCER IN PREGNANCY

The diagnosis of breast cancer in pregnancy is uncommon, with an incidence of 1 in 3000 to 10,000 pregnancies, but it presents difficult decisions for the patient, oncologist and obstetrician. Close liaison between the oncologist and obstetrician is essential. The interests of both the mother and child need to be taken into account. In females age 30 years or younger, 10% to 20% of cases may be associated with pregnancy or within 1 year postpartum.

Histology is similar to age and stage-matched nonpregnant controls. Most tumours are high grade, and lymphovascular invasion is common. Lymph node involvement is reported to be as high as 79%. Most tumours (>70%) are ER negative.

Management will be influenced by the stage of pregnancy, the preference of the patient and the stage of the disease. There is no level I evidence on pregnancy and breast cancer. There are guidelines (e.g. Royal College of Obstetrics and Gynaecology (RCOG, 2011)). However, it should follow as far as possible the protocol for nonpregnant patients. A subsequent pregnancy after the diagnosis of breast cancer does not adversely affect prognosis. Indeed, there is some evidence that it may have a favourable effect on survival.

Ultrasound is used initially to image a breast lump. A tissue diagnosis should be obtained by ultrasound-guided biopsy. With adequate fetal shielding, mammography should not be harmful. However, the increased density of the breast during pregnancy may obscure the radiological signs of malignancy. Staging for metastases should only be undertaken if there is a high level of clinical suspicion and should be restricted to chest radiograph and liver ultrasound. MRI scanning can be used safely.

Continuing the pregnancy should take into account the prognosis, treatment and future fertility between the patient, partner and multidisciplinary team. In the first trimester, termination may be considered and followed by standard treatment, depending on the wishes of the patient.

Surgery can usually be safely performed during all trimesters. In general, this is delayed until at least the 12th week of gestation because, before this point, the risk of spontaneous abortion is highest. Breast-conserving surgery or mastectomy is carried out, depending on tumour features and breast size. Sentinel node biopsy is recommended if preoperative axillary ultrasound and needle biopsy are negative. Radioisotope scintigraphy is allowable because it does not cause significant uterine irradiation. However, blue dye should be avoided because its effects on the foetus are unknown. If the axilla is positive, axillary lymph node dissection should be performed. Reconstruction should be delayed to avoid prolonged anaesthesia. In the first trimester, adjuvant chemotherapy is contraindicated because there is a high risk of foetal abnormality. However, in the second trimester, it is safe (when foetal oncogenesis is complete). Anthracyclines in combination with cyclophosphamide followed by taxanes are most commonly used. A standard 5HT3 antagonist and dexamethasone are used as antiemetics. Growth factors are also permitted during pregnancy. Tamoxifen and trastuzumab are contraindicated in pregnancy but may be used after delivery. No adjuvant RT is given until after the delivery of the baby.

Most patients can proceed to term with natural or induced delivery followed, if indicated, by postoperative RT (with the same criteria as in the nonpregnant patient).

Hormonal therapy, if indicated, should be started after delivery, and after chemotherapy has been completed.

Pregnancy per se does not appear to impair the prognosis of breast cancer for females diagnosed in pregnancy when compared with non-pregnant controls matched for age and stage. However, because pregnancy-associated breast cancer occurs in younger females with many adverse risk factors conferring a higher risk of metastasis (high grade, ER negative), such females may be expected to have a poorer prognosis.

BREAST CANCER IN MALES

Breast cancer in males is rare, only representing 0.5% to 1% of all breast cancer cases per year. Most cases occur in an older age group than in females, typically occurring over the age of 60 years. It has its own biological and clinical features, distinct from female breast cancer. In the largest series to date, the EORTC 100085/TBCRC/BIG/NABCG international male breast cancer program of 1822 patients, the median age was 68.4 years. Of these, 56% were node negative and 48% TI. Nearly 85% were invasive ductal carcinomas, just over half were grade 2, 99% were ER positive, 81% PgR positive and over 96% androgen-receptor (AR) positive; 41% were luminal A-like, 48% luminal B-like HER2 negative, 8% luminal B-like, HER2 positive and <3% triple negative basal. Like female breast cancer, histological grade was not associated with clinical outcome. In males under the age of 50 years, breast cancer-specific mortality was higher. Overall and recurrence survival were superior in strongly ER-, PgR- or AR-positive patients.

In some cases, there is a genetic predisposition. A variable proportion of cases (3%–20%) carry a mutation of the BRCA2 gene. A family history of male breast cancer is a major predisposing factor to female breast cancer. In addition, BRCA2 mutations are associated with an increased risk of other cancers such as lymphomas, laryngeal and kidney cancer.

Presentation is typically with locally advanced disease, often affecting the nipple. Fixation to the chest wall is common. The advanced state of the local disease is in part probably as a result of the limited amount of breast tissue that the tumour has to invade and the lack of awareness among males that they can develop breast cancer.

The rarity of the tumour means that there are no trials of adjuvant therapy. The specific metabolic and endocrine context of male breast cancer suggests that treatment should not be directly extrapolated from that of female breast cancer. In males, 80% of circulating oestrogen is generated from peripheral aromatisation of androgens. The testes account for the other 20%. If aromatisation alone is inhibited, a feedback loop of luteinising hormone (LH) and follicle-stimulating hormone (FSH) production may develop, resulting in increased hormonal testicular production. As a result, it is recommended that aromatase inhibitors are only used in combination with LHRH agonists. If the disease is operable, simple mastectomy (because there is little breast tissue) and sentinel node biopsy is preferred, proceeding to axillary node clearance if node positive. The principles of postoperative RT and chemotherapy apply as per female breast cancer. For ER-positive patients, tamoxifen is safe, both in the adjuvant and metastatic settings. For ER-negative disease, chemotherapy is recommended. The outcome of the disease is usually poor, with a 5-year survival rate of about 65%, reflecting the commonly advanced nature of the disease at presentation.

FOLLOW-UP OF EARLY BREAST CANCER

The main goals of follow-up are:

1. Detection of locoregional or metastatic recurrence, second primary tumour and contralateral breast cancer
2. Assessment and treatment of complications of treatment
3. Encouragement of compliance with therapy
4. Psychosocial support
5. Maintenance and monitoring of response to treatment and treatment-induced morbidity and to facilitate rehabilitation

Clinical trials have failed to show an improvement in patient outcomes from more intensive versus less intensive follow-up for systemic recurrence. There is no evidence that the early detection of asymptomatic disease at distant sites improves survival or quality of life. Routine imaging apart from mammography is not recommended as part of follow-up care.

From the patient's perspective, reassurance that there is no evidence of recurrence or of progressive disease is probably the most important. Most of the evidence suggests that, at least for females treated for operable breast cancer, most recurrences, whether after breast conservation or mastectomy, present symptomatically. It is probable that a policy of annual mammography to detect local recurrence in the conserved or contralateral breast and rapid access to the breast/oncology clinic for females with new symptoms would be much more cost-effective.

The priorities are the detection of local recurrence that can be treated by mastectomy and of contralateral breast cancer. The risk of contralateral breast cancer is three to five times that of the normal population. Guidelines on optimal duration of follow-up vary considerably. NICE recommends annual mammography for 5 years.

Although distant relapses peak in the first 5 years of follow-up, recurrence rates within the treated breast remain constant at 1% to 1.5% per year for at least 10 years. This argues that the frequency of follow-up does not need to be any more frequent in the early years after completion of treatment than in later years. Most studies of follow-up show that multiple clinical visits are of little value in detecting recurrence. In a study from Edinburgh of 1312 females followed up for 10 years after breast-conserving surgery and postoperative RT treated between 1991 and 1998, only 15 relapses were detected clinically (Montgomery et al., 2007). Following mastectomy, local recurrences on the chest wall are most common in the first 2 years after mastectomy, and 80% of the chest wall and axillary recurrences occur within the first 5 years. NICE recommends annual mammography of the contralateral breast for 5 years.

A new trend is patient-managed or patient-initiated follow-up. There are no regular appointments, but patients may be contacted regularly by their specialist breast care nurse or the patient may contact the clinician if they have concerns about anything. Most patients are discharged from follow-up after 5 years, with their general practitioner taking over their care. Females who still lie within the UK screening age group (i.e. age <69 years) should be returned to the 3-yearly breast-screening program. For females over age 70 years, further follow-up should be decided on an individual basis between the patient and their surgeon/oncologist.

CLINICAL OUTCOMES IN BREAST CANCER

Clinical outcomes have improved steadily over the past three decades due to a combination of factors: breast screening and better surgery, RT and systemic therapy. A large study of 500,000 females with early breast cancer diagnosed in England from 1993 to 2015 shows that crude annual breast cancer mortality has fallen from 14.4% (95%, CI 14.25–14.6) for females diagnosed between 1993 and 1999 to 409% (95% CI 4.8–5.0) for those diagnosed between 2010 and 2015 (Fig. 27.39). Adjusted annual breast cancer mortality fell in nearly every patient group over time, twofold for ER-negative disease and threefold for ER-positive disease (lower-left panel of Fig. 27.39). For more than 60% of females diagnosed between 2010 and 2015, the risk of dying from breast cancer in the first 5 years was 3% or less, and for 90% of those diagnosed in the same period the risk of dying from breast cancer was less than 10%. For a 60-year-old female with a screen-detected breast cancer smaller than 20 mm, low grade, node negative and HER2 negative, the estimated 5-year breast cancer mortality risk would be 0.2%. Most patients with early breast cancer will be long-term survivors (Taylor et al., 2023).

Local relapses after breast-conserving surgery have fallen from around 5% at 5 years two decades ago to around 2% to 3% currently. The Edinburgh Breast Conservation series of over 1812 patients typifies these improvements. It includes patients presenting through the breast-screening program or symptomatically, and treated between 1990 and 1998. The actuarial overall survival (deaths from all causes) is 88.5% at 5 years, 77.2% at 10 years, 65.9% at 15 years and 55.8% at 20 years. At 10 years, the cumulative risk of ipsilateral breast relapse was 8.4% (.84% per year). The time to ipsilateral breast tumour recurrence is shown in Fig. 27.46.

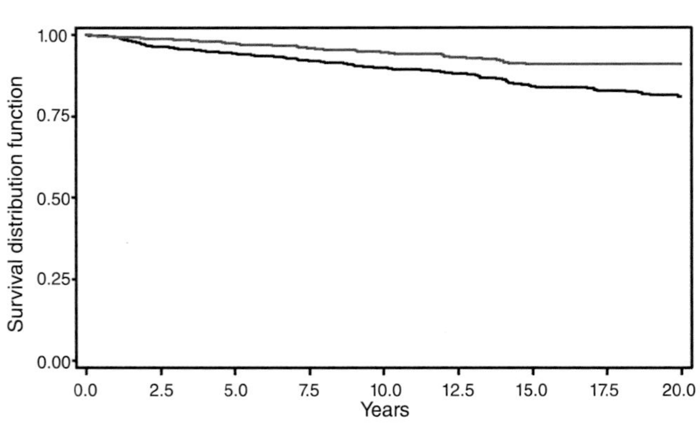

Fig. 27.46 Time to ipsilateral breast tumour recurrence by screened or symptomatic presentation. (Reproduced with permission from Kunkler IH, Kerr GR, Thomas JS, et al. Impact of screening and risk factors for local recurrence and survival after conservative surgery and radiotherapy for early breast cancer: results from a large series with long-term follow-up. *Int J Radiat Oncol Biol Phys.* 2012;83(3):829–838.)

Life expectancy from the time of diagnosis of advanced and metastatic disease has improved, with many long-term survivors over 5 years with HER2-positive breast cancer controlled by trastuzumab.

ACKNOWLEDGMENTS

I would like to thank Professor Mike Dixon, consultant surgeon, and Dr Caroline Michie, consultant medical oncologist, for their very helpful comments on the manuscript.

FURTHER READING

Biganzoli L, Cardoso F, Beishon M, et al. The requirements of a specialist breast centre. *Breast.* 2020;51:65–84. https://doi.org/10.1016/j.breast.2020.02.003

Burnstein HJ, Curigliano G, Loibl S, et al. Estimating the benefits of therapy for early-stage breast cancer: the St. Gallen International Consensus Guidelines for the primary therapy of early breast cancer 2019. *Ann Oncol.* 2019;30(10):1541–1557. https://doi.org/10.1093/annonc/mdz235

Cardoso F, Costa A, Senkus E, et al. 3rd ESO-ESMO International consensus guidelines for advanced breast cancer (ABC 3). *Ann Oncol.* 2017;28(1):16–33. https://doi.org/10.1093/annonc/mdw544

Chainitikun S, Saleem S, Lim B, Valero V, Ueno NT. Update on systemic treatment for newly diagnosed inflammatory breast cancer. *J Adv Res.* 2021;29:1–12. https://doi.org/10.1016/j.jare.2020.08.014

Cortés J, Kim S-B, Chung W-P, et al. Trastuzumab deruxtecan versus trastuzumab emtansine for breast cancer. *N Eng J Med.* 2022;386:1143–1154. https://doi.org/10.1056/NEJMoa2115022

Darby SC, Ewertz M, McGale P, et al. Risk of ischemic heart disease in women after radiotherapy for breast cancer. *N Eng J Med.* 2013;368:987–998. https://doi.org/10.1056/NEJMoa1209825

Debien V, De Caluwé A, Wang X, et al. Immunotherapy in breast cancer: an overview of current strategies and perspectives. *NPJ Breast Cancer.* 2023;9(1):7. https://doi.org/10.1038/s41523-023-00508-3

Duma M-N, Baumann R, Budach W, et al. Heart-sparing radiotherapy techniques in breast cancer patients: a recommendation of the breast cancer expert panel of the German Society of Radiation Oncology. *Strahlenther Onkol.* 2019;195:861–871. https://doi.org/10.1007/s00066-019-01495-w

Early Breast Cancer Trialists' Collaborative Group (EBCTCG); Darby S, McGale P, et al. Effect of radiotherapy after breast-conserving surgery on 10-year recurrence and 15-year breast cancer death: meta-analysis of individual patient data for 10,801 women ssin 17 randomised trials. *Lancet.* 2011;378(9804):1707–1716. https://doi.org/10.1016/S0140-6736(11)61629-2

Early Breast Cancer Trialists' Collaborative Group (EBCTCG); Davies C, Godwin J, et al. Relevance of breast cancer hormone receptors and other factors to the efficacy of adjuvant tamoxifen: patient-level meta-analysis of randomised trials. *Lancet.* 2011;378(9793):771–784. https://doi.org/10.1016/S0140-6736(11)60993-8

Early Breast Cancer Trialists' Collaborative Group (EBCTCG). Aromatase inhibitors versus tamoxifen in early breast cancer: patient level meta-analysis of the randomised trials. *Lancet.* 2015;386(10001):1341–1352. https://doi.org/10.1016/S0140-6736(15)61074-1

Early Breast Cancer Trialists' Collaborative Group (EBCTCG). Long-term outcomes for neoadjuvant versus adjuvant chemotherapy in early breast cancer: meta-analysis of individual patient data from ten randomised trials. *Lancet Oncol.* 2018;19(1):27–39. https://doi.org/10.1016/S1470-2045(17)30777-5

Early Breast Cancer Trialists' Collaborative Group (EBCTCG). Increasing the dose intensity of chemotherapy by more frequent administration or

sequential scheduling: a patient-level meta-analysis of 37,298 women with early breast cancer in 26 randomised trials. *Lancet*. 2019;393(10179): 1440–1452. https://doi.org/10.1016/S0140-6736(18)33137-4
Early Breast Cancer Trialists' Collaborative Group (EBCTCG). Aromatase inhibitors versus tamoxifen in premenopausal women with oestrogen receptor-positive early-stage breast cancer treated with ovarian suppression: a patient-level meta-analysis of 7030 women from four randomised trials. *Lancet Oncol*. 2022;23(3):382–392. https://doi.org/10.1016/S1470-2045(21)00758-0
Early Breast Cancer Trialists' Collaborative Group (EBCTCG). Anthracycline-containing and taxane-containing chemotherapy for early-stage operable breast cancer: a patient-level meta-analysis of 100,000 women from 86 randomised trials. *Lancet*. 2023;401(10384): 1277–1292. https://doi.org/10.1016/S0140-6736(23)00285-4
Early Breast Cancer Trialists' Collaborative Group (EBCTCG); McGale P, Taylor C, et al. Effect of radiotherapy after mastectomy and axillary surgery on 10-year recurrence and 20-year breast cancer mortality: meta-analysis of individual patient data for 8135 women in 22 randomised trials. *Lancet*. 2014;383(9935):2127–2135. https://doi.org/10.1016/S0140-6736(14)60488-8
Elshof LE, Schaapveld M, Schmidt MK, Rutgers EJ, van Leeuwen FE, Wesseling J. Subsequent risk of ipsilateral and contralateral invasive breast cancer after treatment for ductal carcinoma in situ: incidence and the effect of radiotherapy in a population-based cohort of 10,090 women. *Breast Cancer Res Treat*. 2016;159(3):553–563. https://doi.org/10.1007/s10549-016-3973-y
Gandhi A, Coles C, Makris A, et al. Axillary surgery following neoadjuvant chemotherapy—multidisciplinary guidance from the Association of Breast Surgery, faculty of clinical oncology of the Royal College of Radiologists, UK Breast Cancer Group, National Coordinating Committee for Breast Pathology and British Society of Breast Radiology. *Clin Oncol (R Coll Radiol)*. 2019;31(9):664–668. https://doi.org/10.1016/j.clon.2019.05.021
Grantzau T, Mellemkjær L, Overgaard J. Second primary cancers after adjuvant radiotherapy in early breast cancer patients: a national population based study under the Danish Breast Cancer Cooperative Group (DBCG). *Radiother Oncol*. 2013;106(1):42–49. https://doi.org/10.1016/j.radonc.2013.01.002
Harbeck N, Gnant M. Breast cancer. *Lancet*. 2017;389(10074): 1134–1150. https://doi.org/10.1016/S0140-6736(16)31891-8
Hellman S. Karnofsky Memorial Lecture. Natural history of small breast cancers. *J Clin Oncol*. 1994;12(10):2229–2234. https://doi.org/10.1200/JCO.1994.12.10.2229
Hurvitz SA, Hegg R, Chung W-P, et al. Trastuzumab deruxtecan versus trastuzumab emtansine in patients with HER2-positive metastatic breast cancer: updated results from DESTINY-Breast03, a randomised, open-label, phase 3 trial. *Lancet*. 2023;401(10371): 105–117. https://doi.org/10.1016/S0140-6736(22)02420-5
Kunkler IH, Williams LJ, Jack WJL, Cameron DA, Dixon JM. Breast-conserving surgery with or without irradiation in early breast cancer. *N Engl J Med*. 2023;388(7):585–594.
Lal S, McCart Reed AE, de Luca XM, Simpson PT. Molecular signatures in breast cancer. *Methods*. 2017;131:135–146. https://doi.org/10.1016/j.ymeth.2017.06.032
Levy A, Rivera S. 1-Week hypofractionated adjuvant whole-breast radiotherapy: towards a new standard? *Lancet*. 2020;395(10237): 1588–1589. https://doi.org/10.1016/S0140-6736(20)30978-8
Lewis P, Brunt AM, Coles C, et al. Moving forward fast with FAST-Forward. *Clin Oncol (R Coll Radiol)*. 2021;33(7):427–429. https://doi.org/10.1016/j.clon.2021.04.007
Lievens Y, Guckenberger M, Gomez D, et al. Defining oligometastatic disease from a radiation oncology perspective: an ESTRO-ASTRO consensus document. *Rad Oncol*. 2020;148:157–166. https://doi.org/10.1016/j.radonc.2020.04.003
Loibl S, Poortmans P, Morrow M, Denkert C, Curigliano G. Breast cancer. *Lancet*. 2021;397(10286):1750–1769. https://doi.org/10.1016/S0140-6736(20)32381-3
Meattini I, Becherini C, Boersma L, et al. European Society for Radiotherapy and Oncology Advisory Committee in Radiation Oncology Practice consensus recommendations on patient selection and dose and fractionation for external beam radiotherapy in early breast cancer. *Lancet Oncol*. 2022;23(1):e21–e31. https://doi.org/10.1016/S1470-2045(21)00539-8
Miglietta F, Bottosso M, Griguolo G, Dieci MV, Guarneri V. Major advancements in metastatic breast cancer treatment: when expanding options means prolonging survival. *ESMO Open*. 2022;7(2):100409. https://doi.org/10.1016/j.esmoop.2022.100409
Montgomery DA, Krupa K, Jack WJL, et al. Changing pattern of the detection of locoregional relapse in breast cancer: the Edinburgh experience. *Br J Cancer*. 2007;96(12):1802–1807. https://doi.org/10.1038/sj.bjc.6603815
Morrow M. Surgery and prophylactic surgery in hereditary breast cancer. *Breast*. 2022;62(Suppl 1):S63–S66. https://doi.org/10.1016/j.breast.2021.12.010
NICE (National Institute for Health and Care Excellence). *Early and locally advanced breast cancer: diagnosis and management. NICE Guidelines (NG101)*. Manchester, UK: NICE; 2018. Last updated 14 April 2025. https://www.nice.org.uk/guidance/ng101
Offersen BV, Boersma LJ, Kirkove C, et al. ESTRO consensus guideline on target volume delineation for elective radiation therapy of early breast cancer. *Radiother Oncol*. 2015;114(1):3–10. https://doi.org/10.1016/j.radonc.2014.11.030
Piroth MD, Baumann R, Budach W, et al. Heart toxicity from breast cancer radiotherapy. *Strahlenther Onkol*. 2019;195(1):1–12. https://doi.org/10.1007/s00066-018-1378-z
Poortmans PM, Weltens C, Fortpied C, et al. Internal mammary and medial supraclavicular lymph node chain irradiation in stage I–III breast cancer. (EORTC 22922/10925): 15-year results of a randomised phase 3 trial. *Lancet Oncol*. 2020;21(12):1602–1610. https://doi.org/10.1016/S1470-2045(20)30472-1
Recht A. Breast cancer: stages 1–11. Eds.. In: Tepper JE, Foote RL, Michalski JM, eds. *Gunderson & Tepper's Clinical Radiation Oncology*. 5th ed. Philadelphia, Elsevier; 2021.
Recht A, Comen EA, Fine RE, et al. Postmastectomy radiotherapy: an American Society of Clinical Oncology, American Society for Radiation Oncology, and Society of Surgical Oncology focused guideline update. *J Clin Oncol*. 2016;34(36):4431–4442. https://doi.org/10.1200/JCO.2016.69.1188
Royal College of Obstetricians and Gynaecologists. *Pregnancy and breast cancer. Green-top guideline No. 12*. London, UK; 2011. https://www.rcog.org.uk/media/2q4jb0kz/gtg_12.pdf
Sauter E, Razaq W. Metastatic breast cancer: symptoms, diagnosis and treatment. *BMJ Best Practice*. https://bestpractice.bmj.com/topics/en-gb/718?q=Metastatic%20breast%20cancer&c=suggested. Last updated 24th April, 2025.
Schmid P, Cortes J, Dent R, et al. Event-free survival with pembrolizumab in early triple-negative breast cancer. *N Engl J Med*. 2022;386(6):556–567. https://doi.org/10.1056/NEJMoa2112651
Strauss JB, Chmura SJ, Oligometastatic breast cancer. *Sem Rad Oncol*. 2022;32(3):282–290. https://doi.org/10.1016/j.semradonc.2022.01.008
Swain SM, Baselga J, Kim S-B, et al. Pertuzumab, trastuzumab and docetaxel in HER2-positive breast cancer. *N Engl J Med*. 2015;372(8):724–734. https://doi.org/10.1056/NEJMoa1413513

Taylor CW, Nisbet A, McGale P, Darby SC. Cardiac exposures in breast cancer radiotherapy: 1950s–1990s. *Int J Rad Oncol Biol Phys.* 2007;69(5):1484–1495. https://doi.org/10.1016/j.ijrobp.2007.05.034

Taylor C, McGale P, Probert J, et al. Breast cancer mortality in 500,000 women with early invasive breast cancer diagnosed in England, 1993–2015: population based observational cohort study. *BMJ.* 2023;381:e074684. https://doi.org/10.1136/bmj-2022-074684

Thomsen MS, Berg M, Zimmermann S, et al. Dose constraints for whole breast radiation therapy based on the quality assessment of treatment plans in the randomised Danish Breast Cancer Group (DBCG) HYPO trial. *Clin Transl Radiat Oncol.* 2021;28:118–123. https://doi.org/10.1016/j.ctro.2021.03.009

Tutt ANJ, Garber JE, Kaufman B, et al. Adjuvant olaparib for patients with BRCA1- or BRCA2-mutated breast cancer. *N Eng J Med.* 2021;384(25):2394–2405. https://doi.org/10.1056/NEJMoa2105215

Van Seijen M, Lips EH, Thompson AM, et al. Ductal carcinoma in situ: to treat or not to treat, that is the question. *Br J Cancer.* 2019;121(4):285–292. https://doi.org/10.1038/s41416-019-0478-6

von Minckwitz G, Huang C-H, Mano MS, et al. Trastuzumab Emtamsine for residual invasive HER2-positive breast cancer. *N Engl J Med.* 2019;380:617–628.

Watase C, Shiino S, Shimoi T, et al. Breast cancer brain metastases—overview of disease state, treatment options and future perspectives. *Cancers (Basel).* 2021;13(5):1078. https://doi.org/10.3390/cancers13051078

Whelan T, Levine M, Sussman J. Hypofractionated breast irradiation: what's next? *J Clin Oncol.* 2020;38(28):3245–3247. https://doi.org/10.1200/JCO.20.01243

Yates LR, Knappskog S, Wedge D, et al. Genomic evolution of breast cancer metastasisss and relapse. *Cancer Cell.* 2017;32(2):169–184. https://doi.org/10.1016/j.ccell.2017.07.005

28

Gynaecological Cancer

Aspazia Spyrou, Hersha Patel, Adrian Franklin and Alexandra Stewart

CHAPTER OUTLINE

ANATOMY

The female reproductive organs lie within the pelvis and include the vulva, vagina, uterus, fallopian tubes and ovaries. These are represented in Figs. 28.1 and 28.2.

INCIDENCE OF GYNAECOLOGICAL CANCER

The incidence of gynaecological cancer in England from 2016 through 2018 is shown in Table 28.1. The incidence of cervical cancer has declined markedly since 1978. This falling trend has been accelerated by the success of cervical screening and the successful initiation of the human papilloma virus (HPV) vaccination program (Fig. 28.3). However, cervical cancer is the most important female cancer in much of the developing world, including South Asia, sub-Saharan Africa and South America. In the past decade, the incidence of carcinoma of the body of the uterus has remained stable in the United Kingdom.

CARCINOMA OF THE CERVIX

Causes of Cervical Neoplasia

In virtually all cases of cancer of the cervix, there is evidence that the tumour is associated with infection with HPV, particularly types 16 and 18. The virus produces proteins that bind to the products of two important tumour suppressor genes, p53 and RB1. Risk factors associated with cervical cancer are those that promote sexual transmission of the virus, such as a lower age of first intercourse and an increased number of sexual partners. There is a lower incidence of cervical carcinoma in females using barrier methods of contraception. Male behaviour is also important, with a higher incidence of cervical cancer seen in the partners of males whose previous partners have developed cervical cancer. Smoking and immunosuppression are also associated with cervical cancer. Cervical neoplasia is more common in females who are HIV positive. HPV vaccination commenced in the United Kingdom in females age 13 to 14 years from 2008 and extended to include males in 2019. There has been a reduction in the rates of cervical neoplasia since then. The rates of cervical cancer dropped by 34% in females age 16 to 18 years, by 62% in those age 14 to 16 years and by 87% in those age 12 to 13 years. The corresponding risk reduction for CIN3 rates were 39% for those offered the vaccine between the ages of 16 and 18, 75% for between the ages of 14 and 16 and 97% between the ages of 12 and 13.

Pathology of Cervical Cancer

Viral infection of the cervix may lead to premalignant change, which is called *dysplasia (dyskaryosis)*. This can be detected in exfoliated cells removed during a cervical smear. Cervical dysplasia is graded mild, moderate or severe. The terms *CIN1*, *CIN2* and *CIN3* are histological terms used to describe increasing degrees of dysplasia, that is, mild, moderate and severe, in biopsy material. In some females, there is a progression from mild to severe dysplasia and then invasive cancer. This often takes many years to develop and is associated with HPV infection, which can be detected during cervical screening. Treatment of premalignant disease is highly effective. In most cases, dysplasia is self-limiting; patients with moderate or severe dysplasia are offered excisional treatment using large loop excision of the transformation zone. Ablative therapy may be used in selected cases. Even the most

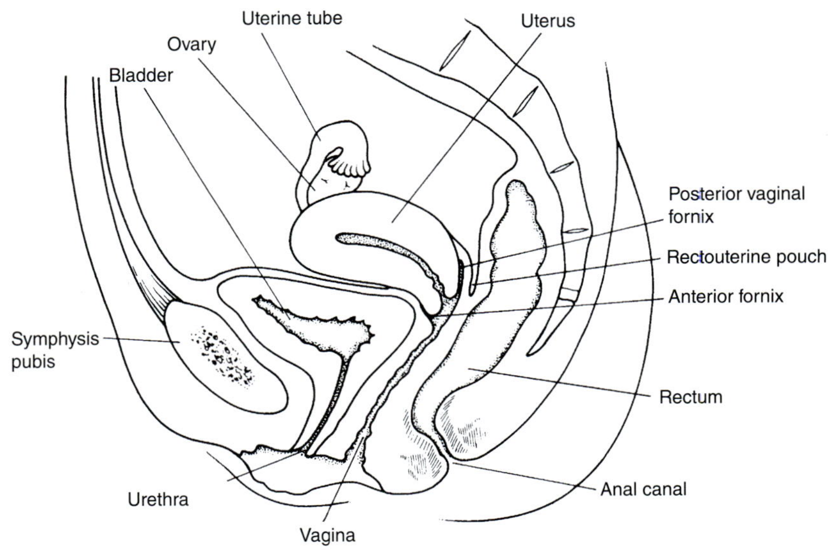

Fig. 28.1 Sagittal section of the uterus and its relations. (Modified from Ellis H. *Clinical Anatomy* (5th ed.). Blackwell; 1975.)

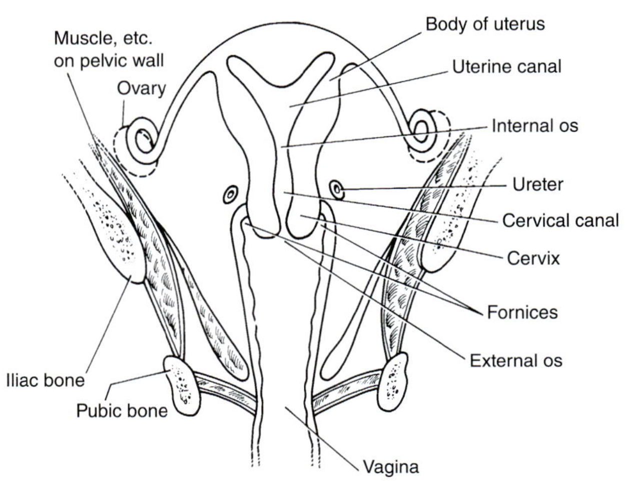

Fig. 28.2 Coronal section of the uterus and vagina. Note the important relationship of the ureter to the cervix.

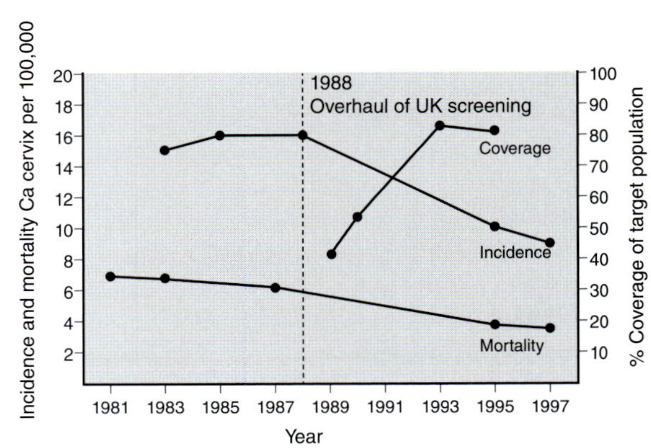

Fig. 28.3 Impact of 1988 overhaul of cervical screening program on incidence and mortality of cervical cancer in the United Kingdom.

TABLE 28.1 Incidence of Gynaecological Cancer in the United Kingdom 2016 Through 2018

	Number of Cases	Incidence per 100,000
Site	Per Annum	Females
Vulva	1372	4.0
Cervix	3197	10.0
Body of uterus	9700	30
Ovary	7495	23

severe form of dysplasia, CIN3, will only progress to invasive cancer in 20% to 40% of females if left untreated. Between 80% and 90% of cases of invasive cancer of the cervix are squamous carcinomas, which have seen an overall reduction in incidence rate of 24% in females in the United Kingdom (2017–2019). The majority of the remainder are adenocarcinoma or adenosquamous tumours. There is evidence that the incidence of adenocarcinoma is increasing among younger females. Significant increases in cervical adenocarcinoma have been seen in Europe, with at least a 2% per year increase in Finland, Slovakia, Slovenia and the United Kingdom. Cervical adenocarcinoma is associated with a poorer prognosis and higher rates of metastases, especially in the ovaries. Some studies indicate that adenocarcinoma of the cervix may have a worse prognosis than squamous cancer when treated with radiotherapy (RT). Carcinoma of the cervix spreads predominantly by direct invasion or through the lymphatic system. Initially, the tumour spreads into the uterus, vagina or parametrium. Later it can infiltrate the bladder or rectum. The tumour spreads to the iliac and then paraaortic lymph nodes (Fig. 28.4). Blood-borne spread is less common and may lead to liver, lung or bone metastases.

Symptoms and Investigations of Cervical Cancer

Premalignant changes are usually asymptomatic. The cardinal symptom of invasive cervical cancer is irregular vaginal bleeding. This may be bleeding after intercourse, bleeding in between periods or postmenstrual bleeding. Sometimes the presenting symptom is a brown vaginal discharge. Pain is usually a symptom of advanced disease and suggests spread to adjacent organs around the cervix. Backache may be associated with paraaortic lymph node spread.

Accurate staging of cervical cancer is essential so that appropriate treatment can be planned. Patients with cervical cancer are staged clinically according to the International Federation of Gynecology and Obstetrics (FIGO) staging system (Table 28.2). Staging traditionally required an examination under anaesthesia (EUA), with digital and visual examination of the cervix and vagina in combination with

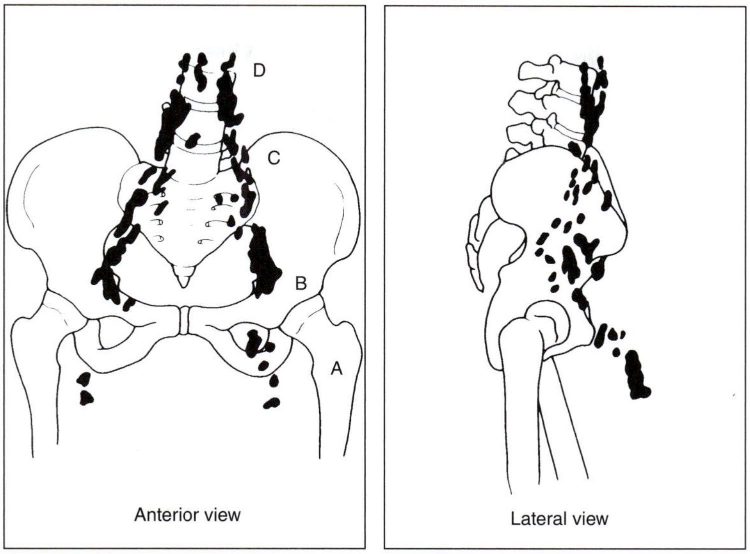

Fig. 28.4 Lymphatic drainage of the cervix: (A) obturator, (B) internal, external and common iliac; (C) lateral sacral; and (D) paraaortic. (From Souhami RL, Tobias JS. *Cancer and Its Management*. Blackwell; 1986.)

sigmoidoscopy and cystoscopy. However, this can be quite subjective, especially in determining parametrial invasion, so staging is now predominantly performed using imaging with a magnetic resonance imaging (MRI) scan of the abdomen and pelvis (Figs. 28.5–28.7) and a positron emission tomography-computed tomography (PET/CT) scan of the body (Fig. 28.8), with EUA often reserved for potentially operable cases.

Treatment

Stage is the most important factor related to outcome. However, tumour size is also an important prognostic feature. Typical survival figures are listed in Table 28.3. The prognosis for locally advanced disease has improved following the widespread use of combined chemotherapy and radiation treatment (Figs. 28.9 and 28.10).

Surgical Treatment of Stage I Disease

The surgical treatment of precancer and cancer of the cervix should take into account fertility. Stage I tumours are subdivided according to tumour size. The prognosis is excellent for Stage IA1 patients, and the challenge is to avoid overtreatment. A cone biopsy or simple hysterectomy offers many of these patients a nearly 100% chance of cure. The prognosis is also very good for Stage IA2 patients. The optimum management of this group has not been clearly defined. The management options vary from cone biopsy or trachelectomy to simple or modified

TABLE 28.2 International Federation of Gynaecology and Obstetrics 2018 Staging: Carcinoma of the Cervix Uteri

Stage I		• Lateral extent of the carcinoma is no longer considered in distinguishing between FIGO Stage IA and IB carcinomas • If margins of loop are involved, patient is allocated to Stage IB1
	IA1	Measured stromal invasion <3 mm in depth
	IA2	IA2: Measured stromal invasion ≥3 mm and <5 mm in depth
	IB1	Invasive carcinoma ≥5 mm depth of stromal invasion and <2 cm in greatest dimension
	IB2 (see Fig. 28.9)	Invasive carcinoma ≥2 cm and <4 cm in greatest dimension
	IB3	Invasive carcinoma ≥4 cm in greatest dimension
Stage II		
	IIA	Involvement limited to the upper two-thirds of the vagina without parametrial involvement
	IIA1	Invasive carcinoma <4 cm in greatest dimension
	IIA2	Invasive carcinoma ≥4 cm in greatest dimension
	IIB (see Figs. 28.5 and 28.6)	With parametrial involvement but not up to the pelvic wall
Stage III		
	IIIA	Tumour involves lower third of the vagina, with no extension to the pelvic wall
	IIIB (see Figs. 28.16 and 28.17)	Extension to the pelvic wall and/or hydronephrosis or nonfunctioning kidney
	IIIC	Involvement of pelvic and/or paraaortic lymph nodes, irrespective of tumour size and extent; Add notation of r (imaging) and p (pathology)
Stage IV		
	IVA (see Figs. 28.11 and 28.12)	Spread of the growth to adjacent organs
	IVB (see Figs. 28.18–28.20)	Spread to distant organs

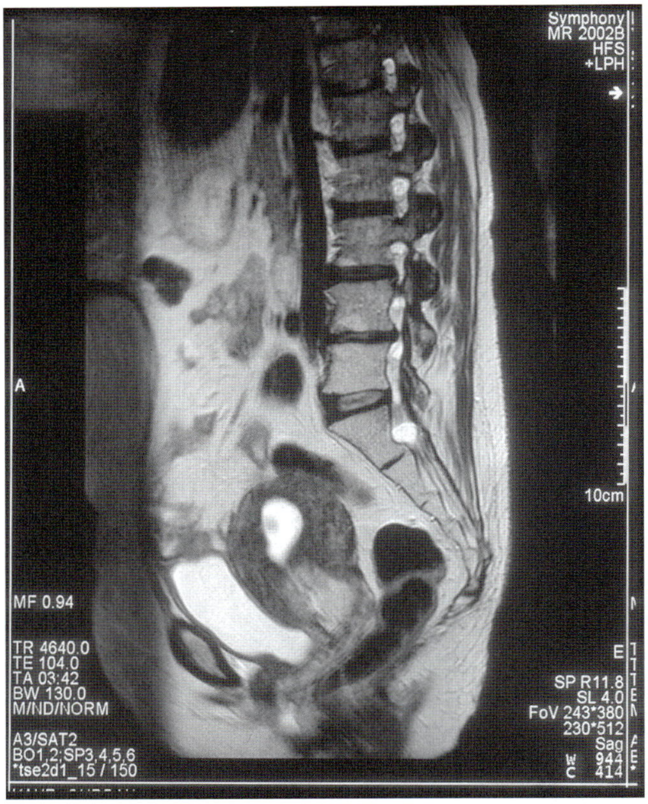

Fig. 28.5 Large cervical tumour in endocervical canal.

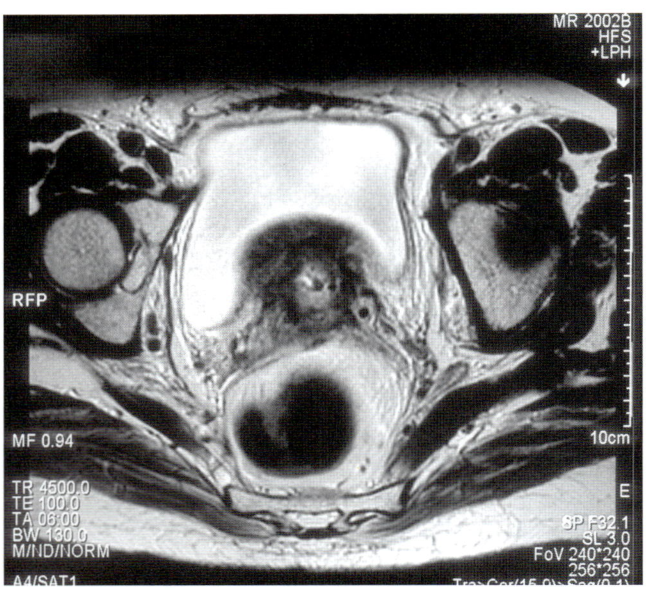

Fig. 28.6 Cervical tumour extending into the right parametrium.

radical hysterectomy. Minimally invasive surgery (MIS) has been shown to be associated with many benefits, including reduced postoperative morbidity, improved recovery and reduced inpatient stay.

Selected Stage IB patients (generally those with tumours <4 cm) may be treated by radical hysterectomy with bilateral pelvic lymph node dissection. Usually, such patients are relatively slim, fit and often premenopausal. A two-stage approach is used by some whereby bilateral pelvic lymph node dissection is performed initially via an MIS approach, and if the histology from the lymph nodes is negative, a second procedure is performed for the radical hysterectomy. This

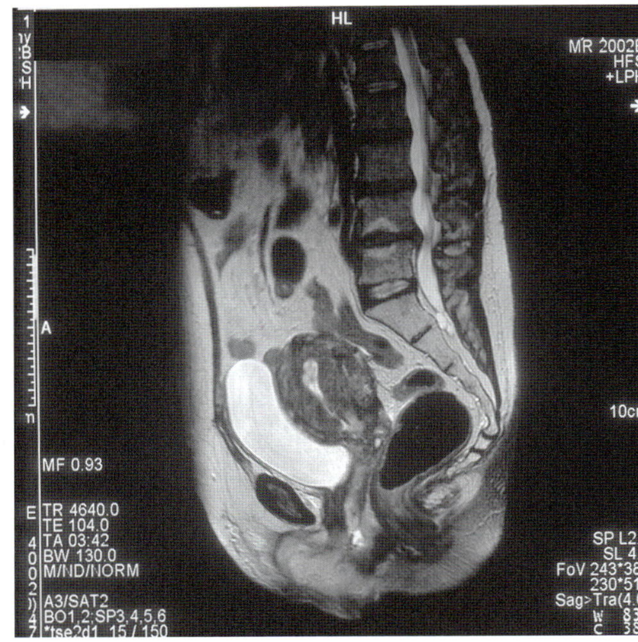

Fig. 28.7 Residual tumour in endocervical canal.

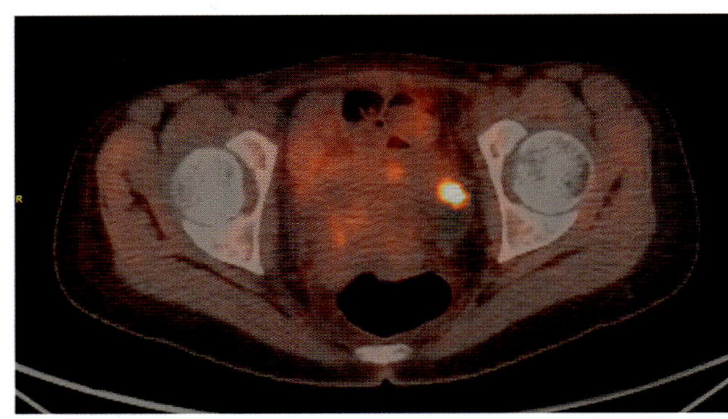

Fig. 28.8 Positron emission tomography scan showing avid uptake of fluorodeoxyglucose in left pelvic lymph node containing metastatic cervical cancer.

TABLE 28.3 Carcinoma of the Cervix: Cancer-Specific 5-Year Survival

Stage	Overall 5-Year Survival (%)
IA1	97–100
IB2	95–97
IB	80–90
IIA	70–75
IIB	65–75
IIIA	40–50
IIIB	45–50
IVA	15–25
IVB	5–10

approach avoids the morbidity associated with dual therapy in the node-positive cohort. Further, for low-risk tumours smaller than 2 cm in size, there is some evidence to support the role of sentinel lymph node sampling. However, data on the long-term safety of this approach are awaited from ongoing prospective studies (SENTIX NCT02494063; SENTICOL III NCT03386734).

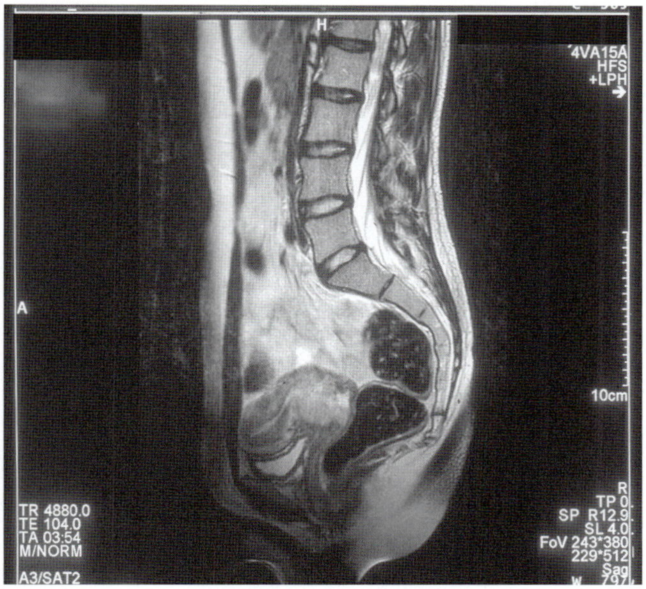

Fig. 28.9 Large Stage IB2 cervical tumour before treatment.

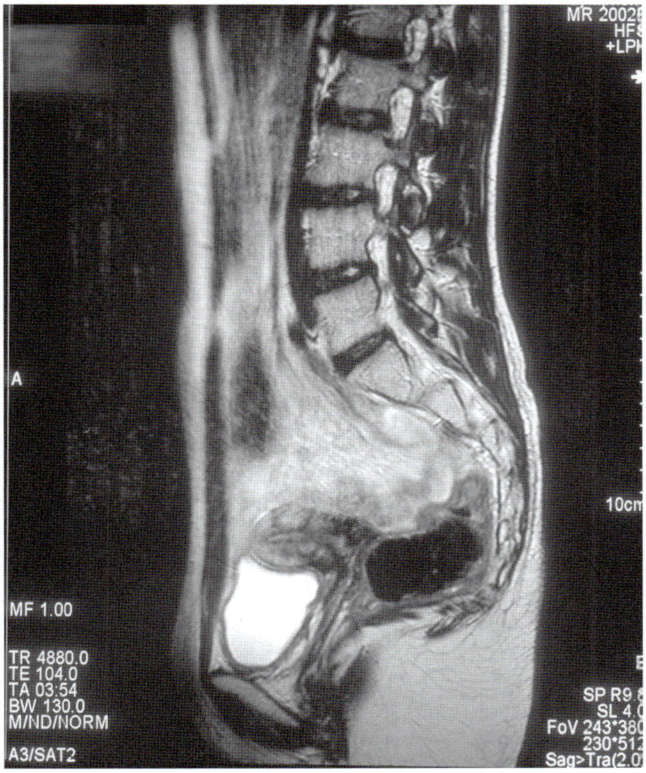

Fig. 28.10 Complete regression after chemoradiotherapy of tumour shown in Fig. 28.9.

The surgical approach to performing a radical hysterectomy (removal of the uterus, cervix, parametrium and upper vagina) has been a topic of debate following the publication of a large randomised controlled trial (LACC Trial) and an epidemiological study, both of which reported inferior oncological outcomes with the MIS approach compared to open surgery. However, the trial was not powered to look at the low-risk group, that is, those with tumour size smaller than 2 cm and no lymphovascular space invasion (LVSI), and the robotic surgical arm was underrepresented. Therefore, the MIS approach can be used in selected low-risk cases in high-volume centres with prospective data collection on survival outcomes.

TABLE 28.4 Sedlis Criteria for Adjuvant Radiotherapy Post Hysterectomy in Early Cervical Cancer, Including Predicted 3-Year Recurrence Risk Between Squamous Cell Carcinoma and Adenocarcinoma

Sedlis Intermediate Risk Factor Combinations	SCC: Predicted 3-Year Recurrence Risk	AC: Predicted 3-Year Recurrence Risk
LVSI positive, deep one-third invasion, any tumour size	38%	22%
LVSI positive, middle one-third invasion, size ≥2 cm	23%	39%
LVSI positive, superficial one-third invasion, size ≥5 cm	18%	45%
LVSI negative, middle/deep one-third invasion, size ≥4 cm	28%–40%	30%–38%

AC, Adenocarcinoma; *LVSI*, lymphovascular space invasion; *SCC*, squamous cell carcinoma.

RT is an alternative for early-stage patients unwilling to undergo surgery or unfit for a radical operation. The standard of care for patients with Stage IB3 and above is concurrent chemoradiotherapy (CRT), although selected patients with Stage IIA disease with early involvement of the vaginal vault may be suitable for treatment by radical hysterectomy.

The only large randomised trial (Landoni et al., 1997) of RT and surgery in operable cervical cancer showed equivalent disease-free and overall survival for both modalities. The number of serious complications was higher in the surgical arm, particularly lymphoedema. However, this study was performed in an era before modern radiological imaging, so a high proportion of surgical patients (nearly two-thirds) received postoperative RT.

Postoperative Radiotherapy

RT is given after surgery if there is an increased risk of local recurrence. Indications after radical surgery include positive surgical excision margins, parametrial extension and lymph nodes involved by tumour. The modified Sedlis criteria use a combination of tumour size, tumour grade and vascular invasion to guide when postoperative RT can be offered (Table 28.4). Treatment may be external beam radiotherapy (EBRT) with or without brachytherapy (intracavitary treatment) to the upper one-third of the vagina. Concomitant chemotherapy has been shown to improve long-term survival in clinical trials.

Non-surgical Treatment of Stage I-IVA

RT remains the mainstay of treatment of patients with Stages IB3 to IVA disease (Figs. 28.11–28.13). There are three components to a radical RT treatment: EBRT, brachytherapy and concomitant chemotherapy.

An important change in the delivery of EBRT in cervical cancer was the introduction and use of intensity modulated radiotherapy (IMRT) (Fig. 28.14). The transition from three-dimensional conformal RT to IMRT allowed a significant reduction in acute and chronic gastrointestinal (GI) and haematological toxicities. The challenge with IMRT has been the potential for a geographical miss from both inter- and intrafractional movement seen within the cervix and the uterus. The positions of both are heavily influenced by daily variation of bladder

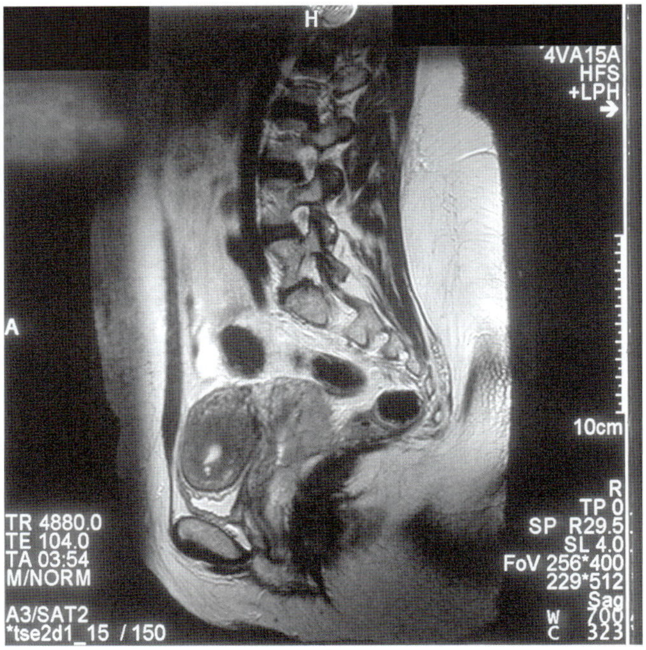

Fig. 28.11 Sagittal view of large cervical tumour involving rectum, Stage IVA before treatment.

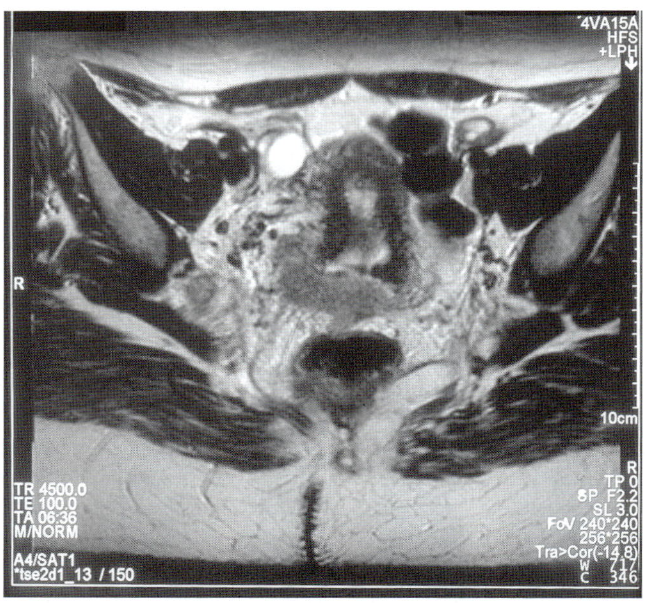

Fig. 28.12 Axial view of large cervical tumour involving rectum, Stage IVA before treatment.

and rectal filling and tumour regression during RT. Allowance is made for organ movement during the course of treatment by formation of an internal target volume (ITV). The ITV is generated by combining the clinical target volume (CTV) contoured on a full and then an empty bladder. Such an approach utilises cone beam computed tomography (CBCT) for daily soft-tissue matching to identify any potential geographical or near misses. The volume of lymph nodes irradiated depends on primary tumour size and the presence or absence of lymph nodes on MRI or PET/CT imaging.

Adaptive strategies have been developed, using either a plan-of-the-day approach or online adaptive radiotherapy (OART) using daily replanning with CT or MRI guidance. Adaptive radiotherapy (ART) allows reduced planning target volume (PTV) margins while ensuring adequate coverage of the CTV. However, it is more labour intensive than standard IMRT. A plan-of-the-day approach requires a variety of plans (usually three to five) to cover a range of predicted CTV positions, with plan selection at the time of treatment. Adaptation with OART is time and labour intensive, with daily optimisation of plans requiring image acquisition, daily contouring of the target volume and organs at risk (OARs) and daily reoptimisation of the plan. MRI LINAC-guided RT (MRgRT) in the context of OART offers many advantages in the treatment of gynaecological cancers. The image quality is superior, the delineation can be precise and functional assessment of tumour response is possible. However, MRgRT comes with technical challenges, including the time required for image acquisition and the fact that the MRI LINAC is unable to rotate the couch within the MR bore, meaning that patient setup errors are accounted for by virtual couch shifts. CBCT-guided OART is an attractive option, as this modality is widely used in RT departments and is faster and requires fewer infrastructure changes. This technique uses artificial intelligence (AI) to contour the OARs on the daily CBCT and uses machine learning to propagate the target volumes on the CBCT depending on the anatomy of the day.

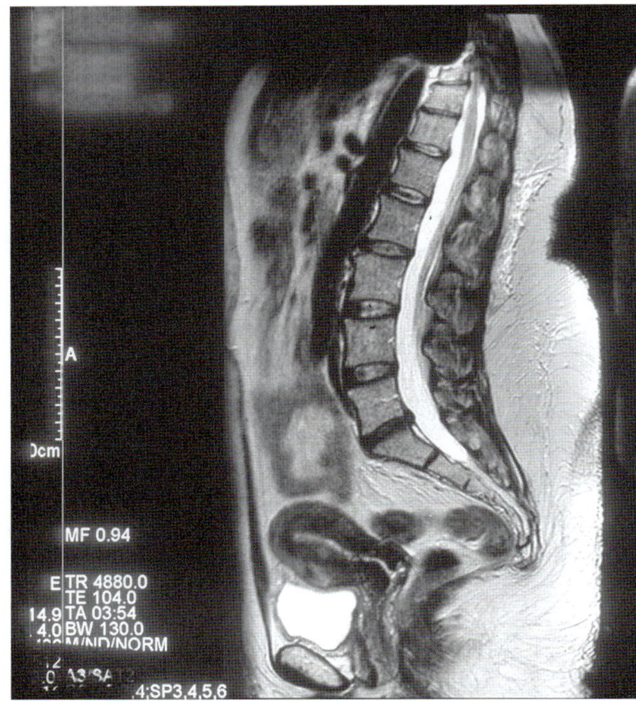

Fig. 28.13 Complete response after treatment without a rectovaginal fistula.

Brachytherapy

Brachytherapy is the highly focal delivery of radiation utilising applicators placed against or inside the tumour. It allows very high doses to be given to the cancer with sparing of the surrounding OARs in the pelvis, particularly the bladder, rectum and sigmoid colon. Rather than prescribing treatment to an arbitrary point such as Manchester point A, modern practice follows an individual approach. This treatment is called image-guided adaptive brachytherapy (IGABT). The prescribed radiation dose is adjusted to incorporate the cervix and any residual tumour demonstrated after EBRT and chemotherapy on an MRI scan taken just before brachytherapy, and it considers the dose received by nearby OARs. Typically, a central tube is placed in the uterine canal and an applicator is placed against the cervix (Fig. 28.15). A combination of intracavitary and interstitial treatment when needles are inserted into the tumour through a ring applicator, or ovoids

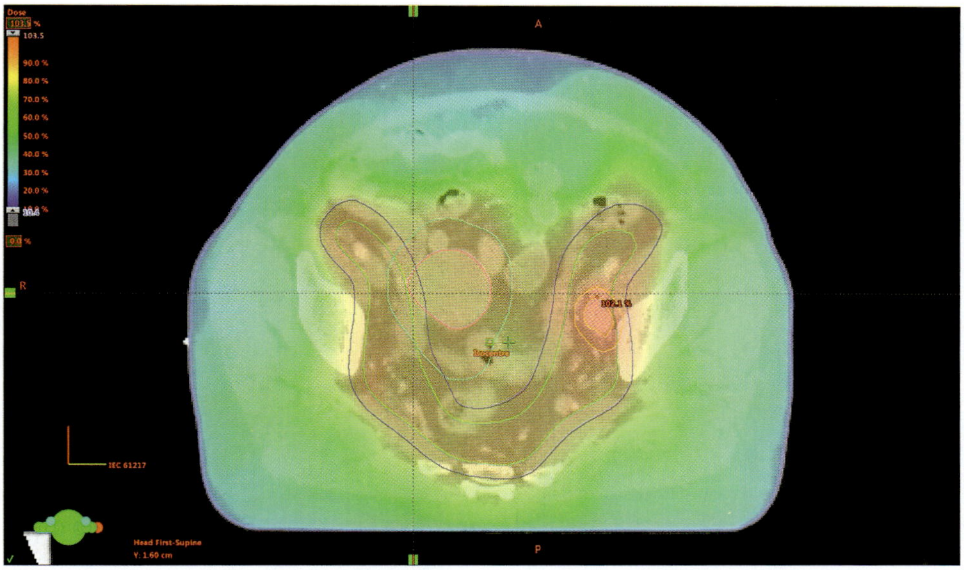

Fig. 28.14 *U*-shaped intensity modulated dose distribution to treat pelvic lymph nodes, avoiding the small bowel.

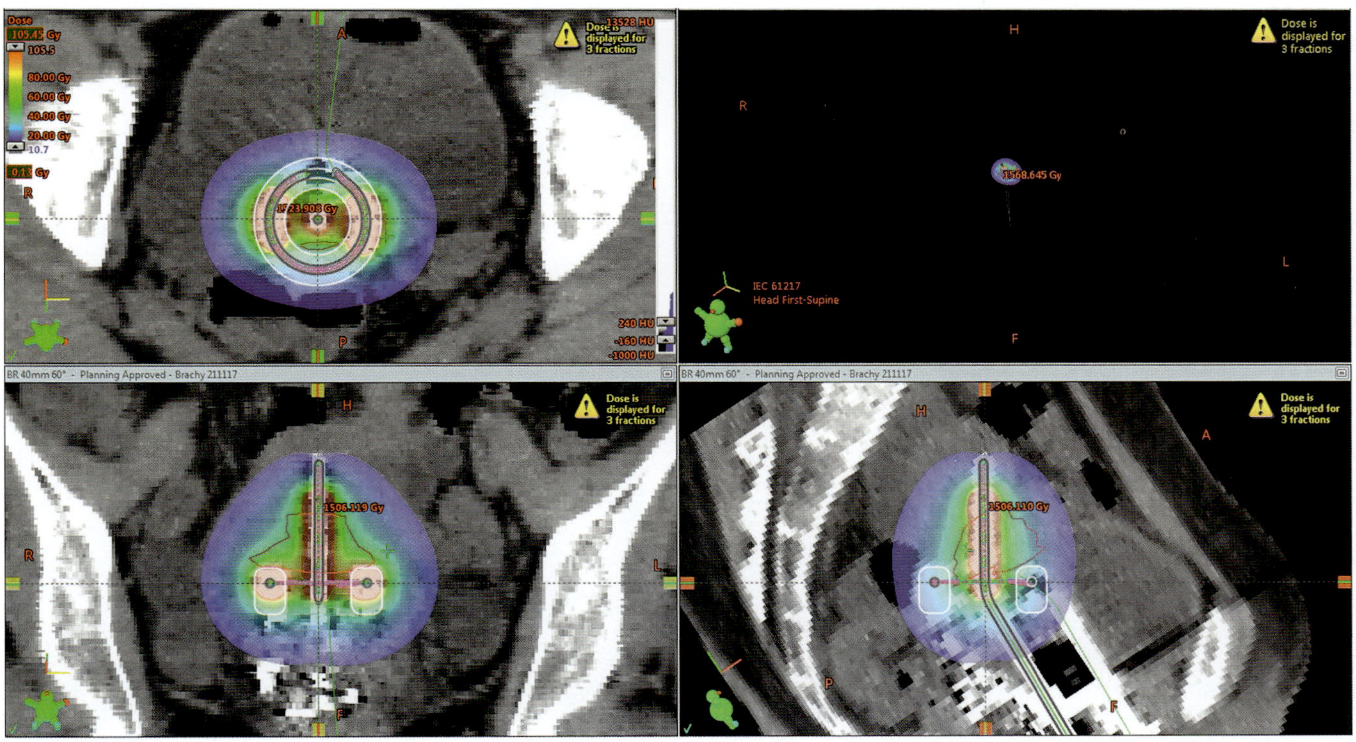

Fig. 28.15 Computed tomography scan showing a central tube in the uterus and a ring applicator placed against the cervix.

(intracavitary/interstitial brachytherapy), has been shown in the retro-EMBRACE study to improve local control compared with the use of a standard intracavitary applicator, without any increase in toxicity. For larger tumours with more extensive lateral extension, a full interstitial implant may be required. Treatment is administered over a few minutes, usually using a high dose rate (HDR) iridium source.

For the purpose of dosimetry, the EBRT dose is combined with the brachytherapy dose using the linear quadratic formula as 2-Gy equivalents (EQD2). The minimum doses received by the most irradiated tissue volumes of the OARs are calculated over an area of 2 cm^2 ($D2cm^3$). Further information is available in the International Commission on Radiation Units and Measurements (ICRU) Report 89. Ideally, both EBRT and brachytherapy should be completed in fewer than 56 days, because cervical tumours can repopulate during gaps in treatment.

Concomitant Chemotherapy

The addition of chemotherapy to RT in the treatment of carcinoma of the cervix improves prognosis. A Cochrane metaanalysis of individual trial patient data demonstrated that concomitant chemotherapy reduces the odds of death by 31% (hazard ratio (HR) .69) with an absolute all-stage improvement in survival by 10% (Figs. 28.16–28.20). Cisplatin given weekly (40 mg/m^2) is the regimen of choice. The number of cycles given to patients is particularly important, especially if they are high risk, that is, they have positive nodes or advanced FIGO

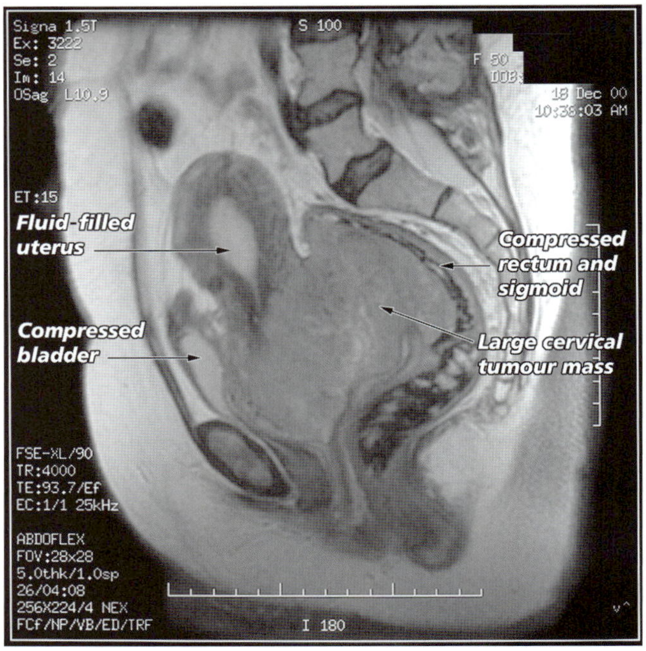

Fig. 28.16 Large Stage III cervical tumour fixed to both pelvic sidewalls and involving the vagina. The tumour is compressing on both the bladder and rectum.

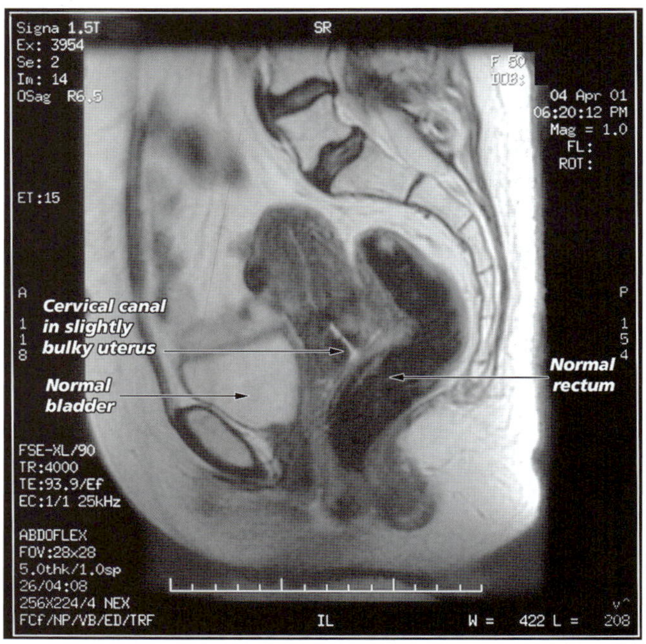

Fig. 28.17 Large Stage III tumour 3 months after chemoradiotherapy. Complete response. This patient was discharged from the clinic in 2007, 7 years after treatment.

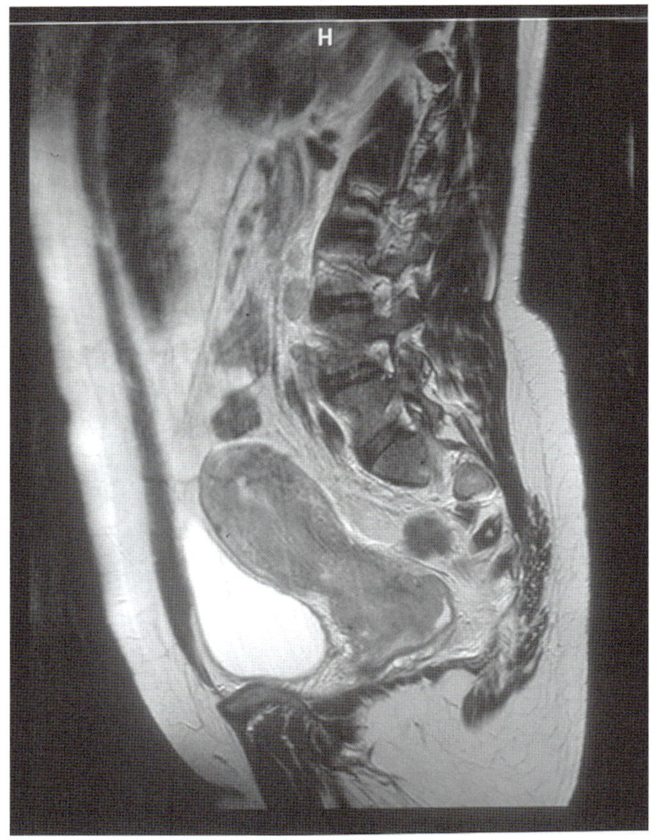

Fig. 28.18 Stage IVB cervical tumour involving virtually the whole of the uterus plus the upper vagina with paraaortic node metastases.

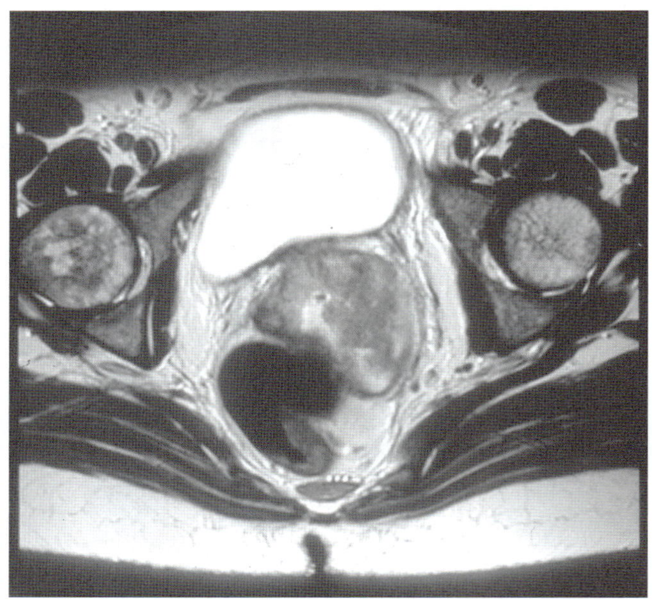

Fig. 28.19 The same tumour as Fig. 27.18 extending around the rectum.

staging IB3 or IIB or higher, or tumour larger than 4 cm and outside the cervix. Administration of 5 to 6 cycles at 100% dose can reduce the risk of distant metastases. The EMBRACE 1 study demonstrated that patients with high-risk disease who receive four or fewer chemotherapy cycles compared to those who receive five or more chemotherapy cycles are at higher risk of systemic relapse.

Complications of Treatment

During EBRT, patients may develop diarrhoea, which can be reduced by agents such as loperamide. The risk of nausea and vomiting is increased by the addition of chemotherapy, but it responds to antiemetics such as ondansetron. RT for cervical cancer gives a risk of serious late complications of treatment such as bladder or rectal fistulae. This is increased by the addition of chemotherapy. However, modern adaptive EBRT and IGABT techniques are leading to a decrease in acute and late toxicity, which will greatly improve survivorship. The site with the highest incidence of Grade III toxicity is the vagina. In part, this occurs when the

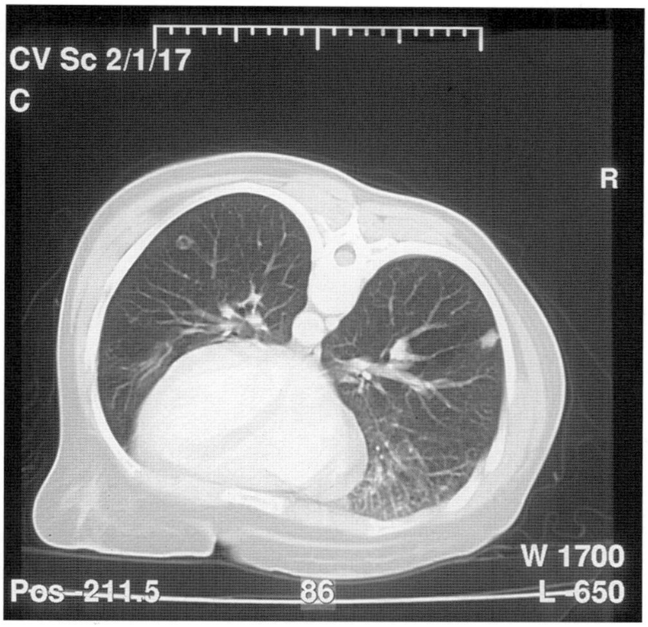

Fig. 28.20 Patient shown in Fig. 27.18, with pulmonary metastases and lymphangitis.

vagina is extensively involved by tumour, because it heals with fibrosis leading to stenosis, but direct radiation effect is also involved. The regular use of vaginal dilators reduces the incidence of vaginal stenosis.

Future Trends

The GCIG INTERLACE trial examined induction chemotherapy prior to concurrent CRT in locally advanced cervical cancer. Patients were randomised to receive either standard CRT with weekly cisplatin or 6 weekly treatments with carboplatin AUC 2 and paclitaxel 80 mg/m^2 followed by the CRT in week 7. The study included 500 patients with Stage IB1/2 to IVA mainly of squamous cell carcinoma. Early results showed that adding induction chemotherapy resulted in a 5-year progression-free survival of 73% compared to 64% with CRT alone ($p = 0.013$). Full results are awaited.

The prospect and benefit of immunotherapy in cervical cancer have been explored by the KEYNOTE-826 trial. This was a phase III randomised double-blind placebo-controlled trial in recurrent, persistent or metastatic cervical cancer. It compared pembrolizumab plus chemotherapy with or without bevacizumab against placebo plus chemotherapy with or without bevacizumab as a first-line therapy. Pembrolizumab was used in patients whose tumours expressed PD-L1 and who had a combined positive score of 1 or more. The addition of pembrolizumab was associated with prolonged progression-free survival and overall survival.

The EMBRACE II study explores radiation dose and clinical outcomes using both IMRT and IGABT. Amongst its aims are to increase the tumour and target doses in patients with a large, high-risk CTV (CTVHR) and/or residual GTV at brachytherapy, decrease the tumour and target doses in patients with a limited size CTVHR and limited or no residual GTV at brachytherapy, and decrease the EBRT and brachytherapy doses to the vagina while decreasing the dose to adjacent OARs, particularly in patients with limited size CTVHR.

CARCINOMA OF THE ENDOMETRIUM

The causes of endometrial cancer are multifactorial. Physiological conditions and diseases that expose the endometrium to high levels of oestrogen are important in the development of this condition. These include early menarche, late menopause, nulliparity, polycystic ovarian disease and, rarely, oestrogen-producing ovarian tumours. Patients who are obese have a greater risk of endometrial cancer as adrenal steroids are metabolised to oestrone and oestrogen in adipose tissue. Both oestrogen-only hormone replacement therapy (HRT) and tamoxifen (used in the treatment of breast cancer) can lead to endometrial hyperplasia and endometrial cancer. It has been shown that up to 25% of endometrial cancers in patients under age 60 years may be caused by a hereditary defect in DNA mismatch repair genes such as Lynch syndrome. The possibility of developing endometrial cancer is 40% to 60% in patients with Lynch syndrome. Typically, patients are younger, with lower body mass index, endometrioid type endometrial cancer and lower uterine segment involvement.

Pathology

Endometrial cancer is pathologically examined and surgically staged (Table 28.5). In all stages, the grade of the lesion, the histological type and the presence of LVSI must be recorded. Molecular classification testing should be performed in all patients with endometrial cancer for prognostic risk-group stratification and factors that might influence adjuvant and systemic treatment decisions. Most tumours are adenocarcinoma of endometrioid type (EEC). Atypical types, such as clear cell or serous papillary tumours, mesonephric-like, GI mucinous, undifferentiated and carcinosarcomas, carry a worse prognosis and are considered high grade. The grade of endometrial cancer is dependent on solid areas; low grade is 1% to 5%, intermediate grade is 6% to 50% and high grade is greater than 50% solid. The presence of unusual nuclear atypia should prompt an evaluation for p53 mutation and consideration of serous carcinoma. Immunohistochemistry evaluation will aid with further histopathological differentiation.

There are four molecular classifications that have been proposed by the Cancer Genome Atlas and verified by PORTEC 3: (1) POLE/ultramutated (irrespective of grade, POLE-mutated endometrial cancers carry excellent prognosis); (2) p53 mutation, which is associated with unfavourable prognosis (most of these cancers are serous, but 25% are EECs or carcinosarcomas); (3) microsatellite instability high/hypermutated, which is associated with intermediate prognosis; and (4) no specific molecular profile (NSMP), which has low somatic number alterations and is associated with low mutational burden and an intermediate prognosis. The oestrogen receptor (ER) status also affects the prognosis. There is a small subset of patients defined as multiple classifiers whereby they have more than one molecular feature. In such cases, where there is POLE mutation or MMRd simultaneously with p53 mutations, these patients should not be considered p53-mutant; rather, the POLE mutations or MMRd trumps the molecular profiling, therefore giving them a favourable or intermediate prognosis, respectively. In addition, tumour grade, LVSI and depth of invasion into the myometrium are useful predictors of pelvic node spread. Serous pathology and Stage III endometrial cancer show a significantly higher risk of recurrence and therefore benefit from additional adjuvant therapy.

Routes of Spread

Tumour may extend beyond the endometrial cavity to involve the cervix, vagina or, less commonly, parametrium. Distant spread is first to pelvic lymph nodes; very rarely is there spread directly to paraaortic nodes without pelvic nodal involvement. Positive peritoneal cytology is linked to a poorer outcome, especially with serous pathology. Haematogenous spread is unusual.

Treatment

The mainstay of treatment for locally advanced endometrial cancer is primary surgery in the form of a simple hysterectomy and bilateral salpingo-oophorectomy with peritoneal washings.

TABLE 28.5 International Federation of Gynaecology and Obstetrics 2023 Staging: Carcinoma of the Endometrium

Stage I	
IA	Disease limited to the endometrium OR nonaggressive histological type, i.e. low-grade endometrioid, with invasion of less than half of the myometrium with no or focal lymphovascular space involvement (LVSI) OR good prognosis disease
IA1	Nonaggressive histological type limited to an endometrial polyp OR confined to the endometrium
IA2	Nonaggressive histological types involving less than half of the myometrium with no or focal LVSI
IA3	Low-grade endometrioid carcinomas limited to the uterus and ovary
IB	Nonaggressive histological types with invasion of half or more of the myometrium, and with no or focal LVSI
IC	Aggressive histological types limited to a polyp or confined to the endometrium
Stage II	
IIA	Invasion of the cervical stroma of nonaggressive histological types
IIB	Substantial LVSI of nonaggressive histological types
IIC	Aggressive histological types with any myometrial involvement
Stage III	
IIIA	Invasion of the uterine serosa, adnexa, or both by direct extension or metastasis
IIIA1	Spread to the ovary or fallopian tube (except when meeting Stage IA3 criteria)
IIIA2	Involvement of the uterine subserosa or spread through the uterine serosa
IIIB	Metastasis or direct spread to the vagina and/or to the parametria or pelvic peritoneum
IIIB1	Metastasis or direct spread to the vagina and/or the parametria
IIIB2	Metastasis to the pelvic peritoneum
IIIC	Metastasis to the pelvic or paraaortic lymph nodes or both
IIIC1	Metastasis to the pelvic lymph nodes
IIIC1i	Micrometastasis
IIIC1ii	Macrometastasis
IIIC2	Metastasis to the paraaortic lymph nodes up to the renal vessels, with or without metastasis to the pelvic lymph nodes
IIIC2i	Micrometastasis
IIIC2ii	Macrometastasis
Stage IV	
IVA	Tumour invasion of the bladder and/or bowel mucosa
IVB	Abdominal peritoneal metastasis beyond the pelvis
IVC	Distant metastasis, including metastasis to any extra- or intraabdominal lymph nodes above the renal vessels, lungs, liver, brain or bone

MIS is the recommended route of surgery, as it is associated with significantly reduced intra- and postoperative morbidity without compromising oncological outcomes. Furthermore, robotic-assisted MIS is associated with a lower conversion rate to open surgery compared to conventional 'straight stick' laparoscopy, particularly in the clinically obese population.

Lymph node staging should be performed in patients with intermediate- and high-risk features. A metaanalysis of clinical trials demonstrated that there is no survival benefit to full lymphadenectomy. Clinically enlarged nodes should be removed at the time of hysterectomy. Sentinel lymph node biopsy (SLNB) is an adequate alternative to systematic lymphadenectomy for staging purposes, showing high sensitivity and negative predictive value. SLNs in endometrial cancer are identified by injecting indocyanine green (ICG) or blue dye and radioactive tracer Tc99m into the cervix with both superficial and deep injections and then using near infrared light, in the case of the ICG dye, to visualise the sentinel node after opening the tissue planes. If a sentinel node is not identified, guidelines advise that a full lymphadenectomy on that side should be performed.

There is increasing evidence supporting SLNB in the group considered to be low risk to rule out occult lymph node metastases. Studies have found up to 6% lymph node involvement in the low-risk group on SLNBs. The ESGO-ESTRO-ESP guidelines allow an approach of SLNB in all patients with endometrial carcinoma, which is endorsed by FIGO. An SLNB should be performed in association with pathological ultrastaging as it will increase the detection of micrometastases and isolated tumour cells in lymph nodes. Although micrometastases are treated as lymph node positive, the clinical significance of isolated tumour cells in the low-risk group remains uncertain and long-term data are awaited. Staging omental biopsy is taken for those with serous histological subtypes. Patients with low-risk tumours require no adjuvant treatment. Pelvic RT may be given as an alternative to surgery as postoperative adjuvant treatment or to treat nodal or vault recurrence.

Radiotherapy Alone

Patients who are treated with RT alone are surgically inoperable, usually due to intercurrent illness. Five-year survival of 72% has been reported in patients treated by two intrauterine caesium insertions. The use of HDR brachytherapy in the nonoperative setting is now well established. A lot of information has been extrapolated from cervical cancer HDR and used in the context of endometrial cancer. To achieve better control in the range of 85% to 95%, image-guided brachytherapy should be used. In inoperable patients, combination treatment of EBRT and HDR brachytherapy is an option that should be considered. HDR brachytherapy can be especially useful in patients with multiple comorbidities as treatment times are significantly reduced from several days to multiple fractions over several minutes each. HDR brachytherapy alone in these patients has been shown to improve overall survival as well as disease-free survival. Doses are recommended in the Royal College of Radiologists (RCR) dose fractionation document.

Adjuvant Therapy

Selected patients may benefit from adjuvant treatment (Table 28.6). Traditionally, the decision for adjuvant treatment was based on the

TABLE 28.6 **Adjuvant Treatment of Endometrial Cancer**

	Histology	Stage	Grade	Lymphovascular Space Invasion	Molecular	Adjuvant Treatment
Low Risk	Endometrioid	IA	1/2	No/focal	MSS/NSMP	None
	Any	I/II	Any			
Intermediate Risk	Endometrioid	IA	3	No/focal	MSS/NSMP	Vaginal brachytherapy (Omit for patients aged <60 years)
	Endometrioid	IB	1/2	No/focal	MSS/NSMP	
	Endometrioid	II	1	No/focal	MSS/NSMP	
	Endometrioid	IA (no invasion)	Any	Any	P53mut	None
High-Intermediate Risk	Endometrioid	1A/1B	Any	Substantial		External beam radiotherapy
	Endometrioid	1B	3	Any		
	Endometrioid	II	1	Substantial		
	Endometrioid	II	2/3		MSS/NSMP	
High Risk	Any	Any	Any (myometrium invasion)	Any	P53mut	Chemotherapy/ radiotherapy
	Serous Undifferentiated MMMT	Any	Any	Any	Any	
	Any	III/IVA	Any	Any	Any	

degree of LVSI, stage and grade. However, in the modern era, molecular profiling is also used to aid decision-making in the adjuvant setting. Both the PORTEC-1 trial and the ASTEC trial examined the role of routine postoperative pelvic EBRT versus surveillance alone for patients with intermediate-risk endometrial cancer (Grade I myometrial invasion >50%, Grade II myometrial invasion >50%, Grade III myometrial invasion <50%). There was a statistically significant decrease in pelvic recurrence in the EBRT arm but no overall survival benefit. Certain higher-risk factors for recurrence were identified as Grade III, over 50% myometrial invasion and age over 60 years. The PORTEC-2 study examined the higher-risk intermediate group further randomising to pelvic EBRT or vaginal vault brachytherapy alone. An identical survival and very similar local recurrence rates were demonstrated at 3 years after treatment, but brachytherapy patients had fewer radiation-induced side effects and better quality of life. Substantial LVSI was seen as a risk factor for pelvic recurrence. Brachytherapy is easy to administer via a vaginal cylinder that can be inserted without an anaesthetic.

Patients with high-risk features may benefit from adjuvant EBRT. A metaanalysis showed postoperative EBRT increased survival by 10% for patients with Stage I poorly differentiated tumours penetrating more than halfway through the myometrium. The pelvic target volume includes the internal iliac, external iliac and obturator lymph nodes plus the upper aspect of the vagina. Brachytherapy in addition to EBRT reduces the risk of vaginal recurrence and improves survival in patients with Stage II (involvement of cervix) tumours.

The PORTEC-3 trial examined the role of CRT followed by chemotherapy versus EBRT alone in high-risk endometrial cancer patients. The groups that showed the largest survival benefit to combined treatment were those with Stage III disease (79% versus 69%) and those with serous pathology (71% versus 53%). With the advent of molecular classification, the PORTEC-2 cohort was reanalysed to define which molecular factors conferred low, intermediate or high risk of recurrence. Treatment stratification based on these factors is under investigation in different clinical trials, such as PORTEC-4 and RAINBO.

Treatment of Recurrent or Metastatic Disease

RT can be used with curative intent if patients develop an isolated pelvic recurrence. In previously unirradiated patients, 5-year survival rates of 50% to 80% have been reported in those with isolated vaginal vault recurrence, although this falls significantly in patients with pelvic sidewall disease. Brachytherapy is indicated in suitable central recurrences and IMRT or stereotactic radiotherapy for nodal recurrences. This can be dose escalation following EBRT or as sole therapy for reirradiation.

The role of systemic anticancer treatment in advanced endometrial cancer is rapidly evolving. Traditional chemotherapy can be used, but the use of targeted treatments and immunotherapy is becoming more defined with multiple trials ongoing, led by the molecular profiling of tumours.

The first-line systemic treatment for relapsed or metastatic disease is paclitaxel and carboplatin. The response rate to carboplatin is between 25% and 35%, and it may be the drug of choice for elderly unfit patients. A phase II trial combining pembrolizumab with lenvatinib demonstrated good antitumour effect in previously treated endometrial cancer. Further investigation within a phase III randomised study, KEYNOTE-775, demonstrated a statistically significant increase in progression-free survival (7 months versus 4 months) and overall survival (18 months versus 11 months) with lenvatinib plus pembrolizumab when compared with single-agent chemotherapy with doxorubicin or paclitaxel, regardless of MSI status. Everolimus targets the mammalian target of rapamycin (mTOR) and can overcome hormone resistance. When combined with letrozole, it can achieve a greater than 30% response rate in recurrent EEC or in those with disease-progression EEC who received two prior lines of chemotherapy.

Patients with microsatellite instability traditionally had a worse prognosis, with higher rates of chemotherapy resistance. However, there is increasing evidence that they respond much more favourably to immunotherapy. KEYNOTE-158 demonstrated the benefit of pembrolizumab monotherapy in treating noncolorectal MMRd cancers. Two randomised phase III trials, RUBY and KEYNOTE-868, demonstrated a statistically significant progression-free survival advantage with the addition of immune checkpoint inhibitors (ICIs), dostarlimab and pembrolizumab, respectively, to standard chemotherapy with carboplatin/paclitaxel followed by ICI maintenance in MMRd patients. RUBY is the only phase III trial to show a statistically significant overall survival improvement in primary advanced or recurrent endometrial cancer. A median overall survival of 44.6 has been demonstrated for those patients who receive dostarlimab in combination with chemotherapy versus 28.2 months for those who receive chemotherapy alone. Although this needs to be investigated further, the RUBY trial also suggested that up to 3 years of immunotherapy could be an ideal treatment duration. Trastuzumab and carboplatin plus paclitaxel can prolong progression-free survival when compared with chemotherapy alone in Stage III HER2neu overexpressed serous endometrial cancers. Bevacizumab combined with chemotherapy showed improved overall survival in a phase II study (34 versus 22.7 months; $p < 0.039$).

Treatment can be challenging in patients with metastatic or locally advanced disease who are not medically fit for chemotherapy. Some endometrial cancers exhibit progesterone and/or oestrogen receptors. About one-third of patients with endometrial cancer will show an objective response to progestogenic hormones such as megestrol acetate. Alternative options are the aromatase inhibitors tamoxifen and fulvestrant. In the PARAGON trial, there was a 7% response rate and 44% clinical benefit seen in a small cohort of patients with the use of anastrozole. These patients had recurrent endometrial cancer that was receptor positive. Response rates tend to be higher in patients with well-differentiated tumours. A single-arm phase II trial showed a high response rate as well as clinical benefit with the combination of letrozole and everolimus.

Results of Treatment

The majority of patients suffer from Stage I cancers. Five-year survival for patients with Stage IA grade 1 or 2 disease is over 90% with increasing treatment options. This falls to about 70% for patients with Stage IB grade 3 disease. Reported 5-year survival for patients with Stage II disease is between 60% and 85%, and Stage III disease is between 40% and 75%, depending on the treatment modality and the degree of histological differentiation of the tumour.

Future Trends

Research is centred on less toxic forms of chemotherapy and molecular targeted agents for use in the small group of high-risk cases requiring additional treatment after surgery. There is ongoing research investigating immunotherapy options and targeted treatment. The Wee1 molecule is one of the most important gatekeepers exerting its effects at the G2/M phase of the DNA repair cycle. Given that in p53-mutated cancers the G1 checkpoint is impaired, inhibiting the Wee1 molecule and therefore the G2 checkpoint within the same cell cycle will lead to miotic catastrophe and death. Wee1 inhibitors are therefore being investigated in p53-mutated endometrial cancer. A phase I trial using Adavosertib in patients with recurrent endometrial cancer and previously treated with platinum-based chemotherapy demonstrated an overall response rate of 29.4%. A larger phase II trial is underway to further investigate this. The SIENDO study has shown the potential use of Selinexor in advanced and recurrent p53 wild-type endometrial cancer. Through all the latest advances and future directions, it is imperative to emphasise that correct patient selection is of paramount importance in improving patient outcomes.

SARCOMAS OF THE UTERUS

The most common true sarcoma of the uterus is a leiomyosarcoma, which is a rare tumour arising from the smooth muscle of the uterus. Metastatic spread through the bloodstream, especially to the lungs, is common. Primary treatment is surgical in the form of a hysterectomy and bilateral salpingo-oophorectomy. In common with other soft-tissue sarcomas, adjuvant chemotherapy delays but does not prevent the development of distant metastases. The overall 5-year survival is 30% to 40%.

CANCER OF THE OVARY

Aetiology

Ovarian cancer is the seventh most common cancer in females in the United Kingdom, but it carries the greatest mortality rate of all gynaecological cancers. Epithelial ovarian cancer is more common in females who have never been pregnant or who had an early menarche or late menopause. Conversely, the incidence of ovarian cancer is reduced in females who have had multiple births, and there is good evidence that oral contraceptives reduce the incidence of this disease. The protective effect of birth parity and oral contraceptives is probably through suppression of ovulation. A case control study showed that females who have not had an ovulation cycle for 8.7 years have a fourfold reduction in ovarian cancer. This protective effect is not secondary to menstrual disorders. Preterm labour increases the risk of ovarian cancer, and giving birth to a male infant is associated with a twofold increase in the risk of mucinous ovarian cancer. Endometriosis-associated ovarian cancer has been documented in various studies. Endometriosis is defined as presence of endometrial tissues outside the uterine cavity. It remains unclear, however, how a benign condition such as endometriosis causes malignant transformation. About 5% of ovarian cancers are familial. The most important hereditary syndromes are associated with carriage mutations of the BRCA1 complex on chromosome 17 and the BRCA2 complex on chromosome 13. The BRCA1 and 2 genes are also associated with breast, colon and endometrial cancers. Familial tumours tend to develop at a younger age than sporadic cancers. Females with two or more first-degree relatives who have developed ovarian cancer or one relative who has developed breast cancer and one other relative who has developed ovarian cancer before the age of 50 may be offered genetic counselling and testing for mutations in the BRCA1 and 2 genes. These patients also may be offered screening for breast cancer. There is no effective screening available for ovarian cancer, and therefore females with known BRCA mutations may be offered risk-reducing surgery after they have completed their family. BRCA1 and BRCA2 mutation carriers have an increased lifetime risk of developing ovarian cancer of around 44% and 17%, respectively. More sophisticated risk predictor calculators can be used to produce individualised risks based on personal risk factors, family history, genetic testing for high- and moderate-risk genes, polygenic scores and mammographic density. Standard risk-reducing surgery for ovarian cancer involves removal of both tubes and ovaries, and this is believed to reduce the risk of ovarian cancer by 96%. There is growing evidence that ovarian cancer originates from fallopian tube secretory cells, and therefore there are studies looking at offering removal of tubes only followed by delayed removal of ovaries, to preserve hormonal function in the premenopausal population. Risk-reducing surgery is usually offered to females after completion of their family, between age 35 and 40 years for BRCA1 carriers and between age 40 and 55 years for BRCA2 carriers.

Pathology

Benign or malignant ovarian tumours may be solid or cystic. Some benign ovarian cysts may exceed 30 cm in diameter and weigh many kilograms. About 10% of ovarian tumours may be classified as borderline. These are tumours that have some histological features of malignancy but lack stromal invasion.

Malignant ovarian tumours are subdivided into epithelial, germ cell and sex cord. Some 85% of ovarian tumours are classified as being of epithelial origin. The most common type of ovarian cancer is high-grade serous, which accounts for about 70% of all cases. Mainly by studying the ovaries and fallopian tubes from patients with BRCA1/2 mutations undergoing prophylactic oophorectomy, a considerable amount has been learned about the origin of these tumours. In fact, they originate from malignant transformation of cells in the fimbria of the end of the fallopian tubes. Malignant cells then implant into the surface of the ovary and into the peritoneal cavity. This explains why many ovarian cancers are at an advanced stage by diagnosis.

Unlike high-grade serous tumours, clear cell and mucinous malignant tumours often present with Stage III to IV disease.

Method of Spread

Ovarian cancer tends to be a disease of the abdominal cavity and rapidly spreads across the peritoneal cavity to involve the omentum. There may also be multiple peritoneal deposits, particularly in the subdiaphragmatic areas. These peritoneal deposits may produce large volumes of ascitic fluid. A potentially fatal consequence of peritoneal disease is intestinal obstruction. The cancer may also spread to pelvic and paraaortic lymph nodes, the liver and pleural cavity by direct spread or via the bloodstream. Involvement of lung parenchyma is less common. Metastasis to other sites, particularly bone and brain, is rare, though it is increasing in prevalence as patients live longer due to an array of therapeutic agents.

Clinical Features

There are no typical symptoms of ovarian cancer. Females may complain of abdominal bloating or nonspecific GI symptoms, and often present through a GI pathway. One of the first signs may be the discovery of a large pelvic mass or ascites. The UK NICE guidelines were revised in August 2023 and stated that any female over age 50 years who presents with symptoms suggestive of irritable bowel syndrome (IBS) within the past 12 months, or has had symptoms of abdominal bloating, fullness, abdominal pain and/or increased urine frequency more than 12 times per month, should be investigated for ovarian cancer.

Investigations and Staging

Investigations in most cases are for a pelvic mass with or without ascites. The tumour marker CA125 is elevated (>35 international units per litre) in about 50% of patients with early-stage disease and 80% of patients with more advanced-stage disease. HE4 is another useful biomarker, especially when CA125 is negative. CT scanning of the abdomen is excellent for demonstrating primary tumour with significant peritoneal spread and involvement of the omentum. CT scanning can also show the degree of spread to adjacent organs and is useful for predicting operability. Between 60% and 70% of patients have spread beyond the pelvis at diagnosis and are placed in Stage III or IV. FIGO staging of this disease is listed in Table 28.7.

Needle biopsy under CT control from the primary tumour or omental metastases can confirm the diagnosis in inoperable cases. Ascites may have to be drained to relieve discomfort and shortness of breath. Ascitic and pleural fluid should always be examined cytologically for the presence of malignant cells.

Treatment

Surgery

The role of surgery may be both diagnostic and therapeutic. The aim of surgery for ovarian cancer is to fully stage presumed early-stage disease and to achieve complete cytoreduction in more advanced cases. The standard approach is via a midline laparotomy, and staging would include total hysterectomy, bilateral salpingo-oophorectomy, supracolic omentectomy, pelvic and paraaortic lymph node dissection and peritoneal biopsies. For advanced-stage ovarian cancer, studies have

TABLE 28.7 International Federation of Gynaecology and Obstetrics 2021 Staging: Carcinoma of the Ovary

Stage I	IA	Tumour limited to one ovary (capsule intact) or fallopian tube; no tumour on ovarian or fallopian tube surface; no malignant cells in ascitic fluid or in peritoneal washings
	IB	Tumour limited to one or both ovaries (capsule intact) or fallopian tubes; no tumour on the surface of ovary or fallopian tube; no malignant cells in ascitic fluid or in peritoneal washings
	IC	Tumour limited to one or both ovaries or fallopian tubes, plus any of the following:
	IC1	Surgical spill
	IC2	Capsule ruptured before surgery or tumour on the surface of the ovary or fallopian tube
	IC3	Malignant cells in ascitic fluid or in peritoneal washings
Stage II		
	IIA	Tumour involving one or both ovaries or fallopian tubes with pelvic extension (below pelvic brim) or peritoneal cancer
	IIB	Extension and/or implants on other pelvic intraperitoneal tissues
Stage III	Tumour involving one or both ovaries or fallopian tubes or peritoneal cancer with microscopically confirmed peritoneal metastases outside the pelvis and/or metastasis to the retroperitoneal lymph nodes	
	IIIA1i	Positive retroperitoneal lymph nodes only (histologically proved) Metastasis ≤10 mm in largest dimension
	IIIA1ii	Metastasis >10 mm in largest dimension
	IIIA2	Microscopic extrapelvic (beyond the pelvic brim) peritoneal involvement, with or without positive retroperitoneal lymph nodes
	IIIB	Macroscopic peritoneal metastases that extend beyond the pelvis and that are ≤2 cm in largest dimension, with or without positive retroperitoneal lymph nodes
	IIIC	Macroscopic peritoneal metastases that extend beyond the pelvis and are >2 cm in largest dimension, with or without metastasis to retroperitoneal lymph nodes (includes extension of tumour to the capsule of the liver and spleen without parenchymal involvement of either organ)
Stage IV	IVA	Pleural effusion with positive cytology
	IVB	Parenchymal metastasis and/or metastases to extraabdominal organs (including inguinal lymph nodes and lymph nodes outside the abdominal cavity)

shown that there is a 5.5% increase in median survival for each 10% increase in maximal cytoreduction. In the advanced ovarian cancer cohort, primary debulking surgery can be offered up front or in the interval setting following three cycles of neoadjuvant chemotherapy. The SCORPION study demonstrated that primary debulking surgery is comparable to neoadjuvant chemotherapy in terms of median progression-free survival and overall survival. The side-effect profile, however, is significantly different. There are numerous nonrandomised studies that indicate that optimal debulking improves prognosis, but there have been no randomised controlled trials comparing aggressive debulking against more conservative surgery.

Ongoing studies are assessing the role of MIS in the management of ovarian cancer. However, it is currently not recommended beyond a trial setting. There is evidence supporting the use of hyperthermic intraperitoneal chemotherapy (HIPEC) in the interval debulking setting. Data from clinical trials have shown both disease-free survival and overall survival were increased without significant impact on morbidity or mortality. However, HIPEC has not been widely adopted into clinical practice, because more evidence is required and because of resource implications.

Chemotherapy

Following surgery, the mainstay of treatment is chemotherapy. Primary debulking surgery is only possible in 40% to 50% of females, given that many patients have bulk residual disease after surgery. Patients with Stage III or IV disease, even after optimal surgery, will rapidly relapse without further treatment, but fortunately, epithelial ovarian cancer is fairly chemosensitive. For the past 20 years, a combination of paclitaxel and carboplatin has been standard chemotherapy. Although 60% to 80% of patients with advanced disease have significant tumour shrinkage after this chemotherapy, the median progression-free survival is only 16 to 18 months, and by 2 years, three-quarters of all patients relapse. In the case of platinum-resistant tumours (<6 months progression-free period), the chemotherapy options are paclitaxel and liposomal doxorubicin with the option of gemcitabine as a third-line consideration. These have an expected therapeutic efficacy of 19% to 28%. Bevacizumab is a monoclonal antibody, which is an antagonist of the tumour growth factor, vascular endothelial growth factor (VEGF). In the NCRN ICON7 trial (2015), the addition of bevacizumab to standard chemotherapy increased progression-free survival in the short term but not ultimate 5-year survival. Bevacizumab should also be considered as an option with standard chemotherapy in platinum-resistant disease. The use of bevacizumab has been superseded by the use of poly ADP ribose polymerase (PARP) inhibitors. Third-line treatments involve the first- and second-line options plus immune checkpoint (PARP) inhibitors. Options such as olaparib, rucaparib, niraparib and talazoparib have represented a turning point in the treatment of ovarian cancer patients with germline mutations within BRCA1 and BRCA2 or refractory to three or more lines of treatment. If there is a BRCA mutation, PARP inhibitors can be used first or second line. The ICON9 trial is examining maintenance therapy in recurrent ovarian cancer and after platinum-based treatment, with olaparib and cediranib versus olaparib alone. This is a randomised phase III trial with the primary objectives being the assessment and efficacy of maintenance treatment with olaparib in combination with cediranib compared to olaparib alone following a response to platinum-based chemotherapy in females with platinum-sensitive ovarian, fallopian tube or peritoneal cancer during first relapse. The results are likely to be published in 2025. Third-line treatments involve the first- and second-line options plus ICIs. The ARIEL 3 trial has shown that rucaparib can be used as maintenance therapy in platinum-sensitive ovarian cancers with or without BRCA1/2 germline mutations. The updated results showed a progression-free survival of 8.2 months with rucaparib versus 4.1 months with placebo.

Radiotherapy

The role of RT is largely palliative and is used to shrink symptomatic ovarian masses, especially tumours causing pain or vaginal bleeding. Clear cell carcinoma is less chemosensitive than the more common serous subtype, and studies have shown an improved survival by the addition of RT to adjuvant chemotherapy in Stages IC and II clear cell patients. Although, it is noted that RT is not the standard and the evidence remains limited.

Results of Treatment of Epithelial Tumours

Ovarian cancer survival has almost doubled in the past 50 years in the United Kingdom. However, the 5-year relative survival for ovarian cancer in females in England, Wales, Scotland and Northern Ireland is below the European average. Thirty-five percent of females diagnosed with ovarian cancer survive their disease for 10 years or more. In addition, 81.2% of females diagnosed with ovarian cancer between the age of 15 and 44 years survive their disease for 10 years or more, compared with 21.5% of females diagnosed between the age of 75 and 99 years.

Future Trends

The use of ICIs is being investigated in advanced and metastatic ovarian tumours. The use of anti-PD-1 (nivolumab and pembrolizumab) and anti-PD-L1 (e.g. atezolizumab) has shown good response in only 10% to 15% of patients. Studies have shown that patients treated with two ICIs have improved and longer-lasting response compared to those treated with only one ICI. Other therapeutic options being investigated are T-cell transfer and chimeric antigen receptor T-cell therapy, therapeutic vaccinations and adoptive cellular therapy.

RARE TUMOURS OF THE OVARY

Sex-Cord Tumours

The most common of the sex-cord tumours are granulosa cell tumours. These display a spectrum of aggressiveness. Some may behave in a benign fashion, and others are extremely aggressive. They are found predominantly in postmenopausal females but can occur at any age, including before puberty. These tumours often produce steroid hormones, particularly oestrogens, which can cause postmenopausal bleeding in older females and precocious puberty in young females. Over 80% of patients present with Stage I disease. Treatment is predominantly by surgery. Bilateral ovarian disease occurs in up to 25% of patients. Usually, both ovaries are removed along with the uterus. A single ovary may be removed in young females with Stage I disease wishing to preserve fertility. Granulosa cell tumours can recur up to 30 years after initial surgery. The site of recurrence is usually within the abdominal cavity or the liver. Metastases from a granulosa cell tumour can be haemorrhagic, leading to internal bleeding. Because of the rarity of this tumour, there have been few comparative studies of chemotherapy, but cisplatin-based regimens such as the BEP regimen (bleomycin, etoposide and cisplatin) or CAP (cyclophosphamide, adriamycin, cisplatin) regimen can offer very useful palliation.

Most of the RT literature comes from the 1970s, but this tumour is more radiosensitive than the more common epithelial cancers. Pelvic RT is sometimes used as an adjuvant after surgery or in the palliation of advanced disease. Pelvic fields are treated with doses of 45 to 50 Gy in 20 to 25 fractions depending on the size of the treated volume. Overall, the prognosis is good in the short term, with 5-year survival of over 80%. A small series of 11 patients treated between 2012 and 2020 demonstrated that stereotactic radiotherapy or IMRT/conformal offers a reduction in tumour of 80% in 3 months and 88% at 12 months, demonstrating ongoing tumour regression. The same series showed two patients achieving a complete response and two with less than 1% residual disease.

Sertoli-Leydig cell tumours are rare. More than half of these tumours produce male hormones that can cause virilisation. The majority of these tumours behave in a benign fashion and present with Stage I disease. Malignant lesions are exceedingly rare.

Germ-Cell Tumours

Dysgerminomas account for 2% to 5% of all ovarian tumours and usually occur in females under age 30 years. Histologically, they are similar to seminoma of the testes in males and tend to spread in a similar way via the pelvic and paraaortic lymph nodes. The majority of tumours present with Stage I disease, although up to 15% of tumours can be present in both ovaries. Surgery is usually aimed at conservation of fertility with removal of only one ovary, but such patients need very close follow-up owing to the risks of developing a further tumour in the remaining ovary.

This tumour is extremely chemosensitive, and fertility is more likely to be preserved following chemotherapy than RT. The BEP regimen is effective if patients relapse after surgery, with a 5-year survival of about 85%. The tumour is quite radiosensitive and, in the past, patients have been treated with wide-field RT with doses between 20 and 40 Gy in 2 to 4 weeks. Good long-term survival has been reported following wide-field RT. It is possible that RT can induce epigenetic reprogramming and influence the hypermethylation status, which contributes to cisplatin resistance in these cancers. This could be an indication for the use of chemotherapy and RT as a reasonable approach, especially after failure of primary systemic treatment. The RT doses being suggested are 60 Gy in 30 fractions or 40 Gy in 5 fractions.

More than 98% of ovarian teratomas are benign, most commonly cystic teratomas or dermoid cysts. Malignant teratomas are rare and have a similar histological appearance to those arising in the testes. The same chemotherapy regimens used to treat the more common testicular teratomas in males are also used in ovarian disease, particularly the BEP regimen. The outlook for such patients is not as good as that for male testicular teratoma patients, with a 5-year survival of about 50%.

TUMOURS OF THE VULVA

There were 1372 new cases of vulvar cancer in the United Kingdom between 2016 and 2018. Vulval cancer mortality rates have decreased by almost two-fifths (38%) in females in the United Kingdom (2017–2019). The prognostic statistics for vulvar cancer are 80% 5-year survival for Stage I, 50% for Stage II, 40% for Stage III and 40% for Stage IV 1 year after diagnosis.

Vulva cancer tends to be a disease in elderly females, with a mean age of diagnosis of approximately 70 years. There is a connection with vulvar skin conditions such as lichen sclerosis and with HPV. Seventy-five percent are squamous carcinoma, and they predominantly metastasise via the lymphatic system to the groin. A Danish cross-sectional study investigated HPV prevalence and p16 positivity in 1200 vulvar cancer cases treated between 1990 and 2017. The study found that HPV and p16 positivity increased to 36%, particularly in the younger patients. Staging considers the tumour size and whether lymph node metastases are present (Table 28.8). The primary treatment for localised vulval cancer without nodal involvement on staging is primary surgery. Surgery consists of radical vulvectomy with groin sentinel lymph node biopsies. For central lesions, bilateral groin sentinel lymph node biopsies are required, and a full groin node dissection would be performed if no sentinel nodes are detected. Adjuvant treatment may be required if micrometastatic deposits are present. The GROINSS V II study demonstrated that inguinofemoral RT is a safe alternative to inguinofemoral lymphadenectomy in vulva cancer patients with SLN micrometastases.

Because many of the females with this disease are elderly and have intercurrent disease, some are not suitable for surgical treatment.

TABLE 28.8 International Federation of Gynaecology and Obstetrics 2021 Staging: Carcinoma of the Vulva

Stage I	Tumour confined to the vulva
IA	Lesions ≤2 cm in size, confined to the vulva or perineum and with stromal invasion ≤1.0 mm, no nodal metastasis
IB	Lesions >2 cm in size or with stromal invasion >1.0 mm, confined to the vulva or perineum with negative nodes
Stage II	Tumour of any size with extension to adjacent perineal structures (one-third lower urethra, one-third lower vagina, anus) with negative nodes
Stage III	
IIIA	Tumour of any size with extension to upper part of adjacent perineal structures, or with any number of nonfixed, nonulcerated lymph node; tumour of any size with disease extension to upper two-thirds of the urethra, upper two-thirds of the vagina, bladder mucosa, rectal mucosa, or regional lymph node metastases ≤5 mm
	Regional lymph node metastases with extracapsular spread
	Regional lymph node metastases >5 mm
IIIB	
IIIC	
Stage IV	
IVA	Disease fixed to pelvic bone, or fixed or ulcerated regional lymph node metastases
IVB	Any distant metastasis including pelvic lymph nodes

However, there are challenges in administering RT to this region. The folds of the groin and vulva lead to loss of skin sparing when EBRT is administered to this region, and patients develop a risk of radiation reactions with moist desquamation. IMRT reduces the possible side effects, including the skin reactions. The latest recommendations advise the use of 66 Gy for definitive or 59.4 Gy for preoperative IMRT with concurrent cisplatin. This is based on the landmark study of the Gynecologic Oncology Group (GOG) 205 trial, which elevated the dose from 47.6 to 57.6 Gy. RT has been shown to reduce pelvic and groin recurrences when given postoperatively in patients with one or more positive lymph nodes. There is also an improvement in 5-year survival. CRT is recommended in fit patients who have inoperable disease. Owing to the toxicity of combination regimens, single-agent cisplatin is the preferred treatment. CRT can shrink inoperable tumours and make such lesions operable. However, wound healing may be impaired.

The most important factor in vulval cancer is the presence of inguinal nodal metastases. Patients without nodal involvement have a 70% to 80% 5-year survival. Survival falls to 30% to 50% for those with involved inguinal lymph nodes (one to more than four positive lymph nodes).

Metastatic disease can be challenging to treat. First-line chemotherapy is usually a platinum-based combination therapy. Several studies have investigated the use of targeted therapies in vulvar cancer. Therapies such as EGFR inhibitors, for example, erlotinib, showed variable results. Although one phase I study that used erlotinib in 41 patients showed a response rate of 67.5%, the duration of this response was short-lived, with progression by 3 months. Several other studies investigated the use of immunotherapy as 73% of vulvar cancers are strongly associated with a PD-L1 expression and 28% of them have a moderate to strong expression. The KEYNOTE-158 study investigated 101 patients with metastatic or unresectable vulvar squamous cell carcinoma who were given pembrolizumab every 3 weeks. Of those, 83% had cancers that were PD-L1 positive. The overall response rate was only 10.9%,

TABLE 28.9 International Federation of Gynaecology and Obstetrics 2018 Staging: Carcinoma of the Vagina

Stage I	The carcinoma is limited to the vaginal wall.
Stage II	The carcinoma has grown through the vaginal wall but not as far as the pelvic wall.
Stage III	The carcinoma can be any size and growing into the pelvic wall and/or growing into the lower one-third of the vagina and/or hydronephrosis.
Stage IV	
IVA	Tumour invades the bladder and/or rectal mucosa and/or direct extension beyond the true pelvis.
IVB	Tumour has spread to distant organs.

although the duration of the response was over 20 months. It is worth noting that even patients with negative PD-L1 status still responded. Further studies are needed to explore these therapies further and to better manage the metastatic/recurrent disease setting in these patients.

TUMOURS OF THE VAGINA

There were 250 new cases of vaginal cancer in the United Kingdom between 2016 and 2018. There have been 110 deaths from vaginal cancer between 2017 and 2019. The staging of vaginal cancer is listed in Table 28.9.

Most vaginal tumours are squamous and tend to occur in females over age 60 years. Surgery as a primary treatment has a limited role, and the majority of patients are treated in a similar fashion to cervical cancer. If the disease is in the lower vagina, the treatment may be closer to vulva cancer treatment. Usually, patients receive pelvic RT, the target volume being the whole vagina and the pelvic lymph nodes. If the patient is fit enough, cisplatin should be given along with EBRT. This would be followed by an intracavity brachytherapy insertion for suitable tumours, or an external beam boost treatment for others. The EMBRAVE study is investigating RT and therapeutic factors in this rare cancer.

CONCLUSION

It is evident that the overall treatment of gynaecological cancers has seen great progress. Cervical cancer RT is seeing the development of adaptive strategies achieving excellent tumour delineation. The molecular profiling of endometrial cancer is allowing for a more personalised approach to treatment aiming to improve prognosis and quality of life simultaneously. The systemic options for ovarian cancer are increasingly expanding, opening more possibilities to patients, even to those with metastatic or recurrent disease. Lastly, it is encouraging to see several more studies investigating treatment options for rarer gynaecological cancers. The next few years are expected to reveal even more advances in systemic and RT treatment possibilities.

FURTHER READING

de Boer SM, Powell ME, Mileshkin L, Katsaros D, Bessette P, Haie-Meder C, Ottevanger PB, Ledermann JA, Khaw P, Colombo A, Fyles A, Baron M-H, Kitchener HC, Nijman HW, Kruitwagen RF, Nout RA, Verhoeven-Adema KW, Smit VT; PORTEC study group. Toxicity and quality of life after adjuvant chemoradiotherapy versus radiotherapy alone for women with high-risk endometrial cancer (PORTEC-3): an open-label, multicentre, randomised, phase 3 trial. *Lancet Oncol.* 2016;17(8):1114–1126.

Fokdal L, Sturdza A, Mazeron R, Haie-Meder C, Tan LT, Gillham C, Šegedin B, Jürgenliemk-Schultz I, Kirisits C, Hoskin P, Pötter R, Lindegaard JC, Tanderup K. Image guided adaptive brachytherapy with combined intracavitary and interstitial technique improves the therapeutic ratio in locally advanced cervical cancer: analysis from the retroEMBRACE study. *Radiother Oncol.* 2016;120(3):434–440.

González-Martín A, Harter P, Leary A, Lorusso D, Miller RE, Pothuri B, Ray-Coquard I, Tan DSP, Bellet E, Oaknin A, Ledermann JA; ESMO Guidelines Committee. Newly diagnosed and relapsed epithelial ovarian cancer: ESMO Clinical Practice Guideline for diagnosis, treatment and follow-up. *Ann Oncol.* 2023;34(10):833–848.

ICRU (International Commission for Radiation Units and Measurements). *Prescribing, recording and reporting brachytherapy for cancer of the cervix.* Oxford, UK: ICRU; 2016 ICRU Report No. 89.

Koh W-J, Greer BE, Abu-Rustum NR, Campos SM, Cho KR, Chon HS, Chu C, Cohn D, Crispens MA, Dizon DS, Dorigo O, Eifel PJ, Fisher CM, Frederick P, Gaffney DK, Han E, Higgins S, Huh WK, Lurain JR III, et al. Vulval cancer version 1.2017, NCCN Clinical Practice Guidelines in Oncology. *J Natl Compr Canc Netw.* 2017;15(1):92–120.

Landoni F, Maneo A, Colombo A, Placa F, Milani R, Perego P, Favini G, Ferri L, Mangioni C. Randomised study of radical surgery versus radiotherapy for stage IB–IIA cervical cancer. *Lancet.* 1997;350(9077): 535–540.

Ledermann JA, El-Khouly F. PARP inhibitors in ovarian cancer: clinical evidence for informed treatment decisions. *Br J Cancer.* 2015;113(Suppl 1):S10–S16.

Ledermann JA, Embleton AC, Raja F, Perren TJ, Jayson GC, Rustin GJS, Kaye SB, Hirte H, Eisenhauer E, Vaughan M, Friedlander M, González-Martín A, Stark D, Clark E, Farrelly L, Swart AM, Cook A, Kaplan RS; ICON6 collaborators. Cediranib in patients with relapsed platinum-sensitive ovarian cancer (ICON6): a randomized, double-blind, placebo-controlled phase 3 trial. *Lancet.* 2016; 387(10023):1066–1074.

Oza AM, Cook AD, Pfisterer J, Embleton A, Ledermann JA, Pujade-Lauraine E, Kristensen G, Carey MS, Beale P, Cervantes A, Park-Simon T-W, Rustin G, Joly F, Mirza MR, Plante M, Quinn M, Poveda A, Jayson GC; ICON7 trial investigators. Standard chemotherapy with or without bevacizumab for women with newly diagnosed ovarian cancer (ICON7): overall survival results of a phase 3 randomised trial. *Lancet Oncol.* 2015;16(8):928–936.

Shelley CE, Barraclough LH, Nelder CL, Otter SJ, Stewart AJ. Adaptive radiotherapy in the management of cervical cancer: review of strategies and clinical implementation. *Clin Oncol.* 2021;33(9):579–590.

Stewart A, Baird P, Dyke E, Powell M, Taylor A, McGivern U, Summers J, Gore A, Cook A, Forrest J, Hanna L. Clinical Oncology: The Royal College of Radiologists expert panel recommendations for radiotherapy treatment for vulval cancer. February 2024. https://www.rcr.ac.uk/media/l1zjohkm/rcr-vulval-cancer-treatment-recommendations.pdf

Vale CL, Tierney JF, Davidson SE, Drinkwater KJ, Symonds P. Substantial improvement in UK cervical cancer survival with chemoradiotherapy: results of a Royal College of Radiologists' audit. *Clin Oncol.* 2010;22(7):590–601.

Wagner MM, van der Zee AGJ, Oonk MHM. History and updates of the GROINSS-V studies. *Cancers (Basel).* 2022;14(8):1956. doi:10.3390/cancers14081956

Zamarin D, Burger RA, Sill MW, Powell DJ Jr, Lankes HA, Feldman MD, Zivanovic O, Gunderson C, Ko E, Mathews C, Sharma S, Hagemann AR, Khleif S, Aghajanian C. Randomized phase II trial of nivolumab versus nivolumab and ipilimumab for recurrent or persistent ovarian cancer: an NRG oncology study. *J Clin Oncol.* 2020;38(16):1814–1823.

29

Cancer of Kidney, Bladder, Prostate, Testis, Urethra and Penis

Aravindhan Sundaramurthy

CHAPTER OUTLINE

KIDNEY

Anatomy

The kidneys lie retroperitoneally on the posterior abdominal wall. They are approximately 11 cm long and 6 cm wide in adults. The left kidney is 1 cm higher than the right. The right kidney is related in front to the liver, the second part of the duodenum and the ascending colon. In front of the left kidney are the stomach, pancreas, descending colon and spleen. On the top of each kidney lies an adrenal gland. Behind the kidneys lie the diaphragm and the 12th rib. On the medial side of the kidney there is an opening, the hilum, through which pass the renal artery and vein, and the ureter. The renal vein drains into the inferior vena cava. The lymphatic drainage is to the paraaortic nodes. The anatomical relationships are shown in Fig. 29.1.

Pathology

The three principal malignant tumours of the kidney are Wilms tumour (nephroblastoma) in children (described in Chapter 34), renal cell carcinoma (RCC) and transitional cell carcinoma (TCC) of the renal pelvis. RCC is the most common adult renal epithelial cancer, accounting for more than 90% of all renal malignancies. The most frequent histological subtype of RCC includes clear cell (75%), papillary (10%) and chromophobe (5%). Other rare subtypes are cystic-solid, collecting duct, medullary, mucinous and Xp11 translocation tumours. Macroscopically, the clear cell RCC appears as a yellowish vascular mass. Microscopically, the tumour cells are large with a foamy or clear appearance to the cytoplasm. The nucleus is small, central and densely staining.

Renal cancer is uncommon, accounting for 3% of all cancers and 1.5% of cancer deaths. Over the past 10 years, the incidence has risen by 23% in males and 29% in females within the United Kingdom, a pattern reflected throughout the world. Overall, there is a 2:1 male-to-female ratio in incidence, and the disease occurs mainly in the fifth to seventh decades of life. The aetiology of RCC is unknown, although smoking and obesity are risk factors. Some 30% of patients present with metastatic disease.

Spread

There is direct spread through the renal substance and into the perinephric fat of the renal bed. The characteristic mode of spread is

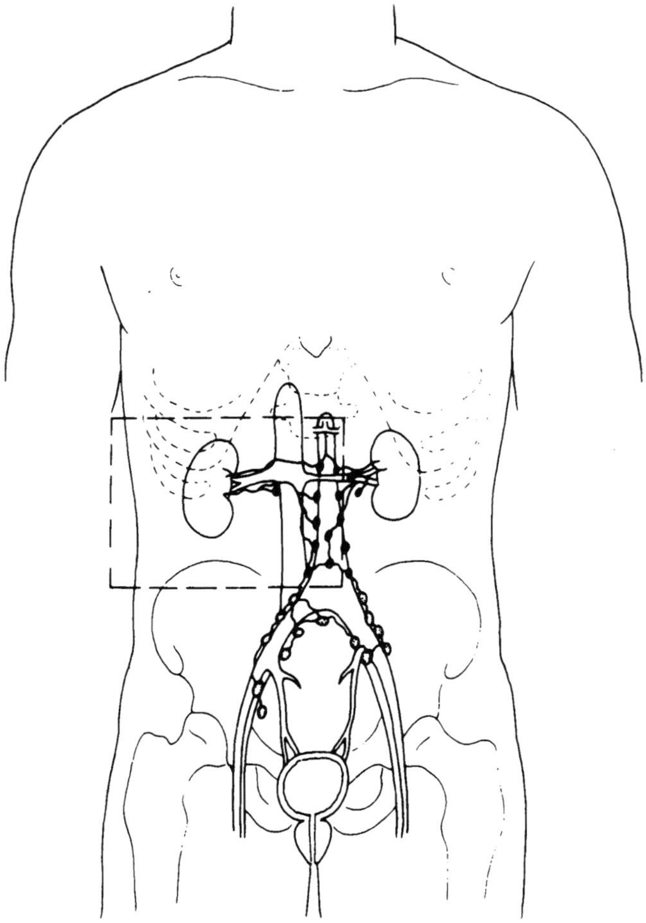

Fig. 29.1 Anatomical relationships of the kidney with lymphatic drainage pathways and typical treatment volume when irradiating the renal bed. (From Souhami RL, Tobias JS. *Cancer and its management.* Blackwell; 1986.)

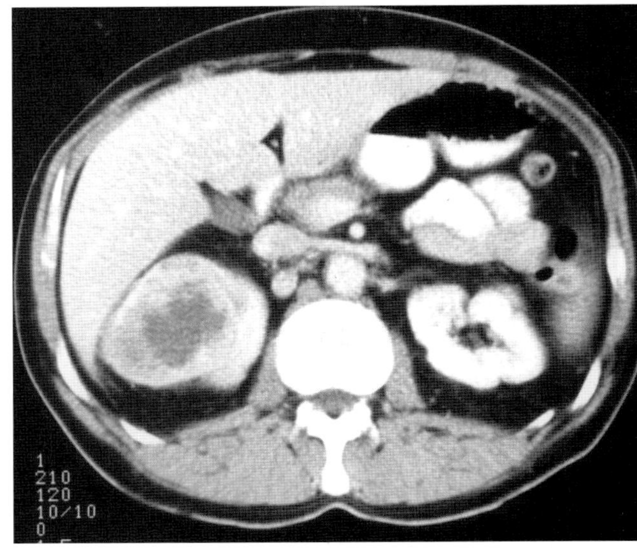

Fig. 29.2 Computed tomography scan showing a typical renal cell carcinoma in the right kidney.

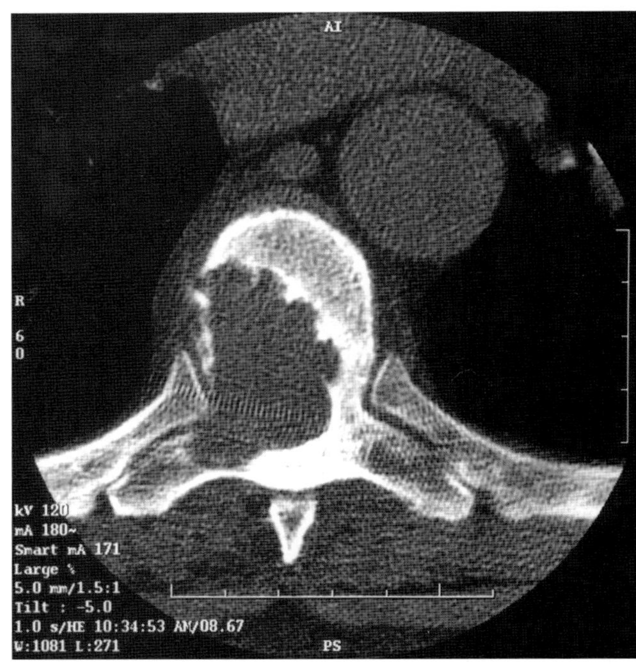

Fig. 29.3 Radiograph showing osteolytic metastasis of the vertebral body from renal cell carcinoma.

permeation along the renal vein and into the inferior vena cava. Tumours may rarely extend up to the right side of the heart, completely blocking the inferior vena cava. Lymphatic spread to local renal hilar and paraaortic lymph nodes, and haematogenous metastatic spread to lung, bone and brain are common. The tempo of metastatic disease may be unpredictable; however, less than 10% of patients remain alive 5 years from diagnosis. Rarely, spontaneous regression of metastases may occur following nephrectomy.

Clinical Features

Presentation is usually with local symptoms. Painless haematuria is the most common, or colicky pain secondary to clots of blood. Other symptoms are aching or a mass in the loin, which may be noticed by the patient. A coincidental finding following radiological imaging of the abdomen is an increasingly common presentation. Distant metastasis may be the first presentation, such as pathological bone fracture, haemoptysis from pulmonary metastases or symptoms of raised intracranial pressure from cerebral deposits. Systemic features such as anaemia, loss of weight and unexplained fever may occur. The kidney may be palpably enlarged.

Investigation and Staging

The urine may contain frank or microscopic evidence of blood. Urine cytology may show malignant cells. Ultrasound and computed tomography (CT) scanning (Fig. 29.2) are helpful in distinguishing between solid and cystic renal masses. Ultrasound may show extension of tumour into the renal vein or inferior vena cava. CT scanning of the chest, abdomen and pelvis may show direct tumour spread, venous and lymph node involvement and soft-tissue metastases in the liver and lung. Angiography is an invasive procedure, and its use is diminishing. It still has a role in demonstrating the renal artery and new vessel formation when the kidney is to be embolised (i.e. material introduced into the renal arterial to cut off its blood supply and cause death of part of or the whole of the kidney). Bone metastases are typically osteolytic (Fig. 29.3).

The Union for International Cancer Control (UICC) TNM 8 staging system is shown in Table 29.1.

TABLE 29.1 Union for International Cancer Control TNM 8 Staging of Primary Renal Tumours

Stage	Clinical Findings
Tumour	
Tx	Primary tumour cannot be assessed
T0	No evidence of primary tumour
T1	Tumour ≤7.0 cm in greatest dimension, limited to the kidney T1a tumour ≤14.0 cm T1b tumour >4.0 cm but ≤7.0 cm
T2	Tumour >7.0 cm in greatest dimension, limited to the kidney T2a tumour >7.0 cm but ≤10.0 cm T1b tumour >10.0 cm but limited to the kidney
T3	Tumour extends into major veins or perinephric tissues but not into the ipsilateral adrenal gland and not beyond the Gerota fascia
T3a	Tumour extends into the renal vein or its segmental branches, or tumour invades the pelvicalyceal system, or tumour invades the perirenal and/or renal sinus (peripelvic) fat but not beyond the Gerota fascia
T3b	Tumour extends into the vena cava below the diaphragm
T3c	Tumour extends into the vena cava above the diaphragm or invades the wall of the vena cava
T4	Tumour invades beyond the Gerota fascia (including the contiguous extension into the ipsilateral adrenal gland)
Nodes	
Nx	Regional lymph nodes cannot be assessed
N0	No regional lymph node metastasis
N1	Metastasis in regional lymph nodes
Metastases	
Mx	Distant metastases cannot be assessed
M0	No distant metastases
M1	Distant metastases
Histological Grading	
Gx	Grade of differentiation cannot be assessed
G1	Well differentiated
G2	Moderately differentiated
G3–4	Poorly differentiated/undifferentiated

Treatment

Surgery is the main treatment for localised renal cell cancer. Radiotherapy (RT) and embolisation have more limited roles. Chemotherapy is of unproven value. Oral tyrosine kinase inhibitors (TKIs) and immunotherapy (programmed death ligand 1; PD-L1 inhibitors) are the first-line therapy for metastatic disease. Immunotherapy is also used as an adjuvant after surgery in RCCs that are at high risk of metastasis.

Surgery

Nephrectomy is indicated for tumours confined to the kidney and/or regional nodes. Extension into the inferior vena cava is not necessarily a contraindication to surgery. T1 tumours (≤7 cm) could be treated with a nephron-sparing surgery or partial nephrectomy if feasible. There are no randomised controlled trials (RCTs) assessing oncological outcomes of laparoscopic versus open radical nephrectomy; however, laparoscopic surgery is associated with less blood loss, less analgesic requirement and a shorter length of stay. Tumours up to T3a could be treated with a laparoscopic approach, and open nephrectomy reserved for stage T3b and higher. Currently, in the era of TKIs and PD-L1 inhibitors, there is debate as to the role of cytoreductive nephrectomy in the presence of metastatic disease. Bulky, symptomatic tumours with small-volume metastases may still be considered for cytoreductive nephrectomy before starting a systemic anticancer therapy at subsequent radiological progression. In selected patients, aggressive surgical removal of the primary tumour together with solitary metastases, particularly in lung and bone, may be followed by up to 35% 5-year survival. Palliative removal of the kidney may be required to control pain or haemorrhage, or if a painful syndrome following embolisation occurs.

Embolisation

Embolisation of the kidney via a catheter inserted into the renal artery may be useful in both operable and inoperable cases. In operable cases, embolisation is indicated where there is concern about blood loss at nephrectomy, for example, in patients who refuse blood transfusion on religious grounds. In inoperable cases, it is effective in controlling renal pain and haematuria. A postembolisation syndrome with pain, ileus and infection may complicate embolisation.

Radiotherapy

RCC is relatively resistant to conventional fraction radiation. Pre- or postoperative RT does not reduce local recurrence where the tumour has spread locally outside the kidney. Its role is palliative to relieve symptoms from the primary tumour or from distant metastases.

There is now a renewed interest in the role of profound hypofractionated RT schedules (stereotactic ablative radiotherapy (SABR)) as a primary treatment modality for small renal masses as well as a metastasis-directed therapy in oligometastatic renal cancers.

Kidney

Target Volume. The whole of the kidney and the regional nodes should be included (see Fig. 29.1).

Technique. A parallel-opposed anterior and posterior pair of fields is used.

Dose and Energy. Dose and energy are 30 Gray (Gy) in 10 daily fractions over 2 weeks (6–15-MV photons) or a single 8 to 10 Gy for haematuria.

Distant Metastases. Palliative RT can be offered for symptomatic bone or nodal metastasis.

Technique. A parallel-opposed field or a single direct field is used.

Dose and Energy. Dose and energy are a single 8 to 10 Gy, up to 30 Gy in 10 daily fractions using 6-to-15-MV photons.

Brain Metastasis. Brain metastasis can be treated, depending upon patient fitness, using 20 Gy in 5 daily fractions to 30 Gy in 10 daily fractions using 6-MV photons using a parallel-opposed field.

Systemic Anticancer Therapy

Chemotherapy has little value in renal cancer. Single-agent vinblastine has a less than 10% response rate. However, other systemic therapy in metastatic renal cancers has progressed in the past decade with the development of various oral TKIs and PD-L1 inhibitors. Currently, the standard-of-care first-line therapy in metastatic renal cancer is combination therapy using TKIs and PD-L1 inhibitors.

TKIs. Currently available TKIs in RCC include sunitinib, pazopanib, tivozanib, cabozantinib, axitinib and lenvatinib. These agents are used either as a monotherapy or in combination with other agents in metastatic renal cancers. TKIs inhibit a number of tumour-cell proliferations and angiogenesis pathways, particularly vascular endothelial growth factor (VEGF) receptors, platelet-derived growth factor (PDGF) receptors and the stem cell receptor c-kit. TKI monotherapies such as sunitinib have been shown to give a longer median progression-free survival (11.9 months versus 5 months) than alpha interferon in a large randomised trial of previously untreated patients with metastatic renal cancer along with a higher objective response rate (31% versus 6%). Diarrhoea, skin marks (hand-foot syndrome) and hypertension are the most common adverse effects. At progression, second-line treatments such as other TKIs (axitinib, cabozantinib), mTOR inhibitors (everolimus) or PD-1 receptor blockers (nivolumab) appear to offer further survival benefit.

Immunotherapy

Earlier studies using interferon-alpha and interleukin-2 (IL-2) to stimulate the body's immunological attack on tumours were associated with marked toxicities such as profound flulike illness with fever, rigors, anorexia, weight loss, myalgia and fatigue. The CheckMate 025 study (a study using the immune checkpoint inhibitor nivolumab) showed that compared with everolimus, an improved median survival of 25 months versus 19.6 months was achieved with nivolumab. Nivolumab is a human monoclonal antibody that binds to the PD-1 receptor, thereby potentiating T-cell response, including antitumour response. Immunotherapy treatments with other combination in first line or as a monotherapy in subsequent lines are currently standard-of-care options in management of metastatic RCC.

Results of Treatment

The outlook of treatment depends on the stage at diagnosis. For tumours confined to the kidney, 5-year survival varies from 50% to 80%. Extrarenal or renal vein invasion, lymph node and blood-borne metastases all confer a poor prognosis. Patients with metastatic disease at presentation have a median survival of only 12 months, with 20% remaining alive 2 years from diagnosis.

BLADDER

Anatomy

The bladder is related anteriorly to the pubic symphysis; superiorly to the small intestine and sigmoid colon; laterally to the levator ani muscle; inferiorly to the prostate gland; and posteriorly to the rectum, vas deferens and seminal vesicles (see Fig. 29.7) in the male, and to the vagina and cervix in the female. At cystoscopy, the bladder mucosa and ureteric orifices can be inspected. Lymphatic drainage is to the iliac and paraaortic nodes.

Pathology

The bladder, ureters and renal pelvis are lined by transitional cell epithelium (urothelium). The same type of tumour may arise anywhere along the urinary tract, but cancers in the renal pelvis and ureter are rare compared with those in the bladder. Prostatic adenocarcinoma and other pelvic tumours are also sometimes secondarily involved with the bladder.

Aetiology

In the majority of cases of bladder cancer, the aetiology is unknown. However, as discussed in Chapter 16, occupational exposure to certain carcinogens has accounted for some cases. The production of aniline dyes and the processing of rubber are associated with 2-naphthylamine, which is now recognised as a procarcinogen. Workers in these industries are now offered regular cytological examination of urine to detect abnormalities or tumours at an early stage.

Smoking is perhaps the most common factor that predisposes to bladder cancer. Bladder cancer is up to six times more common in smokers than nonsmokers and increases in frequency with the number of cigarettes smoked. Phenacetin, formerly used as an analgesic drug, and the cytotoxic alkylating agent cyclophosphamide may give rise to urothelial tumours. Squamous carcinoma tends to be associated with chronic irritation of the bladder, including a parasitic disease, schistosomiasis (formerly known as bilharziasis), which is common in Egypt and Central Africa. Adenocarcinoma occurs on the dome of the bladder in relation to embryological remnants of the urachus, and from the trigone at the bladder base.

Genetic alterations in bladder cancer are common. Deletion of markers on chromosome 9 is an early event. Subsequent mutation in p53 allows cells with DNA damage to proceed through the cell cycle, replicating genetic errors. Loss of the pRB (retinoblastoma) gene product disrupts cell cycling and increases the mitotic index. Patients with both mutations have higher-grade, more advanced disease and a poor response to treatment.

Epidemiology

Bladder cancer is common and accounts for 3% of all new cancers (2015) and 3% of cancer deaths (2014) in the United Kingdom. The male-to-female ratio is 2.5:1, and it has a peak incidence at the age of 75 years. The impact of smoking in females has seen a greater rise in incidence in this group over the past 10 years compared with males. It is twice as common in Caucasians as in those of African descent. Over 90% are TCCs.

Macroscopic Appearance

The chief types on inspection of the bladder are (1) papillary and (2) solid. Multiple growths are common.

Papillary carcinoma has a base with surface fronds. The tumours tend to be multiple and to appear in crops. Confined at first to the mucosa and submucosa, they eventually invade the submucosa, muscle coat and then outside the bladder.

Solid carcinoma is nodular, often ulcerated, grows more rapidly and infiltrates early.

From the point of prognosis, a division can be made between superficial (papillary) and invasive (solid) bladder cancer. Superficial bladder tumours are the most common (80%) and become invasive in 10% to 20% of cases. By contrast, invasive cancer, untreated, carries a very poor prognosis, with less than 10% of patients alive after 2 years. The degree of invasion correlates with the risk of metastatic disease. Invasion of the lamina propria (the layer of tissue between the epithelium and the muscle layer of the bladder), and superficial and deep muscle is associated with 20%, 30% and 60% incidence of lymphatic invasion.

Microscopic Appearance

Benign tumours of the bladder are very uncommon. However, low-grade transitional cell malignant tumours are often erroneously referred to as *papillomas*.

Malignant tumours of the bladder include:

- TCC; papillary and solid variants
- Small cell carcinoma (<1% in the United Kingdom)
- Adenocarcinoma (uncommon)
- Squamous carcinoma (≈5% in the United Kingdom)
- Sarcomas (very rare)

Transitional carcinoma accounts for 90% of bladder cancer and is classified histologically into grades 1 to 3 corresponding to well-, moderately and poorly differentiated tumours. The degree of differentiation is important. Patients with high-grade tumours have a significant risk of dying of their cancer even if it is not muscle invasive and therefore require aggressive management.

After muscle has been invaded, lymphatic spread is to the pelvic and then paraaortic nodes. Blood-borne metastases are common in the lung, liver and bone. Small cell carcinoma of the bladder is rare and has a poor prognosis. Therefore, any amount of small cell histology, even when present with predominantly urothelial elements, is classified as primary small cell bladder cancer, rather than urothelial carcinoma with small cell differentiation.

Clinical Features

The presenting symptom is usually painless frank haematuria. Occasionally, clots of blood are passed and are even more suggestive of the diagnosis. Carcinoma in situ is often associated with dysuria, nocturia and urinary frequency. Papillomatous types grow slowly and may cause no other symptoms for a long time. When aggressive carcinomas invade muscle, there may be urinary frequency, dysuria and pain, especially when there is extravesical (i.e. outside the bladder) spread into the pelvic soft tissues. Bacterial cystitis may be associated with the tumour and may aggravate symptoms.

Obstruction of one or both ureters can occur at any time, with no symptoms at first. Later, there may be upper urinary tract infection, pain in the flank(s) and eventual renal failure from backpressure. In localised bladder disease, clinical examination is usually unremarkable.

Investigation and Staging

Urine

The urine should be examined for red cells, pus cells and bacteria as well as undergoing cytology for malignant cells. Urine cytology is a valuable screening method for industrial workers at risk. Malignant cells are present in the urine of 60% of cases of bladder cancer, particularly the higher-grade tumours. However, negative cytology does not exclude malignancy.

Biochemistry

Serum urea, creatinine and electrolytes are measured for evidence of renal impairment.

Radiology

Radiology is important in the diagnosis and staging of bladder cancer. A CT urogram will determine the site of the tumour in the bladder and exclude a lesion higher up in the renal tract. Obstruction at the lower end of the ureter(s) will be shown by dilatation of the ureter and renal pelvis (hydroureter and hydronephrosis). A CT scan of the chest and abdomen is required to complete radiological staging. Magnetic resonance imaging (MRI) is the more effective modality to demonstrate deep muscle invasion and spread to pelvic lymph nodes.

Cystourethroscopy

Cystourethroscopy is the most important investigation of all. Under general anaesthesia, the urethra and the whole of the bladder are inspected. The number, site, size and character of the tumours are noted and a biopsy is taken. While the patient is relaxed under the anaesthetic, a bimanual examination of the pelvis is made, with a finger in the rectum and the other hand on the lower abdomen. In this way, the tumour may be palpated and any extravesical spread assessed.

Clinical staging of bladder cancer is according to the UICC TNM 8 classification (Fig. 29.4 and Table 29.2).

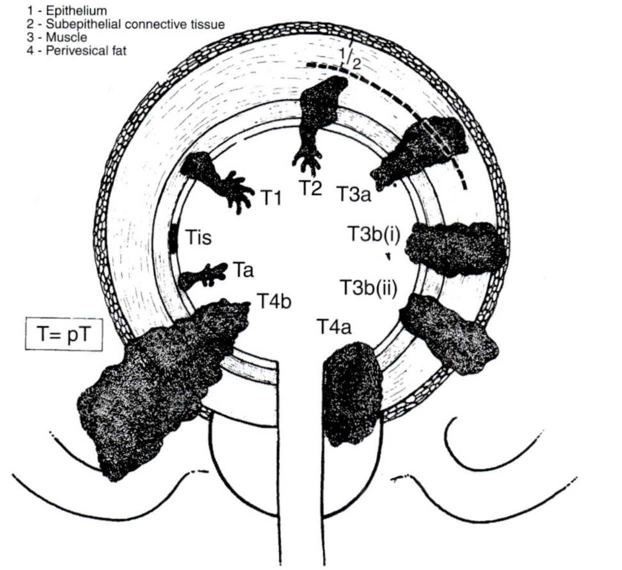

Fig. 29.4 T staging of bladder cancer—Union for International Cancer Control classification. (From Hermanek P, Hutter RVP, Sobin LH (Eds.), *International Union Against Cancer TNM Atlas. Illustrated Guide to the TNM Classification of Malignant Tumours* (4th ed.). Springer-Verlag; 1997.)

TABLE 29.2 Union for International Cancer Control TNM 8 Staging of Bladder Cancer

Stage	Clinical Findings
Tumour	
Tis	Carcinoma in situ
Ta	Papillary noninvasive carcinoma
T1	Invasion into the submucosa but not beyond the lamina propria
T2a	Tumour invades the superficial muscularis propria (inner half)
T2b	Tumour invades the deep muscularis propria (outer half)
T3a	Invasion into the perivesicular tissues microscopically
T3b	Invasion into the perivesicular tissues macroscopically (extravesical mass)
T4a	Tumour invades the prostate stroma, seminal vesicles, uterus or vagina
T4b	Tumour invades the pelvic wall or abdominal wall
Nodes	Regional lymph nodes include both primary and secondary drainage regions; all other nodes above the aortic bifurcation are considered distant lymph nodes
N0	No evidence of nodal involvement
N1	Single regional lymph node metastasis in the true pelvis (hypogastric, obturator, external iliac or presacral lymph node)
N2	Multiple regional lymph node metastasis in the true pelvis (hypogastric, obturator, external iliac or presacral lymph node metastasis)
N3	Lymph node metastasis to the common iliac lymph nodes
Metastases	
M0	No metastases
M1a	Nonregional lymph nodes
M1b	Other distant metastases

Treatment

Treatment will depend on the stage, histology, size and multiplicity of tumours and the age and general medical condition of the patient.

Superficial Tumours Ta, Tis and T1

Superficial tumours are biopsied and removed by transurethral resection (TUR) or diathermy at the time of cystoscopy. Random biopsies of the bladder are carried out to exclude carcinoma in situ. In the majority of patients, these tumours tend to recur rather than invade (≤60% recurrence rate). For this reason, cystoscopic follow-up needs to be lifelong.

In cases of high-grade disease or carcinoma in situ, intravesical BCG should be used to reduce the recurrence rate to 40% and may also delay the rates of progression. Cystectomy is indicated if these measures fail.

Superficial tumours do respond completely to radical RT in over 75% of cases, but there is recurrence in more than 50%. For this reason, radical RT is rarely used in T1 lesions.

Invasive Bladder Cancer (T2 and T3)

Surgery or RT is the standard treatment for invasive bladder cancer.

T2 Tumours. Endoscopic resection (TURBT) alone is inadequate to control T2 tumours. Additional radical treatment with either cystoprostectomy (removal of the bladder and prostate with diversion of the ureters onto the abdominal wall) or radical RT is required. Local practice will determine treatment. Europe and the United States have favored cystoprostectomy as the treatment of choice. In the United Kingdom, radical RT with salvage cystectomy for those patients with persistent or recurrent tumour remains a valid option. This policy has the advantage that the patient has a better chance of tumour control with the bladder intact. If RT fails, there is a 30% chance of successful salvage by cystectomy. By contrast, if primary cystectomy fails, radical RT is rarely successful for recurrent disease. Each policy carries a similar 5-year survival of about 50% to 60%.

T3 Tumours. If bimanual palpation and/or radiological imaging have demonstrated macroscopic extension of disease outside the bladder, cure rates fall to around 40% at 5 years. Such patients are more commonly treated with radical RT than with surgery. Combined modality treatment with concurrent chemotherapy (5-fluorouracil (5-FU) and mitomycin C) and RT appears to improve local control at 2 years in comparison to standard conformal RT alone in patients with T2 to T3 disease.

T4 Tumours. A distinction must be made between T4a and T4b tumours. T4a means tumour penetration into the prostate or vagina. T4a includes both aggressive deeply invasive tumours infiltrating the prostate and less aggressive superficial tumours extending into the prostatic urethra and/or ducts. The latter has a much better prognosis than the former. T4a tumours should be treated radically. T4b tumours are fixed to neighboring structures, are inoperable and should be treated with palliative RT.

Adenocarcinoma and Squamous Carcinoma of the Bladder

Neither adenocarcinoma nor squamous carcinoma of the bladder is very radiosensitive, and they are better treated by cystectomy.

Small Cell Carcinoma of the Bladder

Small cell tumours often present with metastatic disease. Platinum and etoposide combination chemotherapy is the cornerstone in the management of small cell carcinoma. This may be followed by RT to consolidate the response in cases of localised disease. However, the prognosis still remains poor, with 5-year overall survival for all stages combined of approximately 20%.

Neoadjuvant or Adjuvant Chemotherapy

Combination cisplatin-based chemotherapy for two to four cycles before radical therapy improves survival for muscle-invasive TCC by 5% at 5 years. A complete response at cystoscopic reevaluation predicts for better survival, and organ preservation should be considered. Cystectomy and pelvic nodal clearance is indicated for a poor response. Concerns over delaying definitive treatment and chemotherapy-related toxicity exist. Appropriate patient selection for neoadjuvant chemotherapy is important.

To date, all adjuvant chemotherapy studies have failed to recruit adequate patient numbers. The European Organisation for Research and Treatment of Cancer (EORTC) 30994 study is the largest study that managed to recruit 284 patients of the planned 660 and showed only a trend towards better overall survival but a significant improvement in time to treatment failure. A metaanalysis of nine RCTs with 945 patients showed a 22% relative decrease in risk of death with adjuvant chemotherapy. Therefore, four cycles of adjuvant cisplatin-based chemotherapy may be considered in patients with poor prognostic features, such as pT3 or pT4 or node-positive disease, who could not get neoadjuvant chemotherapy.

Radical Radiotherapy

Criteria for accepting patients for radical RT include:

- Age younger than 80 years (unless particularly fit)
- Adequate general medical condition
- No inflammatory bowel disease (IBS) or symptomatic adhesions
- Good bladder function
- Minimal or no carcinoma in situ
- TCC
- Single tumour smaller than 7 cm maximum diameter
- Recurrent T1G3, T2 to T4a
- No metastases

Target Volume. Target volume includes the whole bladder with a 1-to-2-cm margin. The bladder is emptied before CT simulation and before each treatment.

Radiation Planning Technique. The patient is simulated supine with feet in foot stocks and hands elevated onto the chest. The clinical target volume (CTV) includes the whole bladder, and the planning target volume (PTV) is obtained by a 1-to-2-cm expansion. It is a common practice to cover the prostatic urethra in the PTV in view of the risk of local recurrence. The organs at risk (OARs), the rectum and the femoral heads, are contoured on the planning CT scan. An open anterior and two lateral wedged or posterior oblique wedged fields are used, treating isocentrically. However, a four-field technique is employed in occasional cases (Figs. 29.5 and 29.6). A direct lateral field is preferred at our institution, the Edinburgh Cancer Centre, to reduce rectal doses in view of the sharp falloff of the field. With high-energy photon beams such as 15 MV, femoral-head doses are kept below 50% of the tumour dose. The use of conformal therapy techniques is routine and improves treatment-related morbidity in addition to possible dose escalation in the future. In addition, intensity modulated radiotherapy (IMRT) is increasingly being used to treat patients at risk of pelvic lymph node involvement (Fig. 29.7); whether this improves survival, however, is unproven. The use of megavoltage cone beam CT to aid soft-tissue matching has allowed development of different adaptive RT strategies such as 'plan of the day' where pretreatment images are used to select the best fit plan from a library of predesigned treatment plans. The RAIDER study (Randomised phase II trial of Adaptive Image guided standard or Dose Escalated tumour boost Radiotherapy) explores the feasibility of adaptive and dose escalated tumour boost using fiducial markers (Lipiodol) injected around the tumour to aid image guidance.

Dose and Energy. Radical treatment doses are either 55 Gy in 20 daily fractions over 4 weeks (10–15-MV photons) or 64 Gy in 32 daily fractions over 6.5 weeks (10–15-MV photons).

Concurrent Chemotherapy and Radiotherapy

Concurrent chemotherapy with radiation (chemo-rt) should be considered for all patients fit enough to receive it, and it can be given safely after neoadjuvant chemotherapy or on its own. The BC 2001 study (Bladder Cancer, 2001) reported improved local control. Similarly, in an attempt to overcome tumour hypoxia in the bladder, nicotinamide and carbogen in combination with RT within the phase III BCON study has improved local control and survival in comparison with RT

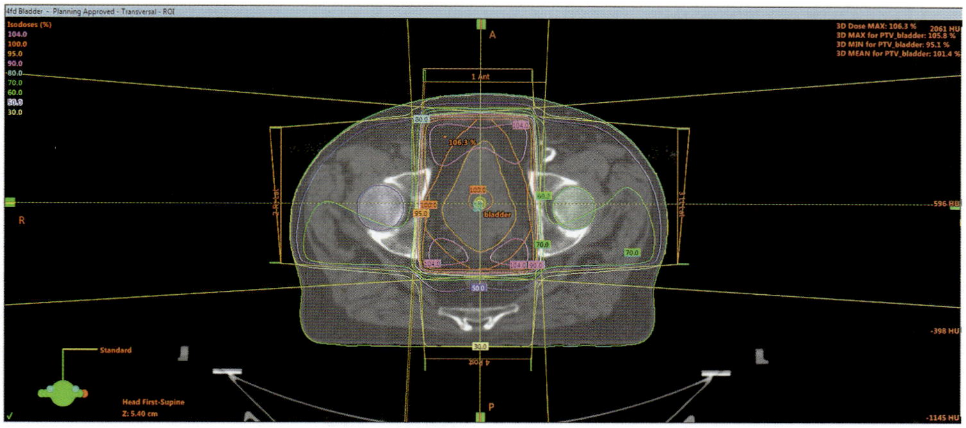

Fig. 29.5 Isodose distribution for radical three-dimensional conformal radiotherapy of the bladder using four fields.

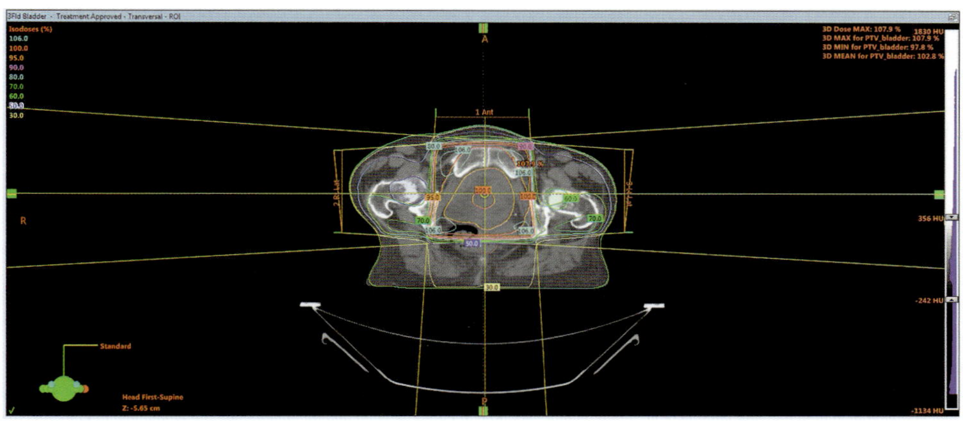

Fig. 29.6 Isodose distribution for radical three-dimensional conformal radiotherapy of the bladder using the anterior and two lateral fields.

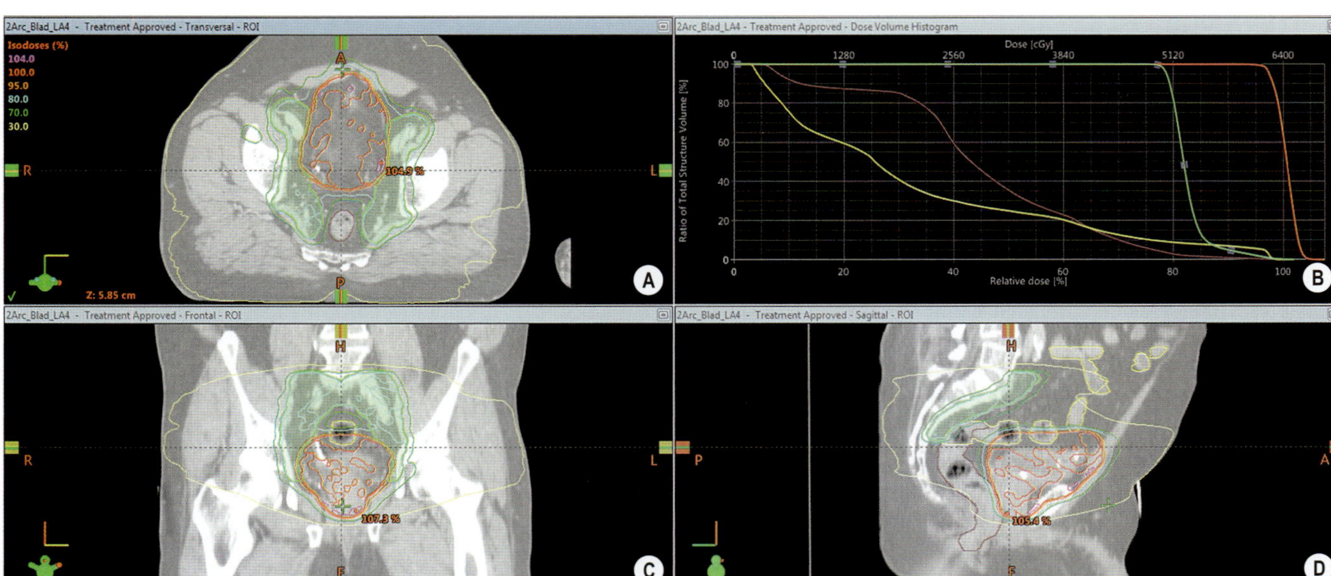

Fig. 29.7 Isodose distribution of a bladder and pelvic nodes radical radiotherapy treatment plan using volumetric arc therapy. (A) Axial view. (B) Dose volume histogram with planning target volume (PTV); bladder in *red*, PTV lymph nodes in *green*, rectum in *brown* and bowels in *yellow*. (C) Coronal view. (D) Sagittal view.

alone. In the United Kingdom, a 5-FU and mitomycin C combination is the most common agent used in chemo-rt.

Radiation Reaction. Before radiation begins, attention is paid to the patient's general condition and nutrition. The patient's hemoglobin level should be maintained over 12 g/dL, by blood transfusion if necessary, because anaemia will reduce the amount of oxygen available to the tumour. It is known that reduced oxygenation in parts of the tumour contributes to resistance to radiation. Urinary infection should be treated with antibiotics. The urine should be made sterile if possible before radiation begins because inflammation has adverse effects on radiation response. However, with an ulcerated mass, this may not be possible until the tumour has shrunk in response to radiation.

Acute Reactions

1. Frequency and urgency, from radiation cystitis during and after the course, are common but not usually serious unless bacterial infection is gross. Painful spasm may require an antispasmodic drug such as oxybutynin or solifenacin. Fluid intake must be strongly encouraged. The patient should be warned that they might pass fragments in the urine (blood clot and tumour) and a little fresh blood.
2. Bowel reactions are also to be expected in almost every case and usually include mild diarrhoea and tenesmus. If they are severe, treatment may have to be suspended or the dosage reduced.

Late Reactions

1. Fibrosis of the bladder may develop. In this case, the bladder wall may be so contracted by fibrosis and the bladder volume so reduced that uncontrollable frequency may make life intolerable. Ureteric diversion may be required.
2. Telangiectasia on the bladder lining may develop, with repeated bleeding. It may be possible to seal them off with the diathermy point at cystoscopy. If they are uncontrolled by this means, cystectomy may be required.
3. Late bowel reactions are similar to those after the irradiation of cancer of the cervix, although less common (<5%). Loops of bowel trapped in the pelvis by adhesions after previous surgery or inflammatory disease are especially at risk. There may be bleeding from telangiectasia on the bowel mucosa, ulceration, and even necrosis and perforation. If conservative measures fail (e.g. steroid enemas), a defunctioning colostomy may be required.

Palliative Radiotherapy

Palliative RT should be considered in the following circumstances: age (>80 years) or poor general condition with either significant local symptoms (e.g. haematuria) or symptomatic metastases, for example, bone and skin.

Technique. The patient is simulated supine with feet in foot stocks and hands by the side. A parallel-opposed anterior and posterior pair of fields is used. The treatment volume includes the bladder with a 2-cm margin or bladder and pelvic nodes if involved.

Dose and Energy. Depending upon the intent of palliation and fitness of the patient, different dose schedules can be considered: 30 Gy in 10 daily fractions over 2 weeks (10–15-MV photons); 21 Gy in 3 fractions over 1 week (10–15-MV photons); or 20 Gy in 5 daily fractions (10–15-MV photons).

For symptoms such as haematuria, a single fraction of 8 to 10 Gy using 10-to-15-MV photons should be considered.

Palliative Chemotherapy and Immunotherapy

Response rates of greater than 50% have been reported using cisplatin-based regimens, such as cisplatin, methotrexate and vinblastine (CMV); methotrexate, vinblastine, doxorubicin and cisplatin (MVAC); or gemcitabine and cisplatin (GC) for metastatic disease. Median survival following chemotherapy depends on sites of disease. Nodal disease carries a relatively good prognosis, with a median survival of 24 months; in comparison, median survival for disease in organs such as the liver remains disappointing, at less than 12 months. Immunotherapy agents targeting the checkpoint pathway are trialed in various studies. Currently, pembrolizumab is approved as a second-line agent in patients with metastatic bladder cancer who have progressed after a prior platinum-containing chemotherapy.

Results of Treatment

The 5-year survival for radical RT is 80% for T1, 55% to 60% for T2, 40% to 45% for T3 and 25% to 30% for T4 tumours.

PROSTATE

Anatomy

The prostate gland lies just below the base of the bladder and in front of the rectum (Fig. 29.8). It resembles a chestnut in size and shape. Through it passes the prostatic urethra. Into the urethra empty the ejaculatory ducts. These carry sperm from the seminal vesicles, which lie behind and to each side of the prostate gland. The prostate is divided into two lobes by a median groove. From a functional point of view, it is divided into a peripheral zone, central zone and transitional zone. It is surrounded by a thin layer of fibrous tissue (true capsule) and a layer of fascia continuous with that surrounding the bladder (false capsule). Between these two layers lies the prostatic venous plexus. Part of the venous drainage is to a plexus of veins lying in front of the vertebral bodies. This may account for the tendency of prostate cancer to spread to the vertebrae.

Pathology

Cancer of the prostate gland is the second most common malignancy in males in the United Kingdom. In total, 47,200 new cases and 11,300 deaths were recorded from 2014 to 2015. There has been a significant rise in the incidence of prostate cancer in the past 20 years as a result of a combination of increased awareness, prostate-specific antigen (PSA) testing and an ageing population with the opportunity to develop the disease.

The exact aetiology of prostatic cancer is unknown. It is most common in the seventh and eighth decades and is rare under the age of 40 years. Marked worldwide variations in incidence exist. In particular, Japan has rates considerably lower than in the United States. A correlation with diet and, in particular, high-fat consumption is directly implicated. Genetic factors have a role; siblings are at increased risk with a

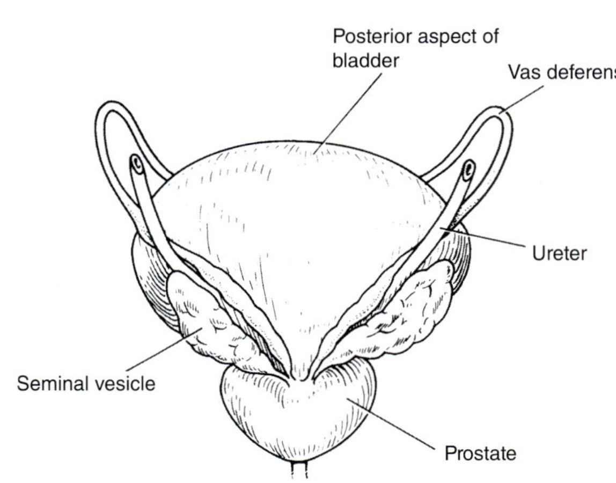

Fig. 29.8 Prostate, seminal vesicles and vas deferens in a posterior view of the bladder. (Modified from Ellis H. *Clinical Anatomy* (5th ed.). Blackwell; 1975.)

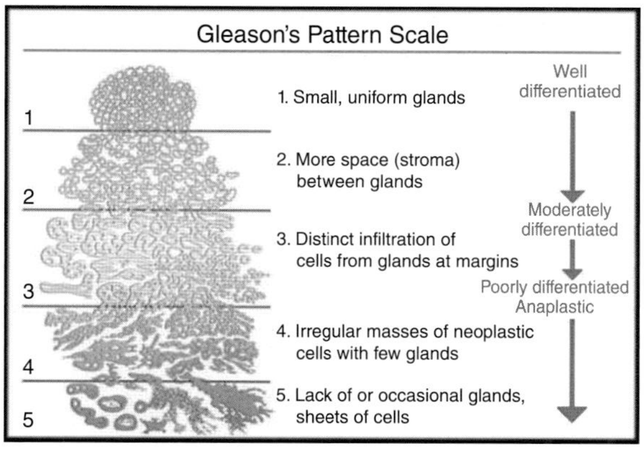

Fig. 29.9 Gleason grading system for carcinoma of the prostate. (From Kirby RS, Brawer MK, Denis LJ (Eds.), *Prostate Cancer Fast Facts* (3rd ed.). Health Press; 2001.)

positive family history, and African Americans have higher levels of disease compared with Americans of European descent. Mutations in the BRCA gene are a risk for developing prostate cancer. Males with BRCA1 mutation are 3.4 times more likely to develop prostate cancer by age 65 years, and this risk is 8.6-fold higher in males with mutation in the BRCA2 gene. Environmental factors include exposure to radiation, heavy metals and chemical fertilisers, although no definitive link has been determined.

Over 95% are adenocarcinomas, 70% arising from the peripheral part of the gland. Other rare histological subtypes include small cell carcinoma, carcinosarcoma, mucinous adenocarcinoma and ductal carcinoma. The ductal and mucinous carcinomas tend to behave similar to conventional prostatic adenocarcinoma, whereas the small cell carcinoma and carcinosarcoma tend to present with metastatic disease frequently and follow an aggressive course. The differentiation of prostate cancer is graded according to the Gleason grading system. It is based on the extent to which the tumour cells are arranged into recognisable glandular structures, with grade 1 tumours forming almost normal glands and grade 5 tumours consisting of sheets of cells (Fig. 29.9). Because of the heterogeneity in prostate cancer, the two most common grades seen are added together to give a Gleason score.

Before the advent of PSA testing, in 75% of cases, the tumour had spread beyond the gland at the time of presentation, and 50% had distant metastases. However, the introduction of PSA screening in countries such as the United States has dramatically reduced the number of patients presenting with advanced disease.

Prostate cancer may spread directly to the bladder, seminal vesicles and rectum. Lymphatic spread is to the obturator and to the presacral, internal and external iliac nodes. Further spread is to the common iliac and paraaortic nodes. It readily invades the pelvic veins and thence the pelvic bones and vertebrae. Bone secondaries are typically of sclerotic type, showing as an increased density on the radiograph because they induce new bone formation.

The natural history of the disease is quite variable. It may be indolent in the elderly patient with a well-differentiated tumour and an incidental finding at postmortem. The disease tends to run a more aggressive course in younger males, particularly with poorly differentiated tumours. Prostate cancer in males with germline BRCA mutation is associated with higher risk of nodal involvement, distant metastasis and poor survival outcomes. Preliminary results from the IMPACT study (Identification of Men with genetic predisposition to ProstAte Cancer: Targeted screening in BRCA 1/2 mutation carriers and controls) suggest a high positive predictive value of PSA screening, and final results of the study are awaited.

Hormonal Sensitivity

The prostate has analogies with the breast and is under hormonal control. Removal of male hormones by orchidectomy, or administration of female hormones (oestrogens), causes shrinkage of the normal gland, and of 80% of tumours.

Prostate-Specific Antigen and Screening

PSA is a glycoprotein that liquefies semen. Approximately 20% of males with PSA levels above the normal range of 4 ng/mL have prostate cancer, and this risk increases to more than 60% in males with a PSA level above 10 ng/mL. PSA levels increase in proportion to the volume of disease and can be used to monitor the response to treatment and development of metastatic disease. PSA has largely superseded the use of an enzyme, acid phosphatase, secreted by normal and malignant prostate tissue, in the diagnosis and assessment of response to treatment.

The benefits of screening for prostate cancer are as yet unproven. The results of two large screening RCTs were conflicting. The European Randomised Study of Screening for Prostate Cancer (ERSPC) improved prostate cancer survival by 20% but at the expense of significant overtreatment. After 13 years of follow-up, 27 males required a prostatectomy to save the life of one additional male. The US-based Prostate, Lung, Colorectal, and Ovarian (PLCO) cancer screening trial did not show a survival advantage; however, many males in the control arm had PSA screening performed outside the study and so reduced any potential benefit to the screening arm. A single PSA screening intervention in the cluster randomisation trial of PSA testing in prostate cancer (CAP trial) did not show a significant difference in prostate cancer mortality after a median follow-up of 10 years compared with standard practice without screening. However, more prostate cancers with a lower grade were detected. The ERSPC study with a mean of 2.1 PSA test per intervention group participant showed a higher cumulative risk of prostate cancer with 3.4 more diagnoses per 1000 person-years over the 13 years of follow-up. In 2017 the US Preventive Services Task Force (USPSTF) revised its earlier recommendation against screening and currently recommends shared decision-making for screening healthy males age 55 to 69 years. At present, there are no plans to introduce a UK mass prostate-screening program; however, there is an informed-choice program where males age 50 years and over can discuss with their doctor and request that their PSA levels be tested.

Clinical Features

The prostate often undergoes benign enlargement, and the early symptoms of cancer may be similar, that is, increased frequency and difficulty of micturition. Haematuria and urinary obstruction can occur. Bone pain or pathological fracture may be the first presenting symptom. Back pressure on the kidneys may cause renal impairment. Sacral, sciatic or perineal pain may occur from infiltration of nerves in the pelvis. Clinical evidence of disease is rare under the age of 45 years.

Diagnosis and Staging

The presence of a hard irregular gland on rectal examination suggests the diagnosis. This should be confirmed by a biopsy of the prostate. Usually, 10 to 12 biopsies of the prostate (5 or 6 from each lobe) are conducted under transrectal ultrasound guidance. Transperineal biopsies could be considered in patients with an anterior gland tumour. Prostatic carcinoma is staged using the TNM classification (Table 29.3). The local stage of the disease is mainly based on digital rectal examination and may be supplemented by ultrasound, CT or MRI scanning. Multiparametric MRI of the prostate is increasingly used both as an initial screening tool and as part of the staging process. The recent Prostate

TABLE 29.3 Union for International Cancer Control TNM 8 Staging of Prostate Cancer

Stage	Clinical Findings
Tumour	
T1	Clinically inapparent tumour not palpable or visible by imaging
T1a	Tumour incidental finding in ≤5% of tissue resected
T1b	Tumour incidental finding in >5% of tissue resected
T1c	Tumour identified by needle biopsy (e.g. because of elevated PSA)
T2	Palpable tumour confined to the gland
T2a	Tumour involves half a lobe or less
T2b	Tumour involves more than half a lobe
T2c	Tumour involves both lobes
T3	Tumour extending through the capsule
T3a	Extraprostatic extension (unilateral or bilateral) including microscopic bladder neck involvement
T3b	Tumour invades seminal vesicle(s)
T4	Tumour fixed or invading adjacent structures
Nodes	
N0	No nodes involved
N1	Regional lymph nodes involved
Metastases	
M0	No distant metastases
M1a	Nonregional lymph node(s)
M1b	Bone(s)
M1c	Other sites

PSA, Prostate-specific antigen.

Magnetic Resonance Imaging Study (PROMIS) has shown that a multiparametric MRI can decrease at least one-quarter of males with raised PSA up to 15 ng/mL from getting a biopsy.

A multiparametric MRI scan, in particular, is helpful in showing the intraprostatic tumour and is a useful tool to assess extracapsular spread, enlarged pelvic nodes and local invasion of the bladder, seminal vesicles and rectal wall. Surgical dissection of the pelvic nodes to assess pelvic node involvement has not gained wide acceptance in the United Kingdom, because it does not improve survival. A bone scan is recommended in view of the high incidence of bone metastases if the PSA is greater than 10 or the Gleason score is 7 or above. Prostate-specific membrane antigen (PSMA) is a promising and specific target for prostate cancer imaging. Positron emission tomography (PET) using novel PSMA agents with CT or MRI scans has gained increasing interest and shows great promise for improving prostate cancer staging, both systemic and local.

Treatment

Localised Prostate Cancer

The overarching goal in the management of prostate cancer is cure with minimal impairment of quality of life. Aggressive treatment of indolent disease exposes patients to the toxicity of treatment, whereas undertreatment may lead to potentially curable disease-causing significant morbidity or cancer-related death. Balancing these issues requires time and experience. Risk classification systems based on PSA, Gleason score and T stage may guide management (Table 29.4).

TABLE 29.4 Prostate Cancer Risk Stratification

Risk Category	
Low risk	T1–T2a and Gleason <7 and PSA <10
Intermediate risk	T2b–T2c or Gleason 7 or PSA 10–20 with no high-risk features
High risk	≥T3 or Gleason 8–10 or PSA >20

PSA, Prostate-specific antigen.

Treatment options include:

- Active surveillance (radical treatment still offered at progression)
- Watchful waiting (noncurative hormonal therapy offered at progression)
- External beam radiotherapy (EBRT)
- Prostate brachytherapy
- EBRT with brachytherapy boost
- Radical prostatectomy

Males with localised disease could be considered for any of the aforementioned treatment options depending upon their fitness, personal preferences and symptoms.

Active Surveillance. The Prostate Testing for Cancer and Treatment study (ProtecT) is the first RCT to determine the optimum treatment for early prostate cancer. The study randomised patients to active monitoring, radical prostatectomy or radical RT. Although the incidence of distant metastasis in the active monitoring arm was approximately double the radical treatment arm, there was no difference in overall survival or prostate cancer-specific survival after a median follow-up of 10 years. The 15-year follow-up data also confirm the lack of difference in the prostate cancer-specific survival rates. The study idea was conceived almost 2 decades ago, and therefore the active surveillance protocol in the study reflects the practice in the late 1990s. Currently, the selection of patients suitable for active surveillance has improved with the advent of multiparametric MRI and transperineal prostate biopsies, and this can potentially improve distant metastasis-free survival. Younger, fitter males with low-risk prostate cancer may be treated with active monitoring initially, with radical treatment offered on progression of disease based on an increase in Gleason grade on repeat biopsy or significant rise in PSA. The philosophy behind this approach is to spare treatment-related toxicity in males who may have indolent disease.

Watchful Waiting. Elderly, medically unfit males with less aggressive histological features may be managed by watchful waiting (with deferred hormonal therapy and/or palliative RT for symptomatic progression).

External Beam Radiotherapy. EBRT in prostate cancer is a noninvasive treatment that has been through significant changes over the past two decades. The Medical Research Council UK Prostate 07 study (PR07) showed an overall survival benefit with the addition of RT to hormones alone in locally advanced prostate cancer. The chance of local control with RT decreases with increasing PSA, grade and stage of disease. Neoadjuvant hormonal therapy for 3 months before RT has demonstrated improved local control in low- and intermediate-risk prostate cancers over RT alone. The hormonal treatment reduces the size of the prostate by 30% and hence the treatment volume. It also reduces the number of tumour cells to irradiate, possibly through synergistic apoptotic mechanisms.

Dose Escalation and Intensity Modulated Radiotherapy. Many randomised trials and single-institution series suggest that dose-escalated RT improves local control and PSA relapse-free survival (a surrogate for actual survival). The Medical Research Council Radiotherapy study (RT01) has demonstrated the safety and efficacy of increasing dose from 64 Gy to 74 Gy in UK institutions. At 10 years, the biochemical progression-free survival was significantly improved to 55% versus 43% in favour of 74 Gy using three-field conformal RT. A study in the Netherlands comparing 68 Gy versus 78 Gy has also shown better progression-free survival at 5 years (64% versus 54%) but no difference in overall survival. The low alpha-to-beta ratio of prostate cancer suggests that prolonged fractionated schedules may not be radiobiologically as efficient as hypofractionation. Two studies using moderate hypofractionation, the CHHiP study (Conventional versus Hypofractionated High-dose Intensity-modulated radiotherapy for Prostate cancer) and the PROFIT study (PROstate Fractionated Irradiation Trial), showed that 60 Gy in 20 fractions is not inferior to dose-escalated RT, 74 Gy or 78 Gy, respectively. This has now been adopted in most UK institutions, offering a moderate hypofractionated regimen of 60 Gy in 20 fractions for patients with low- and intermediate-risk prostate cancer. Hypofractionation in high-risk patients is still debatable, because this subgroup constituted only 12% in the CHHiP study. In the era of dose escalation, either using standard 2 Gy per fractionation or moderate hypofractionation, it is unclear whether there is any extra benefit with addition of neoadjuvant hormonal therapy versus radiation alone in the low- and intermediate-risk cases.

The ability of IMRT to tightly sculpt dose to the prostate, particularly at the prostate-rectal interface, is of particular value. Doses in excess of 80 Gy have already safely been administered with excellent PSA relapse-free survival without additional neoadjuvant hormonal therapy.

For these radiation doses to be delivered, tight treatment margins are required, which in turn requires accurate tumour localisation. Using online portal imaging to localise bony anatomy ensures accurate field setup only. The prostate is a mobile organ, the position of which is influenced by changes in rectal and bladder filling. The two most popular methods of image-guided radiotherapy (IGRT) to ensure accurate treatment delivery are daily megavoltage imaging or kilovoltage imaging of fiducial markers placed within the prostate via transrectal ultrasound or the use of weekly cone beam CT.

Stereotactic Ablative Body Radiotherapy. The PACE study (Prostate Advances in Comparative Evidence) evaluated a dose of 36.25 Gy in 5 fractions in low- and favourable intermediate-risk prostate cancer. The trial was designed as a non-inferiority trial comparing SABR vs. a moderately hypo-fractionated regime of 62 Gy in 20 fractions or 78 Gy in 39 fractions. The prespecified co-primary end point of 2-year late toxicity of the PACE-B arm showed no statistical difference in RTOG GI/GU grade 2 or higher between the two arms of treatment. The 5-year oncological outcome (freedom from biochemical or clinical failure) was not inferior in the 5-fraction (SABR) treatment 95.8% [95% CI, 93.3–97.4] vs control radiotherapy 94.6% [95% CI, 91.9–96.4]. Therefore, SABR to prostate has become one of the standard-of-care treatment options for patients with low-and favourable intermediate-risk prostate cancers.

We also have further evidence for the safety and efficacy of SABR from the HYPRO-RT-PC trial. This phase III randomised trial compared an ultrahypofractionated schedule of 42.7 Gy in 7 fractions over 2.5 weeks versus conventional 78 Gy in 39 fractions. The 5-year outcomes of this noninferiority trial didn't find any difference in biochemical outcome or toxicity.

Prostate Brachytherapy: Low Dose-Rate Seeds. Prostate brachytherapy is now an accepted treatment modality for early prostate cancer. In the traditional preplan technique, the treatment is delivered in two phases. In the first phase, a volume study is performed with the patient in an extended dorsal lithotomy position, usually under a general anaesthetic. A transrectal ultrasound probe mounted on a stepping unit scans the prostate from base to apex in 5-mm slices. On each slice, the prostate is outlined and the volume calculated. Prostate volumes above 50 mL may lead to pubic arch interference at the time of implantation. In these cases, a volume of up to 70 mL may be reduced by 30% and so be suitable for subsequent implantation after 3 months of androgen-deprivation therapy.

Once the volume study has been performed, the images are transferred to the planning computer. The exact seed location and number

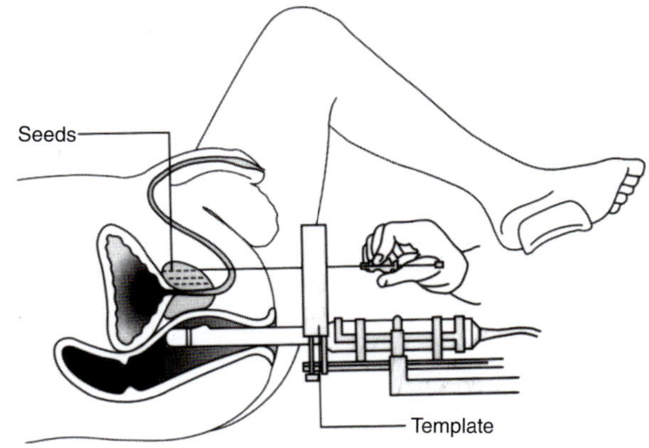

Fig. 29.10 Brachytherapy for early prostate cancer. (From Kirby RS, Brawer MK, Denis LJ (Eds.), *Prostate Cancer Fast Facts* (3rd ed.). Health Press; 2001.)

of needles required to deliver the implant is then determined using three-dimensional planning. The x and y coordinates are provided by the template grid against the perineum, and the z coordinate is set by the transrectal probe position in relation to the base of the prostate. Dose constraints to the rectum and urethra are built into the plan.

The second phase of the procedure is the implant itself. The patient is repositioned as for the volume study, and the prostate position is checked. The brachytherapist guides the implant needles directly into the prostate through a closed transperineal approach (Fig. 29.10). Each needle is loaded with either iodine-125 or palladium-103 seeds. It has been suggested that palladium should be used for higher-grade tumours owing to its greater dose rate. In practice, however, there are no data to demonstrate any difference in PSA relapse-free survival using either isotope. In the United Kingdom, the majority of centres use iodine-125. A dose of 145 Gy to a PTV of the prostate capsule plus 3 mm is delivered. The inverse-square law determines that the dose to the rectum, bladder and neurovascular bundles is very low, with resultant decreased toxicity in comparison to external beam and surgery. The procedure takes approximately 1 hour, and the patient is usually discharged the same day with rapid resumption of normal activity.

An alternative and increasingly popular approach to the two-phase technique is intraoperative planning. With this technique, the whole treatment is delivered in a single visit. The patient is positioned in theatre as before. The brachytherapist places the needles under transrectal ultrasound control into the prostate, usually adopting a modified peripheral loading pattern. A plan is produced based around the needle position. Optimisation of the plan via adjustment of the needle position is performed before loading as an afterloading technique. Whichever technique is adopted, the aim is to deliver a dose of 145 Gy to at least 90% of the prostate (D90) on posttreatment dosimetry.

The appropriate selection criteria are:

- Life expectancy of 10 years
- Organ-confined disease (T1–T2b) on MRI
- PSA less than 20
- Gleason score of 7 or less
- International Prostate Symptom Score (IPSS) less than 20 (a high score indicates marked irritative or obstructive symptoms and predicts for posttreatment urinary retention and significant urinary toxicity)
- Maximum flow rate (Qmax) greater than 10 mL/s (if <10 mL/s, greater risk of posttreatment urinary retention results)
- No previous transurethral resection of the prostate (TURP) (seeds fall into cavity and affect dosimetry)
- Prostate volume 50 mL or less (above this, the risk of pubic arch interference increases)

The major toxicity is radiation-induced urethritis that may last some months. Frequency, dysuria and mild obstructive symptoms are common. Urinary retention and proctitis may be seen in 5% of patients. Patients are routinely placed on an alpha blocker for 3 to 6 months and encouraged to have a high fluid intake. Proctitis is treated as for EBRT. In carefully selected patients, outcomes appear very good, with PSA relapse-free survival of greater than 90% at 10 years of follow-up in good-prognosis patients. Clinical trials comparing radical prostatectomy with prostate brachytherapy have so far not been undertaken.

External Beam Radiotherapy With Brachytherapy Boost. High dose rate (HDR) brachytherapy is increasingly being adopted as a treatment for males with unfavorable intermediate- and high-risk prostate cancer in combination with EBRT. An HDR implant can deliver very high biologically effective radiation doses in a shortened overall treatment time to the tumour, whereas the rapid falloff in dose limits surrounding normal tissue toxicity. HDR brachytherapy as a monotherapy is currently evaluated in trials either as a whole gland approach or a focal approach treating the intraprostatic gross tumour volume (GTV) in the low- and favorable intermediate-risk group.

A single high-dose 15 Gy HDR boost followed by either 37.5 Gy in 15 fractions of external beam to the prostate in unfavorable intermediate-risk prostate cancer or 46 Gy in 23 fractions to prostate and pelvic lymph nodes in high-risk prostate cancer has been commonly used.

Low dose rate (LDR) brachytherapy boost to EBRT is gaining increased acceptance among oncologists since publication of the ASCENDE-RT study (Androgen Suppression Combined with Elective Nodal and Dose Escalated Radiation Therapy). The study compared dose-escalated EBRT 78 Gy versus EBRT 46 Gy to the prostate and pelvic nodes and LDR brachytherapy 110 to 115 Gy boost to the prostate. The brachytherapy boost arm had a superior biochemical control at the cost of late urinary toxicity; prevalence of G3 urinary toxicity at 5 years was 8%. Males with high-risk features but cancer confined to the prostate gland alone are suitable for this approach. It is not feasible to implant LDR seeds into the involved seminal vesicles (SVs), but if the involvement is confined to the SV base alone, an LDR implant could be considered.

Radical Prostatectomy. Patients who are medically fit with organ-confined disease are suitable for surgery. A nerve-sparing radical prostatectomy has improved potency rates postprocedure. Severe incontinence is noted in less than 5% of cases, but a higher proportion may have mild stress incontinence. Positive surgical margins in at least 30% of carefully staged patients are common. Laparoscopic prostatectomy is gaining popularity because of improved surgical visualisation of the urethral anastomosis and neurovascular bundles and potentially shorter inpatient postoperative stay. The use of robotic-assisted laparoscopic prostatectomy can shorten the surgical learning curve and is now available in a number of UK urology centres.

External Beam Radiotherapy Planning

Target Volume. When planning EBRT, if the tumour staging demonstrates that the tumour is confined to the prostate and there is no obvious involvement of the pelvic nodes, the target volume is confined to the tumour and any local extension (e.g. seminal vesicles), with a 1-cm margin of normal tissue around it. At the rectal-prostate interface, a margin of 0.5 cm is satisfactory if using IGRT. The role of additional pelvic RT is unclear; however, an increasing number of protocols treat the pelvis if there is a risk of nodal involvement of at least 15%.

Technique. A three-field technique, with one anterior and two posterior oblique fields at 120 degrees to each other, or one anterior and two wedged lateral fields, is still used in some institutions. Most U. centres offer IMRT using either a multifield-based technique or volumetric modulated arc therapy (VMAT). The patient lies supine with the feet in foot stocks. Localisation is done with a CT planning scan. The bladder should be full to displace the dome of the bladder and small bowel out of the field. CT cuts of 3 to 5 mm are taken through the pelvis. The CTV of prostate ± seminal vesicles is outlined. Difficulty in localisation of the prostatic apex and extension into the bladder are common areas of fault.

In our institution, based on the CHHiP study experience, we treat localised prostate cancer to 60 Gy in 20 fractions.

Technique and Dose Fractionation. A simultaneous integrated boost technique is used to plan and treat two volumes, namely, PTV 57 Gy and PTV 60 Gy, in 20 daily fractions. It is appropriate to change these two volumes to PTV 71 Gy and PTV 74 Gy, respectively, when a total dose of 74 Gy in 37 daily fractions is considered.

The Roach formula (PSA + ((GS−6) × 10)) is used to decide on the extent of seminal vesicle to be included in the CTV 57 Gy (CTV 57 Gy). If the risk of seminal vesicle invasion is 15% or more as per the Roach formula, the base of the seminal vesicle should be included in the CTV 57 Gy. In cases where there is T3b disease (involvement of seminal vesicle), the whole seminal vesicle should be included in the CTV 57 Gy.

The CTV 60 Gy is made of prostate alone or the prostate with involved seminal vesicle (in T3b disease). In general, a margin of 0.5–1 cm is applied to obtain the PTV.

At the Edinburgh Cancer Centre, we use PTV 57 Gy = CTV 57 + 1 cm all round except 0.5 cm posteriorly and PTV 60 Gy = CTV 60 + 0.5 cm all round except 0.3 cm posteriorly.

OARs to be contoured are the rectum (inferior limit—level of ischial tuberosities; superior limit—sigmoid flexure), bladder (whole) and femoral heads.

With IMRT, the volume is shaped to follow the prostate and, in so doing, as much of the normal tissues such as the rectum are avoided. A typical isodose distribution is shown in Figs. 29.11A and B.

Typical OAR dose constraints used for planning are outlined in Table 29.5.

Dose and Energy. Doses administrated are 60 Gy in 20 daily fractions over 4 weeks or 74 Gy in 37 daily fractions over 7.5 weeks.

Acute Reactions. About halfway through a radical course, urinary frequency and, occasionally, dysuria occur. These can often be relieved with an antiinflammatory agent, such as Froben, 50 mg, 3 times daily, and normally settle within 4 weeks of the end of treatment. Diarrhoea and tenesmus from acute proctitis have a similar time course and are treated with a low-residue diet, Fybogel and, on occasion, steroid suppositories.

Late Reactions. Significant late reactions may occur in 3% to 5% of patients. The main late urinary effects are chronic cystitis, urethral stricture or incontinence. Loss of sexual potency also occurs. At 2 years from completion of combined neoadjuvant hormonal therapy and radical RT, 50% of previously potent males will be impotent. Bowel morbidity includes rectal ulceration or stricture and small bowel obstruction. Symptoms are tenesmus, rectal bleeding or incontinence. Proctitis may respond to steroid (Predsol) enemas, but, ultimately, a defunctioning colostomy is required in exceptional circumstances.

Results of Radical Radiotherapy. The 5-year PSA relapse-free survival rates for low-, intermediate- and high-risk prostate cancers are 95%, 85% and 60%, respectively.

Pelvic Lymph Node Irradiation

The treatment of pelvic lymph nodes remains controversial but is increasingly being adopted for high-risk patients within the United Kingdom. A Radiation Therapy Oncology Group (RTOG) trial has shown better progression-free survival when pelvic irradiation (45 Gy in 25 fractions) is combined with definitive irradiation to the prostate

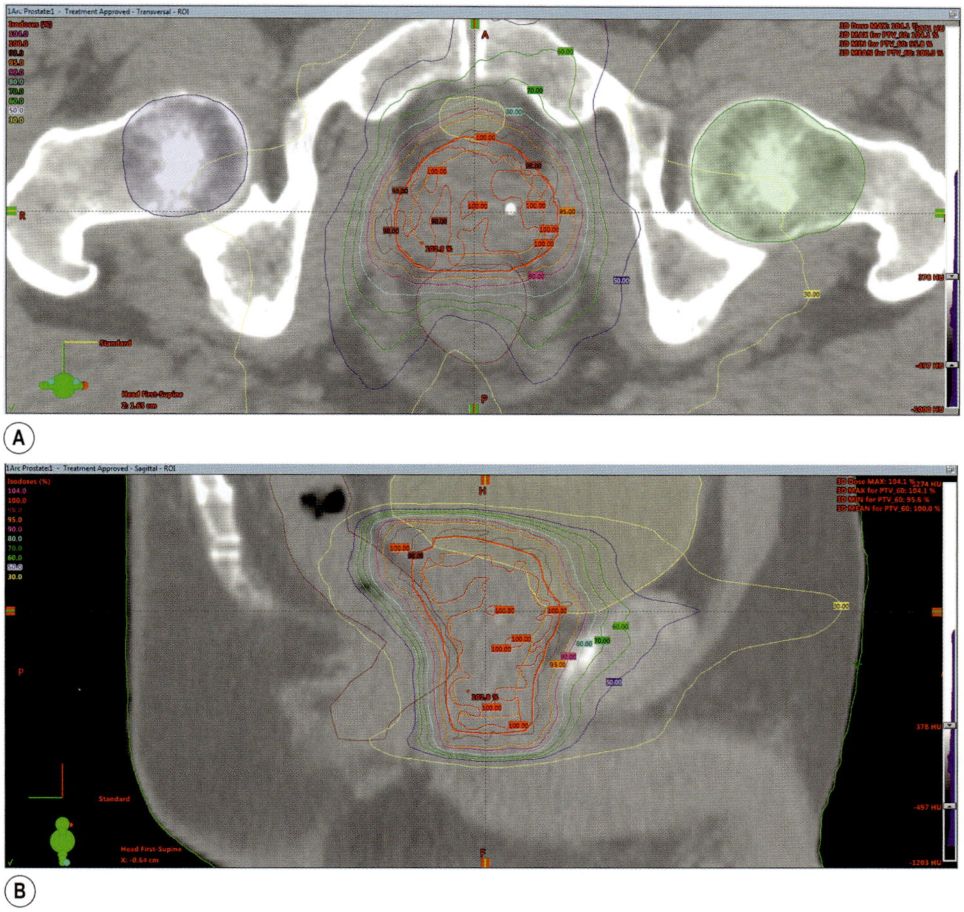

Fig. 29.11 Isodose distribution of a prostate radical radiotherapy treatment plan using volumetric arc therapy. Axial view (A) and sagittal view (B).

(72.2 Gy). Many centres offer whole pelvic RT if the risk of nodal metastases exceeds 15%. The risk of pelvic lymph node involvement is calculated by the following formula:

$$2/3\ \text{PSA} + (\text{Gleason score} - 6 \times 10) \\ = \text{percentage risk of nodal spread}$$

Ideally, the pelvic nodes and the prostate should be treated using an IMRT technique.

Treatment Guide in Prostate Cancer. Treatment based on risk stratification as in Table 29.6 could guide treatment decisions.

TABLE 29.5 Prostate External Beam Radiotherapy Planning Organs at Risk Dose Constraints

Organ	Dose	Target Volume %
Rectum	V100%	3
•	V95%	25
•	V90%	30
•	V75%	50
•	It is recommended that the 60% isodose should not cross the posterior rectal wall.	
Bladder	V100%	25
•	V90%	50

Femoral heads: ≥2 cm³ to receive <70% of dose to isocentre.

Androgen-Deprivation Therapy in High-Risk Prostate Cancer. It is now accepted that for males with locally advanced prostate cancer (T3/4 Gleason score 8–10), longer-term hormonal therapy of at least 2 years improves survival over a shorter 6-month therapy. It is important that hormonal therapy is given concurrently with the RT. In our institution, we offer 3 months of neoadjuvant and concurrent hormonal therapy before stopping the adjuvant hormonal therapy after 2 years if the PSA is 0.1 or less. The definition of treatment failure

TABLE 29.6 Guide to Prostate Cancer Treatment Based on Risk Stratification

Risk Category	Radical Treatment Options to Consider Depending Upon Patient Preference and Other Individual Risks
Low risk	Active surveillance, prostatectomy, EBRT to prostate, LDR monotherapy
Intermediate risk	Prostatectomy, EBRT to prostate, LDR monotherapy, EBRT with seed boost in select patients with unfavourable features such as Gleason 4 + 3
High risk	Prostatectomy in selected patients, EBRT to prostate, EBRT to prostate and pelvic nodes, EBRT to prostate and pelvic nodes with brachytherapy boost
Locally advanced ± nodes	EBRT to prostate, EBRT to prostate and pelvic nodes

EBRT, External beam radiotherapy; *LDR*, low dose rate.

following radical RT is the nadir PSA value posttreatment + 2 ng/mL as per the Phoenix consensus conference definition.

Salvage Radiotherapy

Following surgery, biochemical failure is defined as two consecutive rising PSA levels and a PSA of greater than 0.2 ng/mL. Aim to institute treatment before PSA rises above 0.5 ng/mL. The RTOG 96–01 study shows a 5% improvement in survival at 12 years with the addition of 2 years of bicalutamide, 150 mg. This benefit was more pronounced in patients with a PSA over 0.7.

Technique and Dose/Fractionation Schedule. Technique and dose/fractionation schedule should be as follows:

For prostate bed: 3-field, CT-planned conformal RT using 15-MV photons; 52.5 Gy in 20 daily fractions over 4 weeks (or equivalent) to isocentre for microscopic disease (55 Gy in 20 daily fractions to be considered in cases with macroscopic disease).

For prostate bed and pelvic lymph nodes: 66 Gy in 33 daily fractions using VMAT.

For PTV prostate bed: CTV with 1-cm margin except 0.6 cm posteriorly; 64 Gy in 32 daily fractions.

For PTV pelvic lymph nodes: CTV lymph nodes + 0.5-cm isotropic margin; 52 to 54 Gy in 33 daily fractions.

Metastatic Disease

Androgen-Deprivation Therapy. Most prostatic tumours contain elements sensitive to the androgenic hormone testosterone. Hormonal treatment is designed to reduce levels of testosterone circulating in the blood. This may be achieved in a number of different ways:

1. Removal of the testes, which secrete testosterone (orchidectomy).
2. Chemical compounds, similar to luteinising hormone-releasing hormone (LHRH analogues), which diminish the pituitary production of luteinising hormone (LH) and thus reduce testosterone production; these are administered by a monthly or 3-monthly depot injection.
3. Oral agents, which block the cellular action of androgens (e.g. cyproterone acetate, bicalutamide).
4. Oral oestrogens, for example, diethylstilbestrol (out of fashion because of higher cardiovascular risks and development of newer agents).

About 80% of patients will respond to hormonal therapy. The median duration of response is 18 to 24 months. Early intervention with hormonal therapy reduces complications of the disease, such as pathological fractures; however, it does not appear to improve survival. In general, androgen deprivation is achieved today using either an LHRH analogue or an LHRH antagonist. Antiandrogen monotherapy (bicalutamide 150 mg alone) has shown inferior biochemical outcomes compared with an LHRH agent. Patients who progress on androgen-deprivation therapy (ADT) could be considered for maximum androgen blockade (MAB) with addition of an antiandrogen such as bicalutamide, 50 mg once daily. The median duration of response for patients on MAB is approximately 10 months. Patients with poor fitness who progress on MAB may be considered for low-dose dexamethasone, 0.5 mg instead of the antiandrogen. Fitter patients who progress on an LHRH agent alone or MAB should be offered systemic therapy such as docetaxel or abiraterone or enzalutamide.

Up-front Docetaxel or Abiraterone. Recent evidence from the STAMPEDE study (Systemic Therapy in Advancing or Metastatic Prostate cancer: Evaluation of Drug Efficacy) shows that adding a stronger anticancer agent earlier in the treatment, within 12 weeks of ADT, has improved overall survival in males with metastatic prostate cancer. Consider chemotherapy, six cycles of docetaxel or the CYP17 blocker abiraterone for hormone-naïve new presentation of metastatic prostate cancer.

Agents in Management of Metastatic Castrate-Resistant Prostate Cancer. There are now multiple agents that could be considered for metastatic castrate-resistant prostate cancer (CRPCa). Docetaxel, 75 mg/m^2 once every 21 days with prednisolone, 5 mg twice daily, continuously over 6 to 10 cycles have demonstrated a 3-month survival advantage over mitoxantrone in the TAX 327 (Taxane 327) study. Both abiraterone (CYP17 blocker) and enzalutamide (a novel antiandrogen) have been approved for use either pre- or postdocetaxel in the United Kingdom. Ra-223 is a bone-seeking isotope of radium that has shown to improve survival and pain in symptomatic, bone-only metastatic CRPCa. The dosage for cabazitaxel is 20 to 25 mg/m^2 once every 21 days; up to 10 cycles are approved postdocetaxel in patients with metastatic CRPCa.

Palliative Radiotherapy. RT has a useful role in relieving pain from bone metastases. It can also shrink advanced local disease causing symptoms of outflow obstruction and pelvic nodes causing lymphedema and nerve compression.

Technique. Parallel-opposed fields or single fields are to be considered depending upon the location of the metastasis.

Dose and Energy

1. Prostate: 30 Gy in 10 daily fractions over 2 weeks (10–15-MV photons) using a parallel-opposed field
2. Bone metastases confined to a limited area, for example, lumbar spine: single fraction of 8 Gy or 20 Gy in 5 daily fractions (6–15-MV photons)

Widespread Hemibody Irradiation. Where there are widespread painful bony metastases, hemibody irradiation may be considered to encompass all the painful areas. Improvement in pain control tends to be prompt and may last the few months until death. Treatment of the lower half of the body is better tolerated because the side effects are minimal.

Preparation. The patient is given intravenous fluids and fasted before treatment. Regular antiemetics are given before and after treatment.

Treatment Volume. For the lower half, the field usually extends from the umbilicus to the knees and for the upper half, from the top of the head to the umbilicus. Overlap with the lower field is avoided.

Acute Reaction. Nausea and vomiting occur at the end of treatment and last for up to 6 hours. Lethargy is common. If the upper half is treated, hair loss starts at about 10 days. The mouth becomes dry and taste sensation is altered. The blood count reaches its low point between 10 and 14 days. Hemoglobin, white blood cell and platelet counts are all reduced (pancytopenia) and remain so for up to 8 weeks. Cough and shortness of breath occurring at 6 weeks are usually indicative of radiation pneumonitis. If both halves of the body are treated, an interval of at least 6 weeks is left after the first hemibody irradiation to allow the systemic effects to settle and the blood count to recover.

Technique. The patient is treated supine. Parallel-opposed anterior and posterior fields are used at extended focus skin distance (FSD) (140 cm).

Dose and Energy

For the lower half of body, use an 8-Gy midplane dose in a single fraction (9–10-MV photons).

For the upper half of body, use a 6-Gy midplane dose in a single fraction (9–10-MV photons).

TESTIS

Anatomy

Each testis (the diminutive form *testicle* is also in common use, with its adjective *testicular*) lies within a fibrous capsule (tunica albuginea) inside the scrotum (Fig. 29.12). In the embryo, the testes arise on the

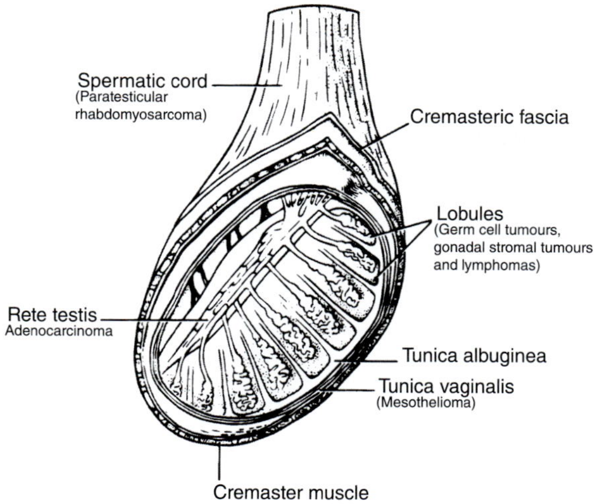

Fig. 29.12 Diagram of testis and spermatic cord indicating sites of tumour origin. Paratesticular rhabdomyosarcoma may arise from connective tissue of the cord or of adjacent structures. (From Williams CJ, Krikorian JG, Green MR. *Textbook of Uncommon Cancer.* Wiley & Sons Limited; 1988.)

posterior abdominal wall and migrate downwards through the inguinal canal to the scrotum.

The testis is divided into 200 to 300 lobules. Each of these contains one to three seminiferous tubules. These drain into the epididymis, which lies on the posterior border of the testis. The lymphatic drainage of the testis is to the paraaortic nodes. Note that the skin of the scrotum drains to the inguinal nodes. To avoid surgical contamination of the scrotal skin, the testis is surgically removed through an inguinal incision.

Aetiology

The main factor predisposing to the development of germ cell tumours of the testis is an undescended testis. This accounts for 10% of cases. The risk is increased fivefold if one testis is maldescended and 12-fold if both are maldescended. However, even if one testis is maldescended, there is an increased risk of testicular cancer in the normally descended testis on the other side. Intratubular germ cell neoplasia or carcinoma in situ is a premalignant condition, which gives rise to malignancy in 50% of patients within 5 years.

Testicular cancer is the most common form of malignancy in males between the ages of 20 and 40 years. The incidence is rising, possibly through increased exposure to environmental oestrogens. Currently, there are about 2300 new cases per year in the United Kingdom (year 2015 figures). Testicular cancer accounts for 0.1% of deaths from cancer. The types of common (germ cell tumours) and rarer tumours and their sites of origin in the testis are illustrated in Fig. 29.12.

Germ Cell Tumours

There are two main tumour types that arise from the germ cells: seminoma and teratoma. Teratoma occurs mainly between the ages of 20 and 35 years, and seminoma between ages 25 and 40 years. Over the age of 50 years, tumours are more likely to be nongerm-cell tumours. These are non-Hodgkin lymphomas and tumours arising from other structures of the testis (Sertoli and Leydig cell tumours). Paratesticular rhabdomyosarcoma (see Fig. 29.12) occurs in infancy and in young adult life.

Seminoma

Seminoma is the most common type of germ cell tumour (60%). It arises from the cells of the seminiferous tubules. Seminoma is solid with a pale cut surface like a potato. There are two principal types: classical and spermatocytic. The characteristic histological feature of classical seminoma is its uniform appearance. The cells are rounded with a central nucleus and clear cytoplasm. The tumour is divided into lobules by a fibrous stroma, associated with a variable infiltration of lymphocytes.

Spread of seminoma may be local to the epididymis and to the spermatic cord, but lymphatic spread is more important. The first group of nodes to be invaded is the upper paraaortic, at the level of the renal hilum. Further lymphatic spread may be upwards to the mediastinum and even to the supraclavicular nodes through the thoracic duct, or downwards to the lower paraaortic and pelvic nodes. If extratesticular tissues of the scrotum are invaded, including the scrotal skin, their draining inguinal lymph nodes may be invaded. Blood-borne spread is much less common.

Spermatocytic seminoma is uncommon and generally seen in older males. The tumour cells show differentiation to spermatocytes, and their behaviour is benign. Metastases are extremely rare.

Teratoma

Teratoma accounts for the remainder of germ cell tumours. Strictly speaking, a teratoma shows differentiation towards all three embryological germ cell layers of ectoderm (e.g. skin, neural tissue), endoderm (e.g. gut, bronchi) and mesoderm (e.g. fat, cartilage). In practice, the British classification applies the term more widely (although American terminology refers to this group as *nonseminomatous germ cell tumours*). Teratomas are subtyped according to their cell constituents as:

- Teratoma differentiated
- Malignant teratoma intermediate
- Malignant teratoma undifferentiated
- Malignant teratoma trophoblastic

Teratoma differentiated (TD) shows cysts lined by various mature-looking epithelium surrounded by smooth muscle, with islands of cartilage and neural tissue. In infants its behaviour is benign, but in adults it is rare and can give rise to metastases. Malignant teratoma undifferentiated (MTU), by contrast, has no recognisable differentiated structures but has undifferentiated rather than carcinomatous tissue. It often has tissue resembling yolk sac (YST), and there are frequently syncytiotrophoblast giant cells. These account for secretion of alpha-fetoprotein (AFP) and human chorionic gonadotrophin (HCG), respectively, which can be measured in the blood and are invaluable as markers of tumour load. MTU has an aggressive clinical behaviour, with early metastasis via lymphatics to paraaortic lymph nodes and blood-borne spread to the lungs. Malignant teratoma intermediate (MTI) has a mixture of differentiated and undifferentiated tissues. Malignant teratoma trophoblastic (MTT) has tissue resembling gestational choriocarcinoma (i.e. syncytiotrophoblast and cytotrophoblast), either throughout or in combination with features of other teratomas. Large amounts of HCG are secreted, and the clinical course is very aggressive, with widespread blood-borne metastases.

Tumour Markers

The two tumour markers, AFP and HCG, are helpful in the diagnosis, staging and monitoring of response to treatment (Fig. 29.13). AFP has a half-life of about 5 days. It is produced by yolk sac elements but is not specific to teratoma. Elevated levels occur in the presence of liver damage. HCG is mainly a marker of trophoblastic neoplasms; it can, however, occur in seminoma. The half-life of HCG is 24 hours and of the beta subunit, 45 minutes. Markers for the presence of seminoma are much less reliable. Serum placental alkaline phosphatase (PLAP) is often raised in the presence of seminoma, particularly if there is bulky disease. However, false-positive and false-negative results for PLAP are common. Lactate dehydrogenase (LDH) is an important nonspecific

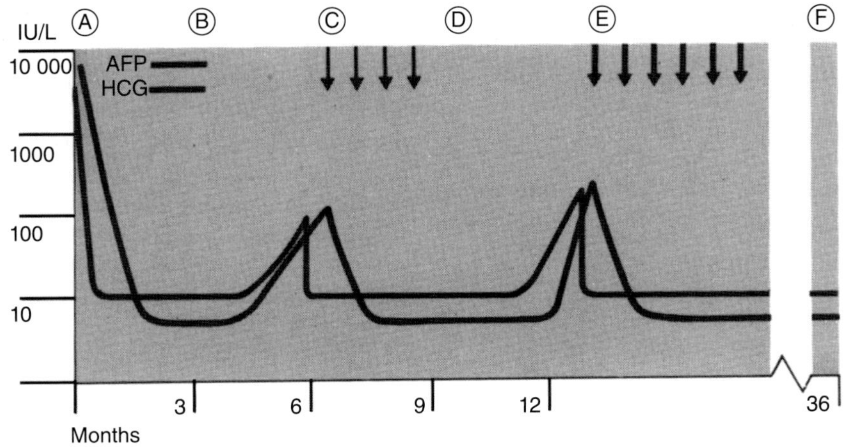

Fig. 29.13 Tumour markers in the management of testicular cancer. (A) Both human chorionic gonadotrophin *(HCG)* and alpha-fetoprotein *(AFP)* are elevated before orchidectomy but fall following operation (HCG more rapidly because of its short half-life). (B) No evidence of recurrence, followed by a rise in marker levels. (C) Combination chemotherapy for recurrence is followed by a fall in levels to normal (D). (E) A further rise in marker levels is treated more intensively, and the patient is disease free at 3 years (F). (From Souhami RL, Moxham J. *Textbook of Medicine*. Churchill Livingstone; 1990.)

marker of disease volume and has been incorporated into the International Germ Cell Consensus Classification (Table 29.7).

Clinical Features

Testicular germ cell neoplasia usually present as a gradually enlarging painless testicular swelling, although atrophy of a testis may occur. The tumour feels hard. Around 30% of patients describe pain in the testis, and an equal number of patients present with a dragging sensation. A small number of patients give a history of trauma. The first symptoms and signs may be of metastatic spread (haemoptysis from lung metastases, back pain from paraaortic metastases, loin pain from ureteric obstruction or neck lymphadenopathy). MTT (choriocarcinoma) may produce gynaecomastia (breast enlargement).

TABLE 29.7 The International Germ Cell Consensus Classification (IGCCC) Prognostic Grouping

Teratoma	Seminoma
Good prognosis with all of:	
Testis/retroperitoneal primary	Any primary site
No nonpulmonary visceral metastases	No nonpulmonary visceral metastases
AFP <1000 ng/mL	Normal AFP
HCG <5000 IU/L	Any HCG
LDH <1.5 upper limit of normal	Any LDH
56% of teratomas	90% of seminomas
5-year survival, 92%	5-year survival, 86%
Intermediate prognosis with all of:	
Testis/retroperitoneal primary	Any primary site
No nonpulmonary visceral metastases	Nonpulmonary visceral metastases
AFP ≥1000 and ≤10,000 ng/mL or	Normal AFP
HCG ≥5000 and ≤50,000 IU/L or	Any HCG
LDH ≥1.5 normal and ≤10 normal	Any LDH
28% of teratomas	10% of seminomas
5-year survival, 80%	5-year survival, 73%
Poor prognosis with any of:	
Mediastinal primary or nonpulmonary visceral metastases	No patients classified as poor prognosis
AFP >10,000 ng/mL or	
HCG >50,000 IU/L or	
LDH >10 normal	
16% of teratomas	
5-year survival, 48%	

AFP, Alpha-fetoprotein; *HCG*, human chorionic gonadotrophin; *IU*, International Units; *LDH*, lactate dehydrogenase.

Diagnosis and Staging

The diagnosis of testicular germ cell neoplasia is made by surgical removal of the testis through an inguinal incision (inguinal orchidectomy) and histological examination. Immunocytochemical stains of the tumour for the presence of AFP and HCG may be positive. Blood levels of AFP and HCG are measured pre- and postoperatively. A chest radiograph is required (for overt lung metastases), together with a CT scan of the thorax (for small-volume lung and mediastinal metastases) and of the abdomen (abdominal nodal and liver metastases).

The Royal Marsden staging classification (Table 29.8), based on the extent of spread and bulk of disease, has been widely used for determining management. Although still useful for seminoma stage II nodal size subgrouping, it has been largely superseded by the International Germ Cell Consensus Classification (IGCCC) prognostic grouping.

TABLE 29.8 The Royal Marsden Hospital Staging Classification of Testicular Tumours

Stage	Clinical Findings
Mk+	Rising serum markers with no other evidence of metastases
I	No evidence of metastases
II	Abdominal node involvement
a	<2 cm in diameter
b	2–5 cm in diameter
c	>5 cm in diameter
III	Nodal involvement above the diaphragm
IV	Extralymphatic metastases
L1	Lung metastases ≤3 in number
L2	Lung metastases >3 in number (all ≤2 cm in diameter)
L3	Lung metastases >3 in number (>2 cm in diameter)

Treatment

Seminoma

Stage I. The majority (70%) present as stage I disease. Approximately 15% to 20%, however, will relapse, 90% of which will be in the paraaortic nodes. There is a slight increased chance of relapse with tumours larger than 4 cm or rete testis invasion. Options include surveillance, prophylactic irradiation or adjuvant chemotherapy.

Surveillance. This is the preferred option for stage I disease for many patients, and the importance of attendance for clinic and follow-up scans should be discussed with the patient. Active surveillance for patients with stage I seminoma results in a relapse rate of 17% and a cause-specific survival of 99.7%. Approximately 2% of stage I seminoma patients on active surveillance will relapse after 2 years, accounting for 9% of all relapses.

Adjuvant Radiotherapy. Depending upon patient preference or if there is concern about subsequent fitness for curative chemotherapy in the event of relapse, adjuvant RT should be strongly considered. Prophylactic irradiation of the paraaortic and if indicated, the ipsilateral pelvic nodes, reduce the relapse rate to 2% to 3%. The Medical Research Council Testicular Cancer Study 18 (MRC TE18) has shown that 20 Gy in 10 daily fractions to the paraaortic strip can safely replace the previous standard of 30 Gy in 15 daily fractions.

Adjuvant Chemotherapy. The Medical Research Council Testicular Cancer Study 19 (MRC TE19) showed that carboplatin prescribed to a dose of area-under-curve (AUC) 7 (based on glomerular filtration rate calculated using ethylenediamine tetraacetic acid (EDTA) clearance) reduces the relapse rate to about the same as RT; however, the duration of follow-up in the TE 19 study is shorter. The site of relapse is often the paraaortic nodes. Hence, follow-up must include CT or MRI scanning of the abdomen.

Spermatocytic seminoma is a different pathological entity to classical seminoma, and no further treatment is indicated following orchidectomy.

Stage IIA. Stage IIA disease (nodes ≤2 cm) can be treated with either postoperative dog-leg RT (30 Gy in 15 fractions) or chemotherapy.

Stage IIB. Based on the Royal Marsden Hospital experience, for stage IIB (nodes 2–5 cm), a single cycle of carboplatin at AUC7 followed by paraaortic RT (30 Gy in 15 fractions) has shown to reduce the relapse rate by less than 10% at 5 years, which is similar to good-prognosis seminomas treated with three cycles of bleomycin, etoposide and cisplatin (BEP) or four cycles of cisplatin and etoposide.

Radiotherapy Target Volume. The upper margin of the paraaortic field is at the level of the junction of the 10th and 11th thoracic vertebrae. The lower limit is the junction of the fifth lumbar vertebra and the first sacral vertebra. Where there has been previous inguinoscrotal surgery, such as hernia repair, the field is extended to cover the ipsilateral pelvic and inguinal nodes (Fig. 29.14). This 'dog-leg'-shaped field is vertical in the paraaortic region and diverges at the level of the junction of the fourth and fifth lumbar vertebrae. The lower limit of the field is the bottom of the obturator foramina and should include the inguinal scar. In addition, previous orchidopexy, removal of the testis through the scrotum or extension of tumour to the tunica vaginalis, requires the ipsilateral scrotum to be irradiated.

Technique. The patient is simulated supine with feet in foot stocks and hands by the side. CT-based simulation and planning allows better visualisation and efficient use of multileaf collimators (MLCs) to shield as much of the normal tissue as possible.

Paraaortic Strip Radiotherapy. It is used for adjuvant RT in stage I seminoma when there is no previous inguinoscrotal surgery. An anterior and posterior pair of fields is used. The patient is simulated supine at normal FSD. The width of the paraaortic field is normally 8 to 10 cm. The field is offset to include the renal hilar nodes on the side of the orchidectomy. The contralateral border is the lateral extent of the pedicle of the vertebral body. Care should be taken not to include more than one-third of the renal substance within the paraaortic fields on either side.

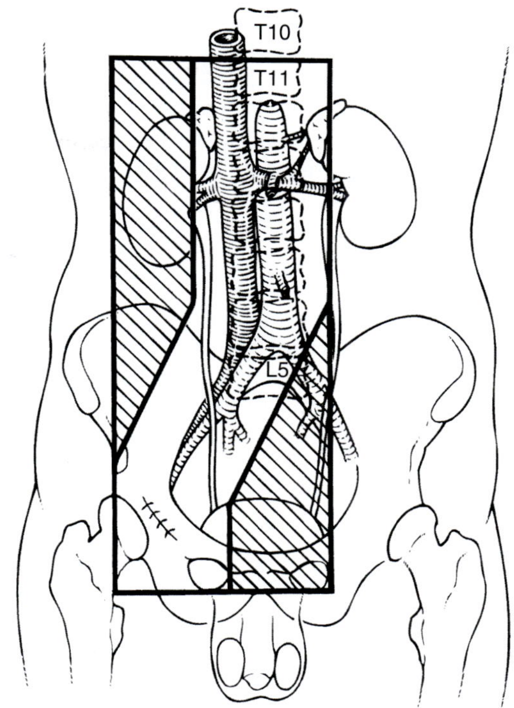

Fig. 29.14 Treatment volume for ipsilateral pelvic and paraaortic (dog-leg) irradiation for testicular seminoma.

Dog-leg Radiotherapy. Used for adjuvant RT in stage I seminoma where patients had previous inguinoscrotal surgery or in stage IIA disease. An anterior and posterior pair of fields is used. The patient is simulated supine throughout, if treatment under couch at an extended FSD (about 140 cm) can be achieved. MLCs protect tissue outside the treatment volume. Care should be taken not to include more than one-third of the renal substance within the paraaortic fields on either side. If there is involvement of the lower paraaortic nodes and risk of retrograde spread to the pelvic lymph nodes, an 'inverted *Y*'-shaped field should be used to treat the paraaortic and pelvic nodes. If the hemiscrotum is to be treated, a direct electron field of appropriate energy or 300-kV x-rays may be used with shielding of the contralateral testis.

Dose and Energy. Seminoma is one of the most radiosensitive of all cancers and can be cured with relatively modest doses. The present standard dose is:

Stage I: 20 Gy in 10 daily fractions over 2 weeks (9–16-MV photons) to the PA strip and consider dog-leg field in cases of scrotal contamination

Stage IIA: 30 Gy in 15 fractions over 3 weeks (9–16-MV photons) using dog-leg field

Stage IIB: 30 Gy in 15 fractions over 3 weeks (9–16-MV photons) to the PA strip 4 to 6 weeks after carboplatin at AUC7

Acute Reaction. About 50% of patients will experience nausea lasting for 2 to 3 hours following treatment. Regular use of a 5-HT_3 antagonist is recommended.

Late Reactions. Late side effects are rare. Dyspepsia occurs in 5% of cases, occasionally with evidence of peptic ulceration. Using the radiation technique and dosage described, the dose to the contralateral testis is very low (<0.5 Gy). Nonetheless, this dose is sufficient to cause a moderate reduction in sperm count for 2 to 3 years, but it is not associated with permanent infertility. There are some concerns about the long-term complications of adjuvant RT, such as second malignancy and hypertension.

TABLE 29.9 Bleomycin, Etoposide and Cisplatin Chemotherapy Regimen

Bleomycin	30,000 units IV infusion	Days 1, 8, 15
Etoposide	100 mg/m^2 IV infusion	Days 1–5
Cisplatin	20 mg/m^2 IV infusion	Days 1–5
Repeated every 21 days		

IV, Intravenous.

Stage IIC, III and IV. Four cycles of combination chemotherapy with BEP (Table 29.9) are recommended for these stages. In good-prognosis seminoma in males age over 40 years or in those with previous chest irradiation, etoposide and cisplatin (EP) may be used to decrease the risks of bleomycin lung.

Results of Treatment. The results of treatment in early-stage seminoma are excellent, reflecting its radiosensitivity: 5-year survival rates by stage are 95% for stage I and 90% for stages IIA and IIB. For more advanced stages, cure rates have improved with the availability of effective combination chemotherapy: 5-year survival for stages IIC and III is 75% and for stage IV, 65%.

Teratoma

Stage I. Teratoma has a higher incidence of extralymphatic spread. In the presence of extralymphatic metastases, irradiating the paraaortic nodes prophylactically may compromise the ability to deliver subsequent combination chemotherapy at desired dosage and frequency. About 30% of patients with stage I disease following orchidectomy will have subclinical metastases and will relapse (80% of whom will relapse in the first 12 months). To avoid overtreatment of the majority of patients, a policy of close surveillance with treatment at relapse is recommended. Patients with lymphatic or vascular invasion are at greater risk of relapse (40%) and are not suitable for surveillance. Such patients are best treated by two cycles of adjuvant combination chemotherapy.

Surveillance. In patients for whom a surveillance policy is adopted, tumour markers, chest x-ray and clinical examination are performed monthly in the first year with 3-monthly CT scans of chest and abdomen. In the second year, follow-up should be 2-monthly with CT scans at 18 and 24 months. Subsequent follow-up should be 3-monthly for the third year, 6-monthly to the fifth year and annually thereafter to 10 years.

Stages II–IV. These stages should be managed by combination chemotherapy (discussed next).

Cytotoxic Chemotherapy. The development of curative combination chemotherapy for advanced testicular cancer in the 1980s has been one of the most important advances in oncology.

The combinations of drugs used for treating seminoma are the same for teratoma. The most effective regimens contain cisplatin. Cisplatin was successfully combined with vinblastine and bleomycin (PVB). Now, vinblastine is replaced by etoposide, which is less myelotoxic, without loss of efficacy. This regimen is known as BEP (see Table 29.9). An attempt to reduce toxicity by replacing cisplatin with carboplatin has proved to be less effective. Before each course of chemotherapy, a number of investigations are carried out to assess fitness to treat, and to modify dosage if necessary, because of the toxicity of the agents. A full blood count is required because of the myelotoxicity of etoposide.

Cisplatin is toxic to the kidney and to hearing. Renal function tests (serum urea, electrolytes and creatinine, 24-hour urine creatinine clearance or formal EDTA GFR) and hearing (audiometry) should be measured before, during and after treatment.

Bleomycin can be toxic to the lung (discussed shortly). Full lung function tests (including gas transfer factor) are carried out before treatment and repeated if toxicity is suspected.

Sperm storage, if available, is desirable for males wishing to father children following chemotherapy because sterility is commonly induced. Normally, an initial sample is examined to count the number and motility of the sperm. If satisfactory, two additional samples are taken for sperm banking. However, chemotherapy, if urgently required, should not be delayed to await this procedure.

Dosage and Scheduling. Normally, four courses of BEP are given at 3-weekly intervals. Patients with good-risk disease can be cured with just three cycles as demonstrated in the MRC TE 20 trial without compromising the 90% overall survival. For those patients in the intermediate- or poor-risk IGCCC groups, survival is 40% to 70%. Efforts to increase the efficacy of chemotherapy schedules through dose intensification and new combinations are ongoing. As yet, there has been no improvement over standard BEP.

Monitoring Response to Treatment. Clinical examination, chest radiograph, tumour markers, full blood count and renal function tests are repeated before each cycle of treatment to monitor the response to and toxicity of treatment.

Following surgery, a fall in tumour marker levels in line with their half-lives usually indicates that there is no residual disease. A slower fall or rising levels suggest residual disease.

It may be necessary to delay the next cycle of chemotherapy or modify its dosage if blood count, renal function or hearing deteriorate below certain thresholds. Every effort should be made to deliver the chemotherapy on schedule, and granulocyte colony-stimulating factor (GCSF) support may be required. Chemotherapy should not be given if the neutrophil count is below 1.0×10^9/L. A CT scan of chest and abdomen is repeated after three cycles to confirm that the disease is responding. Rapid resolution of disease is usual after the first course. Residual 2-to-4-cm masses may, however, persist for several years.

Management of Residual Abdominal Masses. Resection of residual abdominal masses following chemotherapy is indicated for teratoma. Seminoma resection is difficult and usually not indicated, because of a lack of tissue planes and tumour infiltration beyond resection margins. A policy of observation is usually recommended. Resection of residual masses after treatment for teratoma shows that most of them (44%) are the result of differentiated (mature) teratoma or to fibrosis and necrosis (34%). Residual tumour is found in 22% of cases. If recurrence occurs, as it does in 10% to 20% of patients, it is most likely to develop at a site of initial involvement. If surgical expertise is available, resection of residual masses is desirable. It serves both as a diagnostic and therapeutic procedure. Further chemotherapy is indicated if residual disease is found, but the outlook is poor, with less than 50% of such patients remaining free of disease.

Toxicity. In addition to renal damage and ototoxicity (impaired hearing), cisplatin causes severe nausea and vomiting, and peripheral neuropathy. The 5-HT antagonists (ondansetron and granisetron) can reduce nausea and vomiting. Intravenous hydration is required 24 hours before cisplatin is given and for 24 hours afterwards to reduce the risk of renal damage. Nonetheless, the majority of patients will experience temporary renal damage. A 20% to 25% reduction in glomerular filtration rate is usual.

Etoposide causes alopecia and myelosuppression. The incidence of septicemia with etoposide is less than with vinblastine because it is less myelosuppressive.

Bleomycin may cause pneumonitis. Presentation is with progressive dyspnoea. This complication may occur after relatively modest doses (e.g. 200 mg). It can be progressive, is irreversible and carries a 1% mortality. Other side effects are fever, skin rashes, pigmentation and Raynaud's phenomenon.

Results of Treatment. Some 90% of patients with small-volume disease are cured following chemotherapy. For large-volume disease in extralymphatic sites, the probability of survival is reduced to 50% to 70%.

The 5-year survival is 90% for stages I and IA, 70% for stages IIB and III, and 50% to 60% for stage IV.

TESTICULAR LYMPHOMA

Testicular lymphomas are rare (4% of testicular tumours). They are mainly non-Hodgkin lymphomas. Most patients present at an early stage with a unilateral testicular mass; however, bilateral testicular involvement occurs in about 10% of the cases. Clinical features that help differentiate them from germ cell tumours are an older age group (age >50 years), different pattern of metastases, absence of maldescent and absence of gynaecomastia. They are usually of high grade (diffuse large B cell), and contralateral testis and brain are sanctuary sites. Patients initially undergo orchidectomy. The recommended treatment for stages IAE and IIAE are a combination of six cycles of combination chemotherapy using rituximab, cyclophosphamide, doxorubicin, vincristine and prednisolone, commonly called the R-CHOP regimen, and RT to the scrotum (IA) and involved nodes (IIA) and central nervous system (CNS)-directed therapy with either intrathecal methotrexate or high-dose intravenous methotrexate. Treatment of stages III and IV disease is not different from early-stage disease with chemotherapy, CNS prophylaxis and scrotal irradiation.

Dose and Energy

Dose and energy for stage IA are prophylactic RT to the scrotum including remaining testicle to a dose of 30 Gy in 15 fractions over 3 weeks using 6-MV photons or electrons of appropriate energy.

For stage IIA, in addition to scrotal RT, the involved nodal basin should be treated to 30 Gy in 15 daily fractions over 3 weeks (6–15-MV photons) using a parallel-opposed field or three-dimensional conformal technique.

Results of Treatment

With aggressive treatment approaches, the outcome of primary testicular lymphoma is improving. Prognosis is based on a 5-point scoring system, the International Prognostic Index (IPI), which gives 1 point each for stage III/IV disease, raised LDH, performance status 2 or more, age older than 60 years and more than one extra nodal site. Depending upon the IPI score, the 5-year overall survival ranges from 25% to 75%.

URETHRA

Tumours of the urethra are rare and are usually transitional carcinomas. Predisposing factors are as for bladder cancer. Presenting symptoms and signs are pain and haematuria.

Female Urethra

The tumour is twice as common in females as in males. In the proximal third, transitional carcinoma predominates and, in the distal two-thirds, squamous carcinoma predominates. The distal urethra drains to the inguinal nodes and the proximal urethra to the iliac nodes. Presenting features are offensive discharge, bleeding or a mass.

Treatment

Surgery in the form of a cystourethrectomy is perhaps the treatment of choice. In those who are unsuitable, attempts at organ preservation can be considered. For superficial squamous carcinoma of the urethral orifice, three iridium hairpins are an alternative treatment. A dose of 60 to 65 Gy is given in 6 to 7 days. For more proximal lesions, radical external beam irradiation using an anterior and two lateral wedged fields is used. A dose of 55 Gy is given in 20 daily fractions over 4 weeks using megavoltage.

Results of Treatment

The cure rates with surgery and RT are similar, at about 50%.

PENIS

Cancer of the penis is a rare tumour in the United Kingdom with an age-standardised incidence rate of 2.3 and mortality of 0.5 per 100,000 males. The incidence increases with age and is common during the sixth decade of life, although it does occur in younger males. The disease is more common in Southeast Asia, China and Africa. In Uganda, penile carcinoma is currently the most commonly diagnosed male cancer.

Aetiology

Human papilloma virus (HPV) is an important risk factor for penile cancer. However, it remains unclear if an HPV-related penile cancer has a different prognosis compared with non-HPV-related penile cancer. It is less prevalent in communities practising neonatal circumcision, as this removes approximately half of the tissue that can develop into penile cancer. Phimosis is present in up to 50% of cases. Poor penile hygiene is thought to be an important predisposing factor. Other risk factors include smoking, chronic penile inflammation and premalignant conditions such as giant condylomata, erythroplasia of Queyrat, Bowen disease and Paget disease. Squamous cell carcinoma accounts for the majority of the penile cancers, and other rare pathologies include sarcomatoid carcinoma, adenosquamous carcinoma and mucoepidermoid carcinoma.

Clinical Features

These tumours occur as warty growths or, more commonly, as indurated ulcers on the glans or the sulcus at the base of the glans. Symptoms have often been present for 1 year or more before presentation. The first sign may be an infected or bloody discharge from beneath the prepuce. Growth is superficial at first, then by invasion of the penile shaft. If the lesion is visible, the diagnosis is usually obvious. If phimosis hides it, the glans must be exposed by incising and peeling back the prepuce (dorsal slit) or by complete circumcision, under anaesthesia. A biopsy is taken at the same time.

Inguinal and pelvic nodes are the regional drainage basin for the penis. Lymphatic spread first occurs to the inguinal nodes (superficial and deep) and then to the ipsilateral pelvic nodes. Blood-borne metastases are rare and late.

Staging

Both the UICC TNM 8 and Jackson staging systems are in use (Table 29.10). Physical examination is an important part of the diagnostic process, and an MRI can provide valuable information to assess local invasion to aid surgical planning. Conventional cross-sectional imaging such as CT or MRI can be used to assess regional nodes and distant metastatic disease. However, the risk of micrometastatic disease to the draining lymph nodes is 25% even in the absence of clinically palpable disease, and these imaging modalities are often unreliable to detect micrometastatic disease. There are no established tumour markers in penile cancers.

Treatment

Superficial noninvasive disease could be treated with topical chemotherapy such as imiquimod or 5-FU, laser treatment, photodynamic

TABLE 29.10 Union for International Cancer Control TNM 8 and Jackson Staging Systems for Penile Cancer

Stage	Clinical Findings
Tumour	
Tis	Carcinoma in situ (penile intraepithelial neoplasia)
Ta	Noninvasive localised squamous cell carcinoma
T1	Tumour invades subepithelial connective tissue
T1a	Tumour invades subepithelial connective tissue without lymphovascular invasion or perineural invasion and is not poorly differentiated
T1b	Tumour invades subepithelial connective tissue with lymphovascular invasion or perineural invasion or is poorly differentiated
T2	Tumour invades corpus spongiosum with or without invasion of the urethra
T3	Tumour invades corpora cavernosum
T4	Tumour invades other adjacent structures
Nodes	
N0	No palpable or visibly enlarged inguinal lymph nodes
N1	Palpable mobile unilateral inguinal lymph node
N2	Palpable mobile multiple or bilateral lymph nodes
N3	Palpable fixed inguinal nodal mass or pelvic lymphadenopathy, unilateral or bilateral
Metastases	
M0	No distant metastases
M1	Distant metastasis; includes lymph node metastasis outside the true pelvis in addition to visceral or bone sites
Jackson Classification	
I	Tumour confined to the glans or prepuce
II	Tumour extending onto the shaft of the penis
III	Tumour with operable inguinal nodes
IV	Tumour with inoperable metastases

therapy and total or partial glans resurfacing. Surgery and RT are the main treatments for invasive penile cancer. Factors that influence the choice of treatment are the age and general condition of the patient, the extent of the disease, the desire to retain sexual function and the capacity to pass urine in the standing position for young males. In patients with locally advanced disease, cisplatin-based neoadjuvant chemotherapy followed by surgery may be considered for responders.

Surgery

Specialised surgical techniques are now available, which can excise early invasive tumours and reconstruct the penis with a split skin graft for an excellent cosmetic and functional result. More advanced tumours involving the deeper corpora and urethra require amputation of part or the whole of the penis. Although curative if the inguinal nodes are not involved, the procedure is associated with considerable psychological morbidity, especially for young males.

Radiotherapy

Radical RT is still an effective treatment for early penile cancer because it permits the organ to be conserved. However, if there is deep invasion of the shaft, the chances of control by radiation are poor and surgery is preferable. Invasion of the urethra also favors surgery because post-radiation fibrotic stricture is very liable to occur. Circumcision should be considered in appropriate patients if planned for RT because this allows better inspection and staging of the lesion.

Treatment Techniques and Dosage

The choice of technique and energy will depend on the extent and site of the disease. For tumours confined to the glans or the prepuce, superficial, orthovoltage, electron beam or implants are possibilities. For infiltrating tumours or where the inguinal nodes are involved, megavoltage irradiation is required. In general, a total dose less than 60 Gy (2 Gy/fraction) to the primary tumour is associated with higher risk of local recurrence.

Implantation. Brachytherapy for penile cancers is rarely done in the United Kingdom. Tumours greater than 4 cm in any dimension or invading the corpora cavernosa should not be implanted. A recent French study on long-term outcomes with penile brachytherapy suggests a good local control with a local relapse rate of 18.9%, with surgery reserved for local failures. Penile brachytherapy can be done using either an LDR or an HDR implant. In LDR brachytherapy, a two- to three-plane implant should cover the tumour with at least a 1-cm margin. The Paris system of dosimetry is used to guide needle placement at appropriate spacing to cover the lesion with a margin. In general, 12-to-18-mm spacing is acceptable for LDR brachytherapy. LDR brachytherapy is largely superseded by HDR brachytherapy because of advantages of remote afterloading and radioprotection. In an HDR implant, adequate dose coverage could be achieved by dwell position and time adjustment; however, a closer spacing is recommended, generally 10 to 12 mm.

Dose. LDR brachytherapy should be treated with 60 to 65 Gy at 0.5 to 0.6 Gy/h with treatment completed in 5 to 6 days. HDR brachytherapy should be treated with 3.2 Gy twice daily to a total of 38.4 Gy in 6 days.

Superficial or Orthovoltage Therapy. For very small (T1) superficial tumours, 100- or 250-kV x-ray therapy may suffice. A 0.5-cm margin of normal surrounding tissue is included in the treated volume. A dose of 50 Gy is given in 15 fractions over 3 weeks. Alternatively, low-energy (6 MeV) electrons can be used, using an appropriate thickness of Perspex over the lesion to bring up the surface dose to 100%.

Megavoltage

Treatment Volume. If there is evidence of spread onto the shaft of the penis, the whole of the penis should be treated.

Technique. A rectangular wax block with a central cylindrical cavity is made to encompass the penis and ensure homogeneous irradiation of the whole volume. The penis is treated en bloc by a parallel-opposed pair of lateral fields.

Dose and Energy. Doses should be given as 50 to 55 Gy in 20 daily fractions over 4 weeks using megavoltage (4–6 MV) photons or 60 to 66 Gy in 30 to 33 daily fractions over 6 to 7 weeks using megavoltage (4–6 MV) photons.

Acute Reactions. Acute reactions are like skin reactions elsewhere but more marked, and moist desquamation is more common. The urethral reaction causes discomfort and dysuria. If very severe, the reaction may result in acute retention requiring catheterisation.

Late Reactions. Late reactions include telangiectasia, skin atrophy, urethral stricture and necrosis. Urethral dilatation is required for stricture. Necrosis occurs in less than 10% of cases.

Management of Regional Nodes. The management of lymph nodes in clinically node-negative (cN0) patients depends upon stage, grade and presence or absence of lymphovascular invasion. In patients with no palpable nodes, dynamic sentinel node biopsy (DNSB) is promising, with a false-negative rate of 7%. Early lymphadenectomy in clinically node-negative patients improves overall survival compared with delayed lymph node dissection (at the point of recurrence). Uni- or bilateral palpable lymphadenopathy is very likely disease-related, and a block dissection of the groin should be carried out. The use of antibiotics to exclude node enlargement because of infection is discouraged. Following management of the lymphatics, the primary tumour can be addressed with radical RT. There is no value in giving prophylactic groin node irradiation. The only role for RT in the treatment of groin nodes is for palliation. For fixed inoperable nodes, neoadjuvant chemotherapy for downstaging before lymphadenectomy for locally advanced patients can be considered.

Palliative Radiotherapy

Technique. Palliative therapy consists of a simple parallel-opposed pair of fields to the affected groin.

Dose and Energy. Doses should be given as 30 Gy in 10 daily fractions over 2 weeks using 10-to-15-MV photons.

Palliative Chemotherapy. Cisplatin-based chemotherapy can be considered for fit patients. Response rates of 30% to 40% have been reported.

Results of Treatment

Early superficial tumours have a high cure rate: 5-year survival for stage I disease is about 90%. This falls to 60% in stage II and 30% to 40% in stage III.

FURTHER READING

Bolla M, de Reijke TM, Van Tienhoven G, Van den Bergh ACM, Oddens J, Poortmans PMP, Gez E, Kil P, Akdas A, Soete G, Kariakine O, van der Steen-Banasik EM, Musat E, Piérart M, Mauer ME, Collette L; EORTC Radiation Oncology Group and Genito-Urinary Tract Cancer Group. Duration of androgen suppression in the treatment of prostate cancer. *N Engl J Med.* 2009;360(24):2516–2527.

Bolla M, Van Tienhoven G, Warde P, Dubois JB, Mirimanoff R-O, Storme G, Bernier J, Kuten A, Sternberg C, Billiet I, Torecilla JL, Pfeffer R, Cutajar CL, Van der Kwast T, Collette L. External irradiation with or without long-term androgen suppression for prostate cancer with high metastatic risk: 10-year results of an EORTC randomized study. *Lancet Oncol.* 2010;11(11): 1066–1073.

Choueiri TK, Escudier B, Powles T, Mainwaring PN, Rini BI, Donskov F, Hammers H, Hutson TE, Lee J-L, Peltola K, Roth BJ, Bjarnason GA, Géczi L, Keam B, Maroto P, Heng DYC, Schmidinger M, Kantoff PW…METEOR Investigators. Cabozantinib versus everolimus in advanced renal-cell carcinoma. *N Engl J Med.* 2015;373(19):1814–1823.

de Wit R, Roberts JT, Wilkinson PM, de Mulder PH, Mead GM, Fosså SD, Cook P, de Prijck L, Stenning S, Collette L. Equivalence of three or four cycles of bleomycin, etoposide and cisplatin chemotherapy and of a 3- or 5-day schedule in good-prognosis germ cell cancer: a randomized study of the European Organization for Research and Treatment of Cancer Genitourinary Tract Cancer Cooperative Group and the Medical Research Council. *J Clin Oncol.* 2001;19(6):1629–1640.

Dearnaley D, Syndikus I, Mossop H, Khoo V, Birtle A, Bloomfield D, Graham J, Kirkbride P, Logue J, Malik Z, Money-Kyrle J, O'Sullivan JM, Panades M, Parker C, Patterson H, Scrase C, Staffurth J, Stockdale A…CHHiP Investigators. Conventional versus hypofractionated high-dose intensity-modulated radiotherapy for prostate cancer: 5-year outcomes of the randomised, non-inferiority, phase 3 CHHiP trial. *Lancet Oncol.* 2016;17(8):1047–1060.

Escudier B, Eisen T, Stadler WM, Szczylik C, Oudard S, Siebels M, Negrier S, Chevreau C, Solska E, Desai AA, Rolland F, Demkow T, Hutson TE, Gore M, Freeman S, Schwartz B, Shan M, Simantov R…TARGET Study Group. Sorafenib in advanced clear-cell renal-cell carcinoma. *N Engl J Med.* 2007;356(2):125–134.

Hamdy FC, Donovan JL, Lane JA, Mason M, Metcalfe C, Holding P, Davis M, Peters TJ, Turner EL, Martin RM, Oxley J, Robinson M, Staffurth J, Walsh E, Bollina P, Catto J, Doble A, Doherty A…ProtecT Study Group. 10-year outcomes after monitoring, surgery, or radiotherapy for localized prostate cancer. *N Engl J Med.* 2016;375(15):1415–1424. 10.1056/NEJMoa1606220

James ND, Hussain SA, Hall E, Jenkins P, Tremlett J, Rawlings C, Crundwell M, Sizer B, Sreenivasan T, Hendron C, Lewis R, Waters R, Huddart RA; BC2001 Investigators. Radiotherapy with or without chemotherapy in muscle-invasive bladder cancer. *N Engl J Med.* 2012;366(16):1477–1488.

James ND, Sydes MR, Clarke NW, Mason MD, Dearnaley DP, Spears MR, Ritchie AWS, Parker CC, Russell JM, Attard G, de Bono J, Cross W, Jones RJ, Thalmann G, Amos C, Matheson D, Millman R, Alzouebi M…STAMPEDE investigators. Addition of docetaxel, zoledronic acid, or both to first-line long-term hormone therapy in prostate cancer (STAMPEDE): survival results from an adaptive, multiarm, multistage, platform randomised controlled trial. *Lancet.* 2016;387:1163–1177.

James ND, de Bono JS, Spears MR, Clarke NW, Mason MD, Dearnaley DP, Ritchie AWS, Amos CL, Gilson C, Jones RJ, Matheson D, Millman R, Attard G, Chowdhury S, Cross WR, Gillessen S, Parker CC, Russell JM…STAMPEDE Investigators. Abiraterone for prostate cancer not previously treated with hormone therapy. *N Engl J Med.* 2017;377(4):338–451.

Jones WG, Fossa SD, Mead GM, Roberts JT, Sokal M, Horwich A, Stenning SP. Randomized trial of 30 versus 20 Gy in the adjuvant treatment of stage I testicular seminoma: A report on Medical Research Council Trial TE18, European Organisation for the Research and Treatment of Cancer Trial 30942 (ISRCTN18525328). *J Clin Oncol.* 2005;23(6):1200–1208.

Morris WJ, Tyldesley S, Rodda S, Halperin R, Pai H, McKenzie M, Duncan G, Morton G, Hamm J, Murray N. Androgen suppression combined with elective nodal and dose escalated radiation therapy (the ASCENDE-RT Trial): An analysis of survival endpoints for a randomized trial comparing a low-dose-rate brachytherapy boost to a dose-escalated external beam boost for high- and intermediate-risk prostate cancer. *Int J Radiat Oncol.* 2017;98(2):275–285.

Mosconi AM, Roila F, Gatta G, Theodore C. Cancer of the penis. *Crit Rev Oncol Hematol.* 2005;53:165–177.

Motzer RJ, Hutson TE, Cella D, Reeves J, Hawkins R, Guo J, Nathan P, Staehler M, de Souza P, Merchan JR, Boleti E, Fife K, Jin J, Jones R, Uemura H, De Giorgi U, Harmenberg U, Wang J, Sternberg CN, et al. Pazopanib versus sunitinib in metastatic renal-cell carcinoma. *N Engl J Med.* 2013;369(8):722–731.

Motzer RJ, Escudier B, McDermott DF, George S, Hammers HJ, Srinivas S, Tykodi SS, Sosman JA, Procopio G, Plimack ER, Castellano D, Choueiri TK, Gurney H, Donskov F, Bono P, Wagstaff J, Gauler TC, Ueda T…CheckMate 025 Investigators. Nivolumab versus everolimus in advanced renal-cell carcinoma. *N Engl J Med.* 2015;373(19):1803–1813.

Oliver RTD, Mead GM, Rustin GJS, Joffe JK, Aass N, Coleman R, Gabe R, Pollock P, Stenning SP. Randomized trial of carboplatin versus radiotherapy for stage I seminoma: mature results on relapse and contralateral testis cancer rates in MRC TE19/EORTC 30982 study (ISRCTN27163214). *J Clin Oncol.* 2011;29(8):957–962.

Schröder FH, Hugosson J, Roobol MJ, Tammela TLJ, Zappa M, Nelen V, Kwiatkowski M, Lujan M, Määttänen L, Lilja H, Denis LJ, Recker F, Paez A, Bangma CH, Carlsson S, Puliti D, Villers A,

Rebillard X…ERSPC Investigators. Screening and prostate cancer mortality: results of the European Randomised Study of Screening for Prostate Cancer (ERSPC) at 13 years of follow-up. *Lancet.* 2014;384(9959):2027–2035.

Vale C. Neoadjuvant chemotherapy in invasive bladder cancer: a systematic review and meta-analysis. *Lancet.* 2003 Jun 7; 361(9373):1927–1934.

Warde P, Mason M, Ding K, Kirkbride P, Brundage M, Cowan R, Gospodarowicz M, Sanders K, Kostashuk E, Swanson G, Barber J, Hiltz A, Parmar MKB, Sathya J, Anderson J, Hayter C, Hetherington J, Sydes MR…NCIC CTG PR.3/MRC UK PR07 investigators. Combined androgen deprivation therapy and radiation therapy for locally advanced prostate cancer: a randomised, phase 3 trial. *Lancet.* 2011;378(9809):2104–2111.

30

Lymphoma and Disease of Bone Marrow

Thankamma V. Ajithkumar

CHAPTER OUTLINE

LYMPHOMAS

Introduction

Lymphomas present as solid masses arising in lymph nodes or at extranodal sites anywhere in the body, whereas leukaemias and multiple myeloma are diseases primarily of the bone marrow. They are chemo- and radiosensitive and, in contrast to the typical solid tumours, many are curable despite being widespread. Treatments range from simple oral chemotherapy and low-dose radiotherapy (RT) to high-dose chemotherapy, total-body irradiation (TBI) and haemopoietic stem cell transplantation (HSCT). Small molecule inhibitors, monoclonal antibodies and immunotherapy are also entering the clinic.

Lymphomas derive from malignant lymphocytes, with 90% of B-cell and 10% T-cell origin. They are conventionally divided into Hodgkin (HL) and non-Hodgkin (NHL) types. The former, named after Thomas Hodgkin, who described it in 1832, is highly curable, whereas NHL is a diverse group of conditions.

Aetiology and Epidemiology

HL accounts for 0.7% of all cancers and 0.4% of cancer deaths. In the United Kingdom, approximately 2100 new cases of HL are reported each year. It is more common among males (58%). There are two age peaks, from 15 to 35 years and a smaller old-age peak. There is an association between the Epstein-Barr virus (EBV) and higher social class.

Approximately 14,000 new cases of NHL are diagnosed every year in the United Kingdom, and the median age is 55 to 60 years. The incidence of childhood NHL is very low in developed countries, but the incidence is higher in developing countries, particularly of Burkitt lymphoma. Overall, the male-to-female ratio is 1.5:1, although this varies between subtypes.

The causes of most NHL are unknown, but the risk is increased in immunodeficiency syndromes, immunosuppression following organ transplantation, acquired immunodeficiency syndrome (AIDS), autoimmune disorders, coeliac disease and following certain infections or exposure to ionising radiation and carcinogenic chemicals. Characteristic, acquired chromosomal defects include the following translocations involving the immunoglobulin (Ig) genes on chromosome 14q32:

- t(14;18)(q32;q21) in about 80% of follicular lymphoma, involving the BCL2 gene on chromosome 18q21
- t(11;14)(q13;q32) in all cases of mantle-cell lymphoma, involving the Cyclin D1 gene on chromosome 11q13
- t(8:14)(q24;q32) in Burkitt lymphoma, involving the MYC gene on chromosome 8q24

NHL can result from chronic antigenic stimulation of lymphocytes, as in marginal zone lymphoma of mucosa-associated lymphoid tissue (MALT) following *Helicobacter pylori* infection, usually in the stomach or, rarely, following *Chlamydia psittaci* infection. Burkitt lymphoma, initially described in East African children and classically in the jaw, is associated with EBV. A rare but very aggressive type of T-cell NHL is caused by infection with the human T-cell leukaemia virus type 1 (HTLV-1).

Pathological Characteristics

Prognosis and therapy depend on the maturity and subtype of the cell of origin. This is defined by:

1. Morphology: Appearance and arrangement of cells
2. Immunophenotyping: Cellular differentiation (CD) cell surface antigens identified by a panel of antibodies
3. Cytogenetics: Chromosome translocations
4. Molecular biology: Gene expression and genetic mutations

The World Health Organization (WHO) classification includes HL and NHL (Table 30.1). A specialist haematopathologist is essential for accurate categorisation. Morphologically, aggressive NHL can resemble poorly differentiated carcinoma, and indolent NHL may be confused with benign lymphadenopathy.

Hodgkin Lymphoma

HL is characterised by Reed-Sternberg (RS) cells, although these are only 2% to 4% of the cells present. The bulk of the tumour consists of normal reactive lymphocytes, histiocytes, plasma cells, granulocytes and fibroblasts. RS cells are large and multinucleated with prominent eosinophilic nucleoli and express CD30 and CD15. There are two subtypes of HL: classical HL (cHL) and nodular lymphocyte-predominant HL (NLPHL). CHL has an excellent overall survival rate of around 85% at 5 years. NLPHL has a long natural history with distant relapses, more like indolent NHL.

Non-Hodgkin Lymphoma

Follicular lymphoma and diffuse large B-cell lymphoma (DLBCL) comprise 80% of all NHL seen in the West. They are described as indolent and aggressive, respectively, and are grouped with other NHL subtypes, although each is quite distinct.

Aggressive Non-Hodgkin Lymphoma. DLBCL behaves aggressively but is curable in up to 60% of patients. Bone marrow is involved in 10% to 15% of cases. It forms sheets of large cells, often multinucleate with prominent nucleoli. Adverse prognostic markers include expression of p53 and BCL2 proteins and MIB-1 (Ki67). As in Burkitt lymphoma, high proliferation rates (100% MIB-1 staining) are associated with programmed cell death (apoptosis). Pale apoptotic cells in a uniform background of dark blue malignant lymphocytes appear as a starry sky. Thus, at the aggressive end of the spectrum of DLBCL, it may seem and behave like Burkitt or lymphoblastic lymphoma, the truly high-grade types that grow and spread most rapidly but are curable with aggressive treatment. Gene expression profiling of DLBCL cases has identified two major subtypes based on unique gene signatures: germinal centre B-cell like (GCB-DLBCL) and activated B-cell like (ABC-DLBCL). The latter is associated with greater resistance to conventional chemotherapy and worse clinical outcomes.

Mantle cell lymphoma (MCL), characterised by cyclin-D1 and CD5 expression, progresses slowly but has a poor prognosis (median survival 3–4 years) because of chemoresistance. Peripheral T-cell lymphoma is a heterogeneous group of diseases that typically behave aggressively with poor clinical outcomes.

Indolent Non-Hodgkin Lymphoma. In follicular lymphoma, cells arise from lymph node germinal centres and form structures resembling normal follicles. The number of large follicular lymphoma cells seen under the microscope determines the grade. Grade 3b behaves as DLBCL, and grades 1, 2 and 3a behave in a low-grade, indolent way (median survival 7–9 years). It inevitably recurs unless truly localised at diagnosis (15%). It can transform into DLBCL with a poor prognosis. Bone marrow involvement is common (>60%). Marginal zone lymphomas, presumed to arise from the small B cells of nodal or splenic marginal zones, also behave indolently.

Extranodal Non-Hodgkin Lymphoma. DLBCL is the usual type of NHL presenting in the head and neck (Waldeyer's ring, nasal sinuses, thyroid), bone, testis, breast and brain. The marginal zone lymphoma

TABLE 30.1 Simplified Classification of Tumours of Haematopoietic and Lymphoid Tissues Based on the 5th Edition (2022) of WHO Classification of Haematolymphoid Tumours

Precursor B-cell neoplasms

B-cell lymphoblastic leukaemias/lymphomas

Mature B-cell neoplasms

Preneoplastic and neoplastic small lymphocytic proliferations
- Chronic lymphocytic leukaemia/small lymphocytic lymphoma

Splenic B-cell lymphomas and leukaemias
- Hairy cell leukaemia
- Splenic marginal zone lymphoma
- Splenic diffuse red pulp small B-cell lymphoma
- Splenic B-cell lymphoma/leukaemia with prominent nucleoli

Lymphoplasmacytic lymphoma

Marginal zone lymphoma
- Extranodal marginal zone lymphoma of mucosa-associated lymphoid tissue
- Primary cutaneous marginal zone lymphoma
- Nodal marginal zone lymphoma

Follicular lymphoma

Mantle cell lymphoma

Transformations of indolent B-cell lymphomas

Large B-cell lymphomas
- Diffuse large B-cell lymphoma, NOS
- T-cell/histiocyte-rich large B-cell lymphoma
- Diffuse large B-cell lymphoma/high-grade B-cell lymphoma with MYC and BCL2 rearrangements
- Anaplastic lymphoma kinase-positive large B-cell lymphoma
- Large B-cell lymphoma with IRF4 rearrangement
- Lymphomatoid granulomatosis
- Fibrin-associated large B-cell lymphoma
- Fluid overload-associated large B-cell lymphoma
- Plasmablastic lymphoma
- Primary large B-cell lymphoma of immune-privileged sites (central nervous system, vitreoretinal and testis)
- Primary cutaneous diffuse large B-cell lymphoma, leg type
- Primary mediastinal large B-cell lymphoma
- Mediastinal grey zone lymphoma

Burkitt lymphoma

Hodgkin lymphoma
- Classical Hodgkin lymphoma
- Nodular lymphocyte predominant Hodgkin lymphoma

Plasma cell neoplasms

Precursor T-cell neoplasms

T-lymphoblastic leukaemia/lymphoma

Mature T-cell and NK-cell neoplasms

Mature T-cell and NK-cell leukaemias

Primary cutaneous T-cell lymphomas

Intestinal T-cell and NK-cell lymphoid proliferations and lymphomas

Anaplastic large cell lymphoma

Epstein-Barr virus-positive NK/T-cell lymphomas

Mesenchymal dendritic cell neoplasms

Follicular dendritic cell sarcoma

Epstein-Barr virus-positive inflammatory follicular dendritic cell sarcoma

Myofibroblastic tumour

Splenic vascular-stromal tumours

Littoral cell angioma

Splenic hamartoma

predominates in the stomach, orbit, salivary glands, lung and spleen, whereas intestinal lymphoma is commonly of T-cell origin and associated with coeliac disease. NHL may arise in the skin from either B or T cells. Histological diagnosis is often difficult, and clonality studies using IG or TCR rearrangements are needed to distinguish reactive conditions. Mycosis fungoides is a very slowly progressive epidermal tumour of T-cell origin, which may develop a leukaemic form (Sézary syndrome). Anaplastic large-cell lymphoma (ALCL), also of T-cell origin, may arise in the skin or elsewhere and has a good prognosis if CD30 and anaplastic lymphoma kinase (ALK) antigens are expressed. Cutaneous B-cell NHL includes follicular, marginal zone and DLBCL.

Clinical Features

All lymphomatous nodes may spontaneously wax and wane. They have a rubbery consistency and are smooth, multiple, discrete, mobile and painless. These nodes can enlarge to 10 cm or more without fixation or skin involvement, unlike carcinomatous nodes, which invade surrounding structures early. However, patients with aggressive lymphoma can deteriorate rapidly with dehydration, hypercalcaemia, anaemia, infection and damage to critical organs.

HL usually presents with enlarged nodes in the neck (60%), mediastinal mass, axilla (20%) or groin (15%). The spleen (10%) or, rarely, the liver may also be enlarged. Mesenteric nodes, bone marrow and extranodal sites are rarely involved in HL but commonly in NHL. The spread of HL is contiguous, from one lymph node group to the next; in NHL it may not be, and only 10% are localised at presentation.

Three characteristic B symptoms are associated with lymphoma and a worse prognosis: drenching night sweats, weight loss (>10% of body weight in previous 6 months) and fever (>38°C), which may be of a specific periodicity (Pel-Ebstein fever). The disease is staged as A (none of these) or B (any of these). Itching (pruritus) occurs in 12% but is not considered a B symptom. Pain felt in involved lymph nodes after drinking alcohol is a symptom peculiar to cHL.

Approximately 20% of NHL involve extranodal sites. In the head and neck disease, there may be swelling, proptosis or nasal blockage. Thyroid lymphoma presents as a mass with stridor from tracheal compression and sometimes a history of Hashimoto thyroiditis. Primary bone NHL mainly affects proximal long bones and presents with pain, swelling and pathological fracture. Testicular NHL presents at ages 60 to 80 years with a painless, smooth swelling. Bilateral involvement occurs in 20% of patients. NHL of the breast presents with a mass often indistinguishable from carcinoma. Gastrointestinal (GI) lymphoma can present with pain, anaemia or bowel obstruction. Primary cerebral lymphoma presents with raised intracranial pressure or focal neurological deficits, including seizures. In the skin, mycosis fungoides start as erythematous, flat, slightly scaly, itchy lesions on the buttocks, upper thighs or breasts. These develop into thicker plaques and fungating tumours with nodal and visceral involvement. The whole skin may become involved, resulting in generalised erythroderma or l'homme rouge. B-cell cutaneous lymphoma is more likely to present as a discrete fleshy nodular lump with a tendency to ulcerate. Cutaneous ALCL occasionally undergoes spontaneous remission.

Diagnosis and Staging

A formal excision biopsy is preferred and should ideally be sent fresh to the laboratory. Core biopsies are increasingly obtained because of logistical ease but may risk inconclusive results requiring further biopsies. Fine needle aspiration (FNA) is inadequate for accurate diagnosis of lymphoma. There is usually no need to debulk the tumour surgically except when large mediastinal masses compromise the major airways.

TABLE 30.2 Lugano Staging Classification of Lymphoma (2014)

Limited
I: A single lymph node or group of adjacent nodes[a]
IE: A single extranodal lesion without nodal involvement
II: Two or more nodal groups on the same side of the diaphragm
II bulky[b]: Stage II with bulky disease[c]
IIE: Stage I or II nodal diseases with limited contiguous extranodal involvement
Advanced
III: Nodes on both sides of the diaphragm, nodes above the diaphragm with splenic involvement
IV: Additional noncontiguous extra lymphatic disease

[a]Tonsils, Waldeyer's ring and spleen are considered as a nodal disease.
[b]II bulky disease is treated as limited or advanced based on histology and prognostic factors.
[c]Bulky disease for Hodgkin lymphoma is defined as a single nodal mass of ≥10 cm or greater than one-third of thoracic diameter at *any level* of thoracic vertebrae in computed tomography scan. For both Hodgkin and non-Hodgkin lymphoma, the longest diameter as recorded by a designation of X is no longer necessary.
Note: Only Hodgkin lymphoma needs to be assigned A or B status. Splenomegaly is defined as a vertical splenic length of >13 cm.

Staging establishes the extent of the disease using the Ann Arbor classification (Table 30.2), clinical assessment and essential investigations:

1. Blood tests including full blood count, plasma viscosity, serum urea and electrolytes, calcium, liver function, lactate dehydrogenase (LDH), β2-microglobulin and serum Igs.
2. Computed tomography (CT) scan of chest, abdomen and pelvis with intravenous and oral contrast.
3. Positron emission tomography (PET) showing fluorodeoxyglucose (FDG) uptake into areas actively metabolising glucose. Most lymphomas are metabolically very active and so show up clearly.
4. Bone marrow aspirates and a small core of bone (trephine) taken from the posterior iliac crest. This is no longer required in HL and DLBCL, where the absence of PET uptake in bone has been shown to exclude bone marrow involvement adequately.
5. Lumbar puncture for high-risk groups (discussed shortly). Methotrexate 12.5 mg is usually injected at the time of the procedure.

Clinical Prognostic Factors

Prognostically limited stage (stage I–II) HL is classified as favourable or unfavourable based on risk factors, and the EORTC and German Hodgkin Study Group (GHSG) are given in Tables 30.3 and 30.4. The 5-year freedom from progression (FFP) is predicted using the international prognostic score (IPS), which is based on seven factors (albumin <4 g/dL, haemoglobin <10.5 g/dL, male, age ≥45 years, stage IV disease, white blood cell count ≥15,000/mm^3 and lymphocyte count <8% of WBC, or lymphocyte count <600/mm^3). Without any prognostic factors, the 5-year FFP is 84%, which is reduced by approximately 8% with the presence of each factor.

In DLBCL, the international prognostic index (IPI), validated in the pre-rituximab era, remains a widely accepted prognostic score from 0 to 5, with one point for each of the following features:

1. Age 60 years or older
2. More than one extranodal site
3. Stage III or IV disease
4. High LDH
5. WHO performance status 2 to 4

The National Comprehensive Cancer Network (NCCN)-IPI score has been validated in the rituximab era and appears to discriminate

TABLE 30.3 Prognostic Groups in Limited-Disease Hodgkin Lymphoma

Risk Factors	EORTC	GHSG
Age	≥50 years	-
ESR and B symptoms	>50 if A; >30 if B	>50 if A; >30 if B
Mediastinal mass	Mediastinal thoracic ratio (MTR)[a] >0.35	Mediastinal mass ratio (MMR)[b] >0.33
Number of nodal sites[c]	>3	>2
Extranodal lesions	-	any
Definition of prognostic group		
Favourable	Stage I–II without risk factors	Stage I–II without risk factors
Unfavourable	Stage I–II with any risk factors	• Stage I–IIA with any risk factors • Stage IIB with elevated ESR or ≥3 lymph node sites

[a]MTR: Ratio of maximum width of mediastinal mass and intrathoracic diameter at T5-6
[b]MMR: Ratio of maximum width of mediastinal mass and maximum intrathoracic diameter
[c]Nodal site definitions differ between EORTC and GHSG.

TABLE 30.4 Comparison of Supradiaphragmatic Lymph Node Areas According to EORTC and GHSG

EORTC	GHSG
Whole neck including supraclavicular area (right and left)	Whole neck including supraclavicular and *infraclavicular/subpectoral* (right and left)
Axilla *including infraclavicular/subpectoral* (right and left)	Axilla (right and left)
Mediastinum including both hilar nodes	Mediastinum including both hilar nodes

better good- and poor-risk DLBCL. There is an increased risk of central nervous system (CNS) relapse in DLBCL involving the testis, breast and epidural space and in those with raised LDH and more than one extranodal site. Burkitt and lymphoblastic lymphomas carry a significant risk of CNS disease, with treatment protocols including CNS-directed therapy.

Treatment

Initial Management

It is essential to avoid treatment before any biopsy. If awaiting results, steroids may be given (e.g. prednisolone 100 mg daily) to arrest clinical deterioration. In an emergency such as airway obstruction, treatment with RT may be necessary. Urgent chemotherapy can rescue very ill patients despite toxicity. Rapid tumour breakdown can cause tumour lysis syndrome because of the release of cytokines and intracellular products, causing raised serum urate, phosphate and potassium; reduced calcium and impaired renal function; and, rarely, lung function. To prevent this, patients should start allopurinol (300 mg daily), ideally at least 24 hours before chemotherapy, and be very well hydrated. Individuals deemed at very high risk of tumour lysis (very high tumour burden as in Burkitt lymphoma) may receive rasburicase, a synthetic enzyme that breaks down the damaging urate.

Males should be offered sperm storage before chemotherapy. Fertility preservation in females requires ovarian stimulation before egg or embryo storage, which may not be feasible if there is a need to initiate chemotherapy urgently. Preservation of ovarian tissue is under study.

Hodgkin Lymphoma

Historically, extensive field RT was the first curative treatment for stages I–III HL, and chemotherapy (e.g. mustine, vincristine, procarbazine and prednisolone (MOPP)) was used initially for salvage and subsequently as the first treatment. However, cures were achieved at a significant cost of severe toxicities. The intense treatment resulted in up to 10% of patients developing secondary acute myeloid leukaemia and, subsequently, other secondary malignancies, particularly in irradiated areas. Heart disease was also increased. After 10 to 15 years, the risk of death from these causes was greater than from relapse of HL, with many patients rendered infertile. In young females treated with mantle fields, the risk of breast cancer increases with age from 8 years after treatment up to as high as 50% in middle age for those treated in their early teens, or up to 25% if treated at ages 20 to 29 years, and early screening is now offered. Thyroid cancer, colon cancer and sarcomas are also seen. Over the past few decades, treatment approaches have changed significantly, with smaller radiation fields with lower doses to minimise second malignancies and cardiotoxicity.

Limited-Stage Favourable Disease cHL. For limited-stage favourable disease, the GHSG HD10 trial reported a 10-year progression-free survival of 87% with two cycles of Adriamycin (doxorubicin), bleomycin, vinblastine and dacarbazine (ABVD) followed by involved-field radiotherapy (IFRT) of 20 Gy in 10 fractions. Subsequent studies (UK-NCRI RAPID, EORTC/LYSA/FIL H10 and the GHSG HD16 trial) have evaluated the role of early PET scans to guide RT. These studies showed that in patients who achieve complete metabolic response (CMR, defined as a Deauville score of 1–3) after two to three cycles of chemotherapy, progression-free survival is improved by 7% to 12% by adding RT but without an improvement in overall survival. Therefore, the decision to omit RT should be made carefully after a detailed discussion in a multidisciplinary team (MDT) meeting. After discussion, if it is decided to avoid RT, three to four cycles of ABVD should be offered. Patients who do not achieve CMR after two cycles of ABVD should be considered for four cycles for ABVD followed by involved-site radiotherapy (ISRT) (30 Gy in 15 fractions) or, based on the EORTC/LYSA/FIL H10 trial, two cycles of escalated bleomycin, etoposide, doxorubicin, cyclophosphamide, vincristine, procarbazine and prednisolone (eBEACOPP) followed by ISRT (30 Gy in 15 fractions).

Limited-Stage Unfavourable Disease cHL. In the pre-PET era, patients with limited-stage unfavourable disease were treated with four cycles of ABVD followed by IFRT (30 Gy) or two cycles of eBEACOPP followed by two cycles of ABVD (2+2 protocol) with IFRT. The GHSG HD17 study suggests that in patients who achieve a CMR with the 2+2 protocol, RT can be avoided without compromising 5-year progression-free survival (95%). In the H10 trial, patients were randomised to receive four more cycles of ABVD or two more cycles of ABVD plus involved-node radiotherapy (INRT) after achieving CMR with two cycles of ABVD. Patients who did not receive INRT had inferior 5-year progression-free survival (89.6% versus 92.1%) compared with those who received INRT. Patients on the HD17 approach receive the 2+2 protocol followed by surveillance if they achieve CMR at the end of chemotherapy or ISRT (30 Gy) if they do not achieve CMR. Alternatively, using the H10 approach, patients can be treated with two cycles of ABVD followed by an interim PET scan. If patients achieve CMR, the options are either two more cycles of A(B)VD followed by ISRT (30 Gy) or four more cycles of A(B)VD. Those who do not achieve CMR are treated with two cycles of eBEACOPP followed by ISRT (30 Gy).

Advanced Disease cHL. The initial systemic therapy can be two cycles of ABVD or eBEACOPP followed by an interim PET scan.

Patients achieving a CMR after ABVD are treated with four cycles of AVD, and those who do not have a CMR are treated with four cycles of eBEACOPP. Patients achieving a CMR after eBEACOPP are treated with either four cycles of A(B)VD or two more cycles of eBEACOPP. Those who don't have a CMR are treated with four more cycles of eBEACOPP. Patients with residual disease after chemotherapy are considered for consolidation RT. In the GHSG HD15 study, patients with PET-positive residual disease of 2.5 cm or more who received 30 Gy had a 4-year progression-free survival of 86.3%.

Nodular Lymphocyte-Predominant Hodgkin Lymphoma. Approximately 80% of patients with NLPHL present with limited-stage disease, and ISRT alone is curative with a reported 8-year progression-free survival of >90%. Unfortunately, the prognosis of advanced NLPHL is worse than that for cHL, and the indications for RT in the advanced stage are like those for cHL.

RT alone may be the treatment of choice for elderly and unfit patients who are not suitable for chemotherapy. Extended-field RT is used after a partial response to chemotherapy with disease at several sites or where chemotherapy has had to be curtailed, especially in patients who would be unsuitable for HSCT.

High-dose chemotherapy (HDCT) followed by autologous haematopoietic stem cell transplantation (ASCT) is the treatment of choice for patients with primary refractory or relapsed HL. Adding RT may improve outcomes in patients with a focal area of recurrent or refractory disease in a previously unirradiated area.

Non-Hodgkin Lymphoma

Aggressive Non-Hodgkin Lymphoma. The addition of an anti-CD20 human/mouse monoclonal antibody (rituximab) to each cycle of cyclophosphamide, hydroxydaunorubicin, Oncovin (vincristine) and prednisolone once every 3 weeks (R-CHOP) has increased complete response rates from 63% to 76% and 3-year overall survival from 51% to 62% with minimal toxicity. R-CHOP remains the current standard for aggressive NHL. For limited-stage diffuse aggressive B- or T-cell nodal lymphomas, three to four cycles of chemotherapy (R-CHOP) followed by RT yield a 5-year survival of 80% to 90%.

Stage I–II aggressive NHL is treated with four to six cycles of R-CHOP. Patients age 18 to 60 years, with age-adjusted IPI (aaIPI) 0 and nonbulky disease, are offered four cycles of R-CHOP plus two additional infusions of rituximab without RT. Patients age 60 to 80 years with aaIPI 0 and nonbulky disease are treated with four cycles of R-CHOP if an interim PET scan after two cycles shows CMR or six cycles of R-CHOP with ISRT (30Gy) if no CMR after two cycles. Patients younger than age 80 years and with IPI 0–1 are treated with three to four cycles of R-CHOP followed by ISRT (30 Gy) or six cycles of R-CHOP when the risk of RT is greater than additional cycles of R-CHOP. For patients younger than age 80 years with IPI of 2 or higher, six cycles of R-CHOP-polatuzumab vedotin or six cycles of R-CHOP are treatment options. For patients age 80 years and older, a dose of reduced chemotherapy (R-miniCHOP) is considered.

Advanced-stage aggressive NHL is treated with six cycles of R-CHOP-polatuzumab vedotin or six cycles of R-CHOP. More intensive chemotherapy (e.g. R-CODOX-M/R-IVAC) may be considered for younger patients (age ≤50 years) with good performance status and IPI of 3 of higher, particularly those at risk of CNS relapse.

In high-risk groups, prophylactic CNS treatment is given concurrently as intrathecal or high-dose intravenous methotrexate. An interim PET scan (after two cycles of chemotherapy) has been increasingly used to individualise RT indications.

Aggressive lymphomas can also occur in extranodal sites such as the testes, breast, stomach, bones and brain. The optimal management is uncertain. Primary testicular lymphomas are treated with six cycles of R-CHOP, CNS prophylaxis and contralateral testicular RT to reduce the risk of recurrence. Primary breast lymphomas are treated with six cycles of R-CHOP, and CNS prophylaxis and consolidation RT are considered. Primary gastric lymphomas are treated with six cycles of R-CHOP and eradication therapy if *H. pylori* is detected. Primary bone lymphoma is treated with six cycles of R-CHOP followed by consideration for consolidation RT. In primary cerebral lymphoma, the standard treatment is induction chemotherapy with a high-dose methotrexate-based regimen followed by consolidation treatment with high-dose systemic therapy with stem cell rescue if there is a complete response or complete response unconfirmed. Whole brain radiotherapy (WBRT) is an option for consolidation if patients are not suitable for high-dose systemic therapy or have residual disease after induction chemotherapy. WBRT is an effective palliative treatment for patients who are not fit for induction chemotherapy.

At relapse after full-course chemotherapy, HSCT can be curative if chemosensitivity can be shown with salvage regimens (e.g. ICE: ifosfamide, carboplatin, etoposide ± rituximab; GDP: gemcitabine, dexamethasone, cisplatin ± rituximab). Time to relapse is the most important predictive factor, with rituximab refractory disease showing the worst outcome. CAR-T cell therapy is the current standard of care for patients with primary refractory disease or those with relapse within 12 months of first-line treatment. Typically, patients may need bridging systemic therapy, ISRT or both until CAR-T cells are available for infusion.

Burkitt lymphomas are treated with more intensive regimens, such as a cyclophosphamide, vincristine and doxorubicin, with intrathecal methotrexate and cytarabine followed by high-dose intravenous methotrexate (CODOX-M) regimen, which is combined with rituximab and can cure around 50% of patients.

Selected patients with early-stage MCL may be considered for ISRT (24 Gy). For patients younger than age 65 years and with good performance status, an induction chemotherapy regimen containing rituximab, followed by ASCT consolidation, is the standard of care. The Bruton's tyrosine kinase (BTK) inhibitor ibrutinib should be offered during the R-CHOP component of R-CHOP/R-DHAP induction and for 2 years of maintenance if ASCT is not feasible. Patients with refractory and relapsed disease are offered CAR-T using brexucabtagene autoleucel (brexu-cel).

Optimal treatment for peripheral T-cell lymphoma remains unclear, with most patients treated with first-line remission induction chemotherapy (e.g. CHOP). ISRT is considered for patients with early-stage disease and high-dose chemotherapy-conditioned auto-HSCT to consolidate first complete remission.

Indolent Non-Hodgkin Lymphoma. Truly localised (15%) follicular NHL may be cured with RT (24 Gy in 12 fractions) alone. Low doses (4 Gy in 2 fractions) can achieve excellent palliation. In widespread disease, a watch-and-wait approach is acceptable for asymptomatic patients. Immediate treatment with rituximab has not been shown to alter survival but may reduce patient anxiety. On symptomatic progression, chemotherapy (e.g. bendamustine, CHOP, CVP) combined with rituximab or obinutuzumab (anti-CD20 antibodies) is the treatment option. Oral chlorambucil with antibodies may be an option for elderly, less-fit patients.

The PRIMA trial showed that patients who responded to initial systemic therapy, 2 years of maintenance of 2-monthly rituximab, improved 10-year progression-free survival by 16% (51% versus 35%), and 60% of patients in the maintenance arm did not require another line of therapy at 10 years. However, there is no overall survival benefit, and there is concern regarding increased incidence of infection. Therefore, maintenance with anti-CD20 antibody therapy should be considered after discussing the risks and benefits with patients.

At relapse, rebiopsy is advisable to detect high-grade transformation. Selection and timing of treatment depends on the patient's disease-free interval, extent of relapse, age and general condition. Rechallenge with immunochemotherapy is appropriate for patients with long remission periods. Those with short remission periods are considered for rituximab with alternative chemotherapy, and those who are refractory to rituximab are considered for bendamustine in combination with obinutuzumab. High-dose chemotherapy with autologous stem cell rescue is considered for fit patients with relapsed disease who achieve a second or subsequent remission. Patients who haven't previously received maintenance anti-CD20 antibodies and are unsuitable for high-dose therapy are considered for 2 years of maintenance anti-CD20 antibodies.

Marginal zone NHL is described as three types: splenic, nodal and those of MALT origin. Splenectomy is appropriate for the first type; the others respond to the same agents and general approach as follicular NHL. Although the disease pattern is different with more extranodal sites, RT can still be curative for disease truly localised to, for example, the stomach or parotid. Anti-*Helicobacter* therapy is potentially curative in gastric MALT NHL. Gastric MALT can be monitored through regular endoscopies.

Mycosis fungoides has a median survival of 10 years. In the early stages, topical steroids can be used, then often photochemotherapy, using long-wave ultraviolet light with oral psoralens (PUVA). RT can be local or to the whole skin surface using low-energy electrons. Systemic treatments include alemtuzumab (anti-CD52 antibody), which targets T cells. Combination chemotherapy with a CHOP-type regimen is used in visceral disease, but complete response rates are low (20%–25%).

Special Situations

Lymphoma in Children. RT in children causes growth retardation in the treated area, and they are particularly susceptible to second malignancies, so chemotherapy is used alone whenever possible. Lower radiation doses are adequate in paediatric HL, and extranodal presentations are rarer: lymphadenopathy is the presenting feature in 90% of cases.

Lymphoma in Pregnancy. HL is the most common diagnosis. Staging should avoid exposure to ionising radiation, using magnetic resonance imaging (MRI) or ultrasound in preference to CT. RT is potentially teratogenic during the first trimester. A dose higher than 0.1 Gy to the foetus poses a risk of inducing an abnormality. Chemotherapy has an unquantified risk of teratogenesis or carcinogenesis to the foetus.

Termination should be considered if treatment is essential before the early second trimester, if the foetal dose exceeds 0.1 Gy or if chemotherapy is indicated. If the diagnosis is made late in the second or third trimester, it may be possible to postpone treatment until delivery is induced at 32 to 34 weeks. Localised RT above the diaphragm can be safely given, and single-agent chemotherapy may control symptoms in HL for a few weeks. Still, if the disease is life-threatening, combination chemotherapy is best. With ABVD, the risk of carcinogenesis or infertility in the child should be low.

Patients who have been successfully treated for HD should be advised to avoid pregnancy for 2 years after the end of treatment because, after this, the risk of relapse falls markedly. Subsequent pregnancy does not increase the risk of relapse.

Lymphoma in Human Immunodeficiency Virus and Posttransplant. Human immunodeficiency virus (HIV)-associated lymphoma is usually aggressive, presenting with high IPI scores and often CNS disease. Patients are more prone to succumb to infective complications of treatment. NHL is an AIDS-defining illness, but HL is not. Historical survival outcomes were poor but have significantly improved with R-CHOP and the use of highly active antiretroviral therapy (HAART) and are similar to non-HIV lymphoma.

Posttransplant lymphoproliferative disease (PTLD) is an often localised NHL presenting after organ transplantation. It usually remits on the gradual withdrawal of immunosuppressive therapy, but if not, options include rituximab, R-CHOP and ISRT if disease is localised.

MULTIPLE MYELOMA

Multiple myeloma accounts for 2% of all cancers, and about 6000 new cases are diagnosed annually in the United Kingdom. The median age at diagnosis is 62 years, and the male-to-female ratio is 1.5:1. The aetiology is unknown.

Pathology

Myeloma is a tumour of plasma cells, which are Ig-producing B lymphocytes. Their bone marrow microenvironment is increasingly well understood, and new molecular targets for treatment have been identified. Myeloma cells potentiate osteoclast activity and inhibit differentiation of osteoblast precursors, uncoupling bone formation from resorption, so multiple lytic bone lesions are characteristic. They also produce a specific Ig or paraprotein, detectable by immunoelectrophoresis and valuable for diagnosis and treatment monitoring. Although an intact Ig molecule is too large to enter the renal tubules, free light chains (Bence Jones protein) may be produced and are found in the urine. Serum-free light chains can also be quantified in the blood. Normal Igs are reduced, resulting in recurrent infections (immune paresis). In 2%, there is no secreted protein, and the disease is termed *nonsecretory*. Bence Jones only is found in 20%, whereas Ig subtypes are found with frequencies reflecting normal levels, that is, IgG in 50% to 60%, IgA in 20% to 25%, IgD in 2% and IgE and IgM in less than 1%. Paraproteinemia is also found in lymphoma. IgM is associated with Waldenström macroglobulinemia or marginal zone lymphoma. In the normal population, paraproteinemia is found in 1% of those age over 25 years, 3% over 70 years and 25% over 90 years. This is monoclonal gammopathy of uncertain significance (MGUS) and carries an annual risk of 1% of progression to multiple myeloma. Asymptomatic early myeloma is termed *smoldering*.

Clinical Features

The most common presenting feature is bone pain (70%) from a rib or vertebra. The destruction of cortical bone leads to pathological fractures in about 25% and hypercalcemia in 30%. Alkaline phosphatase is normal, and bone lesions are lytic. Spinal cord compression is occasionally the presenting feature and is an emergency. Humoral and cell-mediated immunity are impaired, and recurrent infections are common. Most patients have cytokine-mediated anaemia; pancytopenia due to marrow replacement is uncommon at presentation. One-third have reduced white cell count and platelets. Erythrocyte sedimentation rate (ESR) is raised. Renal failure occurs because of deposition of Bence Jones protein in the renal tubules, dehydration, infection and nonsteroidal antiinflammatory drugs.

If the paraprotein level is high enough, a hyperviscosity syndrome develops, characterised by visual impairment, lethargy and coma. This is most commonly associated with the IgM subtype, as these form larger structures in the blood. Amyloidosis, a deposition of abnormal protein in the kidneys, heart, nerves or other sites, is seen in about 10% of myeloma patients.

A plasmacytoma is a solitary plasma cell mass, usually arising in a rib or vertebra and other bones and soft tissues, with or without a paraprotein. Progression to multiple myeloma is probable but not inevitable.

Diagnosis

The following criteria should be met for the diagnosis:

1. Clonal bone marrow plasma cells 10% or more, or biopsy-proven plasmacytoma

2. One or more of the following multiple myeloma-defining events (MDEs)
   a. Hypercalcaemia, renal impairment, anaemia or bone lesions (CRAB)
   b. Clonal bone marrow plasma cell percentage 60% or higher
   c. Involved-to-uninvolved serum-free light chain ratio ≥100 (involved free light chain (FLC) level must be ≥100 mg/L)
   d. More than one focal lesion on MRI studies (at least 5 mm in size)

Investigations

1. Full blood count.
2. Serum urea, creatinine and electrolytes.
3. Serum calcium.
4. Serum electrophoresis with immunofixation (SIFE) and FLC assay.
5. Urine electrophoresis (increasingly replaced by serum-free light chain quantitation).
6. Bone marrow examination, including fluorescent in situ hybridisation (FISH).
7. Low-dose whole-body CT or positron emission tomography-computed tomography (PET/CT) imaging to assess the extent of bone disease. A conventional skeletal survey is only recommended if resources for advanced imaging are unavailable.
8. MRI of the spine if cord compression is suspected.

Prognostic Factors

Despite improved survival for multiple myeloma, 20% of people have a poor prognosis. Poor prognosis is associated with an increase in the B2-microglobulin level, low serum albumin, high serum LDH and the presence of high-risk chromosomal abnormalities (del (17p), t(4;14) and t(14;16)).

Treatment

Since 2000, patients with multiple myeloma have significantly improved (median survival of 127 months compared with 30 months for patients treated before 2000). Treatment aims to increase survival and improve quality of life by reducing malignant plasma cells in the bone marrow. Patients who are eligible for ASCT typically receive 3 to 6 months of induction therapy using a combination of a proteasome inhibitor (e.g. bortezomib), immunomodulatory drug (e.g. lenalidomide) and steroids (e.g. dexamethasone). Though there are no clearly defined eligibility criteria for ASCT, patients with good performance status and adequate organ function are usually considered. For patients who are not eligible for ASCT, the treatment intent is a continuation of tolerable treatment with minimal risk of discontinuation. Patients not suitable for ASCT but with good performance status are treated with the same induction therapy with or without an anti-CD38 antibody (e.g. daratumumab). In contrast, those with poor performance status are treated with two to three drug combinations. All patients are considered for maintenance therapy with immunomodulatory drugs or proteasome inhibitors.

Prophylactic bisphosphonate therapy is standard for all patients to inhibit bone resorption. Severe hyperviscosity is treated by plasmapheresis, in which some of the patient's plasma is replaced by an appropriate colloid solution (usually albumin) to reduce the paraprotein level. Nephrotoxic agents should be avoided if possible. Dialysis may be required for renal failure. Control of pain and infection is essential.

International Myeloma Working Group response criteria define response to treatment. Complete response requires all the following:

- Disappearance of any soft-tissue plasmacytomas
- Serum and urine M-protein not detected by immunofixation
- Normal FLC ratio (0.26–1.65) if serum and urine M-protein are unmeasurable
- Bone marrow plasma cell percentage less than 5%

Radiotherapy in Myeloma

Solitary plasmacytomas are treated radically with surgery and RT. Radical RT (40–50 Gy) achieves local control in 90% to 100% of patients and a 10-year myeloma-free interval in 45% to 50% of patients.

For diffuse disease, palliative RT relieves bone pain and is often used concomitantly with chemotherapy. Single fractions are commonly utilised, but higher doses may be needed, for example, if there are soft-tissue lesions associated with the bony abnormality or fracture risk. Hemibody treatments (6–8 Gy single dose) are effective for generalised pain in advanced disease, although these are seldom given due to better systemic and bone-directed therapies.

Spinal cord or cauda equina compression may occur at presentation or at any stage of the disease, and it may be caused by extradural disease or a collapsed vertebra. In diffuse disease, urgent RT is often preferable to surgery, but decompression and stabilisation followed by RT is sometimes more appropriate, so surgical consultation should be considered.

LEUKAEMIA

Bone marrow (haemopoietic) stem cells develop into lymphocytes (lymphoid cell line), red blood cells, platelets or granulocytes (myeloid cell line). Cells of all lineages at virtually any stage of differentiation may become malignant.

In acute leukaemia, the marrow fills with immature lymphoid or myeloid leukaemic cells, which displace normal cells and enter the peripheral blood. Untreated, death rapidly results from anaemia, bleeding and immunosuppression.

In chronic leukaemias, which arise from more mature cells, the disease can be stable with few symptoms for many years.

Leukaemia accounts for 2.1% of all cancers and 2.6% of cancer deaths and is more common in males. Described here are:

1. Acute leukaemia
   a. Lymphoblastic
   b. Myeloid
2. Chronic leukaemia
   a. Lymphocytic (chronic lymphocytic leukaemia)
   b. Myeloid (granulocytic) (chronic myeloid leukaemia)
3. Other myeloproliferative disorders

Acute Leukaemia

Acute lymphoblastic leukaemia (ALL) accounts for 80% of paediatric cases and 80% of adult cases. Chapter 34 further discusses ALL.

Acute myeloid leukaemia (AML) increases with age (median age 68 years). It may arise from myelodysplastic syndrome (MDS), a group of clonal stem cell disorders characterised by dysplasia in one or more lineages, ring sideroblasts and bone marrow blasts (if >20%, this becomes AML). Radiation can cause AML, as evidenced by survivors of atomic bombs (20:1) and whole spine irradiation for ankylosing spondylitis (10:1). The risk rises from about 3 years after exposure and peaks at 7 to 8 years.

Some cytotoxic drugs (alkylating agents, etoposide) can induce leukaemia. The risk after MOPP chemotherapy is 3%, and if given with wide-field irradiation for HL, the relative risk is about 6:1. Industrial chemicals, mainly benzene, can also induce AML.

Down syndrome (20:1) shows an inherited predisposition. Ataxia telangiectasias and other DNA repair defect syndromes, such as Bloom syndrome and Fanconi anaemia, all predispose to either ALL or AML, but these are very rare. Infection does not cause leukaemia except in the rare adult T-cell leukaemia/lymphoma syndrome (HTLV1 virus).

Chromosomal abnormalities and translocations are numerous and useful in defining prognostic groups; their absence after treatment verifies remission.

Clinical Features

AML presents with constitutional symptoms, fever, lymphadenopathy, hepatosplenomegaly, bleeding and gingival hypertrophy.

Treatment of Acute Myeloid Leukaemia

Based on cytogenetic and molecular analysis, AML is currently stratified into three prognostic groups: favourable, intermediate and adverse. Conventionally, intensive combination chemotherapy is used to induce remission. Standard regimens involve cytarabine and daunorubicin, plus etoposide, in younger patients. This can achieve an 80% remission rate in patients under age 60 years, but the remission rate is only about 40% in older patients. Relapse is usual without further treatment. Generally, allogeneic HSCT is recommended for patients with an estimated risk of relapse of greater than 35%. Two-thirds of the favourable risk group may be cured. Therefore, transplantation may be reserved for relapse, including those with a promyelocytic disease, where all-trans retinoic acid (ATRA) can induce blast cells to differentiate.

Newer agents are increasingly incorporated into induction therapy to improve outcomes. Approximately 30% of patients with AML have FLT3–ITD or FLT3–TKD mutations. The phase III RATIFY study showed that the addition of the multikinase inhibitor midostaurin to induction chemotherapy improved 4-year overall survival by 7%. The addition of anti-CD33 gemtuzumab ozogamicin to standard induction chemotherapy improved 5-year survival from 55% to 78% in patients with favourable risk core-binding factor leukaemias (t(8;21) or inv(16)).

Long-term cure is possible in younger patients with HSCT, but a cure is very unlikely in older patients or following relapse. Low-dose cytarabine or a hypomethylating agent (e.g. azacitidine or decitabine) is used for patients who are not suitable for intensive chemotherapy, with a median overall survival of less than 1 year. Novel agents are being increasingly investigated for this group of patients. For example, the phase III AGILE study showed that in patients with IDH1-mutated AML, a combination of azacitidine with the IDH1 inhibitor ivosidenib results in better medical survival compared with azacitidine alone (24 months versus 8 months).

Chronic Myeloid Leukaemia

Chronic myeloid leukaemia (CML) is a rare disease that occurs mainly in the fifth and sixth decades. The incidence in the United Kingdom is 1 in 100,000. There is a slight male predominance (1.4:1). In over 90% of cases, the Philadelphia chromosome is present, the result of a translocation from chromosome 22 to chromosome 9, resulting in a fusion BCR-ABL gene whose protein product ($p210^{BCR\text{-}ABL}$) is a tyrosine kinase enzyme essential for malignant transformation. Tyrosine kinase inhibitors (TKIs), such as imatinib (Gleevac), are drugs designed to inhibit these enzymes.

Clinical Features

Presentation is with tiredness because of anaemia or with splenomegaly, which may be massive. The total white cell count is typically between 100 and 500 × 10^9/L, a mixture of myeloid cells at varying stages of differentiation and less than 5% blasts, with this picture reflected in the marrow. The platelet count is normal or raised.

Natural history is of a chronic stable phase lasting an average of 4 to 6 years, though it can be up to a decade, followed by accelerated and terminal blastic phases.

Treatment

In most patients, TKIs are highly effective at inducing both clinical and cytogenetic complete remission in the chronic phase. While imatinib continues to be used widely as the first-line treatment for the chronic phase, second-generation TKIs such as dasatinib, nilotinib and bosutinib are accepted alternatives. Patients who fail to respond to a specific first-line TKI can be switched to an alternative drug within the same class (e.g. ponatinib). Allogeneic HSCT is now only reserved for patients resistant to second-generation TKIs, especially if there is no response to ponatinib. Patients who progress to the accelerated phase are treated with further lines of TKI, which yields a 4-to-5-year major haematological response rate of 45% to 66%. Patients with the accelerated phase at diagnosis have a similar outcome with TKI compared to those in the chronic phase (80%–90% complete cytogenetics response rate, 63%–76% major molecular response rate and 3-year overall survival of 87%–95%). Patients in the blast phase have a poor outcome with a median overall survival of 12 months.

Chronic Lymphocytic Leukaemia

Chronic lymphocytic leukaemia (CLL) is the most common form of leukaemia in the Western world. Its incidence in the United Kingdom is 5 per 100,000, and the male-to-female ratio is 2:1. CLL is usually seen in middle age, and its incidence increases with age. About 5% of cases exhibit some family history of B-cell lymphoproliferative disease, but the nature of the involved gene(s) remains unknown. It is not linked to radiation, chemical exposure or chemotherapy.

Clinical Features

CLL symptoms are mainly caused by anaemia or infection, although diagnosis is often made incidentally on a full blood count. The white cell count is usually between 30 and 300 × 10^9/L and comprises small mature lymphocytes with condensed nuclei and scant cytoplasm. The bone marrow is hypercellular, with an infiltrate composed of mature lymphocytes. Biopsy of enlarged nodes shows monotonous sheets of cells with characteristic proliferation centres.

Enlargement of lymph nodes of the neck and other peripheral sites, spleen and liver is common; staging systems are currently based on the number of enlarged lymph nodes and normal and abnormal cell counts and comprise stages A, B and C (Binet staging).

CLL is slowly progressive, although occasionally, notably with mutations of the p53 gene, resistant to all conventional therapy. In some patients the disease is stable for over 20 years.

Treatment

Most patients have early-stage asymptomatic disease, and treatment is only indicated for symptoms or if critical organs are threatened. The CLL International Prognostic Index (CLL-IPI), based on five factors such as age over 65 years, Rai stage I to IV, serum beta-2 microglobulin higher than 3.5 mg/L, unmutated immunoglobulin heavy chain (IGHV) genes and del17p by FISH or TP53 mutation, is a predictor for time to first treatment. Patients with low- and intermediate-risk CLL-IPI (approximately 70% of patients) are monitored, while high- and very-high-risk patients are offered early intervention. The first-line treatment options for patients who are not suitable for chemoimmunotherapy (CIT) are a combination of venetoclax (a BCL2 inhibitor) and obinutuzumab (anti-CD20) or acalabrutinib (a second-generation BTK inhibitor) irrespective of TP53 status. The treatment options for fit patients with TP53 disruption are acalabrutinib, ibrutinib or venetoclax monotherapy. Fit patients with intact TP53 are considered for venetoclax-obinutuzumab, and those with intact TP53 and mutated IGHV are treated with CIT with the FCR regimen (fludarabine, cyclophosphamide and rituximab). Sometimes CLL can transform into a high-grade lymphoma (Richter transformation) and is treated as DLBCL.

MYELOPROLIFERATIVE NEOPLASMS

Myeloproliferative neoplasms (MPNs) are a related group of disorders, including CML (described earlier), polycythemia vera (PV), essential thrombocythemia (ET) and primary myelofibrosis (PMF). They are slowly progressive, with a median survival of about 10 years. PV (excess red cells) and ET (excess platelets) can lead to myelofibrosis and AML. The exact aetiology of MPN is not known. Patients with a genetic mutation (Janus kinase 2-JAK2) and exposure to a high level of ionising radiation are at risk of developing MPNs. JAK2 mutation can be found in 90% of patients with PV and approximately 50% of patients with ET and PMF.

PV causes pruritus, splenomegaly and gout because of hyperuricemia, and PV and ET cause thromboses, particularly arterial, and less often, haemorrhages.

Patients with low-risk PV (age ≤60 years with no history of thrombotic events) are treated with low-dose aspirin and therapeutic phlebotomy to maintain haematocrit below 45%. Patients with high-risk PV are treated with therapeutic phlebotomy, low-dose aspirin and cytoreductive agents (e.g. hydroxyurea, busulfan).

The median survival of ET is 18 years and is categorised into four groups based on the risk of thrombosis: very low (age ≤60 years, no thrombosis history, JAK2 wild type), low (same as very low but JAK2 mutation present), intermediate (same as low but age >60 years) and high (thrombosis history or age >60 years with JAK2 mutation). The main goal of treatment is prevention of thrombosis. All patients receive low-dose aspirin; high-risk patients are considered for cytoreductive agents (e.g. hydroxyurea, pegylated interferon-α and second-line busulfan). Anagrelide is useful in ET because it prevents the maturation of platelets and is an option for patients who haven't responded to or are intolerant to other treatments.

In PMF, there is bone marrow fibrosis and failure with associated splenomegaly. The current international classification distinguishes 'prefibrotic' (may mimic ET at presentation) from 'overly fibrotic' PMF. Approximately 15% of patients with ET or PV may progress into PMF. Current prognostic scoring is based on mutations and karyotypes. Very-high-risk abnormalities include −7, inv (3), i(17q), +21, +19, 12p- and 11q-. Favourable risk abnormalities include normal karyotype or isolated +9, 13q-, 20q- or 1q abnormalities and loss of Y chromosome. Low- and very-low-risk disease has a good prognosis (10-year overall 56%–92%) and therefore is observed. Patients with very-high and high-risk disease (10-year overall survival 0%–13%) are considered for allogeneic HSCT. Systemic therapy improved anaemia, splenomegaly and other symptoms. Systemic agents include hydroxyurea and JAK2 inhibitors such as ruxolitinib, fedratinib and pacritinib. Splenectomy is considered for drug-refractory splenomegaly. RT helps achieve symptom control in splenomegaly and bone pain. However, in PMF the spleen may be a site of extramedullary haematopoiesis, and even a single dose of RT can cause significant cytopaenias (reported in 10%–30% of patients). Therefore, splenic RT should be carefully titrated starting at a fraction size of 0.1 to 0.5 Gy to avoid life-threatening cytopaenia. Splenic irradiation (to a total dose of 3–10 Gy) before allogeneic stem cell transplantation for myelofibrosis is increasingly used for patients with massive splenomegaly to improve clinical outcomes.

HAEMOPOIETIC STEM CELL TRANSPLANTATION

The term *haemopoietic stem cell transplantation (HSCT)* describes the collection and transplantation of HSC from bone marrow, peripheral blood or umbilical cord blood. HSCT is essential to the delivery of high-dose treatments used increasingly in haematological malignancies and will be referred to throughout this chapter.

Stem cells from the patient's marrow are autologous and allogeneic if donated by another HLA-matched person. Cells are transplanted by infusion through a central venous Hickman line and are then described as the *graft.*

Autografting has a 1% to 2% mortality. Stem cells are harvested from the peripheral blood after stimulating them to proliferate by giving conventional chemotherapy and granulocyte-colony stimulating growth factors (G-CSFs), and they are reinfused after high-dose therapy, which would otherwise be fatally myelosuppressive. Harvesting cells following prior chemotherapy may not be possible, especially with alkylating agents and fludarabine, and this problem has altered first-line treatments. Plerixafor inhibits a molecule in the bone marrow, releasing stem cells into the peripheral blood, and has been shown to increase the success of harvesting procedures.

Allografting has about a 30% mortality, lower with a sibling than with a matched unrelated donor (MUD). Still, it is the only curative option when there is residual disease in the marrow or autografting has failed. High-dose conditioning therapy is given to eradicate the underlying disease and immunosuppress the patient enough to prevent transplant rejection, for example, cyclophosphamide (Cy) 100 mg/kg over 2 days and TBI (Cy/TBI). Chemotherapy may be used alone, for example, cyclophosphamide and busulfan (Bu/Cy). Donor harvesting may be from peripheral blood or directly from bone (multiple punctures under general anaesthesia), which gives a better yield of cells. Allografting has the beneficial effect of donor T lymphocytes recognising residual malignant cells as foreign and destroying them.

Following chemoradiotherapy, the white cell and platelet counts drop within 10 days and recover after 3 to 6 weeks. Intensive support with antibiotics and red cell and platelet transfusions is needed during this period. Graft-versus-host disease (GvHD) occurs when T cells from the donor react with antigenic targets on host cells. It may be acute (jaundice, skin rashes, diarrhoea and weight loss) or chronic (arthritis, liver disease, malabsorption, oral mucositis and sicca syndrome, lung disease, pericardial and pleural effusions, scleroderma, skin rashes) and has a high mortality. The incidence is reduced by immunosuppression with cyclosporin A or tacrolimus and by depleting the donor T cells using monoclonal antibodies such as alemtuzumab (CAMPATH) and antithymocyte globulin (ATG). Blood products are irradiated to kill T lymphocytes, which may precipitate GvHD.

Corticosteroids with or without a calcineurin inhibitor are the first-line treatment for chronic GvHD, and the second-line treatment is extracorporeal photopheresis, pentostatin, rituximab or imatinib. Immunodeficiency due to defects of T-cell and B-cell functions occurs during the first 6 months and for longer in the presence of GvHD. Viral, bacterial and fungal infections may be fatal.

In the event of relapse after transplantation, donor T lymphocytes can be used therapeutically for their graft-versus-disease effect. This is exploited in mini-allografting in patients unfit to undergo a myeloablative transplant: after reduced-intensity conditioning (no TBI), the host normal marrow survives and coexists with the donor marrow, and the donor T cells control the leukaemia.

CHIMERIC ANTIGEN RECEPTOR T-CELL THERAPY

Chimeric antigen receptor (CAR) T-cell therapy is a novel form of immunotherapy using patients' immune cells to treat aggressive cancers. It is a beneficial treatment in patients with relapsed and refractory haematological malignancies. Studies have shown that CD19-directed (CAR) T-cell therapy achieves durable remission in relapsed high-grade lymphomas. CAR T therapy involves several complex steps, such as collecting patients' T cells by plasmapheresis, genetic modification of T cells to have CAR and infusion of CAR T cells. After plasmapheresis of a patient's T cells, it usually takes 3 to 4 weeks to manufacture the autologous (CAR) T cells before infusion. Being aggressive, DLBCL can grow during this period, leading to deterioration in the patient's condition. RT (9–30 Gy in 3–4 Gy per fraction) has been used as bridging therapy while a patient waits for CAR T infusion to reduce tumour burden and maintain performance status. RT is usually given to the bulkiest, rapidly growing disease sites with a 1.5-to-2-cm margin.

RADIOTHERAPY DOSES, TECHNIQUES AND TOXICITIES

RT techniques and doses have constantly evolved over the past three decades, while RT plays a vital role in the multimodality management of haematological malignancies. The RT target volume has shrunk considerably in the past two decades without compromising clinical outcomes. Extended-RT volumes such as Mantle field and inverted-Y are no longer used routinely. IFRT volumes encompass the anatomically involved nodal regions without first-station nodes. Current clinical practice is a further refinement of IFRT as ISRT or INRT. The clinical target volume (CTV) for ISRT encompasses prechemotherapy (or involved nodes if no chemotherapy) with a margin to account for uncertainties in transferring gross tumour volume (GTV) from the diagnostic scan onto the planning CT scan. The CTV for INRT is the prechemotherapy nodal disease in the optimal diagnostic image. However, using INRT requires acquiring the baseline diagnostic image in the RT treatment position with the exact breathing instructions and precision of coregistration of the diagnostic image with the planning CT scan. It is challenging for many departments to reproduce the essential requirement for INRT; therefore, ISRT is the standard volume for modern lymphoma RT.

Megavoltage is used (a 4–10-MV photon bolus may be needed to ensure an adequate dose to superficial nodes or any skin involvement). Children, teenagers and young adults, especially those with mediastinal lymphomas, may be considered for proton beam therapy to minimise the risk of late cardiac and lung toxicities.

Hodgkin Lymphoma

- Early-stage favourable risk: 20 Gy in 10 fractions following two cycles of ABVD.
- Early-stage unfavourable risk: 30 Gy in 15 fractions to involved node/site following four cycles of ABVD.
- Patients with early or advanced disease may have RT decisions made based on functional imaging results such as PET/CT after three cycles of ABVD. Still, the omission of RT is generally not advised if there was bulky disease at diagnosis.
- RT alone (stage I–II disease in patients who decline or are unfit for chemotherapy): 30 to 34 Gy in 15 to 20 fractions to extended or at least to IFRT.
- Palliative treatment: Depending on the clinical situation, there are options of 8 Gy in a single fraction, 20 Gy in 5 fractions or 30 Gy in 10 fractions.

Non-Hodgkin Lymphoma

Diffuse Large B-Cell Lymphoma

- Radical: postchemotherapy, 30 Gy in 15 daily fractions over 3 weeks to involved node/site.
- RT alone (stage I–II disease in patients who decline or are unfit for chemotherapy): 30 to 40 Gy in 15 to 20 fractions to the involved field.
- Palliative: 20 to 30 Gy in 5 to 10 fractions to the involved field is usual. Large single fractions, for example, 8 Gy, may be appropriate for bone.

Indolent Lymphoma: Follicular and Marginal Zone

- Radical: Generally, RT alone, 24 Gy in 12 fractions, is usually adequate to the involved field or modified involved site. If chemotherapy has been given, treat the involved site/nodes. If bulky or at a site at risk of organ impairment, consider 30 Gy.
- Palliative treatment: 4 Gy in 2 fractions can give prolonged remission.

Treatment Techniques

IFRT

CTV encompasses all pretreatment macroscopic and PET-positive diseases within the anatomical nodal region. When chemotherapy has considerably shrunk the disease away from critical organs such as the lung, spinal cord or kidney, CTV should be modified to avoid these organs (Figs. 30.1 and 30.2).

ISRT

ISRT, initially developed for HL, is the currently accepted technique for almost all lymphomas, providing appropriate optimal diagnostic images showing the initial extent of the disease. The International Lymphoma Radiation Oncology Group has produced consensus guidelines (see the section titled Further Reading) for ISRT. The RT volume for nodal ISRT should be defined as follows:

- GTV: The radiologically visible enlarged nodes or disease on the diagnostic scan before chemotherapy (prechemotherapy GTV) or surgery (presurgery GTV). For PET avid histological subtypes, it is the PET+ disease at diagnosis.
- CTV: Craniocaudally (to follow the direction of lymph nodes and lymphatic flow), a 15-mm margin is added to the GTV by hand in line with the direction of the nodal compartment (treatment planning expansion tools overestimate or distort the margin) and axially. The CTV stays within/extends up to the boundaries of the nodal compartment in the axial plane based on published nodal

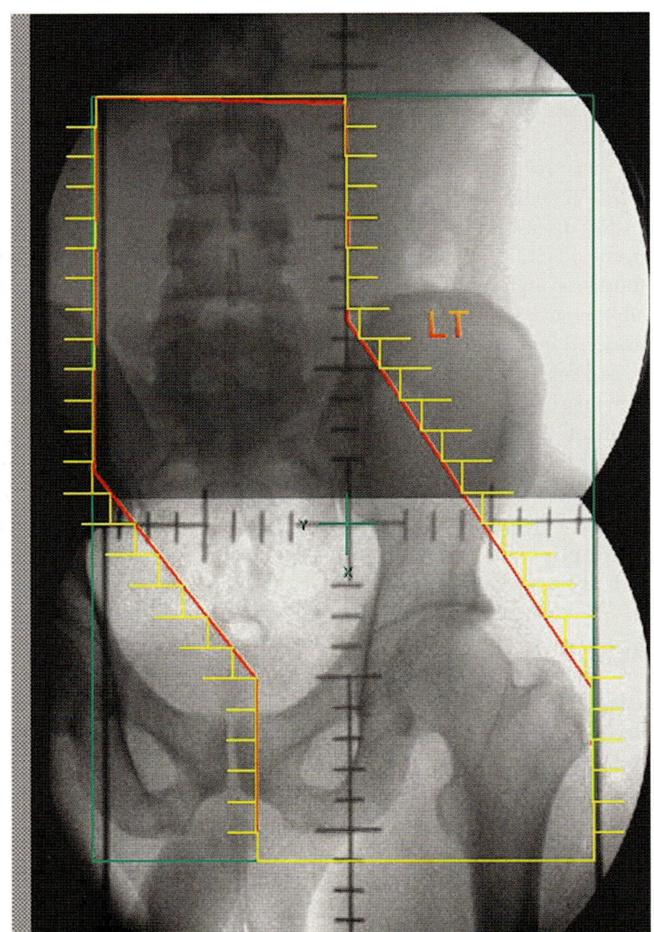

Fig. 30.1 Involved-field radiotherapy for disease involving lower para-aortic and left iliac and inguinal nodes.

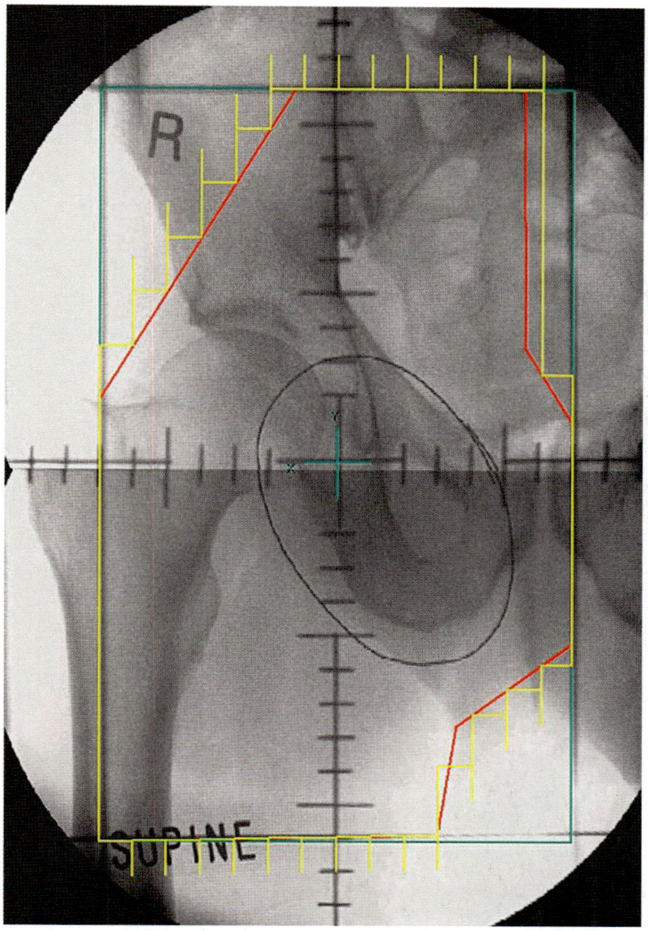

Fig. 30.2 Involved-field radiotherapy for disease involving right pelvic and inguinofemoral nodes.

atlases (Figs. 30.3 and 30.4). The CTV should be edited to avoid uninvolved organs, natural barriers and air cavities. Where there is no residual mass, the volume describes the lymph node chain in the space bounded by other structures, such as muscle, large vessels, lung and bone. Volumes are irregular in shape, and a good knowledge of anatomy is required to define them with standard atlases, radiological opinion, prechemotherapy PET scans and contrast-enhanced CT scans for planning. A margin is added to the CTV to give the required PTV according to the site, setup error, likely movement and local departmental practice, and might vary from 3 to 4 mm to 1.5 cm.

Extranodal Sites

ISRT for extranodal sites following chemotherapy is CT-planned in a similar way to involved nodes. The CTV may define the whole organ, for example, the stomach, spleen or thyroid, where no adjacent nodes were involved, or part of a node chain may need to be outlined in addition.

Head and Neck. The patient is immobilised in a supine shell, and CT planning is used.

Waldeyer's Ring. Although Waldeyer's ring can be considered one site for staging purposes, the entire volume need not be treated if localised disease, such as unilateral tonsillar involvement, is present. The single structure can be outlined with appropriate margins based on prechemotherapy volumes. For extensive involvement and partial response to chemotherapy, larger fields may be considered, but this can lead to considerable toxicity.

Thyroid. The thyroid gland is included with or without cervical lymph node chains, depending on whether nodes are involved at diagnosis. As for a head and neck tumour, immobilisation and CT planning are adopted.

Orbit. The whole orbit is treated using CT planning. For small lateral and conjunctival indolent NHL, a single beam may suffice. Beams are angled to avoid the other eye (Figs. 30.5–30.7).

Nasal Sinuses. Planning is the same as for carcinoma (Figs. 30.8 and 30.9)

Brain. A parallel pair of lateral beams treats the whole brain. As meningeal involvement is likely, the fields are extended down the neck to the C2/3 vertebrae and should cover the posterior orbit and facial nerve root as for ALL (Figs. 30.10 and 30.11).

Gastrointestinal Lymphoma. For gastric NHL, plan on using oral contrast and treating the stomach empty. CT planning can help spare the kidneys or spinal cord, especially for large postchemotherapy residual abdominal masses.

Bone. The volume should include the whole of the affected bone or, in cases of long bones, a prechemotherapy disease with a 1.5-to-2-cm margin. A parallel-opposed pair of fields may be adequate, shielding soft tissues with a 2-cm margin. Tomotherapy, VMAT or IMRT can also be used.

Breast. The whole breast is included as the CTV. Uninvolved lymph nodes do not need to be treated. This is planned with tangents as per breast carcinoma irradiation.

Spleen. The CTV is the edge of the spleen. CT planning may help minimise the dose to the kidney.

Toxicity

Acute Side Effects. All treatments cause tiredness, temporary hair loss and mucositis in the treated area from 2 weeks into treatment and for several weeks afterwards. Dry mouth and altered taste are usual where salivary tissue has to be treated and may last after bilateral high-neck fields.

Late Effects. The organs most subject to late effects are the thyroid, lung, heart and spinal cord. There is an increased risk of solid tumours in irradiated areas.

Thyroid. Up to 30% of patients develop clinical or biochemical hypothyroidism several years after bilateral neck treatment, requiring thyroxine replacement therapy.

Lung. Symptoms, if any, are seen after about 6 weeks and include dry cough and dyspnoea, which usually settle with steroids (prednisolone 40–60 mg/day). Clinically, significant late effects are rare with modern RT.

Cardiac. Radiation-induced cardiac disease used to occur in less than 5% of patients after mantle treatment and less with involved fields, although data are scarce. It can rarely present as transient pericarditis within a few months of treatment or much later as cardiomyopathy or premature coronary artery disease.

Bone. Avascular necrosis of the femoral head occurs in 2% of patients with Hodgkin lymphoma, particularly following chemotherapy and steroid treatment, but RT to the hip is a contributory factor. Symptoms of hip pain develop on average about 2 years following the start of chemotherapy. Total hip replacement may be necessary. The humeral head may also be affected if it cannot be shielded.

Fertility. Pelvic RT with lymphoma doses will cause infertility in most young people: for males, sperm banking is effective, but for females, surgical oophoropexy and, if possible, cryopreservation of ovarian tissue is advised. Hormone replacement therapy (HRT) should be prescribed for premature menopause.

Growth. Growth retardation in children after RT includes limited height, but also, for instance, thinning of the neck muscles and shortening of the clavicles from neck treatment.

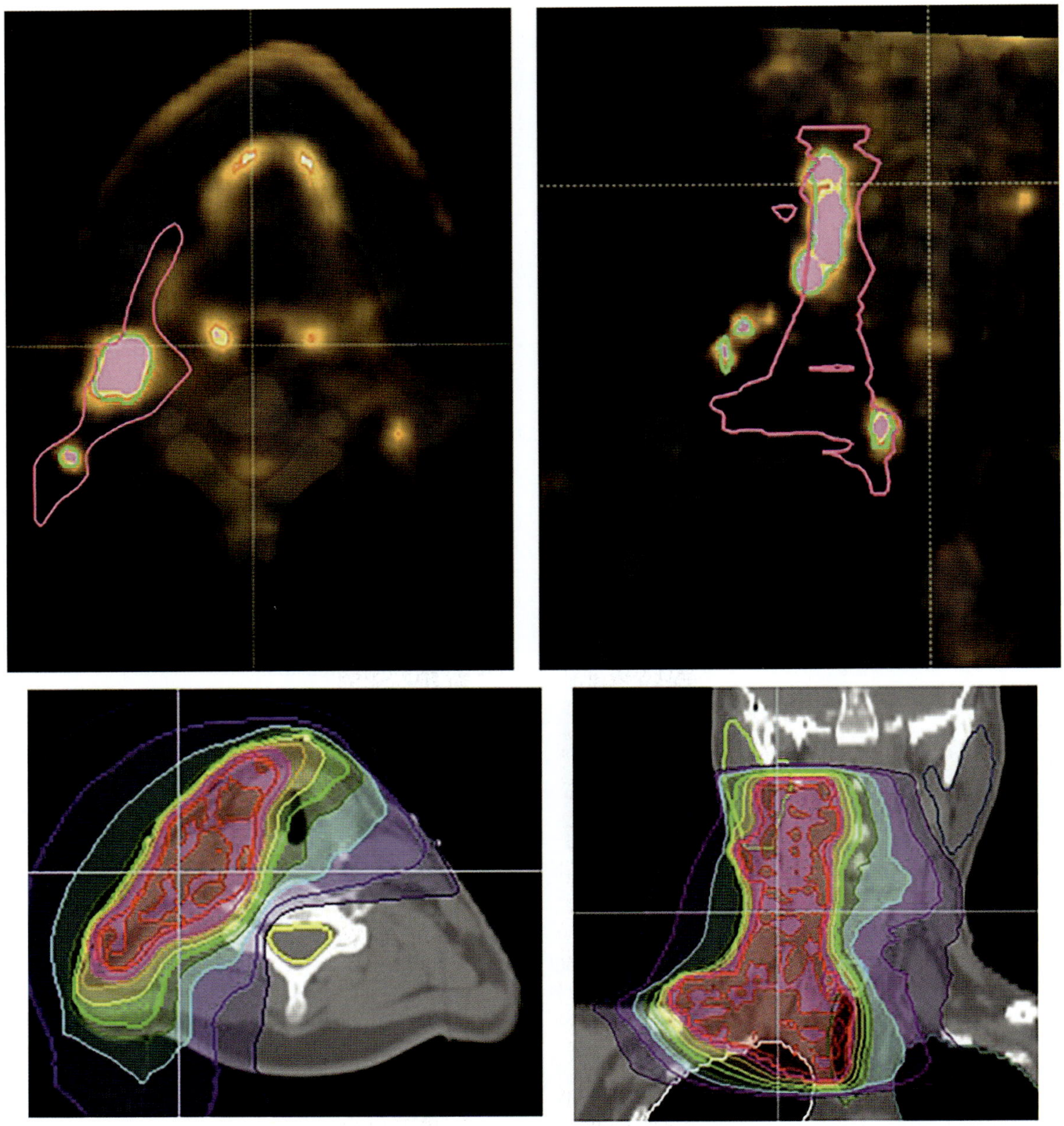

Figure 30.3 Involved-site radiotherapy for a favourable-risk Hodgkin lymphoma involving right neck, right supraclavicular fossa and upper paratracheal nodes.

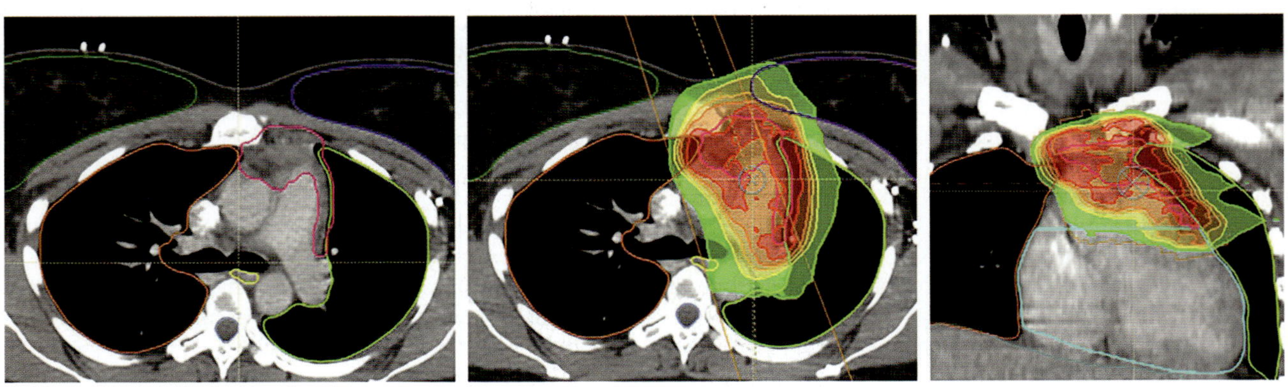

Figure 30.4 Consolidation involved-site radiotherapy for a primary mediastinal high-grade non-Hodgkin lymphoma.

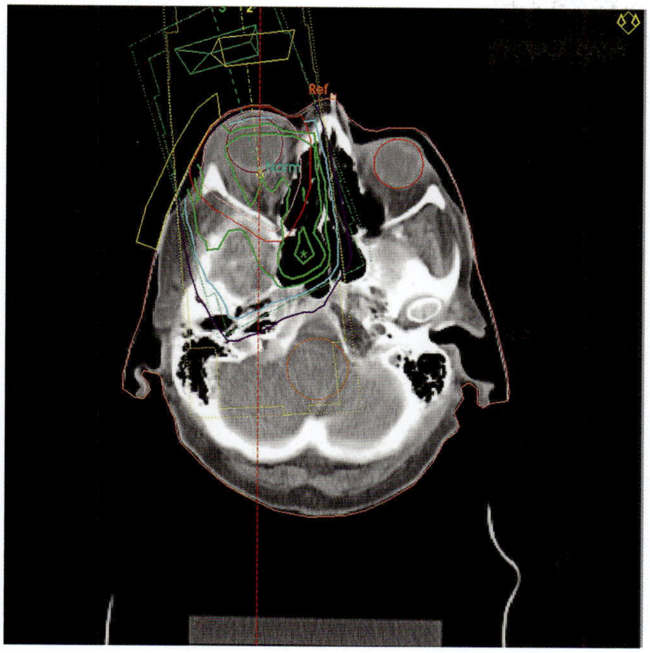

Fig. 30.5 Orbital lymphoma with anterior mass: Axial view of sagittal beams and bolus.

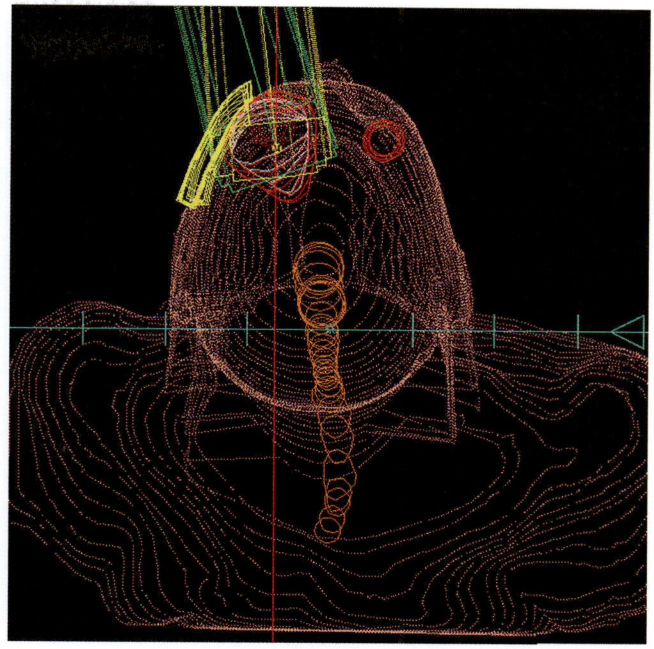

Fig. 30.7 Orbital lymphoma: Outline view of volume and beam arrangement.

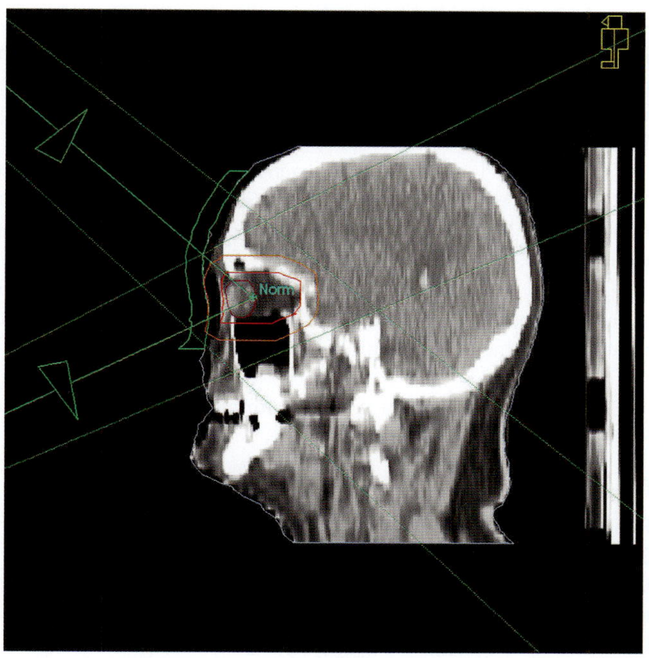

Fig. 30.6 Orbital lymphoma: Sagittal view of anterior-wedged pair of angled beams.

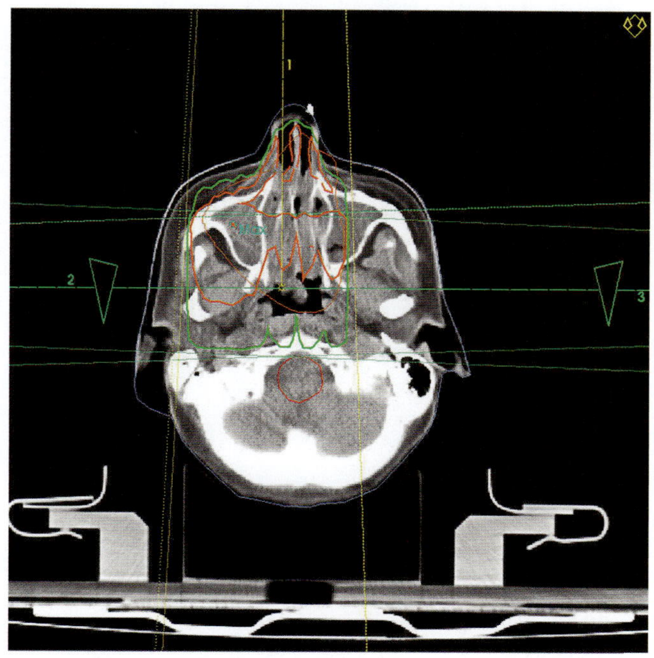

Fig. 30.8 Nasal natural killer/T-cell lymphoma: Three-field plan.

Total Body Irradiation Before Transplantation

Total body irradiation is given to a dose of 13.2- to 4.4-Gy midplane dose in 8 twice-daily fractions over 4 days (6-MV photons) or 12 Gy in 6 fractions over 3 days. Current trials generally determine doses and schedules.

Technique. Techniques vary in detail from centre to centre. Some have machines dedicated to extended field treatment for TBI, and increasingly, VMAT and tomotherapy are being used (Fig. 30.12).

Using a LINAC at extended focus to skin distance (FSD) (about 4 metres), a lateral beam can treat the whole patient, who is then turned 180 degrees for the other side.

Thermoluminescent dosimeters (TLDs) are positioned at regular intervals along each side of the body, and tissue compensators can be conveniently attached to a rectangular Perspex screen placed alongside the patient. Typically, 1-mm, 8-mm and 6-mm brass compensators are placed over the head, neck and thorax, respectively. Doses are measured at each fraction to adjust arm position and compensators, if necessary, to ensure dose homogeneity within around 5%.

Side Effects. Side effects are more familiar with single-fraction than with fractionated TBI and include:

1. Pneumonitis. Lungs are the dose-limiting organs. Because pneumonitis commonly occurs following bone marrow transplantation

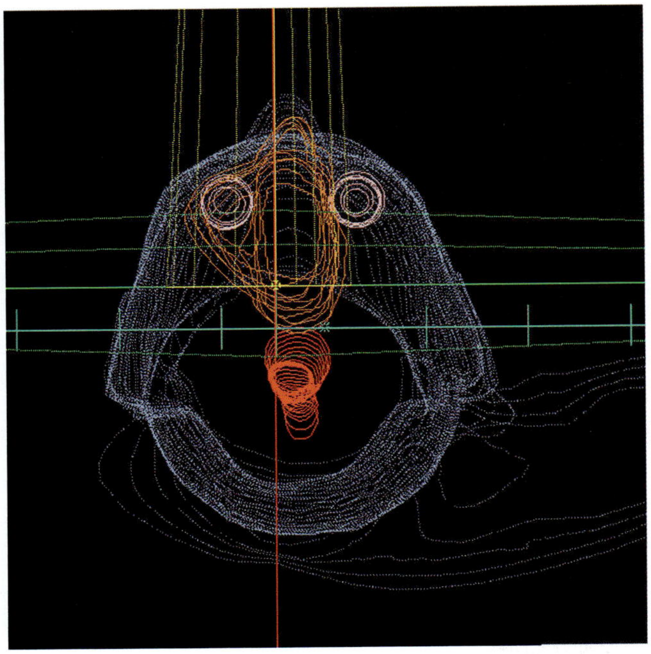

Fig. 30.9 Nasal natural killer/T-cell lymphoma: Volume and critical structures—contralateral eye and brainstem.

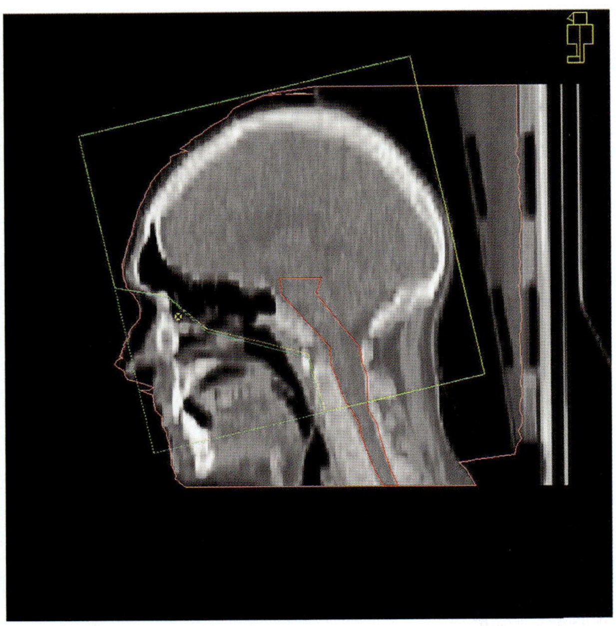

Fig. 30.10 Whole brain and meninges down to C2/3 for acute lymphoblastic leukaemia.

in the absence of radiation, the role of TBI in its causation is difficult to assess.

2. Cataracts. The incidence of cataracts is about 20% between 3 and 6 years.
3. Hepatic venoocclusive disease. This is seen in up to 25% of patients but is usually mild. However, the mortality of established disease is high (30%).
4. Infertility. In females under age 25 years, periods may return, but permanent sterility is expected in others. Males are rendered azoospermic and should have sperm frozen.
5. Hypothyroidism. Hypothyroidism occurs in up to 30%.
6. Growth delay. Growth hormone secretion may be impaired, especially if previous cranial irradiation has been given.
7. Second malignancy.

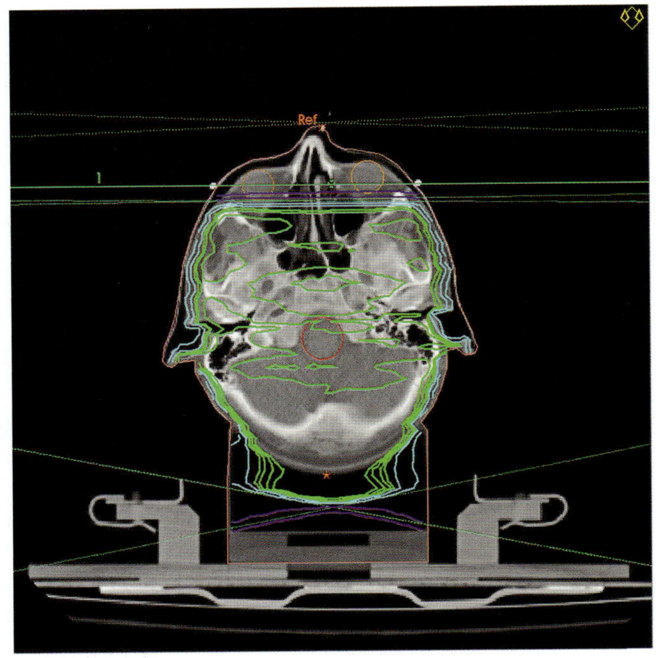

Fig. 30.11 Computed tomography plan for acute lymphoblastic leukaemia.

Splenic Radiotherapy

Splenic RT is used in myeloproliferative disorders, mainly CML and myelofibrosis, to shrink an uncomfortably large spleen and to improve blood counts by reducing splenic consumption; this is a delicate balance as counts will initially drop.

Dose. If there is extramedullary haematopoiesis, the dose is 0.25 to 0.5 Gy/day, up to a total dose of 1 to 10 Gy with 4-to-6-MV photons. A higher dose per fraction, 1 to 1.5 Gy, can be used for other causes of splenomegaly.

Target Volume. While the CTV is the whole spleen, irradiation of the entire spleen is unnecessary to achieve shrinkage and symptomatic benefit. The kidney is dose limiting but can tolerate 20 Gy, so treatment can be repeated.

The spleen is outlined on the CT planning scan, and a parallel pair is often adequate.

Myeloma

Radical treatment of solitary plasmacytoma is 40 to 50 Gy in 20 to 25 fractions (Fig. 30.13). For solitary bone plasmacytoma, CTV is GTV+ 10–15 mm margin. If there is uncertainty regarding the extent of bone involvement, the whole bone should be included in CTV (e.g. vertebrae). For solitary extramedullary plasmacytoma, a margin of 10–15 is added to GTV to get CTV. Surgical nails may be included in the CTV if they traverse the tumour, to prevent surgical seeding.

Palliative Treatment of Multiple Myeloma

Spinal Deposits. 8 Gy single fraction with a posterior beam to cover abnormal bone(s) plus one vertebra on either side, about 8 cm width to include the transverse processes of the vertebrae, wider to include any paravertebral mass.

Soft Tissue Mass/Spinal Cord Compression/Pathological Fracture/ Severe Pain. 20 Gy in 5 fractions. Consider 30 Gy in 10 fractions, for example, soft tissue with extensive bone destruction when the disease is mainly in one area.

Rib Deposits. 8 Gy single fraction. Orthovoltage or electron treatment can be used on the painful area with a 1.5-to-2-cm margin along the rib.

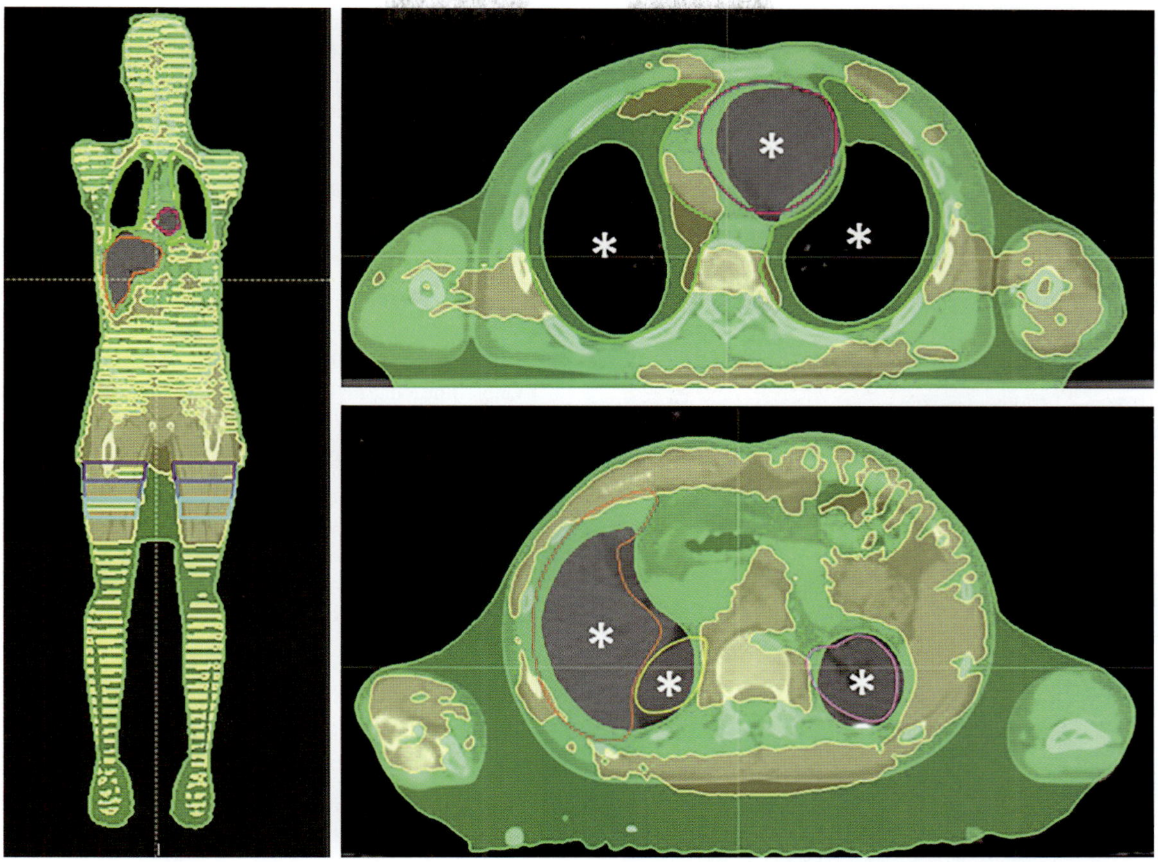

Figure 30.12 TBI using tomotherapy showing dose-sparing of the heart, lungs, kidneys and liver. (*)

Hemibody Radiotherapy for Widespread Deposits. This is now rarely used because systemic treatment options have increased. If treating both in sequence, a gap of 6 weeks is necessary for blood count recovery.

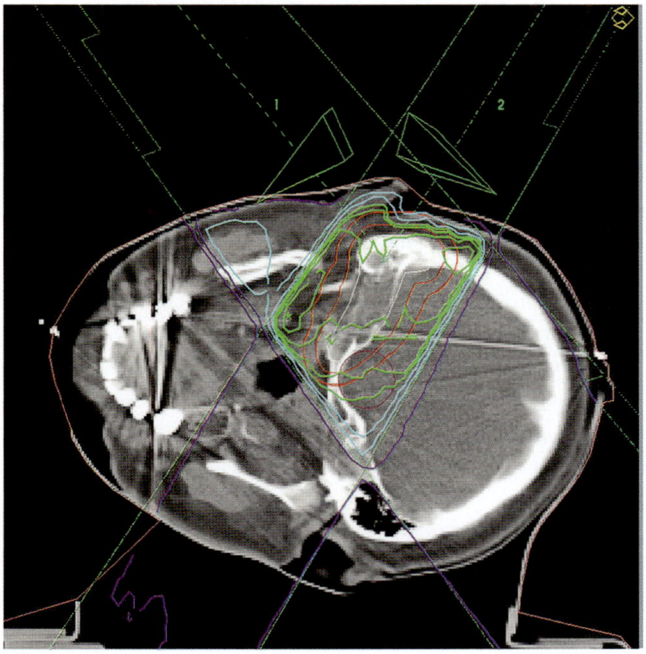

Figure 30.13 Plasmacytoma of petrous bone: Lateral-wedged pair of angled beams.

Position. Supine with arms folded across the chest, hands on shoulders.

Upper half: 6 Gy single fraction—chin to umbilicus, wide enough to cover shoulders.

Lower half: 8 Gy single fraction—umbilicus to maximum field size inferiorly and width to cover iliac bones.

Technique. Extended FSD (140 cm) and anteroposterior parallel beams.

Acute side effects. Nausea and vomiting are prevented with, for example, ondansetron 1 hour before RT, dexamethasone 4 mg twice daily and metoclopramide 10 mg as needed. Pneumonitis is rare at 6 Gy but has an increasing incidence above this dose in the whole lungs.

Diarrhoea occurs in one-third of patients 3 to 5 days after lower hemibody treatment and is controllable with codeine or loperamide.

Pancytopenia is common and contributes to lethargy. Blood and platelet transfusions may be required.

Mycosis Fungoides

Local

Use 10 Gy in 5 daily fractions or 8 Gy in a single fraction for small lesions. Higher doses may be needed for the tumour stage.

Use 80 to 120 kV for superficial lesions and 220 to 300 kV, or electrons of appropriate energy, for plaque or tumour stage.

Total-Skin Electron Therapy

Total-skin electron beam therapy (TSEBT) is a specialised treatment offered in regional centres, and techniques vary.

Doses can vary, but typically, they are 12 Gy in 8 fractions over 2 weeks with an 8-Gy boost in 2 fractions over 2 days or the more conventional 30 Gy in 20 fractions over 5 weeks.

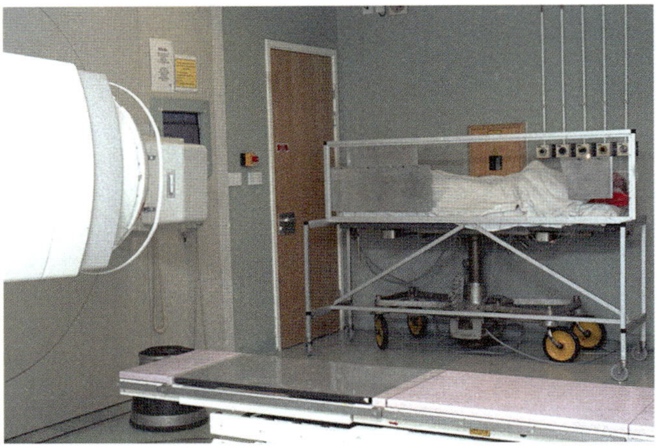

Figure 30.14 Machine head and patient showing extended focus to skin distance.

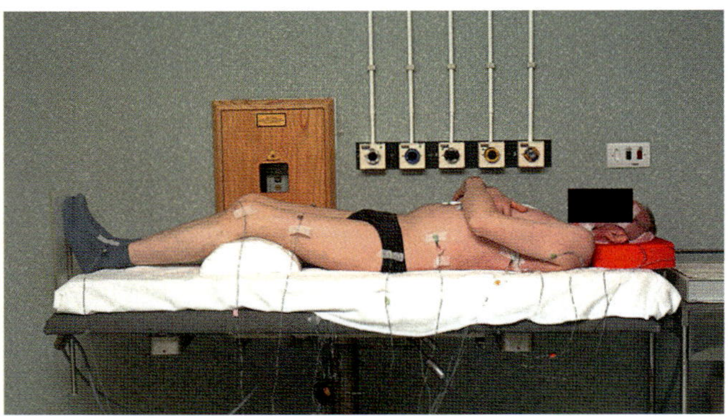

Fig. 30.15 Patient with dosimeters placed and ready for treatment.

Four fields can cover the whole body at an extended source-to-surface distance (SSD) (120 cm) with the patient supine. Lead shielding is applied to protect the eyes and the fingernails. If the eyelids are involved, a lead internal eye shield is used. If 5- or 8-MeV electrons are used, Perspex is used to reduce the depth of penetration. Skin in folds (e.g. axilla and groin) is spared with this technique and may be marked for separate treatment when skin erythema develops. This can be minimised by positioning patients carefully.

Temporary alopecia and nail loss are followed by permanent skin atrophy, oedema and radiodermatitis (Figs. 30.14 and 30.15).

CHEMOTHERAPY REGIMENS AND TOXICITIES

Most chemotherapy regimens cause myelosuppression and the risk of life-threatening neutropenic sepsis. Chemotherapy typically causes alopecia. There is also the risk of infertility, particularly in males, although this is more commonly encountered with intensive regimens. The problems of nausea and vomiting (mainly because of anthracyclines, dacarbazine and mustine) have been transformed by new antiemetics in the HT3 blocker class (ondansetron, granisetron). Anthracyclines cause cardiomyopathy if a high cumulative dose has to be given, but this is rarely a problem with first-line treatment. The vinca alkaloids (vincristine, vinblastine) cause peripheral neuropathy and constipation. Bleomycin can rarely cause pulmonary fibrosis, which can be fatal. Oral chlorambucil alone is the least acutely toxic treatment used; it does not cause alopecia or much nausea but, like other alkylating agents (cyclophosphamide, melphalan, mustine), causes some irreversible toxicity to bone marrow and gonads.

Hodgkin Lymphoma

Doxorubicin, Bleomycin, Vinblastine and Dacarbazine

The ABVD drug regimen is as follows:

Doxorubicin (adriamycin) 25 mg/m^2 intravenously (IV)	Days 1 and 15
Bleomycin 10,000 units/m^2 IV	Days 1 and 15
Vinblastine 6 mg/m^2 IV	Days 1 and 15
Dacarbazine 375 mg/m^2 IV	Days 1 and 15
Repeated every 28 days	

Acute toxicity is marked. Alopecia is common, but patients also experience nausea, myelosuppression, constipation, painful veins, pulmonary fibrosis from bleomycin, which is fatal in 1% to 30% of patients and highest in elderly patients. However, there is minimal risk of infertility or leukaemia with ABVD, so this is standard treatment.

Escalated BEACOPP

Escalated BEACOPP is an intensive first-line treatment suitable for unfavourable-risk patients. The regimen is as follows:

Bleomycin 10,000 units/m^2 intravenously (IV)	Day 8
Etoposide 200 mg/m^2 IV	Days 1–3
Doxorubicin (adriamycin) 35 mg/m^2 IV	Day 1
Cyclophosphamide 1250 mg/m^2 IV	Day 1
Vincristine (oncovin) 1.4 mg/m^2 (max 2 mg) IV	Day 8
Procarbazine 100 mg/m^2 orally	Days 1–7
Prednisolone 40 mg/m^2 orally	Days 1–14
Repeated every 21 days	

Non-Hodgkin Lymphoma

Diffuse Large B Cell, T Cell-Rich, B Cell, Follicular Grade 3b (and for T-Cell Lymphomas)

Use CHOP alone without rituximab for T-cell lymphoma.

R-CHOP. Side effects include alopecia, nausea, myelosuppression, peripheral neuropathy, antibody reaction, steroid effects and cardiomyopathy. The regimen is as follows:

Rituximab 375 mg/m^2	Day 1
Cyclophosphamide 750 mg/m^2 intravenously (IV)	Day 1
Doxorubicin 50 mg/m^2 IV	Day 1
Vincristine 1.4 mg/m^2 (max. 2 mg) IV	Day 1
Prednisolone 50 mg/m^2 orally	Days 1–5
Repeated every 21 days	

In those assessed to be at high risk of CNS disease, prophylaxis by intrathecal or systemic intravenous methotrexate can be given within 3 to 4 cycles.

CNS Prophylaxis

Methotrexate × 4 doses
1 g/m^2 IV on day 14
or 12.5 mg IV on day 1 or 2
with each of first 4 cycles

Burkitt Type, Lymphoblastic (Some DLBCL If 100% MIB-1 Staining)

R-CODOX-M/R-IVAC. This is an intensive myelosuppressive regimen with CNS treatment. The regimen is as follows:

R-CODOX-M

Rituximab 375 mg/m²	Day 1
Cyclophosphamide 800 mg/m² intravenously (IV) on day 1 and 200 mg/m² IV on days 2 and 3	Day 1–3
Vincristine 1.5 mg/m² (max. 2 mg) IV	Day 8
Doxorubicin 40 mg/m² IV	Day 1
Methotrexate 3 gm/m² IV	Day 10

Intrathecal treatment:

1. Cytarabine 70 mg day 3
2. Methotrexate 12 mg day 15

R-IVAC

Rituximab 375 mg/m² intravenously (IV)	Day 1
Ifosfamide 1.5 g/m² (with Mesna)	Days 1–5
Etoposide 60 mg/m² IV	Days 1–5
Cytarabine 2 g/m² IV	Days 1 and 2

Intrathecal treatment:

Methotrexate 12 mg day 5

Relapsed Non-Hodgkin Lymphoma

(R)IVE, (R)ICE

Rituximab
Ifosfamide
Etoposide (Vepesid) in IVE or carboplatin in ICE
Epirubicin in IVE or carboplatin in ICE
Reinduction regimens to minimise bulk and mobilise stem cells for harvesting

BEAM

Busulfan
Etoposide
Cytosine arabinoside (Ara-C)
Melphalan

Myeloablative Regimen. Oral etoposide: 50 mg twice daily for 10 days, every 3 to 4 weeks: palliative single agent

Myeloma

CTD

Cyclophosphamide
Thalidomide
Dexamethasone

CTD is a generally well-tolerated oral regimen. Specific side effects include pulmonary fibrosis (cyclophosphamide), neuropathy, thrombosis, teratogenesis and thyroid dysfunction (thalidomide).

Bortezomib

Bortezomib is a proteasome inhibitor with various sites of action. The main side effects include neuropathy and thrombocytopenia.

Lenalidomide

Lenalidomide is a novel analogue of thalidomide with similar side effects as bortezomib, but neuropathy is less likely.

Acute Myeloid Leukaemia

DA

Daunorubicin
Cytarabine (Ara-C)

DA is significantly myelosuppressive. It commonly causes mucositis (oral ulcers, diarrhoea) and, more rarely, conjunctivitis and cardiomyopathy.

FURTHER READING

Bales JR, Kim HT, Portillo R, Patel C, McAfee S, Dey B, Spitzer T, Chen Y-B, El-Jawahri A, DeFilipp Z, Hobbs GS, et al. Splenic irradiation prior to allogeneic hematopoietic cell transplantation for patients with myelofibrosis. *Bone Marrow Transplant.* 2023;58(4):459–461.

Cheson BD, Fisher RI, Barrington SF, Cavalli F, Schwartz LH, Zucca E, Lister TA; Alliance, Australasian Leukaemia and Lymphoma Group; Eastern Cooperative Oncology Group; European Mantle Cell Lymphoma Consortium; Italian Lymphoma Foundation; European Organisation for Research; Treatment of Cancer/Dutch Hemato-Oncology Group; Grupo Español de Médula Ósea; German High-Grade Lymphoma Study Group; German Hodgkin's Study Group; Japanese Lymphorra Study Group; Lymphoma Study Association…United Kingdom National Cancer Research Institute. Recommendations for initial evaluation, staging, and response assessment of Hodgkin and non-Hodgkin lymphoma: the Lugano classification. *J Clin Oncol.* 2014 Sep 20;32(27):3059–3068.

Constine LS, Yahalom J, Ng AK, Hodgson DC, Wirth A, Milgrom SA, Mikhaeel NG, Eich HT, Illidge T, Ricardi U, Dieckmann K, Moskowitz CH, Advani R, Mauch PM, Specht L, Hoppe RT. The role of radiation therapy in patients with relapsed or refractory Hodgkin lymphoma: guidelines from the International Lymphoma Radiation Oncology Group. *Int J Radiat Oncol Biol Phys.* 2018;100(5):1100–1118.

Cowan AJ, Green DJ, Kwok M, Lee S, Coffey DG, Holmberg LA, Tuazon S, Gopal AK, Libby EN. Diagnosis and management of multiple myeloma: a review. *JAMA.* 2022;327(5):464–477.

Cross NCP, Ernst T, Branford S, Cayuela J-M, Deininger M, Fabarius A, Kim DDH, Polakova KM, Radich JP, Hehlmann R, Hochhaus A, Apperley JF, Soverini S. European LeukemiaNet laboratory recommendations for the diagnosis and management of chronic myeloid leukemia. *Leukemia.* 2023 Nov;37(11):2150–2167.

DiNardo CD, Erba HP, Freeman SD, Wei AH. Acute myeloid leukaemia. *Lancet.* 2023 Jun 17;401(10393):2073–2086.

Döhner H, Wei AH, Appelbaum FR, Craddock C, DiNardo CD, Dombret H, Ebert BL, Fenaux P, Godley LA, Hasserjian RP, Larson RA, Levine RL, Miyazaki Y, Niederwieser D, Ossenkoppele G, Röllig C, Sierra J, Stein EM, Tallman MS, et al. Diagnosis and management of AML in adults: 2022 recommendations from an international expert panel on behalf of the ELN. *Blood.* 2022 Sep 22;140(12):1345–1377.

Follows GA, Barrington SF, Bhuller KS, Culligan DJ, Cutter DJ, Gallop-Evans E, Kassam S, Osborne W, Sadullah S, Townsend W, Uttenthal BJ, Collins GP; British Society for Haematology. Guideline for the first-line management of classical Hodgkin lymphoma—a British Society for Haematology guideline. *Br J Haematol.* 2022 Jun;197(5):558–572.

Fox CP, Chaganti S, McIlroy G, Barrington SF, Burton C, Cwynarski K, Eyre TA, Illidge T, Kalakonda N, Kuhnl A, McKay P, Davies AJ. The management of newly diagnosed large B-cell lymphoma: a British Society for Haematology Guideline. *Br J Haematol.* 2024 Apr;204(4):1178–1192.

Hoskin PJ, Díez P, Williams M, Lucraft H, Bayne M; participants of the Lymphoma Radiotherapy Group. Recommendations for the use of radiotherapy in nodal lymphoma. *Clin Oncol (R Coll Radiol).* 2013;25(1):49–58.

Illidge T, Specht L, Yahalom J, Aleman B, Berthelsen AK, Constine L, Dabaja B, Dharmarajan K, Ng A, Ricardi U, Wirth A; International Lymphoma Radiation Oncology Group. Modern radiation therapy for nodal non-Hodgkin lymphoma—target definition and dose guidelines from the International Lymphoma Radiation Oncology Group. *Int J Radiat Oncol Biol Phys*. 2014;89(1):49–58.

Rajkumar SV. Multiple myeloma: 2022 update on diagnosis, risk stratification, and management. *Am J Hematol*. 2022 Aug;97(8): 1086–1107.

Sive J, Cuthill K, Hunter H, Kazmi M, Pratt G, Smith D; British Society of Haematology. Guidelines on the diagnosis, investigation and initial treatment of myeloma: a British Society for Haematology/UK Myeloma Forum Guideline. *Br J Haematol*. 2021 Apr;193(2):245–268.

Specht L, Yahalom J, Illidge T, Berthelsen AK, Constine LS, Eich HT, Girinsky T, Hoppe RT, Mauch P, Mikhaeel NG, Ng A; ILROG. Modern radiation therapy for Hodgkin lymphoma: field and dose guidelines from the International Lymphoma Radiation Oncology Group (ILROG). *Int J Radiat Oncol Biol Phys*. 2014;89(4): 854–862.

Tefferi A. Primary myelofibrosis: 2023 update on diagnosis, risk-stratification, and management. *Am J Hematol*. 2023 May;98(5): 801–821.

Walewska R, Parry-Jones N, Eyre TA, Follows G, Martinez-Calle N, McCarthy H, Parry H, Patten PEM, Riches JC, Hillmen P, Schuh AH. Guideline for the treatment of chronic lymphocytic leukaemia. *Br J Haematol*. 2022 Jun;197(5):544–557.

Yahalom J, Illidge T, Specht L, Hoppe RT, Li Y-X, Tsang R, Wirth A; International Lymphoma Radiation Oncology Group. Modern radiation therapy for extranodal lymphomas: field and dose guidelines from the International Lymphoma Radiation Oncology Group. *Int J Radiat Oncol Biol Phys*. 2015;92(1):11–31.

31

Tumours of the Central Nervous System

Pinelopi Gkogkou, Sarah J. Jefferies and Fiona Harris

CHAPTER OUTLINE

INTRODUCTION

Primary tumours of the central nervous system (CNS) are relatively uncommon: the overall annual incidence of primary CNS tumours is around 3% of new cancer cases, with approximately 12,300 newly diagnosed patients in the United Kingdom each year. Although accounting for only 2.6% of cancer deaths, brain tumours lead, on average, to a greater loss of life per patient than any other adult tumour, and the effect on the individual with a primary CNS tumour is frequently devastating. Primary CNS tumours affect patients of all ages, from childhood to old age, and there is a rising incidence from middle age onwards. In childhood, they are the most common solid tumours (as opposed to leukemias).

There are a huge range of outcomes for patients with primary CNS tumours, from almost guaranteed cure in some conditions (e.g. germinoma) to almost guaranteed fatality in others (e.g. glioblastoma isocitrate dehydrogenase wild type grade 4 (GBM IDH WT grade 4)). For patients with CNS tumours, a holistic approach is always required, and for many, involvement of palliative care services at an early stage is highly desirable. For many patients, driving is forbidden after the diagnosis of brain tumour (see later).

Tumour Types

Overall, about 80% of CNS tumours are primary and 20% secondary, but this is dependent on exactly how the patient populations are defined and collated. Patients presenting with cerebral metastases are generally seen and looked after by site-specific specialist teams based on the tissue of origin.

The major types of primary tumour are given in Table 31.1. The majority of primary tumours are gliomas, of which two-thirds are GBM IDH WT grade 4 (Fig. 31.1), making this the most common type of primary CNS tumour in adults. Gliomas in general and GBM IDH WT in particular are devastating tumours, and their management is best conducted by a multidisciplinary team with access to all specialties and appropriate support services. Although gliomas represent the largest proportion of primary brain tumours, over one-third of new referrals are for other tumour types, requiring equivalent expertise and knowledge in management.

Gliomas are graded according to the World Health Organization (WHO) classification, which was significantly updated in 2021. They are graded from 1 to 4, where 4 is the most malignant. Grade 1 and grade 2 gliomas together are termed low grade. Grade 1 tumours are more typical of childhood but occasionally occur in adults. The grade 2 tumours are (1) the oligodendroglioma, IDH mutant and 1p/19q codeleted; and (2) the diffuse astrocytoma, IDH-mutant and1p/19q non-codeleted. Grade 3 and grade 4 tumours together constitute high-grade gliomas (HGGs). Grade 3 IDH mutant gliomas may also be called *anaplastic* (e.g. anaplastic astrocytoma or anaplastic oligodendroglioma),

TABLE 31.1 A Simplified Classification of the Major Categories of Brain Tumour

Intrinsic tumours (i.e. those arising within the brain substance)
Gliomas, glioneuronal tumours and neuronal tumours
Adult-type diffuse gliomas
Astrocytoma, IDH mutant
Oligodendroglioma, IDH mutant and 1p/19q codeleted
Glioblastoma, IDH wild type
Ependymal tumours
Extrinsic tumours of the brain covering
Meningioma
Other tumours
Pituitary adenoma and craniopharyngioma
Vestibular schwannoma
Skull base chordoma and chondrosarcoma
Metastases to the CNS
Metastases to the brain and spinal cord parenchyma
Metastases to the meninges

CNS, Central nervous system; *IDH*, isocitrate dehydrogenase.

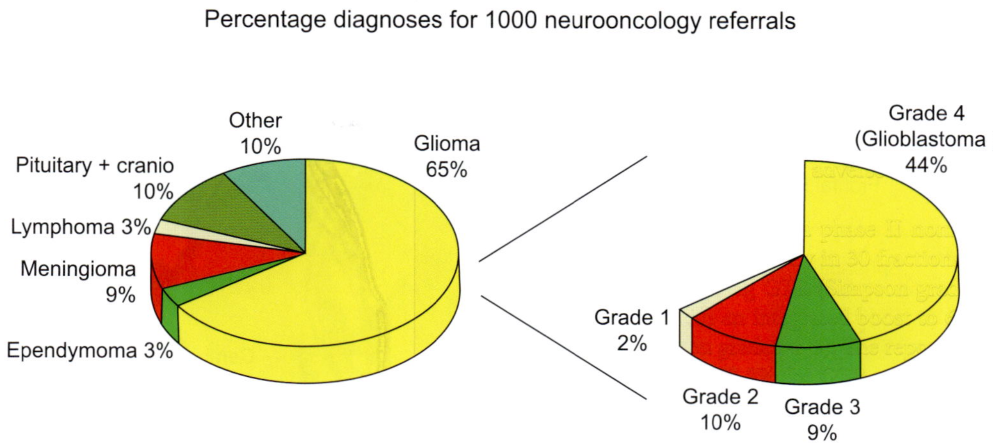

Fig. 31.1 Frequency of the main tumour types. Percentages of different grades of glioma. Grade 4 glioma is glioblastoma. (Courtesy Professor NG Burnet, Oncology Department, Cambridge, UK.)

and grade 4 gliomas are known as *glioblastoma IDH WT* and *astrocytoma IDH WT*.

Gliomas arise from astrocytes and oligodendrocytes, cells which nourish and support neurons. Primary tumours of neurons alone are extremely uncommon, though they do exist (e.g. neurocytoma). There are a surprisingly large range of very rare tumours within the brain, but apart from those mentioned explicitly in Table 31.1 and described in this chapter, their overall management and outcome can generally be inferred from their grade and molecular biology.

Gliomas have a slight male predominance, at 55%. Meningiomas are more common in females than males at a ratio of 2:1. There are only two definite aetiological factors for the development of brain tumours: exposure to ionising radiation and genetic predisposition. Genetic syndromes including Li-Fraumeni syndrome, neurofibromatosis types 1 and 2, Gorlin syndrome, tuberous sclerosis, Cowden disease, Turcot syndrome and von Hippel-Lindau disease are known to predispose to the development of gliomas, generally at a younger age than in the general population. Rare cases are *familial*, defined as two or more gliomas diagnosed in first- or second-degree relatives. However, the majority of CNS tumours are sporadic.

Metastatic disease within the CNS may arise from primary tumours at almost any site. However, certain cancers have a propensity to metastasise to the brain. Lung cancer accounts for 60% of metastases, followed by breast cancer (15%), melanoma (6%–11%) and renal cancer (1%–4%). Other tumours causing metastases include those in the colon, pancreas and ovary. Metastases are usually multiple but occasionally can be solitary.

Anatomy of the CNS

Anatomy is the key to understanding the presentation and spread of neurological tumours and concepts about treatment, particularly radiotherapy (RT) and surgery.

Anatomy of the Brain

Tissues of the Brain

Within the brain substance itself, tissue is divided into grey matter and white matter. Grey matter covers the surface folds of the brain (gyri) and broadly is the location of active neurons. White matter lies below grey matter and contains fibres which communicate with other parts of the brain and body, equivalent to electrical cabling. At a cellular level, the brain is composed of neurons and of cells designed to support the structure and function of those neurons, that is, the glial-supporting cells. In right-handed patients, the left hemisphere is almost invariably dominant.

The frontal lobe is very large, extending back to the central sulcus, which divides it from the parietal lobe. The motor cortex sits immediately in front of the central sulcus. More anteriorly, the frontal lobe is responsible for intellect, motivation and emotional response. Damage to the frontal lobes can affect intellectual performance, including reasoning, memory, the initiation of activity and insight. The medial frontal lobe is particularly important for these activities, and damage to both medial frontal lobes is extremely destructive to the intellect. The motor speech centre (Broca's area) lies in the dominant frontal lobe (see Fig. 31.2).

The parietal lobe extends from the central sulcus posteriorly onto the occipital lobe, and it too is large. The parietal lobe has large areas which are silent, that is, with no obvious functional activity as yet understood. Immediately behind the central sulcus is the sensorimotor cortex, which deals predominantly with reception of sensory information. In reality, there are other areas adjacent to both the motor and sensory cortices which support those functions. At the most posterior part of the cerebral hemisphere is the occipital cortex, which deals with central processing of visual information. The optic radiation connects the optic tracts to the occipital cortex and runs through the temporal

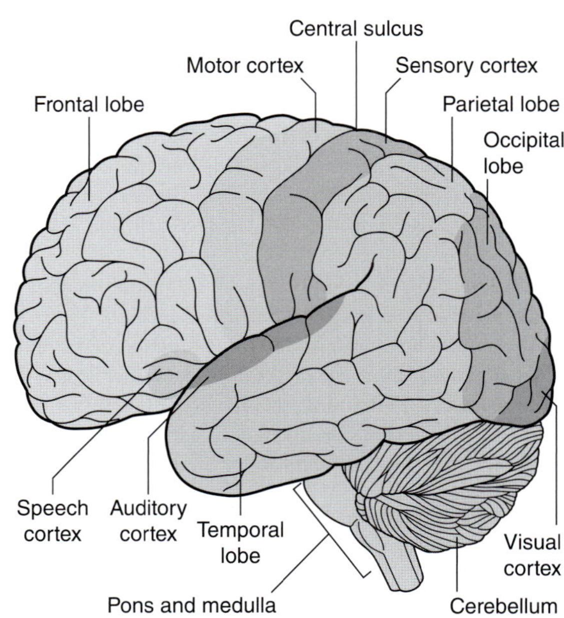

Fig. 31.2 The major anatomical divisions of the brain.

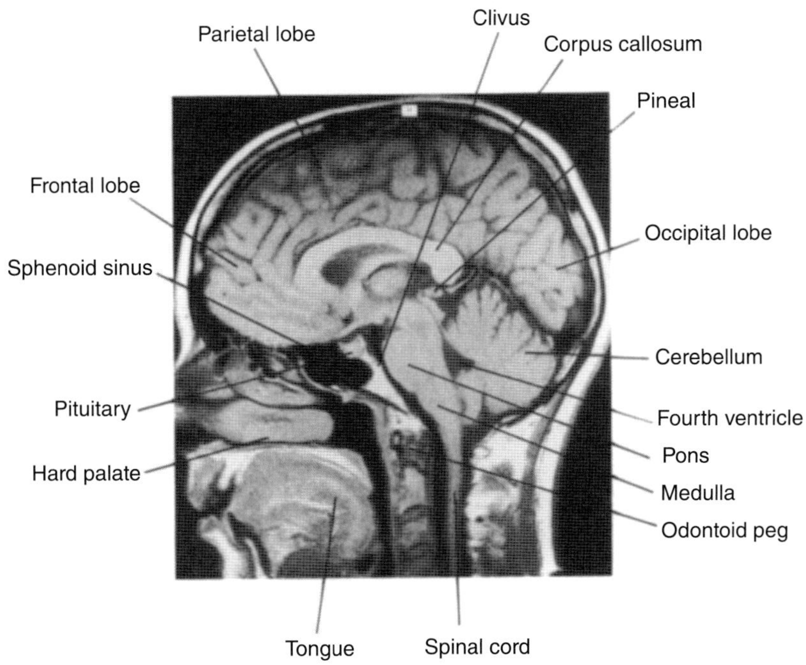

Fig. 31.3 Normal anatomy of the central nervous system. Magnetic resonance midline sagittal section. (Courtesy Dr L Turnbull, MRI Unit, Sheffield, UK.)

and parietal lobes. Tumours lying at any point along that pathway can therefore affect vision.

Inferiorly and laterally, with its tip in the middle cranial fossa, lies the temporal lobe. The medial part is involved in short-term memory. In the dominant hemisphere, the temporal lobe is the location for one of the speech centres, the auditory cortex.

The pons and medulla together form the brainstem. These have processing functions, important functional centres such as the respiratory centre, and carry all motor and sensory information between the cerebral cortex and spinal cord (Figs. 31.2 and 31.3). Even small lesions within the brainstem have very severe neurological effects. The function of the cerebellum is the subconscious control of movement. Damage to the cerebellum therefore leads to ataxia and other difficulties with coordinated movement.

The lobes of the brain communicate through extensive pathways of white matter. These run from front to back, side to side and up and down through the brain. Tumours which spread through white matter tracts (especially the gliomas) therefore have access to pathways which can allow them to disseminate extensively. The corpus callosum (see Fig. 31.3) is the major route of side-to-side communication between the two cerebral hemispheres. HGGs lying medially in the hemisphere often involve this structure, thus allowing spread into the opposite hemisphere.

Functional imaging, especially magnetic resonance imaging (MRI), has demonstrated that damage to particular areas of the brain, for example, the motor cortex, can lead to some function being taken over by other areas, provided that the rate of damage is slow. This is the concept of *neuroplasticity*. In the adult, this can occur in only a modest way but can explain why, in some circumstances, patients do not lose all the neurological function that might be anticipated from the tumour site.

Anatomy of the Cerebral Spinal Fluid Pathways and Hydrocephalus

The major cerebral spinal fluid (CSF) structures are shown in Fig. 31.4. CSF is produced by the choroid plexus within the two lateral ventricles and flows into the third ventricle anteriorly through the foramen of

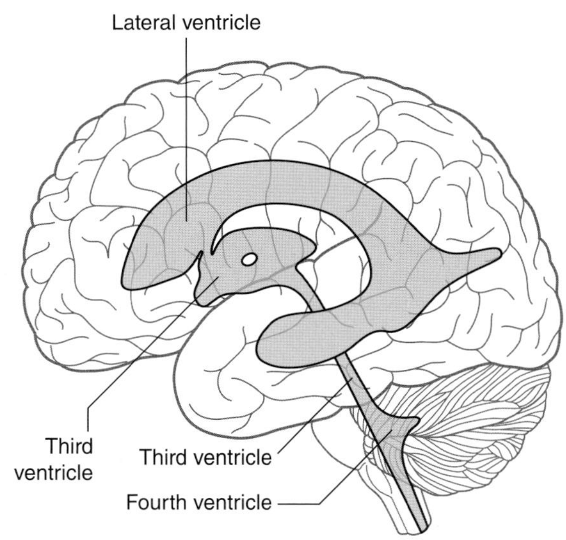

Fig. 31.4 The ventricular system, showing the cerebral spinal fluid pathways. See text for further details.

Munro (Fig. 31.4). CSF exits the third ventricle posteriorly through the aqueduct and flows into the fourth ventricle. From there, CSF leaves the fourth ventricle through three foramina (the foramina of Luschka laterally and the foramen of Magendie in the midline) to surround the outside of the brain. A small amount also passes down the central canal in the spinal cord. CSF is actively absorbed by the arachnoid granulations which protrude into the major venous sinuses, especially the superior sagittal sinus at the vertex of the skull. The CSF canals are lined by ependymal cells, from which ependymomas arise. These tumours are therefore related in space to the ventricular system.

Disturbance in the flow or absorption of CSF causes hydrocephalus. Obstruction of the flow before the exit foramina in the fourth ventricle leads to obstructive hydrocephalus. Obstruction of the arachnoid granulations leads to communicating hydrocephalus.

Tumours most commonly cause obstructive hydrocephalus. This is normally the result of obstruction in the fourth ventricle by tumours growing in or around the ventricle (such as medulloblastoma or ependymoma) or within the cerebellum (most commonly metastases). The next most common location for obstruction is the aqueduct, from compression by tumour tissue in adjacent brain or the pineal gland. More proximal obstruction can also occur at the foramen of Munro, usually from infiltrative HGG, causing hydrocephalus in one or both lateral ventricles.

Communicating hydrocephalus can be caused directly by tumour when extensive meningeal involvement occurs. This is almost always metastatic (most commonly from breast cancer) and it is rare. A more common cause of communicating hydrocephalus is blood in the CSF, resulting from surgery or a spontaneous bleed directly from a tumour. Blood can occlude the pores in the arachnoid granulations. Often this resolves spontaneously, but occasionally a CSF shunt (such as a ventriculoperitoneal (VP) shunt) must be inserted. Infection can also result in this through the same mechanism.

Anatomy of the Skull and Meninges

The skull itself is divided into three fossae. The frontal fossa contains the frontal lobe, the middle cranial fossa contains the temporal lobe and the posterior cranial fossa contains the cerebellum. The cerebellum is divided from the cranial contents by the tentorium cerebelli ('tent'), except for an aperture through which the brainstem passes. The cerebral hemispheres are divided by the falx cerebri. These two structures are composed of layers of tough meninges and are designed to dampen movements of the brain which might otherwise be damaging to the delicate brain substance. They are relatively rigid. The falx and tentorium cannot be infiltrated by gliomas and so present efficient barriers to their spread. Meningiomas, on the other hand, can spread along their surface, and their potential direction of spread can be anticipated by understanding this anatomy.

The meninges consist of three layers. The outer dura mater (usually known simply as dura) is a tough membrane which acts like a periosteum; it is the part visible on imaging and forms the falx and tent. Below and closely applied to the dura is the arachnoid mater. Below this lies the pia mater, a thin, delicate layer which covers every surface and fold of the brain substance. In some places, there is a space (the subarachnoid space) between the arachnoid and pia that is crossed by thin strands with a cobweb-like appearance (hence the origin of the name *arachnoid*). The dura lines the whole cranial cavity, including the skull base. In some areas the dura splits to form venous channels, such as the superior sagittal sinus, and the cavernous sinuses. It also forms two important folds, the tentorium cerebelli and the falx cerebri, which are continuous with the dura covering the skull vault and skull base.

CLINICAL FEATURES: PRESENTATION OF BRAIN TUMOURS

Presenting symptoms and signs of CNS tumours are manifold; patients may present with one or more classes of symptoms, as follows.

Specific Focal Neurological Deficit

CNS tumours may cause local damage, leading to specific deficits dependent on the location of the tumour. For example, a meningioma affecting the motor cortex will produce weakness and stiffness in a limb, depending on which part of the motor cortex is affected. A GBM affecting the frontal lobe produces intellectual, motivational and memory problems. Symptoms and signs can thus indicate the site of the tumour, which will then be confirmed by imaging. Tumours arising in eloquent areas typically present earlier than those in silent areas of the brain because they produce symptoms when smaller. Tumours which grow slowly, for example, meningiomas, often have an insidious onset with relatively mild symptoms and signs and may be surprisingly large when detected. Tumours which grow rapidly and destructively, such as GBMs, produce symptoms and signs which often appear to commence abruptly.

Symptoms and signs relating to specific parts of the brain are:

- Frontal lobe: Intellectual impairment and personality change
- Parietal lobe: Sensory or visual inattention
- Frontotemporoparietal lobe: Speech disturbance, especially dysphasia
- Occipital lobe: Visual field defects
- Brainstem: Cranial nerve defects, sensory or motor disturbance
- Cerebellum: Loss of coordination of movement

Epileptic Seizure

Almost all CNS tumours have the potential to cause epileptic seizures (and can be a consequence of the craniotomy required to treat them). These can take a number of forms, including generalised grand mal seizures, Jacksonian motor seizures, sensory seizures and petit mal absence attacks. Seizures are typically associated with slow-growing, low-grade gliomas (LGGs), especially oligodendrogliomas. A seizure can often be an early presenting feature of a tumour, and thus the presence of seizures is associated with a slightly improved survival in patients with HGG. However, a recurrence or worsening of a seizure following first-line treatment usually indicates disease progression. The efficacy of anticonvulsant medication depends on age, gender, organ dysfunction, comorbidity and cotherapies. Most patients are controlled with simple antiepileptic medication, but the advice of a neurologist is invaluable in managing complex or treatment-resistant seizures. Seizure control can be improved by surgical resection, RT and chemotherapy. Older antiepileptic drugs such as phenobarbital, carbamazepine or phenytoin stimulate the synthesis of hepatic cytochrome P450 enzymes and can affect the metabolism of concomitant drugs. Nonenzyme-inducing antiepileptic agents such as levetiracetam, lacosamide or clobazam are preferred due to fewer drug–drug interactions and improved adverse effect profiles. For patients who never had a seizure, routine anticonvulsant prophylaxis is not recommended. The use of antiepileptic drugs perioperatively is common, but evidence for this practice is scant.

Raised Intracranial Pressure

Raised intracranial pressure (ICP) typically produces a triad of symptoms and signs: headaches, generally worse in the morning; nausea and vomiting; and papilloedema (oedema of the optic disk). Raised ICP most commonly arises as the result of obstructive hydrocephalus and is therefore particularly associated with tumours in the posterior fossa. It can also be associated with drowsiness, mild confusion and (sometimes) personality change. In severe cases it can be followed by stupor and coma, hemiparesis or quadriparesis, respiratory abnormalities and eventually cardiopulmonary arrest. Management of elevated ICP depends on the patient's physical condition. CSF drainage should be attempted as appropriate, along with surgical removal of the lesion. Occasionally, other medical options (e.g. mannitol) need to be explored. Osmotic diuretics (mannitol) can be used in the acute situation to relieve pressure before commencing more definitive treatment. The first-line management in reducing ICP and symptomatic relief of symptoms is corticosteroids (e.g. dexamethasone). It is important that any patient likely to develop increased ICP should be educated regarding the warning symptoms of the same, including persistent headaches and vomiting, and know whom to contact if they develop these.

Nonspecific Symptoms

Nonspecific symptoms are common and typical of CNS tumours. Such symptoms may be very difficult to identify as significant in the early phase of the illness. Headache, which may be local or generalised but not related to raised ICP, occurs in some patients. The other characteristic symptom, particularly of HGG, is tiredness. Early symptoms may be frustratingly nonspecific, and a patient who complains of vague headache, tiredness and feeling off-color is not likely to be investigated for a primary CNS tumour.

PRINCIPLES OF MANAGEMENT

Although most patients come to oncology with a definitive diagnosis, it is important for oncologists to contribute to the multidisciplinary management of CNS patients.

Diagnosis: A Combination of History, Imaging and Pathology

It is always helpful to combine information from the patient's history and examination findings with imaging results and histology in determining the definitive diagnosis. The history and physical signs, especially the duration and any family history, may indicate a likely diagnosis or help indicate whether the condition is a high-grade malignancy rather than a low-grade or benign tumour.

Typically, the diagnosis is suggested by computed tomography (CT), which is quicker to acquire in an emergency setting than MRI, although MRI gives a much better diagnostic yield. In some tumour types, such as vestibular schwannoma (acoustic neuroma), imaging is definitive; in other cases, imaging offers only a differential diagnosis. Advanced imaging techniques such as functional MRI (fMRI) and diffusion tensor imaging have enriched presurgical evaluations by improving differential diagnosis and facilitating better surgical planning. Additionally, newer uses of perfusion imaging, susceptibility-weighted imaging (SWI), spectroscopy and positron emission tomography (PET) are proving to be helpful in distinguishing between tumour progression and treatment-related inflammatory changes, which is a common clinical challenge. Classical difficulties arise in distinguishing glioma from primary cerebral lymphoma and solitary metastasis from abscess or small glioma. Benign lesions can also have imaging appearances suggestive of malignancy. Biopsy therefore is crucial to establishing a definitive diagnosis.

Some CNS tumours, especially gliomas, are rather heterogeneous, and it is understood that biopsy material may not necessarily be representative of the whole tumour. Occasionally it may contain necrotic material only. Thus clinical history and imaging appearances must also be considered in defining the exact diagnosis.

Principles of Neurosurgery

The acquisition of histological material to define the diagnosis is extremely important. However, in many cases, there is also a role for a more extensive procedure to debulk or remove the tumour and relieve pressure effects (see sections on individual tumours). Surgical decompression improves symptoms quickly, allows reduced steroid doses and facilitates RT, especially in patients with HGGs. Although maximum debulking of the tumour is a positive prognostic factor, gliomas are not cured by excision, due to infiltration of tumour cells far beyond the visible lesion. The aim of neurosurgery therefore should be to obtain as maximal a resection as is possible without the patient acquiring new or worsening neurological deficit. Resection of lesions located in eloquent areas of white matter is not always the best treatment option, as it can cause permanent neurological deficits and reduce quality of life. Use of techniques such as fluorescent 5-ALA (5-aminolevulinic acid hydrochloride), which permits intraoperative identification of anaplastic foci and thus improves the extent of surgical resection by allowing previously nonvisible tumour to be seen and awake craniotomy with accompanying functional monitoring, have improved the safety of tumour resections. Occasionally, HGGs grow with a cystic component to the tumour. If fluid reaccumulates, a small catheter can be placed into the cyst and attached to a subcutaneous (Ommaya) reservoir. By inserting a needle through the skin, fluid can be aspirated without the need for a further surgical procedure. This is not a long-term solution, as the fluid often reaccumulates rapidly and by its proteinaceous nature can block the reservoir. Patients who present with or develop hydrocephalus may need a shunting procedure to redirect the flow of CSF. In adults, this is usually done with a VP shunt. Some patients with obstructive hydrocephalus can be successfully treated by a third ventriculostomy, avoiding the need for a shunt. In this procedure a perforation is made in the floor of the third ventricle, allowing CSF to escape and circumventing the obstruction.

Performance Status in the Treatment Decision

Performance status is an important predictor of outcome, including survival, particularly for patients with glioma (Table 31.2). It also indicates how well the patient is likely to tolerate treatment. This is an important factor when recommending a treatment program. The choice can be radical treatment, palliative treatment or active supportive care. For patients with disabling neurology, especially those with GBM, supportive care may be the most appropriate option.

Principles of Radiotherapy Planning for CNS Tumours

The fundamental principles of RT planning and treatment delivery apply to CNS tumours. These include accurate and reproducible immobilisation,

TABLE 31.2 WHO Performance Status, Glasgow Coma Scale and Karnofsky Performance Status

The WHO Performance Status is useful in assessing patient capabilities, especially with respect to activities of daily living. The Glasgow Coma Scale (GCS) is a measure of conscious level.

WHO Performance Status

0: Able to carry out all normal activity without restriction
1: Restricted in physically strenuous activity but ambulatory and able to carry out light work
2: Ambulatory and capable of all self-care but unable to carry out any work; up and about >50% of waking hours
3: Capable of only limited self-care; confined to bed or chair >50% of waking hours
4: Completely disabled. Cannot carry out any self-care; totally confined to bed or chair

Karnofsky Status

Normal, no complaints	100
Able to carry on normal activities. Minor signs or symptoms of disease	90
Normal activity with effort	80
Care for self; unable to carry on normal activity or to do active work	70
Requires occasional assistance but able to care for most of their needs	60
Requires considerable assistance and frequent medical care	50
Disabled; requires special care and assistance	40
Severely disabled; hospitalisation indicated though death nonimminent	30
Very sick; hospitalisation necessary, active supportive treatment necessary	20
Moribund	10
Dead	0

high-quality imaging to localise the tumour and critical normal structures, and the use of either three-dimensional conformal RT or preferably, intensity modulated radiotherapy (IMRT), typically with rotational techniques including tomotherapy and volumetric modulated arc therapy (VMAT). Brain tumours are characterised by irregular shapes which change in three dimensions. IMRT combined with image guidance has facilitated optimal RT, especially for tumours considered difficult to treat due to their location (e.g. meningiomas of the skull base, gliomas located near the orbit and the brainstem). Proton treatment is now being more widely used, generating highly conformal and complex dose distributions in these anatomic locations and allowing for dose escalation, especially in the management of radioresistant tumours (see Chapter 37). The other key clinical consideration in CNS tumour treatments is reduction of RT toxicity, especially to serial structures such as the brainstem and optic pathway. Lower doses to the whole brain can also be achieved with highly conformal RT delivery. IMRT does not increase the integral dose to the healthy brain and thus can lead to reduced acute and late neurotoxicity, which is especially relevant with the addition of chemotherapy for some tumours in patients with increased overall survival. The benefits of IMRT can be maximised with the addition of image-guided radiotherapy (IGRT), which can result in reduced margins and lead to further reduction of the total cumulative dose to normal untreated tissues (integral dose–total energy). IGRT allows for correction of both systematic (treatment preparation) and random (treatment delivery) errors. Immobilisation devices include thermoplastic shells, an Orfit shell or a relocatable stereotactic head frame. The optimal treatment position depends on the location of the tumour and the immobilisation devices available. A supine position is more comfortable for the patient. Using couch extensions, such as an 'S' frame or a relocatable stereotactic radiotherapy (SRT) head frame, allows treatment of posterior lesions with the patient supine.

For craniospinal irradiation (CSI), IMRT plus IGRT should be considered the standard of care, achieving reduced dose to organs at risk (OARs) and better target dose homogeneity than older techniques.

Most planning is based on CT because this delivers exact patient geometry and position without distortion and because CT density is required for accurate dosimetry calculation. Intravenous contrast may be used to enhance discrimination of the target. However, in most circumstances, tumours are less well demonstrated on CT than on MRI; thus fusing CT and MR images should be considered an essential modality for planning and will likely obviate the need for contrast with a CT scan. All efforts should be made to perform the MR imaging in the treatment position. The MR images are then coregistered with those of the CT scan.

The correct choice of MRI sequence must be made to optimise definition of the tumour. T1-weighted MRI (T1W) with contrast enhancement provides information on tumour extent; however, the appearances can be influenced by areas of blood–brain barrier breakdown. T2-weighted (T2W) and fluid-attenuated inversion recovery (FLAIR) images can help identify nonenhancing components of the tumour. The FLAIR sequence is helpful in LGGs and in demonstrating progression of the tumour in secondary GBMs.

Target delineation in the context of brain tumours should incorporate the use of contrast-enhanced three-dimensional T1-weighted and T2/FLAIR sequences. In particular, three-dimensional sequences prove especially beneficial when there is residual nonenhancing tumour tissue. It is of utmost importance that the MRI protocol guarantees both adequate image quality and spatial resolution, as emphasised in reference. Nonetheless caution must be exercised when relying on T2/FLAIR sequences for planning purposes. These signals lack specificity and can represent various conditions, such as oedema, inflammation, postoperative ischemic changes or gliosis, rather than tumour infiltration. Furthermore, T2/FLAIR signal characteristics can exhibit significant fluctuations over short periods, influenced by factors such as tumour mass effect, postoperative oedema and steroid treatment.

Utilising the entire T2/FLAIR hyperintense signal to define the clinical target volume (CTV) may result in an excessively large target volume that could surpass the tolerance of normal brain tissue. Nevertheless T2/FLAIR signal alterations can serve a valuable role in identifying regions suspected of tumour infiltration. These abnormalities indicative of tumour infiltration may include cortex or deep grey nuclei infiltration, mass effect characterised by gyral thickening and sulcal effacement, ventricular compression and/or corpus callosum thickening. On the other hand, oedema typically follows natural white matter tracts, respects the cortex and is closer to the CSF signal than the tumour, which tends to be denser.

In addition to conventional MRI sequences (T1, T2 and FLAIR) that aid in defining the structural boundaries of the tumour, perfusion- and diffusion-weighted MRI can provide insights into regional blood volume and microstructural architecture. MR spectroscopy can offer additional molecular and metabolic information. However, the roles of functional and metabolic MRI in target delineation for GBM are not firmly established, and currently these techniques should primarily be utilised within the context of prospective clinical trials rather than routine GBM delineation.

Apart from MRI, metabolic PET imaging is increasingly becoming an integral part of clinical practice. Unlike (18F)-2- fluorodeoxyglucose (FDG), which is commonly used for staging extracranial cancers, radiolabelled amino acids exhibit minimal uptake in the normal brain, facilitating superior delineation of brain tumours, especially gliomas. Frequently employed amino acid tracers include (11C-methyl)-L-methionine (MET), O-(2-(18F)-fluoroethyl)-L-tyrosine (FET), 3,4-dihydroxy-6-(18F)-fluoro-L-phenylalanine (FDOPA) and anti-1-amino-3-(18F)fluorocyclobutane-1-carboxylic acid (fluciclovine). A crucial feature of these tracers is their capacity to penetrate the intact blood–brain barrier. This characteristic proves particularly advantageous in delineating glioma regions that do not exhibit enhancement on MRI. These tracers may therefore be suitable for RT planning. The use of FET PET as a valuable additional tool for target delineation could be helpful. However, it is still undergoing investigation, and practical and financial considerations may limit its routine use.

CT and MRI are complementary. Although MRI is in general the better modality for showing tumour, CT is extremely useful to determine the exact position of the bone, extent of bone involvement or barriers to spread of a noninvasive tumour which is limited by bone. MRI sequences (such as diffusion weighted and diffusion tensor imaging) can be used to help distinguish tumour cell density and fractional anisotropy at resection margins in LGGs. MR perfusion measures cerebral blood volume in tumours and can be used to identify the best area to obtain a biopsy, as it can help in distinguishing malignant activity from tumour necrosis. MR spectroscopy and PET imaging can provide information on the metabolic activity of the tumour. They can also be helpful in tumour grading and in differentiating between response to treatment and necrosis. In some meningiomas that have been completely resected, coregistration with the preoperative MRI may be helpful in determining the location of the tumour and possible spread. PET scanning can be useful for planning in some circumstances, using methionine (an amino acid) or DOTATOC (1,4,7,10-tetraazacyclododecane-N^{I},N^{II},N^{III},N^{IIII}-tetraacetic acid (D)-Phe^{1}-thy^{3}-octreotide).

Planning Volumes

The International Commission on Radiation Units and Measurements (ICRU) Report 83 sets guidelines on planning IMRT and offers useful recommendations for planning volumes. The definitions of GTV, CTV and PTV as outlined in ICRU 83 should be used for planning purposes. Imaging shows the extent of the GTV. For GBMs, early recurrence after the operation is common and can even be visible in the MRI RT planning scan. New imaging approaches mentioned earlier could be used for gliomas and meningiomas to improve target volume definition and aid in individualisation of treatment. Historical data are used to define a CTV margin around the GTV, which is typically the same in all patients with that tumour type. Following isotopic growth from the GTV, the CTV is edited to account for anatomical barriers of tumour spread (e.g. bone and dural reflections). The PTV margin is designed to account for uncertainties in planning and treatment and has systematic (i.e. 'treatment preparation') and random (i.e. 'treatment delivery') elements. The margin should be added based on the recipe formula outlined in the British Institute of Radiology 2003 report 'Geometric Uncertainties in Radiotherapy' and incorporated into ICRU 83. Most departments know what margin they can achieve with the immobilisation techniques and machine specificities they have.

Doses should be estimated to all OARs close to the PTV. These should be outlined at the time of treatment planning to allow the physicists to provide a dose to each critical structure, thus determining whether this remains within accepted limits or not. IMRT with IGRT should be considered astandard practice because this reduces dose to normal tissues, in turn reducing complications in patients by reducing the volume of tissue, especially brain, receiving a high dose, or avoiding exposure to sensitive structures such as the hypothalamus and pituitary gland (conformal avoidance). Cone beam imaging or its equivalent should be used to confirm positioning for treatment. Three-dimensional RT can be used in the palliative setting to increase the conformity of the dose in comparison to older techniques and to protect critical structures.

Normal Tissue Tolerance to Radiotherapy

Normal tissue tolerance is an important concept. It embodies both the risk of a complication and the severity of its effect on the patient. The relevance also depends on the clinical setting: a higher risk of normal tissue damage might be accepted in a patient with a highly malignant tumour requiring a high RT dose who has only a low chance of long-term survival than is reasonable in a patient with a benign tumour. The dose that is considered safe may therefore vary from one condition to another. Another important factor is the addition of chemotherapy and biological agents to RT in the treatment of CNS tumours. These may affect the tolerance of normal brain, the brainstem and the optic pathway, though detailed information is lacking. It is known that drugs such as methotrexate (MTX) used for primary CNS lymphomas (PCNSLs) can induce radiation damage.

There is almost certainly a volume effect in normal tissue tolerance of CNS structures, as in other parts of the body. This means the larger the volume irradiated, the lower the safe dose. The CNS is also particularly sensitive to the dose per fraction, and many of the dose-fractionation schedules used are designed to take advantage of this. The best available data are presented in the detailed QUANTEC reports.

Tolerance of the brain itself (to avoid necrosis) is in the region of 54 to 60 Gy in approximately 30 fractions, depending on the volume treated and dose per fraction. A volume effect also exists for intellectual damage. Using three-dimensional conformal RT, intellectual damage in adults is uncommon with doses up to 54 Gy in 30 fractions. The brainstem is said to have a slightly lower tolerance than brain substance, approximately 54 Gy in 30 fractions (or 55 Gy in 33 fractions). Smaller volumes of the brainstem (1–10 mL) could receive a maximum dose of 59 Gy using conventional fractionation of 2 Gy per fraction. QUANTEC suggests a change in α/β ratio for normal brain of 2.9 Gy in comparison to the 2.0 Gy used in Emami's original report.

The optic nerves and chiasm are also thought to be more sensitive than brain parenchyma. For benign tumours in this region, a dose of 45 Gy in 25 fractions to 50 Gy in 30 fractions should be safe, with a risk of blindness which is virtually zero. Optic neuropathy should be avoided with doses less than 55 Gy as a primary criterion and less than 60 Gy as secondary criterion, according to the QUANTEC report. The incidence of optic neuropathy is approximately 7% for doses of 66 Gy.

The pituitary gland and hypothalamus have a much lower tolerance for hormonal dysfunction, which may occur in 80% of patients receiving RT. There is probably little effect for doses under 20 to 24 Gy, but adults in whom these structures receive 40 to 60 Gy have a significant long-term risk of hypothalamic–pituitary axis (HPA) dysfunction. The cells most sensitive to RT are those that secrete growth hormone (GH), followed by gonadotropin hormones, adrenocorticotropic hormone (ACTH) and thyroid stimulating hormone (TSH). The frequency and severity of symptoms correlate to the total dose, the dose per fraction and the age of the patient at the time of irradiation, although the exact details of the dose–response relationships are not known. It is important that patients who receive high doses of RT to the HPA have long-term follow-up. Early replacement therapy should be started as required to avoid the development of endocrinological syndromes.

The lacrimal gland shows reduced tear output after doses over about 20 Gy (similar to salivary glands). Doses over 40 Gy can cause dry eye syndrome, whereas doses over 57 Gy can lead to permanent atrophy and fibrosis of the lacrimal gland.

The lens of the eye should not develop cataract after doses less than 5 to 6 Gy delivered over 30 fractions. There is a 50% risk of cataract after a dose of 15 Gy. Therefore the recommended maximum dose for adults should range between 5 and 10 Gy. The middle and inner ears are also sensitive structures, and there are reports of hearing loss in adults with doses to the cochlea ranging between 45 and 50 Gy.

The risk of permanent alopecia depends on the dose to the hair follicles in the dermis. The risk is very low with doses below 10 to 15 Gy, but 50% of patients will develop permanent alopecia after 43 Gy (in 30 fractions) to the scalp. This dose is difficult to estimate routinely because the hair follicles normally fall within the buildup region.

The spinal cord has a tolerance of approximately 50 Gy in 30 fractions. This may be a conservative estimate and in some circumstances, higher doses may be appropriate, such as for GBM of the spinal cord. New evidence suggests that an α/β ratio of 0.87 Gy may be more appropriate for the cervical spinal cord. This ratio is low, meaning that larger fractions can cause more severe effects.

The hippocampus (dentate gyrus) contains neural stem cells which aid cognitive function. The delineation of the hippocampus as an OAR is advisable, although there is no consensus on what the tolerance radiation dose to this area should be. Suggestive dose restrictions, with the aim to avoid impairment in memory function, are 7.3 Gy to 40% of the bilateral hippocampus, but not to exceed 9 Gy to 100% of the hippocampus, with maximal hippocampal dose not exceeding 16 Gy in 30 fractions. The ipsilateral hippocampus is included in the PTV area in the majority of the glial tumours, so efforts usually concentrate on sparing the contralateral hippocampus where feasible.

The retina should have doses restricted to less than 45 Gy to avoid the risk of radiation retinopathy.

The cochlea, which is a spiral-shaped organ surrounding the modiolus, contains the endolymphatic receptor system consisting of hair cells that detect sound vibrations. Various studies conducted on adult patients have aimed to establish a correlation between the mean dose of radiation received by the cochlea and the development of sensorineural hearing loss. They have reported a significant increase in the risk of hearing loss when the mean cochlear dose exceeds 45 to 50 Gy.

Principles of Steroid Therapy

Steroids, generally oral dexamethasone, are used to treat oedema in the brain caused by tumour or surgery. A daily dose of dexamethasone of 16 mg, in 2 divided doses (twice daily), is considered the highest useful dose in most circumstances. Patients on anticonvulsant drugs, which increase the metabolism of dexamethasone, occasionally benefit from higher doses in the palliative setting. Mild to moderate symptoms, such as headache or sensory deficits, can be managed with dexamethasone 4 to 8 mg daily without a loading dose. Once- or twice-daily dosing is typically sufficient, with the last dose at lunchtime to prevent the insomnia typically associated with steroid use. The lowest dose required for symptom control should be administered, and tapering off corticosteroids should be attempted as soon as appropriate. A slow taper (e.g. dose reduction every 7–10 days) is recommended to identify the minimal steroid dose required to control neurological symptoms and to reduce the risk of adrenal insufficiency. Bone protection should be considered for patients who require long-term steroids.

Dexamethasone has important side effects which can impact seriously on quality of life. These include increased appetite, weight gain, muscle weakness, gastric irritation, diabetes, cerebral atrophy, reduced taste and smell, osteoporosis, infections and mood disturbances. Myopathy is a common complication of corticosteroid use in patients with brain tumours. Patients with steroid-induced myopathy may report difficulty when rising from a seated position and when climbing stairs. Symptoms may resolve after steroid discontinuation. Rarely, it may cause psychosis, which is very distressing and difficult to manage. Patients should be managed with the minimum possible dose. For reduction, the dose must be tailed off slowly and not stopped abruptly. Patients should also be issued a steroid card.

In patients requiring RT where significant ICP remains, steroid is needed and may need to be increased during the treatment course. However, there is no absolute indication for steroids during RT. In patients in whom surgery has relieved ICP, none may be necessary, and it is possible to reduce steroid doses during a course of RT.

Driving After a Diagnosis of CNS Tumour

Many patients with primary CNS tumours are not allowed to drive following the diagnosis. This is because there is a risk of seizure as the result of the tumour. There is also a small risk of seizure following craniotomy, whatever the underlying condition. In particular, patients with HGGs have their driving licences revoked for 12 months to 2 years, timed from the completion of treatment.

INDIVIDUAL TUMOUR TYPES

HIGH-GRADE GLIOMAS

Pathology and Clinical Features

GBM IDH WT, CNS WHO grade 4 is the most common primary CNS tumour in adults (see Fig. 31.1), representing 54% of malignant brain tumours. In the WHO 2021 classification of brain tumours, GBM falls under grade 4 gliomas and encompasses two distinct categories: astrocytoma IDH WT and diffuse hemispheric glioma with H3G34 mutation. However, when a tumour displays the histological features of a grade 2 or 3 glioma but is found to be IDH WT through sequencing, further analysis becomes necessary. If there is evidence indicating the presence of the genetic alterations telomerase reverse transcriptase (TERT) promoter mutation, epidermal growth factor receptor (EGFR) gene amplification or gain of an entire chromosome 7 combined with loss of an entire chromosome 10 (7+/10−), the tumour is managed as a GBM IDH WT. Furthermore, GBM IDH WT tumours can be further subdivided into those with or without MGMT promoter methylation. This not only serves as a predictive factor for the likelihood of responding to temozolomide chemotherapy but also carries independent prognostic significance irrespective of temozolomide use. The presence of methylation in the O6-alkylguanine DNA alkyltransferase (MGMT) gene is particularly valuable as it inactivates the gene responsible for breaking down temozolomide, thereby enhancing the drug's efficacy. MGMT methylation status is a critical factor guiding treatment decisions, especially in elderly patients.

It's important to note that the presence of a TERT promoter mutation negatively impacts prognosis and is identified in approximately 74% of GBM cases. Additionally, testing for the amplification of EGFR is common and is detected in about 40% of GBM cases. Grade 3 gliomas include anaplastic astrocytoma, anaplastic oligodendroglioma and pleomorphic xanthoastrocytoma and together with grade 4 tumours are collectively known as HGGs. In grade 3 tumours, the reclassification distinguishes between astrocytomas and oligodendrogliomas based on the presence or absence of 1p19q codeletion. These tumours are classified as either (1) oligodendroglioma, IDH-mutant, 1p19q codeleted, CNS WHO grade 3 (formerly known as anaplastic oligodendroglioma) or (2) astrocytoma, IDH mutant, 1p19q non-codeleted, CNS WHO grade 3 (formerly known as anaplastic astrocytoma). In cases where immunohistochemistry for IDH1 R132H is negative, sequencing of IDH1 codon 132 and IDH2 codon 172 should be conducted for all WHO grade 2 and 3 diffuse astrocytic and oligodendroglial gliomas, as well as for all GBMs in patients under age 55 years. Anaplastic astrocytomas, anaplastic oligodendrogliomas and anaplastic oligoastrocytomas frequently exhibit mutations in the IDH1 and IDH2 genes, with a prevalence ranging from 55% to 80%. These IDH mutations are often associated with codeletion of the 1p and 19q chromosome arms (1p19q codeletion) as well as MGMT promoter methylation. In the context of anaplastic gliomas, the presence of WT IDH1 and IDH2 without mutations is associated with a heightened risk of aggressive disease. Anaplastic oligodendrogliomas, which require codeletion of chromosomes 1p and 19q for diagnosis, tend to have extended survival compared to non-codeleted tumours, primarily due to their heightened responsiveness to treatment, particularly alkylating chemotherapy.

HGGs, especially GBMs, are efficient at spreading through the brain, predominantly following white matter tracts (see earlier discussion and Fig. 31.3). Spread across the midline, principally through the corpus callosum, is a major route for invasion. HGGs grow with an expanding, destructive process. Beyond the gross tumour, malignant cells infiltrate widely. This infiltration occurs at a microscopic level and so currently cannot be imaged. The extent of invasion varies among individuals. The gross tumour is typically surrounded by a zone of extensive oedema. Steroid treatment reduces oedema and may improve neurological function. However, there is no method to restore function which has been lost as a result of the destruction of neural tissue by the tumour.

Despite the wide infiltration, HGGs typically recur at the primary site. There is thus no survival advantage in irradiating the whole brain. HGGs very rarely metastasise outside the CNS.

HGGs area difficult to manage for a number of reasons:

1. They cause significant damage to neurological function, meaning that a proportion of patients will never be of a performance status that correlates with benefit from treatment.
2. They are resistant to all treatment modalities, including RT and chemotherapy.
3. They diffuse infiltration through the brain, frequently crossing the midline to involve the contralateral brain.

Presentation and radiology were described earlier. A typical GBM is shown in Fig. 31.5.

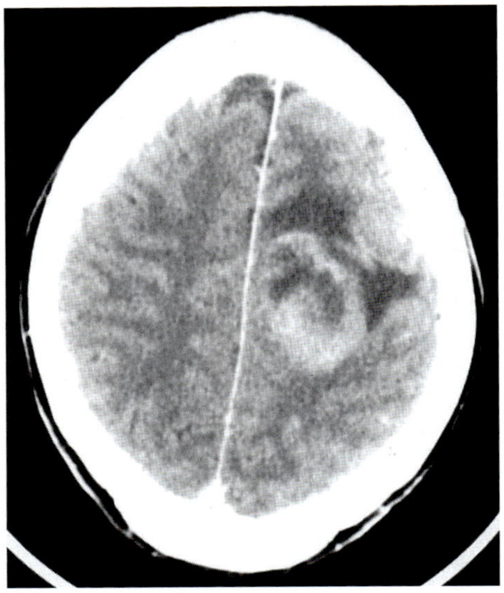

Fig. 31.5 Computed tomography scan with contrast of a patient with a glioblastoma, showing a contrast-enhancing mass with central necrosis and surrounding oedema.

Treatment

Management options may be radical, palliative or active supportive care only (Table 31.3). The decision depends on patient status, patient age, tumour location and patient preference. Patients with poor neurological condition are unlikely to benefit from radical treatment, and older patients tolerate the neurological effects of both the tumour and the treatment less well. For these patients the option of shorter-course palliative treatment may be most suitable. For elderly patients or those with very poor neurological function, quality of life is not improved by any available therapy. Referral for expert palliative and supportive care is therefore the most appropriate management.

Histological diagnosis is highly desirable, provided further treatment will be given, and can be used as a predictive or prognostic factor as well as aid in patient selection for clinical trials.

For radical treatment, debulking surgery is preferred where possible. It extends survival and, equally importantly, it relieves mass effect. In turn, this improves neurological functioning, reduces steroid requirements and facilitates RT. Early postoperative MRI, within 24 to 48 hours, demonstrates the extend of any residual gross tumour; it is very useful for comparison with the RT planning MRI.

In the case of GBM IDH WT astrocytoma grade 4, for young, fit patients the addition of chemotherapy with oral temozolomide concomitantly to RT and then adjuvantly for 6 cycles has been shown to significantly extend survival. The treatment for anaplastic astrocytoma (without 1p19q codeletion) has been guided by the CATNON study and consists of RT (59.4 Gy in 33 fractions) followed by 12 months of temozolomide. Patients with anaplastic oligodendroglioma (1p19q codeleted) should be offered RT (54–59.4 Gy in 30–33 fractions) with adjuvant PCV (procarbazine, lomustine (CCNU), and vincristine) for 6 cycles.

The outcome of patients with HGG is very variable. The three most important prognostic factors for better outcome are younger age, good performance status, including good cognitive status, and extent of surgery. In terms of age, patients under age 40 years have the best outlook, those under age 60 years do less well and those over age 70 years fare badly. The extent of surgical resection has prognostic value as it improves survival and might increase the efficacy of adjuvant treatments. Patients with brainstem HGG, in whom even a biopsy attempt is hazardous, do particularly badly. Presentation with epilepsy provides a small survival advantage, but this is almost certainly simply the result of the patient presenting earlier in their illness pathway.

TABLE 31.3 Suggested Criteria for Choice of Treatment in Patients With High-Grade Glioma

Radical radiotherapy	Age <70 (younger in some centres) or chemoradiotherapy
Performance status 0 or 1	
No significant neurological deficit remaining	
Palliative radiotherapy	Age ≤70 and performance status 0 or 1
Age <70, with a significant deficit	
Supportive care	Severe residual deficit, e.g. hemiplegia
Intellectual impairment	

Note: The patient's choice should be considered in all cases. Where appropriate, agreement from the patient's relatives is also valuable, especially for the supportive care option.

In rare cases, HGG can be very extensive, affecting the whole of the hemisphere or even the majority of the cerebrum. This used to be known as gliomatosis cerebri. It normally responds to RT and although often not much of the normal brain can be spared, RT can improve the neurological deficit in some patients.

Radiotherapy

Target Volume

The patient should be immobilised in a shell and positioned supine with the chin in a neutral position. Postoperative imaging is required to demonstrate the true extent and position of residual tumour after decompression. MRI produces superior definition of tumour, and the T1-weighted plus gadolinium (T1W+Gd) and T2/FLAIR sequences should be coregistered to the planning CT.

The ESTRO-EANO group have produced guidelines for RT target volume definition based on protocols used in the studies they have designed and run. The recommendation of ESTRO-EANO is to aim to deliver 60 Gy in 30 fractions in a single phase.

The GTV is defined as the visible contrast-enhancing edge of tumour, shown most clearly on MRI using T1W+Gd contrast. For the definition of the GTV in the context of resected tumours, it is advisable to define the GTV by considering the resection cavity, if it exists, along with any remaining enhancing tumour areas visible on contrast-enhanced T1-weighted MRI scans. It is important to note that peritumoural oedema should not be included in the GTV. The GTV should encompass all regions that show postoperative contrast enhancement. Some of these areas may actually represent postsurgical infarction or gliosis and therefore should be edited out of the GTV. Thus a comparison of planning MRI scans with preoperative scans and postoperative diffusion-weighted imaging (DWI) can help differentiate postoperative vascular changes from residual tumour. Although there are no available data indicating that incorporating perifocal oedema into the target volume leads to improved outcomes, changes observed in T2/FLAIR images may indicate areas of tumour infiltration. If this is the case, they should be encompassed within the CTV.

The utilisation of perfusion- and diffusion-weighted MRI techniques and amino acid PET tracers such as MET, FET, and FDOPA can aid in the detection of tumour infiltration in areas that go beyond those revealed by conventional MRI. These advanced imaging methods can be particularly valuable in precisely defining suspected nonenhancing tumour regions.

While PET imaging is not a standard part of GBM target delineation, its adoption is recommended based on findings from early-phase clinical trials, and available data support its utilisation for enhancing target delineation accuracy.

Some of the newly classified categories of molecular HGG do not demonstrate the same imaging characteristics as classical GBM, appearing as nonenhancing lesions on MRI. Obviously in these cases the GTV should encompass both the resection cavity and any remaining tumour that is either visible in T1c sequences or hyperintense on T2/FLAIR.

The GTV is expanded isotropically to reach the CTV. The CTV is defined as including the GTV along with an additional margin to account for potential microscopic tumour spread. Based on studies that have examined recurrence patterns and tumour infiltration, it is recommended to apply a margin of 15 mm in all directions to encompass likely tumour extension. Currently, there is a consensus against intentionally including the subventricular zone in the CTV.

The CTV does not have to extend beyond the inner table of the skull, which is best shown on CT using the bone window. Margins should be reduced at anatomical barriers such as the skull (0 mm, using the bone window), ventricles (5 mm), falx (0 mm), tentorium cerebelli (0 mm), visual pathways/optic chiasm and brainstem (each 0 mm), provided the tumour is distant from the white matter tracts extending to these regions (e.g. midbrain). No margin reduction should be applied at the corpus callosum or cerebral and cerebellar peduncles. In molecularly defined GBMs, similar margins should be applied.

The precise CTV-PTV margin should be determined based on the specific fixation technique used by the institution and local quality assurance measurements. Ideally, each department should conduct an audit of their setup results and implement the margin recommended by their data. As a general guideline, daily IGRT and modern treatment machines offer the opportunity to reduce the PTV margin, thereby sparing nearby healthy tissues. A PTV margin of 3 mm is strongly recommended, but a range of 2 to 5 mm is considered acceptable depending on the institution's IGRT program. There is evidence that employing a 2-mm PTV margin along with daily IGRT and VMAT can yield similar progression-free and overall survival outcomes compared to three-dimensional conformal RT with wider margins in a substantial cohort of GBM patients. This suggests that a 2-mm margin may be sufficient in certain institutional settings.

Outline critical normal structures, including the eyes, lenses, lacrimal glands, cochlea, pituitary and hypothalamus. It is essential to outline the optic structures. The delineation of the contralateral hippocampus should be considered in terms of sparing the organ; however, there is not sufficient evidence to support recommendations on hippocampal sparing.

Technique

IMRT with image guidance should be considered as the standard of care. It achieves the best target dose conformity and homogeneity and optimum critical normal tissue sparing.

Dose and Energy

Factors which need to be considered when assessing the optimum dose and fractionation for patients with GBM IDH WT include performance status, age, cognitive impairments, volume of residual disease (and surrogate of steroid dose), location of tumour and comorbidities. Shorter-course schedules are recommended for those over the age of 70 years. Some trials have used 65 years of age as the cutoff for 'elderly' whereas others have used 70 years of age. Consequently, the optimal management of people between age 65 and 70 years needs to be assessed on a case-by-case basis. Concurrent and adjuvant temozolomide has been shown to improve overall survival in patients with methylated GBM IDH WT. The addition of temozolomide may be considered in patients with unmethylated tumours, but the survival gain is more marginal. The gold standard fractionation scheme for fit, younger patients is a dose of 60 Gy delivered in 30 fractions of 2 Gy each with concurrent daily oral temozolomide. Alternatively, a shorter fractionation schedule of 40 Gy in 15 fractions may be considered for elderly and/or frail patients with smaller tumours.

Grade 4 IDH-mutated glioma was previously classified as GBM but was given a new classification in WHO 2021 in recognition that it has a better prognosis (median survival around 36 months compared to 14 months for GBM IDH WT). The optimal management of this new subgroup has not been tested in clinical trials, but as they were included in prior GBM trials they are managed according to the aforementioned protocols.

Summary

Patients with good performance status (KPS 80–100) and age less than 70 years with minimal residual tumour should receive 60 Gy in 30 daily fractions over 6 weeks +/– temozolomide (grade A).

Patients with moderate performance status (KPS 60–70) or age over 70 years should receive 40 Gy in 15 fractions over 3 weeks +/– temozolomide (grade A).

Patients with poor performance status (KPS 50–60) may be considered for shorter-course treatments such as 34 Gy in 10 fractions (grade B) or 30 Gy in 6 fractions on alternate days (grade C) or best supportive care.

Chemotherapy for Radical Treatment of Glioblastoma

Using the protocol from the EORTC trial, oral temozolomide is given in two blocks, the first one daily (including weekends), concomitant with radical RT, and the second one for 5 days each month as an adjuvant treatment following RT:

Concomitant with radical RT: Continuous daily dose of 75 mg/m^2 (i.e. 7 days per week), starting on the first day of RT and finishing on the last day.

Adjuvant treatment following RT: Commencing 28 days after completion of RT, temozolomide daily for 5 days, at a dose of 150 to 200 mg/m^2. This is repeated 4-weekly for 6 cycles.

Grade 3: IDH Mutant Non-Codeleted

The management of grade 3 IDH mutated non-codeleted gliomas (anaplastic astrocytoma) has been assessed in the CATNON trial. This study gave patients 59.4 Gy in 33 fractions and then assessed the use of concurrent and/or adjuvant temozolomide. Though the final analysis is awaited, initial analysis of the data demonstrates significant improvement in overall survival with the use of adjuvant temozolomide. However, to date there is no survival gain from the use of concurrent temozolomide.

Grade 3: IDH Mutant Codeleted

Two RT trials examined giving patients 59.4 Gy in 33 fractions with or without adjuvant/neoadjuvant PCV, and both demonstrated an improvement in overall survival with the addition of chemotherapy.

For most patients with grade 3 codeleted gliomas, immediate postoperative RT and chemotherapy is recommended, though for some with minimal residual disease and only foci of anaplasia, active surveillance may be an appropriate management strategy.

Side Effects

Acute

Acute tiredness is almost invariable, though it is of variable severity. It appears to be related to the volume treated. It increases during the course, has a fluctuating pattern and may be at its worst shortly after completion of RT. Early delayed somnolence is rare in adults.

Hair loss occurs in about the third week after treatment starts. Hair washing has no effect on hair loss or scalp reactions, provided it is carried out carefully. With 54 Gy, hair regrowth is almost normal in most patients; with 60 Gy, at least some hair loss is usually permanent. Erythema and soreness of skin can occur, particularly if the pinna is included in an entry port. If the external auditory canal is irradiated, this gets sore and crusted, and the wax becomes more viscid and difficult to remove. If the ear drum and middle ear are irradiated, secretory otitis media (glue ear) may result, but this usually settles spontaneously. Inner ear damage is uncommon. In patients treated for HGG, headache and nausea are uncommon. Seizures occasionally worsen during RT: dexamethasone is useful, and anticonvulsants should be reviewed.

Late

If the hypothalamus and pituitary have been irradiated, hormone failure may occur after a minimum of 1 to 2 years, but it may occur later. Routine pituitary function tests are therefore appropriate in the few patients who are long-term survivors. Although the most important late effect in the brain is radionecrosis, this is an extremely uncommon clinical event. The QUANTEC report suggests that there is a possibility of 5% and 10% risk at 5 years of symptomatic radionecrosis applying the standard fractionation at doses of 72 Gy (range 60–84 Gy) and 90 Gy (range 84–102 Gy), respectively, that is, significantly higher than used routinely.

Deterioration During Radiotherapy

Some patients deteriorate during RT. This is usually due to increased oedema, possibly as a result of tumour cell necrosis. It is usually treatable with an increase in dexamethasone dose. Occasionally, a cystic component can enlarge and warrants neurosurgical intervention such as aspiration and insertion of an Ommaya reservoir. A few patients deteriorate during RT due to tumour progression. In these cases it is appropriate to switch to palliative fractionation (discussed shortly), making an appropriate dose change according to the dose already delivered, or to stop RT altogether.

Results of Treatment

In a randomised trial of patients with GBM, the addition of oral temozolomide chemotherapy extended survival significantly: median survival was extended from 12 months to 14.5, and 2-year survival increased from 10% to 26%. Anaplastic (grade 3) gliomas with IDH mutation were found to have an improved median survival of 14.7 years compared with 6.8 years for those that did not carry the mutation. The prolonged overall survival and disease-free survival with the addition of temozolomide in the CATNON trial are shown in Fig. 31.6.

Elderly Patients

The EORTC 26062 trial showed that a palliative dose of RT (40 Gy in 15 fractions) in addition to concomitant and maintenance temozolomide offered a modest increase in median survival (9.3 versus 7.6 months, $p = 0.001$) compared with RT alone for both groups (mMGMT and unmethylated). The maximum benefit was for patients older than age 70 years, particularly those with tumours that express MGMT methylation.

In addition, a prospective trial which compared 40 Gy in 15 fractions to 25 Gy in 5 fractions over 1 week supported that the short course was not inferior in terms of survival.

The outlook for patients with HGG who receive palliative RT is poor, with a median survival of only 140 days (just under 5 months) from first presentation in oncology. However, a small number of patients survive for much longer, with a few remaining alive for over 2 years. Those patients deemed unfit for palliative RT have a median survival of only 6 weeks.

Reirradiation

There is increased interest in the use of reirradiation, particularly in patients who have relapsed after a reasonable interval of local control (usually >12 months). Schedules utilised vary depending on tumour biology, interval from initial presentation and tumour volume. There is one randomised phase II trial (RTOG 1205) which randomised patients to bevacizumab with or without reirradiation, giving 35 Gy in 10 fractions. Although there was no improvement in overall survival, the proportion of patients with progression-free survival at 6 months was significantly higher in the reirradiation arm. In the United Kingdom, a schedule of 35 Gy in 10 fractions is being increasingly used, particularly for GBM. A UK trial is underway comparing reirradiation with palliative chemotherapy (BRIOCHE) which will hopefully provide more evidence on the impact of reirradiation on survival.

LOW-GRADE GLIOMAS

Pathology and Clinical Features

LGGs represent about 12% of the total number of cases referred to oncology (see Fig. 31.1). The patients typically present at a younger age than those with high-grade gliomas, with a peak incidence between ages 35 and 44 years. Although LGGs present in similar ways to other primary tumours, seizure is a much more common presenting complaint than with other tumours. Grade 2 oligodendrogliomas are particularly likely to present with epilepsy. In some patients the diagnosis is an incidental finding after imaging for unrelated symptoms. The course of the illness is extremely variable. Some LGGs appear never to progress, and others may take a decade or more to do so. However, some tumours show evidence of disease progression from the time of diagnosis, driven by malignant transformation related to the accumulation of genetic mutations.

LGGs are characterised by a mutation in the IDH gene family. A separate subtype of oligodendrogliomas is classified by the losses of the whole arm of the 1p and 19q chromosomes (1p/19q codeletion). Astrocytomas have intact 1p and 19q chromosomes but loss of ATRX. In grade 2 diffuse gliomas, the mutations in either IDH1 or IDH2 are present in 80% of the cases. When these tumours progress, they may do so in their original form, but they may also undergo further genetic mutation causing transformation to a higher grade, grade 3 or even GBM. This occurs in about half of the patients who progress and is not itself caused or influenced by RT. Grade 2 oligodendrogliomas altering to higher-grade tumours are categorised as grade 3 anaplastic oligodendrogliomas. When grade 2 astrocytomas transform to a higher grade, they can become either grade 3 anaplastic astrocytomas or GBMs.

A metaanalysis showed that the presence of neurological deficits, a rapid onset of symptoms (less than 30 weeks), an astrocytic subtype and a tumour larger than 5 cm in diameter carries a worse prognosis. According to a long-term analysis of the RTOG 9802 trial, half of the low-risk patients (age younger than 40 years) included in the study who underwent only gross total resection (GTR) relapsed at 5 years, indicating that active surveillance with MRI is a possible option in this group. For the high-risk group (age >40 years in addition to the aforementioned features), the addition of chemotherapy with PCV and RT to surgery offered a greater benefit in overall survival. The benefit was highest in the subgroup with 1p19q codeletion. These patients, regardless of histology and molecular profile, are offered RT and PCV in addition to surgery. Two ongoing trials (RTOG 0424 and EORTC 22033-26033) add temozolomide to RT and report a benefit in overall survival as well an improvement in progression-free survival in those with IDH-mutated astrocytoma without 1p19q codeletion.

The role of surgery was controversial, but with the improvement in surgical techniques and careful patient selection, the evidence is that,

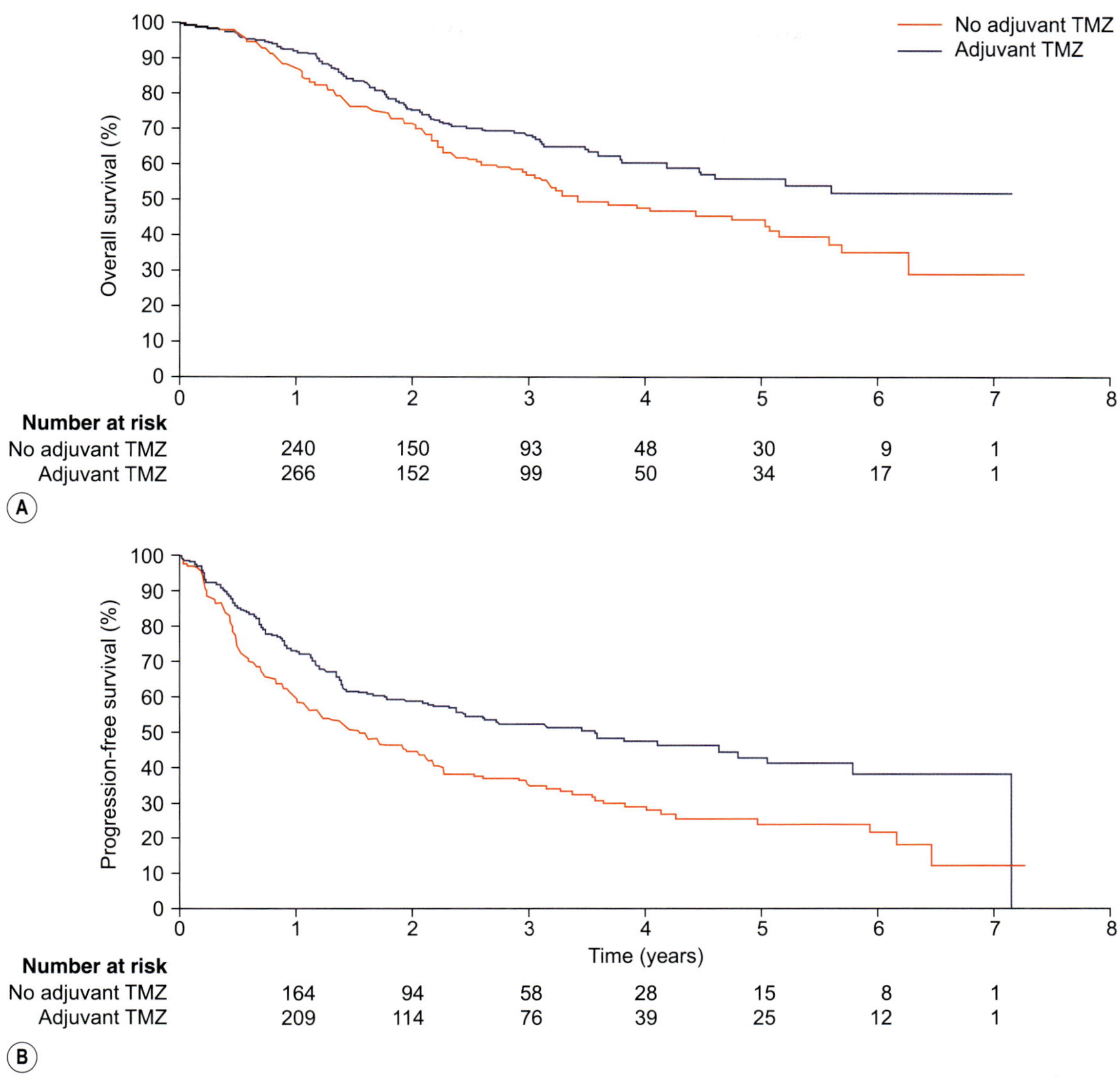

Fig. 31.6 Kaplan Meier Overall Survival and Progression Free Survival curves in patients treated with or without adjuvant temozolomide as per CATNON Trial (A) Overall survival. (B) Progression-free survival. *TMZ,* Temozolomide.

similar to HGG, the extent of resection can improve prognosis. For patients who are asymptomatic. a period of surveillance may be helpful initially. If a tumour is in eloquent brain or is large, the decision to perform surgery should take into consideration possible cognitive deficits that may be a consequence of surgery.

RT is indicated for patients with disease progression, demonstrated by worsening neurology, worsening epilepsy or imaging evidence of growing disease. Pathological diagnosis is mandatory before RT is undertaken. In patients with progressive disease, RT almost certainly delays tumour progression and death. Whether RT actually cures some patients is not known. RT improves epilepsy in about 50% of patients with LGG. In rare circumstances, it can be used to try to improve intractable epilepsy in a patient with LGG.

In patients without demonstrable progression, the timing of RT is less critical. There is excellent information that survival is unaffected by the timing of RT, whether it is given immediately or later when progression occurs, but any neurological deficit cannot be reversed by treatment.

LGGs grow with a diffuse infiltrative pattern and without destruction of involved brain. Therefore patients may have functioning brain within the tumour, even though the tumour may be very large. This imposes a fundamental limitation on surgery for LGG. Neurological deficits caused by LGGs frequently improve following RT. It is therefore appropriate to consider patients for RT even if they have neurological deficits, which is entirely the opposite of HGGs.

On imaging with CT, tumours are typically large and with low density. Oligodendrogliomas often have areas of calcification, which give a characteristic speckled appearance and is helpful in suggesting a preoperative diagnosis. On MRI, LGGs show a low signal on T1W and absence of contrast enhancement. The tumour is usually best delineated using a T2W or FLAIR sequence where CSF and oedema appear white. This correlates with the low density seen on CT. A typical LGG is shown in Fig. 31.7.

Radical Treatment

Target Volume

The patient should be immobilised in a shell and new imaging obtained. MRI produces optimal localisation of the tumour, especially the T2W or FLAIR sequence. This should be coregistered with the planning CT. The GTV is defined as the full extent of visible abnormality demonstrated on the T2W or FLAIR MRI. This volume is often very large. For patients who have undergone surgery, the GTV should include the postoperative residual disease. A CTV margin of approximately 1.5 cm

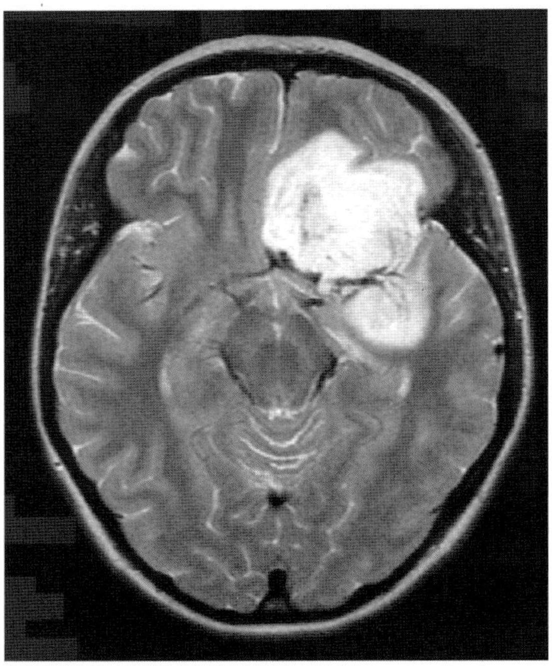

Fig. 31.7 T2-weighted magnetic resonance imaging scan of a large grade 2 astrocytoma. Oedema within the tumour has a high signal *(appears white)*. This region would be considered the gross target volume. Cerebral spinal fluid between the folds of the brain is also *white*. On computed tomography, this area would be shown as a low-density region.

can be used, smaller than for HGG. The CTV does not have to extend beyond the inner table of the skull, which is best shown on CT. The CTV should be grown isotropically to its PTV, with an appropriate margin; 0.3 to 0.5 cm is common.

Technique

An IMRT solution is optimal for these patients, aiming to achieve good dose homogeneity in the target and reduce the dose to normal tissues and OARs. A thermoluminescent dosimeter (TLD) is recommended to estimate doses to the lens.

Dose and Energy

Two studies examining dose escalation in patients with grade 2 gliomas (EORTC: 45 Gy in 25 fractions versus 60 Gy in 30 fractions, and RTOG: 50.4 Gy in 28 fractions versus 64.8 Gy in 36 fractions) failed to demonstrate an improvement in survival and showed increased toxicity in the dose escalation arms. Consequently, lower doses are recommended, although recent trials have used 50.4 Gy in 28 fractions.

Grade 2: IDH mutated codeleted: 50.4 Gy in 28 fractions (or 45 Gy in 25 fractions or 54 Gy in 30 fractions) with adjuvant PCV 205 (grade A)

Grade 2: IDH mutated non-codeleted: 50.4 Gy in 28 fractions (or 45 Gy in 25 fractions or 54 Gy in 30 fractions) with adjuvant PCV 159 (grade A) or adjuvant temozolomide (grade D)

Side Effects

Acute and late effects are similar to HGG. Seizures may worsen during RT. Dexamethasone is useful, and anticonvulsants should be reviewed. Late hypothalamic and pituitary dysfunction is an important issue in long-term follow-up, particularly because the prognosis is much more favourable than HGG. In addition, the higher survival rates seen with LGG tumour have revealed the impact of side effects related to cognitive decline and memory deficits, endocrine deficits and secondary malignancies. There is an emerging need to address the quality of life for these patients as an important issue due to long-term survival.

Chemotherapy in LGG

The EORTC conducted a study that compared initial RT (50.4 Gy in 28 fractions) to chemotherapy (temozolomide) and revealed superior progression-free survival for patients with non-codeleted tumours managed with RT.

Analysis of long-term results from a trial involving patients with grade 2 glioma over age 40 years or those with more than 2 cc residual disease compared RT alone (54 Gy in 30 fractions) to RT with adjuvant PCV chemotherapy. This analysis demonstrated a significant increase in overall survival with the addition of adjuvant PCV, particularly for IDH-mutated tumours with or without 1p19q codeletion. Consequently, there is a growing trend to consider RT and adjuvant chemotherapy earlier for patients meeting these criteria. The optimal chemotherapy for non-codeleted tumours remains debated, as there has been no trial of adjuvant temozolomide in this group.

Results of Treatment

In younger cohorts with grade 2 IDH-mutant gliomas characterised by minimal residual tumour burden and no neurological symptoms attributable to the tumour, an observational approach based on serial MRI assessments may be suitable. This conservative management strategy aims to delay the onset of treatment-related side effects such as fatigue and cognitive deficits. Subsequent analyses from trials such as NRG Oncology/RTOG 9802 have identified a survival benefit in patients with high-risk features (those age ≥40 years or those with subtotal resections) when a chemotherapy regimen comprising procarbazine, lomustine and vincristine is added to RT. This regimen significantly extends overall survival, especially in subgroups with IDH-mutant 1p/19q codeleted gliomas, as evidenced by reduced mortality risk. Long-term data from trials such as EORTC 26951 and RTOG 9402 further support the efficacy of adjunctive chemotherapy alongside RT in managing anaplastic oligodendroglial neoplasms. These trials also highlight the potential for long-term disease control, with a significant portion of patients with 1p/19q codeleted tumours achieving progression-free survival over a 20-year period. Consistency in therapeutic effectiveness is observed in IDH-mutant tumours without 1p/19q codeletion, reinforcing the utility of the procarbazine, lomustine and vincristine regimen, as confirmed by RTOG 9802 results. Temozolomide is another viable option, as demonstrated by the CATNON Intergroup trial, which showed improved overall survival after RT in anaplastic gliomas without 1p/19q codeletion. Ongoing research aims to compare the efficacy of temozolomide to the PCV in newly diagnosed 1p/19q codeleted gliomas.

The oligodendroglial subtype has a better prognosis (median survival 10–15 years) than the astrocytic subtypes (median survival 6 years). Multimodality therapy increases median overall survival (13.3 years in patients treated with both chemotherapy and RT versus 7.8 years in patients receiving RT alone). Ten-year disease-free survival is 51% in patients receiving both treatments and 21% in patients receiving only RT.

EPENDYMOMA (INTRACRANIAL)

Pathology and Clinical Features

Intracranial ependymoma is a rare primary tumour more commonly seen in children than adults. The incidence of ependymomas is 1.8% of all primary CNS tumours, with male predominance. It is thought to be derived from ependymal cells that line the ventricular system.

It arises most often in the posterior fossa, though it can be supratentorial or spinal. Typically, posterior fossa lesions present as the result of obstructive hydrocephalus and increased ICP, causing multiple cranial nerve palsies, neck stiffness and head tilt when they infiltrate the upper portion of the cervical cord. In accordance with the 2021 WHO classification, the classification of ependymomas is now based on a combination of histological, molecular and anatomical features spanning three tumour locations: supratentorial, infratentorial and spinal. Ependymomas are grouped by their morphological characteristics and their molecular profiles, with each anatomical site having its own subgroup. Molecular features can be determined through DNA methylation–based classification and fusion gene analysis. WHO CNS5 now recognises two molecularly defined types of supratentorial ependymoma: one characterised by ZFTA fusion (formerly known as C11orf95, considered more representative of the tumour type due to its fusion with various partners) and another featuring YAP1 fusion. Similarly, there are two molecularly defined types of PF ependymoma, referred to as group PFA and group PFB, as well as a spinal tumour subtype defined by the presence of MYCN amplification. Presently, there are 10 recognised ependymoma subtypes, with two of them, ST-YAP1 and posterior fossa group A, primarily occurring in infants and young children.

Supratentorial ependymomas in adults may fall into the subcategories of subependymoma (ST-SE) or ZFTA fusion ependymoma (ST-ZFTA, formerly known as RELA fusion). These are typically graded as WHO 2 or 3 tumours. Posterior fossa subependymoma (molecular subgroup PF-SE), much like its supratentorial counterpart (ST-SE), exhibits a balanced genome and an excellent prognosis. In contrast, posterior fossa group B often displays chromosomal instability and is graded WHO 2 or 3, with a 5-year progression-free survival rate of 73% and an overall survival rate of 100%.

Imaging demonstrates a contrast-enhancing tumour adjacent to the fourth ventricle but away from the midline. The range of enhancement is related to the tumour grade. There is surrounding oedema, and typically there are enlarged ventricles above. Supratentorial ependymomas present in the same way as other cerebral primary tumours. On imaging, the appearances are very similar to HGG. In addition, ependymomas can present with a cystic component, calcification and/or intratumoural haemorrhage. Spread may occur in the CSF in patients with newly diagnosed ependymoma, so craniospinal MRI of the spine is necessary to stage the patient and CSF cytology is mandatory following surgery.

Treatment

Maximum surgical resection is the aim, as it increases 10-year survival rates in low- and high-grade tumours to 80% and 50%, respectively. Subtotal resection increases the risk of tumour recurrence and CSF dissemination. In the case of persistent hydrocephalus despite tumour resection, shunting or endoscopic ventriculostomy should be performed. However, in posterior fossa tumours, encasement of the cranial nerves and brainstem vasculature might limit the extent of tumour resection. Subependymomas and grade 1 and 2 tumours which undergo complete surgical resection are unlikely to relapse. Current standard practice dictates that adjuvant RT should be offered to patients diagnosed with anaplastic ependymomas classified as WHO grade 3. However, the results from retrospective studies are inconclusive when it comes to assessing the benefits in terms of progression-free survival and overall survival for using RT in cases of grade 2 ependymomas, particularly those that have undergone GTR. In instances of extensive residual disease following subtotal resection, RT can be considered for patients with WHO grade 2 ependymomas.

Postoperative focal RT is recommended for all grade 3 ependymomas and for grade 2 tumours that were incompletely resected. However, it is worth noting that in a subset of posterior fossa group B tumours, the need for postoperative RT may not be universal and should be further investigated.

Although ependymoma can spread through the CSF, there is good evidence that prophylactic craniospinal RT confers no advantage, because spinal seeding is unlikely to happen if the primary tumour does not recur locally. CSI is used only if there is proof of spinal seeding.

Intracranial subependymoma is a rare entity. Surgical removal offers long-term survival. However, poorly defined resection borders have been associated with a shorter progression-free survival. A second-look surgery could be an option that should be considered, and postoperative RT might be offered after subtotal or partial resection.

Target Volume

The patient should be immobilised in the conventional way, preferably supine in an 'S' frame, to allow for posterior beams. Pre- and postoperative MRI T1-weighted images should be coregistered with the CT planning images.

For posterior fossa tumours, the standard treatment volume should include the postsurgical bed with a margin of 1 to 2 cm for all low- and high-grade supratentorial tumours. Coregistration with the preoperative imaging may help ensure that all at-risk tissue is included.

Supratentorial ependymomas should be treated along similar lines to HGG, using postoperative MRI T1W+Gd to define the GTV as any residual postoperative enhancing tumour. The CTV requires a margin of 1.0 to 2.0 cm (dependent on grade), grown isotropically, which can be edited along the skull. An appropriate PTV should be added.

Technique

In adults, the posterior fossa is best treated with IMRT to reduce the dose to OARs. This achieves the best conformation to the posterior fossa target volume.

Dose and Energy

Single phase: 55 Gy in 33 daily fractions over 6.5 weeks. An alternative is 54 Gy in 30 fractions, treating daily over 6 weeks.

For grade 2 ependymoma, 54 to 59.4 Gy in 30 fractions is recommended following incomplete resection.

For grade 3 (anaplastic) ependymomas, 60 Gy in 30 fractions over 6 weeks is recommended, regardless of the extent of the resection.

Chemotherapy

Chemotherapy does not play a role in the initial treatment of adult ependymoma and should only be contemplated when dealing with recurrent cases where no local treatment options such as surgery, RT or radiosurgery are available.

Results of Treatment

Ependymoma is curable in approximately 50% of cases. Infratentorial lesions have shown improved survival compared to supratentorial, which are usually of high grade.

CNS LYMPHOMA

Pathology and Clinical Features

PCNSL is non-Hodgkin lymphoma arising in the brain, typically of the diffuse large (high-grade) B-cell type. PCNSL accounts for approximately 3% of all primary CNS tumours (see Fig. 31.1). The incidence may be increasing. It affects patients of all ages; however, the incidence rises with age, with the majority of patients over age 60 years. Myelosuppression predisposes to the development of PCNSL, and this was one of the early AIDS-defining diagnoses.

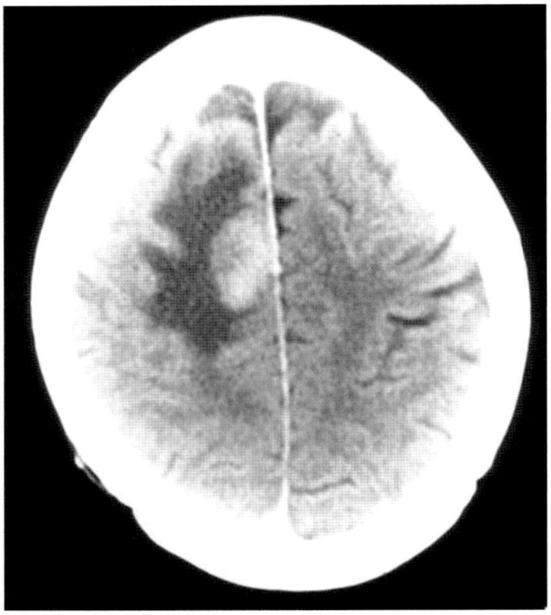

Fig. 31.8 Primary central nervous system lymphoma (PCNSL) in the cerebral hemisphere, shown on computed tomography. A homogeneously enhancing mass can be seen. In approximately two-thirds of cases, PCNSL presents as a single mass; in one-third it is multifocal. A definitive diagnosis will require biopsy, to distinguish between high-grade glioma, metastasis and PCNSL. Note the similarity to Fig. 31.5.

Presentation is the same as other primary tumours arising within the brain substance and typically includes headache, neurological deficit often including intellectual decline, seizure, signs of elevated ICP and visual symptoms if affecting the eyes. Onset of symptoms is usually quite rapid. 'B' symptoms (see Chapter 30) are not a feature of PCNSL.

On imaging, typical appearances are of a homogeneously enhancing mass, often in a periventricular location and often presenting on precontrast T1W images as iso- or hypointense and on T2W images as hyperintense (Fig. 31.8). The most common location is supratentorial. In approximately two-thirds of cases, PCNSL presents as a single mass; in one-third it is multifocal. The disease can spread within the brain, especially in the subependymal layer around the ventricular system, but it is rare for it to metastasise outside the CNS. Metastases to the brain from peripheral lymphoma are also rare.

Management Principles

Biopsy, using a navigation-guided surgical technique, is necessary to prove the diagnosis, but resection should not be undertaken if a diagnosis of PCNSL is suspected, because it does not improve the prognosis and carries a greater risk of neurological deficit. In addition to biopsy, other investigations should be performed, including CT imaging of the chest, abdomen and pelvis to exclude systemic lymphoma and, where needed/indicated, MRI of the spine and CFS cytology. All patients must undergo neurocognitive evaluation and eye examination.

Steroids are cytotoxic to lymphomas (as with peripheral lymphomas). Therefore, if dexamethasone is given for symptom relief before a biopsy is performed, the lesion may disappear temporarily. The inclusion of lymphoma in the radiological differential diagnosis thus provides an important contribution to management.

Optimum management of these tumours is a matter of debate. PCNSL is highly sensitive to chemotherapy and radiation, and the goal of treatment is cure, although approximately 33% to 60% of patients will relapse.

Late neurotoxicity associated with the combination of chemotherapy, especially MTX (alone or in combination with other drugs) with RT, is a significant problem. This occurs commonly, especially in older people, and can be severely disabling or even fatal. Choice of optimal treatment therefore currently depends on the age and general health of the patient. For patients with a good performance status, high-dose MTX-based chemotherapy is recommended, without RT. MTX should be administered at a dose of 3.5 g/m^2 IV on day 1 and cytarabine at a dose of 2 g/m^2 IV on days 2 and 3. This is repeated 3-weekly for four cycles. It is a well-tolerated treatment that improves survival from 33 to 60 months and increases response rates to 94%.

Radical Treatment: Full-Dose Radiotherapy

Proposals have been introduced to modify radiation treatment parameters with the aim of reducing the risk of neurotoxicity caused by radiation exposure while ensuring its continued effectiveness. These considerations encompass various factors, including the overall radiation dosage, size of radiation fractions, specific volume targeted by radiation, strategies aimed at preserving the hippocampus and utilisation of neuroprotective medications.

In the context of whole brain radiotherapy (WBRT), the conventional radiation dose typically falls within the range of 36 to 40 Gy, with protective measures for the eyes initiated after reaching 30 Gy, or at 36 Gy if there is any intraocular disease present. No additional advantages have been observed with higher radiation doses. Recent focus has shifted towards investigating the efficacy of reduced-dose WBRT, an area of exploration currently underway in the RTOG 1114 randomised phase II trial. Preliminary results from this trial suggest that the addition of low-dose WBRT (administered as 23.4 Gy in thirteen 1.8-Gy fractions) to the R-MPV-A regimen may enhance progression-free survival in patients diagnosed with PCNSL. It is important to note that, at the time of reporting these results, there was no significant increase in the rates of neurotoxicity. Nevertheless comprehensive studies involving neuropsychological assessments and neuroimaging are still ongoing. The full findings of these studies are pending and will provide a more comprehensive understanding of the impact of radiation-induced neurotoxicity in PCNSL, which can manifest several years after the completion of treatment.

Radiotherapy Planning and Target Volumes

PCNSL is a multifocal disease, and the RT field should cover the whole brain area. After chemotherapy, a boost is not recommended. For CTV, the inferior border should be the C2–C3 or C1–C2 intervertebral space.

The posterior aspect of the orbit should be covered (if the eyes were initially affected from the disease) to ensure that the retina, whole eyeball and optic nerves are included in the treated volume. They should be treated to a dose of 30 to 36 Gy.

Weighted opposed lateral fields are typically employed and are modulated to deliver a homogeneous dose. The isocenter is placed anteriorly; it should bisect the bony canthi to allow for a potential future isocentric match to an ocular field, because the eyes are occasionally an isolated site of relapse and future ocular fields may have to be added later.

RT techniques have evolved dramatically over decades from a parallel opposed two-field technique to three-dimensional conformal RT techniques. For three-dimensional conformal RT, the GTV is the grossly visible tumour in postcontrast T1-weighted MR images. PET, if available, may be used for delineation to improve accuracy. The whole brain and the sites harbouring the potential microscopic disease, including the posterior part of the orbit and the upper two cervical vertebrae, as mentioned earlier, are included in the CTV. The PTV is created as per standard protocols. The tumour boost is delineated, adding a 1.5-to-2-cm margin to the gross tumour. The margin around the GTV to define the boost volume CTV seems to differ from one series to another, and the impact of these margins in terms of local control has not been assessed in prospective studies. If the boost is planned after chemotherapy, the postchemotherapy GTV can be used to contour the boost volume. Three-dimensional conformal RT is a preferred technique, with the isocenter of the WBRT field being placed anteriorly near the orbit. In the modern era, there is widespread use of IMRT which can be utilised for the simultaneous integrated boost technique if a higher dose is planned for the gross disease. The CTV is expanded isometrically to a PTV to account for setup errors. The commonly used dose per session of radiation therapy is 1.8 Gy per day. Although no specific studies have targeted this dosage, research involving smaller doses or twice-daily hyperfractionation has not shown any variance in patient outcomes. The necessity for traditional WBRT coverage is underscored by the frequency of widespread disease, CSF and eye involvement and the pervasive nature of brain involvement observed in postmortem studies. Thus it's recommended to maintain radiation fields down to the lower edge of the C2 vertebra, ensuring that the meninges and the back two-thirds of the orbit are included in the treatment area. Additionally, a retrospective analysis has indicated a higher rate of tumour recurrence outside the treatment zone when using margins less than 4 cm, in contrast to margins of 4 cm or more (83% versus 22%).

Localised Unifocal Disease

RT is rarely used and is therefore not described.

Palliative Radiotherapy

This may be necessary for patients with poor performance status.

Target Volume and Technique

Immobilise and irradiate the whole brain with a single phase, as per palliative RT for metastases.

Dose

Severe forms of treatment-associated neurotoxicity have been reported with whole brain doses greater than 30 Gy, and patients treated with daily fractions less than 1.8 Gy are less likely to develop delayed toxicity. Moreover, recent phase III trials have included reduced-dose RT with MTX-based chemotherapy. Hence the total dose is recommended as follows:

- Standard-dose WBRT as monotherapy: 36 Gy in 1.8 Gy per fraction, with a sequential boost of 9 Gy to the gross disease
- Reduced dose WBRT as consolidation treatment: 23.4 Gy in 1.8 Gy per fraction in patients with complete response after induction chemotherapy; a sequential boost of 12.6 Gy in patients with partial response or
- WBRT of 30 Gy in 1.5 Gy per fraction ± simultaneous integrated boost up to 40 Gy if the response was partial to systemic therapy

  A variety of dose schedules can be utilised:

  30 Gy in 10 fractions, treating daily, over 2 weeks

  20 Gy in 5 fractions, treating daily, over 1 week

  30 Gy in 6 fractions, treating on alternate days over 2 weeks (as for HGG)

In patients age 70 years or younger, induction chemotherapy followed by consolidative high-dose chemotherapy plus autologous stem cell transplantation (ASCT) or WBRT has been associated with a significant improvement in overall survival. ASCT is the most preferred treatment option, as WBRT, especially with a dose of greater than 30 Gy, is occasionally associated with risk of permanent, irreversible neurotoxicity.

Elderly Population

At present, most major centres recommend deferring WBRT until the time of progression. The application of WBRT in the treatment of PCNSL remains under evaluation. This is particularly true for elderly patients who face a significantly high risk of suffering from delayed neurotoxic effects. Improvements in the rates of positive responses to initial chemotherapy treatments could lead to a standardised implementation of lower doses of WBRT or the employment of different consolidation methods. For each clinical scenario, it is critical to tailor the approach to the individual circumstances of the patient, carefully weighing the immediate benefits of the treatment against the potential for long-term toxicity and the subsequent effects on the patient's functional capabilities and overall quality of life.

Results of Treatment

The major prognostic factors for better survival are younger age, especially younger than age 60 years, excellent performance status and chemotherapy. Suitability for chemotherapy is strongly determined by performance status. Localised disease, rather than a multifocal pattern, also carries a better prognosis. Long-term survival is poor, especially in patients over age 60 years, which comprises the majority of patients with PCNSL. In a series of unselected cases, the median survival was only 8 months, with a 5-year survival of 6%. The prognosis could be determined by the use of algorithms introduced in recent trials. Factors related to poor prognosis in terms of survival are over age 60 years, performance status greater than 1, high CSF protein concentration, involvement of deep regions of the brain and elevated LDH serum level. The Memorial Sloan Kettering Cancer Center (MSKCC) prognostic model recommends three prognostic classes (class 1: age <50 years; class 2: age >50 years and KPS 70; class 3: age >50 years and KPS <70), with significantly different overall survivals (8.5 years, 3.2 years and 1.1 years for classes 1, 2 and 3, respectively).

GERMINOMA

Clinical Features and Management Principles

Germinomas are rare in adults, but they present like other primary tumours. They frequently arise in the suprasellar region or the region of the pineal gland, close to the (CSF) aqueduct (see Fig. 31.4), and therefore the symptoms and signs of hydrocephalus are common presenting features. Some patients require a shunt. They should be curable in almost every case.

Germinomas spread through the CSF and therefore require RT to the whole craniospinal axis. Different tumours show a wide range of growth rates, but a few grow extremely fast, leading to neurological deterioration taking place over days or even hours. If a patient has metastatic spread to the optic chiasm, rapid progression may threaten vision and may require urgent treatment with RT. This type of disease does not respond well to steroid treatment.

In adults the standard treatment for intracranial germinoma should be RT. The total dose is modest, and the toxicity profile in adults is excellent because growth is complete. There is therefore no advantage in considering an alternative strategy of reduced-dose RT together with chemotherapy in adults, at least at the present time.

Recent studies in children have raised the question of whether the volume to be irradiated should be the entire craniospinal axis or the local ventricular RT only. Germinomas are also sensitive to chemotherapy, but chemotherapy alone is associated with a roughly 50% chance of relapse.

Postoperative imaging of the head and preoperative imaging of the spine (and head), together with CSF examination, measurement of plasma and CSF tumour markers AFP and BHCG, are all useful to have prior to planning treatment. Germinomas produce AFP but not beta-HCG.

Treatment

Target Volume

Phase 1 should treat the whole craniospinal axis, and this is most effectively planned from CT. The technique is largely the same as for paediatric craniospinal RT (see Chapter 34).

For phase 2 the primary site is treated to a higher dose. This should be localised using CT-to-MR coregistration, and the imaging must be carried out before RT starts, because the tumour is extremely radiosensitive and may disappear within a few days of starting RT. The GTV is the contrast-enhancing tumour. The CTV margin can be small, for example, 1 to 2 cm, grown isotropically. The PTV should be grown from the CTV, with a standard margin such as 0.3 to 0.5 cm.

Any sites of metastatic disease can also be boosted in this phase. Occasionally, the whole craniospinal axis must be treated to the phase 2 dose (discussed shortly).

Technique

Technique for phase 1 is as for paediatric craniospinal RT (see Chapter 34). For phase 2, use an appropriate beam arrangement, usually with IMRT.

Dose and Energy

Phase 1, craniospinal axis: 25 Gy in 15 daily fractions in 3 weeks, using megavoltage x-rays

Phase 2: 15 Gy in 9 fractions in 2 weeks, to boost the primary site and any sites of metastasis

If necessary, in the case of extensive metastatic spread, it is possible to treat the whole craniospinal axis to 40 Gy in 24 fractions, provided that the full blood count is carefully monitored. If urgent RT is required while the craniospinal plan is being prepared, this can be done using a parallel pair of lateral fields. A few fractions (e.g. 5 Gy in 3 fractions) are normally sufficient to prevent clinical deterioration. It is probably best, in adults, to simply consider this as an extra dose added to the two phases described earlier.

If chemotherapy is used, a whole ventricular approach to RT can be utilised instead, thus minimising the volume irradiated and resulting in reduced acute and late toxicity. There are several good ventricular atlases that can be used to assist with outlining, but the principles are to cover the entire CSF drainage, including the prepontine space. The dose would then be 24 Gy.

Results of Treatment

The cure rate is almost 100%, which applies even if metastatic disease is present at diagnosis. Regular follow-up is required, particularly to recognise any endocrine deficiencies early.

MEDULLOBLASTOMA

The management of medulloblastoma in adults follows the general principles of this disease in children. Because adults have already achieved full height and brain maturity, there is less need to reduce the whole craniospinal axis dose. A survival advantage has been shown for the addition of chemotherapy in children, and this has been replicated in a metaanalysis of adults with medulloblastoma too.

The management of paediatric medulloblastoma is described in Chapter 34.

Dose and Energy (Adults)

Phase 1, craniospinal axis: 36 Gy in 20 fractions

Phase 2: 18 Gy in 10 fractions

MENINGIOMA

Pathology and Clinical Features

Patients with meningioma present with a mixture of symptoms and signs. Headache is common. As with other primary tumours, meningiomas may also cause confusion and intellectual impairment, resulting from compression of the frontal lobes; 20% of patients have seizures. Occasionally, patients may present with specific cranial nerve palsies, which is different from glial tumours.

The majority of meningiomas arise sporadically. However, they may be associated with previous radiation treatment, for example, cranial RT used for childhood leukaemia. The incidence of meningiomas is notably higher in females, with rates of around 12.76 per 100,000, compared to 5.79 per 100,000 in males, and can be associated with genetic conditions predisposing to cancer, including neurofibromatosis type 2. Benign meningiomas normally express progesterone receptors (PR) but not estrogen receptors (ER), and this may account for occasional reports of change during pregnancy or in patients using HRT. More malignant tumours typically become less well differentiated and lose this expression.

Meningiomas arise in the coverings of the brain and so can occur at any intracranial site. However, the two most common sites are the vertex of the skull and the greater wing of the sphenoid bone. Tumours at the vertex can usually be fully resected. Those on the sphenoid wing are resectable if they lie laterally. Medial sphenoid wing tumours usually involve the cavernous sinus, which normally precludes complete resection.

Meningiomas rank as the predominant type of primary CNS tumour among adults, with over 90% classified as benign (WHO grade 1) and typically manageable without intervention or treatable through surgical or targeted radiation methods. They are graded 1, 2 (atypical) and 3 (anaplastic). Only about 5% of these tumours are categorised as atypical (WHO grade 2), and 1% to 2% are considered malignant or anaplastic (WHO grade 3). Grading historically has been based on morphological features, but it has long been recognised that there are lesions where the behaviour is not accurately reflected by this approach alone. Consequently, the new WHO 2021 grading incorporates some molecular markers, such as mutations in the TERT promoter, deletions in CDKN2A/B and the absence of histone 3 lysine 27 trimethylation, which have been linked to a poorer prognosis. Sophisticated genomic or combined molecular-morphological assessments have proven to be more accurate than conventional WHO histopathological grading in forecasting patient outcomes.

Meningiomas may also infiltrate through the foramina and fissures of the skull base, and the extensions should be followed in outlining the GTV. On imaging, tumours are of similar density to the surrounding brain. Usually they are solitary lesions. Sometimes they cause surrounding oedema. With contrast, they normally enhance vigorously and homogeneously (Fig. 31.9). They may cause hyperostosis of the surrounding skull. Calcification, best seen on CT, is characteristic of very slow-growing tumours. It is typical to have meningeal enhancement extending away from the site of a meningioma, and this does not necessarily indicate tumour spread. Rather, this 'tail' is a useful diagnostic feature. Additional images that can help improve target delineation include (1) T2-weighted high-resolution gradient and fast spin echo sequences with and without fat suppression and (2) FLAIR sequences. Specifically, T2-weighted sequences can also be useful to assess the extent of peritumoural oedema and dural tail abnormalities. In addition, extraaxial growth can be verified on T2-weighted images by CSF cleft interposed between the tumour and the parenchyma. CT is valuable for the detection of calcification of varying degrees within the tumour and hyperostosis of adjacent bone. Methionine (an amino acid) and DOTATOC (an octreotide analogue) PET tracers have a role in the diagnosis of complex meningiomas. In selected cases, PET imaging, mainly with DOTATOC or DOTANOC tracers, helps improve target volume definition, for example, in patients with large tumours infiltrating the parapharyngeal soft tissues or for those located in the bony structures which are difficult to distinguish on MRI and CT.

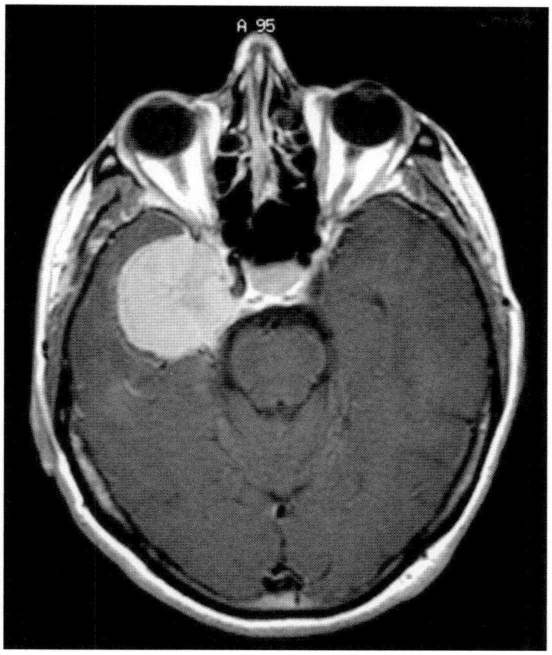

Fig. 31.9 Magnetic resonance imaging (T1W+Gd) of meningioma arising from the 0 medial wing of the sphenoid ridge. The cavernous sinus is involved. A small 'tail' of contrast enhancement can be seen in the meninges anteriorly in the middle fossa. The tumour was managed by subtotal resection and postoperative radiotherapy.

Treatment

The choice of treatment depends on the size, shape, location and grade of the meningioma. The optimal treatment for grade 1 meningiomas is radical surgical resection, which improves local control. The patient's performance status, comorbidities and wishes need to be taken into consideration before a decision to operate is made. RT is reserved for incompletely resected tumours if there is evidence of growth and no further surgical option or for growing unresectable lesions.

There are three main RT techniques used in the treatment of meningiomas: conventional fractionation, which delivers 1.8 to 2.0 Gy daily using VMAT or fractionated stereotactic radiotherapy (fSRT); single-session radiosurgery (SRS); and hypofractionated SRS, which administers doses larger than 5 Gy per session. Treatment method selection is influenced by the location and size of the tumour. Tumours located near vital structures, such as the optic nerves and chiasm, are typically treated with conventional fractionation to stay within safe dose limits for single sessions (e.g. the chiasm can only tolerate less than 10 Gy in a single session or less than 25 Gy across 5 sessions). Studies indicate that single-fraction SRS may be less effective for tumours larger than 7.5 to 10 cm^3. The likelihood of side effects such as treatment-related oedema increases with the size of the tumour, which is why conventional fractionation is generally preferred for tumours larger than 3 cm. Unlike RT, chemotherapy is not a treatment option for meningiomas.

Optic nerve meningiomas cause visual deterioration. These tumours are normally diagnosed entirely on imaging. In these patients, surgery, including biopsy, can further damage vision. RT is effective in stabilising the disease, and some patients (about one-third) experience an improvement in vision. RT is thus the treatment of choice for optic nerve meningioma to prevent visual deterioration and ptosis.

For grade 2 meningiomas, the exact role of adjuvant RT following surgery is uncertain. They have a recurrence rate in the region of 40% at 5 years, and RT is often recommended to try to avoid or delay this. A large trial (ROAM) comparing early adjuvant RT (60 Gy in 30 fractions) with observation alone is currently underway. Patients with WHO grade 2 meningiomas have a higher risk of tumour recurrence after complete resection (Simpson grades 1–3), necessitating a careful assessment of the benefits of adjunctive RT versus its potential for inducing long-term adverse effects such as neurocognitive impairment.

The RTOG 0539 study, a phase II nonrandomised clinical trial, involved administering 54 Gy in 30 fractions to patients with grade 2 meningiomas following GTR (Simpson grades 1–3) and an escalated dose of 54 Gy with an integrated boost to 60 Gy in cases of subtotal resection (Simpson grades 4–5). The reported 3-year progression-free survival rates were 93.8% for GTR and 57.1% for subtotal resection, respectively. Concurrently, the EORTC's phase II trial (22042) delivered 60 Gy in 30 fractions for patients with GTRs (Simpson grades 1–3), supplemented with a 10-Gy boost for those with subtotal resections (Simpson grades 4–5), and culminated in a 3-year progression-free survival rate of 88.7%, which surpassed the a priori projected progression-free survival of 70%.

The role of stereotactic radiosurgery (SRS) in the management of grade 2 meningiomas remains contentious due to the requisite margin expansions—most current standard RT protocols stipulate a 1-cm margin from the GTV to the CTV to mitigate local recurrence risk. The optimal dosimetric parameters and fractionation schemes for SRS in this context have not yet been established.

For grade 3 meningiomas, the recommendation is for surgical resection with radical intent, providing neurological deficit can be avoided. Adjuvant high-dose RT should follow, to minimise the risk of recurrence. The timing of RT appears to be an important factor; if given following the initial resection, it may improve survival. Anaplastic meningiomas are rare (<3% of meningiomas, though this will increase with the new molecular classification), so data on optimal management are limited. Retrospective studies show that, although reduced after adjuvant RT, the risk of recurrence both locally and in other areas of the meninges remains high, and though dose escalation has been considered, whether or not this approach is beneficial is yet to be established.

Radiotherapy Target Volume

The patient should be immobilised in a shell or relocatable stereotactic head frame. If resection has been carried out, postoperative imaging is required. A current MRI scan should be used for planning, coregistered with the planning CT scan. Both modalities are helpful for target volume delineation. MRI using a T1W sequence with gadolinium contrast produces optimal localisation of the tumour; CT shows the limits of meningioma extension up to bone or, in uncommon cases where the tumour involves the bone, the extent of the invasion. Bone invasion should be assessed on bone windows. CT also shows the foramina and fissures of the skull through which meningiomas can spread. The preoperative MRI, coregistered, can be very helpful in defining the CTV margin.

The GTV is defined as the visible edge of contrast enhancement on MRI, plus relevant skull boundaries. If resection has been carried out, coregistration with the preoperative MRI is very helpful. This shows the original location of the tumour and therefore the meningeal surfaces into which spread might occur (i.e. the CTV). The majority of meningiomas originate from the dura mater. A significant consideration in treatment planning is whether the 'dural tail'—a strip of dura mater that appears radiographically enhanced and extends from the main body of the meningioma—ought to be included in the GTV. This dural tail, discernible on postgadolinium T1-weighted MRI scans, predominantly constitutes vascularised dura and occasionally contains microscopic aggregations of meningioma cells within the dura contiguous to the tumour. The question of whether the dural tail contributes to a higher likelihood of tumour recurrence compared to other areas of the dura surrounding the main tumour mass is still subject to discussion. However, current evidence does not strongly indicate that the dural tail is a more frequent site of recurrence.

In line with the protocols of the RTOG 0539 and EORTC 1308 clinical trials, only the dural tail that appears visibly thickened should be marked as a target for radiation and thus included in the GTV. Conversely, a linearly enhanced or nonenhancing thickened dura that extends from the meningioma is typically not incorporated into the GTV. A similar approach is adopted for bone involvement; the GTV should include bone that is directly invaded by tumour and bone that is clearly hyperostotic, as identified by CT scans with bone window settings to enhance the precision of target delineation, in accordance with the aforementioned trials.

In the case of 'en plaque' meningiomas, which are characterised by widespread and extensive dural invasion often extending beyond the cranial confines to areas such as the calvarium, orbit and soft tissues, all dural thickening and enhancement observed should be encompassed within the GTV to ensure comprehensive treatment coverage.

There is very little hard evidence for the size of the CTV margin that should be used; thus suggestions are provided. For an individual tumour, the growth pattern may suggest whether a small or large margin is needed. Many meningiomas show a more invasive pattern of growth, with extension along adjacent meningeal layers. Any such (imaged) extension should be outlined in the GTV. Where histology is available, this can be incorporated into the margin decision. Thus the CTV includes any gross tumour, the postoperative tumour bed if resection has been undertaken, plus areas of extension along the meninges, and any hyperostotic bone changes or frank bone invasion if present. It does not need to include a large margin of adjacent brain. It is not necessary to expand the CTV isotropically.

It is helpful to outline critical normal structures, including the eyes and lenses, the pituitary and the optic nerves and chiasm. The following margins are recommended:

Grade 1: CTV = GTV + 0.5 cm.

Grade 2: Along the meninges CTV = GTV + 1 cm, reduced to 0.5 cm at natural barriers to spread, and 0.3 to 0.5 cm into adjacent brain tissue (unless there is evidence of invasion when a larger margin should be added).

Grade 3: Along the meninges CTV = GTV + 1.5 to 2.0 cm and limited by barriers to spread, as with grade 2. The margin should include any invasion of the brain.

In some cases it is worth contouring the hippocampi. Other structures, such as the parotid gland, may be relevant for very inferior lesions.

Technique

IMRT should be used with image guidance.

Dose and Energy

For grades 1 and 2, the prescribed dose delivered with 6-MV photons in a single phase is:

- 50 Gy in 30 fractions over 6 weeks
- 50.4 Gy in 28 fractions over 6 weeks
- 55 Gy in 33 fractions over 6.5 weeks

For grade 3 the dose is 60 Gy in 30 fractions over 6 weeks, with VMAT at 60 Gy in 30 fractions over 6 weeks (grade B).

The dose may vary according to which critical structures are contained within the CTV and PTV. Although there is no formal evidence of dose response in grade 3 tumours, it is widely accepted that higher doses in the region of 60 Gy in 30 fractions should be used.

Side Effects

Acute effects are the same as for glioma irradiation. In terms of late effects, if the hypothalamus and pituitary have been irradiated, hormone failure may occur years after treatment, so routine pituitary function tests are necessary during follow-up. Intellectual function should not be affected over and above changes already caused by the tumour (and surgery). In cases where high eye doses cannot be avoided, such as optic nerve meningiomas, cataract may develop (as discussed earlier). Retinopathy can be observed with doses to the eyeball exceeding 50 Gy.

Results of Treatment

RT improves the outcome in patients for whom surgery is either impossible or incomplete. The results of subtotal resection plus RT are equivalent to complete surgical excision and may be safer for the patient. Meningiomas grow slowly, so follow-up needs to be carried out over a long period, at least 10 to 15 years, to define the outcome.

Age does not appear to be prognostic and should not be considered a bar to radical RT. Tumours which are larger or of higher grade have a higher chance of earlier relapse. In addition, it is likely that tumours with a high number of active cells in the mitotic cycle have a higher probability of early relapse, assessed by MIB-1 (Ki67: Tumour Proliferation Index).

In general, meningiomas do not change in size after RT, although a few do shrink modestly. However, it is important for the patient to understand that no change after treatment represents a successful outcome. Neurological deficits, such as cranial nerve palsies, do not usually improve. The exception is with optic nerve meningiomas: about one-third of patients experience some improvement in vision, even if there is no change in the size of the lesion on imaging.

Overall control rates for patients with meningioma are good. Survival after surgery and RT for benign meningiomas (i.e. grades 1 and 2) is around 80% to 90% at 5 years and 50% to 80% at 10 years. For patients with inoperable tumours treated with RT alone, control rates are probably on the low end of these ranges. However, patients with malignant meningiomas (i.e. grade 3) have a poor outlook, with 5-year survival rates around 30% to 60%, that is, about half the survival of patients with benign tumours.

PITUITARY TUMOURS

Pathology and Clinical Features

Pituitary tumours are virtually always primary adenomas of the anterior pituitary gland itself. Other primary tumours are exceedingly rare, and metastatic deposits involving the pituitary fossa, although well described, are uncommon. Pituitary lesions account for 15% of intracranial tumours and the majority are benign adenomas, but around one-third invade local structures.

Pituitary adenomas can be divided into secretory tumours that produce excess hormone and nonsecretory ones that do not. Secretory adenomas most commonly produce an excess of a single hormone, usually GH, causing acromegaly; ACTH, which causes Cushing disease; or prolactin, leading to hyperprolactinaemia. Production of TSH is uncommon. Patients with secretory tumours usually present with the effects of excess hormone production and a small tumour confined to the pituitary fossa. In many cases, hormone levels can be controlled medically, but surgery produces the quickest reduction of hormone levels in secreting tumours and is often curative. New endoscopic techniques have made surgery even more effective at removing tumour. These tumours may require intervention due to their secretion of hormones or because of the pressure they exert on nearby structures, including the optic chiasm. Surgery is typically the first line of treatment (or dopamine agonists in the case of prolactinomas), with RT being considered for specific situations such as:

- Recurrent or growing nonsecretory tumours postsurgery
- Tumours with unfavourable pathological characteristics, for example, a Ki67 index higher than 3% (refer to Raverot 2018)
- Secretory tumours that continue to show high hormone levels despite comprehensive hormonal suppression
- Individuals who are not suitable candidates for surgery due to their medical condition

While RT can lower hormone levels, this process is slow, typically taking several months to years, making it ineffective for immediate management. There is growing interest in using SRS for tumours larger than 3 mm and smaller than 3 cm. This may enhance the chances of biochemical remission, but the evidence is limited to reports from individual centres, and there are little data on tumour size and follow-up durations.

Nonsecretory tumours typically present with symptoms and signs of optic chiasm compression. Occasionally, they present with pituitary failure and are sometimes associated with headache. Surgical decompression results in immediate relief of pressure on the optic tract, and vision often improves by the time the patient wakes from the anaesthetic. Extension of tumour to the lateral walls of the pituitary fossa and cavernous sinus cannot be removed surgically and is a frequent site for residual tumour.

After complete removal, RT is usually not required. However, a proportion do recur, so adequate follow-up is essential. The indications for RT are relative, and patients are best managed through a multidisciplinary team. The decision regarding RT should be individual to the patient, taking into account extensive residual tumour, invasion of the cavernous sinuses laterally, uncontrolled elevated hormone levels and evidence of progression of tumour after surgery alone. If the patient is young and has normal pituitary function, the risk of inducing a second tumour with RT outweighs the apparent benefit. Patient preference is also important. If recurrence does occur in a patient managed by surveillance, a second operation may be desirable if the optic chiasm is compressed, before proceeding to RT.

In considering a patient for RT, it is important to ensure that the patient's hormone status is stable, and pre-RT documentation of the visual fields is required.

Treatment

Target Volume

The patient should be immobilised in a shell. A relocatable stereotactic frame may also be used. A current (postoperative) coregistered MRI (T1W+Gd) with a slice thickness of 1 mm helps define the GTV, including any involvement of the cavernous sinuses and suprasellar extension. CT shows the bony anatomy well, especially inferiorly, where it is helpful to identify the floor of the fossa.

The target is based on residual tumour bulk, which most commonly involves the cavernous sinuses. Some tumours have residual suprasellar extension, even after surgery, and this must be included in the GTV. Reviewing the GTV on a coronal view can be helpful in confirming coverage, especially superiorly and inferiorly. In cases where patients have undergone multiple surgeries, using preoperative and postoperative T1-weighted MR images with fat suppression can be beneficial to differentiate surgical aftereffects from the tumour itself, including any fat or biomaterial deposits. If MRI use is not advised, a thin-slice CT scan with contrast of the pituitary area should be undertaken before and after the introduction of contrast material. Pituitary adenomas do not infiltrate at a microscopic level, so no CTV margin is required for this; however, a margin of 2 to 3 mm may be added in the case of invasive and aggressive pituitary tumours to encompass all potential areas of microscopic tumour infiltration, for example, fast-growing tumours invading the cavernous sinus. The whole extent of the original tumour (preoperative imaging) should be included in the CTV.

Critical normal structures, especially the optic nerves, chiasm and tracts, should be outlined so that the dose distribution and the dose volume histograms (DVHs) for these can be reviewed.

Technique

IMRT should be used, with image guidance. Stereotactic RT/radiosurgery may be a choice for some patients with tumours less than 2.5 cm in maximum diameter, while the tumour target should be at least 2 to 3 mm from the optic chiasm. The dose can be delivered in a single fraction, offering higher convenience to the patient. However, there is currently no evidence that IMRT is superior to fractionated treatment.

Dose and Energy

The standard treatment is 45 Gy in 25 daily fractions over 5 weeks, with megavoltage x-rays. In cases with negative features such as significant size or extensive local invasion, an increased dose ranging from 50.4 to 54 Gy, applied at 1.8 Gy per session, might be considered.

A slightly higher dose is sometimes recommended for Cushing disease and for very large adenomas, such as 50 Gy in 30 fractions (as for craniopharyngioma). Higher doses may be used when treating secreting pituitary adenomas; doses up to 54 Gy may be used for large aggressive pituitary tumours and carcinomas.

In current clinical practice, single-fraction SRS at doses of 13 to 16 Gy and 16 to 25 Gy is a feasible approach to treating patients with nonfunctioning and secreting pituitary adenomas less than 2.0 to 2.5 cm in size at safe distance from the optic chiasm, respectively. Few studies report on fractionated SRS, usually 21 Gy in 3 fractions or 25 Gy in 5 fractions, showing tumour control rates consistent with those observed after single-fraction SRS. The NHS England commissioning guidelines also state that hypofractionated SRT (2–5 fractions) can be considered in patients with nonfunctional adenomas where the optic tract is involved, for example, 25 Gy in 5 fractions. This was restricted to nonfunctional lesions due to lack of evidence in functional lesions. For larger lesions and/or those involving the anterior optic pathway, fractionated RT, including either SRT or IMRT, is usually recommended.

Side Effects

With rotational IMRT, there is no hair loss. Use of fixed fields may lead to hair loss in the entry portals, usually over the temples, which will regrow. Some patients experience mild nausea and loss of appetite during RT, which is easily controlled with simple antiemetics. In some patients where the PTV extends rather inferiorly, ear symptoms occur as the result of acute irritation and blockage of the eustachian tube. Patients may report mildly reduced hearing, with bubbling in the ears and, sometimes, mild unsteadiness. These symptoms are due to fluid in the middle ear (secretory otitis media), which is unable to drain down the blocked eustachian tube, and settle spontaneously.

For patients already requiring hydrocortisone replacement, it is often sensible to increase the dose, typically by 50% or doubled. A few patients can be managed without this increase, although it may be needed later in the course. Tiredness is a good measure of the dose of steroid required in this patient group. RT does increase the risk of HPA dysfunction, requiring hormone replacement. However, damage to the HPA is the result of the combination of tumour and surgery as well as RT. HPA dysfunction is dependent upon RT dose. In all, one-half to three-quarters of patients require hormone replacement after surgery and RT. Patients should be followed up regularly in the endocrinology clinic.

The risk of late RT damage to the optic nerves should be negligible with a dose of 45 Gy in 25 fractions. Therefore, if visual deterioration occurs after RT, it is important to look for a cause other than RT. Cataract should not occur with standard techniques.

Any RT treatment carries risk of late secondary tumours. In patients treated for pituitary adenoma, the risk is roughly 1% per decade of follow-up after treatment. Of the tumours caused, about half are benign, typically meningiomas, and about half are malignant, for example, GBM or sarcoma. Because the risk is cumulative with time, this is especially important in younger patients.

Results of Treatment

Postoperative RT produces very high rates of control. Overall, tumour control rates should be around 95% at 10 years and 90% at 20 years. However, control of hormone secretion is poorer, with only 60% to 90% achieving control of hypersecretion. The time to hormonal normalisation is dependent primarily on preirradiation levels.

CRANIOPHARYNGIOMA

Pathology and Clinical Features

The incidence of craniopharyngiomas is 0.13 to 0.18 per 100,000, constituting 1% to 4% of tumours in adults. Disease peaks are seen at age 5 to 14 years and age 65 to 74 years. In adults, it typically presents with symptoms and signs related to raised ICP, compression of the optic chiasm and optic nerves or reduction in pituitary hormone secretion. When these tumours are very extensive, pressure on the frontal lobes or involvement of the hypothalamus can cause behavioural disturbance.

Craniopharyngiomas are thought to arise from cells derived from the embryological structure known as the Rathke pouch, which extends from the embryonic pharynx to form the anterior pituitary gland. Craniopharyngiomas are normally cystic, with a thin wall and a solid component. The craniopharyngioma itself is lined by epithelium (reflecting its origin), which produces the cyst fluid. At both a macroscopic and microscopic level, the wall of the cyst projects into spaces in the surface of the brain, to which it can be strongly adherent.

On CT, flecks of calcification are often seen. On MRI the cyst has almost unique signal characteristics, being those of neither CSF nor brain; both the cyst wall and solid regions are easily seen on T1W sequences and are enhanced with gadolinium. When opened surgically, thick viscous fluid is often seen, with the macroscopic appearances of machine oil and containing microscopic cholesterol crystals accounting for the MRI appearance.

Surgery is the initial treatment modality for most patients with a craniopharyngioma; complete resection is associated with a 5-year tumour growth control of 70% to 90% in adult and pediatric series, although aggressive surgical management is associated with a high risk of complications, particularly relating to hypothalamic damage. Limited surgery followed by radiation is an alternative to aggressive surgical treatment and is associated with comparable outcome and lower risk of long-term sequelae. Enlargement of the cystic component prior to or after RT is an indication for further surgical intervention.

RT is recommended for virtually all adult patients after both subtotal resection and apparently gross tumour resection to reduce recurrence rates. The recurrence rates following surgery alone, even after apparently complete removal, are high. Because this can increase neurological deficits, which are often found in patients with this disease already, the risk and consequences of recurrence greatly outweigh the risks from RT.

Treatment

Target Volume

The patient should be immobilised in a shell, or a relocatable stereotactic frame may be used. CT should be acquired, along with a coregistered MRI (T1W+Gd). In most circumstances, coregistration with the preoperative MRI is also helpful as a guide to the CTV.

RT for craniopharyngioma is more difficult to plan than for pituitary adenoma. The tumour is very adherent at both a macroscopic and microscopic level, and all parts of the brain with which the original tumour was in contact need to be irradiated, which is where coregistration of the preoperative MRI is useful. However, resection decompresses the tumour and reduces the mass effect, thereby shifting the anatomy. Thus neither preoperative nor postoperative imaging exactly represents the location of the target, so the internal anatomy of the brain must also be considered in the planning. The GTV is defined as the visible lesion on postcontrast T1-weighted and T2-weighted MRI sequences with a 1-to-2-mm slice thickness to ensure the accuracy of target delineation. The solid portion of craniopharyngiomas is more precisely contoured using the contrast-enhanced three-dimensional T1-weighted images, whereas fast spin-echo T2-weighted images with and without fat suppression allow for better visualisation of cystic components of the tumour.

The CTV should contain any postoperative gross tumour, the surface of the preoperative gross tumour and a margin for any potential microscopic residual disease. It is appropriate for the CTV to adjust according to any brain shifts that occur following decompression, based on anatomical changes. Generally, the CTV is defined as the GTV plus an additional margin of 0.3 to 0.5 cm.

The PTV margin should be grown isotropically, depending on the immobilisation method used, usually PTV = CTV + 0.3–0.5 cm. As for pituitary adenoma, the lenses, optic nerves, chiasm and tracts, together with the lacrimal glands and brainstem, should be outlined so that the dose distribution and the DVHs for these structures can be reviewed.

Technique

IMRT with image guidance as per pituitary adenoma. TLD measurements of the eye doses should be made.

Dose and Energy

50 to 55 Gy in 30 to 33 daily fractions over 6 weeks, with megavoltage x-rays

Side Effects

Side effects are similar to those for pituitary adenoma. Most patients have significant endocrine dysfunction requiring replacement before RT, and many are pan-hypopituitary. Unlike pituitary adenoma, many will also require desmopressin replacement to compensate for loss of posterior pituitary gland function. For patients already taking hydrocortisone replacement, it is sensible to increase the dose. The major difference in side effects compared to pituitary adenoma is the small but important risk of visual deterioration during RT as a result of the cystic component reaccumulating fluid and compressing the optic chiasm. Patients should be warned to report any visual disturbance the same day, and an urgent MRI is needed. If cyst recurrence is confirmed, immediate neurosurgical referral for operation should be made to try to preserve vision. Reaccumulation of cyst fluid is unrelated to RT itself but may occur coincidentally during the postoperative phase when RT is being given. In children it is a normal practice to perform one or more MRI scans during RT to ensure that the target volume has not increased in size. This has not yet become a standard practice in adults, but it should be considered, at least in selected cases.

The risk of late RT damage to the optic nerves should be very small with a dose of 50 Gy in 30 fractions. The risk of second tumour formation is similar to patients with pituitary adenoma, but this risk is very much less than the risk of recurrence of the craniopharyngioma if RT is not given.

Results of Treatment

RT following surgery produces high rates of control. Using doses of 50 to 55 Gy in 25 to 33 daily fractions of 1.67 to 2.0 Gy with either photons or protons, several large retrospective series report tumour control rates of 85% to 95% and survival rates of 90% to 100% at 5 years. Limited surgery plus RT produces local control rates as good as those from radical surgery, with lower neurological morbidity. Clinical follow-up should include endocrinology, ophthalmological assessment and imaging.

Prognostic factors include the size of the tumour and age at presentation, with a worse prognosis in older patients. There is no benefit in overall survival from GTR. Incomplete resection may produce a better quality of life. Postoperative RT is superior to surveillance after non-radical resection in terms of progression-free survival.

VESTIBULAR SCHWANNOMA

Pathology and Clinical Features

Vestibular schwannoma (VS) is a common cause of unilateral deafness, with a population incidence in the range 0.5 to 2 per 100,000 per year. Patients commonly experience tinnitus, despite losing hearing. Rarely, a VS can be large enough at presentation to compress the brainstem, causing disturbance of balance. Some (approx. 5%) are associated with the genetic condition of neurofibromatosis type 2 (NF-2), which may present with bilateral VS.

The principles of VS management are to reduce mass effect, while preserving facial nerve function and hearing where possible. The three optimal treatment pathways for VS are surgery, SRS/SRT and a wait-and-scan policy. As the VS is in close proximity to anatomical structures such as the cochlea, the brainstem and cranial nerves VII and VIII, treatment can lead to changes in balance, communication and appearance, reducing quality of life. Treatment choice depends on tumour size and location, comorbidities and patient wishes. For the patient with VS secondary to NF2, different management is required. Surgical management is the cornerstone for these patients. RT can have a role in management, especially in those who are elderly and in high-risk surgical candidates.

Small tumours can be managed with a wait-and-scan policy, and some stabilise spontaneously for long periods of time. Observation policy should be followed in elderly patients and in patients with comorbidities and high surgical risk. Active treatment is only required with disease progression. SRS can be performed using a Gamma Knife or LINAC-based solution. SRS is indicated in unilateral tumours with maximum diameter less than 3 cm and no brainstem compression. SRS enables patients to return to normal activities more quickly, and the cost is lower than that of surgery. Very large tumours may be too big to resect safely and therefore are considered for FSRT.

Surgical intervention is the preferred initial approach for the removal of a symptomatic growth or to mitigate the risk posed by a potentially critical increase in mass, and this method may be applicable to smaller growths as well. Achieving either a gross total or a near total removal of the tumour often results in local control rates ranging from 80% to 90%. In surgical centres with extensive experience, patients with minor lesions and intact hearing initially have a 50% to 75% likelihood of maintaining their hearing over 5 years, which decreases to 25% to 50% over 10 years. The occurrence of long-term facial paralysis postsurgery is estimated to be between 3% and 15%. RT is known for its high efficacy and minimal adverse effects. It is a reliable and noninvasive treatment option for VS, and it can be administered as either single-session SRS or multisession fractionated SRT, depending on the lesion's size. Rates of local control appear similar for both surgery and RT, using either FSRT or SRS. Surgery has the attraction of removing the tumour and avoiding the small risk of an RT-related second tumour but has the disadvantages of a small operative mortality, protracted rehabilitation, a risk of facial nerve damage and hearing loss depending on the surgical approach. RT avoids a major surgical procedure, has a lower rate of serious morbidity (and mortality) and a lower rate of facial nerve damage, at the expense of the tumour remaining in situ. Patient preference must be considered, and this group of patients is typically very well informed. Hearing preservation rates are in the range of 60% to 90%, with patients with useful hearing prior to RT having the highest chance to fully preserve their hearing function.

Treatment

Here, only the technique for FSRT will be described; SRS is a highly specialised technique which should be studied in more specific texts.

Target Volume

The patient should be immobilised in a beam direction shell or relocatable stereotactic frame. RT should be fully conformal or use IMRT, based on CT planning with coregistered T1W+Gd MRI (see Fig. 31.10). The tumour is not well shown on CT, but the internal

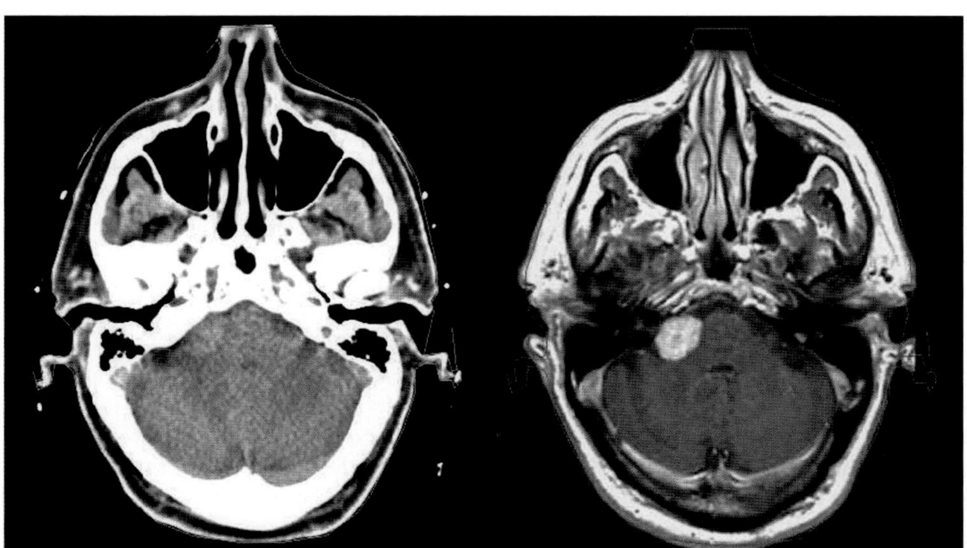

Fig. 31.10 Planning computed tomography scan and coregistered magnetic resonance image of a vestibular schwannoma

auditory meatus (IAM) is clearly visualised. On MRI the tumour is obvious, and extension into the IAM is apparent. For GTV delineation, thin-slice CT and MRI with and without contrast enhancement are recommended. The GTV is represented by the lesion visible on isotropic contrast-enhanced three-dimensional T1-weighted sequences with 1-mm slice thickness. Additional sequences are represented by high-resolution three-dimensional T2-weighted sequences (e.g. CISS/FIESTA) and may improve the visualisation of cisternal segments of the lower cranial nerves and their relationship with the tumour. For contouring, bony CT windows are helpful because the enlargement of the vestibular canal can make the tumour volume visible. Provided the coregistration accuracy is high, no CTV margin is required. The PTV should be grown isotropically with an appropriate margin.

It is helpful to outline the pituitary so that a low dose can be confirmed. The cochlea is bound to lie within the PTV and should be outlined to determine the dose delivered, particularly in patients who still have some hearing on that side. The eyes, specifically the lenses, should be outlined to ensure that the tolerance dose is not exceeded, as should the ipsilateral parotid gland.

Technique

IMRT, rotational or with fixed fields, should be used and provides an excellent solution. Small volumes may also be treated with multiple arcs.

Dose and Energy

50 Gy in 30 daily fractions over 6 weeks, with 6-MV photons

Some centres have used higher doses, in the range of 54 to 57.6 Gy, in 1.8-Gy fractions. Some hypofractionated schedules have also been designed, using lower doses in 12 fractions only. These doses exceed brainstem tolerance and are only suitable for small lesions. Preservation of cranial nerve function may be better with the slightly lower dose (50 Gy) and dose per fraction, but this needs to be formally evaluated. The variation in local control with dose also needs investigation. Although the hearing preservation rate is lower in patients with neurofibromatosis, a lower dose is not recommended.

Side Effects

Acute side effects include hair loss in the (fixed) field entry portals, and there may be mild erythema of the skin. The skin within the external auditory meatus may also become irritated and, in the longer term, the wax may become thicker and more tenacious. Some patients experience mild nausea, which is easily controlled with simple antiemetics. A proportion of patients also experience some disturbance of balance, due to vestibulocochlear irritation. This resolves after RT, though this may take several weeks.

Late effects include hearing loss and cranial nerve dysfunction. Hearing preservation rates are in the region of 75% with both FSRT and SRS but also depend on tumour size and dose in SRS series. Preservation of some useful hearing may be higher, and has been suggested to be as high as 90%, in FSRT series. Patients with NF-2 have a higher risk of losing their hearing, with a preservation rate of only 60%. Both FSRT and SRS series report facial neuropathy risks in around 1% (including facial paralysis, spasm and dysgeusia), and ontological symptoms in 1% to 3% of patients (including tinnitus, hearing loss, vertigo and imbalance). Other less prominent side effects reported are hydrocephalus and pituitary treatment failure. There is a risk of late second tumour following RT, most relevant in younger patients. By analogy with the data from pituitary patients, and considering the small, lateralised volume, this is expected to be rather less than 1% per decade after treatment.

Results of Treatment

Local control rates after FSRT or SRS are excellent, with a 5-year local control rate of 90% to 99%, with the preservation of hearing in 50% to 79% of cases, facial nerve preservation in 95% to 100% of cases and trigeminal nerve preservation in 80% to 99% of cases. This is equivalent to microsurgery results, though a direct comparison has never been attempted. The radiological average response after 6 years of follow-up shows a tumour volume decrease in about half of patients. Tumour regrowth can occur, and salvage surgery may be an option.

CHORDOMAS AND LOW-GRADE CHORDOSARCOMAS

Pathology and Clinical Features

These are rare tumours of the skull base and spine, with a median age at presentation of 60 years. Chordomas are twice as common as chondrosarcomas. Chordomas and chondrosarcomas are distinct pathological entities, but given that they share common features, they can be considered together. Both are difficult to resect and require very high doses of RT to achieve local control. Chordomas can metastasise. Chordomas arise in the skull base, typically near but not in the midline, and along the whole length of the spine. The skull base, upper cervical spine and sacrum are the most common locations. Low-grade chondrosarcomas may present at any age but are most common in older adults. They also occur in the skull base, arising from bony or cartilaginous elements. Usually they are located in the parasellar area, cerebellopontine angle or paranasal sinuses but may also arise in the clivus. Both types of tumour typically present with pain, headache or cranial nerve palsies. Chordomas grow slowly but have a high tendency for local recurrence, and metastases can occur in 30% to 40% of patients; common sites of spread include the lungs, bones and lymph nodes. Outcome is generally poorer than low-grade chondrosarcoma.

Treatment

The mainstay of treatment is maximal tumour debulking. En bloc resection is the recommended treatment, with 5-year local recurrence-free survival rates of more than 50%. However, en bloc resection with R0 margins for skull base chordomas and chondrosarcomas (negative microscopic margin of 1 mm or greater of normal tissue around the tumour) is very rarely achievable, despite major advances in cytoreductive surgical interventions. Surgery should be practised in referral centres because the quality and extent of surgery are the principal determinants of outcome, together with tumour size, quality of RT and patient age. Modern endoscopic techniques have dramatically improved resection and reduced morbidity. Complete resection with negative margins is the optimal treatment option as it increases progression-free survival and overall survival. In all tumours, adjuvant RT should be offered. Bimodality treatment improves local control and DFS, particularly in skull base tumours. Postoperative RT should also be considered for patients with partially resected tumours. There is good evidence that doses of more than 65 to 70 Gy are required.

Best results have been achieved using RT with proton or carbon ion RT, which appear to be able to deliver higher doses than x-rays with safety. Metal used to reconstruct and stabilise the skull base or spine is considered by many to be a contraindication to protons or carbon ion therapy. Efforts are now being made to avoid using metal implants in patients with chordoma and chondrosarcoma. They require referral to a specialist proton beam therapy (PBT) centre. Patients with metal implants or those requiring palliative RT should be treated with IMRT. In palliative cases, it is often worth attempting high-dose treatment because responses may be durable.

Target Volume

Most patients will be seen and treated in a PBT or carbon ion centre. For those patients not able to receive PBT, high-dose image-guided IMRT is required. Effective immobilisation is vital. Imaging should include the coregistration of preoperative and postoperative MRI, both T1 with contrast and T2 sequences, the latter often showing the original tumour well. A specific diagnostic bone window CT is helpful to identify intraosseous disease.

The GTV should include the surgical cavity and residual macroscopic disease. The CTV should encompass all potential areas at risk of microscopic spread of disease and is typically based on preoperative tumour volume and postoperative residual tumour and resection margins. The PTV depends on the immobilisation and image guidance protocol and is usually 0.3 to 0.5 cm, with protons usually requiring larger margins than photon stereotactic techniques.

Technique

Image-guided IMRT is essential. The relevant OARs should be carefully delineated. For the neural OARs, a PRV also should be outlined, in respect to dose constrains to the brainstem, the spinal cord and the optic apparatus.

Dose and Energy

Doses up to 70 to 76 Gy in 1.8-to-2.0-Gy fractions for chordomas; lower doses for chondrosarcomas

Chondrosarcoma grade 1 to 3: 65 to 70 Gy in 39 fractions over 8 weeks

These doses should also be used for high-dose palliation. The spinal cord maximum surface dose can be as high as 58 Gy in 39 fractions.

Results of Treatment

The extent of surgical resection is significant and the volume of any residual gross tumour is prognostic. Chondrosarcomas can be controlled in over 90% of cases and metastasise very rarely. Chordomas are less well controlled, with local control rates of only 50% to 80%. Of those chordomas that recur, local failure is the major problem, occurring in 95% of patients. Metastatic disease is found in 20%. This can be manifest as widespread dissemination or involvement of regional lymph nodes. No effective treatment is available for patients who recur.

SPINAL CORD TUMOURS: PRIMARY

Pathology and Clinical Features

The majority of these tumours are intrinsic, predominantly ependymomas or astrocytomas. GBMs are rare. Intrinsic tumours compress the spinal cord from within and often produce some permanent neurological damage. Primary spinal cord tumours typically present with a mixture of sensory and motor impairment related to the site of tumour involvement. Less commonly, they present with pain. Improvement in microsurgical techniques has led to excellent outcomes with regards to preservation of neurological function.

Grade 1 ependymomas of myxopapillary type are one of the most common primary tumours affecting the lower end of the spinal cord itself (the conus medullaris) and the lumbosacral nerve roots. Many of these tumours can be removed completely and will not require RT. If there is residual disease, they can be observed in the first instance and if progression occurs can be irradiated at that point. Astrocytomas are usually high grade and require RT; they account for 40% to 50% of the intramedullary spinal cord tumours. Surgical debulking is a reasonable option for high-grade tumours. GBMs are usually irradiated but have a bleak outlook.

Occasional extrinsic tumours also occur: meningiomas arise from the coverings of the cord; schwannomas and neurofibromas arise in nerve roots. These extrinsic tumours compress the spinal cord. Surgical removal relieves the compression, and the deficit often recovers. Surgery alone is usually curative.

Treatment: Radical

In adults, RT can improve disease control, survival and neurological function and quality of life where there is postoperative residual disease in higher-grade tumours.

Target Volume

Treatment planning is based on CT coregistered with preoperative and postoperative MRI. Sometimes spinal curvature is so different that the MRI will not coregister reliably, but the key issue is the longitudinal extent of the tumour, which can be measured from the vertebral levels.

The GTV includes the residual tumour visible on the T1 enhancing abnormality on MRI or the tumour on T2/FLAIR images in low-grade gliomas. The postoperative cavity should be included in the GTV.

Longitudinally, the CTV should include the oedema on a T2-weighted MRI with a margin of 1.5 cm for low-grade tumours and 2 to 3 cm for high-grade tumours around the GTV to include any subclinical spread. Axially, the CTV includes the whole spinal canal. The PTV uses an additional 0.5-to-1.0-cm margin to account for setup error, depending on the immobilisation technique.

CT planning allows normal tissue structures to be delineated, such as the esophagus, thyroid and oral cavity in patients with cervical tumours; the lungs, esophagus and heart in those with thoracic tumours; and the kidneys and possibly ovaries in patients with lumbosacral tumours.

Technique

Supine positioning is now conventional, and IMRT should be used to provide increased dose homogeneity.

Dose and Energy

50 to 54 Gy in 30 fractions, treating daily, over 6 weeks, with megavoltage photons

This is a reasonable estimate of safe cord tolerance in a patient with spinal cord tumour. For patients with GBM of the spinal cord, the higher dose of 54 Gy in 30 fractions is appropriate.

Side Effects

Side effects of treatment are usually mild and depend on tumour location. It is unusual for neurological function to deteriorate and, if this does happen, it can be managed by increasing the steroid dose. Some esophagitis may occur in patients with cervical or upper thoracic tumours, but it is normally mild. Patients with lumbar or lumbosacral tumours may experience nausea or mild diarrhoea, but these symptoms can be managed effectively with simple medication.

Myelopathy is possible with doses exceeding the spinal cord tolerance. For doses up to 50 Gy, the incidence of myelopathy is less than 0.5%, and it is 1% to 5% for doses high than 60 Gy. Radiation myelopathy can present acutely or chronically. Acute myelopathy, known as Lhermitte syndrome, is reversible; symptoms include sudden tingling and electric shock-like sensation radiating to the hands and feet on neck flexion. It does not progress to late myelopathy and is uncommon when treating spinal tumours. Chronic myelopathy presents as loss of sensor and motor function and is usually irreversible.

Treatment: Palliative

A few patients require palliative treatment and are managed in a similar way to a metastatic cord compression.

Results of Treatment

Ependymomas have a better prognosis than astrocytic tumours. Grade 1 lesions are cured in most patients, and grade 2 tumours are cured in the region of 50% of patients. Higher-grade ependymomas are rare but, as expected, have a worse prognosis. Astrocytomas have a worse prognosis, grade for grade, than ependymomas. GBMs of the cord have an appalling prognosis. Recurrence often occurs within a few weeks or months of treatment and may include dissemination through the CSF. Favourable prognostic factors are younger age at presentation, the absence of neurological deficits at diagnosis and lower grade. The 5-and 10-year survival rates for spinal ependymomas range between 66% to 100% and 62% to 91%, and for primary spinal astrocytomas between 60% to 100% and 40% to 75%, respectively.

CEREBRAL METASTASES

Clinical Features and Management Principles

The majority of patients with cerebral metastases have multiple lesions (Fig. 31.11), and around 80% occur in the cerebrum. Those in the cerebellum may cause hydrocephalus. Many patients also have active extracranial disease, which is relevant in assessing prognosis and treatment options, including suitability for SRS. Occasionally, the first presentation is with metastasis, and biopsy may be important in establishing the diagnosis. Intraaxial metastases have similar presentation to primary tumours (discussed earlier).

Metastatic spread may also cause diffuse meningeal disease, infiltrating widely over the surface of the brain. Leptomeningeal disease may present with confusion, photophobia and neck stiffness, or it may cause cranial nerve palsies from involvement of meninges at the base of the brain. Metastatic disease may also affect the bones of the skull, which is common in prostate cancer. Involvement of the skull base typically produces cranial nerve palsies, by compression of the nerves as they pass through the skull.

Patients with single or multiple cerebral metastases are almost always incurable. The treatment objective is therefore palliative, and additional supportive care should be instituted. Steroid treatment is normally appropriate to reduce surrounding oedema. Unless the patient is in the end stage of their disease, it is helpful for the patient to be restaged to assess the extent and aggressiveness of the disease, to guide systemic treatment and inform prognosis. It is usually appropriate for the patient to be managed by the relevant site-specific team. As well as palliative RT, chemotherapy and hormonal therapy may be helpful.

As treatment options multiply and patients survive for longer with disease, more and more patients are being considered for aggressive management of brain metastases. There is now NHS England direction for patient selection when considering SRS to treat oligometastatic brain metastases. Patients must have controlled or controllable extracranial disease, have KPS greater than 70, have a prognosis of more than 6 months and have a total lesion volume less than 20 cc (the European Association of Neuro-Oncology (EANO) recommends 15 cc). Where these criteria are fulfilled, SRS has been shown to control 80% of intracranial disease at 12 months following treatment.

Unfortunately, this only covers a small fraction of patients, leaving a large number who need to be managed palliatively with dexamethasone for symptom control and possibly the use of WBRT.

WBRT in the Management of Patients With Brain Metastasis

WBRT is the most common treatment for multiple metastases. However, it is important to note that certain patient subgroups may not derive significant benefit from it. The QUARTZ trial conducted by the Medical Research Council found that individuals with NSCLC and a limited life expectancy did not experience an improvement in overall survival or quality of life when treated with WBRT as compared to receiving best supportive care.

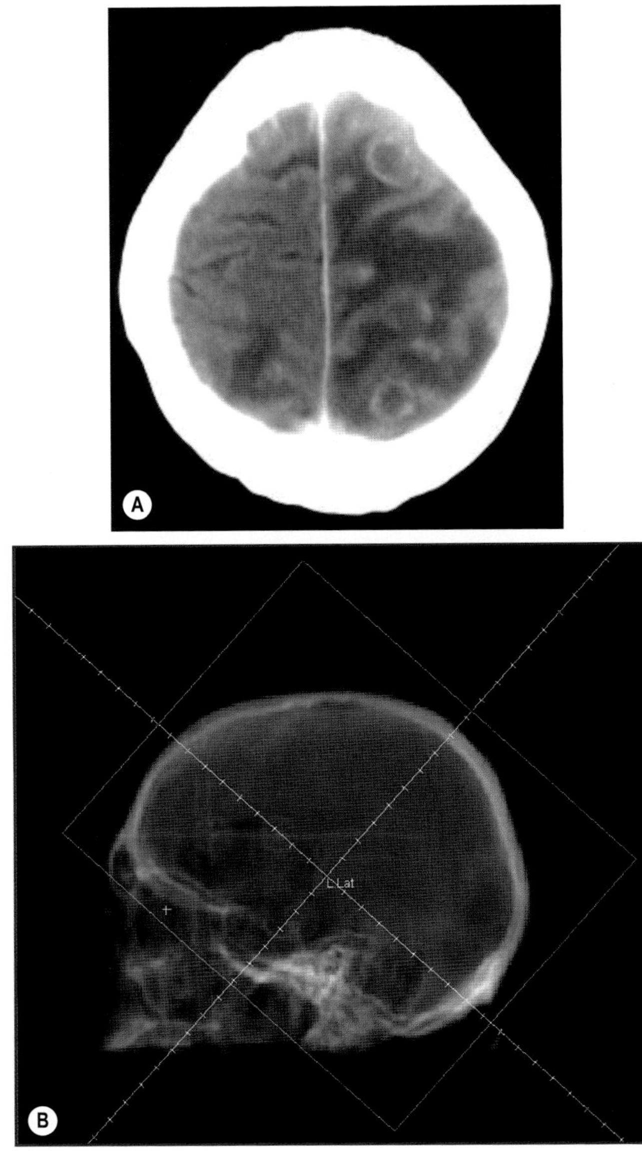

Fig. 31.11 (A) Computed tomography scan of a patient showing multiple cerebral metastases from nonsmall cell lung cancer, surrounded by oedema. Three deposits are seen in the left hemisphere, and another single lesion is visible in the right cerebral hemisphere, posteriorly. Oedema is seen around each deposit. (B) Field for whole brain irradiation, showing adequate coverage around the skull, including at the skull base. The collimator angle allows sparing of dose to the eyes and pharynx.

Several randomised trials have explored various RT regimens for patients with multiple brain metastases. Most of these trials have utilised 30 Gy delivered in 10 fractions as the control arm, but only one small study, involving 70 patients, compared 6-month survival after 30 Gy in 10 fractions to that after 20 Gy in 5 fractions and found no statistically significant difference. Additionally, an RTOG study from 1980 compared three different regimens: 40 Gy in 15 fractions, 30 Gy in 10 fractions and 20 Gy in 5 fractions. The median survival for all three groups fell within the range of 3.2 to 3.5 months ($p > 0.05$). Consequently, there is currently insufficient evidence to support the assertion that 20 Gy in 5 fractions is either inferior or superior to 30 Gy in 10 fractions. Furthermore, increasing the dose beyond 30 Gy in 10 fractions has not shown any survival benefit.

To mitigate the risk of neurocognitive decline associated with WBRT, methods such as hippocampal sparing can be employed, provided that no lesions are located in close proximity to the hippocampus. A randomised controlled study investigating the concurrent use of the glutamate receptor antagonist memantine did not achieve its primary endpoint of reducing cognitive function decline and therefore did not receive approval from the National Institute for Health and Care Excellence (NICE) in the United Kingdom.

Patients With One to Three Brain Metastasis

Both surgical resection and SRS improve local control within the brain for patients with oligometastatic disease. Surgical resection is particularly useful for patients with posterior fossa tumours causing hydrocephalus. The decision to undertake surgical resection or stereotactic RT should be made through the neurooncology multidisciplinary team and is based on the location and size of the mestastasis(es) and other patient factors. Some patients may be of sufficiently poor performance status that even simple palliative RT may not be of value. For meningeal disease, that is, carcinomatous meningitis, in addition to palliative RT, intrathecal MTX may be of symptomatic benefit. Neurosurgery may be considered for palliation of symptoms related to mass effect, haemorrhage or hydrocephalus.

A randomised trial comparing cavity SRS to WBRT after resection of metastases in patient with one to three lesions reported better neurocognitive function and quality of life in the SRS arm. The WBRT arm did not show any improvement in survival. Two further trials showed that SRS is superior to observation after surgical resection in achieving local control in patients with one to three lesions. This benefit was higher in cases with a single lesion, and SRS proved to be a safe treatment. The benefit was highest for cavities smaller than 2.5 cm.

Hypofractionated, focal brain RT can be considered as an alternative to SRS for brain metastasis. The delivery of high-dose RT to the surgical cavity improves local control. The side effects are acceptable, while larger tumours can be treated.

Postoperative Radiotherapy

Evidence from two randomised trials indicates that adding surgery to WBRT offers an overall survival advantage for patients with a solitary metastasis and a good performance status (level 1a). A third trial which did not demonstrate an overall survival benefit may have been influenced by the inclusion of a high proportion of patients with poor performance status. Surgical resection without subsequent adjuvant WBRT comes with a twofold increased risk of cavity recurrence. SRS administered to the surgical cavity has shown comparable overall survival rates and less neurocognitive decline compared to adjuvant WBRT and is generally the preferred approach.

At present, SRS to the surgical cavity following the complete resection of cerebral metastases is not recommended by NHS England due to the absence of evidence showing improvement in overall survival when compared to observation alone. Nevertheless, when there is evidence of residual or recurrent disease, SRS or some form of postoperative RT is warranted. Preoperative SRS aims to address challenges related to contouring the surgical cavity. International trials have been initiated comparing preoperative and adjuvant SRS, and we await the results of these (trial identifiers: NCT03741673, NCT04503772).

Treatment

Palliative Radiotherapy

Target Volume and Technique

Whole Brain Irradiation. The patient should ideally be immobilised in a shell. The whole brain should be treated, both cerebrum and cerebellum, because part of the objective is to treat micrometastases. The standard beam arrangement is a parallel pair of lateral opposing fields. The collimator should be rotated to follow the base of the skull to avoid the eyes. Sufficient margin should be allowed to adequately treat the whole brain effectively (see Fig. 31.11).

Skull Base Irradiation. The beam arrangement is also a parallel pair of lateral opposing fields. Under normal circumstances, when it is necessary to treat the bones through which the cranial nerves pass, the field should extend from the outer canthus down and back to the posterior edge of the foramen magnum. This will cover cranial nerves II to XII.

Postoperative Hypofractionated Radiotherapy

There is no consensus as to the appropriate dose, and this is still an area for further research. The GTV includes the remaining tumour, or tumour bed, defined as the enhancing disease in the T1W MRI scan. The CTV includes the surgical cavity as outlined in the planning MRI scan, with a small margin. The PTV should be expanded according to the immobilisation used.

Dose and Energy

A variety of dose schedules are available:

30 Gy in 10 fractions, treating daily, over 2 weeks.

20 Gy in 5 fractions, treating daily, over 1 week.

12 Gy in 2 fractions, treating on consecutive days or up to 1 week apart. This should be avoided if there is a very heavy burden of metastases, to avoid coning with the high dose/fraction.

Hypofractionated Radiotherapy

Dose 30 Gy in 5 fractions over 5 days

Side Effects

Side effects are the same as for palliative RT for HGG. Acutely these include headache, nausea, fatigue and hair loss. Late effects relate mostly to neurocognition and quality of life.

Stereotactic Radiosurgery

SRS delivers a high dose of RT in a single fraction or fewer than 5 fractions to a very small volume with high precision. Single doses are typically in the range of 18 to 21 Gy depending on the tumour size. This is delivered with stereotactic localising technique using the stereotactic frame or specialised shell for immobilisation of the patient. The outcome is similar to the outcome of surgery, with lower cost (except in the posterior fossa), and is achieved irrespective of the delivery platform (LINAC based, Gamma Knife or CyberKnife).

There are constraints in delivering this treatment in relation to critical normal structures and the size of the lesion. The maximum diameter should be no larger than 3 cm in longest diameter, tumour volume less than 10 mL and total cumulative volume 15 mL or less, and patients should fulfil the commissioning criteria outlined earlier. Lesions that are located near the optic apparatus (less than 5 mm away) or in the brainstem, pons or medulla cannot be treated with SRS.

Findings from the HyTEC report indicate that single-session treatments resulting in more than 12-Gy exposure to volumes of healthy tissue beyond the tumour (5 cm^3, 10 cm^3 or more than 15 cm^3)

correspond to radionecrosis rates of roughly 10%, 15% and 20%, respectively. As such, for tumours larger than 2 to 3 cm, those situated near vital organs, or when the volume receiving more than 12 Gy exceeds 10 cm^3, a fractionated or staged radiosurgery regimen should be contemplated. Reports highlighted better local control and a reduced incidence of radiation necrosis in metastases over 2 cm in diameter treated with a fractionated schedule of 27 Gy delivered in 3 consecutive daily doses, as opposed to a single session. Another frequently employed hypofractionated schedule is 30 Gy given over 5 daily sessions, and a regimen of 35 Gy across 5 days has been tested in prospective studies as well.

Dose Recommendations

Single-fraction SRS based on lesion diameter:

- Less than 20 mm: 21 to 24 Gy, single dose (grade B)
- 21 to 30 mm: 18 Gy, single dose (grade B)
- 31 to 40 mm: 15 Gy, single dose (grade B) (consider hypofractionated SRS)

Hypofractionated SRS:

- 24 to 27 Gy in 3 daily fractions
- 30 Gy in 5 daily fractions
- 35 Gy in 5 daily fractions

Target Volume and Technique

SRS is a highly specialist technique and beyond the scope of this chapter.

Results of Treatment

Where patients have controlled extracranial disease and low-volume intracranial metastases, the disease control rate is 80% at 12 months. Good patient selection ensures that most of those who undergo treatment appear to benefit in terms of palliation of symptoms. For patients with meningeal disease, the prognosis is much worse.

SPINAL CORD COMPRESSION

Pathology and Clinical Features

Metastatic epidural spinal cord compression (MESCC) is a common oncological emergency. It occurs in 3% to 6% of patients presenting with malignancy, and it can occur in up to 20% of patients with breast, prostate and lung cancer. Almost 60% of cases involve the thoracic spine. The pathology of MESCC is related to direct invasion or extrinsic compression in vertebral bodies, obstruction of the vertebral venous plexus resulting in cord oedema and further tumour growth. In most cases it affects more than one vertebral body. Almost 90% of patients present with pain either localised to a vertebra or in a radicular distribution. Other common symptoms include motor weakness, sensory loss and autonomic dysfunction. Sphincter disturbance and urine incontinence are usually late presentations. Permanent motor and neurological dysfunction may develop after the initial back pain. MESCC may rarely be the initial presentation of a cancer diagnosis. A detailed history and focused neurological examination should be performed, and MRI scanning is necessary to establish a diagnosis. However, if patients cannot undergo an MRI or if MRI is contradicted, CT myelography can be used.

Management Principles

The treatment of spinal metastases is palliative, although some patients may achieve prolonged survival. The aim of the treatment should be pain relief, maintenance of neurological function, durable local tumour control, mechanical stability and quality of life.

Steroids

Steroids should be considered in all cases: randomised studies have proved that there is neurological improvement after their use. However, high doses of steroids can cause serious adverse effects including gastric ulcers and infections. Dexamethasone 16 mg daily is most frequently prescribed, which can be continued throughout the RT course and then tapered depending on the clinical situation.

Surgery and Radiotherapy

The combination of decompression surgery and RT has been evaluated in one phase III and one phase II study. Both showed improvement in mobility, with some patients even regaining the ability to walk, improved pain control and better quality of life. Surgery should be considered in patients with a single site of vertebral metastasis, vertebral collapse at presentation, good performance status and life expectancy of more than 3 months. In addition, surgery should be considered in cases of worsening neurological symptoms, new neurological findings during RT, disease recurrence within a prior radiation site and spinal instability.

External Beam Radiotherapy

Palliative RT is used to prevent neurological deterioration, improve the neurological and ambulatory function and for pain relief. RT should be delivered within 24 hours of symptom commencement. There is no consensus on the ideal RT regimen. Two randomised trials with a primary endpoint of maintenance of neurological function compared different radiation doses and showed that 8 to 10 Gy in a single fraction is noninferior to multiple fractions (20 Gy in 5 fractions). Nonetheless a metaanalysis showed that better local control was achieved in patients with a soft-tissue mass component when longer fractionation was prescribed. In patients with good prognosis where preserving their neurological function and mobility is critical, a longer scheme should be considered. However, in patients with poor prognosis, poor performance status and paraplegia, where the objective is pain control, a single fraction should be prescribed.

Target Volume and Technique

Careful correlation with the diagnostic MRI is essential. Typically, a direct posterior field is used, but two lateral opposing fields can be considered when treating the C-spine, provided the shoulders are not in the beam. Traditionally, one vertebra above and one below the affected area are also included in the target to account for possible epidural extensions. The dose should be kept below the tolerance dose of the spinal cord.

Dose

30 Gy in 10 fractions, treating daily, over 2 weeks
20 Gy in 5 fractions, treating daily, over 1 week
8 Gy in 1 fraction, single fraction

Stereotactic Body Radiation Therapy

In many centres, SBRT is used in the treatment of selected cases with cord compression. This technique requires precision in mobilisation and image guidance allowing for pretreatment confirmation and advanced radiation treatment planning. The aim of treatment is to provide a high dose of ablative radiation to improve local control. SBRT treats only the lesion, sparing most of the adjacent tissue, and is usually delivered in a single fraction. Published data suggest that SBRT can offer complete pain control in more than 50% of patients and improves disability. The role of SBRT in patients with oligometastatic disease is also of particular interest.

Results

Factors that influence the outcomes include rate of symptom development, neurological impairment at diagnosis, certain tumour types and response to therapy.

FURTHER READING

Baumert BG, Hegi ME, van den Bent MJ, von Deimling A, Gorlia T, Hoang-Xuan K, Brandes AA, Kantor G, Taphoorn MJB, Hassel MB, Hartmann C, Ryan G, Capper D, Kros JM, Kurscheid S, Wick W, Enting R, Reni M, Thiessen B, et al. Temozolomide chemotherapy versus radiotherapy in high- risk low-grade glioma (EORTC 22033-26033): A randomised, open-label, phase 3 intergroup study. *Lancet Oncol.* 2016;17(11):1521–1532.

Combs SE, Baumert BG, BendszusM Bozzao A, Brada M, Fariselli L, Fiorentino A, Ganswindt U, Grosu AL, Lagerwaardm FL, Niyazi M, Nyholm T, Paddick I, Weber DC, Belka C, Minniti G. ESTRO ACROP guideline for target volume delineation of skull base tumours. *Radiother Oncol.* 2021;156:80–94.

Eekers DBP, Di Perri D, Roelofs E, Postma A, Dijkstra J, Ajithkumar T, Alapetite C, Blomstrand M, Burnet NG, Calugaru V, Compter I, Coremans IEM, Harrabi S, Iannalfi A, Klaver YLB, Lambrecht M, Romero AM, Paulsen F, Timmermann B, et al. Update of the EPTN Atlas for CT- and MR-based Contouring in Neuro-Oncology. *Radiother Oncol.* 2021 Jul;160:259–265. doi:10.1016/j.radonc.2021.05.013

Hoang-Xuan K, Deckert M, Ferreri AJM, Furtner J, Gallego Perez-Larraya J, Henriksson R, Hottinger AF, Kasenda B, Lefranc F, Lossos A, McBain C, Preusser M, Roth P, Rudà R, Schlegel U, Soffietti R, Soussain C, Taphoorn MJB, Touitou V, et al. European Association of Neuro-Oncology (EANO) guidelines for treatment of primary central nervous system lymphoma (PCNSL). *Neuro Oncol.* 2023 Jan 5;25(1):37–53. doi:10.1093/neuonc/noac196

Lambrecht M, Eekers DBP, Alapetite C, Burnet NG, Calugaru V, Coremans IEM, Fossati P, Høyer M, Langendijk JA, Romero AM, Paulsen F, Perpar A, Renard L, de Ruysscher D, Timmermann B, Vitek P, Weber DC, van der Weide HL,…work package 1 of the taskforce. European Particle Therapy Network" of ESTRO. Radiation dose constraints for organs at risk in neuro-oncology; the European Particle Therapy Network consensus. *Radiother Oncol.* 2018;128(1):26–36.

Louis DN, Perry A, Wesseling P, Brat DJ, Cree IA, Figarella-Branger D, Hawkins C, Ng HK, Pfister SM, Reifenberger G, Soffietti R, von Deimling A, Ellison DW. The 2021 WHO Classification of Tumours of the Central Nervous System: A summary. *Neuro Oncol.* 2021 Aug 2;23(8):1231–1251. doi:10.1093/neuonc/noab106

Niyazi M, Andratschke N, Bendszus M, Chalmers AJ, Erridge SC, Galldiks N, Lagerwaard FJ, Navarria P, Munck AF, Rosenschöld P, Ricardi U, van den Bent MJ, Weller M, Belka C, Minniti G. ESTRO-EANO guideline on target delineation and radiotherapy details for glioblastoma. *Radiother Oncol.* 2023 Jul;184:109663. doi:10.1016/j.radonc.2023.109663

Perry JR, Laperriere N, O'Callaghan CJ, Brandes AA, Menten J, Phillips C, Fay M, Nishikawa R, Cairncross JG, Roa W, Osoba D, Rossiter JP, Sahgal A, Hirte H, Laigle-Donadey F, Franceschi E, Chinot O, Golfinopoulos V, Fariselli L, et al. Short-course radiation plus temozolomide in elderly patients with glioblastoma. *N Engl J Med.* 2017;376(11):1027–1037.

Raverot G, Burman P, McCormack A, Heaney A, Petersenn S, Popovic V, Trouillas J, Dekkers OM; European Society of Endocrinology. European Society of Endocrinology Clinical Practice Guidelines for the management of aggressive pituitary tumours and carcinomas. *Eur J Endocrinol.* 2018 Jan;178(1):G1–G24. doi: 10.1530/EJE-17-0796. Epub 2017 Oct 18.

Rudà R, Bruno F, Pellerino A, Ependymoma Soffietti R. Evaluation and management updates. *Curr Oncol Rep.* 2022 Aug;24(8): 985–993. doi:10.1007/s11912-022-01260-w

van den Bent MJ, Baumert B, Erridge SC, Vogelbaum MA, Nowak AK, Sanson M, Brandes AA, Clement PM, Baurain JF, Mason WP, Wheeler H, Chinot OL, Gill S, Griffin M, Brachman DG, Taal W, Rudà R, Weller M, McBain C, et al. Interim results from the CATNON trial (EORTC study 26053-22054) of treatment with concurrent and adjuvant temozolomide for 1p/19q non-co-deleted anaplastic glioma: A phase 3, randomised, open-label intergroup study. *Lancet.* 2017;390(10103):1645–1653.

32

Eye and Orbit

Thankamma V. Ajithkumar

CHAPTER OUTLINE

ANATOMY

The orbit is defined by bony margins and is conical in shape. It contains the eye, the optic nerve, the recti and the oblique extra-ocular muscles. The optic nerve exits from just below the centre of the back of the eye and extends to the optic foramen at the apex of the orbit posteriorly. The globe is composed of three layers: an outer fibrous layer called the sclera; a middle layer that is vascular and composed of the choroid, the ciliary body and the iris; and an inner neural layer, the retina. The vascular choroid covers the inner surface of the sclera. The sclera is continuous anteriorly with the cornea, a transparent membrane covering the iris and pupil. The anterior-posterior diameter of the eye is 24 mm, and the lens is 5 mm from the anterior surface. These measurements vary little amongst individuals.

The movement of each eye is performed by six muscles (four recti and two oblique muscles) and directed by three cranial nerves, the IIIrd, IVth and VIth. The VIth cranial nerve supplies the lateral rectus muscle that moves the eyeball laterally. The medial, superior and inferior recti elevate, depress and move the eyeball inwards, whereas the inferior oblique moves the eyeball upwards and outwards. These four muscles are supplied by the IIIrd cranial nerve. The superior oblique, which moves the eye downwards and outwards, is supplied by the IVth cranial nerve.

The eyelids have multiple layers. The skin of the eyelids is the thinnest in the body (<1 mm), and tarsal plates are 28 to 29 mm long and 1 mm thick. The tarsal plate is 10 mm in height in the upper lid and 3.5 to 5 mm in the lower lid. The membrane lining the inner surface of the eyelids is the conjunctiva, which courses over the anterior surface of the globe and extends to the corneoscleral junction. Tears are secreted by minor lacrimal glands situated mainly on the lower eyelid and can be supplemented by the lacrimal gland situated in the upper lateral part of the orbit. They drain into the nose through the nasolacrimal duct.

PRINCIPLES OF RADIOTHERAPY TO THE EYE

The chosen radiotherapy (RT) technique will be determined by whether radical or palliative treatment is being given; tumour factors such as histology, radiosensitivity and location; and patient factors such as fitness and comorbidity. Brachytherapy can be used for some ocular melanomas and retinoblastomas, which are described in the relevant sections in this chapter.

For fractionated external beam radiotherapy (EBRT), the patient should have a comfortable setup, which is likely to make fractionated treatment more reproducible and appropriate immobilisation. For palliative treatment a simple thermoplastic immobilisation shell will suffice. For radical treatment the shell (thermoplastic or Perspex) should be made with appropriate quality assurance to keep systematic and random movement errors to an absolute minimum so as to avoid sensitive, normal structures with more accuracy. It is often difficult to protect any one part of the eye, particularly the lens and cornea, as the substructures are so small, although internal eye shields can be used to protect the lens when treating skin tumours close to the eye. Internal eye shields should not be used if they cover the tumour target volume.

When superficial x-rays or electrons are used, the target volume or field is marked directly onto the shell. Beam data are used to choose an appropriate energy and to decide whether tissue-equivalent bolus is required to increase the surface dose. A lead cutout is made to define the field shape.

A computed tomography (CT) scan is performed with the patient immobilised in the treatment shell for megavoltage EBRT. CT slices should be no more than 3 mm thick. Intravenous contrast can help in defining adjacent vessels and enhancing tumour. Target volumes are defined on the CT data set, and appropriate organs at risk (OARs) are contoured. A simple parallel-pair beam arrangement will provide good target coverage with minimal morbidity for low-dose treatments where the bilateral orbit is the target volume. In more complex situations, inverse planned intensity modulated radiotherapy (IMRT) is recommended to be able to balance target coverage with appropriate normal tissue sparing. Noncoplanar beams can be helpful in avoiding the lacrimal gland and minimising the dose to uninvolved parts of the eye. Careful attention should be paid to eye care throughout treatment, and regular reviews should be performed by the ophthalmologist and radiation oncologist during the course of RT.

RADIATION AND OCULAR MORBIDITY

The Lens

Of all the tissues in the body, the lens is one of the most sensitive to RT. Cataracts have been reported at doses as low as 2 Gy. However, it should be remembered that they invariably occur without RT over the age of 70 years and are associated with various common diseases, such as diabetes, and medications, such as steroids. The appearance and region of the cataract can help in deciding their causation. Radiation cataracts are caused by damage to cells in the anterior central area of the lens, which then start to form a cataract at the back of the lens centrally (posterior subcapsular cataract). The total dose, energy of radiation, volume of the lens, health of the eye and concomitant disease are all factors that play a part in cataract formation. When high doses are given with β-irradiation eye plaques, usually for treatment of posterior choroidal melanomas, cataracts often will not occur, because of the rapid falloff of dose (as opposed to the historical use of cobalt plaques). After EBRT, fractionated doses of over 10 Gy are likely to cause detectable lens opacities, usually occurring within 2 to 3 years of RT. Fig. 32.1 shows a radiation cataract. Treatment of a cataract is by surgical removal with or without placement of posterior intraocular lenses, although if the eye is dry (most commonly as a result of RT damage to the lacrimal glands) and there is a risk of retinal damage, the success of surgery may be affected.

The Sclera and Retina

The sclera is radioresistant because it is avascular and can tolerate doses of up to 100 Gy by radioactive eye plaques to a small area. Above this dose there is a risk of necrosis. The retina can tolerate doses of 50 Gy, but, above this, retinal damage is manifest by haemorrhages, exudates and atrophy. The macula is the most sensitive area of the retina, and doses here should be minimised or avoided, if possible, when using radioactive eye plaques. Similarly, as the dose increases above 50 Gy, there is an increasing likelihood of optic atrophy.

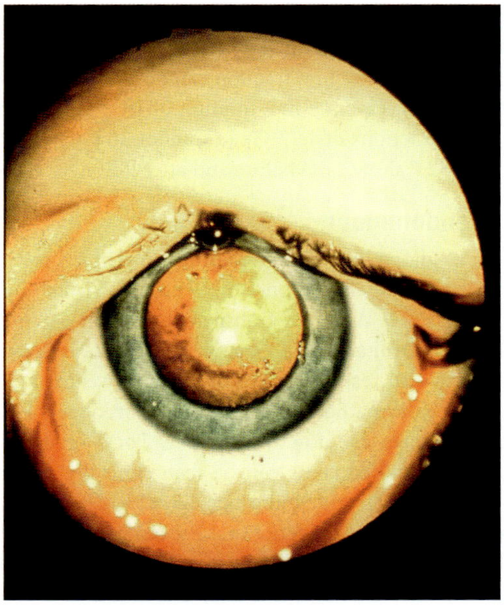

Fig. 32.1 A radiation cataract.

The Cornea and Lacrimal Apparatus

These structures usually tolerate doses of up to 50 Gy well, depending on RT technique, energy, fractionation and attention to good eye care. RT will result in erythema of both skin and conjunctiva and local irritation. If megavoltage RT is used, these reactions will be reduced due to buildup and skin sparing. Tear production is from the minor lacrimal glands mainly located on the lower eyelid and supplemented by the major lacrimal gland in the upper lateral part of the orbit, anteriorly. The major lacrimal gland should be contoured as an OAR in RT planning in an attempt to reduce the dose to below 30 Gy to preserve tear production as much as possible. With a lacrimal gland dose of above 30 Gy, patients may require hypromellose eye drops (artificial tears) and Lacri-Lube. Doses of 50 Gy and above result in more serious problems.

Stenosis or occlusion of the nasolacrimal duct due to a tumour adjacent to the inner canthus will result in a weeping eye (epiphora). There is evidence that this does not happen due to RT alone if it is carefully fractionated and the tumour has not already comprised the function of the duct. Fig. 32.2 (before RT) and Fig. 32.3 (after RT) illustrate a basal cell carcinoma treated with superficial RT in this region. Radiation-induced nasolacrimal duct stenosis is treated surgically with either

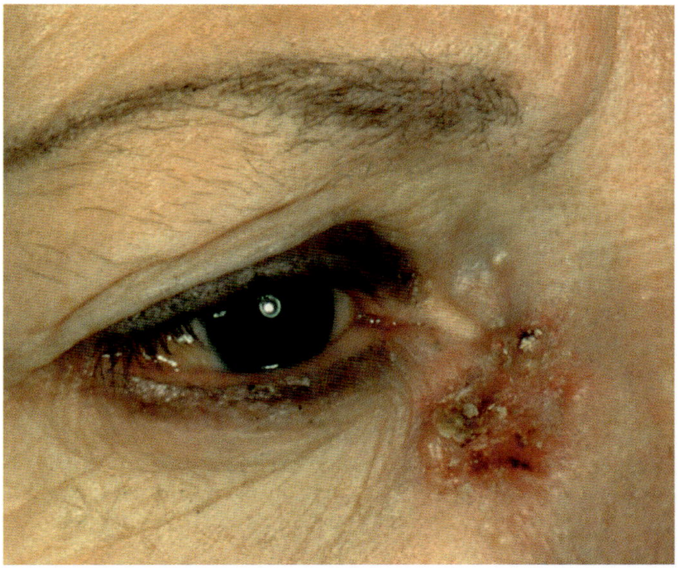

Fig. 32.2 Basal cell carcinoma before radiotherapy.

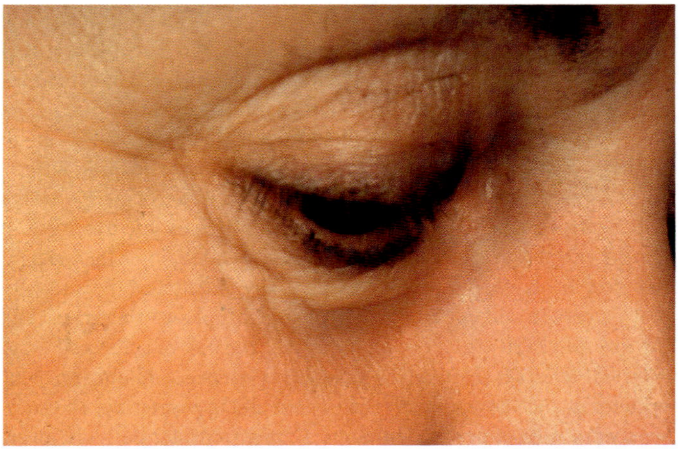

Fig. 32.3 Basal cell carcinoma 4 months after radiotherapy with superficial x-rays.

dacryocystorhinostomy (DCR) or conjunctival DCR, the outcome of which could be affected by the severity of canalicular and nasal mucosal scarring.

Developing a dry eye is very uncomfortable and may result in loss of vision. Corneal damage occurs, partly due to reduced sensation. Punctate keratitis and oedema lead to corneal ulceration, scarring, infection and impairment of vision. If high-dose RT is given, the involvement of an ophthalmologist to give advice and eye protection and to ensure good eye care is imperative during the course of RT. This will aid in achieving patient comfort, maximising vision and minimising late complications. Keratinisation of the cornea is a late complication and occurs after doses in excess of 50 Gy. Rarely, it leads to secondary revascularisation.

The Optic Nerves and Chiasm

The tolerance of optic nerves and chiasm depends primarily on the total dose and dose per fraction used. Radiation-induced optic neuropathy (RION) is very uncommon when the maximum dose to the nerve is less than 55 Gy. The risk is 3% to 7% for doses of 55 to 60 Gy, though most reported incidences of RION in this range have involved doses of 59 Gy and above. Recent studies suggest that a single dose of RT of less than 12 Gy could lead to RION in 1% of patients, whereas a dose above 15 Gy following stereotactic radiosurgery could lead to RION in more than 75% of patients. There is evidence that RION is more common in elderly patients. While concomitant chemotherapies, particularly those with radiosensitising effect, could increase the risk of RION, the data on whether diabetes or hypertension influences risk are inconsistent.

BENIGN CONDITIONS

Thyroid Eye Disease

Thyroid eye disease (TED) is an autoimmune process causing eyelid retraction, proptosis, myopathy and exophthalmos. Most people with TED have Grave's disease and are hyperthyroid at diagnosis, but it can also occur in people without current or prior hyperthyroidism or in Hashimoto thyroiditis. Orbital fibroblasts are thought to express autoantigens such as the thyrotropin receptor. Autoantibodies produced in Grave's disease interact with the autoantigens to activate the orbital fibroblasts, producing cytokine and inflammation of the orbital muscles and fat. Most TED is mild and can be managed by controlling thyroid function, smoking cessation, good eye care and selenium supplements.

The natural history of TED is variable, but an initial active inflammatory phase is often followed by a spontaneous improvement over 1 to 2 years and then a chronic phase due to residual fibrosis and scarring. Moderate to severe active TED occurs in about 5% of cases and is defined as a disease having a sufficient impact on daily life to justify systemic steroids. There is usually radiological evidence of orbital fat, muscle expansion, diplopia and significant exophthalmos. Fig. 32.4 shows bilateral medial rectus swelling from TED.

High-dose intravenous steroids are the recommended initial treatment for moderate to severe active TED and are effective in 77% to 88% of patients. Orbital RT is recommended as a second-line treatment. It is more effective at improving ocular motility and diplopia than exophthalmos. Trials show that RT synergistically potentiates the effects of oral glucocorticoids. It is a relatively straightforward treatment, and the low doses (20 Gy) required mean that the risk of acute and long-term side effects is small. Many patients experience mild inflammatory symptoms, such as conjunctival irritation and eye-watering, and transient worsening of ocular symptoms if concurrent steroid is not given. Careful technique should enable the lens dose to be well below 10 Gy, though patients should be consented for cataract formation. The risk of a radiation-induced second malignancy is about 0.2%. Microvascular retinal abnormalities have been detected after TED RT, so radiation is contraindicated in people with diabetic retinopathy or severe hypertension. The mechanism of action is thought to be antiinflammatory, reducing lymphocyte infiltration and fibrosis.

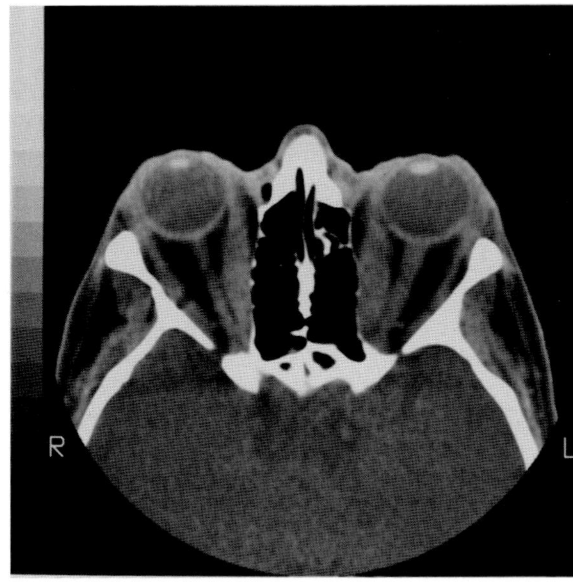

Fig. 32.4 An axial computed tomography slice showing bilateral medial rectus swelling due to thyroid eye disease.

Although dysthyroid eye disease is occasionally unilateral, it is usually recommended to treat both eyes. Patients are immobilised in a thermoplastic shell, and CT is planned. The target volume is the orbital fat and extraocular muscles. Using anything more complex than paired unmodulated lateral radiation fields has no real dosimetric advantage. Beam sizes of up to 5 cm in each direction are chosen to encompass both orbits so that 50% of isodose is through the anterior pituitary. The fields are angled slightly posteriorly or are half-beam blocked to prevent divergence through the contralateral lens. This angulation posteriorly is usually on the order of 5 degrees except where there is marked asymmetrical proptosis. Fig. 32.5 shows a typical beam arrangement and isodoses. The usual dose is 20 Gy in 10 fractions over 2 weeks, though 10 Gy in 5 fractions over 2 weeks has also been used. One study has reported that a regimen of 1 Gy per week over 20 weeks is equally effective and better tolerated. If the patient is not being given steroids concomitant with RT, the first fraction can occasionally cause oedema to worsen. For this reason, a first fraction of 1 Gy is sometimes used, followed by 11 fractions of 1.73 Gy (a total of 20 Gy in 12 fractions). Figs. 32.6 and 32.7 show TED before and after RT.

Orbital Pseudotumour

Also known as idiopathic orbital inflammation, orbital pseudotumour is a rare diagnosis of exclusion once other causes of inflammation such as lymphoma, TED, Wegener granulomatosis and sarcoidosis have been ruled out. Orbital pseudotumour usually causes pain behind the eye and can also result in proptosis, eyelid swelling and diplopia. Improved molecular pathology diagnostic techniques mean accurate alternative diagnoses are now often made. Focal or diffuse inflammation of the orbital contents can be seen clinically or on imaging. A biopsy is necessary to rule out other diagnoses. It is usually treated with steroids, but there is evidence that RT can be effective if there is a relapse after steroids or if they do not work. Twenty Gy in 10 fractions is used with a technique similar to TED for bilateral disease or for diseases similar to orbital lymphoma or unilateral disease. In a systematic

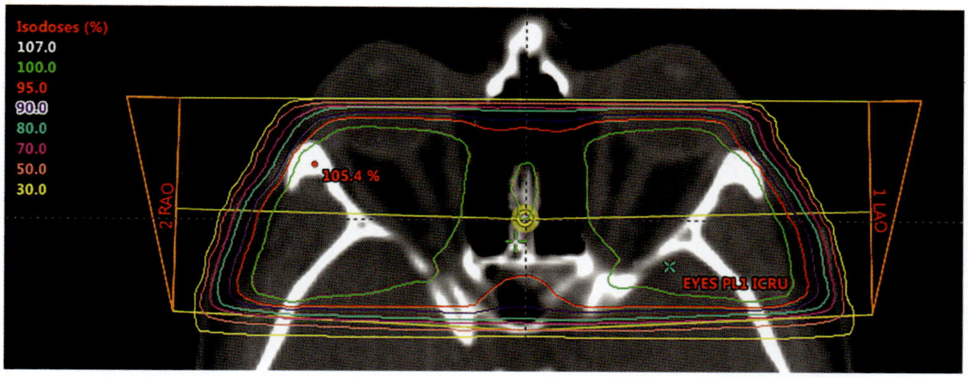

Fig. 32.5 Lateral beams to treat thyroid eye disease and corresponding isodoses.

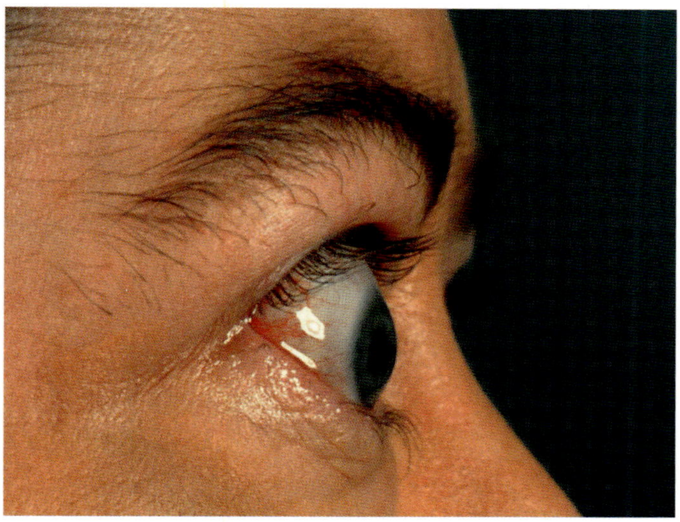

Fig. 32.6 Thyroid eye disease before radiotherapy.

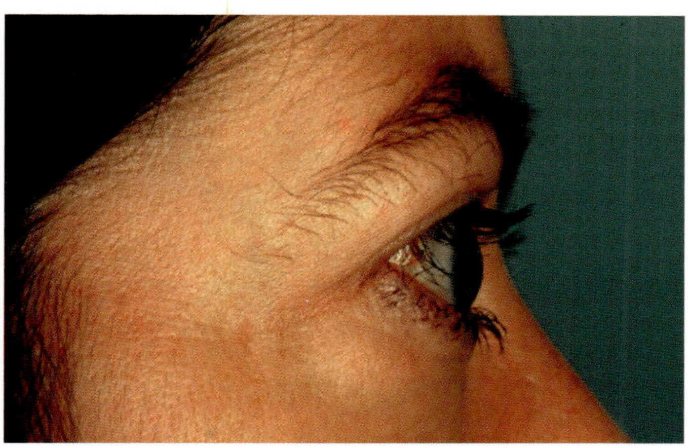

Fig. 32.7 Thyroid eye disease after radiotherapy.

review, the response rate after RT was 74% to 100% with a median recurrence rate of 10%.

MALIGNANT TUMOURS

Primary tumours can be classified as arising from the skin and adnexa, orbit or intraocularly. Basal cell carcinomas (BCCs) and squamous cell carcinomas (SCCs) are skin tumours commonly arising on the face, especially around the eye and lower eyelid. In contrast, lacrimal gland and nasolacrimal duct tumours are rare, as are orbital tumours. Rhabdomyosarcoma of the orbit is a tumour of childhood. It is usually embryonal and is discussed in further detail in Chapter 34. Intraocular tumours are rare, with retinoblastoma occurring in the very young and melanoma occurring in adults. The choroid is the most common site in the eye for metastatic disease.

PRIMARY MALIGNANT TUMOURS

Primary tumours of the eye and orbit can be classified according to their primary location:

1. Skin and adnexa
   a. BCC of the skin
   b. SCC of the skin
   c. Lacrimal gland cancer
   d. Nasolacrimal duct cancer
   e. Miscellaneous
2. Orbital tumours
   a. Lymphoma
   b. Melanoma (conjunctival)
   c. Rhabdomyosarcoma
   d. Optic nerve glioma
3. Intraocular
   a. Melanoma (choroidal and iris)
   b. Retinoblastoma

Skin Cancers Involving the Eyelid

Periocular skin cancers should be managed by a team with dermatology, ophthalmology, plastic surgery and oncology expertise given the many critical structures close to the tumour and the importance of achieving local tumour control.

BCCs are the most common skin tumours and frequently occur on the face, especially around the eye. The incidence is higher in those who have a lot of sun exposure and so is related to outside occupations. They grow slowly and so may be neglected, but, if left, will invade, ulcerate and destroy tissue locally. The ulcerating BCC in Fig. 32.8 had extended into the orbit and frontal lobe. The lower eyelid is the most common site for a periorbital BCC. They usually present as a slow-growing reddish nodule, sometimes with a pearly surface or central ulceration. Clinically, they can be very difficult to differentiate from SCCs, which can also occur in this location, so a biopsy should be carried out. When BCCs occur near the inner canthus, the nasolacrimal duct may be affected, causing the patient to complain of a watery eye.

For BCCs and SCCs, local excision, often with Mohs surgery for margin control and oculoplastic reconstruction, is usually preferred to RT as long as the patient is fit enough and good cosmetic and functional outcomes are expected. RT remains an effective technique with a 90% cure

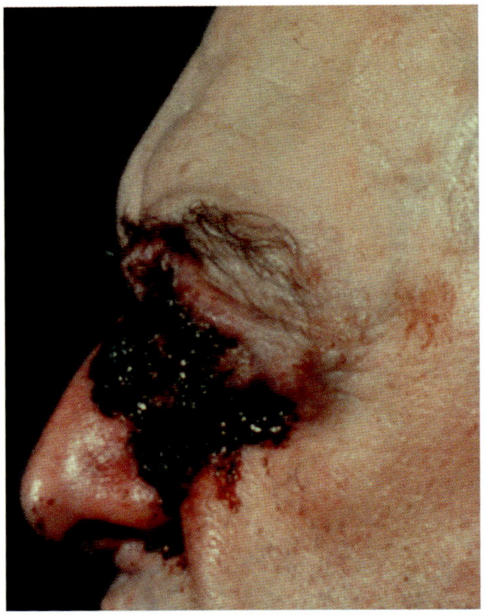

Fig. 32.8 A basal cell carcinoma destroying local structures.

rate using superficial (50–150 kV) or deep (>150–300 kV) x-rays or low-energy electrons. Kilovoltage is preferred as the bowing of isodoses at depth and lateral scatter make shielding of critical structures more difficult with electrons. RT to the upper eyelid should be avoided as it can cause fibrosis of the tarsal plate, leading to corneal exposure and ulceration.

The target volume is the visible tumour with a 5-to-10-mm margin depending on size, histological subtype and how well-defined the tumour is. A lead cutout is made to shield adjacent structures. An internal eye shield should be inserted for each treatment to protect the cornea and lens when the treated area is right next to the eye or involving the eyelid. The eye shield is essentially a lead contact lens coated on the inside with liquid paraffin to reduce friction and is inserted after local anaesthetic eye drops have been instilled.

Various dose-fractionation schedules can be used, such as 32.5 to 35 Gy in 5 fractions, 45 Gy in 10 fractions over 2 to 3 weeks, 50 Gy in 15 to 20 fractions over 3 to 4 weeks and 55 Gy in 20 fractions over weeks. Tumours that are thought to extend to deeper structures may need to be treated with MV photons using an IMRT/VMAT (volumetric modulated arc therapy) technique and a longer course of fractionated RT (≥20 fractions). Conjunctival oedema (chemosis) due to RT is uncommon if treatment is reasonably fractionated and the nasolacrimal duct is not stenosed by the tumour.

Lacrimal Gland and Nasolacrimal Duct Cancer

Lacrimal gland and nasolacrimal duct carcinomas are rare, locally invasive and difficult to treat. Surgical excision, appropriate reconstruction and postoperative RT are usually required to maximise local control. Orbital exenteration should be considered if there is destruction of the orbital wall or tumour in the orbital cavity, but with modern surgical and RT techniques, preservation of a functioning eye should be the treatment goal. Careful multidisciplinary discussion involving ophthalmologists; ear, nose and throat (ENT) specialists; head and neck reconstructive surgeons; and oncologists is essential to achieve this, also taking into account the wishes of the patient.

Tumours Arising From Adjacent Structures

Maxillary sinus tumours can invade the orbit through the orbital floor, whereas ethmoid sinus tumours can infiltrate through the thin lamina papyracea. Surgery and postoperative RT is usually recommended. Radiation doses of 60 Gy or more in 1.8 to 2 Gy per fraction are required. Because this exceeds the tolerance dose of many orbital structures, excellent immobilisation, meticulous target volume and OAR delineation are essential, particularly if an exenteration has not been carried out. Conformal planning usually using IMRT/VMAT will provide the best compromise between giving an appropriate dose to the planning target volume (PTV) and limiting the risk of acute and late side effects.

As in other sites, rare primary tumours can occur around the eye. Angiosarcomas respond rapidly to RT but, despite high doses, also recur locally and regionally.

Lymphoma

Orbital lymphoma may affect the conjunctiva, eyelid, lacrimal gland or retrobular contents. Fifteen percent are bilateral, although disease in the contralateral eye may be metachronous. Presentation may be due to a typically discrete erythematous conjunctival lesion, minor eye discomfort, a mass most often involving the major lacrimal gland, ptosis, chemosis, diplopia, exophthalmos and a red eye. A magnetic resonance imaging (MRI) or CT scan of the orbits should be performed, even for conjunctival lymphoma, as the tumour sometimes tracks around the globe and involves the orbital cone. The conjunctival extent of a superficial tumour is best determined by careful ophthalmic assessment. Biopsies will confirm the histological subtype with low-grade marginal-zone lymphomas being most common, although follicular lymphoma and diffuse large B-cell lymphoma (DLBCL) are sometimes seen. A CT scan or a positron emission tomography-computed tomography (PET/CT) scan of the whole body should be performed to look for other sites of disease that are often found in high-grade lymphomas. A management plan should be recommended by the radiation oncologist, haematologist and ophthalmologist, taking the patient's preferences into account. RT is an effective sole treatment for low-grade tumours confined to the orbit and is also used as consolidation after systemic therapy for high-grade lymphoma.

If the lymphoma is confined to the conjunctiva, the target volume is the entire ipsilateral conjunctiva under the upper and lower eyelids but not the posterior orbital contents. This can usually be treated with a direct superficial x-ray or electron beam using a 5-cm circular lead cutout to define the field edge, remembering that the size of the eyeball is very consistent amongst individuals. The eye should be shut during treatment, but some bolus may still be required when using electrons to bring the conjunctiva surface dose to 90%. Figs. 32.9 and 32.10 show a low-grade marginal zone lymphoma of the conjunctiva before and after RT.

For more extensive orbital lymphomas, the clinical target volume (CTV) is the whole orbit including the retrobulbar space, lacrimal

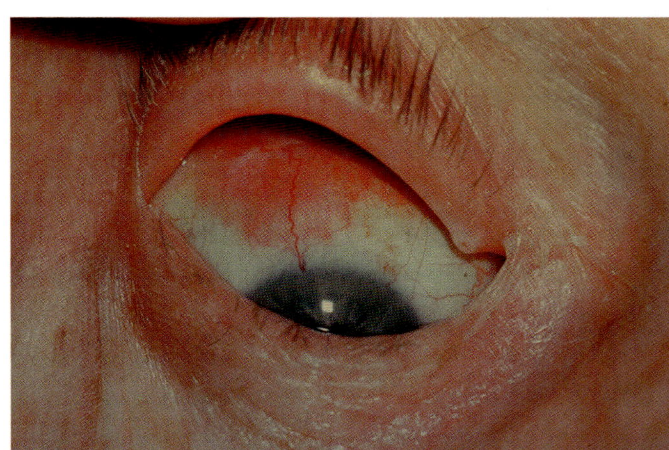

Fig. 32.9 Marginal zone lymphoma of the conjunctiva before radiotherapy.

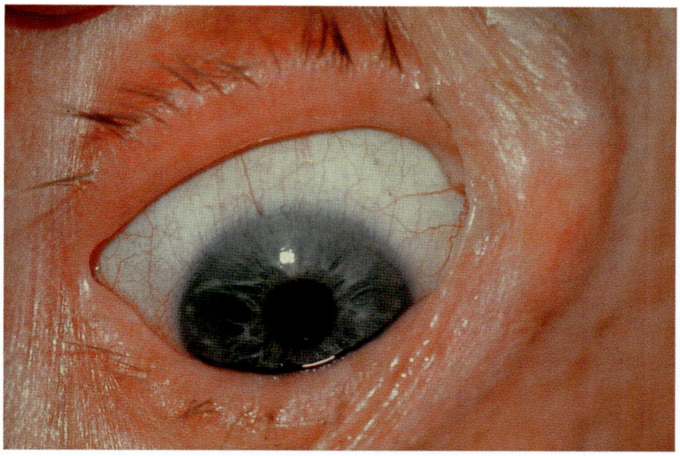

Fig. 32.10 Marginal zone lymphoma of the conjunctiva after radiotherapy.

gland and conjunctiva. Having immobilised the patient, a CT scan with no more than 3 mm thick slices is obtained, on which the CTV is delineated. A small PTV margin is added based on department error data. There will be minimal intrafraction motion, so CTV-PTV margins of 3 to 4 mm should be possible. Superior and inferior oblique beams usually provide good coverage of this conical volume and have the advantage of completely avoiding the contralateral eye. If there is bilateral disease, a parallel-pair technique similar to that used in TED will provide good coverage, or each eye can be planned and treated separately if treating curatively.

For low-grade lymphoma, a dose of 24 Gy in 12 fractions is recommended. Consolidation RT for DLBCL requires 30 Gy in 15 fractions, with higher doses of up to 36 Gy sometimes used for macroscopic residual disease after chemotherapy or if the patient is unable to receive chemotherapy. With these higher doses, it may be appropriate to try to reduce dose to the cornea by treating with the eye open and to limit the higher-dose target volume to visible disease, rather than treating the whole orbit to more than 30 Gy. Figs. 32.11 and 32.12 show DLBCL of

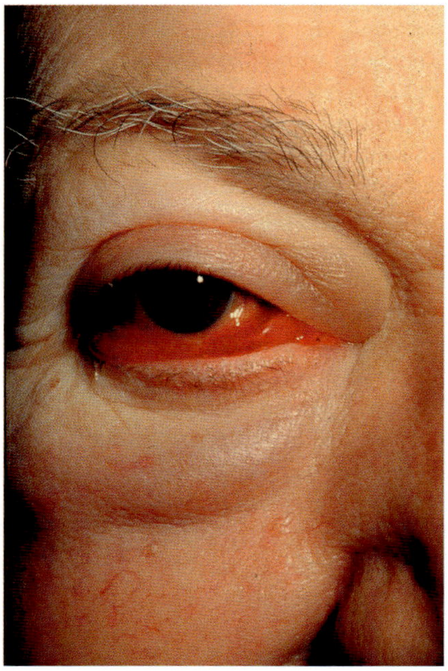

Fig. 32.11 Diffuse large B-cell lymphoma of the orbit before radiotherapy.

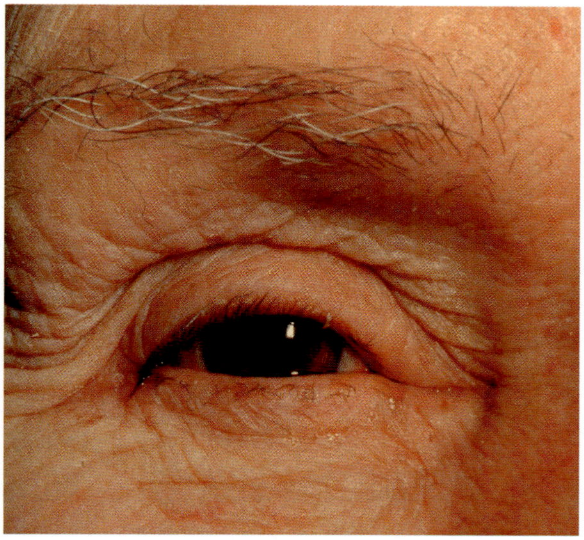

Fig. 32.12 Diffuse large B-cell lymphoma of the orbit after radiotherapy.

the orbit before and after RT. Fig. 32.13 shows a typical beam arrangement and isodoses used to treat a unilateral orbital lymphoma.

Ocular Melanoma

Melanoma is the most common primary intraocular tumour in adults, with an incidence of 1 per 1 million annually. In adults, it most frequently affects the uveal tract, especially the choroid.

It is not uncommon for asymptomatic patients to be referred by an optician who, at a routine eye test, has detected a pigmented lesion in the fundus. Some of these lesions will be choroidal nevi, but some will be melanomas. It may be difficult to distinguish between the two, particularly for a small melanoma, and so the patient may be initially managed conservatively with 6-monthly assessments. Other patients may present with visual loss that may be associated with retinal detachment. Pain does not often occur and may indicate a large tumour. Tumours arising from the iris and conjunctiva are clearly visible and so are noticed by the patient or their family. Fig. 32.14 shows a melanoma of the iris, and Fig. 32.15 illustrates a melanoma of the conjunctiva.

An expert ophthalmic assessment is mandatory by a clinician experienced in this field and will include direct and/or indirect ophthalmoscopy, ocular ultrasound and fluorescein angiography. This may be supplemented by MRI for large tumours that may be considered for local resection to assess extraocular extension.

Melanomas of the eye are often detected when they are very small and may measure under 5 mm at their base and 1 mm in height. They grow slowly and so initial treatment may be observation to confirm the diagnosis. Some patients present with metastases, particularly involving the liver. Others develop metastatic disease up to 15 years later, and the risk increases with the size of the ocular tumour at presentation. Patients with anteriorly placed tumours in the uveal tract are at higher risk than those with posterior choroidal melanomas. Cytogenetic subtypes with different metastatic risk profiles are now recognised, helping to predict recurrence rates and determine surveillance strategies. The diagnosis is usually made by expert ophthalmic assessment, and biopsy is not required before treatment.

Choroidal melanoma treatment using radioactive eye plaque brachytherapy, originally with ^{60}cobalt, has now been superseded by ^{106}ruthenium, ^{90}strontium, ^{103}palladium or ^{125}iodine and used for a long time. Studies have therefore shown that eye preservation has not adversely affected survival. Indeed, some even considered it to improve survival by possibly an immunoprotective mechanism. Brachytherapy is contraindicated in tumours with more than 5-mm extraocular

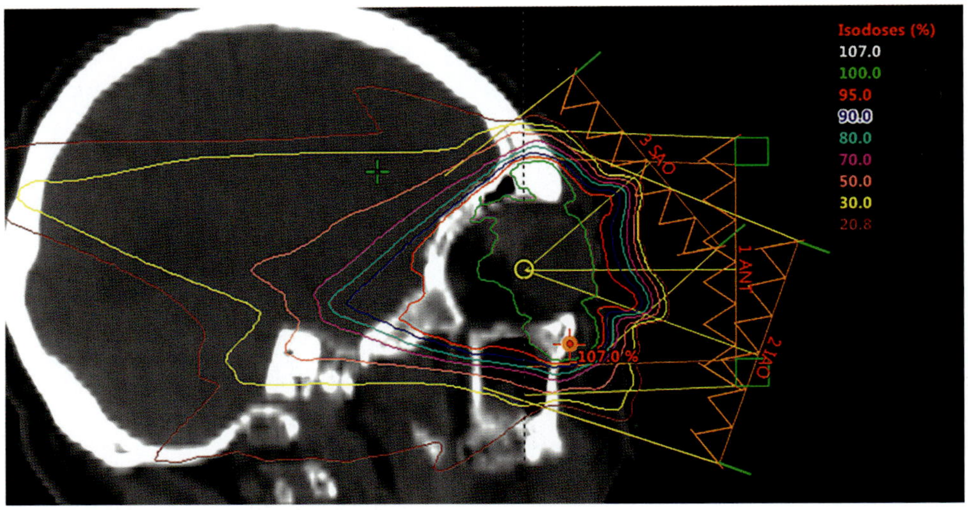

Fig. 32.13 Sagittal view of beam arrangement and isodoses used to treat a unilateral orbital lymphoma.

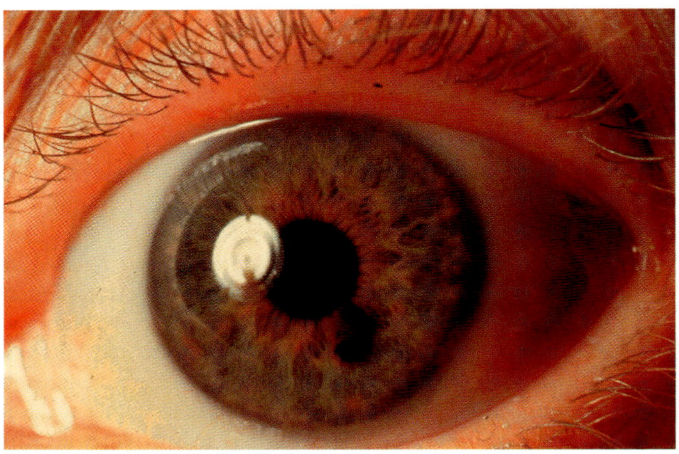

Fig. 32.14 Melanoma of the iris.

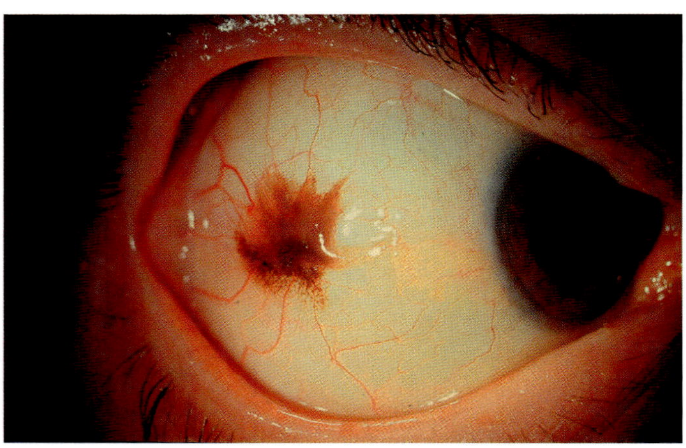

Fig. 32.15 Melanoma of the conjunctiva.

extension where the basal diameter is too large for brachytherapy, in blind painful eyes or in patients with no light-perception vision. In these situations, surgery is preferred, sometimes with an enucleation.

^{106}Ruthenium is a beta emitter, which is suitable for tumours smaller than 6 mm deep. It comes in a range of ready-made shapes and sizes. ^{103}Palladium and ^{125}iridium are low-dose gamma emitters that are custom-made with a 2-mm margin around the tumour. A notch can be created in the plaque when the tumour is close to the optic nerve to reduce the dose at this site. The tumour is visualised by transpupillary or transocular illumination of the globe and marked on the adjacent sclera with a 2-to-3-mm margin with tissue dye. The plaque is sutured in place to cover this target volume and removed after 5 to 7 days.

It is unclear whether the dose to the base or apex of the tumour is important and radiation dose prescriptions vary between centres, though a dose of 70 to 100 Gy to the tumour apex is most commonly used.

Fractionated proton therapy (60 Gy in 4 fractions or 70 Gy in 5 fractions) can also be used to treat uveal melanoma with 5-year local control rates of 95% in most series, though the anterior eye structures will receive some radiation dose with this technique. In a recent meta-analysis, the 5- and 10-year overall survival after proton beam therapy for choroidal melanoma is 73% and 39% respectively. The 5-year metastasis free survival was 76%. The incidence of glaucoma after proton therapy ranged from 18% to 27%. The incidence rates of optic neuropathy and cataracts ranged from 13–64% and 27–40% respectively. Fractionated stereotactic radiotherapy (fSRT) is also sometimes used which is also reported to be equally effective as proton beam therapy. However, in one study, more patients after fSRT developed vitreous haemorrhage compared with proton beam therapy (18.3% vs. 3.3%). There has never been a trial comparing these approaches.

Conjunctival and iris melanomas are treated by local excision, sometimes with adjuvant plaque brachytherapy once the conjunctiva has healed. A handheld ^{90}strontium applicator is used to deliver 50 Gy in 5 daily fractions to the surface, or 60 Gy in 4 fractions once a week. Due to the size of the tumour, enucleation may be the only option.

Unfortunately, patients very occasionally present with very extensive, neglected tumours that are inoperable. Palliative RT can produce a useful regression of extensive tumour. High-dose fractionated RT must be used, either with weekly fractions of 6 Gy or daily treatment of 60 Gy or more over 6 weeks.

The advent of targeted therapies such as the MEK inhibitor, selumetinib, immunotherapy and hepatic perfusion techniques holds the promise of changing the prognosis for systemic disease, which usually presents in the liver. As long as the patient is well enough to consider therapy for liver metastases, 6-monthly screening with nonionising radiation such as MRI or ultrasound is recommended.

Retinoblastoma

Retinoblastoma is a rare tumour occurring in the very young, usually in children under the age of 2 years. It is usually caused by a heritable or nonheritable mutation in the RB1 tumour-suppressor gene on chromosome 13. In the hereditary form, often both eyes are affected. Parents or family may notice a white reflex in the pupil, which usually indicates a large tumour, or a squint and difficulty in fixation. Early detection is key and has enabled cure rates of 95%. Extension into the orbit or perforation of the globe is very unusual but very serious with respect to prognosis, as these patients are incurable. In advanced disease, rarely seen in patients in Europe at initial presentation, metastases may occur to the central nervous system (CNS) and the bone marrow.

Retinoblastoma is exceptional with respect to oncological management in that a biopsy for confirmation of the diagnosis is never performed and, indeed, is contraindicated because of the high risk of spread of tumour cells outside the globe. Therefore, the diagnosis is a clinical one made in specialised centres with great expertise in retinoblastoma and characterised by appearances on bilateral indirect binocular ophthalmoscopy under general anaesthetic. Even when enucleation is performed for a large tumour and/or a nonseeing eye, previous biopsy should not have been carried out.

Early tumours (International Intraocular Retinoblastoma Classification (IIRC) group A) can be treated with focal cryotherapy or laser therapy. Groups B, C and D tumours are treated with intravenous chemotherapy and sometimes additional focal treatments as for group A or occasionally with brachytherapy. Chemotherapy usually includes carboplatin, etoposide and vincristine. There are also techniques to deliver chemotherapy directly into the ophthalmic artery or vitreous cavity. Group E tumours are usually treated with enucleation and adjuvant chemotherapy.

Brachytherapy uses ^{106}ruthenium or ^{125}iodine plaques, both of which are beta emitters and therefore not so penetrating. They are sutured onto the back of the globe overlying the tumour, its position outlined by transillumination. For ^{125}iodine, a dose of 40 Gy is given over 4 to 5 days, depending on the activity of the plaque at time of use, and is prescribed to the apex of the tumour, which has been measured by ultrasound.

EBRT used to be the principal eye-conserving therapy, but it is now used only to salvage eyes when other treatments have not worked. In such cases, brachytherapy techniques, which enable the orbit to be treated by intraconal delivery systems containing ^{125}iodine, and proton therapy both have the advantage of reducing radiation dose to extraorbital structures. This is particularly important as radiation increases the risk of second malignancy in heritable retinoblastoma.

METASTASES

Secondary deposits to the eye via the bloodstream are common but often not clinically evident or recognised. The most frequent site of ocular metastases is the vascular choroid, leading to retinal detachment. Therefore, the presentation may be an oncological emergency due to sudden loss of vision. It usually occurs in patients known to have malignancy, especially from breast or lung cancer. Other tumours that metastasise less frequently are urogenital and upper gastrointestinal (GI) tumours. Orbital metastases usually indicate widespread metastatic disease and, consequently, a poor prognosis, except in some patients with breast cancer. Patients may have brain metastases as well. If the full fundal examination is carried out, asymptomatic metastases are not infrequently found, often involving the contralateral eye. Choroidal metastases have a characteristic appearance, with a yellow raised honeycomb lesion. RT should be given to try to preserve vision. Prostate cancer metastases can involve the orbit, usually due to expansion from a bone deposit resulting in visual disturbance or loss, diplopia, ptosis or exophthalmos.

The patient lies prone on a headrest, with the head supported and immobilised using a beam-directional thermoplastic shell. Choroidal deposits can be treated by a single anterior megavoltage photon field or a lateral field angled 5 to 10 degrees posteriorly. If an anterior field is used, the eye is treated open to take advantage of the skin-sparing effect of megavoltage to reduce the dose to the cornea and lens. In breast cancer, choroidal metastases are often multiple and/or bilateral, so both eyes should be treated using parallel-opposed lateral fields similar to those used in TED. A dose of 20 Gy in 5 daily fractions over 1 week with megavoltage RT is usually the most appropriate, but 30 Gy in 10 fractions can be used in people with a good prognosis for their underlying cancer.

ACKNOWLEDGMENT

The editors acknowledge the excellent contribution from Tom Roques and Adrian Harnett, the authors of this chapter in the previous edition.

FURTHER READING

American Brachytherapy Society–Ophthalmic Oncology Task Force. The American Brachytherapy Society consensus guidelines for plaque brachytherapy of uveal melanoma and retinoblastoma. *Brachytherapy*. 2014;13(1):1–14.

Ataídes FG, Silva SFBR, De Campos Baldin JJCM. Radiation-induced optic neuropathy: literature review. *Neuroophthalmology*. 2020;45(3): 172–180.

Bartalena L, Kahaly GJ, Baldeschi L, et al. The 2021 European Group on Graves' Orbitopathy (EUGOGO) clinical practice guidelines for the medical management of Graves' orbitopathy. *Eur J Endocrinol*. 2021;185(4):G43–G67.

Fionda B, Pagliara MM, Lancellotta V, et al. The role of radiotherapy in orbital pseudotumor: a systematic review of literature. *Ocul Immunol Inflamm*. 2022;30(5):1162–1167.

Kahaly GJ, Rösler HP, Pitz S, Hommel G. Low- versus high-dose radiotherapy for Graves' ophthalmopathy: a randomized, single blind trial. *J Clin Endocrinol Metab*. 2000;85(1):102–108.

Nathan P, Cohen V, Coupland S, et al. Uveal melanoma UK national guidelines. *Eur J Cancer*. 2015;51(16):2404–2412.

Royal College of Radiologists. *Recommendations for using radiotherapy for benign disease in the UK*. Royal College of Radiologists; 2023. https://www.rcr.ac.uk/our-services/all-our-publications/clinical-oncology-publications/recommendations-for-using-radiotherapy-for-benign-disease-in-the-uk/

Schwarcz RM, Coupland SE, Finger PT. Cancer of the orbit and adnexa. *Am J Clin Oncol*. 2013;36(2):197–205.

Stannard C, Sauerwein W, Maree G, Lecuona K. Radiotherapy for ocular tumours. *Eye (London)*. 2013;27(2):119–127.

Yahalom J, Illidge T, Specht L, et al. Modern radiation therapy for extranodal lymphomas: field and dose guidelines from the International Lymphoma Radiation Oncology Group. *Int J Radiat Oncol Biol Phys*. 2015;92(1):11–31.

33

Sarcomas

Gail Horan, Sarah Prewett and Thankamma V. Ajithkumar

CHAPTER OUTLINE

SOFT-TISSUE SARCOMAS

Soft-tissue sarcomas (STSs) are malignant tumours arising from supporting connective tissues anywhere in the body. These structures (fibrous tissue, fat, blood vessels, smooth and skeletal muscle, tendons and cartilage) are derived embryologically from the mesoderm. Tumours of peripheral nerves are also included in the classification of STS. Despite arising from a wide variety of tissues, adult-type STSs have many similarities in pathology, clinical findings and behaviour. However, paediatric-type STSs, such as rhabdomyosarcoma and soft-tissue Ewing sarcoma, are distinct because of their cytogenetics and differing treatment approaches. The principles of treatment outlined in this chapter mainly apply to adult-type STSs.

Pathology

STSs are rare, representing 0.4% of all cancers and 0.3% of cancer deaths. The incidence is about 0.6 per 100,000 population per year. However, they constitute 6% of tumours in children under age 15 years. Most occur in those age 40 to 70 years, but peak age of incidence varies according to histological subtypes. The gender ratio is virtually the same.

The aetiology is unknown in the majority of cases. In a minority of cases, genetic factors, previous radiotherapy (RT), chronic lymphoedema, chemotherapy and an association with viral infections are identified. The incidence of STS is significantly higher in children treated with both chemotherapy and RT (SIR 113) compared with RT alone (SIR 19). Radiation-induced sarcomas commonly occur within previously irradiated areas (especially for benign angiomas). The common types of radiation-induced sarcomas are undifferentiated pleomorphic sarcoma and osteosarcoma.

Genetic syndromes associated with STSs include Li-Fraumeni syndrome (osteosarcoma, rhabdomyosarcoma and Ewing sarcoma), Gardner syndrome (intraabdominal desmoid tumours), tuberous sclerosis and von Recklinghausen disease (malignant nerve sheath tumours and rhabdomyosarcoma). Rarely, STSs may occur in the children of mothers with early-onset breast cancer.

Sarcomas are associated with numerous genetic abnormalities. The first demonstrated specific gene abnormality associated with malignant transformation in people was the loss of the retinoblastoma (RB), a tumour suppressor gene. There are alterations to the RB gene in up to 70% of STSs. Chromosome translocations are the most common genetic abnormality and are seen in virtually all cases of Ewing sarcoma (primitive neuroectodermal tumours). Translocation of 11:22 is the most common in Ewing sarcoma, occurring in 85% of cases. In more than 90% of synovial sarcomas, there is a chromosome 18 translocation. Such cytogenetic abnormalities may be useful diagnostically and may be of prognostic significance. It is noteworthy that translocations tend to occur most commonly in high-grade tumours.

The 2020 World Health Organization (WHO) classification is extremely complex, and a simplified version listing malignant tumours by their tissue of origin is presented in Table 33.1.

Although histological grade and the size of tumour continue to dictate management and prognosis, molecular pathology is increasingly used to guide management, especially the choice of systemic therapy. MDM2 gene amplification in liposarcoma, NTRK, CIC and BCOR sarcoma are all examples where molecular pathology is key to confirming a diagnosis. The grading system for sarcoma described by Trojani is in regular use both in the United Kingdom and internationally (Table 33.2). Low-grade tumours have a recognisable pattern of differentiation, relatively few mitoses and no necrosis. High-grade tumours include all examples of certain subtypes (e.g. alveolar soft part), tumours with little or no apparent differentiation and those with necrosis and a high mitotic rate. The tumour size is also important, and those over 5 cm are much more likely to recur locally or give rise to distant metastases.

TABLE 33.1 Simplified Version of the WHO Classification (2020) of Sarcomas

Fat
Intermediate: Atypical lipomatous tumour/well-differentiated liposarcoma
Malignant: Liposarcoma
Fibrous Tissue
Intermediate: Desmoid-type fibromatosis, lipofibromatosis, dermatofibrosarcoma protuberans, solitary fibrous tumour, etc.
Malignant: Fibrosarcoma, myxofibrosarcoma, sclerosing epithelioid fibrosarcoma
Smooth Muscle
Leiomyosarcoma
Skeletal Muscle
Embryonal rhabdomyosarcoma
Alveolar rhabdomyosarcoma
Pleomorphic rhabdomyosarcoma, spindle cell/sclerosing rhabdomyosarcoma
Blood Vessels
Intermediate: Haemangioblastomas, Kaposi sarcoma
Malignant: Angiosarcoma, epithelioid hemangioendothelioma
Gastrointestinal Stromal Tumours
Bone
Osteogenic sarcoma, chondrosarcoma, giant cell tumours, chordoma, fibrosarcoma of bone, angiosarcoma of bone
Nerve Sheath
Malignant peripheral nerve sheath tumours, epithelioid malignant nerve sheath tumour, malignant granular cell tumour
Sarcomas of Uncertain Differentiation
Synovial sarcomas
Epithelioid sarcomas
Alveolar soft part sarcomas
Desmoplastic small round cell tumour, PEComa
Undifferentiated small round cell sarcomas
Ewing sarcoma
Round cell sarcoma with EWSR1-non-ETS fusions
CIC-rearranged sarcomas
Sarcoma with BCOR genetic alterations

PEComa, Perivascular epithelioid cell neoplasms; *WHO*, World Health Organization.

Natural Spread

Initial spread from the primary site is into adjacent tissue and along tissue planes between structures such as muscle bundles. STSs do not possess a true capsule but are often surrounded by a pseudo capsule of compressed surrounding tissues. This apparent encapsulation may tempt the surgeon to try to shell out the tumour. Local recurrence from residual tumour at the periphery is then very likely (≥90% within 2 years). Lymph node spread is infrequent, whereas blood-borne spread is common, giving rise to distant metastases, predominantly in the lungs.

TABLE 33.2 Grading System for Adult Soft-Tissue Sarcoma

Score	Tumour Differentiation	Necrosis	No. of Mitoses/10 HPF
1	Well	Absent	<0
2	Moderate	<50%	10–19
3	Poor	≥50%	≥20

The total scores are 2–3 for grade 1, 4–5 for grade 2 and ≥6 for grade 3 tumours.

Clinical Features

Approximately 40% of STSs occur in the upper and lower limbs. Of these, about 75% occur at or above the knee. Some 10% of sarcomas arise in the upper half of the body. Of the sarcomas of the trunk, 10% occur in the retroperitoneum and 20% in the chest or abdominal wall. Presentation with locally advanced disease is common, particularly with intraabdominal sarcomas, which may reach a very large size.

The history is usually of a painless lump developing over a few weeks or months and occasionally over years. Pain may occur from pressure on local structures, for example, nerves and joints. Occasionally, nonmetastatic effects are seen (e.g. hypoglycaemia in malignant fibrous histiocytoma).

Diagnosis and Staging

Patients with a suspected STS should have an initial ultrasound examination or a referral to a specialist multidisciplinary team (MDT) for a triple assessment (clinical history, imaging and biopsy). An initial ultrasound may rule out benign lesions.

Triple Assessment

Clinical history and examination are to assess the position of the primary lesion (superficial or deep to the fascia), any involvement of bone, vascular or neural invasion and regional nodal involvement, although the latter is uncommon. Patients with suspicious ultrasound or clinical features should have a magnetic resonance imaging (MRI) scan of the affected region (Fig. 33.1). Plain x-ray is useful to rule out bony involvement or risk of fracture.

A biopsy is required in all cases. Although in 90% of cases, adequate histology can be achieved by a percutaneous core needle biopsy, where an incisional biopsy is required, care should be taken to make the incision longitudinal so that any subsequent radical surgery or postoperative radiation fields can include it. This is particularly important where preservation of limb function is a major consideration. Inappropriate biopsy can compromise the feasibility of limb conservation surgery and the chances of local control and cure as a result of inadvertent contamination of uninvolved tissue planes. The biopsy should therefore be carried out only in a specialist sarcoma centre or by the surgeon who will undertake the definitive resection. If computed tomography (CT)-guided biopsy is needed, for example, for impalpable deep-seated lesions, there is also potential for needle track contamination. Close liaison with the surgeon and clinical oncologist is needed to plan the best route of biopsy.

Staging Investigations

Other investigations include a full blood count, liver function tests, imaging of the tumour-bearing region (Fig. 33.1) and CT of the chest to rule out lung metastases (Fig. 33.2). Chest x-ray may be appropriate for staging in patients with very low risk of lung metastases (e.g. those with atypical lipomatous tumours) and those who are frail with small low-grade lesions. CT of the abdomen/pelvis may be considered for tumours of the lower extremities and histological subtypes with a risk of soft-tissue metastases such a myxoid liposarcoma. A positron emission tomography–computed tomography (PET/CT) scan is useful in selected diagnoses such as Ewing sarcoma, where it can detect bone marrow involvement, or clear cell sarcoma, rhabdomyosarcoma or synovial sarcoma, where it can detect nodal spread. A whole body MRI scan in the diagnostic staging of myxoid liposarcomas can detect extrapulmonary metastases.

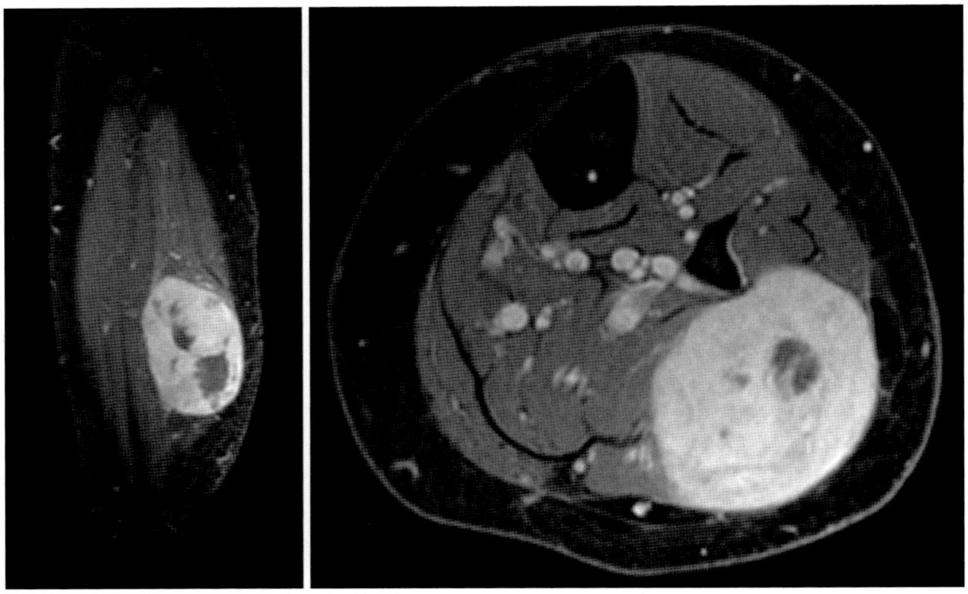

Fig. 33.1 Magnetic resonance imaging scan showing soft-tissue sarcoma with necrosis/cystic areas arising from the lateral gastrocnemius muscle. The lesion extends to the lateral border of the fibula. Histology confirmed undifferentiated spindle cell/pleomorphic sarcoma.

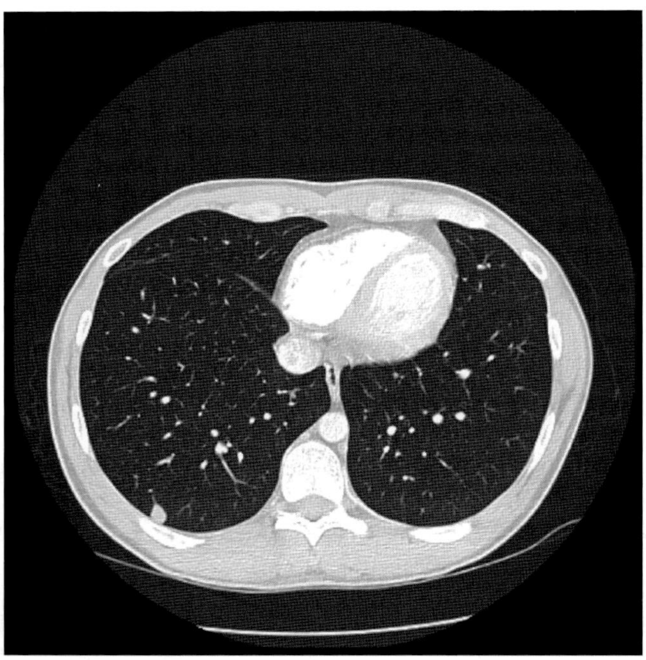

Fig. 33.2 Computed tomography scan of the chest demonstrating a subpleural metastasis in the right lower lobe from a soft-tissue sarcoma.

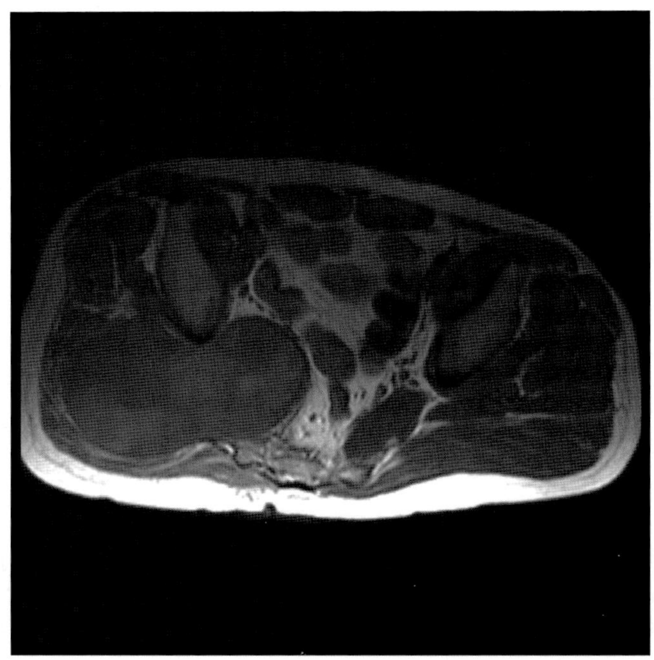

Fig. 33.3 Magnetic resonance imaging scan showing a large, heterogeneous, dumbbell-shaped mass passing through the sciatic notch in the right side of the pelvis. Histology confirmed a malignant peripheral nerve sheath tumour.

A CT scan and MRI (Fig. 33.3) are important in defining the local extent and operability of the tumour. MRI is the imaging modality of choice for limb sarcomas because it provides good contrast between the tumour and adjoining normal tissues and is particularly useful to assess involvement of the neurovascular bundle. It also provides better multiplanar versatility in planning surgery and RT. CT can be helpful in exclusion of cortical erosion of bone. CT is also useful in confirming any subsequent local recurrence, particularly in deep-seated abdominal/pelvic tumours, and can be used as part of a surveillance program where indicated. CT/MRI of the brain may be considered in histological subtypes with a high risk of brain metastases (e.g. alveolar soft part sarcoma and clear cell sarcoma). Staging of STS is shown in Tables 33.3 and 33.4.

Management

An MDT is required because surgery, RT and chemotherapy may all have a role to play, depending on the stage, site, grade and size of the tumour. A dedicated sarcoma MDT allows treatment to be carefully coordinated and minimises the number of surgical procedures necessary.

TABLE 33.3 Staging System for Soft-Tissue Sarcomas[a] (Union for International Cancer Control TNM Classification, 2017)

Primary Tumour (T)	
T1	≤5 cm in greatest dimension
T2	>5 cm but not >10 cm in greatest dimension
T3	>10 cm but not >15 cm in greatest dimension
T4	>15 cm in greatest dimension
Regional Nodes (N)	
N0	No lymph node spread
N1	Involvement of regional lymph nodes
Distant Metastases (M)	
M0	No distant metastases
M1	Distant metastases

[a]Applicable to the extremities, superficial trunk and retroperitoneal sarcomas. The staging for the head and neck and thoracic and abdominal visceral sarcomas differs.

TABLE 33.4 Stage Grouping for Soft Sarcoma (Union for International Cancer Control 2017) (Taking Into Account Histopathological Grade[a])

Stage IA	T1	N0	M0	G1
Stage IB	T2–4	N0	M0	G1
Stage II	T1	N0	M0	G2–3
Stage IIIA	T2	N0	M0	G2–3
Stage IIIB	T3–4	N0	M0	G2–3
	Any T	N1	M0	Any grade
Stage IV	Any T	Any N	M1	Any grade

[a]Grade 1 is considered low grade, and grades 2–3 are high grade.

Surgery

Surgery is the initial treatment of choice for localised sarcomas, and the aim of the surgery is to achieve a wide local excision (margin ≥1 cm where possible) (Fig. 33.4). The resection should include all the skin and subcutaneous tissue near the tumour, any previous excision or biopsy scars and areas containing blood clot from previous biopsies. Metallic clips at the margins of the excision are helpful in planning postoperative irradiation. If there is a positive margin, a reexcision should be attempted to achieve a clear margin provided this will not result in excess morbidities. Based on histological margins, resections are categorised as intralesional, marginal, wide or radical (Table 33.5).

A complete microscopic excision in limb sarcomas leads to a 5-year local control of more than 90%, whereas with incomplete resection, the local control rates are in the range of 60% to 80%. The extent of the resection will depend upon the site of the tumour. For example, a complete microscopic resection can be challenging for tumours in the head and neck, the pelvis and the retroperitoneum.

Conservative surgery (e.g. limb conservation) has evolved significantly in the past few years. Modern surgical techniques including biological and endoprosthetic reconstructions have increased the chances of limb preservation and improved the quality of life of sarcoma survivors. Computer-assisted surgical techniques have improved the rates of margin-negative resections and therefore are valuable in complex locations such as the pelvis. Amputation for extremity sarcomas is thus only indicated in the following situations:

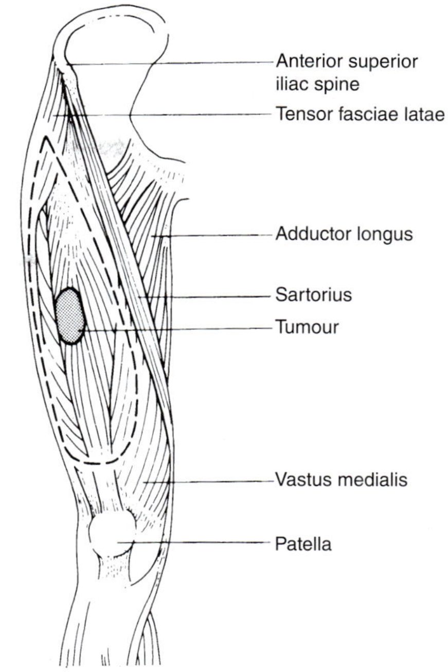

Fig. 33.4 Compartmentectomy. The diagram illustrates the wide surgical excision of soft tissue situated, in this case, in the rectus femoris. (Reproduced with permission from Souhami R, Tobias J. *Cancer and Its Management*. Blackwell; 1986.)

TABLE 33.5 Types of Resections Based on Histological Margins

Type	Description
Intralesional	Surgical plane runs through the tumour. Highest risk of local recurrence.
Marginal	Surgical plane runs through the pseudocapsule. High risk of local recurrence.
Wide	Surgical plane in normal tissue outside the tumour but within the same compartment. Low risk of recurrence.
Radical	Compartmental excision of the tumour. Lowest risk of recurrence.

- When serious radiation-induced morbidity would result from attempting radical RT
- In some distal limb sarcomas, where a below-knee amputation may be more functional than a lower limb with the combined local morbidity of surgery and RT
- When there is recurrent disease not suitable for limited resection or adjuvant RT

Radiotherapy

Adjuvant RT. Patients who have an amputation do not require RT. Completed excised (R0 resection) low-grade tumours of less than 5 cm also do not need further therapy. Postoperative adjuvant RT is indicated in the following circumstances to reduce the probability of local recurrence:

- Limb-conserving wide-excision or limited surgery
- Inadequate margin, tumour extends to cut edge (R1 resection) or macroscopic residual disease (R2 resection) and further excision is not possible

- Any high-grade tumours (2 or 3)
- Tumours 5 cm or more in any dimension and most tumours deep to the fascia
- Virtually all tumours in the head and neck (because a complete excision is unlikely)
- After surgery for recurrent sarcoma if not previously irradiated

Postoperative RT (60–66 Gray (Gy)) is conventionally delivered with external beam (photons, electrons or, more recently, protons, at least in a selected population). In a randomised trial, intraoperative brachytherapy with iridium-192 (42–45 Gy over 4–6 days) resulted in a higher 5-year local control rate (80%) compared with no further therapy (65%) for high-grade tumours ($P = .0025$). Brachytherapy did not improve local control in low-grade lesions. There are no randomised trials comparing brachytherapy with external beam irradiation. Brachytherapy should only be carried out in specialist units undertaking a substantial number of procedures.

Preoperative Radiotherapy. Preoperative RT has the advantage that the tumour is well oxygenated and intact. It may also allow coverage by smaller radiation fields and use of lower doses (50 Gy) without reducing local control. These advantages have to be balanced against the disadvantages of difficulties in interpreting pathology following irradiation and an increased risk of wound complications.

Both pre- and postoperative RT give similar local control rates but different toxicity profiles. Preoperative RT is associated with increased wound complications and a better limb function, whereas postoperative RT is associated with increased late complications such as fibrosis, oedema, joint stiffness and bone fractures. Preoperative RT is considered in the following situations:

- Borderline operable tumours (to improve chances of R0 resection)
- Tumours with anticipated marginal resection (e.g. sites such as paranasal sinuses, skull base and retroperitoneum)
- Tumours close to neurovascular structures
- In situations where larger postoperative RT volume might lead to significant late toxicities

Primary (Radical) Radiotherapy. Radical RT alone is indicated for patients unfit for surgery but otherwise in reasonable general condition, those who refuse surgery or where the anatomical site precludes it (e.g. the head and neck and the retroperitoneum). RT is contraindicated for tumours located in areas that tolerate RT poorly, for example, to the Achilles tendon, especially in young and active patients, because rupture may occur.

Palliative Radiotherapy. In advanced sarcoma, palliative RT is useful in controlling pain, stopping bleeding and so on. However, often little benefit is seen with single-dose (8–10 Gy) RT, and usually, patients need higher doses (e.g. 30 Gy in 10 fractions) for a meaningful clinical benefit.

Chemotherapy

In the past few decades, improvements in both surgery and RT have led to marked improvements in local control and a subsequent decrease in the incidence of amputation. Although adjuvant chemotherapy has significantly improved the clinical outcome of paediatric-type STS, the role of adjuvant chemotherapy in adult-type STS remains controversial. Doxorubicin and ifosfamide are the only chemotherapeutic agents that consistently have a greater than 20% response rate against STS. Two large metaanalyses and an EORTC trial failed to show clinically significant benefit with routine adjuvant chemotherapy using these agents. The Sarcoma Meta-Analysis Collaboration reported improvements in local and distal recurrence rates with doxorubicin-containing adjuvant regimens but a statistically nonsignificant trend towards improvement in overall survival (4% at 10 years). A second updated metaanalysis showed an improved overall survival (absolute risk reduction of 11%). However, the subsequent EORTC study, 62931, and a pooled analysis of two large randomised trials (EORTC 62771 and 62931) failed to show improved survival with adjuvant chemotherapy.

There is no clear evidence to show that preoperative chemotherapy offers a significant survival advantage, but this may be used in patients with initially inoperable tumours. A recent Italian Sarcoma Group study suggests that neoadjuvant chemotherapy with anthracycline and ifosfamide improves relapse-free and overall survival in patients with high-risk STS of the extremity and trunk, but long-term results are awaited.

Single-agent doxorubicin is the treatment of choice for locally advanced inoperable and metastatic STS. The highest rate of response (37%) has been seen with doses of 60 to 75 mg/m^2 3 times weekly, with a 6-month progression-free survival of 45%. Even though the EORTC 62012 study reported a higher response rate with a combination of doxorubicin and ifosfamide compared with single-agent doxorubicin alone (26% versus 14%, $P < .0006$), there was no difference in median overall survival (14.3 months versus 12.8 months, $P = .076$). Therefore, combination chemotherapy may be considered in selected clinical situations such as in life-threatening progressive disease and preoperatively to downstage a large, locally advanced chemosensitive tumour to facilitate a curative resection.

Recent studies have highlighted that some agents are more effective, in particular, histological subtypes. For example, ifosfamide-containing regimens are more active in synovial sarcoma, taxanes and liposomal doxorubicin in angiosarcoma, and trabectedin in liposarcoma and synovial sarcoma.

Retroperitoneal Sarcomas

Retroperitoneal sarcomas (RPSs) are often huge, causing dramatic distortion of the patient's contour, but rarely present as an emergency. The tumours are often dedifferentiated liposarcomas or leiomyosarcomas and as such have a characteristic radiological appearance (Fig. 33.5). In these circumstances, preoperative biopsy may be eschewed, but if radiological appearance is doubtful, a biopsy is mandated.

Surgery may require en bloc resection with removal of many organs such as the spleen, one kidney, the tail or body of the pancreas or segments of the large and/or small bowel. The placement of surgical clips around narrowly excised tumour areas can guide the clinical oncologist. The dose of postoperative RT is necessarily limited, and more than 50 Gy is unlikely to be achievable. At 5 years, up to 50% of patients develop local or intraabdominal recurrence.

With the evolution of high-precision RT techniques that can spare radiosensitive organs such as the kidney and spinal cord, interest in the use of preoperative RT has been rekindled recently. An EORTC study (STRASS trial) randomised 266 patients with RPS and pelvic STS to surgery alone or preoperative RT (50.4 Gy in 28 fractions) followed by surgery 4 to 8 weeks later. Results did not show any improvement in abdominal recurrence-free survival with preoperative RT compared with surgery alone, and thus preoperative RT is not considered the standard of care.

Radiotherapy Technique

Position, Immobilisation and Localisation Imaging

Positioning and immobilisation are challenging for extremity sarcomas, and the clinical oncologist should carefully evaluate the position of the limb, taking into consideration the radiation beam arrangements. Stability of the limb is best assisted by a shell and appropriately positioned bolus bags. The scar may be marked out during the planning scan, especially in situations where there is a need to apply bolus

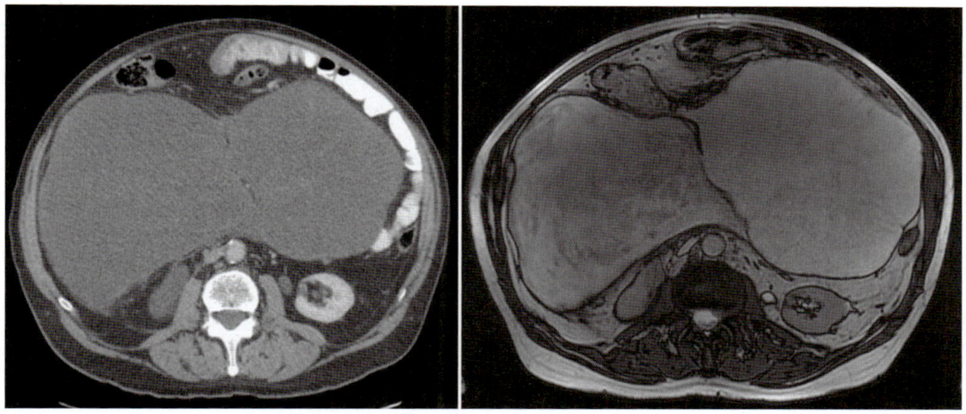

Fig. 33.5 Computed tomography scan showing a bilobulated cystic retroperitoneal mass, and on magnetic resonance imaging the lesion has high T2 signal intensity with multiple septations and low-signal components. Histology showed dedifferentiated liposarcoma.

to ensure that it receives the maximum dose to minimise the risk of scar recurrence. However, routine application of bolus to the scar is not recommended. Sagittal lasers are especially useful in lining up the limbs.

Target Volume

Definition of the target volume requires information from the surgeon, pathologist and radiologist. The surgeon should be encouraged to place radiopaque clips at the margins of the resection. The pathologist should comment on the adequacy of the resection. The radiotherapist needs to discuss with the radiologist the position of the tumour, local extent and any residual disease as seen on CT and MRI.

Most sarcomas tend to spread in the axial plane of the limb (major fascial planes, bone and interosseous membranes). For this reason, the margins of the radiation field must be generous in the craniocaudal directions. In the transverse plane, there can be greater confidence that local structures are not breached and field margins can be tighter. For nonextremity lesions, the orientation of the fields should follow the planes of the local musculature, while including the local fascial planes.

Currently, preoperative three-dimensional conformal RT is given as one phase and postoperative and radical treatment in two phases. The 2-year interim results of a randomised controlled trial (Volume of Radiotherapy for Extremity Sarcomas (VORTEX)) evaluating the role of postoperative single-phase smaller-field RT compared with the standard two-phase RT did not report any difference in grade 2 or higher long-term toxicities or limb function. Retrospective and phase II studies suggest that intensity modulated radiotherapy (IMRT) has a potential to significantly reduce long-term toxicities of subcutaneous fibrosis, joint stiffness and oedema. In the United Kingdom, the IMRiS trial is evaluating the role of IMRT in terms of the feasibility in non-extremity sarcomas and the improvement in long-term and functional effects in extremity sarcomas.

For the purposes of planning, the gross tumour volume (GTV) should be defined, with a margin around it to include the tissues at risk of microscopic involvement, to create the clinical target volume (CTV). The planning target volume (PTV) is based on departmental data and generally involves an expansion of the CTV by 5 to 10 mm isotropically. Care is taken to avoid irradiating the whole circumference of a limb to reduce the likelihood of lymphoedema as a late complication. This is achieved by leaving a longitudinal strip of unirradiated tissue outside the volume (normal tissue corridor) or restricting dose to this corridor (Fig. 33.6).

The following section gives a summary of these target volumes in various clinical settings.

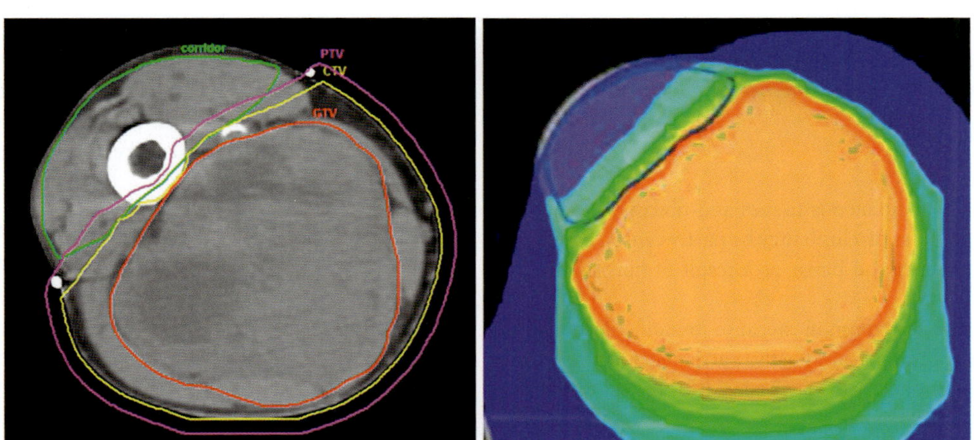

Fig. 33.6 Planning computed tomography (CT) scan showing target volumes and a corridor of radiotherapy avoidance area to avoid late lymphoedema. Planning CT showing the sparing of corridor. *CTV*, Clinical target volume; *GTV*, gross tumour volume; *PTV*, planned target volume.

Preoperative Single-Phase Extremity Tumours. GTV: Tumour on gadolinium-enhanced T1-weighted (W) imaging (just the lesion and not oedema)

- CTV = GTV with 3-to-4-cm longitudinal expansion and 1.5-to-2-cm expansion in all other directions.
- Edit the CTV (ideally using T2W) to include the peritumoural oedema, which is often most pronounced in the longitudinal direction.
- Edit the CTV to stay within bones, fascia and skin (unless infiltrated).

Postoperative Two-Phase Extremity Tumours

Phase I. Reconstruct GTV, defined on the gadolinium-enhanced T1W preoperative imaging fused with the postoperative planning CT scan (just the lesion and not oedema)

- CTV1: GTV + 2 cm axially (unless an intact fascial/bone boundary) and GTV + 5 cm superiorly and inferiorly – Cover biopsy and drain sites and scar.
- Inclusion of any seroma, lymphocoele or haematoma should be based on a discussion with surgeons.
- In case of an unplanned surgical resection, the surgical bed CTV should include residual disease, all disturbed muscle compartments and involved tissues.
- Edit CTV to stay within bones, fascia and skin (unless infiltrated).

Phase II

- CTV2: Same transaxial volume – GTV + 2 cm superiorly and inferiorly.

Radiation Dose

Preoperative Radiotherapy. Single phase: 50 Gy in 1.8 to 2 Gy per fraction

Postoperative Radiotherapy. Phase I: 50 Gy in 1.8 to 2 Gy per fraction

Phase II: 10 to 16 Gy in 2 Gy per fraction. If gross residual disease, increase dose up to a total of 70 Gy if within the tolerance dose of neighbouring critical organs.

Radical Radiotherapy. 66 Gy in 33 daily fractions over 6.5 weeks or 70 Gy in 35 fractions over 7 weeks, if within the tolerance dose of neighbouring critical organs

Retroperitoneum. 50.4 Gy in 28 fractions over 5.5 weeks

Head and Neck. 66 Gy in 33 daily fractions over 6.65 weeks

Radiotherapy Side Effects

Acute Reactions

Skin reactions are often a problem. This is because very high doses are needed in the boost volume and are sometimes given to graft areas. Dry desquamation normally develops and is treated as for other skin reactions. Moist desquamation is more likely to occur in the axilla, groin and perineum and is treated with hydrocortisone cream or ointment. If there is secondary infection, Flamazine (silver sulfadiazine) can promote healing.

Late Reactions

Atrophy of the skin and subcutaneous tissues and fibrosis within the muscles are common. Stiffness of a limb may be partly caused by fibrosis of the intermuscular septa and partly as a result of fibrosis in the joint capsule.

Osteoporosis of bone is common because bone is frequently included in the target volume. Occasionally, particularly if the bone is invaded by tumour, radionecrosis may occur. In the ribs, this may cause pathological fractures.

Proton Therapy

Protons have a similar relative biological effectiveness (RBE) to photons. The advantage of protons is a reduction of dose to critical structures, such as the spinal cord or underlying bone. Proton therapy has potential clinical benefits for tumours located in the head and neck, spinal and paraspinal regions, pelvis, thorax and abdomen, but confirmatory results are still awaited.

Results of Treatment

Conservative surgery and RT can achieve over 90% local control and 5-year survival in stage 1 disease. For stage 2 disease, local control is 85% to 90% and survival is 65% to 90%. For stage 3, local control is similar to stage 2 but survival is lower, 85% (3A) and 45% (3B). If there is only microscopic residual disease following surgery, overall survival is 65%, falling to 30% when there is gross residual disease.

BONE TUMOURS

Benign and malignant tumours may arise in bone. The pathological classification is shown in Table 33.6. Bone tumours represent 0.4% of all cancers. Primary bone tumours are rare and account for only 1% of bone neoplasia. The vast majority of bone lesions are secondary deposits. The main bone-forming malignant tumour is osteosarcoma and cartilage-forming is chondrosarcoma. Malignant tumours arising from the bone marrow are myeloma, Ewing sarcoma, and lymphoma (see Chapter 30).

Osteosarcoma (Osteogenic Sarcoma)

Osteosarcoma is the most common and most malignant primary bone tumour. It arises in bone-forming cells (osteoblasts) and is most common between the ages of 10 and 20 years. There is a second peak incidence in the elderly as a complication of Paget disease of bone. The male-to-female ratio is 1.6:1.

The cause of adolescent-type tumour is unknown. There is an increased incidence (400-fold) of osteosarcoma in patients with bilateral retinoblastomas, presumably because of the same genetic abnormality or mutation of the Rb tumour suppressor gene developing outside the irradiated areas. Li-Fraumeni syndrome, Werner syndrome and Rothmund-Thomson syndrome are also risk factors.

Pathology

Osteosarcoma is most common near the knee in the metaphysis of the distal femur or proximal tibia. In the elderly, its distribution matches Paget disease.

Macroscopically, the tumour is usually haemorrhagic. It expands the bone, destroying both the cortex and the medulla. The periosteum is frequently raised, giving rise to the radiological features of Codman triangle, where the raised periosteum meets the cortex. Extension into the soft tissue follows.

Blood-borne metastases to the lungs occur early. Bone metastases, though less frequent, also occur. Microscopically, there are malignant osteoblasts laying down small pieces of irregular osteoid tissue. The

TABLE 33.6 Classification of Bone Tumours

A. Tumours forming bone
1. Benign: e.g. osteoma
2. Malignant: osteosarcoma
B. Tumours forming cartilage
1. Benign: e.g. enchondroma
2. Malignant: chondrosarcoma
C. Giant cell tumour (generally benign)
D. Tumours of the bone marrow: myeloma, lymphoma, Ewing sarcoma
E. Other tumours

two common histological varieties are osteoblastic and telangiectatic (containing irregular blood vessels). A third variety is parosteal sarcoma. It arises from the surface of the bone and does not involve the medullary cavity.

Clinical Features

The most common presenting feature is pain, usually with swelling and a limp. Sometimes pathological fracture may follow minor trauma. Rarely, cough, dyspnoea and pneumothorax may indicate lung involvement.

Diagnosis and Staging Investigations

Plain radiographs and CT scan (Fig. 33.7A) of the affected part may show the typical features of bone destruction and soft-tissue extension. The cortex may be raised with a sunburst appearance. Full blood count, liver function tests and lactate dehydrogenase (LDH) are required. All patients should have a chest radiograph and CT scan of the chest to rule out lung metastases.

MRI of the involved bone with adjacent joints is essential for staging (Fig. 33.7B). CT is also helpful in assessing whether the capsule of a limb joint has been breached. Whole body bone scintigraphy may show increased uptake at the site of the tumour, in the adjacent bone (as a result of increased vascularity), in bone metastases and in bone-forming metastases in soft tissues. Whole body MRI and PET scan (especially for craniofacial sarcomas) may be considered for staging and response assessment.

A biopsy should be carried out to confirm the diagnosis. It is important that the position of the biopsy is chosen so that the whole biopsy scar can be excised with the tumour to include potentially surgically contaminated tissue along the track of the biopsy. Ideally, both biopsy and definitive surgery should be performed by the same surgical team. The endoprosthesis must be planned several weeks ahead of limb-sparing surgery (Fig. 33.7C).

Treatment

The management of osteosarcoma requires a multidisciplinary approach including orthopaedic surgeon, oncologist, pathologist and physiotherapist. Current treatment for localised disease is over 6 to 9 months involving 10 weeks of neoadjuvant chemotherapy followed by surgery and adjuvant chemotherapy.

Chemotherapy. Neoadjuvant and adjuvant chemotherapy are an important part of the treatment of osteogenic sarcoma. Chemotherapy has reduced the frequency of pulmonary metastases, which used to occur in 80% of cases. Although neoadjuvant chemotherapy does not improve survival compared with postoperative chemotherapy alone, early chemotherapy can shrink the primary tumour, leading to rapid improvement in symptoms, and can also treat micrometastases. Undoubtedly, neoadjuvant chemotherapy has reduced the rate of amputation in this disease. Although only about 10% of inoperable tumours are rendered operable by neoadjuvant chemotherapy, in many more cases, surgery is much easier owing to the reduction of the tumour allowing for the insertion of an endoprosthesis and sparing of the limb. The most accepted neoadjuvant chemotherapy regimen is high-dose methotrexate, doxorubicin and cisplatin (MAP). A good response to neoadjuvant chemotherapy is an independent good prognostic factor and the degree of viable tumour at surgery being related to ultimate survival. In the EURAMOS1 trial, patients ($n = 2260$) received 2 cycles of induction chemotherapy with

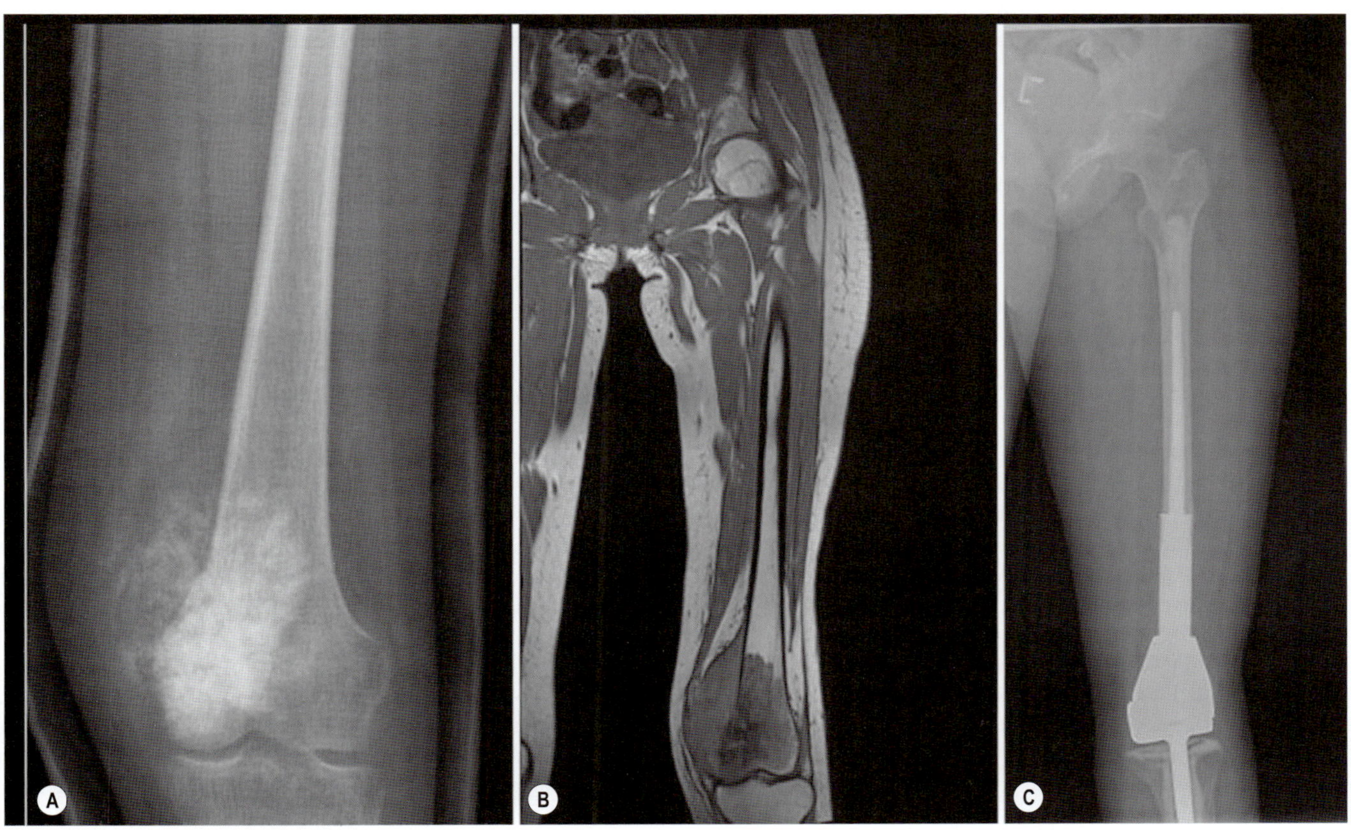

Fig. 33.7 (A) Osteosarcoma involving distal left femur with cortical destruction and extensive osteoid matrix. (B) Magnetic resonance imaging showing destructive lesion in the femur with extensive soft-tissue component. (C) Patient had neoadjuvant chemotherapy followed by limb-conservation surgery.

MAP followed by surgery. Patients (n = 1334) were randomised after surgery based on histological response (<10% viable tumour in the resected specimen: good response versus ≥10% viable tumour: poor response). Early results showed no improvement in event-free survival with the addition of interferon (IFN)-α-2b to MAP in patients with good histological response. In patients with poor histological response, the addition of ifosfamide and etoposide to MAP did not improve event-free survival. Patients with metastatic disease are also treated with a MAP regimen and 30% of patients are long-term survivors.

Low-grade central and parosteal sarcomas do not need adjuvant chemotherapy as they usually have a low-malignant potential.

Surgery. Surgery is aimed at removing the whole tumour with adequate margins to allow for functional preservation. Limb preservation involves removing the tumour and replacing the bone defect with a custom-made artificial prosthesis. Careful preoperative assessment is necessary, and referral to a specialist centre is essential. To obtain adequate margins, the prosthesis incorporates an artificial joint as well as femoral and tibial components (see Fig. 33.7C). Although pathological fracture increases the risk of local recurrence, it does not preclude a conservative surgery. However, contraindications to limb conservation may include poor radiological response after chemotherapy and situations such as extensive soft-tissue infiltration and/or invasion of neurovascular bundles when a safe complete resection is not possible.

Resection of Lung Metastases. Lung metastases are occasionally isolated and, in the absence of metastases elsewhere, surgical resection should be considered. Results are best if lung metastases develop after a long disease-free interval. Surgery is contraindicated if there is pleural involvement. A 5-year survival of up to 40% has been reported following resection of pulmonary metastasis.

Radiotherapy. There is no routine role for RT. In the following situations, RT may be indicated either to improve progression-free interval or to achieve symptom control:

- Unresectable tumours (e.g. the head and neck, vertebrae, ilium and sacrum). However, proximity of critical structures, such as the spinal cord, often limits the dose that can be delivered.
- Positive resection margin and further surgery not possible and/or poor response to chemotherapy (<90% necrosis).
- Intralesional resection or contaminated margin, with no further surgery planned.
- A displaced pathological fracture of bone at the primary site.
- Palliation of pain from the primary tumour in the presence of metastatic disease or bony metastases.

Target Volume

Gross Tumour Volume

- Primary RT: Visible tumour on planning CT scan/MRI
- Postoperative GTV: Areas of risk based on preoperative imaging, operation notes and histopathology report
- CTV = GTV + 2 to 3 cm (ensure inclusion of scar with 0.5-to-1-cm margin in postoperative situation)
- PTV = GTV + 5 to 10 mm

Technique. Three-dimensional conformal RT or advanced RT techniques such as IMRT, image-guided radiotherapy (IGRT) or particle therapy may be needed if tumours are near critical organs. Beam arrangements vary with the site of the primary. For tumours arising in a vertebra, a posterior oblique wedged pair with or without an unwedged direct posterior field provides a satisfactory dose distribution. For the ilium, parallel-opposed fields suffice. An optimised parallel-opposed pair of fields is suitable for limb primaries.

Dose and Energy. Megavoltage is required. The choice of dose will be determined by critical organ tolerance. For primary RT and postoperative macroscopic disease, the suggested dose is 60 to 66 Gy in 1.8-to-2-Gy fractions and for adjuvant microscopic disease, 60 Gy in 1.8-to-2-Gy fractions. In the spine above L2, the dose should be limited by spinal cord tolerance to 47.5 Gy in 25 daily fractions over 5 weeks. Palliative fractions include 30 Gy in 10 daily fractions over 2 weeks, 40 Gy in 15 fractions over 3 weeks and 6 Gy once every week for 5 to 6 weeks.

Results of Treatment

With multimodality treatment, the survival of osteosarcoma has improved from 10% to 20% to approximately 60%. Patients with poor histological response to neoadjuvant chemotherapy, pathological fracture and elevated alpha-fetoprotein (ALP) or LDH have a poor prognosis. Osteoblastic and telangiectatic tumours have a similar prognosis. Parosteal sarcomas have a better prognosis and may be cured by surgery alone.

Ewing Sarcoma

Ewing sarcoma is the second most common primary bone tumour. In the United Kingdom, its incidence is 0.6 per million. The peak age is between 10 and 15 years. It is slightly more common in males.

Pathology

Ewing sarcoma probably arises from connective tissue within the bone marrow. The most common sites in order of frequency are the pelvis, femur, tibia, fibula, rib, scapula, vertebra and humerus. In contrast with osteogenic sarcoma, a higher proportion of these tumours occurs in the flat bones of the trunk. About 40% occur in the axial skeleton. Microscopically, there are sheets of uniform undifferentiated, small, deeply staining round cells. The tumour needs to be distinguished from other small round-cell tumours, including non-Hodgkin lymphoma, Hodgkin disease, neuroblastoma and metastatic carcinoma. Some 90% of tumours have 11:22 chromosome translation.

There is local spread along the marrow cavity, causing bone destruction. However, the epiphyseal plates are rarely breached. Blood-borne spread is early and common. Spread to the central nervous system (CNS) may occur, usually late in the course of the disease.

Clinical Features

Presentation is usually with a rapidly developing and painful swelling. Neurological symptoms may accompany this if there is nerve compression. Fever occurs in about 30% of patients. Approximately 25% of patients have detectable metastatic disease at presentation (10% lung, 10% bone/bone marrow and a combination of sites for the remaining).

Diagnosis and Staging

Full blood count may show anaemia (leukoerythroblastic if there is bone marrow infiltration) and a mildly raised white cell count. Erythrocyte sedimentation rate (ESR) is often moderately elevated. Liver function tests may be abnormal (raised LDH or alkaline phosphatase).

A biopsy of the tumour is required. As in osteogenic sarcoma, care is taken to ensure that the biopsy lies within the incision for any later proposed definitive surgical procedure. Plain radiographs of the primary are taken in two planes (usually anteroposterior and lateral). In long bones, this may show the typical multilayered onion-skin appearance of the periosteal reaction and often a large adjacent soft-tissue mass. Pathological fracture occurs in 5% of patients (less frequently

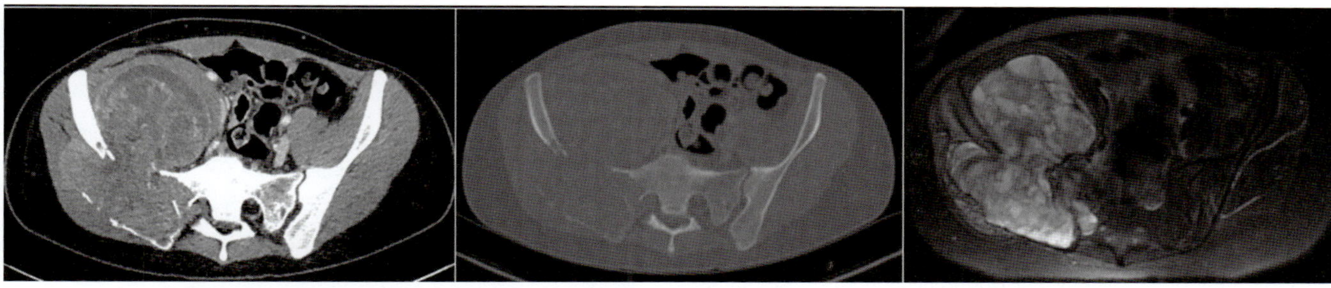

Fig. 33.8 Ewing sarcoma arising from the right pelvis showing a large soft-tissue mass and extensive destruction of right ilium.

than osteogenic sarcoma). CT scanning gives more detail of the local extent of the tumour and is useful in planning the site for a biopsy and subsequent surgery (Fig. 33.8). MRI is superior to CT in assessment of the extent of infiltration within the medullary canal. A fluorodeoxyglucose (FDG)-PET scan may be sufficient for screening of bone and bone marrow metastases. Because pulmonary metastases are common, a CT scan of the chest is mandatory.

Treatment

The choice of treatment will depend largely upon the site of the primary. A close liaison is required between the orthopaedic surgeon and oncologist. Similar to osteogenic sarcoma, treatment should only be carried out by an experienced team. The current treatment duration for localised disease is 8 to 9 months comprising 9 cycles of neoadjuvant chemotherapy followed by local therapy and further adjuvant chemotherapy. Patients with metastatic disease are treated similarly to localised disease. Patients with lung metastases may be considered for whole lung RT, even though firm data on survival advantage are lacking.

Chemotherapy. Ewing sarcoma is a chemosensitive tumour, and chemotherapy before surgery or RT has been shown to improve local control and reduce the incidence of distant metastasis. The Euro-Ewings 2012 trial showed superior results with dose-intense chemotherapy with vincristine, doxorubicin and cyclophosphamide, alternating with ifosfamide and etoposide. This is given neoadjuvantly for 9 cycles and then is followed by treatment to the primary site. This may be surgery or RT, or both, depending on the location of the tumour. Subsequently, 5 cycles of adjuvant chemotherapy are delivered to complete the planned course. In patients with pulmonary metastatic disease, high-dose chemotherapy with autologous stem cell rescue does not add any additional benefit to conventional chemotherapy with whole lung radiation.

Surgery. Surgery should be as radical as possible, with limb preservation and aimed at removing all tissues initially involved by the tumour, irrespective of response to neoadjuvant chemotherapy. Expendable bones may be completely removed (e.g. rib or fibula). With advances in expandable implants, limb conservation is possible, even in growing children. Historically, telescopic prosthetic implants were lengthened periodically to match the growth of the unaffected limb by turning a mechanism using an Allen key through a small incision. Currently, noninvasive expandable implants are being increasingly used.

Where radical surgery to a limb would cause major functional impairment, a conservative approach may be adopted with the addition of postoperative RT. Similarly, in axial bones, incomplete surgery following postoperative RT is acceptable.

Radiotherapy. Unlike osteogenic sarcoma, Ewing sarcoma is radiosensitive. Preoperative RT is indicated if there is a poor response to chemotherapy and when a marginal resection is anticipated. Preoperative RT is also useful in locations such as the pelvis and ribs, where a treatment response facilitates subsequent surgery. Radical RT is indicated for inoperable lesions or when surgery would be disabling. Postoperative RT is indicated in the following situations:

- Inadequate (<1 mm) or positive margin.
- Microscopic or macroscopic residual disease and further surgery not feasible.
- All tissues involved by the tumour at diagnosis have not been excised, even if the surgical margins are negative.
- A poor histological response (≤90% necrosis) to neoadjuvant chemotherapy even if the surgical margins are negative.
- A displaced pathological fracture of bone at the primary site and all contaminated tissue are not excised.
- Tumour in locations where complete surgery is difficult, for example, the spine and paraspinal sites, rib tumours with pleural effusion, the pelvis and sacrum, and the head and neck.

RT is contraindicated if there are concerns about high risk of late toxicities, impaired wound healing and an increased risk of metallic prosthesis infection.

Target Volume. If a total dose of 54 Gy or more is needed, a shrinking-field approach based on the pretreatment tumour volume is adopted.

Extremity Tumours

- Phase I: GTV is tumour at diagnosis, including scars after biopsy and resection. A margin of 3 to 5 cm in craniocaudally and 2 cm axially is added to derive the CTV. If there is extensive intramedullary involvement or skip lesions, and the whole bone should be irradiated. An unirradiated strip of normal tissue containing lymphatics outside the tumour-bearing area is left, if possible, to avoid constrictive fibrosis.
- Phase II: Phase II CTV is phase I GTV with a 2-cm margin craniocaudally and a 1-to-2-cm margin in other directions.

Nonextremity Tumours. The CTV is a prechemotherapy tumour with a 2-cm margin in all directions. Smaller margins are allowed if the tumour hasn't invaded the anatomical boundaries of critical structures (e.g. eye, optic apparatus). If tumours that were protruding into body cavities (e.g. chest or abdomen) have regressed after chemotherapy, the residual tumour with a smaller margin is treated to minimise radiation toxicities.

Technique. The choice of technique will vary with the site of the primary. High-precision RT techniques such as IMRT and particle-beam therapy are useful to deliver higher dose to a target with optimal sparing of normal structures. For the limbs, a parallel-opposed wedged pair of fields or three-dimensional conformal RT usually suffices. For pelvic primaries, it may be possible to surgically displace the bowel out of the radiation field by inserting an absorbable mesh or a spacer. For rib primaries, electrons of appropriate energy may be used to diminish the dose to the underlying lung. A parallel-opposed pair of fields encompassing both lung fields is used for whole lung RT. In the United Kingdom, children with localised Ewing sarcoma are treated with proton therapy if RT is indicated.

Dose and Energy. RT is delivered using megavoltage, photons, electrons or proton therapy. High-proton therapy is increasingly used for tumours located near critical structures and/or in children and young adults.

- Preoperative: 50.4 Gy in 28 fractions in a single phase. If there are concerns about organ tolerance or wound healing, this dose can be reduced to 45 Gy in 25-Gy fractions.
- Postoperative: 54 Gy in 30 fractions delivered as two phases (phase I: 45 Gy in 25 fractions and phase II: 9 Gy in 5 fractions).
- Radical RT: 54 Gy in 30 fractions delivered as a single phase. A boost of 5.4 Gy in 3 fractions may be considered.
- Whole lung RT: 15 Gy in 10 fractions for patients younger than age 14 years or 18 Gy in 12 fractions for patients age 14 years and older.

Radiotherapy Side Effects. Both the acute and late reactions are the same as for STS and depend on the site of irradiation and the total dose to the normal tissue.

Results of Treatment

The outcome is better for patients with tumours of the peripheral rather than central skeleton. Up to 90% disease-free survival for peripheral tumours and 65% for central (axial) tumours has been achieved. There is overall 5-year survival of 60% to 70% for localised tumours and 20% to 40% for metastatic disease. Local recurrence occurs in about 10% to 15% of long-bone primaries and 25% to 30% of pelvic tumours. The higher recurrence rate in the pelvis is probably because of the larger tumour size and the difficulty of irradiating the tumour homogeneously without damaging surrounding normal tissues.

Chondrosarcoma

Chondrosarcomas are malignant tumours of cartilage. They may arise in benign enchondromas or be malignant from the start. Adults age 30 to 50 years are affected. The most common sites in order of frequency are the pelvis (50%), femur, humerus and scapula.

Macroscopically, the tumour is bulky, lobulated and semitranslucent. Microscopically, it is a sarcoma containing cartilage. Differentiation is variable. Poorly differentiated tumours (mesenchymal chondrosarcomas) behave more aggressively. In the well-differentiated form, spread is slow, locally. Blood-borne metastases occur late to the lungs.

Clinical Features

Presentation is usually with a slowly progressive painless swelling, which eventually becomes painful.

Diagnosis and Investigation

A biopsy is required. Plain radiography shows bone destruction and commonly abnormal flecks of calcification. An MRI scan helps define the local extent (Figs. 33.9A and B).

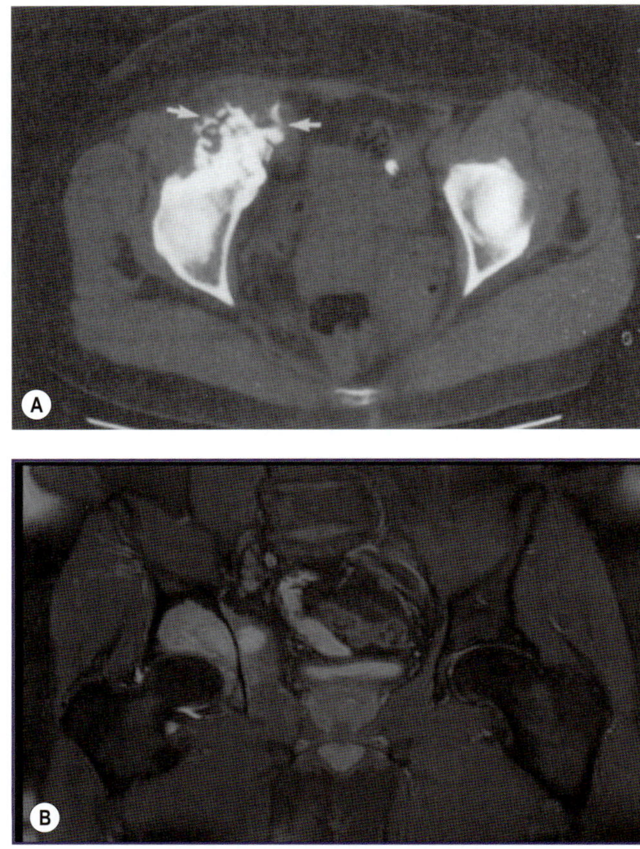

Fig. 33.9 (A) Computed tomography scan of the pelvis showing a chondrosarcoma of the ileum *(arrows)*. Note the flecks of calcification. (Courtesy Dr R Nakielny, Sheffield, UK.) (B) Magnetic resonance imaging showing a lesion in the right acetabulum with extraosseous extension. Patient underwent right pelvectomy and histology showed dedifferentiated chondrosarcoma.

Treatment

Radical surgery is the treatment of choice, except for low-grade central limb chondrosarcoma, which may be treated with curettage alone with or without adjuvant therapy (e.g. high-speed burring, thermal cauterisation and bone cementation with polymethylmethacrylate). Limb preservation may be possible. It is a very radioresistant tumour. An exception is chondrosarcomas of the facial bones and the base of skull, where a combination of surgery and RT offers long-term control. RT has a palliative role for the relief of local symptoms, such as pain, and relatively high doses are required even for palliative effect.

Radiotherapy

Technique. A parallel-opposed wedged pair of fields or three-dimensional conformal RT is suitable for the long bones. Three-dimensional conformal RT using a three-field technique (anterior and posterior wedged fields with an open lateral field) for pelvic tumours may limit the dose to the bowel.

Dose and Energy. 60 Gy in 30 daily fractions over 6 weeks at megavoltage (4–6-MV photons)

Chemotherapy. By and large, chondrosarcomas are chemoresistant, although there has been a renewal of interest in chemotherapy recently using the same agents that have been very useful in osteogenic sarcoma, particularly for the mesenchymal subtypes. However, the increase in overall survival following chemotherapy is small.

Results of Treatment

Five-year survival is about 50% over the age of 21 years but falls to 35% under that age. Younger patients tend to have tumours in the pelvis, where radical surgery is more difficult than in long bones. They also have more poorly differentiated tumours that metastasise more frequently.

Undifferentiated Pleomorphic Sarcoma of Bone

This heterogeneous group of tumours constitutes 2% to 5% of bone tumours. It usually occurs in adults age 30 to 50 years, and the common sites are ends of long bones. These are typically high-grade tumours with rates of metastases as high as 50%. The treatment approach is the same as for osteosarcoma, consisting of neoadjuvant chemotherapy followed by wide excision.

Secondary Tumours in Bone

The majority of bone tumours are of metastatic origin. They represent 15% to 20% of the workload of an RT department. The most common primary sites are breast, lung, prostate, myeloma and kidney. The prognosis of bone metastases is generally poor, though the course of the disease may be relatively slow over a period of years, for example, in some patients with breast cancer. Patients presenting with bone metastases from prostate or breast cancer may live for years while this tumour is hormone sensitive. Good symptomatic relief by a combination of analgesics according to the WHO analgesic ladder and local RT can be achieved in most cases.

Clinical Features and Investigation

The usual presentation is with pain caused by pressure on the periosteum or on nerve roots as they emerge from the spinal canal (Fig. 33.10). Early diagnosis is important before bone destruction has advanced so far as to cause pathological fracture (Fig. 33.11) or spinal cord compression.

Plain radiographs of the symptomatic area may show the deposits (osteolytic or osteosclerotic or both) or a pathological fracture. However, a metastasis in a vertebral body has to have reached a size of about 2 cm before it will be visible on a radiograph.

A radioisotope bone scan is helpful in detecting bone metastases too small to be visible on plain radiographs and to detect deposits elsewhere in the skeleton. Multiple bone metastases are common, predominantly in the spine, ribs, pelvis and upper femur. CT scanning of areas of the spine and sacrum where plain radiographs and bone scan are equivocal or normal may show bone destruction. If there is no known primary site, a CT-guided biopsy may be necessary.

Treatment

The treatment of bone metastases includes analgesics, RT, bisphosphonates and, occasionally, surgery. Treatment is aimed at relieving pain

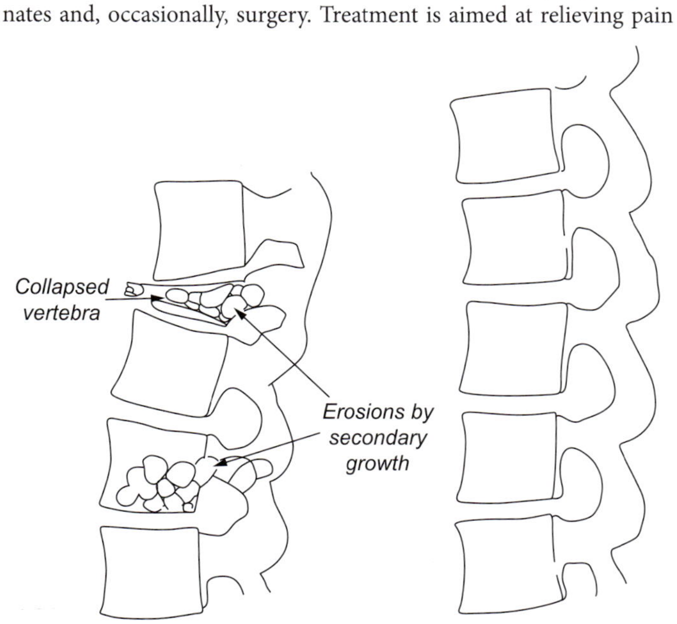

Fig. 33.10 Diagrammatic radiological appearances of normal vertebral column and secondary deposits from cancer (e.g. breast).

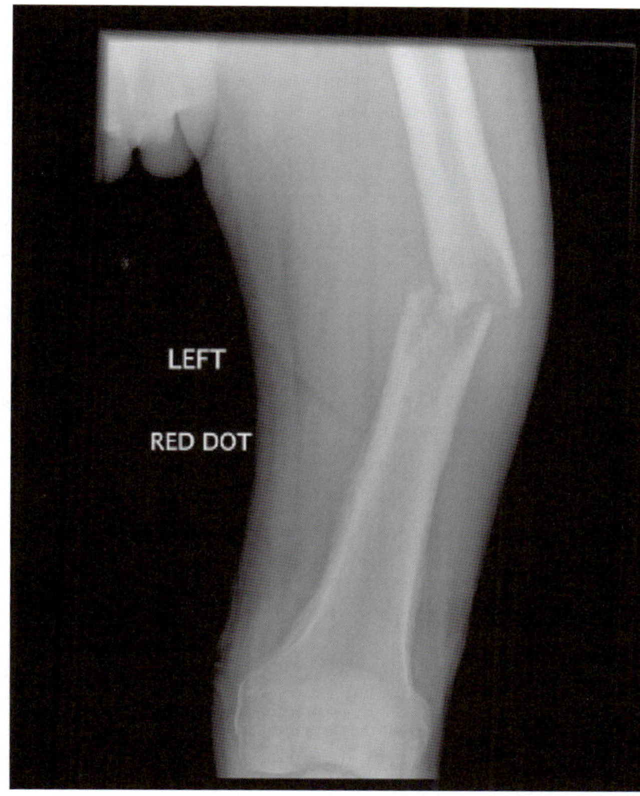

Fig. 33.11 A pathological fracture of the mid-left femur. The patient had metastatic nonsmall cell lung cancer. A femoral pin was inserted and the femur irradiated.

as simply and quickly as possible. Patients should always be given adequate analgesia, escalating according to the WHO analgesic ladder. The choice of treatment will depend on the site of the pain and its severity, complications such as spinal cord compression or pathological fracture, the presence of hypercalcaemia, the underlying tumour and the general condition of the patient.

Numerous randomised clinical trials and metaanalyses have shown that a single fraction of 8 to 10 Gy is as effective for relieving pain as a regimen of 30 Gy in 10 fractions when analgesic effect is measured at 6 weeks after treatment. The duration of pain relief after a single fraction is not known, but it is very easy to repeat the treatment. Depending on the site of the tumour, up to 90% of patients may have a marked diminution of pain following a single radiation fraction and up to 54% may have complete pain relief. Single fields are usually adequate for vertebral, sacral and rib deposits. Obese patients with lumbar metastasis should be treated with parallel-opposed fields. Kilovoltage radiation offers practical treatment advantages in the treatment of cervical spine lesions. Patients can be treated sitting in a chair, which is very useful if the neck is painful or the patient is wearing a supportive collar. Because the absorption of kilovoltage x-rays in bone is greater than megavoltage, the exit dose is small with less mucositis. Similarly, rib lesions can easily be treated using 300-kV x-rays. Parallel-opposed fields are usually used for tumours in the pelvis, long bones and base of skull. Usually, field sizes are generous, particularly in the spine. Fields usually include the uninvolved vertebra above and below the target lesions. In the treatment of long-bone metastases, margins of 3 to 5 cm are added beyond visible lesions to deal with occult disease.

In the past, patients with relatively radiosensitive tumours with widespread analgesic-refractory painful bone metastases (e.g. myeloma) were treated with hemibody irradiation (typically, single doses of 6 Gy are given to the upper and 8 Gy to the lower body). Doses greater than 6 Gy to the upper hemibody can induce an acute pulmonary reaction and pulmonary oedema. Hemibody RT is seldom used now because of the widespread availability of effective analgesics, bisphosphonates and radioisotopes.

Bisphosphonates are usually given intravenously every 3 weeks and are effective by preventing further osteoclastic resorption of bone. Pain relief is durable. The main side effect is hypocalcaemia. Radioisotopes are either β-emitters (strontium-89 and samarium-153) or α-emitters (radium-223). Compared with β-emitters, the rate of myelosuppression is less with radium-223.

Although single-dose palliative RT is the standard of care for patients with multiple metastases, there is an argument for giving higher doses (e.g. 40 Gy in 15 fractions) to a select group of patients. This may include patients with solitary nonspinal bone metastasis or metastases in up to 3 vertebrae from breast, renal or thyroid cancers. Studies of stereotactic body RT of a single dose of 15 to 24 Gy or a fractionated regimen of 13 to 35 Gy in 3 to 5 fractions report local disease control in up to 95% of cases and pain control in more than 80% of cases.

Pathological Fracture

If there is a pathological fracture or plain x-ray showing a lesion at risk of a pathological fracture of a long bone, an orthopaedic opinion should be sought on the feasibility of reducing and stabilising the fracture or preventing it. Pinning a fracture usually provides prompt pain relief and a return to mobility. Although there is no clear evidence for RT after pinning of a long bone, many clinicians prefer to give single-dose RT (8–10 Gy) to the whole bone.

If there is evidence of spinal cord compression, surgical decompression of the cord may be necessary prior to fractionated RT. Steroids should be given to patients with pain from nerve root infiltration and spinal cord compression. If patients are too unwell for even single fractions of RT, their pain should be controlled medically.

FURTHER READING

Ajithkumar TV, Hatcher H. Multidisciplinary management of sarcomas—where are we now? *Clin Oncol (R Coll Radiol)*. 2017;29(8):467–470.

Baldini EH, Wang D, Haas RLM, et al. Treatment guidelines for preoperative radiation therapy for retroperitoneal sarcoma: preliminary consensus of an international expert panel. *Int J Radiat Oncol Biol Phys*. 2015;92(3):602–612.

Bhattacharya IS, Hoskin PJ. Stereotactic body radiotherapy for spinal and bone metastases. *Clin Oncol (R Coll Radiol)*. 2015;27(5):298–306.

Bielack SS, Smeland S, Whelan JS, et al. Methotrexate, doxorubicin, and cisplatin (MAP) plus maintenance pegylated interferon alfa-2b versus MAP alone in patients with resectable high-grade osteosarcoma and good histologic response to preoperative MAP: first results of the EURAMOS-1 good response randomized controlled trial. *J Clin Oncol*. 2015;33(20):2279–2287.

Dangoor A, Seddon B, Gerrand C, Grimer R, Whelan J, Judson I. UK guidelines for the management of soft tissue sarcomas. *Clin Sarcoma Res*. 2016;6:20.

ESMO/European Sarcoma Network Working Group. Soft tissue and visceral sarcomas: ESMO Clinical Practice Guidelines for diagnosis, treatment and follow-up. *Ann Oncol*. 2014;25(Suppl 3:III):102–112.

ESMO/European Sarcoma Network Working Group. Bone sarcomas: ESMO clinical practice guidelines for diagnosis, treatment and follow-up. *Ann Oncol*. 2014;25(Suppl 3:III):113–123.

Euro-Ewing Radiotherapy Guidelines. Chapter XVII. In: EUROpean Ewing tumour working initiative of national groups Ewing tumour studies. 1999. EE 99 Amended Version. 2006. https://www.skion.nl/workspace/uploads/ee99_amended_treo__2006_02_14.pdf

Ford SJ, Almond LM, Gronchi A. An update on non-extremity soft tissue sarcomas. *Clin Oncol (R Coll Radiol)*. 2017;29(8):516–527.

Frisch S, Timmermann B. The evolving role of proton beam therapy for sarcomas. *Clin Oncol (R Coll Radiol)*. 2017;29(8):500–506.

Gerrand C, Athanasou N, Brennan B, et al. UK Guidelines for the management of bone sarcomas. *Clin Sarcoma Res*. 2016;6:7.

Gronchi A, Ferrari S, Quagliuolo V, et al. Full-dose neoadjuvant anthracycline + ifosfamide chemotherapy is associated with a relapse free survival (RFS) and overall survival (OS) benefit in localized high-risk adult soft tissue sarcomas (STS) of the extremities and trunk wall: interim analysis of a prospective randomized trial. *Ann Oncol*. 2016;27(Suppl. 6:vi552–vi587).

Haas RLM, Delaney TF, O'Sullivan B, et al. Radiotherapy for management of extremity soft tissue sarcomas: why, when, and where. *Int J Radiat Oncol Biol Phys*. 2012;84(3):572–580.

Hatcher H, Benson C, Ajithkumar T. Systemic treatments in soft tissue sarcomas. *Clin Oncol (R Coll Radiol)*. 2017;29(8):507–515.

Jeys L, Morris G, Evans S, Stevenson J, Parry M, Gregory J. Surgical innovation in sarcoma surgery. *Clin Oncol (R Coll Radiol)*. 2017;29(8):489–499.

Judson I, Verweij J, Gelderblom H, et al. Doxorubicin alone versus intensified doxorubicin plus ifosfamide for first-line treatment of advanced or metastatic soft-tissue sarcoma: a randomised controlled phase 3 trial. *Lancet Oncol*. 2014;15(4):415–423.

Le Cesne A, Ouali M, Leahy MG, et al. Doxorubicin-based adjuvant chemotherapy in soft tissue sarcoma: pooled analysis of two STBSG-EORTC phase III clinical trials. *Ann Oncol*. 2014;25(12):2425–2432.

Marina NM, Smeland S, Bielack SS, et al. Comparison of MAPIE versus MAP in patients with a poor response to preoperative chemotherapy for newly diagnosed high-grade osteosarcoma (EURAMOS-1): an open-label, international, randomised controlled trial. *Lancet Oncol*. 2016;17(10):1396–1408.

O'Sullivan B, Davis AM, Turcotte R, et al. Preoperative versus postoperative radiotherapy in soft-tissue sarcoma of the limbs: a randomised trial. *Lancet*. 2002;359(9325):2235–2241.

Pervaiz N, Colterjohn N, Farrokhyar F, Tozer R, Figueredo A, Ghert M. A systematic meta-analysis of randomized controlled trials of adjuvant chemotherapy for localized resectable soft-tissue sarcoma. *Cancer*. 2008;113(3):573–581.

Pisters PW, Harrison LB, Leung DH, Woodruff JM, Casper ES, Brennan MF. Long-term results of a prospective randomized trial of adjuvant brachytherapy in soft tissue sarcoma. *J Clin Oncol*. 1996;14(3):859–868.

Prewett S, Horan G, Hatcher H, Ajithkumar T. Borderline sarcomas and smooth muscle tumours of uncertain malignant potential. *Clin Oncol (R Coll Radiol)*. 2017;29(8):528–537.

Reddy KIA, Wafa H, Gaston CL, et al. Does amputation offer any survival benefit over limb salvage in osteosarcoma patients with poor chemonecrosis and close margins? *Bone Joint J*. 2015;97-B(1):115–120.

Sarcoma Meta-analysis Collaboration. Adjuvant chemotherapy for localised resectable soft-tissue sarcoma of adults: meta-analysis of individual data. *Lancet*. 1997;350(9092):1647–1654.

Tap WD, Jones RL, Van Tine BA, et al. Olaratumab and doxorubicin versus doxorubicin alone for treatment of soft-tissue sarcoma: an open-label phase 1b and randomised phase 2 trial. *Lancet*. 2016;388(10043):488–497.

Trojani M, Contesso G, Coindre JM, et al. Soft-tissue sarcomas of adults; study of pathological prognostic variables and definition of a histopathological grading system. *Int J Cancer*. 1984;33(1):37–42.

Whelan JS, Burcombe RJ, Janinis J, Baldelli AM, Cassoni AM. A systematic review of the role of pulmonary irradiation in the management of primary bone tumours. *Ann Oncol*. 2002;13(1):23–30.

Whelan JS, Bielack SS, Marina N, et al. EURAMOS-1, an international randomised study for osteosarcoma: results from pre-randomisation treatment. *Ann Oncol*. 2015;26(2):407–414.

Yang JC, Chang AE, Baker AR, et al. Randomized prospective study of the benefit of adjuvant radiation therapy in the treatment of soft tissue sarcomas of the extremity. *J Clin Oncol*. 1998;16(1):197–203.

34

Paediatric Oncology

Thankamma V. Ajithkumar

CHAPTER OUTLINE

INTRODUCTION

Cancer in childhood is uncommon. In the United Kingdom, approximately 1500 children under age 15 years develop cancer each year. Approximately 1 child in 500 will develop cancer before age 15 years. According to Cancer Research UK (CRUK), there were 1838 cases and 260 deaths per year from 2016 to 2018. The range of childhood cancers differs significantly from that seen in the adult population (Table 34.1).

The evolution of the multidisciplinary care of children with cancer has been one of the success stories of modern oncology. Paediatric oncology collaborative groups have successfully entered many children into clinical trials. In North America, clinical research has been coordinated via the Pediatric Oncology Group (POG), Children's Cancer Group (CCG), Intergroup Rhabdomyosarcoma Study Group (IRSG) and National Wilms Tumour Study Group (NWTS). In 1999, these groups were amalgamated to form the Children's Oncology Group (COG), the world's largest paediatric oncology collaborative group.

In the United Kingdom, 22 Children's Cancer and Leukaemia Group (CCLG) paediatric oncology centres coordinate treatment. Increasingly, collaboration is across European boundaries, with clinical trials coordinated via the European network of the International Society of Paediatric Oncology (SIOP-E).

Currently, approximately 80% of children treated for cancer can expect to be long-term survivors. For most diseases, this has been brought about mainly as a result of the incorporation of chemotherapy as part of a multimodality approach, including surgery and radiotherapy (RT). Since the introduction of chemotherapy into treatment programs in the 1960s and 1970s, the proportion of children surviving cancer has demonstrated this gratifying increase.

Approximately 40% to 50% of children with cancer receive RT as a component of their treatment. RT is an important treatment modality in local tumour control, and most paediatric tumours are radiosensitive. Cure or long-term survival, however, often comes with a cost as a result of the long-term sequelae of treatment. Long-term effects of RT include impaired bone and soft-tissue growth, impaired neuropsychological development as a result of irradiation of the central nervous system (CNS) and radiation-induced malignancies. Increasing awareness of long-term effects in the 1970s and 1980s led to a general decline in the use of RT. However, more recently it has become evident that chemotherapy is also associated with long-term side effects, including late myocardial damage due to anthracyclines, nephrotoxicity due to cisplatin or ifosfamide, and secondary leukaemia related to many chemotherapeutic agents including alkylating agents. The overall aim of paediatric oncology programs is to maximise the chance of cure with the minimum chance of long-term effects of treatment. Continued vigilance for the long-term effects of treatment is essential. This is ideally performed in the setting of dedicated long-term follow-up clinics and employing national treatment-related guidelines for long-term follow-up, such as those produced by the CCLG and SIOPE.

The administration of chemotherapy and RT for children must be undertaken only in specialised oncology centres treating relatively large numbers of children. In the United Kingdom, these centres are affiliated with the CCLG. The multiprofessional paediatric RT team should include a specialist paediatric therapy radiographer, a nurse

TABLE 34.1 **Comparison of Common Cancers in Children, Teenagers and Young Adults (15–24 years) and Adults in the United Kingdom**

Children (0–14 years)	Teenagers and Young Adults (15–24 years)	ADULTS (≥24 YEARS) Male	Female
Leukaemia (31%)	Lymphoma (20%)	Prostate cancer (24%)	Breast cancer (28%)
Central nervous system tumours (25%)	Germ cell tumours (15%)	Lung cancer (13%)	Lung cancer (13%)
Lymphoma (10%)	Skin cancer (15%)	Colorectal cancer (13%)	Colorectal cancer (11%)
Soft-tissue sarcoma (6%)	Central nervous system tumours (12%)	Bladder cancer (4%)	Uterine cancer (5%)
Neuroblastoma (6%)	Leukaemia (9%)	Skin cancer (4%)	Skin cancer (4%)
Kidney tumours (6%)	Soft-tissue sarcoma (5%)	Non-Hodgkin lymphoma (4%)	Ovarian cancer (4%)
Bone tumours (4%)	Thyroid cancer (5%)	Kidney cancer (4%)	Non-Hodgkin lymphoma (3%)
Germ cell tumours (3%)	Bone tumours (4%)	Head and neck cancer (4%)	Pancreatic cancer (3%)
Retinoblastoma (3%)	Cervical cancer (3%)	Oesophageal cancer (3%)	
		Pancreatic cancer (3%)	
		Leukaemia (3%)	

specialist, a play specialist and a dedicated anaesthesia team. Young children, particularly those under age 3 to 4 years, find it very difficult to lie still for RT planning and delivery, especially when an immobilisation headshell is required. Adequate sedation to ensure immobilisation is challenging to achieve without it persisting for several hours, and it is not feasible for this to be administered daily for each fraction of RT. Because of the importance of immobilisation, short-acting general anaesthesia, such as propofol, is frequently required for children under age 3 to 4 years. The daily fasting for this results in surprisingly little disruption to nutrition. An experienced play therapist can be beneficial in preparing the child for RT and may avoid the need for daily anaesthesia for some children.

TOXICITY OF RADIOTHERAPY FOR CHILDREN

RT side effects are due to disruption of the normal cell cycle, resulting in injury or death of cells with consequent inflammatory and fibrotic changes. While side effects of RT and their management are the same as for adults, many children will also receive chemotherapy along with radiation, resulting in a higher incidence and severity of acute reactions. In addition, children have immature tissues with high stem cell populations, which are more sensitive to radiation, and thus side effects may include impairment of tissue growth and maturation.

Side effects are categorised arbitrarily as:

- Acute (early) effects: Those appearing during or within 6 weeks of completion of RT (e.g. mucositis, dermatitis, vomiting, diarrhoea)
- Subacute effects: Those developing more than 6 weeks after but within 3 months of completion of treatment (e.g. somnolence syndrome)
- Late effects: Those occurring after 3 months of treatment (e.g. growth impairment, neurocognitive dysfunction)

Acute Effects

Fatigue, anorexia, erythema, mucositis, nausea, diarrhoea and other side effects occur in children as in adults and are generally managed by similar means (Chapter 35). Children receiving RT to areas of bone marrow-bearing bone (e.g. craniospinal radiotherapy (CSRT), whole abdominal radiotherapy) are at risk of bone marrow suppression. The risk is higher when myelosuppressive chemotherapy is used concurrently. Therefore, all children at risk of bone marrow suppression should have at least weekly blood counts, and appropriate corrective measures should be taken to complete RT within the intended overall time.

Subacute Effects

Liver

A large proportion of the liver may need to be irradiated when treating Wilms tumour. Radiation hepatopathy may occur 1 to 3 months following RT and consists of hepatomegaly, jaundice, ascites, thrombocytopenia and elevated transaminases. A risk factor is the administration of actinomycin-D following hepatic irradiation for the treatment of Wilms tumour. Long-term dysfunction is rare, and the risk is dose related.

Lung

The whole lungs may receive RT as part of total-body irradiation (TBI) or in the treatment of pulmonary metastases from Wilms tumour or Ewing sarcoma. Mild radiation pneumonitis consists of a dry cough and mild dyspnoea. The risk of pneumonitis is related to dose and radiation volume. Radiation pneumonitis is the dose-limiting toxicity for TBI. It is essential to consider potential interactions between chemotherapeutic drugs and lung irradiation, particularly to avoid lung irradiation in association with busulfan.

Central Nervous System

The somnolence syndrome occurs in at least 50% of children approximately 6 weeks after cranial irradiation and is probably related to temporary demyelination. Clinical features are irritability, reversal of sleep pattern, loss of appetite and exacerbation of tumour-associated symptoms. It is a transient self-limiting effect and fully recovers within 6 weeks. Corticosteroids may shorten the duration of symptoms.

Lhermitte's syndrome consists of an electric shock-like symptom radiating down the spine and into the limbs. It may follow radiation to the upper spinal cord, for example, following mediastinal RT for lymphoma. Within the first 2 months following RT for brain tumours, children may experience a transient deterioration of neurological symptoms and signs.

Long-Term Effects

Late effects are much more important in children than in adults. The extent and severity of these effects depend on the age at RT, the dose and volume of the organ irradiated and the use of concurrent chemotherapy.

Musculoskeletal

Impairment of bone growth and associated soft-tissue hypoplasia can be one of the most apparent and distressing long-term effects, particularly when treating the head and neck region. For example, a dose above 18 Gy to the craniofacial region can cause significant cosmetic and functional deformity, including micrognathia, which can lead to problems with dentition.

Age at the time of treatment, radiation dose and volume impact the severity of musculoskeletal effects. Careful consideration of the late musculoskeletal effects of radiation is essential when planning RT for children.

The epiphysial growth plates are also very radiation sensitive and excluded from the RT field whenever possible. RT of the epiphyseal plates in long bones can cause a reduction in bone length, and it can occur at a dose of 10 to 15 Gy in children younger than age 3 years and at a dose of more than 25 Gy in children older than age 3 years. Hip irradiation can cause a slipped capital femoral epiphysis, especially in children under age 4 years treated with 25 Gy and avascular necrosis (>30 Gy; at a lower dose if concurrent steroids or chemotherapy are given). Therefore, high-precision techniques may be helpful to keep the RT dose below tolerance when these areas cannot be excluded from radiation volume. When irradiating the spine, an essential principle of paediatric RT is that if the minimum vertebral dose is lower than 18 to 20 Gy, the dose gradient across the vertebra should be no greater than 3 Gy to minimise long-term kyphoscoliosis. When the dose is more than 18 to 20 Gy, the growing part of any vertebra adjacent to the treatment volume is irradiated to a uniform dose of 18 to 20 Gy to avoid late risk of kyphoscoliosis due to nonuniform dose.

Central Nervous System

Paediatric radiation oncology typically involves a significant amount of time devoted to the treatment of children with brain tumours, and consideration needs to be given to the toxicity of therapy.

Radionecrosis is rare below 60 Gy and generally occurs with a latency of 6 months to 2 years. It results from a direct effect on glial tissue. It is very unusual to have to deliver a dose of 60 Gy to any part of the CNS for a child, and for the most radical treatment for brain tumours, it is uncommon to exceed a dose of 50 to 54 Gy. The clinical effects of radionecrosis vary according to the site within the CNS and are most devastating in the spinal cord.

Necrotising leukoencephalopathy may be seen when cranial irradiation is followed by high-dose methotrexate to treat leukaemia. Clinical features include ataxia, lethargy, epilepsy, spasticity and paresis.

Neuropsychological effects. The effects of cranial RT are now well established. Data from children treated with prophylactic RT for leukaemia have demonstrated that compared to siblings, children given 24 Gy prophylactic cranial irradiation show a fall in IQ of approximately 12 points. Recent Pediatric Normal Tissue Effects in the Clinic (PENTEC) data suggest that 36 Gy to 10% of brain results in a 5% risk of IQ less than 85%. This risk increases with the percentage of brain irradiated and the total dose. An important risk factor for the incidence and severity of neuropsychological long-term effects is the age at RT. This has driven the investigation of treatment approaches that do not include RT for children below the age of 3 years. Other factors include the impact of direct and indirect tumour-related parameters, treatment parameters with neuropsychological long-term effects worse for whole brain compared with partial brain irradiation, concomitant use of some chemotherapeutic agents, premorbid patient characteristics, such as intelligence, and the quality of catch-up education.

Kidney

Long-term effects on renal function are usually seen 2 to 3 years following a course of RT. The risk increases following a dose greater than 14.5 Gy to both kidneys. The severity is related to the dose received. When mild, it consists of hypertension (5% risk of hypertension if dose to whole kidney is >9.6 Gy). When more severe, following a higher dose, renal failure may ensue.

Endocrine

Endocrine deficiencies following RT are common. The risk of growth hormone and other pituitary hormone deficiencies following pituitary irradiation for CNS tumours is of particular concern. If the whole pituitary-hypothalamic axis receives 22 Gy, there is a 20% risk of central hypopituitarism. Following RT to the thyroid, the incidence of elevated thyroid-stimulating hormone (TSH) is 44% after a mean dose of 30 Gy.

Reproductive

The germinal epithelium is susceptible to the effects of low-dose irradiation in male children. In adult males, transient oligospermia is seen after 2 Gy, but slow recovery can occur after 2 to 5 Gy.

In female children, the oocytes are also sensitive. Subsequent pregnancy is rare after 12 Gy whole body irradiation, but anecdotal cases of pregnancy after bone marrow transplantation (BMT), including whole body irradiation, have been reported.

TOLERANCE OF CRITICAL ORGANS TO RADIOTHERAPY

Critical organ tolerance frequently limits the dose of radiation that can be given. Table 34.2 lists the important organs at risk (OARs) and their tolerance doses if given in 1.8-to-2-Gy fractions based on the PENTEC consortium recommendations.

CHEMOTHERAPY/RADIOTHERAPY INTERACTIONS

Interactions between radiation and chemotherapy are complex and poorly understood. However, they can be exploited to attempt to improve disease-free survival. The most frequently employed mechanism in paediatric oncology is spatial co-operation, whereby chemotherapy and RT are combined to exploit their differing roles in different anatomical sites. Examples are the use of radiation for local control of a primary and chemotherapy for subclinical metastatic disease, such as in the treatment of Ewing sarcoma.

Chemotherapy and RT may be combined to increase tumour cell kill without excess toxicities. An example is the use of combined chemotherapy and RT for children with Hodgkin lymphoma. It may be possible to reduce the intensity of both treatment modalities to maintain disease control rates while reducing long-term morbidity. When using combined modality therapy, the aim is to improve the therapeutic ratio. Many protocols for children involve the use of concurrent chemotherapy and RT. It is essential to be vigilant for additional early- or long-term morbidity. Clinically significant chemotherapy/RT interactions are often unpredictable, and their mechanisms are poorly understood. Actinomycin-D and cisplatin increase the slope of the radiation dose-response curve, and actinomycin-D inhibits the repair of sublethal damage (SLD). Clinical interactions include enhanced skin and mucosal toxicity when radiation is followed by actinomycin-D (the recall phenomenon); enhanced bladder toxicity when chemotherapy is combined with cyclophosphamide; enhanced CNS toxicity from combined radiation and methotrexate, cytosine arabinoside or busulfan; and enhanced marrow toxicity from wide-field irradiation and many myelotoxic chemotherapeutic agents. In the case of the effect of combined radiation and anthracyclines, such as doxorubicin on the heart, doxorubicin has its effect on the myocytes and radiation on the vasculature.

RADIOTHERAPY QUALITY ASSURANCE

Because most childhood cancers have a high cure rate, it is important to achieve local tumour control and avoid a geographical miss. Avoiding unnecessarily large field sizes is also important to minimise long-term effects.

All RT departments must deliver the highest possible standard of RT for all patients, including children. Many RT departments have adopted quality systems. In several studies, particularly those

TABLE 34.2 **Normal Tissue Tolerance Doses Based on the Pediatric Normal Tissue Effects in the Clinic (PENTEC) Consortium 2024**

Organ	Endpoint (% risk)	Dose and Volume
Whole brain	Symptomatic necrosis (5%)	59 Gy to any part
Whole brain (reirradiation)	Symptomatic necrosis (5%–7%)	112 Gy to any part
Optic apparatus	Optic neuropathy (5%)	57 Gy D_{max}
Retina	Retinopathy (5%)	42 Gy D_{max}
Lens	Cataract (50%)	Mean 9 Gy
Pituitary	GH deficiency (5%)	D100% 15 Gy
	ACH deficiency (20%)	D100% 34 Gy
	Central hypopituitarism (20%)	D100% 22 Gy
Spinal cord	Myelopathy (rare)	D1cc <50.4 Gy without chemotherapy
		D1cc <45 Gy with chemotherapy
Cochlea	Hearing loss (<5%)	Mean <35 Gy
Both parotid glands	Acute grade >2 xerostomia (32%)	Mean 35–40 Gy
	Chronic grade >2 xerostomia (13%–32%)	Mean 35–40 Gy
Thyroid gland	Clinical hypothyroidism (7%)	Mean 20 Gy
Lung	Symptomatic (grade 2) late pneumonitis (<5%)	V27 <20%
Heart	Any cardiac disease (3.8%)	Mean 20 Gy
Liver	Hepatic sinusoidal obstructive syndrome (6.1%)	D100% 10 Gy
Kidney	Grade 3–5 chronic kidney disease (5%)	Whole kidney 14.5 Gy
Testes	Oligospermia at 1 year (>90%)	Mean >1 Gy
	Low testosterone level (25%)	Mean 0.2–12 Gy
Ovaries	Ovarian failure (1.5%)	2 Gy

ACH, Adrenocorticotropic hormone; *GH*, growth hormone.
From Constine LS, Marks LB, Milano MT, et al. A user's guide and summary of Pediatric Normal Tissue Effects in the Clinic (PENTEC): radiation dose-volume response for adverse effects after childhood cancer therapy and future directions. *Int J Radiat Oncol Biol Phys.* 2024;119(2):321–337.

employing CSRT for medulloblastoma (MB), the delivery accuracy of RT has impacted tumour control and patient survival. In many North American paediatric multicentre studies, RT quality, including beam data, dose prescription, planning films and verification films, are reviewed centrally in the Imaging and Radiology Core Cooperative (IROC) situated in Providence, Rhode Island. In Europe, the Quality and excellence in radiotherapy and imaging for Children and adolescent with cancer across Europe in Clinical trials (QUARTET) project provides QA review for prospective clinical trials.

LEUKAEMIA

One of the early successes of paediatric oncology was improving the survival of children with acute lymphoblastic leukaemia (ALL). Currently, more than 85% to 90% are long-term survivors. Leukaemias account for the most frequent group of paediatric malignancies. Approximately 80% have ALL, and 20% have acute nonlymphoblastic leukaemia (ANLL), usually acute myeloid leukaemia (AML) or, rarely, chronic myeloid leukaemia (CML).

Current treatment for ALL is stratified according to risk status based on presenting white count and cytogenetic profile and has different phases:

1. Remission induction: This is an intensive chemotherapy approach to destroy a maximum number of leukaemic cells. This phase lasts 4 to 6 weeks. Children also receive CNS prophylaxis with intrathecal chemotherapy.
2. Consolidation with CNS prophylaxis: Cranial RT is no longer employed except for patients presenting with CNS involvement by leukaemia.
3. Maintenance: This is usually based on a continuous low-dose antimetabolite drug such as 6-thioguanine, with a total duration of therapy of approximately 2 years.

During the 1960s and 1970s, the routine use of prophylactic whole brain radiotherapy (WBRT) and intrathecal methotrexate reduced the risk of CNS relapse to less than 10%. WBRT may be employed for patients who present with CNS involvement (Fig. 34.1). Patients are immobilised in a headshell and treated with opposed lateral beams using 4 to 6 MV (megavoltage), which may be centred on the outer canthus to minimise divergence into the contralateral lens. Shielding will cover the face, dentition, nasal structures and lenses. The clinical target volume (CTV) includes the intracranial meninges extending inferiorly to the lower border of the second or third cervical vertebra. Attention should be paid to including the cribriform fossa, temporal lobe and skull base in the CTV. It is often challenging to spare the lenses when the posterior orbit is included to avoid ocular relapses. The CTV is localised with lateral computed tomography (CT) simulation. The prescribed dose in UK protocols is 24 Gy in 15 fractions of 1.6 Gy daily.

Male children who suffer a testicular relapse are treated with testicular RT (Fig. 34.2). The technique employed is an anterior field, generally electrons. The CTV includes both testes, the scrotum and the inguinal canal superolaterally as far as the deep inguinal ring, with shielding of nontarget skin and perineum. The prescribed dose is 24 Gy in 12 fractions of 2.0 Gy daily.

As for adults, children with ANLL are treated with intensive multidrug chemotherapy, which can achieve a survival rate of 60%. BMT is frequently employed for children with a human leucocyte antigen (HLA)-matched sibling. A survival rate of 65% can be achieved for children in first complete remission treated with BMT as consolidation therapy for AML.

Total-Body Irradiation

TBI is an important technique, usually with high-dose cyclophosphamide (cyclo-TBI) as the conditioning regimen for adults and children before BMT. Bone marrow donors for BMT are generally HLA-matched

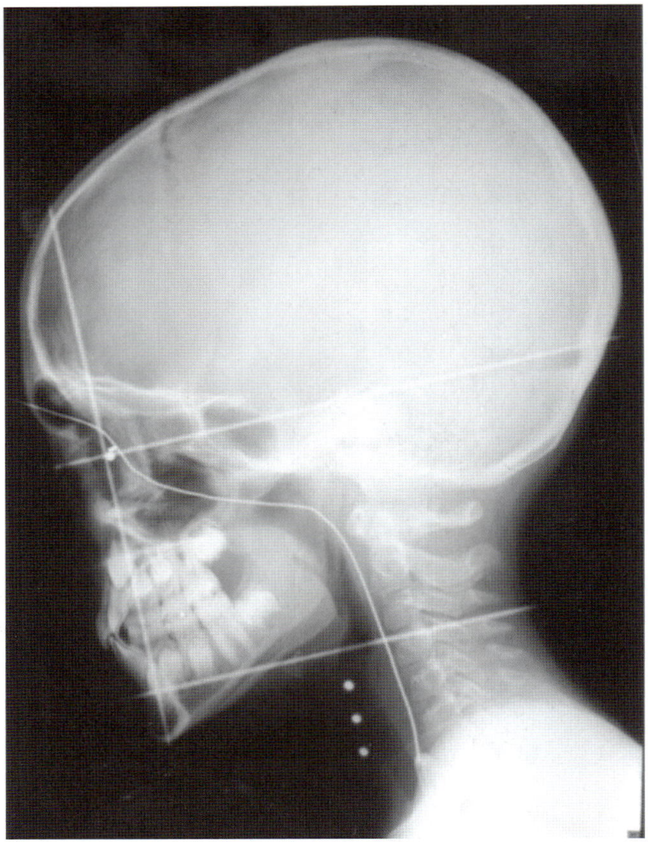

Fig. 34.1 Simulator film of whole brain field for acute lymphoblastic leukaemia central nervous system prophylaxis.

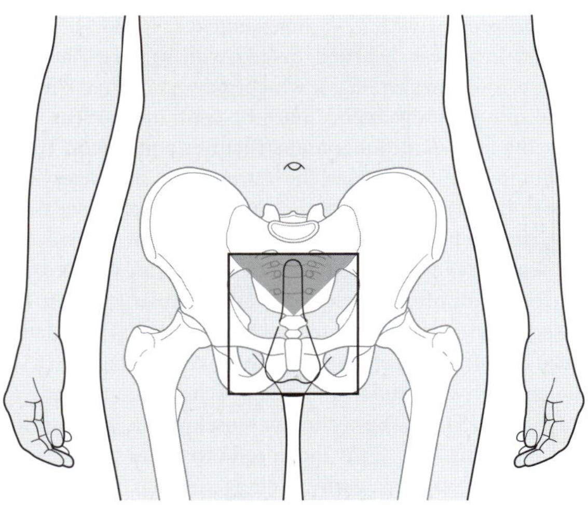

Fig. 34.2 Diagram of the field for testicular radiotherapy.

siblings. However, increasingly, volunteer unrelated donors from donor panels donate marrow, resulting in a significant increase in the number of patients for whom BMT can be considered. TBI is indicated as part of the conditioning regimen for allogeneic BMT in children with progressive, refractory and relapsed ALL or AML.

Techniques for TBI have evolved in different departments, depending on the availability of treatment facilities. Modern linear accelerator design and field sizes allow large anterior and posterior fields to be used. TBI dosimetry is usually based on in vivo measurements.

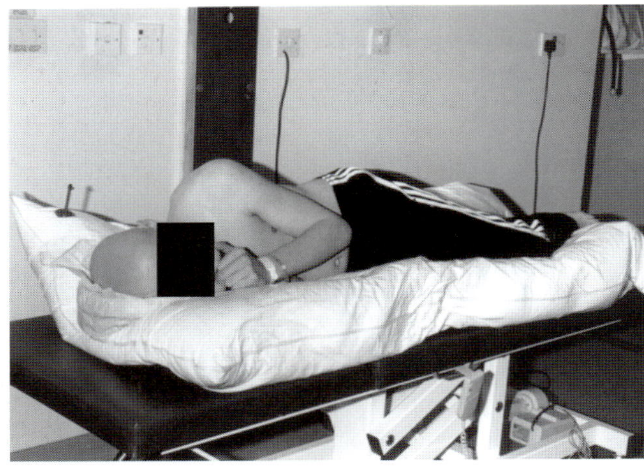

Fig. 34.3 Total-body irradiation technique.

The TBI technique developed in Leeds is provided as an example. The patient lies in the lateral position in an evacuated polystyrene immobilisation bag. Hands are placed under the chin to provide lung compensation (Fig. 34.3). Alternatively, volumetric modulated arc therapy (VMAT) or tomotherapy can also deliver TBI (Fig. 30.12). With tomotherapy, children shorter than 140 cm can be treated without any junctions in the treatment field. Dosimetry is determined using in vivo measurements performed at a test dose of 0.2 Gy for each field. For such a large and complex target volume, it is not feasible to adhere to the International Commission on Radiation Units and Measurements (ICRU) 50 guidelines of a range of −5% to +7%; a range of −10% to +10% is more realistic. The TBI dose for children is 13.2 to 14.4 Gy in 8 fractions of 1.8 Gy twice daily with a minimum interfraction interval of 6 hours. Recent clinical trials use a dose of 12 Gy in 6 fractions over 3 days treated twice daily, and a 2-Gy single fraction is given as part of a reduced-intensity cord transplant.

For children with ALL, many centres advise a cranial boost in addition to the TBI to reduce the risk of CNS relapse. Planning for the cranial boost is the same as for prophylactic cranial irradiation. Unlike the standard TBI dose, policies for the cranial boost vary amongst individual centres. A typical regimen for the cranial boost would be 5.4 Gy in 3 daily fractions.

Morbidity of Total-Body Irradiation

Acute effects include nausea and lethargy during TBI, mucositis, diarrhoea, erythema and parotitis in the first few weeks following treatment and somnolence approximately 6 weeks after TBI. Long-term effects of TBI include impaired growth because of a direct effect from irradiation of epiphyses and also as a growth hormone deficiency. There is also a risk of cataracts, hypothyroidism and, in some studies, the possibility of renal impairment. TBI is generally not considered for children under the age of 2 years, and instead, a conditioning regimen with two drugs, busulfan and cyclophosphamide (Bu-Cy), is generally employed.

HODGKIN LYMPHOMA

The age incidence of Hodgkin lymphoma spans the older paediatric age range through the adolescent and young adult age ranges. The overall survival rate for children with Hodgkin lymphoma is at least 90%, and an important aim is to maintain this excellent overall survival rate while reducing long-term treatment effects. These include the late musculoskeletal effects of RT, such as impaired bone growth resulting from direct irradiation of the epiphyses and infertility from alkylating agents and procarbazine. Wide-field RT, such as the mantle technique, has been avoided in children for several decades. In Europe a

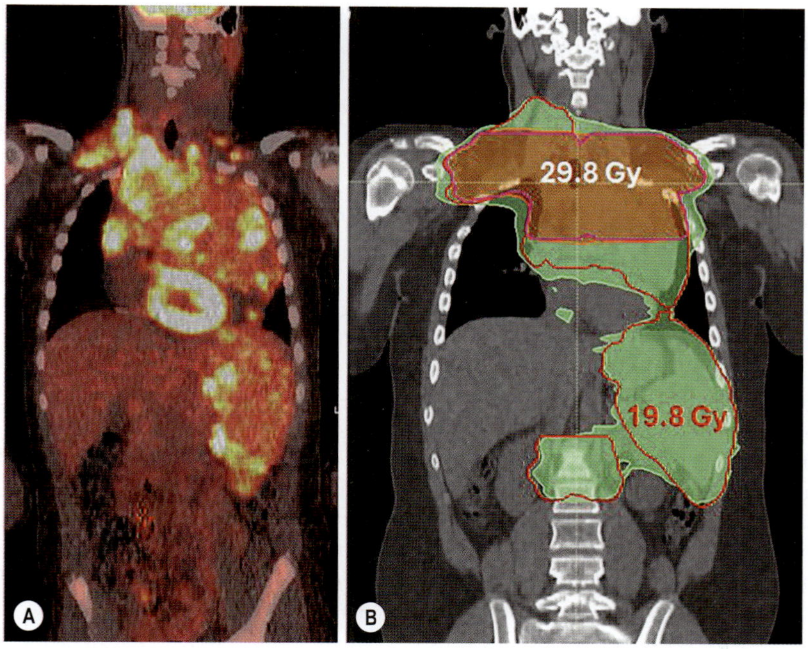

Fig. 34.4 (A) Diagnostic positron emission tomography scan in Hodgkin lymphoma showing extensive disease involving lower neck, mediastinal, splenic and paraaortic (not visible on this scan) nodes. (B) Involved-site radiotherapy to sites of initial (19.8 Gy) and residual disease (29.8 Gy).

chemotherapy approach is taken with response assessment by positron emission tomography (PET) scanning, which is now established as a predictor for patients who require RT. Consolidation RT is selectively employed for children whose response on PET scans is suboptimal.

In the Euronet PHL C1 study, all children with inadequate response after induction chemotherapy received modified involved-field RT (all initially involved nodes with a 1-to-2-cm margin) to a dose of 19.8 Gy in 11 fractions over 2.2 weeks. In addition, children with a poor response and/or bulky residual disease after consolidation chemotherapy received boost RT (10 Gy in 5 fractions) to a target volume of residual mass with a 1-to-2-cm margin (Fig. 34.4). This study led to a reduction in the rate of RT use from 85% to 55% without compromising cure rates. The RT rates are anticipated to be further reduced in the recently completed Euronet PHL C2 trial, which has more intensified chemotherapy.

NON-HODGKIN LYMPHOMA

A different spectrum of non-Hodgkin lymphoma (NHL) is seen in children compared with adults. Follicle centre cell lymphoma and diffuse large B-cell lymphoma, common in adults, are uncommon in childhood. Most children have T-cell lymphoblastic lymphoma, Burkitt, Burkitt-like or anaplastic large-cell lymphoma. Survival rates have improved in recent years, and more than 80% survive long term. Patients are treated by intensive multiagent chemotherapy, including CNS prophylaxis with intrathecal chemotherapy, and there is no routine role for RT in their management. However, children with T-cell lymphoblastic lymphoma, which is managed according to the same principles as ALL, may be considered for BMT with TBI. RT is an effective palliation for advanced chemo-resistant disease. RT is given to a target volume encompassing the symptomatic disease with a margin of 1.5 to 2 cm to a dose of 8 Gy single or 20 Gy in 5 fractions.

NEUROBLASTOMA

Neuroblastoma (NB) is the most common solid tumour of childhood. NB is generally a disease of very young children. Approximately one-third are less than 1 year of age at presentation. NB arises in neural crest tissue in the autonomic nervous system, usually in the adrenal area, but can occur anywhere from the neck to the pelvis. The majority of children present with widespread metastases, including bones, marrow, lungs and liver. The prognosis for individual clinical groups varies considerably and is related to several prognostic factors. The prognosis is better for young children age less than 1 year at presentation and is worse for children whose tumours have amplification of the oncogene Myc-n. Deletion of the short arm of chromosome 1 has emerged as an important prognostic factor, with a worse prognosis for those with 1p deletion. Hyperdiploid tumours have a better prognosis. Management is now stratified according to risk grouping. Patients in the best-risk group with localised disease have a survival rate of greater than 90% following surgery alone. The majority are treated with intensive chemotherapy using drugs such as vincristine, cisplatin, carboplatin, etoposide and cyclophosphamide. The 5-year event-free survival of children with low-risk disease is greater than 95% and with intermediate-risk, 80% to 95%. Five-year overall for children with high-risk disease is poor and is less than 50%.

For good-risk patients, RT is unnecessary. RT is considered in intermediate and high-risk diseases. Adjuvant RT to the tumour bed and residual primary tumour is given to children over age 18 months with undifferentiated or poorly differentiated tumours and with intermediate-risk disease. Intermediate risk is defined as:

- Limited disease without the involvement of vital structures (L1) with mycN amplification OR
- MycN nonamplified tumours in children over age 18 months with locoregional tumours with the presence of one or more image-defined risk factors (L2): tumour involving two body compartments, encasing major blood vessels, extending to the skull base or intraspinal space or infiltrating adjacent organs OR
- MycN nonamplified tumours in children under age 12 months with metastatic disease OR
- MycN nonamplified tumours in children age 12 to 18 months with metastatic disease without segmental chromosomal abnormalities

Though the predominant relapse pattern is metastatic rather than local in patients with high-risk disease, RT is given to maximise the probability of local tumour control.

High-risk disease is defined as:

- Myc amplification with L2 disease or MS disease (metastatic disease in children under age 18 months with metastases confined to skin, liver and/or bone marrow) OR
- Metastatic disease in children age 12 to 18 months with segmental chromosomal abnormalities OR
- Metastatic disease in children over age 18 months

With current intensive chemotherapy, some patients with metastases at presentation can hopefully be cured, and local tumour control becomes essential, employing a combination of surgical resection and postoperative RT. In the recent European High-Risk NB protocol, the dose for postoperative RT to the tumour bed was 21 Gy in 14 fractions. In planning postoperative RT for NB, care has to be taken to consider dose limits to OARs, particularly the liver and kidneys, the function of which may have been compromised by high-dose chemotherapy. The CTV is derived by adding a 5-mm margin to the virtual gross tumour volume (GTV) derived from preoperative images after chemotherapy. Traditionally, RT is given using an opposed anterior-posterior beam with multileaf collimator (MLC) shaping, and more recently, intensity modulated radiotherapy (IMRT) techniques have been used.

Meta-iodobenzylguanidine Therapy for Neuroblastoma

Most NBs take up the guanethidine analogue, meta-iodobenzylguanidine (MIBG). MIBG can be conjugated with iodine radionuclides for imaging and targeted RT. Generally, 123I-MIBG is the radionuclide used for diagnostic imaging. High-activity 131I-MIBG (typically 3.7–7.4 GBq) can be used for targeted therapy. In a UK multicentre study, a response rate of 30% has been achieved for children with residual NB following first-line chemotherapy. However, MIBG therapy is available in only a limited number of specialist paediatric oncology centres.

WILMS TUMOUR (NEPHROBLASTOMA)

Wilms tumour is an embryonic renal tumour that generally presents as a large abdominal mass, sometimes with pain or haematuria. It may be genetically associated with aniridia (congenital absence of the iris) and other inherited syndromes, such as Beckwith-Wiedemann syndrome (variable features including macrosomia or hemihypertrophy, macroglossia and omphalocele). The WT1 gene is located on chromosome 11 and is a tumour-suppressor gene. If both copies of the gene are lost by mutation, Wilms tumour may arise.

The median age at diagnosis is between 3 and 3.5 years. Patients are staged according to histopathological findings following nephrectomy. Table 34.3 shows the National Wilms Tumour Study Group (NWTS) staging system for Wilms tumours. Tumours are bilateral in 4% to 8% of cases (stage 5).

TABLE 34.3 National Wilms Tumour Study Group Staging System

Stage	Clinicopathological Features
I	Tumour confined to within renal capsule, completely excised
II	Tumour invading outside renal capsule, completely excised
III	Residual abdominal tumour—positive margins, tumour rupture, involved nodes
IV	Haematogenous metastases
V	Bilateral disease

The current long-term survival rate for Wilms tumour is more than 80%. Treatment aims to maintain this high survival rate while attempting to reduce the long-term side effects of therapy. There is a significant difference between treatment approaches in Europe and North America. The North American approach is immediate nephrectomy with staging and postsurgical adjuvant treatment based on histological examination of the primary tumour. Wilms tumour histology is referred to as favourable (FH) or unfavourable (UH) because of anaplasia.

Postoperative chemotherapy is given using the drugs vincristine, actinomycin-D and doxorubicin; the number of drugs and duration depend upon the staging.

The European approach, based on SIOP studies, has been preoperative chemotherapy to downstage the primary, reducing the surgical morbidity, particularly tumour rupture at surgery, and the number of children requiring postoperative RT. In the SIOP 2001 study, children received preoperative chemotherapy with actinomycin-D and vincristine, with delayed nephrectomy, after 6 weeks of preoperative chemotherapy. Postoperative adjuvant therapy was based on subsequent pathological staging and allocation of risk status (good-risk versus intermediate-risk versus poor-risk histology). There was a randomisation for intermediate-risk patients to receive or not receive doxorubicin. This aimed to determine whether doxorubicin could be omitted, thus reducing the risk of late cardiac sequelae. The trial results demonstrated that avoiding doxorubicin in this patient group was safe, and it now forms the basis of current management. Currently, 15% of children receive RT.

Based on postoperative histopathology in Europe, stage I to III disease is grouped into low-, intermediate- and high-risk disease, and metastatic disease as standard and high risk. In children with stage I disease (tumour limited to the kidney and completely excised), low- and intermediate-risk stage II (tumour extending beyond the kidney and completely excised) and low-risk stage III (residual tumour, node positive, rupture or renal/inferior vena cava involvement), adjuvant RT is not recommended. Postoperative RT is indicated in children with stage II high-risk disease (defined as diffuse anaplasia, clear cell sarcoma or malignant rhabdoid tumour) and all patients with stage III disease. These patients receive flank RT except when there is a tumour rupture or macroscopic peritoneal disease when whole abdominopelvic RT is indicated. In stage IV disease, the indication for local RT is similar to stage II to III, but RT to metastatic sites is also indicated.

Current standard radiotherapeutic management involves opposing anterior-posterior beams with MLC shaping. The CTV for flank RT includes the preoperative extent of the tumour and kidney following preoperative chemotherapy, with a margin of 1.0 cm. Fields extend across the midline to irradiate the entire width of the vertebral body homogeneously to minimise the risk of kyphoscoliosis (Figs. 34.5 and 34.6). For patients with intermediate-risk histology, the dose is 14.4 Gy in 8 fractions of 1.8 Gy daily, and for high-risk histology, 25.2 Gy in 14 fractions of 1.8 Gy. There is a boost to macroscopic residual disease: 10.8 Gy in 6 fractions of 1.8 Gy. For future European trials, it is proposed that rather than using parallel-opposed fields, a retroperitoneal CTV should be planned based on the anatomical site where disease recurrence is considered possible and considering the surgeon's assessment of the site of risk of recurrence.

Whole abdominopelvic RT has considerable acute and long-term morbidity and is considered for those who present with extensive intraabdominal tumour spread or generalised preoperative or perioperative tumour rupture. For patients with intermediate-risk histology, the dose is 15 Gy in 10 fractions, and for high-risk histology, 19.5 Gy in 13 fractions. There is a boost to macroscopic residual disease: 10.8 Gy in 6 fractions. The mean dose to the contralateral kidney should be limited to 12 Gy.

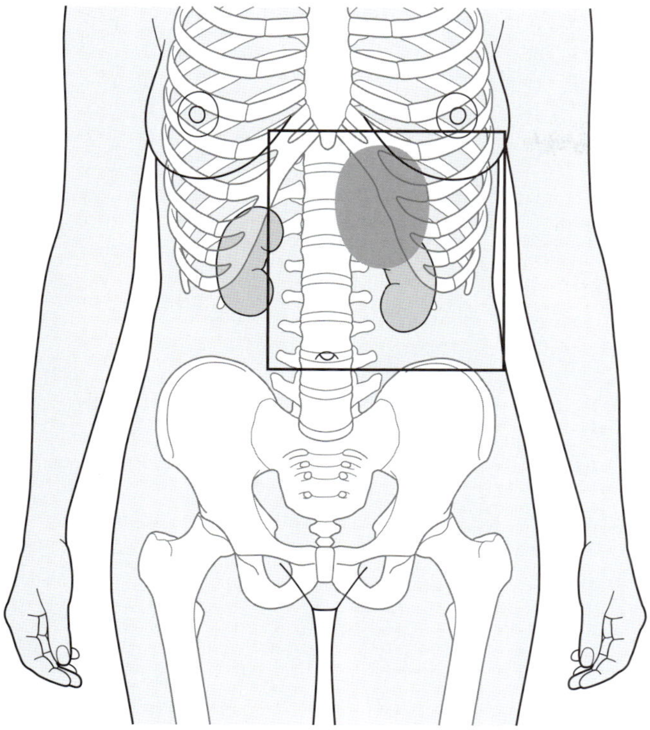

Fig. 34.5 Diagram of flank radiotherapy field for Wilms tumour.

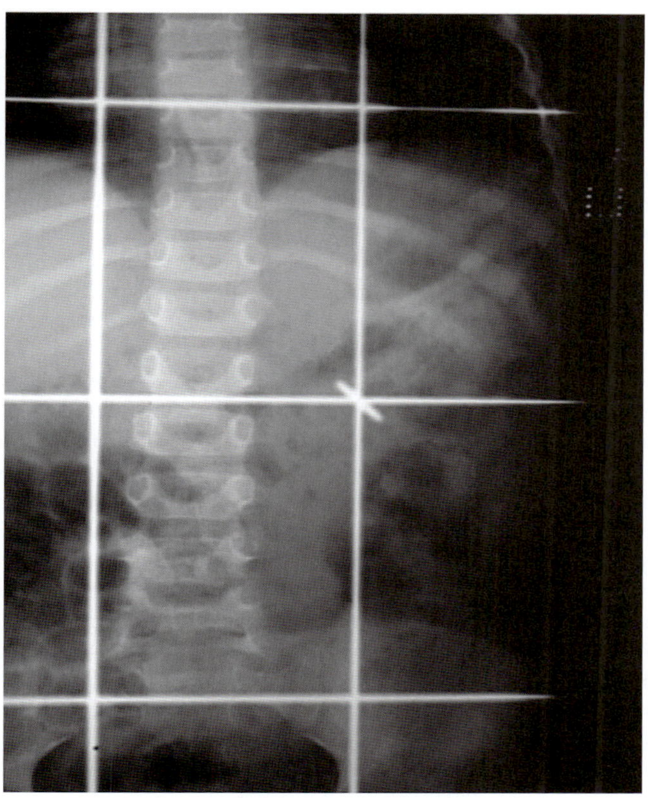

Fig. 34.6 Wilms tumour flank radiotherapy.

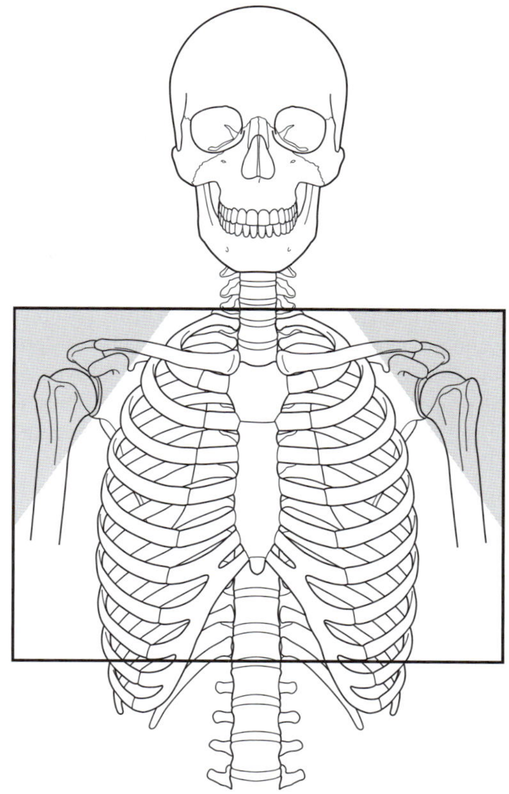

Fig. 34.7 Diagram of the whole lung radiotherapy field.

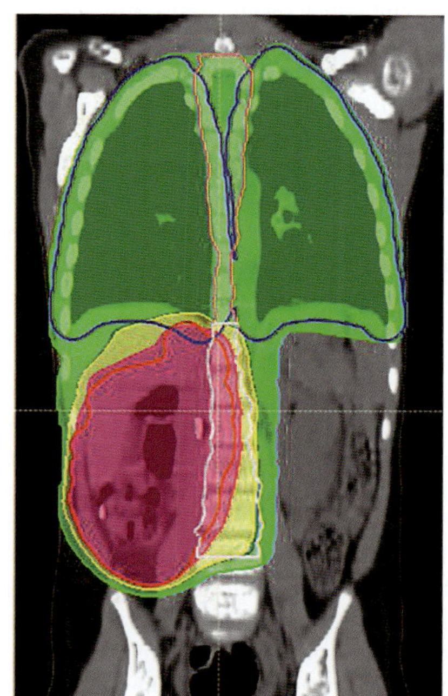

Fig. 34.8 Right flank (25.2 Gy) and whole lung radiotherapy (15 Gy) for metastatic Wilms tumour. All growing vertebrae in the treatment field received a uniform dose to avoid kyphoscoliosis.

For children presenting with pulmonary and liver metastases, which do not resolve completely after chemotherapy, whole lung RT (Figs. 34.7 and 34.8) and whole liver RT, respectively, are indicated. The whole lung target volume includes the costophrenic recess, and the lower border generally extends to the lower border of the 12th thoracic vertebra. The humeral heads are shielded. For patients with intermediate-risk histology, the dose is 12 Gy in 8 fractions and 15 Gy in 10 fractions for high-risk histology. The boost to macroscopic disease is 10 to 12 Gy in 1.5 Gy per fraction for intermediate-risk disease and 15 to 20 Gy in 1.5 Gy per fraction for high-risk disease. The CTV for whole liver RT is the whole liver with a margin of 0.5 to 1 cm. For patients with intermediate-risk histology, the dose to the whole liver for intermediate-risk disease is 14.4 Gy in 8 fractions with a boost of 10.8 Gy in 6 fractions if there is a macroscopic disease, and high-risk disease is 19.8 Gy in 11 fractions with a boost of 16.2 Gy in 9 fractions to the macroscopic disease.

RHABDOMYOSARCOMA

Rhabdomyosarcoma (RMS), the most common soft-tissue sarcomas in children, may arise at any site, although they tend to have a predilection for sites in the head and neck (45%) and urogenital regions (35%). These include head and neck sites such as the orbit, nasopharynx and middle ear and urogenital tract sites such as the bladder, prostate and vagina. Tumours that arise in sites such as the nasopharynx and middle ear have the propensity for base of the skull and intracranial invasion and are referred to as parameningeal RMS. The median age at presentation is 5 years.

There are two main histopathological subtypes: alveolar (15%) and embryonal RMS (70%). Generally, embryonal RMS occurs in younger children and has a better prognosis, whereas alveolar RMS occurs in older children and has a poorer prognosis. Eighty percent of alveolar RMS have a specific chromosomal translocation that results in the fusion of the PAX3 or PAX7 gene with FOXO1. The fusion-negative alveolar RMS has a prognosis similar to embryonal RMS.

In many European countries, including the United Kingdom, children have been treated according to the SIOP series of studies. The basis of these has been the use of intensive chemotherapy to improve survival and reduce the use and intensity of local therapy with surgery and RT, thus minimising long-term effects. The strategy for this series of studies includes stratifying patients within risk groups based on histological subtype (embryonal versus alveolar histology), stage of disease and primary tumour site. Patients with localised disease are categorised into low-risk, standard-risk, high-risk and very high-risk groups based on fusion status, the International Rhabdomyosarcoma (IRS) group, the site of disease (favourable sites are genitourinary, non-parameningeal head and neck, orbit or biliary), age (favourable age is >1 year to <10 years), nodal status and size (<5 cm in the longest diameter is favourable). There are three IRS groups: group I, primary complete resection; group II, microscopic residual tumour or primary complete excision but with node positive; and group III, macroscopic residual disease.

Surgery and RT are essential in achieving optimal local disease control. Patients in the low-risk category, that is, those with localised tumours that are microscopically completely resected, are treated with chemotherapy using actinomycin-D and vincristine for 9 weeks. Standard-risk tumours are those that are locally more extensive but at selected favourable sites, the vagina, uterus or paratestis, and are treated with ifosfamide, vincristine and actinomycin-D. High-risk tumours include other incompletely resected tumours, including all those arising in parameningeal sites (nasopharynx, middle ear) and those with involved lymph nodes. The 3-year event-free survival for children with low-risk disease is 90%, standard risk is 70% to 80%, high-risk is 50% to 55% and very high risk is 30% to 40%. Children with lung and bone metastases have a poorer outcome: a 3-year event-free survival of less than 30%.

Although there are risks of local and metastatic recurrences, local tumour control is an essential consideration in managing RMS. RT is an important modality for many patients, improving local control and overall survival. Radical RT is considered when there is inoperable residual disease after induction chemotherapy. Adjuvant RT is indicated in patients with any risk factors for local recurrence, such as a positive resection margin (R1 or R2) after surgery, node-positive disease, fusion-positive disease or metastatic disease.

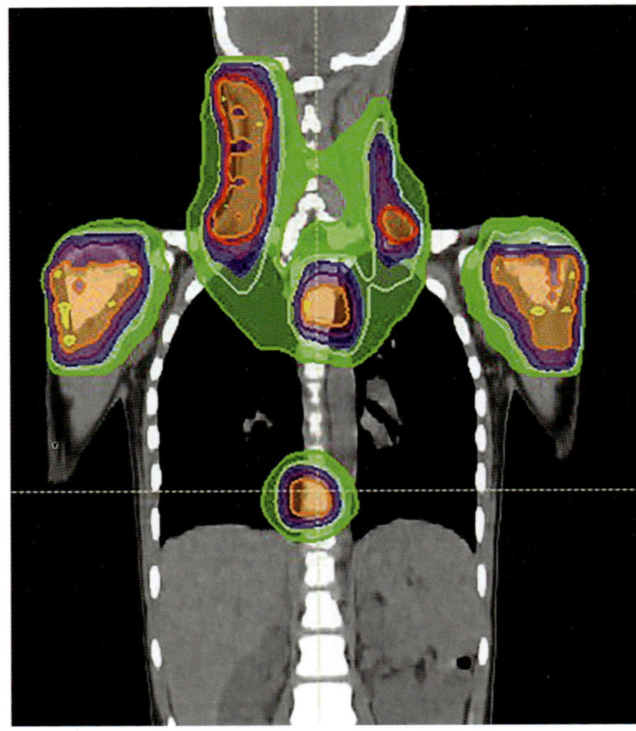

Fig. 34.9 Radiotherapy to primary and metastatic sites for rhabdomyosarcoma of the neck with multiple bone metastases (both humeral heads and spine).

Patients with inoperable residual disease are treated with radical RT in two phases or using a simultaneous integrated boost (SIB). In phase I, 41.4 Gy in 23 fractions is delivered to a target volume encompassing pretreatment disease. In phase II, 9 Gy in 5 fractions is delivered to the posttreatment primary disease and bulky node volume. Adjuvant or preoperative RT is given in 41.4 Gy in 23 fractions. The same dose is also suitable for metastatic sites of disease (Fig. 34.9). Planning of RT requires meticulous attention to detail, and proton therapy or IMRT/VMAT/tomotherapy is used to minimise RT dose to adjacent normal tissue.

Brachytherapy may be considered for a few highly selected children with RMS, usually with limited tumours arising in the head and neck, vagina, bladder or prostate. However, in the United Kingdom, the main area where brachytherapy has been successfully employed has been for the treatment of primary RMS arising in the vaginal vault. Brachytherapy can provide a means of local tumour control with reduced morbidity compared with external beam radiotherapy (EBRT). However, for a child to be suitable for brachytherapy, the tumour must be sufficiently localised to achieve local control with a small planning target volume (PTV) suitable for brachytherapy rather than a larger volume suitable for only EBRT (typically 2–3 cm). If brachytherapy is being considered for primary genitourinary tract tumours, discussion amongst oncologists and surgeons at an early stage is essential, followed by a joint examination under anaesthesia (EUA). Both low dose rate (LDR) and high dose rate (HDR) afterloading brachytherapy techniques have been used with equal success. Most young children require sedation or general anaesthesia during treatment, and HDR brachytherapy has been evaluated in several centres internationally.

The European Paediatric Soft Tissue Sarcoma Group (EpSSG) Frontline and Relapsed Rhabdomyosarcoma (FaR-RMS) trial addresses a number of RT questions. Patients with predicted R0/R1 resection after induction chemotherapy will be randomised to receive either preoperative or postoperative RT. Patients with a higher local failure risk (defined as disease in an unfavourable site and/or age ≥18 years) will be randomised to receive preoperative RT. They will be treated with either 41.4 Gy or 50.4 Gy. Those randomised to receive postoperative RT will be treated with 50.4 Gy or 59.4 Gy. The randomisation for patients with unfavourable metastatic disease will be either for RT to metastatic sites or no RT.

EWING SARCOMA AND PERIPHERAL PRIMITIVE NEUROECTODERMAL TUMOUR

Ewing sarcoma of bone is predominantly a disease of adolescents, having its peak incidence in the early teenage years. The 5-year overall survival is 60% to 70% for localised disease and 20% to 40% for metastatic disease. Chapter 33 gives a detailed description of Ewing sarcoma.

Peripheral primitive neuroectodermal tumour (pPNET) is a rare aggressive variant of small round cell carcinomas arising from the neural crest cells. pPNET is part of the Ewing sarcoma family of tumours and has a chromosomal translocation, t(11;22) (q24;q12). The management principles are similar to those of Ewing sarcoma.

OSTEOSARCOMA

Osteosarcoma is the most frequent bone tumour of childhood, occurring between the ages of 10 and 20 years. The most frequent primary sites are the lower femur and upper tibia, with approximately 65% developing around the knee. Less frequent sites include the humerus, fibula, sacrum, spine, mandible and pelvis. Before the advent of effective chemotherapy, approximately 80% of patients died because of the progression of lung metastases. Currently, a survival rate of approximately 55% can be achieved using intensive adjuvant chemotherapy. Most primary tumours can be resected and the affected bone replaced by a titanium endoprosthesis, thus avoiding an amputation. The most frequently employed chemotherapy regimen is the combination of high-dose methotrexate, cisplatin and doxorubicin.

RT has only a minor role in the management of osteosarcoma. However, it is probably not as radioresistant as previously thought. RT is indicated in the following situations:

- Positive resection margin and further surgery feasible and/or a poor response to chemotherapy (<90% necrosis)
- Unresectable tumours (e.g. in the head and neck region, the vertebrae and the pelvis)
- Intralesional resection or contaminated margin with no further surgery feasible or planned
- Palliative setting (e.g. local or metastatic deposits causing symptoms)

In curative settings, the dose has to be as high as normal tissues will tolerate, that is, 60 to 70 Gy if possible. RT can be employed for the local palliation of metastases, using a relatively high dose such as 40 Gy in 15 fractions.

CENTRAL NERVOUS SYSTEM TUMOURS

Tumours of the CNS account for approximately 20% to 25% of malignant childhood tumours and are the leading cause of death from childhood cancer. Approximately 420 children develop CNS tumours each year in the United Kingdom. However, individual tumour types are uncommon, and experience in managing each type is limited. The overall 5-year survival rate is approximately 75%; however, the burdens of survivorship are high, and the majority of survivors experience sequelae from either the tumour or therapy or, very frequently, a combination of both.

Specialised paediatric neurooncology multidisciplinary teams manage children with CNS tumours and their families.

RT for children with CNS tumours is technically challenging. Many children require CSRT, one of the most complex techniques in most oncology departments.

Long-Term Effects of Radiotherapy for Central Nervous System Tumours

Of greatest concern are the long-term neuropsychological effects of RT on the CNS, particularly for very young children. Other factors include the direct and indirect effects of the tumour itself and the effects of surgery. One of the most important factors increasing the risk and severity of long-term neuropsychological sequelae is the young age at diagnosis. For children younger than age 3 years at diagnosis, RT is delayed, if possible, by the use of chemotherapy.

Children receiving CSRT will frequently experience dose-dependent spinal shortening as a direct effect of irradiation of the spine. For many children the hypothalamic/pituitary axis has to be included in the irradiated volume. This often results in growth hormone deficiency, but other endocrine deficiencies, such as thyrotrophin-releasing hormone (TRH) or adrenocorticotrophic hormone (ACTH) deficiency, may occur. TRH deficiency is relatively easily managed by thyroid hormone replacement, but ACTH deficiency may require life-long steroid replacement therapy, which may be problematic.

Chemotherapy for Central Nervous System Tumours

Chemotherapy also has an established role for the majority of paediatric CNS tumours. Secreting intracranial germ cell tumours (GCTs) are routinely treated with chemotherapy. Adjuvant chemotherapy improves the outcome for standard-risk MB compared with RT alone and is also used for high-risk diseases. The use of chemotherapy can delay the need for RT for very young children, particularly those with low-grade astrocytoma and ependymoma.

Low-Grade Gliomas

Low-grade gliomas (LGGs) comprise the most frequent group of children's CNS tumours (see Table 31.1). The most frequent histological types are WHO grade 1 (pilocytic) and grade 2 (usually fibrillary), with other varieties, such as ganglioglioma and oligodendroglioma, much less frequent. The presence of neurofibromatosis type 1 (NF1) predisposes to the development of these tumours. LGGs may undergo long periods of quiescence, even when not completely resected. It is also clear that LGGs are more chemosensitive than previously thought. Following treatment of LGG, the 5-year survival rate is relatively high at approximately 80% to 85%, but late relapse is not uncommon.

Initial treatment usually involves a complete surgical resection if it is safe. This is usually more straightforward for tumours in the cerebellum, where complete resection is generally feasible, compared with those from the optic tract or optic chiasm. Because of the considerable risk of surgery in this area, tumours with typical features on MRI scanning of a hypothalamic/optic tract astrocytoma are not necessarily biopsied, as many consider the risk of the procedure (i.e. visual deterioration) outweighs the risk of an incorrect diagnosis.

Following initial maximal surgical resection, patients with grade 1 tumours are observed. Patients with clinical or radiological evidence of progression, those with severe symptoms or those with a threat to vision receive nonsurgical treatment. If further surgery is not possible, nonsurgical treatment is indicated. Systemic therapies are used to delay or prevent the need for RT. The optimal timing of RT is not known but is generally considered in children age 8 to 10 years when there are no other options for treatment. Using the drug combination of carboplatin and vincristine, the majority of children with LGG can achieve either a response or stabilisation of previously progressive tumours. RT yields a 10-year event-free survival of more than 70% and overall survival of more than 95% for LGGs.

RT for LGGs is based on careful imaging for target volume definition. The technique will depend upon the tumour site and anatomy. A volume-based planning technique using IMRT/VMAT or proton beam therapy delivers homogeneous RT to the PTV and minimises the dose of nontarget tissues and OARs. The CTV includes the GTV and, in the case of surgical resection, any brain tissue previously surrounding the tumour with a margin in potential areas of spread of 0.5 cm. Patients are immobilised in a supine immobilisation device. The extent of the GTV is localised using T2 or fluid-attenuated inversion recovery (FLAIR) images on the MRI scan. For planning, CT/MRI fusion should be employed. The RT dose is specified to the ICRU reference point. In international studies, the prescribed dose is 54 Gy in 30 fractions of 1.8 Gy daily. For patients with a spinal cord primary requiring RT, the dose is 50.4 Gy in 28 fractions of 1.8 Gy.

High-Grade Gliomas

Unlike in adults, where high-grade gliomas (HGGs) comprise the most frequent group of primary CNS tumours, HGGs are uncommon in childhood. As with HGGs arising in adults, the outlook is generally abysmal, and survival rates are currently approximately 20% at 5 years. Infants under age 3 years typically do better than older children, resulting in outcomes similar to those of young adults. Treatment is based on surgical resection and postoperative RT, generally 54 Gy in 30 fractions. Current management is based on concurrent and adjuvant temozolomide chemotherapy together with focal radical RT using a similar regimen to the current standard approach for adults with glioblastoma. A recent European trial of adding bevacizumab to standard treatment with RT and temozolomide failed to achieve additional survival benefits. Identifying the potential for novel systemic agents to improve outcomes is an essential priority for these patients.

Brainstem Glioma

This group of brain tumours comprises a heterogeneous mix of tumours arising in the midbrain, pons and medulla. They are classified as focal (5%–10%), dorsal exophytic (10%–20%), corticomedullary (5%–10%) and diffuse intrinsic tumours (75%–85%). Focal, dorsal exophytic and corticomedullary tumours are generally LGGs. Surgical excision is the treatment of choice, with RT reserved for inoperable tumours.

The majority of children with brainstem gliomas have diffuse intrinsic pontine gliomas (DIPGs), which, when subject to biopsy, have generally been shown to be high-grade astrocytomas. They can be diagnosed by their typical MRI appearance (Fig. 34.10). A biopsy procedure, such as a stereotactic biopsy, is often considered to be risky. Diffuse midline gliomas, H3K27M mutant, occur in the thalamus, brainstem, spinal cord and other midline structures. The prognosis for DIPG and H3K27M mutant gliomas is poor. Because of these tumours' frequent relatively short history, RT often needs to be commenced quickly. Although RT results in the improvement of neurological symptoms for approximately 70% of children, median survival is about 9 months, and there are very few long-term survivors. The management of these children remains a significant challenge, and domiciliary palliative care usually has to be introduced at a relatively early stage.

Patients are generally treated with a relatively straightforward technique with CT planning. The CTV includes the GTV as defined on the diagnostic MRI scan with a margin of 2 cm along potential areas of spread superiorly, inferiorly and posteriorly along the brainstem. Patients are treated supine in a Perspex or thermoplastic shell with CT simulation. The acceptable dose regimens are 54 Gy in 30 fractions of 1.8 Gy daily for low-grade tumours and 39 Gy in 13 fractions for DIPG. Children with progressive DIPG after 6 months of initial treatment may be considered for a short course of reirradiation, such as 20 Gy in 10 fractions, to provide an additional period of palliation.

Ependymoma

Ependymomas arise from the intracranial or spinal ependymal lining. Historically, management was with surgical excision, followed by RT, which was generally craniospinal for those with posterior fossa primaries or high-grade histology. However, it is now generally recognised that, although there is a risk of leptomeningeal metastases at relapse, this risk does not appear to be modified using CSRT. The overall 5-year survival rate is approximately 50% to 60%. In most studies, prognostic factors include the extent of resection and tumour grade. The current European SIOP ependymoma trial recommends that, for completely resected tumours, postoperative focal RT (59.4 Gy in 33 fractions) should be given using a CTV margin of 1.0 cm. For incompletely resected tumours, an initial trial of chemotherapy using vincristine, cyclophosphamide and etoposide is employed, with further evaluation of postchemotherapy resectability (so-called second-look surgery). The predominant site of relapse is postoperative RT within the surgical bed, and it is important to try to achieve a complete or near-complete resection. Several studies report a 3-to-4-year overall survival of 30% to 40% with reirradiation to a dose of 54 Gy in 30 fractions.

Embryonal Tumours

MB is a primitive neuronal tumour that arises in the cerebellum, usually from the vermis. It has a propensity for metastatic spread via the cerebral spinal fluid (CSF) (leptomeningeal). MB is both radiosensitive and chemosensitive. Primitive neuroectodermal tumour (PNET)

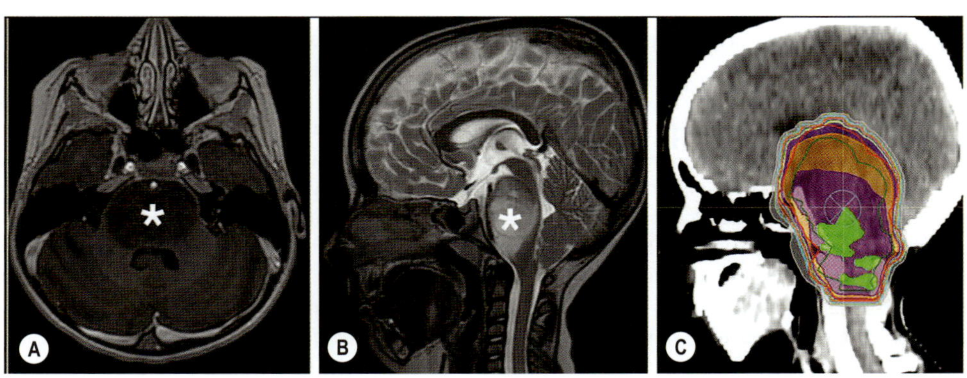

Fig. 34.10 Axial (A) and sagittal (B) views of diffuse pontine glioma (*) on diagnosis magnetic resonance imaging scans. (C) Dose distribution of conformal planning using opposed lateral beams.

arises elsewhere in the CNS, usually the supratentorial cerebral cortex, but sometimes the pineal area (pineoblastoma). Supratentorial PNET has a significantly worse prognosis (approximately 40%–50% 5-year survival versus 60%–70% for MB).

MBs are managed by maximal surgical resection followed by CSRT and a boost to the primary site. Postoperative treatment is based on the risk group: standard risk (two-thirds of patients) and high risk. Patients with more than 1.5 cm^2 postoperative residual disease, evidence of metastases at diagnosis or anaplastic large cell histology are considered high risk. Children younger than age 3 to 5 years are generally treated with a chemotherapy-only approach.

Patients with standard-risk disease are treated with craniospinal irradiation (CSI) (23.4 Gy) with a boost (30.6 Gy) followed by adjuvant chemotherapy with cisplatin, lomustine and vincristine. The boost RT is given to the posterior cranial fossa or the tumour bed with a 1-to-2-cm margin. This approach yields a 10-year overall of 81% and an event-free survival of 76%. Patients with high-risk disease are treated with CSI (36–39.6 Gy) with a boost to the posterior cranial fossa (to a total dose of 54–55.9 Gy) and focal spinal disease (to a total dose of 45–54 Gy) with concurrent or adjuvant chemotherapy. This approach yields a 5-year event-free survival of 50% to 70%.

Since the 1990s in North America, it has been a standard practice to employ adjuvant chemotherapy (vincristine, lomustine and cisplatin) following RT, and this has now become a standard practice in clinical practice and trials.

Current trials evaluate risk-adapted treatments based on histological subtypes of MB and molecular biological tumour parameters. In 2016 the WHO classification (2016) recognised four molecular subgroups of MB, namely, the Wingless (WNT), Sonic Hedgehog (SHH), group 3 and group 4. The WNT subgroup is characterised by a very good prognosis compared with the other subgroups, with long-term survival of over 90%. Most WNT subgroup MBs have classical histology, with these tumours demonstrating beta-catenin nucleopositivity, *CTNNB1* gene mutations (90%) and monosomy 6 (86%). WNT MB can occur at all ages but is infrequent in infants, and less than 5% of children have metastasis at diagnosis. Although overall MB is more common in males, the male-to-female (M:F) ratio for the WNT subgroup is approximately 1:1.

The SHH MB subgroups include *TP53*-mutant and *TP53*-wildtype subgroups. They are named after the sonic hedgehog signalling pathway, which is considered to drive tumour initiation in most cases. The frequency of SHH subgroups of MB is bimodal and frequent in infants under age 3 years and in adults. The M:F ratio is approximately 1:1. Most nodular/desmoplastic MBs are included within the SHH subgroup. However, around 50% of SHH subgroup MB have other histological subtypes, including classical, large cell/anaplastic and MBEN varieties. Approximately 20% of children present with metastasis at diagnosis. The prognosis for SHH appears similar to group 4 (see later) and intermediate between WNT and group 3.

Group 3 MB represents the subgroup of MB with the worst prognosis. Most MBs in group 3 are classical MB and include the majority of large-cell/anaplastic tumours. They occur more commonly in males than females (2:1) and arise in infants and older children but rarely in adults. They frequently (40%–50%) present with leptomeningeal metastases. Group 3 MB is typically characterised by high-level amplification of the *MYC* proto-oncogene, and almost all cases exhibit aberrant *MYC* expression.

Patients with group 4 MB have an intermediate to good prognosis, similar to patients with SHH tumours. They include classical and large cell/anaplastic histologies. Group 4 tumours account for approximately 30% to 40% of MB cases. This subgroup represents the archetypal MB, for example, a 7-year-old male child with a classical histology MB. The M:F ratio is approximately 2:1.

Improvements in understanding the molecular mechanisms of MB tumourigenesis are emerging as important factors in clinical trial design, leading to a tailored approach for different histological and molecular biological subtypes. Collaborative clinical trial groups are developing studies that will prospectively investigate therapy stratification according to pathological, biological and more traditional clinical parameters. In particular, clinical studies are beginning to involve cautiously lowering the treatment intensity for patients with WNT MB and maintaining intensity for those in group 3. Studies suggest that WNT-pathway MB can be treated with a reduced dose of CSRT, 18 Gy, rather than the more conventional 23.4 Gy. For patients with group 3 MB, the priority is to improve outcomes by intensification of treatment.

Studies of Altered Fractionation for Medulloblastoma/ Primitive Neuroectodermal Tumour

Hyperfractionated radiotherapy (HFRT) involves the use of a larger number of small fractions, usually delivered twice daily. Long-term normal tissue effects are related to fraction size, and the aim of HFRT is to improve the therapeutic ratio by increasing the antitumour effect, reducing long-term effects on the CNS or a combination of both.

A multicentre French study employing a CSRT dose of 36 Gy and a primary tumour dose of 68 Gy has also produced encouraging results. The use of HFRT was evaluated in the European PNET-4 randomised study. The PNET-4 study aimed to assess whether the use of HFRT could improve survival without an increase in long-term effects. Conventionally fractionated RT, employing a craniospinal dose of 23.4 Gy followed by 30.6 Gy to the posterior fossa, was compared with an HFRT regimen. The HFRT dose per fraction was 1 Gy, given twice daily with a minimum interval of 8 hours. The craniospinal dose was 36 Gy, with a second phase of 24 Gy to the whole posterior fossa and a final phase of 8 Gy to the tumour bed. The outcome of this trial was that there was no benefit for HFRT with respect to tumour control or survival, and conventional daily fractionation of 1.67 to 1.80 Gy remains the standard of care. The current SIOP high-risk MB trial compares conventional fractionation with HFRT.

Craniospinal Radiotherapy

CSRT is one of the most complex RT techniques delivered in oncology departments. The shape of the CRT is complex, including the entire cranial and spinal meninges. Traditionally, the technique employed lateral-opposed cranial fields, with one or more posterior spinal fields carefully matched onto the lower border of the cranial fields. Shielding of the face, dentition, nasal structures and lenses is necessary. In the past two decades, significant developments have been made in advancing techniques for CSRT to achieve maximum homogeneity within the CTV and normal tissue sparing. A range of technological solutions are available for the delivery of CSRT, including IMRT, VMAT, and tomotherapy. Proton beam therapy achieves maximal normal tissue sparing, particularly from the exit dose to organs anterior to the spine.

The CTV includes the entire arachnoid space, which consists of intracranial and spinal meninges extending inferiorly to the lower border of the thecal sac. Great care is taken to include the cribriform fossa, temporal lobe and base of the skull. This should include the extensions of the meninges into the cranial nerve foramina, including the intraorbital optic nerve in the cranial CTV and the extensions of CSF along the nerve root laterally in the spinal CTV. In children the cribriform fossa frequently lies between the lenses (Fig. 34.11A). In many series of patients treated for MB, the cribriform fossa has been the site for isolated recurrence in a significant minority of patients. Treating the

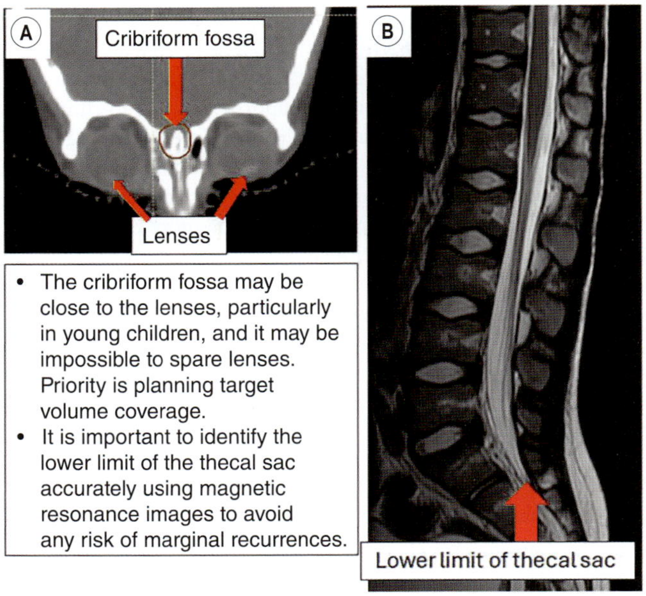

Fig. 34.11 Illustrations of the closeness of the cribriform fossa to the lenses (A) and lower limit of the thecal sac on T2-weighted magnetic resonance imaging scan (B).

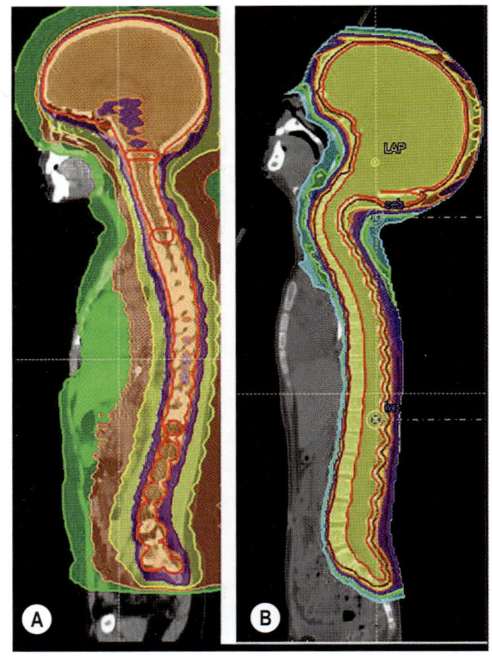

Fig. 34.12 A comparison of dose distribution for craniospinal radiotherapy using photons (A) and protons (B) showing optimal sparing of normal tissues outside planning target volume by protons.

CTV and adequately shielding the lenses may not always be possible, so priority is given to treating the CTV. Current management involves the use of cisplatin chemotherapy, which carries the risk of ototoxicity. In planning CSRT, the dose to the middle and inner ears is minimised without compromising the dose to the CTV.

The lower border of the spinal field has generally been placed at the lower border of the second sacral vertebra. However, there is evidence that the lower border of the thecal sac varies, and planning of the lower border of the spinal field should be based on MRI scanning (Fig. 34.11B). Patients are treated in a Perspex headshell, generally in the supine position, which is more comfortable and safer in the case of the requirement for anaesthesia than the traditional prone position. For example, the body may be immobilised in an evacuated polystyrene bag. The prescribed dose depends upon the clinical scenario. Currently, 23.4 Gy in 13 fractions of 1.8 Gy daily is employed for standard-risk MB and 36 Gy in 20 fractions for high-risk MB.

Meticulous attention to detail in the planning and delivery of CSRT is essential, and accuracy contributes to the chances of curing MB and other PNETs. It is necessary to avoid areas of underdose at field junctions and partially shield any part of the intracranial or spinal meninges.

When planning the primary tumour boost for MB, it is generally accepted that the CTV should encompass the surgical cavity and any residual tumour, with a 1-to-1.5-cm margin for standard-risk MB. The aim is to deliver a total dose of 54 to 55.8 Gy in 1.8 Gy per fraction to the tumour bed. The CTV is the whole posterior fossa or tumour bed for high-risk MB, delivering 19.8 Gy in 11 fractions. Whenever facilities are available, proton beam therapy is the technique of choice (Fig. 34.12).

Intracranial Germ Cell Tumours

Intracranial GCTs account for approximately 30% of paediatric GCTs, and most patients are age 11 to 20 years. Histological appearance is similar to their gonadal counterparts, and tumours arise in midline locations such as the suprasellar or pineal regions. Diagnosis is based on clinical presentation, tumour markers (β-HCG and AFP in serum and CSF), CSF cytology and imaging. A biopsy is not attempted if tumour marker-positive disease (AFP >50 IU/L or hCG in serum or CSF >50 IU/L) and radiological appearances are typical of intracranial GCTs. Biopsy is attempted in all cases of uncertain diagnosis.

For therapeutic purposes, GCTs are categorised as germinoma and nongerminoma. Nongerminoma is diagnosed if there is a raised serum/CSF level of AFP greater than 25 IU/L and β- hCG greater than 50 IU/L in Europe and greater than 100 IU/L in the United States or there is histological evidence of a nongerminatous component.

Germinomas are very radiosensitive. The traditional view has been that CSRT should be employed because of the risk of leptomeningeal metastases. With this approach, more than 90% of germinomas are cured but at a cost of significant late toxicities. Therefore, studies have attempted to reduce the dose and volume of RT by integrating chemotherapy. In the latest SIOPE GCT II trial, patients with localised germinoma are treated with chemotherapy (two cycles of carboplatin and etoposide alternating with two cycles of ifosfamide and etoposide) followed by whole ventricular irradiation (WVI) alone (24 Gy in 15 fractions) if there is a complete response at reassessment after chemotherapy. If there is a partial response, WVI (24 Gy) is followed by a tumour bed boost (16 Gy in 10 fractions) (Fig. 34.13), or if there is a stable disease, surgery is followed by RT. Early results suggest that 24 Gy in 15 fractions achieves excellent cure rates of more than 95% in patients with complete chemotherapy responses. The SIOP CNS GCT 96 study reported 5-year event-free survival and overall survival of 98% in patients with metastatic germinoma treated with platinum-based chemotherapy followed by CSRT (CSI 24 Gy) and a boost to the primary tumour (16 Gy) and site of metastases. Therefore, the current treatment recommendation in metastatic germinoma is CSI, followed by a boost to primary and metastatic sites.

Management of localised nongerminomatous GCTs varies globally. In Europe the current approach is chemotherapy followed by tumour bed RT (54 Gy in 30 fractions), which gives a 10-year overall survival of 67%. Patients with disseminated disease are treated with chemotherapy followed by CSI (30 Gy) and a boost to the primary tumour and macroscopic metastases (24 Gy), which gives a 5-year progression-free survival of 72%.

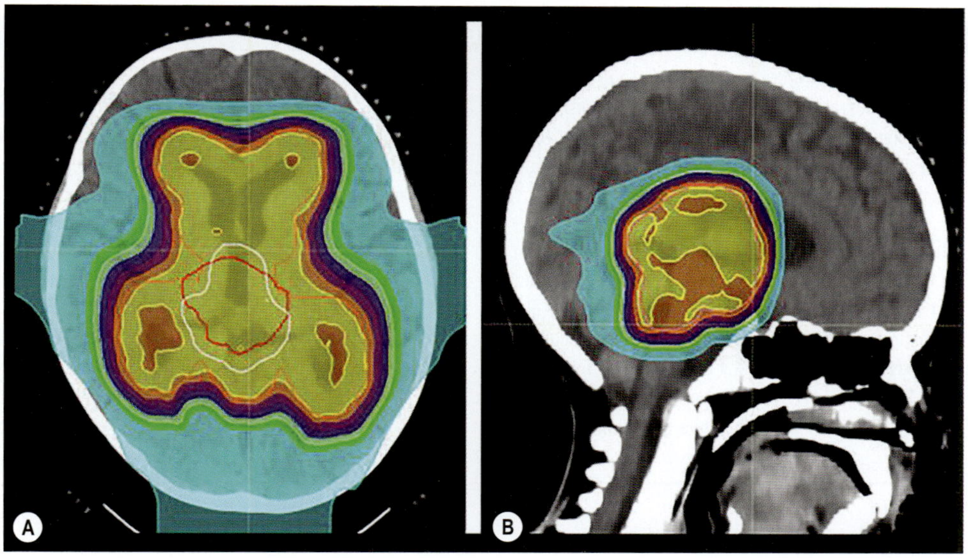

Fig. 34.13 Whole ventricular radiotherapy (A) and tumour bed boost (B) using proton beam therapy for an intracranial germ cell tumour.

Craniopharyngioma

Craniopharyngiomas account for approximately 5% to 10% of intracranial tumours in childhood. These are predominantly cystic tumours that arise in the suprasellar area from remnants of Rathke pouch. Although considered histologically benign, they are often associated with considerable morbidity, such as pituitary deficiencies including diabetes insipidus and disturbances of hypothalamic function such as obesity. They are frequently adherent to adjacent structures within the CNS. There is a significant risk of involvement of the optic chiasm with a risk of visual impairment or blindness. Small craniopharyngiomas may be amenable to complete surgical excision if this can be achieved without risk of damage to the optic chiasm. An alternative approach is to consider partial or subtotal excision of the tumour with postoperative RT. The margin for CTV around the GTV is generally approximately 0.5 cm, with a dose of 50 to 55 Gy in a fraction size of 1.67 to 1.8 Gy. Long-term local control rates of approximately 80% can be achieved with either complete or partial resection and postoperative RT.

Proton Therapy for Paediatric Tumours

Proton therapy has been available for several decades in selected centres, mainly in North America. In the past few years, the proton treatment facilities have exponentially increased globally, so children with potentially curative cancers are treated predominantly with proton beam therapy in developed countries. The modulated Bragg peak can deliver homogeneous irradiation to the target volume while reducing the magnitude and/or extent of the low-dose area beyond. This may be clinically relevant for long-term effects in children. For several decades, proton therapy has had an established role in the treatment of adults with skull base chordomas and chondrosarcomas. This role has now been extended to the treatment of children. In addition, planning studies have demonstrated the potential for improving the therapeutic ratio for RT for tumours either within or adjacent to the CNS and achieving a uniform dose within the target volume, while potentially minimising the severity of neuropsychological sequelae. Chapter 37 deals with proton beam therapy.

CONCLUSION

Paediatric oncology management continues to present many challenges, and RT plays an important role in the treatment of many of these children. They require the highest standards in RT planning and delivery, incorporating modern technical developments. Children present with a wide variety of malignancies, which pose many different problems for the patients themselves and for their families. Thus, management needs to be family centred as well as patient centred. Although cure rates for the majority of childhood cancers have continued to improve over the past decade, this has frequently been achieved with increased intensity of chemotherapy. Compared with adult radiation oncology practice, when planning RT for children, consideration of the long-term effects of treatment is always of paramount importance. Constant vigilance for interactions between chemotherapy and RT is required with the increasing use of concurrent combined modality therapy, including intensive chemotherapy. Therapeutic developments initially investigated in adults, such as hyperfractionation, also require investigation for childhood cancers. Clinicians and parents should be encouraged to recruit children in clinical trials whenever a suitable trial is available (Box 34.1).

BOX 34.1 Summary of Current Paediatric Cancer Trials

Altogether-1 Trial

The objectives of this current UK and European collaborative trial in ALL are to deescalate treatments in children with low-risk ALL without compromising the chances of cure and to escalate treatment in children with high risk to improve the chances of cure. For example, in the low-risk group, children will be randomised to omit doxorubicin in the delayed intensification phase of treatment, whereas in the high-risk group, children will be randomised with the introduction of either two cycles of inotuzumab (anti-CD22 antibody) before the maintenance phase or low-dose 6-Thioguanin (6TG) into the maintenance phase with monitoring of 6TG incorporation into the DNA of leukocytes.

European Paediatric Soft Tissue Sarcoma Group (EpSSG) Frontline and Relapsed Rhabdomyosarcoma (FaR-RMS) Trial

This trial addresses a number of RT questions. In this study, patients with predicted R0/R1 resection after induction chemotherapy will be randomised to receive either preoperative or postoperative RT, and patients with a higher local

(continued)

BOX 34.1 Summary of Current Paediatric Cancer Trials—cont'd

failure risk (defined as disease in an unfavourable site and/or age ≥18 years) will be randomised to receive preoperative RT and will be treated with either 41.4 Gy or 50.4 Gy. Those randomised to receive postoperative RT will be treated with either 50.4 Gy or 59.4 Gy. The randomisation for patients with unfavourable metastatic disease will be either for RT to metastatic sites or for no RT.

SIOP High-Risk Medulloblastoma (SIOP-HRMB) Trial

This is a biomarker-driven randomised clinical trial in high-risk MB evaluating whether the clinical outcome can be improved with hyperfractionated/accelerated radiotherapy (HART) or high-dose therapy with thiotepa followed by conventional RT. Patients with non-WNT histology with any risk factors of metastatic disease, large cell/anaplastic histology, MYC amplification, MYCN amplification or TP53 somatic mutation (both in SHH subgroup tumours only) will be eligible for this study.

Ependymoma-2 Trial

This current SIOP European trial is a randomised trial investigating whether the addition of chemotherapy (vincristine, etoposide, cyclophosphamide, cisplatin) improves the outcome for patients with completely resected intracranial ependymoma treated by complete surgical excision and postoperative RT, 59.4 Gy in 33 fractions. Patients who have inoperable residual disease also receive a stereotactic RT boost (8 Gy in 2 fractions) to the residual tumour.

SIOPEN High-Risk Neuroblastoma 2 (HR-NBL2) Trial

The current SIOPEN High-Risk Neuroblastoma 2 (HR-NBL2) trial involves a comparison of two treatment strategies in three therapeutic phases (induction, high-dose chemotherapy and RT). For local RT, the study will compare standard dose RT (21.6 Gy in 1.8 Gy per fraction) with standard dose (21.6 Gy) plus boost RT (14.4 in 1.8 Gy per fraction) to the residual tumour.

FURTHER READING

Ajithkumar T, Avanzo M, Yorke E, et al. Brain and brain stem necrosis after reirradiation for recurrent childhood primary central nervous system tumors: a PENTEC comprehensive review. *Int J Radiat Oncol Biol Phys*. 2024;119(2):655–668.

Ajithkumar T, Kortmann RD. "Indeed, cure is not enough"—a reflection on paediatric radiation oncology. *Clin Oncol*. 2019;31(3):135–138.

Constine LS, Marks LB, Milano MT, et al. A user's guide and summary of Pediatric Normal Tissue Effects in the Clinic (PENTEC): radiation dose-volume response for adverse effects after childhood cancer therapy and future directions. *Int J Radiat Oncol Biol Phys*. 2024;119(2):321–337.

Faure Conter C, Calaminus G, Nicholson J, et al. Central nervous system germ cell tumor, an archetypal AYA tumor and a model for pediatric and neuro-oncology collaboration, review from the EURACAN domain 10 group. *Front Oncol*. 2022;12:971697.

Gaze MN. Good practice guide for paediatric radiotherapy. *Clin Oncol*. 2019;31(3):139–141.

Inaba H, Mullighan CG. Pediatric acute lymphoblastic leukemia. *Haematologica*. 2020;105(11):2524–2539.

Jackson K, Packer RJ. Recent advances in pediatric medulloblastoma. *Curr Neurol Neurosci Rep*. 2023;23(12):841–848.

Krystal J, Foster JH. Treatment of high-risk neuroblastoma. *Children (Basel)*. 2023;10(8):1302.

Lo AC, Dieckmann K, Pelz T, et al. Pediatric classical Hodgkin lymphoma. *Pediatr Blood Cancer*. 2021;68(Suppl 2):e28562.

Mandeville HC. Radiotherapy in the management of childhood rhabdomyosarcoma. *Clin Oncol (R Coll Radiol)*. 2019;31(7):462–470.

Padovani L, Horan G, Ajithkumar T. Radiotherapy advances in paediatric medulloblastoma treatment. *Clin Oncol (R Coll Radiol)*. 2019;31(3):171–181.

Sait SF, Giantini-Larsen AM, Tringale KR, Souweidane MM, Karajannis MA. Treatment of pediatric low-grade gliomas. *Curr Neurol Neurosci Rep*. 2023;23(4):185–199.

Steinmeier T, Schleithoff SS, Timmermann B. Evolving radiotherapy techniques in paediatric oncology. *Clin Oncol*. 2019;31(3):142–150.

Thorp N, Gandola L. Management of ependymoma in children, adolescents and young adults. *Clin Oncol*. 2019;31(3):162–170.

Tsang DS, Laperriere NJ. Re-irradiation for paediatric tumours. *Clin Oncol*. 2019;31(3):191–198.

van den Heuvel-Eibrink MM, Hol JA, Pritchard-Jones K, et al. Position paper: rationale for the treatment of Wilms tumour in the UMBRELLA SIOP-RTSG 2016 protocol. *Nat Rev Urol*. 2017;14(12):743–752.

35

Care of Patients During Radiotherapy

Heather Reid and Pete Bridge

CHAPTER OUTLINE

INTRODUCTION

Patient Care Principles

When patients are referred for radiotherapy (RT), they will expect that their treatment is planned and delivered in an optimal way. Everyone involved in this process is well aware that patients have a right to expect that they will be well cared for and supported during this time. The quality of this care is dependent on a multiplicity of factors, and the aim should be that it is all-encompassing and holistic, addressing both the physical and emotional needs of patients.

The responsibility of assessing how patients are as they progress through treatment and how they are coping with their treatment belongs to all, as is an acknowledgment of where an individual's skills and expertise start and stop and when patients should be cared for by more appropriate members of the team. It is to be recommended that RT centres adopt a culture that encourages both the philosophy and the mechanisms to facilitate such a team approach, and this team approach should reach out to the interface between primary and secondary care. Coordination of care therefore needs patients and their carers to remain the focus of the process, and this means that they should be kept informed and involved and that their autonomy and rights to be included in the treatment decision-making process are respected at all times.

The most simplistic method of exploring supportive care in RT is to consider any aspect of care that may be experienced by the patient within the physical, psychosocial and spiritual realms, and this chapter will introduce some of the common themes within supportive care of all RT patients. The physical aspects of supportive care in relation to the management of site-specific conditions are addressed in related chapters in this text. In addition, these and the other aspects of care can be explored further in specialist texts that deal with issues relating to palliative care, symptom control and psychosocial interventions.

Assessment of Individual Patient and Carer Needs

To provide care that is appropriate to patients' needs requires first assessing and establishing what those needs are.

Although it is vital that the medical and physical needs of the patient are addressed, it is important to ask patients how they are feeling and coping from an emotional and psychological level. In doing this, consideration should be given to:

- Physical effects of both treatment and disease
- Psychological and social issues
- Sexual function
- Spiritual needs
- Family and carer support
- Access to evidence-based information
- Involvement in decision-making

Many of these symptoms do not sit in isolation and can, indeed, be synergistic. A patient's quality of life is affected not only by the physical and emotional impact of their cancer but also by the treatments prescribed to treat their condition. Because RT causes a degree of damage to the normal tissues of the body and can cause local and systemic side effects, this aspect of their management should be assigned pivotal importance. These side effects can be acute or delayed, with acute (early effects) occurring during radiation treatment and continuing after treatment or in the subsequent weeks and months. Delayed side effects can occur months or even years after treatment. Although side effects of RT are to an extent unavoidable, they can be managed if patients are well supported and appropriate advice is given before and as they progress through treatment. Such support and education should be an essential component of the management process for all patients receiving RT.

The Impact on Staff

In cancer care the main focus is justifiably on the needs of the patient and their families and friends. However, bear in mind that such care does not exist in a vacuum and can pose particular burdens for the health professionals involved. How we react to the pressures of caring is dependent on a multiplicity of factors but mainly includes our interpersonal resources, skills and life experiences. Indeed, many of the influencing factors that patients bring to coping with a diagnosis of a life-threatening illness (see the 'Psychosocial Care' section) also hold true for all of us in terms of our attitudes, beliefs and coping mechanisms as individuals, as well as our training, skills, knowledge and experience as healthcare professionals.

There are particular types of strategies for coping that can be aimed at dealing with preparing staff for many of the intense emotions with which they will be faced. Emotions such as anger, resentment, frustration and grief are often displayed by patients and their families, and communication skills training is particularly helpful and, indeed, desirable to help improve the situation for all concerned. It is also important to challenge unrealistic expectations of professional achievability. Often, healthcare professionals believe their task is to help people get better. However, in cancer care it has to be accepted that this is not always possible. The juxtaposition between the benefits and toxicities of treatment and the concerns about the impact on quality of life for the patient and their family can be issues of great concern and stress for staff, which can result in significant emotional costs to those who feel unsupported in trying to meet clinical demands.

Recognition and understanding of the emotional issues of healthcare professionals working in cancer care is therefore important to help reduce the likelihood of stress. Attention must be paid to providing appropriate training in communication and coping strategies. In addition, a multiprofessional team working together should also aim to provide a supportive atmosphere with peer support and an opportunity to allow staff to share and reflect on their feelings and perceived difficulties in dealing with particular patient cases or complex situations. This would allow them to draw on the expertise and support of others and negate any feelings of isolation and despondency.

Finally, it must be acknowledged that if healthcare professionals are to work effectively with patients and families in cancer care, the emotional costs to them must be recognised and not simply dismissed under the umbrella term of *staff stress*. Appropriate support mechanisms must be established to allow individuals to continue to offer high-quality supportive care without it coming at the cost of staff stress and burnout. In short, if we are to be able to care for our patients, we must also and perhaps first be able to care for ourselves.

PREPARATION FOR RADIOTHERAPY

Prehabilitation

Patients with cancer are not only subjected to the adverse effects of their cancer. Their health, well-being and quality of life can also be negatively impacted by the side effects associated with the treatments used to treat their cancer. Many cancer patients will also present with preexisting comorbidities that can increase their risk of developing side effects and complications while also potentially restricting their suitability for particular treatments. Research demonstrates that optimising a patient's physical and psychological health at the earliest opportunity can make them stronger, increase their endurance and help them fare better during and after treatment.

Prehabilitation is the implementation of an intervention to enhance a patient's functional and psychological capacity in the period between diagnosis and starting treatment. It has many recognised benefits, including improved health and survival outcomes, access to treatment previously unavailable, decreased hospital admissions, reduced direct and indirect healthcare costs associated with cancer, increased patient satisfaction and increased compliance. Cancer prehabilitation is therefore becoming increasingly recognised as an integral part of the cancer treatment trajectory.

The 'waiting period' between diagnosis and treatment can be a difficult time for patients. Engagement in prehabilitation not only offers an opportunity for the patient to improve their functional status but also provides a focus and allows active participation and engagement in their overall care and treatment. This can help the patient feel empowered and promotes some ownership in a situation that can often feel beyond their control. It can not only improve a patient's outcome but also positively impact their experience.

Prior to commencing treatment, it is fundamental to establish the patient's baseline function, identifying any current impairments while considering any anticipated future impairments. Limitations and risk should also be considered and thoroughly assessed, being mindful of any potential adverse effects from the cancer treatment itself or from the intervention. Appropriate interventions can then be recommended and utilised to reduce the incidence and severity of current and future related impairments and improve the patient's health and well-being.

A holistic, tailored approach must be employed, responding to and suiting an individual's needs. There are three levels of intervention: universal (suitable for anyone with cancer and their families), targeted (planned support from an expert) and specialist (for more complex needs, with support from registered professionals). There must also be recognition that these needs and required levels of support are likely to change. Therefore, ongoing monitoring and a proactive approach are essential to gain maximum benefit. Any intervention should also be complemented by additional engagement, education and support to encourage co-operation, adherence and compliance.

Multidisciplinary collaboration is fundamental. The disciplines involved in providing interventions may include a combination of registered professionals including dieticians, physiotherapists, therapy radiographers and psychologists and unregistered professionals such as fitness instructors and healthcare support workers. It can also be beneficial to involve and educate family members/carers as this can help support the patient and improve compliance.

Prehabilitation can be *unimodal*, that is, focusing on exercise only, or *multimodal*, which is multifaceted and includes lifestyle optimisation (smoking cessation, alcohol reduction), physical activity/exercise, nutritional management, well-being support and psychological support. Studies suggest that a multimodal approach may be more effective than a unimodal approach. Prehabilitation can be carried out as a group intervention or on a one-on-one basis. It is worth noting that it can be difficult to quantify the true effectiveness of prehabilitation based on individual outcome measures. As one would expect, on completion of treatment, the patient's functional level is likely to be less than it was prior to starting treatment.

Barriers to compliance with prehabilitation must also be considered when discussing interventions with patients. The patient should be involved in these discussions and the intervention should be realistic, achievable and not negatively impact the patient. One should be mindful of potential barriers such as travel, mobility and financial issues. If these aren't addressed or considered, it will impact the patient's compliance and the intervention outcome will undoubtedly be suboptimal.

Informed Consent

Good, patient-centred communication is associated with important and meaningful health outcomes, including improvements in treatment compliance, satisfaction with care and overall improvements in psychosocial adjustment. Conversely, when patients are dissatisfied and feel unable to speak freely, it reduces the likelihood that they will offer and seek the information necessary for a good, informative exchange. Patients and carers place a lot of importance on face-to face communication with healthcare professionals, which is the usual way information is given at crucial points in a patient's illness and treatment pathway. Effective communication is central to identification of an individual's specific needs and the provision of appropriate support with respect to their needs, age, gender, culture and socioeconomic status. Good communication requires an ability to listen to and hear the person and to engage with them both emotionally and psychologically.

Seeking information is one strategy that many people use to help them cope with the challenges that a cancer diagnosis brings. The provision of appropriate, timely and honest information can make them feel more in control of their situation and can therefore be a key element for many people in managing the experience of cancer. In addition, there is evidence that the psychological distress in patients with serious illness is reduced when they think that they have received adequate information.

It is important to understand that patients are unlikely to have retained all the relevant information they have been given, particularly after one consultation. A best practice is to repeat and reinforce this information at subsequent consultations and treatment visits. Regardless of the amount of information they have retained, patients tend to remember what they were told first, rather than subsequently, so it can be difficult to undo any wrong perceptions and misunderstandings of patients and their carers in relation to this. It is therefore vital that there is consistency in explaining diagnosis, prognosis, treatment and effects.

Patients must understand the particular benefits and risks associated with their site and stage of disease as well as treatment intent and planned rationale to provide informed consent. For example, whether RT is being combined with chemotherapy will affect not only the patient's outcome but also the early and late effects of their treatment, as will whether the patient has had previous surgery. Although the current Department of Health guidelines state that patients should be advised on substantial or unusual risks of treatment, the details of these for site-specific conditions are beyond the scope of this chapter. However, it is worth noting that many cancer centres now include details of both acute and late effects of treatment for specific cancers as an essential element in the consent process. Patients must balance the risks of RT for them and their specific cancer against the risks of not having any treatment at all. It should also be emphasised that, generally, the long-term risks tend to be rare and affect a very small number of people and that, generally, the benefits of RT treatment far outweigh the possibilities of involved risks.

Thus, providing information is pivotal to underpinning a morally and ethically sound consent process. In essence, informed consent requires that patients have had their treatment options, procedures, risks and benefits explained in a way that they can understand so that they can make decisions about their own treatment and care. This is important at all stages in the process but, particularly, at times when stages of illness and treatment options change. Indeed, the law regards giving and obtaining consent to be a process, not a one-off event. It is also important to be aware that a patient may change their mind and withdraw consent at any time; if in any doubt, always check that the patient still consents to treatment.

The National Health Service (NHS) plan pledges that consent must be sought from all NHS patients. Both English and Scottish law state that before you examine, treat or care for competent adult patients you must obtain their consent. The Department of Health's Reference Guide to the consent process offers a comprehensive summary of the law on consent and offers help on frequently asked questions for both health professionals and patients (available at https://www.gov.uk/government/publications/reference-guide-to-consent-for-examination-or-treatment-second-edition). This provides a comprehensive guide and is usually well supplemented by individual health providers producing their own guidelines for use at a local level.

As a general guide, the professional seeking consent should consider whether a patient can understand and weigh the information needed to make the required decision. It is also important to bear in mind that if a patient reaches a decision that appears unexpected, it may not indicate incompetence, but rather a need for further information or explanation. It is advised that it is always best for the actual person who is in charge of treating the patient to seek their consent, although it is acceptable for appropriately trained and knowledgeable colleagues to do this if necessary.

SYMPTOM AND SIDE-EFFECT CARE

Skin Reactions

Radiotherapy-induced skin reactions (RISRs) are one of the most common side effects of treatment, with all patients being at risk of developing some form of reaction during or soon after completing treatment. They can cause distress to some patients and may also be a factor that can limit radiation dose and treatment schedules. Complete prevention of RISRs is unlikely; however, intensity modulated radiotherapy (IMRT) and volumetric modulated arc therapy (VMAT) have the potential to reduce the severity by increasing the number of beams, subsequently reducing the dose contribution from each individual beam.

RISRs have two phases: an initial acute toxicity phase predominantly driven by inflammation and oxidative stress that lead to a temporary cessation in stem cell proliferation, and a late or chronic toxicity effect characterised by fibrosis and its effects. This includes reduced lymphovascular functioning resulting in lymphoedema and poor wound healing from reduced vascularity.

Acute skin reactions include mild erythema, hyperpigmentation and dry-to-moist desquamation occurring more frequently in the head and neck area, breast and chest wall as well as areas with skin folds such as the groin, anal cleft and axilla. With conventional fractionated RT, erythema and hyperpigmentation develop approximately during the third week of treatment and become more pronounced through the remainder of treatment. Dry and/or moist desquamation may develop during the fourth to sixth weeks of treatment. The acute toxicity experienced is lower with hypofractionated schedules than with conventional dose fractionations. Therefore, in practice, consideration must be given to changing techniques and fractionation schedules. For example, in breast cancer RT, there has been a change from a 15-fraction to a 5-fraction schedule, and many patients are not developing skin reactions until after treatment has finished; this requires a different approach to post-RT information and management.

RISRs can be influenced by *intrinsic factors*, such as demographic or disease-related characteristics such as age, hormonal status, infection, smoking, ethnic origin, obesity and preexisting conditions or comorbidities (e.g. diabetes), and *extrinsic factors*, such as concomitant medication use, treatment dose, volume, fractionation, site of treatment, beam energy and use of bolus or immobilisation equipment. The various factors that influence how people react to RT need to be taken into consideration when designing advice to be given to patients.

The use of accelerated radiation dose schedules with concurrent chemotherapy or biological agents will lead to an increase in RISRs. In most departments, this is addressed by offering suitable advice and support while monitoring and recording the severity of these reactions during treatment. The goal of good management is to have a system in place that facilitates the identification of risk and delays the onset of skin reactions. There may also be a benefit to risk-stratifying patients to help identify those at higher risk of developing severe RISRs, allowing appropriate interventions to be introduced in an effort to manage this risk. Consideration should also be given to the patient's current skin care regimen, existing skin conditions, sensitivities and allergies.

TABLE 35.1 Radiation Therapy Oncology Group Grading of Acute Skin Reactions

RTOG 0	RTOG 1	RTOG 2a	RTOG 2b	RTOG 3
No visible change	Faint or dull erythema	Tender or bright erythema with/without dry desquamation	Patchy moist desquamation; moderate oedema	Confluent moist desquamation; pitting oedema

RTOG, Radiation Therapy Oncology Group.

Patients should be provided with information explaining:

- How and why skin reactions occur
- When they are likely to appear
- What they will look and feel like
- How they will be treated
- Where the reaction is likely to occur
- Self-care strategies
- Risk factors

The UK College of Radiographers has produced a clinical practice guideline that outlines a set of evidence-based recommendations to assist radiographers, RT nurses and the wider RT workforce in advising patients how to care for their skin while undergoing a course of radical external beam radiotherapy (EBRT) (excluding proton therapy). They have also produced a radiation dermatitis guideline for RT healthcare professionals. The guidelines were developed systematically using the best available evidence from research and expert opinion and were subjected to peer, professional and lay assessment. The guidelines have recommendations for evidence-based practice; however, they conclude that overall, the current evidence base is not strong enough to either support or refute the use of any particular product for topical application.

Management of skin toxicities can be facilitated by having a patient review process that includes the assessment (baseline, then weekly during and after RT), grading and recording of skin reactions. The most widely used assessment tool is the Radiation Therapy Oncology Group (RTOG) grading system (Table 35.1), although it should be noted that the common toxicity scale tends to be used to assess acute and late effects of skin in clinical trials.

Involving patients in the prevention and care of skin reactions is not only an important element of the management process but also places an emphasis on empowering the patient to use products they are familiar with, while promoting improved comfort. Skin can be exposed to a number of irritants that, if avoided, can lessen the likelihood of a troublesome reaction (Table 35.2). As part of this self-care strategy, patients should be educated and encouraged to reduce irritants to irradiated skin. Recording of patient acceptability/satisfaction and compliance with skin-care advice is also recommended as such information can be used to evaluate the appropriateness of skin-care products for future patients.

Care for radiation skin reactions once they have occurred and what products to recommend in this event require a knowledge of the more general wound care literature. It is important that advice and treatment given to patients is evidence based. Table 35.3 provides some details on skin-care products that can be used. Other sources that may be useful include published national skin-care guidelines.

For some patients, one of the most distressing side effects of chemotherapy or RT to the head is hair loss. A good-quality wig may help maintain the patient's appearance and morale. Scalp-cooling devices may help reduce hair loss if the chemotherapeutic agent is cleared fairly quickly from the blood, although results can vary.

Late skin toxicity symptoms can occur months or years after treatment and include telangiectasias, fibrosis, lymphoedema and cellulitis. The area treated will always be more sensitive to the sun. Therefore, patients should be advised to protect the treated area from sun exposure for life.

TABLE 35.2 Recommendations for Reducing Irritants to Irradiated Skin During a Course of Radiotherapy

Sun exposure	Protect from direct sun exposure: Cover with clothing or shade area. Stress the risk from sun exposure during and following radiotherapy. Sunscreen with both UVA/UVB protection; minimum SPF 50 should be used on previously irradiated skin.
Mechanical irritants (guidelines apply within the treatment fields only)	Minimise friction: Wash or shower gently; avoid using a washcloth; pat dry with a soft, clean towel; wear loose-fitting, soft clothing. Avoid shaving, or shave using an electric shaver. Avoid hair removal creams. Avoid scratching. Avoid rubbing vigorously and massaging. Avoid use of adhesive tape in treatment field. Wash hair gently with usual shampoo if the scalp is in the treatment field, but do not dry with a hairdryer or use hair straighteners or curling tongs.
Chemical irritants	Current guidelines show no evidence for avoidance of using normal shower/washing products unless they begin to cause discomfort or skin is broken. There is no evidence to support not using deodorant; therefore, patient may continue with normal products unless they begin to cause discomfort or skin is broken. Apply only recommended products—check with treatment centre and refer to Table 35.3. Avoid perfume and aftershave if these are to be applied within the treatment area. Use a moisturiser that is SLS-free (see Table 35.3). Use mild detergent to wash clothing.
Thermal irritants	Use water that is not overly hot. Avoid exposure to temperature extremes. Avoid application of ice packs or heat (e.g. heating pad, hot water bottles, sun lamp).

Informed by The Society and College of Radiographers, Practice Guideline Document: Radiation Dermatitis Guidelines for Radiotherapy Healthcare Professionals, 2020. *SLS*, Sodium lauryl sulphate.

Pain

Up to three-quarters of patients with advanced cancer may have some degree of pain, and up to 80% of patients may have pain at multiple sites. The three most common sources of cancer pain are bone metastases, compression of nerves and soft-tissue disease.

Pain has both physical and psychological dimensions. Anxiety or depression may accentuate the perception of pain and lower the pain threshold. Physical conditions such as hypercalcaemia may also physiologically increase the degree of pain. The treatment of hypercalcaemia may be a pain control measure by itself. The basis of pain control is to establish the causes of pain and, if possible, eradicate the source of pain. The patient may benefit from a single RT treatment. However,

TABLE 35.3 Characteristics of Skin-Care Products for Each Stage of Radiation Skin Reactions

No change in skin (RTOG 0)	No intervention required. Use of an SLS-free moisturiser. Advise only for SLS-free moisturiser as in RTOG 1.
Faint or dull erythema (RTOG 1)	An SLS-free moisturiser may be applied to skin within the treatment field and may soothe and moisturise skin. There is no evidence that any one cream may be superior. Therefore, this cannot be stated as a recommendation, and patients can elect to choose their preference. However, SLS-free creams include Zerobase, Diprobase, Aquamax, Aveeno, Cetraben, Epimax, QV Cream and E45.
Tender or bright erythema (RTOG 2a)	Use of urea 10% cream may alleviate pruritus if present. Where a rash is present, hydrocortisone 1% may act as an antiinflammatory. Skin to be reviewed and documented daily.
Patchy moist desquamation (RTOG 2b)	Dressings should be nonadhesive. Hydrogel dressing and nonadhesive dressings such as soft polymer dressings and polyurethane foam film dressings without adhesives may be used. These will depend on local policy.
Moist desquamation (pitting oedema) (RTOG 3)	Choice of dressing is determined by site, amount of exudate and potential need for removal before treatment. Principles of wound management are applicable; dressings of choice should maintain a moist environment in the wound bed; keep the area clean to minimise risk of infection, keep the wound warm to encourage mitotic activity and prevent friction. The wound exudates contain nutrients, enzymes and white blood cells that are important for healing. Maintain clear documentation of wound assessment undertaken and involve a multidisciplinary review approach as per local policies; involve Tissue Viability Team if required.

RTOG, Radiation Therapy Oncology Group; *SLS*, sodium lauryl sulphate.

come what may, the pain should be controlled by suitable analgesia if this is possible.

Ideally, all analgesics should be given by mouth. Mild or moderate pain may respond to simple analgesics such as paracetamol or aspirin. The nonsteroidal group of analgesics, such as diclofenac, may be useful, especially for bone pain. They can, however, cause gastric irritation and should be used with caution in even mild degrees of renal failure. Codeine or dihydrocodeine is useful for moderate pain but, unlike morphine, the dose of these drugs cannot be escalated. Increasing the doses above 60 mg 4 times daily produces toxicity and not an increase in analgesia.

Morphine is still a standard analgesic for severe pain. In patients with normal renal and hepatic function, the metabolic half-life of morphine is 2.5 hours. It therefore needs to be given no less frequently than every 4 hours. Morphine serum levels are stable after six half-lives. Therefore, in practice, morphine doses can be escalated every 12 hours. An initial dose of oral morphine should be chosen according to the patient's age, size and degree of pain. This may vary between 5 and 30 mg. The dose is usually given in the form of either morphine sulphate tablets or an elixir. The dose can be rapidly escalated if necessary. When pain control is achieved, the total morphine dose over 24 hours can then be added up. This is a guide for the prescription of a strong-acting analgesic such as morphine sulphate continuous tablets (MST). These tablets contain morphine in a cellulose matrix that is slowly released over a 12-hour period. If the patient has been receiving 30 mg of morphine elixir every 4 hours, the total morphine dosage in 24 hours is 180 mg. This can be given in the form of 90 mg of MST every 12 hours to provide sustained pain control. If the patient cannot swallow, diamorphine is a useful substitute. This is highly soluble in very small quantities of water and can be given subcutaneously either by intermittent injection or continuously using a syringe driver. Diamorphine has roughly twice the potency of morphine when given by injection and three times the potency of oral morphine.

Virtually all opiates cause constipation and patients should be routinely prescribed a laxative. A common side effect is nausea, but this usually settles within 5 days. Respiratory depression is rarely a problem, but if the patient develops significant respiratory oppression, morphine can be temporarily stopped and restarted at a lower dose. Occasionally, very high doses of morphine can cause myoclonic twitching of limbs. About 10% to 15% of patients are intolerant to morphine because of either prolonged nausea or a dysphoric reaction. Alternative preparations are fentanyl patches, hydromorphone or oxycodone.

In the treatment of neuropathic pain, tricyclic drugs such as amitriptyline or anticonvulsants such as gabapentin, pregabalin or sodium valproate often help symptoms. Occasionally, patients with neuropathic pain may require a nerve block. Sites where this can be carried out are in the intercostal nerves in the ribs, the brachial plexus when this is involved by an apical lung tumour, or the coeliac axis plexus following infiltration by a pancreatic cancer or involvement of the lumbar-sacral nerve plexus by pelvic cancer. These nerve blocks are technically very demanding. Usually a long-acting local anaesthetic is injected to check that the nerve block will bring about adequate analgesia. If the pain is relieved, this could be followed by a further injection using phenol or alcohol to destroy the nerve.

Nausea and Vomiting

There are many causes of nausea and vomiting in advanced cancer patients; these include drug-induced vomiting, renal or hepatic failure, raised intracranial pressure or abdominal RT. These issues can cause a significant threat to the comfort and well-being of patients and impact on quality of life. It is important that patients are monitored for the development of such side effects, that their severity is assessed and that appropriate treatment is instigated. Use of 5HT3 antagonists such as granisetron or ondansetron can reduce RT- or chemotherapy-induced nausea and vomiting. Granisetron 2 mg orally 1 hour before RT can be a very good prophylaxis even for wide-field RT. Where nausea and vomiting are associated with a strong anxiety component, antiemetic drugs with tranquilising properties, such as prochlorperazine or haloperidol, are often useful.

Diarrhoea and Constipation

Diarrhoea is a common side effect of RT to the pelvis and can cause discomfort, distress, dehydration and weight loss. Although some patients may find it difficult to discuss bowel movements, a comprehensive assessment of the condition is essential so that the appropriate pharmacological therapy can be made available. Loperamide (Imodium) is a frequently used standby in the treatment of diarrhoea. Codeine phosphate is especially useful if diarrhoea is associated with colicky abdominal pain. Some patients may report constipation; dietary advice concerning reduction of fibre content and increasing fluids can help with this.

Weight Loss

Anorexia can cause functional limitations as well as significant emotional distress. Anorexia is often multifactorial in origin. The most common cause is the underlying malignancy. It is thought that the cancer stimulates the release of cytokines from the immune system, which induce anorexia. Anorexia, though, may be attributed to treatment (RT or chemotherapy) or to the physical effects of cancer such as pain or intestinal obstruction. Radiation treatment to several different regions (head and neck, gastrointestinal (GI), pelvis, thoracic) can cause anorexia and result in significant weight loss. Treatment-related anorexia may have implications for survival in certain patient populations. In a study of 364 patients receiving preoperative chemoradiation for locally advanced rectal cancer, severe weight loss during chemoradiation was found to impact on survival. Critical weight loss (>10%) was found to be independently associated with worse overall survival in patients with head and neck cancer receiving RT.

Dietetic advice may be helpful. Steroids are the most effective anti-anorexic agents. It is worth trying prednisolone at 30 mg over a 7-day period. If this increases appetite, the dose can be reduced to a maintenance dose of 5 to 10 mg. Progesterones, such as megestrol acetate, do improve appetite; however, they can cause ankle oedema and have been associated with an increased risk of thrombosis.

Guidance on nutritional status and diet for patients undergoing RT can impact positively on patients if it is undertaken in a routine and evidence-based manner. The nutritional status of patients may be adversely affected by not only their disease but also by the impact of their RT. Treatment-induced toxicities such as dry mouth, mucositis, dysphagia, nausea, vomiting, diarrhoea and tenesmus can all impact negatively on nutritional status and, ultimately, on the quality of life of patients. In addition, when patients are referred for RT, they may already have undergone surgical intervention, chemotherapy or both, and they may also be receiving concomitant treatment that could further exacerbate their nutritional status. These factors and the possibility that food intake may be modified during RT make it essential that sound nutritional advice and support are available to ensure that patients have sufficient nutrition to support tissue repair. Patients often have coexisting medical and social conditions that can affect nutritional status, and it is important that these are recognised and their impact incorporated into nutritional planning.

In patients where side effects of treatment commonly jeopardise nutritional status, for example, head and neck, oesophagus, colorectal and pelvis/abdomen, patients must be screened to identify those who need a more in-depth nutritional assessment. Studies demonstrate the benefits that can be gained when early intervention and a proper assessment of nutritional status and requirements are undertaken alongside early nutritional counselling and monitoring of diet. In some patients undergoing RT and/or chemoradiation for head and neck cancer, a percutaneous endoscopic gastrostomy (PEG) tube is surgically inserted into the stomach through the abdominal wall before treatment and is used as a way of introducing foods, fluids and medicines directly into the stomach to maintain good nutritional status. In some instances where nutritional intake has been limited due to treatment-related side effects, a nasogastric (NG) tube may be inserted as an alternative to a PEG tube. This is less invasive and can be done relatively easily, mitigating the risk of any interruption to ongoing treatment.

Advice to patients should, wherever possible, have an evidence base and will be dependent upon the area being treated, the regimen employed and a myriad of other factors. Treatment and advice to patients should therefore be tailored to suit their needs. Identifying the reason for the impaired nutrition is pivotal to its adequate treatment and, although dieticians are the key professionals, this is the responsibility of the multidisciplinary team.

Fatigue

One of the most common symptoms experienced by cancer patients is fatigue. It is described as one of the most distressing symptoms patients experience while receiving radiation; symptoms of fatigue can persist for months to years, affecting quality of life over a long time span. Radiation-related fatigue occurs across a wide range of cancer types and can contribute to depression, anxiety, concentration difficulties, decreased participation in work and recreational activities and difficulty with relationships. In a study by Storey et al. (2007), the group of patients most at risk of chronic cancer-related fatigue were young, female and treated for breast cancer.

Fatigue is a multidimensional phenomenon that makes it difficult to describe. It has been attributed to the illness, as in *cancer-related fatigue*, and as it develops the term *radiotherapy-related fatigue* has been used. Fatigue tends to begin 1 to 2 weeks into treatment and gets worse as treatment progresses, often peaking once RT has finished. Strategies to support staff in supporting patients during RT to manage fatigue have been published.

Patients can describe fatigue in many ways, for example, as feelings of tiredness, exhaustion, lethargy and being overwhelmed by events. Patients should be advised that, although their treatment may cause tiredness, they should try to get enough rest and sleep but also try to continue with some of their daily activities and incorporate some form of physical activity. Potential treatments for fatigue are to correct any nonradiation-related causes of fatigue, for example, anaemia. Treatments for radiation-induced fatigue and data assessing these treatments are limited; however, treatments can be divided into pharmacological and nonpharmacological.

Several nonpharmacological interventions are recommended, and several studies have shown an improvement in fatigue with physical exercise. Macmillan Cancer Support disseminates information, underpinned by research, that promotes the advantages of exercise in helping to alleviate side effects, fatigue and depression as well as overall health benefits. If fatigue is caused by underlying depression or a sleep disorder caused by anxiety, these underlying causes should be treated before using pharmacological treatments such as psychostimulants and corticosteroids.

Cancer treatment-related fatigue generally improves after therapy is complete, but some level of fatigue may persist for months or years following treatment. Research indicates that for at least a subset of patients, fatigue may be a significant issue long into survivorship.

HOLISTIC CARE

Psychosocial Care

It is crucial to remember that patients do not exist with a particular illness in isolation and that the dynamics of family and social relationships that may or may not exist within their own supportive networks may influence the content, context and ability to offer the desired or needed care. The patient should rarely be considered in isolation, and due thought and support should also be given to the needs of close family and carers, as they will also experience many similar feelings to those of our patients. The family is an extended agent of patient care. A cancer illness can have a profound effect not only on the patient but

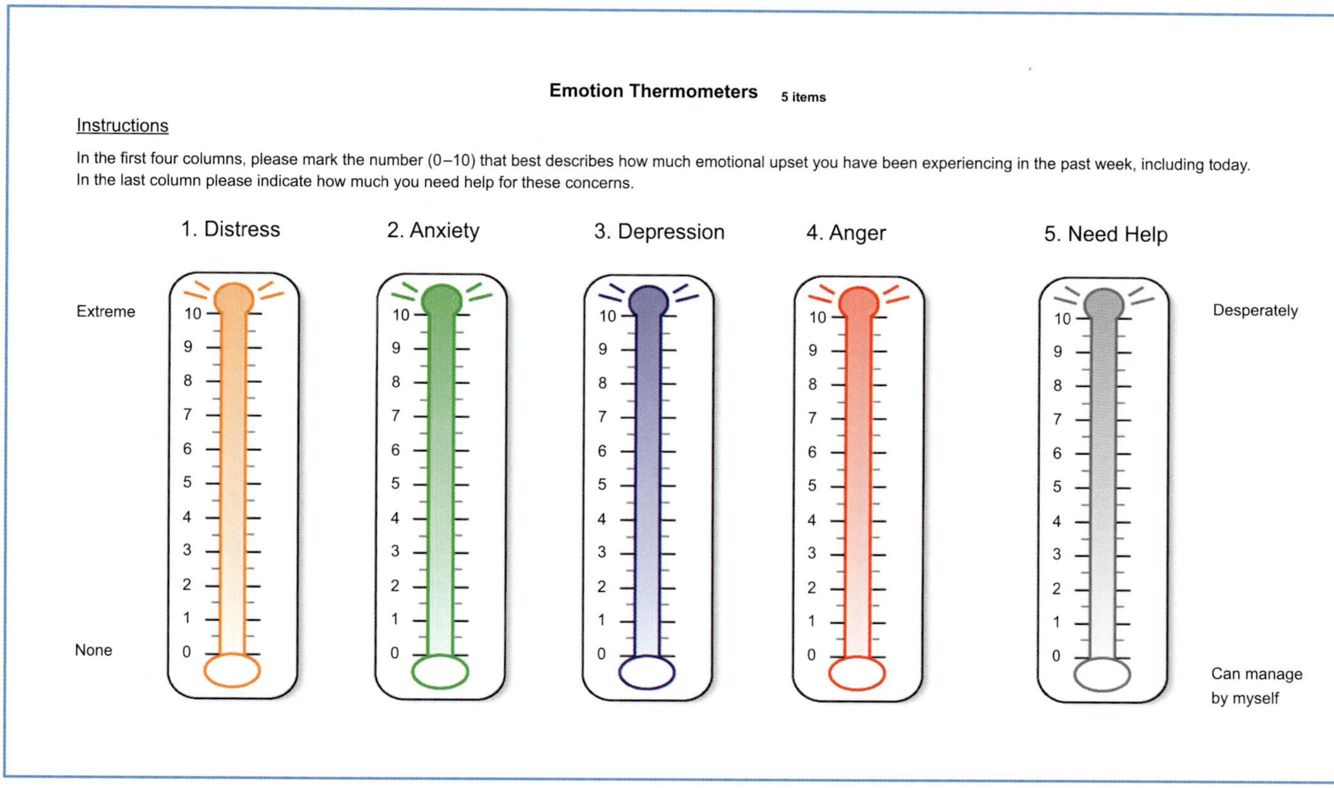

Fig. 35.1 The Emotion Thermometers tool. (Reproduced with permission from Alex M. http://www.psycho-oncology.info/ET.htm)

also on their relatives, and the process of a patient informing their relatives of their illness can be traumatic for all concerned.

Many patients and carers experience a range of psychological and emotional challenges as a result of their diagnosis and subsequent treatment effects. Research suggests that the prevalence of long-term psychological distress in cancer patients ranges from 20% to 66% and is higher than the general population. This was found in a study that screened for psychological distress in very long-term adult survivors of childhood cancer. Distress and psychological complications may be better recognised by using a simple validated screening tool, such as the Emotion Thermometers tool, which identifies patients in need of further psychological evaluation (Fig. 35.1).

At least one-quarter of patients with advanced cancer have significant depression. Virtually all patients with advanced cancer have a feeling of sadness and a sense of loss. Antidepressant medication should be considered sooner rather than later. The selective serotonin reuptake inhibitors, such as fluoxetine or sertraline, are better tolerated than the traditional tricyclic antidepressants. They often work faster than the 3 weeks often quoted. Counselling, relaxation therapy and other measures are also useful adjuncts in the treatment of anxiety and depression.

For the patient coming to terms with a cancer diagnosis, it has become helpful to think of their emotional adjustment as a series of different emotional stages. Barraclough (1999) describes patients initially experiencing shock, numbness or disbelief, often with the bad news seeming too much to take in. This usually short-term denial is then followed by distress as the reality of the situation becomes clear, and is often associated with anger, anxiety, and protest and bargaining. This phase often lasts a number of weeks and can be followed by sadness and depression, again taking several weeks before gradual movement to adjustment and acceptance, taking weeks and even months.

Although this is a useful guide to apply to many situations associated with loss of any kind, it is important to caution against using it as a simple sequential model of what every patient (and their carers) will experience. Although many will react with some of these emotions, we should not expect all to be initially shocked by a diagnosis and then work through all the stages to a final acceptance. Often there are more individual emotions, and they may not occur in any clear order or may overlap or be gone through more than once, particularly in an illness that has remissions and relapses or a series of progressive deteriorations. Heightened anxiety and intensity of these emotions will occur most strongly at diagnosis, during treatment episodes, at times of recurrence and in the terminal phase.

A summary of some of the common responses and influencing factors is illustrated in Fig. 35.2, which aims to illustrate the dynamic that emotional adjustment changes through time and is affected by many different factors that will be highly individualised for each patient. These reactions do not occur in any particular order and are particular to the individual who may move in and out of the different responses as the stimuli change.

In a study by Appleton and Perkins (2017), the authors explore how help is constructed during and following RT for patients with cancer. This study provides the basis for a greater understanding on the part of professionals into the impact of diagnosis and RT treatment on family and friends. In doing so, the study identifies opportunities for the experience of helpers to be recognised and supported by professionals.

Sexual Issues

Sexual issues arising from both functional impairment and psychological sequelae can have a significant impact on the quality of life for both patients and their partners. Responsible healthcare professionals must be proactive in addressing these concerns, providing education and offering a range of interventions to improve patients' sexual function and overall quality of life during and after treatment.

Erectile dysfunction (ED) is a common side effect of RT to the prostate, particularly when combined with androgen deprivation therapy

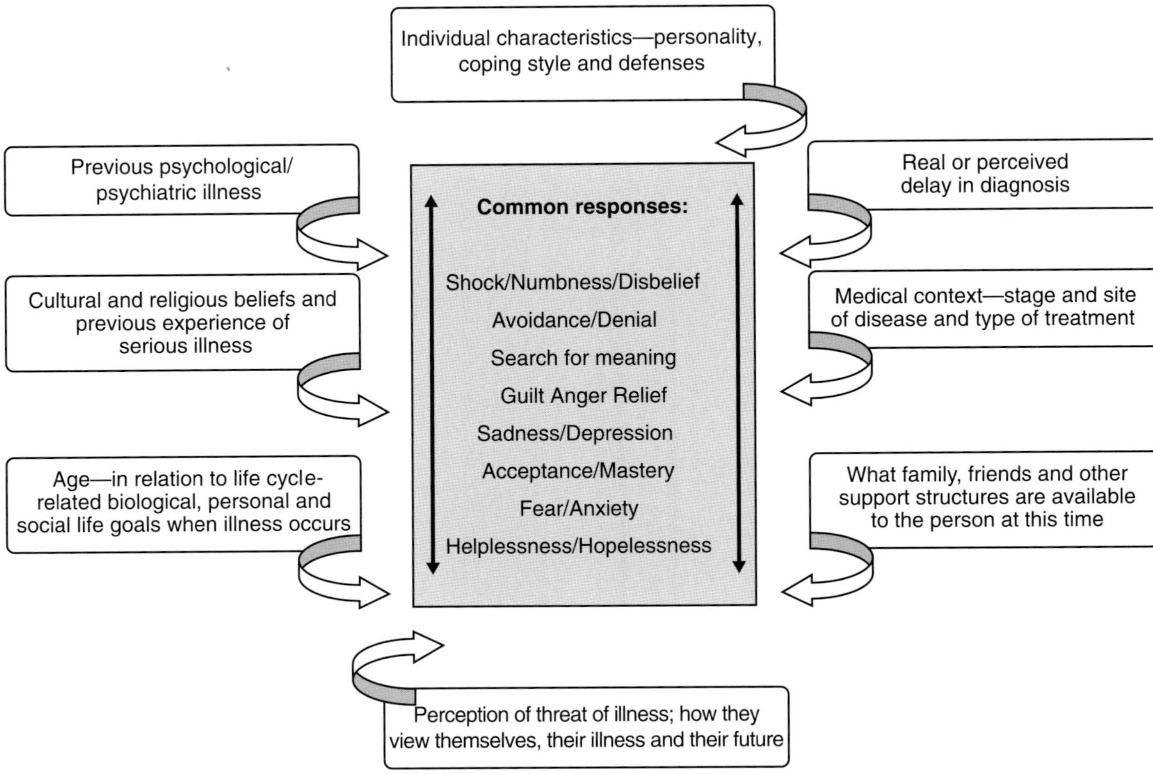

Fig. 35.2 Common responses and influencing factors in a life-threatening illness.

(Li et al., 2023), and is thought to impact up to 70% of patients. Radiation damage to blood vessels and nerves as well as changes to the hormonal environment within the body can cause ED throughout radical prostate management and beyond if not addressed by healthcare professionals (Doherty and Bridge, 2019). Maintenance of ED can be preserved even after androgen deprivation by prescribing low daily doses of medications such as PDE5 inhibitors (e.g. Viagra). These drugs can also be highly effective in treating ongoing ED following treatment. Limited evidence (Nicolai et al., 2021) suggests that physical interventions such as vacuum erectile devices and rings can help achieve and sustain erections, although patients can find these cumbersome to use.

Vaginal dryness and stenosis (narrowing) can occur following pelvic RT for gynaecological cancers. These effects can make sexual intercourse painful and difficult. Regular use of vaginal dilators and moisturisers are often recommended to manage these issues (Tahseen et al., 2023).

Radiation can damage the urinary and bowel systems, causing issues such as incontinence or frequent urination. These problems can affect sexual confidence and comfort. While pelvic floor physical therapy can help address incontinence and pelvic pain, the psychological impact of incontinence cannot be underestimated. Evidence (Ralph and Richardson, 2019) has also indicated that rectal irradiation arising from RT to the prostate can cause issues for males who engage in anal intercourse and patients should be advised regarding this.

Many sexual issues arising from RT, and indeed from cancer diagnoses, are strongly linked to psychological well-being. As discussed earlier, the physical and emotional stress associated with cancer treatment, along with anxiety, depression and body image concerns, can cause psychological issues and can also contribute to reduced libido. Counselling and support groups are often beneficial in addressing these emotional challenges, but it is vital that healthcare professionals engage in open and honest discussions with patients and partners about their expectations, anxieties, potential side effects and possible remedies as early as possible.

Spiritual Needs

Increasingly, research is demonstrating the importance of spiritual care. It is especially important when patients and their carers face a life-threatening condition. Defining spirituality is challenging—to a degree it is intangible—but it can be said to encompass those facets of an individual that give a sense of purpose and meaning to life. Contemporary medical literature supports the importance of spirituality for patients and proposes that strong spiritual beliefs can aid individuals when fighting illness. It has been suggested that spiritual well-being can have a positive effect on a patient's coping skills and their quality of life and can promote feelings of peace and acceptance. There are those, however, who identify the dangers of the spiritual challenge when patients ask, 'Why me?'

Patients need to be supported to find coping mechanisms during their illness, and the spiritual dimension may help in this process. There is a recognition that meeting spiritual needs is important, and policies to develop and implement spiritual care in our centres are now being advised. A study by Murray et al. (2004) concluded that spiritual issues were significant for many patients in their last year of life and their carers and that many healthcare professionals lack the necessary time and skills to uncover and address such issues. There is a growing body of evidence that suggests providing interventions that can have a positive impact on spiritual well-being among patients can also increase spiritual well-being among family caregivers of cancer patients. Addressing a patient's spirituality can be a challenge, but communicating at this level can be a positive experience for healthcare professionals as well as patients.

Financial Impact

There are practical implications of illness, and a patient and their family may have difficulties in terms of their financial and employment status, as well as disruption caused by changes in their role and family dynamics. A patient with cancer may be the main breadwinner for the family. Therefore, their illness may cause acute financial problems. Medical social workers and the Department for Work and Pensions may be able to provide financial support both from the state and from charitable bodies.

SURVIVORSHIP

Posttreatment Care

During and after cancer treatment, a wide range of services to provide the patient with physical, psychological and social support should be available. The most important single individual in this process is the general practitioner. The general practitioner needs to be apprised of the patient's progress, the likely side effects of cancer treatment and what can be done at home to treat these side effects. They also need to be informed of the patient's likely prognosis. This is especially true if the treatment is palliative, because the general practitioner has a key role to play in the provision of continuing care and is often the gatekeeper to appropriate services. Another key aspect of ongoing care is the wide range of specialist nursing services. Increasingly, specialist nurses are attached to multidisciplinary teams in areas such as breast, gynaecological and central nervous system cancer. They have multiple roles in giving the patient specialist advice and psychological support. As well as providing advice on symptom control and emotional support for both patient and family, these nurses also play an important liaison role as links between the patient, the general practitioner and hospital services. District nurses play an important role in at-home care, providing basic services such as bathing, dressing of wounds and giving medicines by injection.

Patients may also require the help of prosthetic services. Other cosmetic prostheses that are important include replacements for eyes and sometimes ears or noses. Prosthetic limb fitters may be required to provide replacement limbs following amputation.

Palliative Care

In a regional oncology centre, up to 50% of the work is treatment of advanced disease. Patients may be judged incurable from the outset, and the aim of treatment is the relief of physical and psychological distress. Subsequently, patients who were thought initially to be in the curable category may develop advanced disease and may require the same type of care. Oncology centres will have developed their own systems of care to support these patients, and this should interface well with their home or hospice care. Ideally, patients should be cared for at home with the help of the general practitioner and district nurses. Macmillan specialist nurses make a significant contribution to this process and, increasingly, organisations such as Marie Curie provide hospice-at-home services.

Patients who have symptoms that cannot be controlled at home or whose nursing care is too complex may need admission to hospital or, ideally, to a specialist hospice. Hospices provide a more homey, less institutional and quieter environment than the noisy, busy hospital ward. The higher staff-to-patient ratio gives more time for patients to talk about their illnesses. The hospice team has the distinctive knowledge and skills needed to provide spiritual and emotional support for patients at this challenging time. Often, after symptoms have been controlled, patients may be able to return home, perhaps to return to the hospice at a later date. Such patients while at home can be helped by attendance at the hospice day centre. As well as checking that the patient's symptoms are controlled, hospice day centres provide a social environment for patients and can allow other family members a respite from care to continue employment. One of the main aims of a hospice is symptom control. These include pain, anorexia, nausea, vomiting, dysphasia, dyspnoea and lack of energy.

Patient-Reported Outcome Measures

Patient-reported outcome measures (PROMs) are being used increasingly to assess the impact of RT on quality of life and treatment outcomes (NHS, 2021). PROMs are self-reported tools completed by patients that often include assessments of pain, fatigue, nausea and specific cancer-related symptoms. They can offer valuable insights into various aspects of well-being that are more challenging to collect via traditional follow-up mechanisms, including physical, emotional and social dimensions. Research is ongoing into the use of online platforms or mobile apps to help gather these data as 'ePROMS' (Payne et al., 2023), along with innovative use of devices such as smart watches (Amaro et al., 2023) to provide additional metrics.

One of the primary applications of PROMs following RT is the evaluation of treatment efficacy and potential side effects. Patients use PROMs to report their symptoms and functional status, enabling clinicians to assess whether treatment goals have been met and to identify any treatment-related toxicities. By routinely collecting PROM data, clinicians can make timely adjustments to treatment plans and provide more effective symptom management. PROMs inherently facilitate a patient-centred approach to care, empowering patients to voice their concerns and preferences. Clinicians can utilise PROM data to tailor treatment plans, supportive care interventions and rehabilitation strategies to address the individual needs and priorities of each patient. This personalised approach contributes to improved patient satisfaction and overall treatment experiences (Girgis et al., 2018). For cancer survivors, the monitoring of their quality of life over the long term is crucial. PROMs can assist in tracking survivors' well-being and detecting late treatment-related side effects.

In the realm of clinical trials, PROMs provide objective data on the impact of RT interventions (Oliver et al., 2023). These additional data can help researchers compare treatment arms, evaluate the effectiveness of new therapies and gain insights into the patient experience during trials. PROMs are increasingly playing a pivotal role in the development of evidence-based guidelines and treatment protocols.

FURTHER READING

Amaro PF, Bridge J, Davies L, et al. Interim analysis of patient recruitment, compliance and experience using smart watches for cardiac monitoring following curative-intent radiotherapy to the thorax. *Lung Cancer*. 2023;178(Supplement 1):S63–S64. https://doi.org/10.1016/S0169-5002(23)00573-1

Appleton L, Perkins E. The construction of help during radiotherapy: redefining informal care. *Psycho-Oncology*. 2017;26(12):2057–2062.

Barraclough J. *Cancer and Emotion: A Practical Guide to Psycho-Oncology*. 3rd ed. John Wiley & Sons, New York; 1999.

Bower JE, Ganz PA, Desmond KA, et al. Fatigue in long-term breast carcinoma survivors: a longitudinal investigation. *Cancer*. 2006; 106(4):751–758.

Breitbart W. Spirituality and meaning in supportive care: spirituality- and meaning-centered group psychotherapy interventions in advanced cancer. *Support Care Cancer*. 2002;10(4):272–280.

De Laage A, Allodji R, Dauchy S, et al. Screening for psychological distress in very long-term adult survivors of childhood cancer. *Pediatr Hematol Oncol*. 2016;33(5):295–313.

Doherty W, Bridge P. A systematic review of the role of penile rehabilitation in prostate cancer patients receiving radiotherapy and androgen deprivation therapy. *J Med Imag Radiat Sci*. 2019; 50(1):171–178.

Erridge SC, McCabe M, Porter MK, Simpson P, Stillie AL. Prospective audit showing improved patient-assessed skin toxicity with use of betamethasone cream for those at high risk of radiation dermatitis. *Radiother Oncol*. 2016;121(1):143–147.

Faithfull S, Wells M. *Supportive Care in Radiotherapy*. Churchill Livingstone, New York; 2003.
Girgis A, Durcinoska I, Koh E-S, et al. Development of health pathways to standardize cancer care pathways informed by patient-reported outcomes and clinical practice guidelines. *JCO Clin Cancer Inform*. 2018;2:1–13.
Gosselin TK, Schneider SM, Plambeck MA, Rowe K. A prospective randomized, placebo-controlled skin care study in women diagnosed with breast cancer undergoing radiation therapy. *Oncol Nurs Forum*. 2010;37(5):619–626.
Hojan K, Kwiatkowska-Borowczyk E, Leporowska E, et al. Physical exercise for functional capacity, blood immune function, fatigue, and quality of life in high-risk prostate cancer patients during radiotherapy: a prospective, randomized clinical study. *Eur J Phys Rehabil Med*. 2016;52(4):489–501.
Kleeberg UR, Suciu S, Bröcker EB, et al. Final results of the EORTC 18871/DKG 80-1 randomised phase III trial. rIFN-alpha2b versus rIFN-gamma versus ISCADOR M versus observation after surgery in melanoma patients with either high-risk primary (thickness >3 mm) or regional lymph node metastasis. *Eur J Cancer*. 2004;40(3):390–402.
Koontz BF. *Radiation Therapy Treatment Effects: An Evidence-Based Guide to Managing Toxicity*. Springer, New York; 2018.
Langius JAE, Zandbergen MC, Eerenstein SEJ, et al. Effect of nutritional interventions on nutritional status, quality of life and mortality in patients with head and neck cancer receiving (chemo)radiotherapy: a systematic review. *Clin Nutr*. 2013;32(5):671–678.
Langius JAE, Bakker S, Rietveld DHF, et al. Critical weight loss is a major prognostic indicator for disease-specific survival in patients with head and neck cancer receiving radiotherapy. *Br J Cancer*. 2013;109(5):1093–1099.
Li X, Fu R, Ni H, et al. Effect of neoadjuvant therapy on the functional outcome of patients with rectal cancer: a systematic review and meta-analysis. *Clin Oncol (R Coll Radiol)*. 2023;35(2):e121–e134. https://doi.org/10.1016/j.clon.2022.07.003
Lin J, Peng J, Qdaisat A, et al. Severe weight loss during preoperative chemoradiotherapy compromises survival outcome for patients with locally advanced rectal cancer. *J Cancer Res Clin Oncol*. 2016; 142(12):2551–2560.
Lloyd-Williams M. *Psychological issues in palliative care*. Oxford University Press, Oxford; 2018.
Mitchell AJ, Baker-Glenn EA, Granger L, Symonds P. Can the distress thermometer be improved by additional mood domains? Part I. Initial validation of the Emotion Thermometers tool. *Psycho-Oncology*. 2010;19(2):125–133.
Morley L, Tse K, Cashell A, Sperduti A, McQuestion M, Chow J. Dosimetric impacts on skin toxicity for patients using topical agents and dressings in radiotherapy. *J Radiother Prac*. 2016;15: 314–321.
Murray SA, Kendall M, Boyd K, Worth A, Benton TF. Exploring the spiritual needs of people dying of lung cancer or heart failure: a prospective qualitative interview study of patients and their carers. *Palliat Med*. 2004;18(1):39–45.
NHS (National Health Service). *NHS Long term plan: cancer*. Leeds, UK: NHS; 2021. https://www.longtermplan.nhs.uk/online-version/chapter-3-further-progress-on-care-quality-and-outcomes/better-care-for-major-health-conditions/cancer
Nicolai M, Urkmez A, Sarikaya S, et al. Penile rehabilitation and treatment options for erectile dysfunction following radical prostatectomy and radiotherapy: a systematic review. *Front Surg*. 2021;8:636974. https://doi.org/10.3389/fsurg.2021.636974
Oliver LA, Hutton DP, Hall T, et al. Amplifying the patient voice: a survey of practitioners' use of patient-reported outcome measures across radiotherapy providers in England. *Clin Oncol (R Coll Radiol)*. 2023;35(3):199–208. https://doi.org/10.1016/j.clon.2022.11.004
Payne A, Horne A, Bayman N, et al. Patient and clinician-reported experiences of using electronic patient reported outcome measures (ePROMs) as part of routine cancer care. *J Patient Rep Outcomes*. 2023;7(1):42. https://doi.org/10.1186/s41687-023-00544-4
Ralph S, Richardson C. EP-2206 How long should men abstain from receiving anal sex following treatments for prostate cancer? *Radiother Oncol*. 2019;133:S1216. https://doi.org/10.1016/S0167-8140(19)32626-X
SCoR (Society and College of Radiographers). Skin care advice for patients undergoing radical external beam megavoltage radiotherapy. 2020. https://www.sor.org/getmedia/53bd52ff-679e-48de-82a0-dc8dae570896/2020_version_4_final_practice_guideline_radiotherapy_skin_care_llv1.pdf
Storey DJ, Waters RA, Hibberd CJ, et al. Clinically relevant fatigue in cancer outpatients: the Edinburgh Cancer Centre symptom study. *Ann Oncol*. 2007;18(11):1861–1869.
Tahseen R, Ahmed Y, Tariq M, Abrar S, Ali N. Compliance and clinical efficacy of vaginal dilator after radiotherapy for cervical and endometrial malignancies. *Ecancermedicalscience*. 2023;17:1545. https://doi.org/10.3332/ecancer.2023.1545
Zabora J, BrintzenhofeSzoc K, Curbow B, Hooker C, Piantadosi S. The prevalence of psychological distress by cancer site. *Psycho-Oncology*. 2001;10(1):19–28.

36

Medical Complications of Malignant Disease and Treatment

Kiran Purushothaman and Thankamma V. Ajithkumar

CHAPTER OUTLINE

Cancer can cause a wide variety of medical and metabolic problems. These can be caused by the physical presence of the tumour obstructing structures such as the bile duct or a ureter, secretion of fluid into a body cavity (e.g. pleural effusion) or local invasion of adjacent structures. Cancer and its treatment frequently predispose the patient to infection due to immunosuppression and, more recently, immune-related adverse effects from immunotherapy. In addition, cancer may cause constitutional disturbances, which are not attributed to the local effect of the tumour but are the consequence of secreted tumour products resulting in paraneoplastic syndromes. This chapter discusses the problems caused by effusions, thrombosis, infection and paraneoplastic syndromes (Table 36.1) in malignancy and immune-related adverse events (irAEs).

EFFUSIONS SECONDARY TO MALIGNANT DISEASE

Normally, the pleural, pericardial and peritoneal spaces contain only a few millilitres of fluid to lubricate the inner and outer surfaces of these membranous coverings. However, in cancer the normal capillary and lymphatic vessels can become damaged or obstructed, and the hydrostatic pressures that regulate the transfer of fluid from one compartment of the body to another can be disturbed. A buildup of fluid at any of these three sites can cause unpleasant symptoms, which may require treatment. Although effusions are usually a sign of advanced malignancy and treatment is only palliative, intervention is usually indicated as it can provide clinical benefit and improve quality of life.

Pleural Effusions

The most common malignancy to cause a pleural effusion is carcinoma of the lung. In addition, metastasis from carcinoma of the breast, other adenocarcinomas and lymphoma may also be implicated. Clinical detection is not normally possible until at least 500 mL has accumulated and, typically, a symptomatic effusion comprises 1000 to 4000 mL of fluid. This is usually straw coloured but may be bloodstained. Associated symptoms include increasing shortness of breath, a dry cough and sometimes pain as it increases in size. Diagnosis is usually made clinically and confirmed by imaging (chest x-ray and computed tomography (CT) scan). Incidental small effusions may also be detected on imaging performed for other indications in patients with a diagnosis of cancer. Ultrasound and/or CT may help distinguish pleural fluid from a solid pleural mass or thickening and determine the most appropriate management strategy.

Fluid drainage is required to relieve symptoms when symptomatic or when there is a significant mass effect from the effusion. This can be performed through a needle inserted into the pleural space, typically under ultrasound guidance, to increase the success rate and reduce the risk of complications. This can be particularly helpful when the effusion is loculated. Pleural aspiration alone is recognised to be associated with a high risk of recurrence of the effusion, and therefore, to reduce the risk of recurrence and for the management of larger pleural effusions, drainage using an intercostal tube is often undertaken. Here, a small-bore chest tube is attached to an underwater sealed drainage system, acting as a one-way valve. A chest drain allows controlled drainage of larger pleural effusions, reducing the risk of reexpansion pulmonary oedema.

To prevent recurrence of the effusion, either effective treatment of the underlying cancer is required or the effusion should be drained to dryness and the lung should be allowed to reexpand before pleurodesis is performed. Talc is the most commonly used sclerosant for pleurodesis. This is usually injected into the pleural space via the chest drain, resulting in inflammation of the pleural surfaces to encourage sticking together of the two layers and the development of fibrosis.

This will prevent recurrence of the effusion in 50% to 75% of patients. Pleurodesis may also be performed via thoracoscopy (video-assisted thoracoscopy or pleuroscopy), and this may be particularly useful when a histological diagnosis is required. In some patients with recurrent pleural effusions despite attempts at pleurodesis or where there is lung entrapment or obstruction by the tumour, an indwelling pleural catheter may be placed. The patient or

TABLE 36.1 Endocrine and Paraneoplastic Manifestations of Malignancy

System	Manifestation
Endocrine	Hypercalcaemia caused by parathyroid hormone-related peptide Water retention caused by inappropriate antidiuretic hormone secretion Cushing syndrome caused by the adrenocorticotrophic hormone Hypoglycaemia caused by insulin-like proteins/somatomedins Gynaecomastia caused by human chorionic gonadotrophin Thyrotoxicosis caused by human chorionic gonadotrophin
Neurological	Peripheral neuropathy Cerebellar ataxia Dementia Transverse myelitis Myasthenia gravis Eaton-Lambert syndrome
Haematological/ vascular	Anaemia Thrombophlebitis Thromboembolism Disseminated intravascular coagulation Polycythemia Nonbacterial endocarditis Red cell aplasia
Musculoskeletal	Polymyalgia rheumatica Arthralgia Clubbing Hypertrophic pulmonary osteoarthropathy
Dermatological	Pruritus Various skin rashes
Renal	Nephrotic syndrome

carer is then able to drain pleural fluid at home using the indwelling pleural catheter.

Pericardial Effusions

Pericardial effusions are much less common than pleural effusions. Again, the same tumour types are usually responsible. Pericardial effusions may accumulate slowly or suddenly and can present with a spectrum of severity, from mild asymptomatic effusions detected incidentally on imaging to presentation with haemodynamic compromise. Normally, 10 to 50 mL of pericardial fluid is present within the pericardial sac. However, the pericardium can stretch to accommodate an increase in pericardial volume, which is greater if the effusion develops slowly. If there is a sudden and rapid increase in the pericardial volume, this may impair cardiac filling and result in cardiac tamponade.

Less than 1% of cancer patients will develop a symptomatic collection of pericardial fluid. When they occur, symptoms include shortness of breath, chest pain and fullness. Nonspecific symptoms may include cough, weakness, palpitations and loss of appetite. Occasionally, symptoms caused by local pressure effects may occur, such as nausea and dysphagia, which are attributed to effects on the diaphragm and oesophagus, respectively. Clinical findings that may be associated with cardiac tamponade are sinus tachycardia, elevated jugular venous pressure, oedema and pulsus paradoxus.

The diagnosis of a pericardial effusion is made based on clinical signs and confirmed by cardiac echocardiography. This allows assessing the size of the pericardial effusion and the haemodynamic effects. When there is evidence of haemodynamic compromise, urgent drainage of the pericardial fluid is required unless the patient is in the terminal phases of the disease process. Immediate intervention is not required for a pericardial effusion without haemodynamic compromise. Percutaneous pericardial drainage is technically more difficult than pleural drainage and is performed under echocardiographic or fluoroscopic guidance to ensure the safe placement of the drainage catheter. Surgical pericardiectomy and drainage are less commonly performed but may be required for the management of recurrent pericardial effusions. Treatment of the underlying malignancy will usually prevent recurrence.

Peritoneal Effusions (Ascites)

In cancer, ascites is most commonly caused by widespread peritoneal seedling metastases that exude protein-rich fluid. However, liver metastases and hypoalbuminaemia or portal hypertension may also result in the development of ascites. Ascites is most commonly caused by advanced carcinomas of the ovary, gastrointestinal (GI) tract, breast and pancreas. Lymphoma may also cause chylous ascites.

Patients present with abdominal distension, pain, early satiety and shortness of breath caused by diaphragm splinting. The presence of ascites can be confirmed by ultrasound and cytological examination. Therapeutic paracentesis, usually performed under ultrasound guidance or following ultrasound marking of a safe site, can relieve symptoms. An indwelling tunneled catheter drain can be placed for recurrent symptomatic malignancy-related ascites, enabling fluid to be drained at home.

Drainage of the fluid should be performed slowly, not exceeding a rate of 500 mL per hour. Drainage to dryness of ascites is not realistic, and therefore sclerosants are much less effective for ascites than for pleural effusions and are not commonly used. Diuretics are rarely effective in relieving established ascites. Intraperitoneal administration of chemotherapy is sometimes beneficial, and agents, such as mitoxantrone and carboplatin, have been used successfully. For recurrent ascites, surgical procedures should be considered if medical treatments have failed to control the underlying disease. A peritoneovenous shunt can be inserted, which drains the fluid through a one-way valve into the venous system. Interestingly, despite the drainage of large numbers of malignant cells into the circulation, metastatic disease in the lungs and other sites does not appear more common.

The most effective method of controlling ascites, though, is treatment of the underlying malignancy using systemic chemotherapy and/or targeted therapies. Ascites can be abolished often in ovarian cancer because response rates are high, but it may be more difficult to control in GI tumours because response rates to chemotherapy are comparatively low.

VENOUS THROMBOSIS

The risk of venous thromboembolism (VTE) in patients with cancer is increased between fourfold and sevenfold because of the presence of a hypercoagulable state. This may involve the interaction of several factors, including tissue factors, inflammatory cytokines and platelets. Furthermore, additional risk factors include the anatomical position of the tumour, hospital admission, the presence of a central venous catheter and treatment-related factors such as surgery, chemotherapy and targeted therapies such as antiangiogenesis agents.

Thrombosis can present in various forms, such as deep vein thrombosis, pulmonary embolism, arterial thrombosis, superficial thrombophlebitis and hepatic venoocclusive disease. It may also be the presenting feature of malignancy. In approximately 4% of patients diagnosed with an unprovoked VTE, cancer is diagnosed within 1 year following their diagnosis.

Treatment and duration of VTE will depend on the balance of the risk of recurrence of VTE and the risk of bleeding, in which anticoagulation may be contraindicated, such as active bleeding or a platelet count of less than 30×10^9/L. Direct-acting oral anticoagulants (DOACs) have replaced low molecular weight heparin (LMWH) to treat VTE in cancer patients. The choice of DOACs is apixaban (10 mg twice daily for 7 days, followed by 5 mg twice daily) or rivaroxaban (15 mg twice daily for 21 days, followed by 20 mg once daily). When DOACs are not suitable (e.g. creatinine clearance <15 mL/min, high bleeding risk), the recommendation is either LMWH (e.g. dalteparin) for at least 5 days followed by dabigatran or edoxaban or LMWH concurrently with vitamin K antagonist (VKA., e.g. warfarin) for at least 5 days or until INR is at least 2.0 in 2 consecutive readings followed by VKA alone. In patients with active cancer, anticoagulation is recommended for 3 to 6 months.

METABOLIC AND ENDOCRINE MANIFESTATIONS OF MALIGNANCY

Hypercalcaemia

Hypercalcaemia is a complication in around 5% of patients with advanced malignancy and is particularly common in patients with carcinomas of the breast, lung and multiple myeloma. Three mechanisms are involved. First, metastatic cancer cells in bone stimulate osteoclasts, the normal bone cells that resorb (break down) bone, to destroy bone more quickly than the osteoblasts, the normal bone cells that build bone and repair the damage. Second, the tumour may secrete proteins, such as parathyroid hormone-related protein (PTHrP), into the circulation, which have similarly destructive effects on the bone and promote the kidney to reabsorb more calcium from the urine than is appropriate. Finally, dehydration, which occurs due to the diuretic effect of an increased calcium load on the kidney, worsens the situation, and tubular damage to the kidney, as commonly occurs in multiple myeloma, may also be important.

Hypercalcaemia causes many symptoms, including lethargy, nausea, thirst, constipation and drowsiness. Because the symptoms are nonspecific and commonly encountered in many patients with advanced cancer, the diagnosis can be easily missed. As a result, a high index of suspicion is required. However, the diagnosis is often identified by routine biochemical testing, which usually includes the measurement of serum calcium. The serum calcium level that causes symptoms varies from one patient to another and according to the speed of onset. Patients are better able to tolerate slowly developing hypercalcaemia than a sudden rise. However, most patients will have symptoms when the serum calcium exceeds 3.0 mmol/L.

Appropriate treatment will rapidly improve the patient's condition and relieve the unpleasant symptoms. This can be reliably achieved without side effects by rehydration of the patient and inhibition of bone breakdown by one of the class of drugs called *bisphosphonates*. Rehydration should be with normal saline, typically requiring 3 to 6 L over 24 to 48 hours. Rehydration reduces serum calcium and relieves many symptoms but is rarely sufficient treatment, and the benefits are usually short-lived over a few days. A single, 15-minute intravenous (IV) infusion of 4 mg zoledronic acid, one of the potent bisphosphonates now readily available, will restore the serum calcium to normal in around 90% of patients with a duration of action of approximately 3 to 4 weeks. Zoledronic acid is the most commonly used agent and has the highest probability of success, but pamidronate (≤90 mg depending on serum calcium every 3–4 weeks), ibandronate (2–4 mg IV every 3–4 weeks) and clodronate (1.6–3.2 g orally daily) are also effective in the majority of cases. Repeated IV infusions are usually required every 3 to 4 weeks unless successful systemic therapy can be instituted. For this reason, patients should be closely monitored every few weeks following a diagnosis of hypercalcaemia. Recurrent hypercalcaemia, despite regular bisphosphonates, has a very poor prognosis and may be a terminal event.

Syndrome of Inappropriate Secretion of Antidiuretic Hormone

This syndrome (abbreviated as SIADH) results in fluid retention by the kidney and is characterised by low serum sodium. This causes weakness and confusion, occurring most commonly in patients with small cell lung cancer. Treatment is by fluid restriction, drugs such as demeclocycline or a vasopressin receptor antagonist (e.g. conivaptan, tolvaptan), which inhibit the action of antidiuretic hormone (ADH), and chemotherapy for the underlying malignancy.

Other Endocrine Manifestations of Malignancy

Many cancers produce hormones and peptides with biological activity. These include adrenocorticotrophic hormone (ACTH), which may result in the features of Cushing syndrome, hypoglycaemia from production of insulin-like substances and gynaecomastia from tumour production of human chorionic gonadotrophin (HCG).

Hyperuricaemia and Tumour Lysis Syndrome

An acute metabolic disturbance may result from the rapid destruction of a tumour following chemotherapy. This is particularly likely to occur in childhood leukaemia and chronic lymphocytic leukaemia, lymphomas with bulky disease, germ-cell malignancies or small cell lung cancer. As chemotherapy destroys the cancer, the cells release products of nitrogen metabolism, especially urea and urate, plus large amounts of potassium and phosphate into the circulation. The high urate concentration may result in urate crystal formation in the kidneys and lead to acute renal failure. A high potassium level is the most dangerous component of tumour lysis syndrome and may cause cardiac dysrhythmias and even sudden death. An increased phosphate level may bind with calcium, resulting in tetany due to hypocalcaemia. The syndrome can be prevented by prescribing allopurinol or rasburicase to prevent the production of large amounts of urate and IV fluids to encourage the kidneys to excrete the products of cell breakdown. Ideally, these interventions should be commenced 1 or 2 days before chemotherapy.

INFECTION

Infections are a major cause of death in cancer. Not only do they occur frequently, but they are often more severe than in other patients, are less responsive to therapy and are often related to organisms that, in normal health, would not cause any problem. The susceptibility of cancer patients to infection results from the suppression of host defence mechanisms produced by the disease and its treatment. Infections are particularly frequent when the neutrophil count is suppressed by chemotherapy. In susceptible populations, granulocyte colony-stimulating factor (G-CSF) may be prescribed during a chemotherapy cycle to reduce the risk of neutropenia and the length of neutropenia associated with treatment, reducing the risk of severe infection.

However, advanced cancer and treatment are also associated with impaired neutrophil and lymphocyte function, depressed cell-mediated and humoral immunity, and skin and mucous membrane damage, allowing organisms to enter the bloodstream more easily. *Escherichia coli*, pseudomonas, staphylococci and streptococci are the most frequent bacterial pathogens. Viruses, such as herpes simplex and herpes zoster (shingles), fungi, particularly *Candida*, and protozoal infection of the lungs with pneumocystis are important nonbacterial causes of infection requiring specific treatment. Most of the infecting organisms come from within the patient, for example, gut bacteria, and while sensible precautions are taken regarding personal hygiene, infections transmitted from family or healthcare staff are of minor importance.

If patients develop an infection while neutropenic, urgent admission to the hospital is usually required, blood and urine cultures taken and, where clinically indicated, sputum, throat or wound swabs sent for culture. Treatment with broad-spectrum IV antibiotics should be commenced immediately after taking the necessary cultures because untreated septicaemia can be rapidly fatal. The choice of antibiotics varies according to the clinical situation and the individual hospital policy. It may change from year to year as directed by the type of local pathogens and patterns of resistance. In some patients, IV fluids, inotropic support and high-dependency care may be required. Occasionally, even in specialist cancer centres, and despite efficient and aggressive treatment of infection, patients still die from overwhelming infection following chemotherapy.

PARANEOPLASTIC SYNDROMES

Neurological

Cancers, particularly small cell lung cancer, as well as cancers of the ovary, uterus, breast and Hodgkin lymphoma, are associated with several neurological syndromes, which are unrelated to direct compression or infiltration of neural tissue. The mechanisms that give rise to these problems are poorly understood. They are uncommon and usually are possible to diagnose only by excluding the presence of malignant disease in the central nervous system (CNS) or around nerve roots. The syndromes include numbness and weakness as a result of sensory and motor peripheral neuropathies, respectively, paralysis from spinal cord damage, unsteadiness from cerebellar degeneration, the most common form of paraneoplastic disease associated with small cell lung cancer, dementia from cerebral damage and a form of muscle weakness that resembles myasthenia gravis. These neurological conditions may be the first manifestation of cancer. Sadly, treatment for the underlying cancer frequently fails to produce much neurological improvement.

Hypertrophic Pulmonary Osteoarthropathy

Lung cancer is the principal cause of this condition, in which the bones of the forearms and shins become inflamed and painful. Plain radiographs show characteristic appearances, and usually the patient has a nail deformity known as clubbing. Antiinflammatory drugs relieve many symptoms, and the condition may improve if the underlying tumour can be removed or destroyed.

Other Paraneoplastic Syndromes

A variety of general effects of cancer are sometimes described as *paraneoplastic phenomena*, and almost every organ in the body can be affected by one of these syndromes. Fever, cachexia, anaemia, thrombophlebitis and clotting disorders are all relatively common and may be the presenting symptoms of malignancy. In addition, arthritis, skin rashes, itching, muscle inflammation and renal impairment are uncommon but well-recognised complications of malignant disease. Each should be treated symptomatically, although the increased risk of thromboembolism may warrant prophylactic anticoagulation.

IMMUNE-RELATED ADVERSE EVENTS

Immune checkpoint inhibitors (ICIs) have changed the cancer treatment landscape, with proven effectiveness in most cancers. This has led to an exponential increase in the use of these medicines and therefore irAEs. Broadly, there are two categories of immunotherapy drugs, one targeting programmed cell death protein 1 (PD-1) or programmed death-ligand 1 (PD-L1) and the other targeting cytotoxic T-lymphocyte-associated protein 4 (CTLA-4).

Prompt recognition of these complications is important. Principles of management include immediate cessation of immunotherapy and treatment with immunosuppressants or immune-modulating drugs. Patients who develop severe toxicities (grade 3–4) on ICI are usually not considered for rechallenge with immunotherapy, but patients who have minimal side effects (grade 1–2) could be rechallenged once steroids or immune-modulating medicines are tapered off.

Spectrum of irAEs

ICIs disrupt the body's immune balance and reduce T-cell tolerance, leading to a spectrum of AEs (Fig. 36.1). These common effects occur in 90% of patients treated with anti-CTLA-4 and 70% of patients treated with anti-PD-1/PD-L1. Severe (grade 3–4) toxicities occur in 21% of patients. The side effects of immunotherapy treatment are different from chemotherapy and have a distinct presentation regarding timing and duration of toxicities (Fig. 36.2). The general principles of management of irAEs are illustrated in Fig. 36.3.

The following section discusses common irAEs.

Skin

Immune-related cutaneous adverse events (ircAEs) are the most common side effects of ICI therapy (>50% for all grades) but are rarely severe and usually do not necessitate treatment discontinuation. Grade 3 to 4 skin reaction occurs in 3% to 5% of patients, which warrants treatment discontinuation. Table 36.2 gives the management according to the grade of the toxicity.

Gastrointestinal Toxicities

Common GI toxicities are enterocolitis, hepatitis and gastritis. Enterocolitis is the most common form of GI toxicity. It may develop after weeks or months of ICI treatment. The median onset time is shorter with anti-CTLA-4 (1 month after first infusion) than with anti-PD-1 (2–4 months after first infusion).

The hallmark symptoms of enterocolitis are diarrhoea and abdominal pain; other symptoms include fever, vomiting and mouth or anal ulcerations. Investigations include stool analysis to exclude infection and flexible sigmoidoscopy or colonoscopy with biopsy to confirm anti-CTLA-4-induced enterocolitis. Early flexible recto sigmoidoscopy or ileocolonoscopy with biopsies is strongly recommended in patients with suspected enterocolitis of a grade higher than 1. Endoscopic assessment is useful to accurately assess the severity of toxicity, as clinical presentation may not correlate with endoscopic and radiological findings and outcomes. Endoscopic features have a prognostic value. Colonic ulcerations, particularly those larger than 1 cm and/or deeper than 2 cm, and extensive colitis are features of the high-risk group associated with a lower rate of steroid response. Early introduction of infliximab or vedolizumab in high-risk groups can significantly reduce the chances of hospitalisations and the duration of steroid treatment. When endoscopy is not feasible, the estimation of faecal calprotectin (a marker for mucosal damage) and its normalisation is useful for clinical management. The management approach to enterocolitis is given in Table 36.3. Patients treated with a steroid or immunosuppressive drug treatment for more than 6 weeks or with infliximab prophylaxis should be considered for *Pneumocystis carinii* infection.

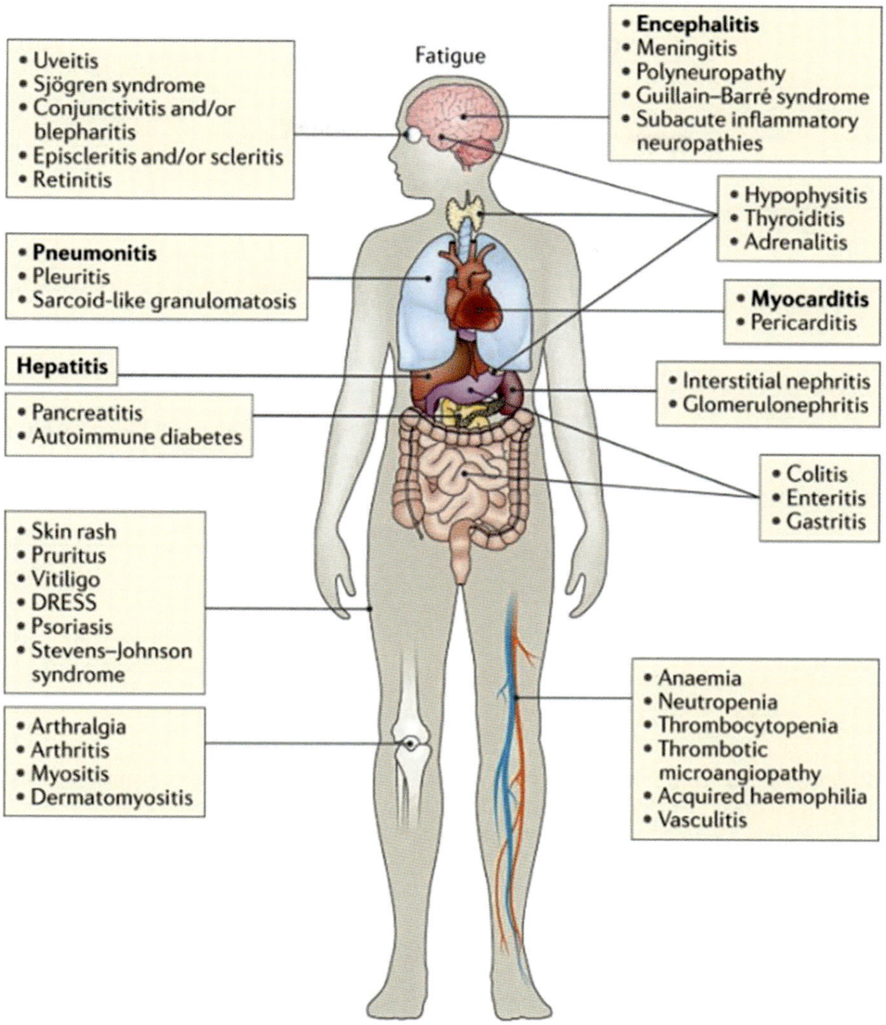

Fig. 36.1 Spectrum of immune-related adverse events. (Martins F, Sofiya L, Sykiotis GP, et al. Adverse effects of immune-checkpoint inhibitors: epidemiology, management and surveillance. *Nat Rev Clin Oncol.* 2019;16(9):563–580. https://doi.org/10.1038/s41571-019-0218-0)

Hepatotoxicity

Approximately 5% to 10% of patients develop hepatotoxicity with single-agent immunotherapy (~2% grade 3) and 13% to 30% with a combination (~5% grade ≥3). A liver biopsy is often helpful in ruling out other causes. The most common pathology finding is lobular hepatitis with necrosis, either spotty or confluent. Management of immune-related hepatotoxicity is given in Table 36.4.

Endocrinopathies

Thyroid Disorders. Primary hypothyroidism is the most common immune-related endocrinopathy, usually occurring within 3 months of therapy. It may be preceded by a subclinical hyperthyroid state. Hypothyroidism is treated with replacement therapy. In symptomatic hyperthyroidism, immunotherapy should be temporarily withheld until recovery.

Hypophysitis. Patients present with headache and visual disturbance due to an enlarged pituitary gland. Patients with severe headaches and visual disturbance should be started on IV methylprednisolone 1 mg/kg after sending blood for pituitary function tests.

Pneumonitis. Immune-related pneumonitis is a group of heterogeneous diseases. Although it is rare, it can be serious and life-threatening, particularly when patients develop acute interstitial pneumonitis/diffuse alveolar damage syndrome. Many cases are subclinical, with the most common symptoms of new or worsening cough, shortness of breath, increased oxygen requirement, chest pain and/or fever. The clinical management of pneumonitis is given in Table 36.5.

Cardiac Toxicity

While immune-related cardiotoxicity is rare, mortality rates are extremely high (35%–50%). When myocarditis is suspected, the patient should be admitted and started on high-dose (methyl)prednisone (1–2 mg/kg). In the case of an inadequate response, consider adding another immunosuppressive drug (e.g. MMF or tacrolimus). Patients should be managed jointly with input from cardiologists.

Neurological Toxicity

Immune-related neurotoxicities can present with a spectrum of central and peripheral neurological symptoms. The commonly reported toxicities are encephalitis, myelitis, demyelinating disease (including optic neuritis), meningitis and vasculitis. In the case of mild neurological AEs, withhold ICI and do a clinical workup (e.g. magnetic resonance imaging (MRI) scan, lumbar puncture) to define the nature of neurotoxicity. In the case of deterioration or severe neurological symptoms, patients should be admitted and started on methyl

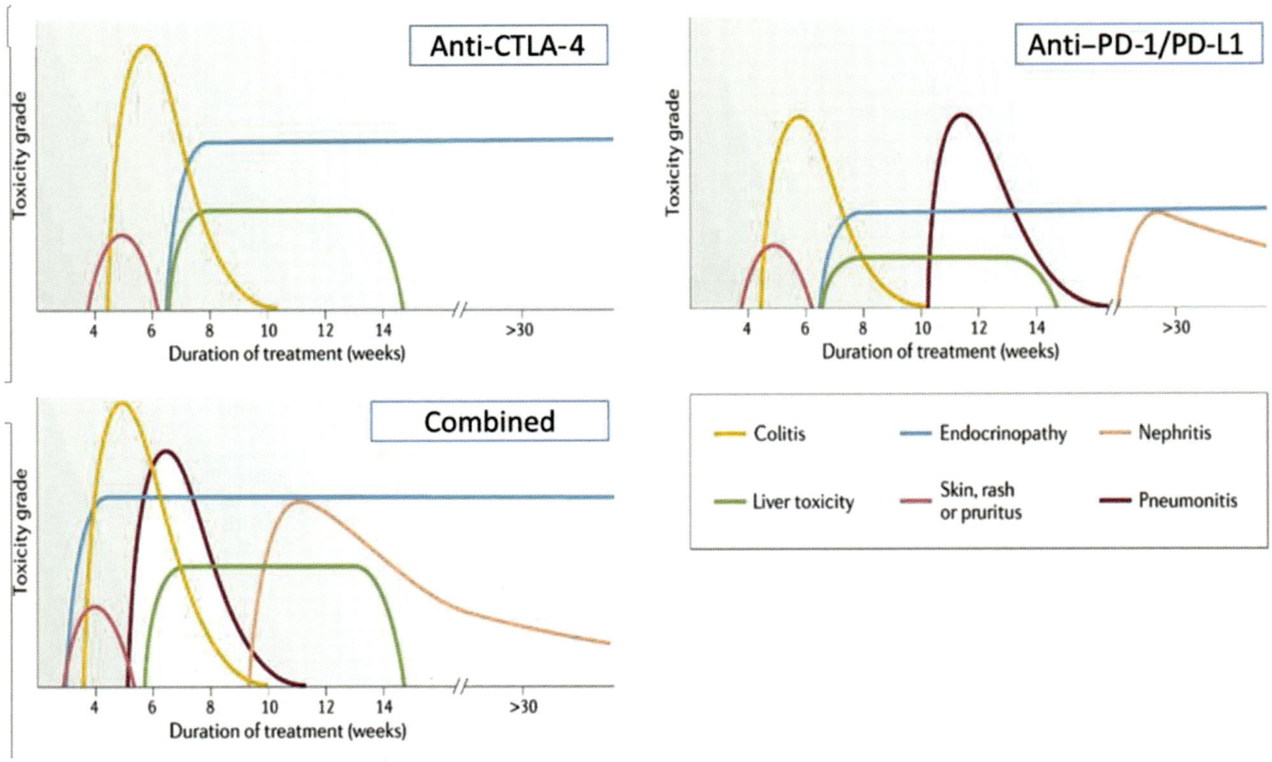

Fig. 36.2 Onset and duration of immune-related adverse events. *CTLA-4*, Cytotoxic T-lymphocyte-associated protein 4; *PD-1*, programmed cell death protein 1; *PD-L1*, programmed death-ligand 1. (Martins F, Sofiya L, Sykiotis GP, et al. Adverse effects of immune-checkpoint inhibitors: epidemiology, management and surveillance. *Nat Rev Clin Oncol.* 2019;16(9):563–580. https://doi.org/10.1038/s41571-019-0218-0)

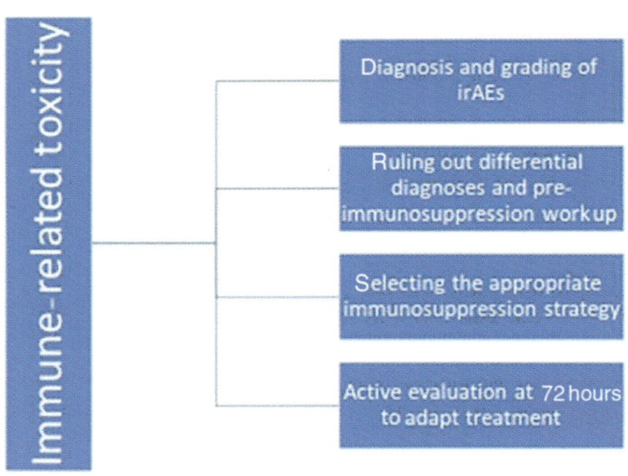

Fig. 36.3 General principles of management of immune-related adverse events. *irAEs*, Immune-related adverse events.

prednisone 1 to 2 mg/kg IV, and specialist neurology advice should be sought.

Musculoskeletal Toxicities

The common immune-related musculoskeletal AEs are inflammatory arthritis (IA), myositis and polymyalgia-like syndrome. For mild arthralgia, start nonsteroidal antiinflammatory drugs (NSAIDs), and if there is no improvement, low-dose steroids (10–20 mg prednisone) is considered. High-dose steroids are needed for severe polyarthritis.

Renal Toxicity

From 3% to 5% of patients develop immune-related nephrotoxicity, commonly acute kidney injury related to acute interstitial nephritis.

TABLE 36.2 Management of Immune-Related Adverse Events According to the Grade of Toxicity

Grading of Toxicity	Management
Grade 1: Macules or papules involving <10% of the body-surface area	Continue immune checkpoint inhibitors. Topical emollients, topical corticosteroids, oral antihistamines Provide advice regarding sun protection and avoidance of skin irritants, e.g. soap-free and perfume-free body wash.
Grade 2: Macules or papules involving 10%–30% of body-surface area; limiting instrumental activities of daily living	Consider holding immune checkpoint inhibitors. High-potency topical corticosteroids (e.g. betamethasone dipropionate 0.05% ointment, Betnovate cream 0.122%); oral antihistamines (e.g. cetirizine, loratadine) If refractory, initiate oral prednisolone (0.5–1 mg/kg) and taper over >4 weeks. (Reduce the prednisolone dose by 10 mg for 5 days as toxicity allows until the dose is 10 mg/day. Then, reduce by 5 mg for 5 days, then stop.) Restart immune checkpoint inhibitors when grade 1 and prednisolone <10 mg.

(continued)

TABLE 36.2 Management of Immune-Related Adverse Events According to the Grade of Toxicity—(cont'd)

Grading of Toxicity	Management
Grade 3: Macules or papules involving >30% of body-surface area; limiting self-care	Hold immune checkpoint inhibitors. High-potency topical corticosteroids, oral antihistamines If refractory, initiate oral prednisolone (0.5–1 mg/kg) and taper over >4 weeks. Restart immune checkpoint inhibitors when grade 1 and prednisolone <10 mg.
Grade 4: Papulopustular rash with life-threatening superinfection; Stevens-Johnson syndrome, toxic epidermal necrolysis and bullous dermatitis involving >30% of body-surface area requires intensive care.	Permanently discontinue immune checkpoint inhibitors. Seek hospital admission and urgent dermatology review. Intravenous methylprednisolone 2 mg/kg daily. Consider infliximab or tocilizumab if refractory to steroids.

TABLE 36.3 Management of Immune-Related Enterocolitis

Grading of Toxicity	Investigations	Management
Patients with grade 1 toxicity (<4 liquid stools per day) persisting for >14 days	Clinical monitoring	Low-fibre diet, loperamide, continue immune checkpoint inhibitors
Patients with grade 2 toxicity (4–6 liquid stools per day) or abdominal pain or haematochezia or nocturnal episodes	Stool testing for enteropathogens, faecal calprotectin, hepatitis and HIV screening (infliximab is contraindicated if positive), endoscopic evaluation, polymerase chain reaction test for cytomegalovirus	Withhold immune checkpoint inhibitors, oral prednisolone 40–60 mg/day
Patients with grade 3–4 toxicity (≥7 liquid stools per day) or any grade diarrhoea with one of the following: abdominal pain, mucus in stool, dehydration, fever	Same as grade 2	Urgent hospital admission and isolation until infection is ruled out No improvement within 48 hours or worsening should be considered for infliximab 5 mg/kg unless there are contraindications (perforation, hepatitis, sepsis, tuberculosis, etc.).

TABLE 36.4 Management of Immune-Related Hepatotoxicity

Grading of Toxicity	Management
AST or ALT ULN to >3 ULN	Monitor blood and continue immune checkpoint inhibitors.
AST or ALT ULN 3–5 ULN	Withhold immune checkpoint inhibitors. Avoid a hepatotoxic drugs. Provide oral prednisolone (0.5–1 mg/kg) and taper over >4 weeks. Restart immune checkpoint inhibitors when grade 1 and prednisolone <10 mg.
Grade 3: AST or ALT ULN 5–20 ULN Grade 4: AST or ALT ULN >20 ULN	Discontinue immune checkpoint inhibitors. Provide intravenous methylprednisolone 2 mg/kg daily. Seek specialist opinion from a haepatologist. Refractory: Consider mycophenolate mofetil 1000 mg twice daily.

TABLE 36.5 Management of Immune-Related Pneumonitis

Grading of Toxicity	Investigation	Management
Grade 1: Asymptomatic, radiological changes confined to one lobe or less than 25% of lung volume	Computed tomography scan of chest with contrast Screen for viral/opportunistic infections	Consider delaying immune checkpoint inhibitors and monitor symptoms. If they worsen, treat as grade 2.
Grade 2: New or worsening cough, shortness of breath, increased oxygen requirement, chest pain	Computed tomography scan of chest with contrast Infection screen Bronchoscopy with bronchoalveolar lavage	Withhold immune checkpoint inhibitors. Provide antibiotics if suspicious of infection and review in 48 hours. If no repose, provide oral prednisolone. Review in 48 hours. If no improvement, treat as grade 3.
Grades 3 and 4: Severe symptoms, acute respiratory distress syndrome and worsening hypoxia	Urgent admission, test as above, high-resolution computed tomography scan	Specialist respiratory review Discontinue immune checkpoint inhibitors. Intravenous methylprednisolone 1–2 mg/kg daily If no improvement or worsening within 48 hours, consider tocilizumab or infliximab.

It is important to rule out other causes of renal failure. ICI should be interrupted or permanently discontinued based on the severity of the renal insufficiency. If appropriate, all other nephrotoxic drugs should be discontinued, and in severe renal failure, methylprednisolone 1–2 mg/kg is started. Consider renal biopsy and a specialist's opinion to confirm the diagnosis.

ACKNOWLEDGEMENT

The authors acknowledge the contributions of Robert Coleman and Harriet S. Walter, the authors of this chapter in the previous edition.

FURTHER READING

Almuradova E, Cicin I. Cancer-related hypercalcemia and potential treatments. *Front Endocrinol (Lausanne)*. 2023;14:1039490.

Durani U, Hogan WJ. Emergencies in haematology: tumour lysis syndrome. *Br J Haematol*. 2020;188(4):494–500.

Gonnelli F, Hassan W, Bonifazi M, et al. Malignant pleural effusion: current understanding and therapeutic approach. *Respir Res*. 2024;25(1):47.

Haanen J, Obeid M, Spain L, et al. Management of toxicities from immunotherapy: ESMO Clinical Practice Guideline for diagnosis, treatment and follow-up. *Ann Oncol*. 2022;33(12):1217–1238. https://doi.org/10.1016/j.annonc.2022.10.001

Hodge C, Badgwell BD. Palliation of malignant ascites. *J Surg Oncol*. 2019;120(1):67–73.

Ikezoe T. Cancer-associated thrombosis and bleeding. *Int J Hematol*. 2024;119(5):493–494.

Klastersky J, de Naurois J, Rolston K, et al. Management of febrile neutropaenia: ESMO Clinical Practice Guidelines. *Ann Oncol*. 2016;27(suppl 5):v111–v118.

Sardiña González C, Martínez Vivero C, López Castro J. Paraneoplastic syndromes review: the great forgotten ones. *Crit Rev Oncol Hematol*. 2022;174:103676.

Schneider BJ, Naidoo J, Santomasso BD, et al. Management of immune-related adverse events in patients treated with immune checkpoint inhibitor therapy: ASCO guideline update. *J Clin Oncol*. 2021;39(36):4073–4126. https://doi.org/10.1200/JCO.21.01440 Erratum in: *J Clin Oncol*. 2022;40(3):315.

Walker MD, Shane E. Hypercalcemia: a review. *JAMA*. 2022;328(16): 1624–1636.

37

Proton Beam Therapy

Jenny Gains, Amy Colori, Laura Beaton and Richard A. Amos

CHAPTER OUTLINE

INTRODUCTION

Recognising the potential benefit of the physical characteristics of proton beams, physicist Robert R. Wilson first proposed the therapeutic use of protons in 1946. Wilson proposed that the geometric and dosimetric localisation properties of monoenergetic proton beams could be used to target structures inside the body. This led to the first patient treatment with protons in 1954 at the Lawrence Berkeley National Laboratory in California.

Although similar to brachytherapy in its ability to conform to the target, proton beam therapy (PBT) represents a noninvasive way of delivering effective radiotherapy (RT). The early adopters of PBT were neurosurgeons. Proton radiosurgery resulted in a level of precision that was compared with alternative confocal methods, eventually culminating in the development of the Gamma Knife. The first hospital-based PBT facility opened in 1989 at the Clatterbridge Centre for Oncology in the United Kingdom. This facility used a low-energy proton beam specifically for the treatment of ocular diseases. In 1990, Loma Linda University Medical Center in California opened the first hospital-based PBT facility for treating deep-seated tumours.

The number of clinical PBT facilities has continued to grow at an increasing rate over recent decades, with many facilities currently operational or under development globally. According to the Particle Therapy Co-Operative Group, the total number of patients treated with PBT worldwide was approximately 350,000 by the end of 2023. Recently opened National Health Service (NHS) PBT facilities at The Christie Hospital and University College London Hospitals commenced treatment in late 2018 and late 2021, respectively, and have treated approximately 2000 patients between them to date.

In this chapter, we review the physics and technology of PBT and then discuss the major clinical indications in children and adults.

PHYSICS AND TECHNOLOGY OF PROTON BEAM THERAPY

Physical Characteristics of Proton Beams

Protons and other heavier charged particles have a distinctive depth-dose distribution based on the nature of their physical interaction with matter. As a proton beam enters a medium, such as a patient, the protons continuously lose energy along their path as a result of Coulomb interaction. As protons lose energy, they lose momentum, slowing down and becoming more densely ionising before eventually stopping. This gives rise to the characteristic low entrance dose and relatively flat dose plateau, before rising sharply to a maximum, the Bragg peak, and falling to zero at the end of the beam range (Fig. 37.1A). The depth of the Bragg peak is dependent upon the composition of the medium through which the beam is travelling and the energy of the protons. The incident energy of the proton beam is chosen such that the depth of the Bragg peak is coincident with the target being treated.

For a monoenergetic beam, the Bragg peak, or so-called pristine Bragg peak, is typically too narrow to encompass the target. To achieve a high-dose region large enough along the depth direction to cover the target, the range is modulated such that multiple weighted pristine Bragg peaks at various depths are delivered in superposition, creating an extended high-dose region called the *spread-out Bragg peak* (SOBP) (see Fig. 37.1B). For large SOBPs the entrance and plateau doses increase as a result of the superposition of modulated beams, but the highest dose region remains within the SOBP. The main dosimetric advantage offered by proton beams is the lack of exit dose distal to the target, enabling the reduction of integral dose to organs at risk (OARs), potentially reducing risk for radiation-related toxicities (Fig. 37.2).

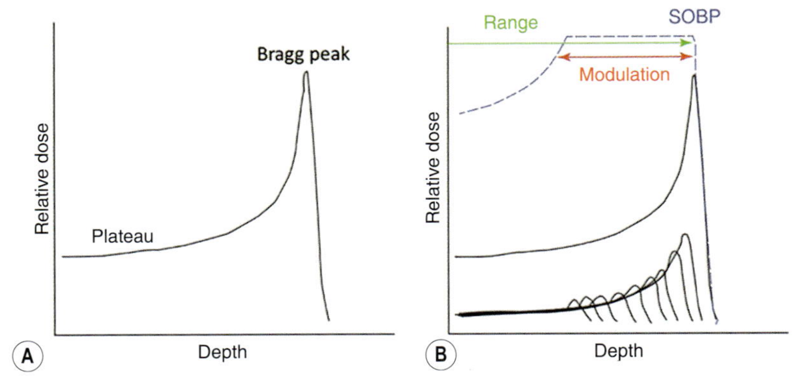

Fig. 37.1 (A) Depth-dose distribution of a monoenergetic proton beam. (B) Superposition of modulated and weighted pristine Bragg peaks resulting in a spread-out Bragg peak. *SOBP*, Spread-out Bragg peak.

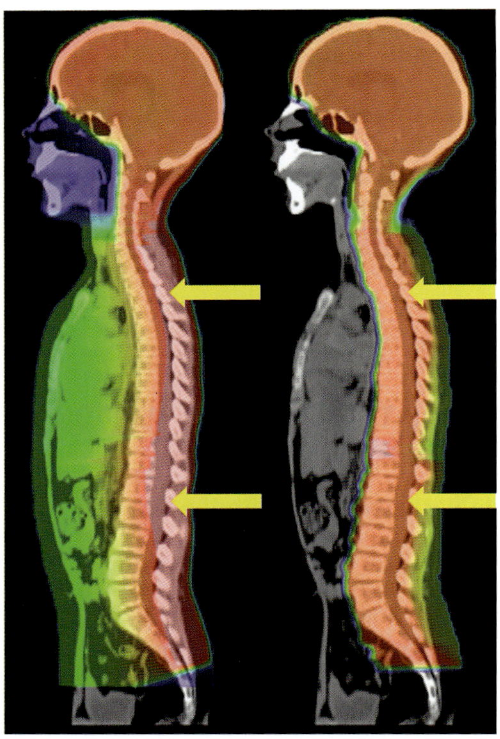

Fig. 37.2 Comparison of dose distributions for craniospinal irradiation using protons (*right*) or x-rays (*left*). The lack of exit dose from the proton beams spares organs at risk anterior to the target.

Proton Therapy Systems Overview

All facilities use either cyclotrons (isochronous cyclotrons or synchrocyclotrons) or synchrotrons to accelerate protons to the required energies for treatment. Protons are then transported along an evacuated beamline using magnetic steering to focus and direct them towards the treatment rooms. Each treatment room consists of either a horizontal fixed beamline or, more typically, a rotating gantry-mounted beamline that enables treatment to be delivered to the patient from any angle. The beamline transports protons into the delivery system, or *treatment nozzle*, which is analogous to the treatment head in a clinical x-ray LINAC. Clinical SOBP beams are then generated using either passively scattered or actively scanned beam delivery systems.

Historically, clinical proton therapy facilities have consisted of one single accelerator serving a number of treatment rooms, typically three to five (Fig. 37.3). In this scenario the proton beam may only be transported into one treatment room at a time, but all rooms can actively set patients up for treatment in parallel, delivering individual proton portals whenever the beam next becomes available. This requires sophisticated scheduling to optimise operational efficiency. However, to democratise access to PBT, equipment suppliers now offer single-room systems and continue to engage in research and development to further reduce associated costs.

Passively Scattered Proton Beams

Early clinical experience with PBT has mostly come from passively scattered proton therapy (PSPT). Passively scattered delivery systems use a number of beam-shaping devices in the treatment nozzle to create a volume of high dose that encompasses and conforms to the target (Fig. 37.4). As the beam passes through the treatment nozzle, it is typically broadened and flattened laterally through a double scattering system. The SOBP is generated by modulation of the beam range, either statically with a ridge filter or dynamically with a rotating range modulator wheel consisting of steps of graduated thickness of degrading material such as poly (methyl methacrylate) (PMMA, also called acrylic or Perspex) or aluminium.

The broad beam is then shaped to conform to the target laterally in the beam's-eye view (BEV) by the use of custom apertures, designed during treatment planning and commonly manufactured from brass.

The distal dose surface of each beam is tailored to conform to the distal shape of the target with a custom range compensator, or bolus. Range compensators are designed during treatment planning to control the depth of penetration along each rayline of the beam, taking into account homogeneities along each path, and are typically manufactured from PMMA or wax.

Active Proton Pencil Beam Scanning

The current state-of-the-art PBT delivery technology is active pencil beam scanning (PBS). All PBT facilities under development and those which have recently come online have adopted PBS technology.

In a PBS delivery system, the narrow pencil-like beam entering the treatment nozzle is magnetically scanned across the target cross section. The energy of the protons is adjusted to vary the depth of dose delivery layer by layer, enabling a three-dimensional pattern of pristine Bragg peaks to be delivered throughout the target volume. This technique is also known as *spot scanning* (Fig. 37.5). Spots are typically delivered across the deepest layer first, with shallower layers scanned subsequently as beam energies are reduced. This technique allows for the delivery of highly conformal and complex three-dimensional dose

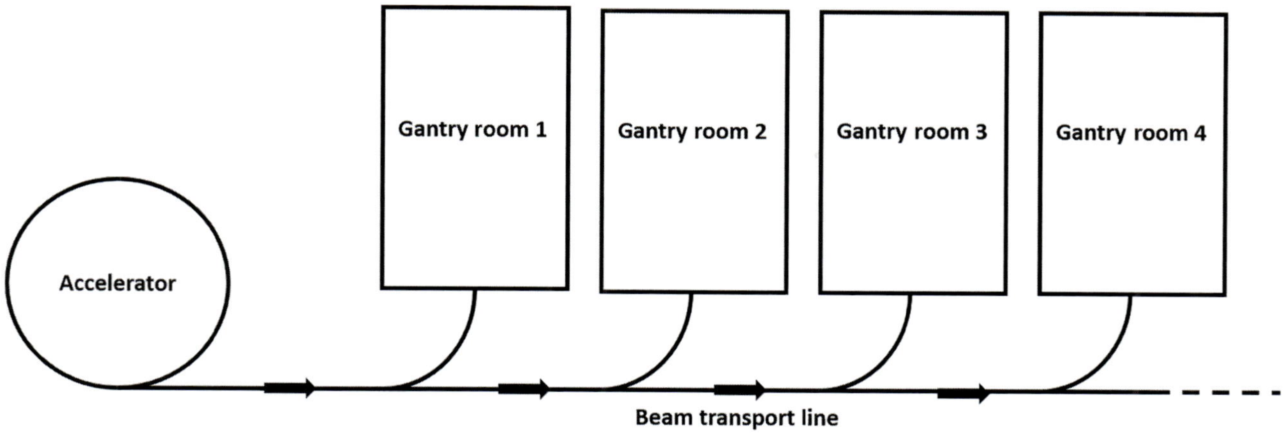

Fig. 37.3 Schematic of a proton beam therapy facility layout with multiple treatment rooms and single proton accelerator.

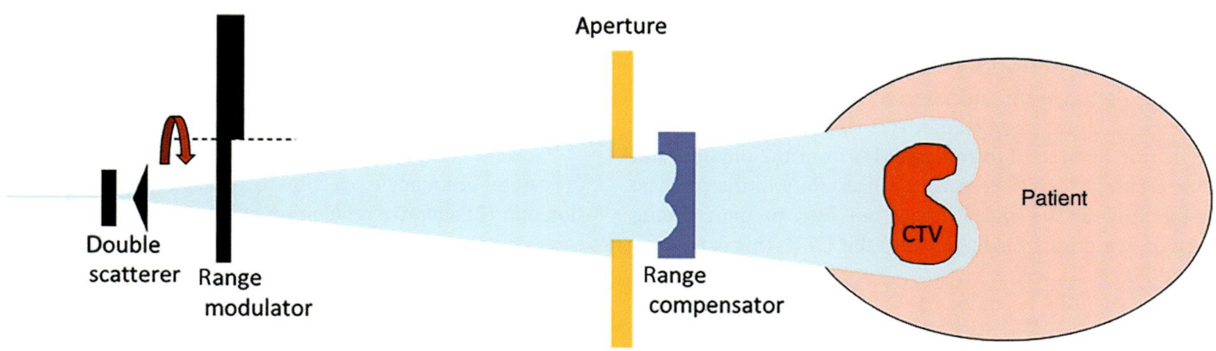

Fig. 37.4 Schematic of a passively scattered proton beam system. *CTV*, Clinical target volume.

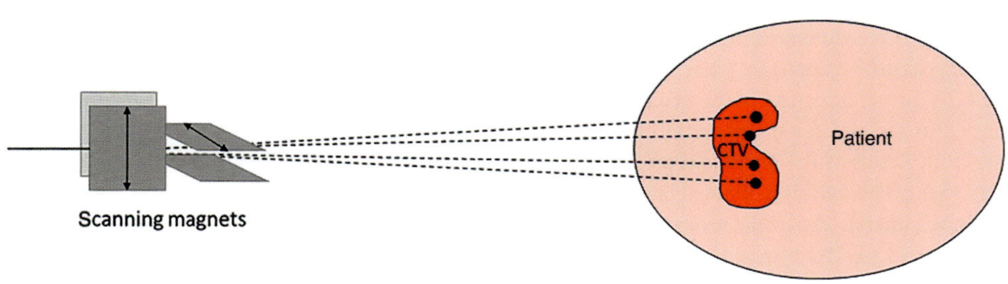

Fig. 37.5 Schematic of a proton pencil beam scanning system.

distributions, not always possible with PSPT. Furthermore, without the need for beam modifiers and patient-specific field shaping hardware, secondary neutron production from nuclear interaction within such devices is removed, sparing the patient from unnecessary exposure.

Sources of Physical and Biological Uncertainties

Although the finite range of protons offers a dosimetric advantage, there are a number of sources of uncertainty that need to be understood and mitigated during the treatment planning and delivery process. Briefly, the major sources of uncertainty in proton therapy are:

1. Range calculation uncertainty
   Proton beam range varies as a function of proton energy and relative stopping power (RSP) of the absorbing material. A significant source of range uncertainty comes from the conversion of Hounsfield units (HU) in the planning of computed tomography (CT) to RSP. This uncertainty in range is approximately 2% for soft tissue and as high as 5% for lung, fat and bone. An average value of 3.5% is assumed for clinical practice. Greater uncertainty exists for high-Z materials such as metallic screws and dental fillings. Traversing these implants should be avoided wherever possible. CT image reconstruction artefacts also increase range uncertainty.
2. Patient position variability
   Proton ranges are highly sensitive to the composition of the media through which the beam traverses and therefore are highly sensitive to patient positioning variability. Daily image guidance is highly desirable to ensure accurate alignment with the machine isocentre as well as alignment of the patient relative to the patient positioning system and immobilisation equipment in the beam path.

3. Anatomical variability
Proton ranges are highly sensitive to intra- and interfractional variations in anatomy. Variations can be caused by respiratory motion, weight loss, tumour shrinkage, bladder filling, bowel gas and changes in sinus filling, to name a few. Mitigation techniques include four-dimensional computed tomography (4DCT)–based planning for respiratory motion; adaptive replanning for weight loss or tumour shrinkage; and careful beam angle selection to avoid traversing anatomy susceptible to variation wherever possible. Mitigating the effect of internal organ motion is particularly important when using dynamic PBS delivery because of the so-called *interplay effect.*
4. Biological uncertainty
The relative biological effectiveness (RBE) of protons is accepted as 1.1 for clinical practice. This is based on a metaanalysis of in vivo and in vitro data obtained in the middle of the SOBP. However, linear energy transfer (LET) increases towards the distal end of the SOBP, with a corresponding increase in RBE. The biological dose is extended distal to the physical range; 2 to 3 mm is a reasonable approximation for this extension.

Treatment Planning and Delivery

Although a single proton beam can deliver a volumetric dose distribution that covers the clinical target volume (CTV), multiple beams from different angles are often used to mitigate risk from the physical and biological uncertainties described earlier. Uncertainty in the physical range and the RBE at the end-of-range can lead to underdosing the CTV and/or overdosing OARs distal to the CTV. This is true for both PSPT and PBS beam delivery.

For an individual SOBP beam for PSPT, the field-shaping aperture is designed to conform dose to the CTV in the plane of the BEV. The aperture is also designed to include the margin around the CTV to account for internal target motion, patient positioning variability and lateral field penumbra. This two-dimensional margin expansion from the CTV is identical in principle to that used for the three-dimensional expansion that gives rise to the planning target volume (PTV) in conventional x-ray RT. However, three-dimensional expansion of this margin is not adequate for proton therapy. The SOBP is designed to also conform dose to the CTV in the direction of the beam, with both distal and proximal margins to account for the physical range uncertainties described earlier. Dimensions of the distal and proximal margins essentially differ from that of the two-dimensional lateral margin, giving rise to a nonuniform volumetric expansion from the CTV. Furthermore, each individual beam in a PSPT treatment plan will have distal and proximal margins that differ from the other beams because range uncertainty depends on each beam's path length. This gives rise to the concept of the beam-specific PTV (bsPTV). Each beam is designed to cover its own bsPTV, and assessment of CTV coverage requires that each beam is evaluated individually. A single PTV cannot be used adequately for reporting and evaluating plan quality. PSPT planning margins are described in greater detail by Zeng et al. (2018).

There are two general categories of PBS-based treatment planning, both using inverse-planning optimisation. The first uses single-field optimisation (SFO), also known as *single-field uniform dose* (SFUD). With SFUD plans, spot scanning patterns from each beam direction are individually optimised to cover the target. This is similar in principle to PSPT planning, and the bsPTV concept applies.

The second category of PBS-based treatment planning uses multifield optimisation (MFO), also known as *intensity modulated proton therapy* (IMPT). With IMPT plans, spot scanning patterns from all beam directions are optimised simultaneously to cover the target. This means that the spot pattern from each individual beam direction does not necessarily cover the target. Although IMPT is a very powerful technique for generating highly conformal and complex dose distributions, the range uncertainty of each individual pencil beam contributing to the combined spot pattern leads to a potential lack of plan robustness. If individual spots over- or undershoot, the dose distribution can become extremely heterogeneous within the target; margin expansion from the CTV cannot account for this.

Robust optimisation has been clinically adopted to improve the robustness of IMPT and SFUD treatment plans. The treatment planner may enter values into the treatment planning software for range uncertainty, typically 3.5%, and positional uncertainty in millimetres. Using these values, the optimisation algorithm will iteratively improve the robustness of the plan given all possible scenarios. In theory, robust optimisation should eliminate the need to plan to a margin expansion beyond the CTV, thus removing the PTV issue altogether.

The complex nature of PBT planning margins, both for PSPT and PBS delivery, often complicates the direct comparison of PBT plans with x-ray RT plans for the purposes of clinical trials. Lowe et al. (2020) have produced UK consensus guidelines for doing this.

An emerging technique for mitigating risk to OARs from the increased RBE at the end of the proton beam range is *LET-based optimisation.* Using increasing LET as a surrogate for increasing RBE, treatment plans may be optimised so as to redistribute higher LET in such a way as to reduce risk to OARs.

General strategies for delivering robust proton plans include (1) careful beam angle selection to avoid anatomy susceptible to variation and (2) adaptive replanning over a course of treatment as necessary. Daily image guidance is paramount for accurate and reproducible patient alignment, and contemporary PBT systems incorporate in-room volumetric imaging. Advanced imaging techniques will play an increasing role for image-guided positioning, target delineation, proton range verification, adaptive replanning and motion tracking.

Emerging Techniques and Technology

There are currently a number of emerging techniques and technologies within the field of PBT. These areas of ongoing research and development aim to improve the clinical efficacy and efficiency of PBT while reducing the financial costs associated with this modality. This section briefly highlights four of these emerging innovations.

Proton FLASH Radiotherapy

The demonstration of significantly reduced toxicity in a mouse model by Favaudon et al. in 2014 by delivering radiation at the ultra-high dose rate (UHDR) of 40 to 60 Gy/s represents a potential paradigm shift for clinical RT. A significant amount of preclinical research, both in vitro and in vivo, has continued around the world over the past decade producing increasing evidence of a normal tissue sparing effect, known as the FLASH effect, at UHDR. The underlying biological mechanisms responsible for the FLASH effect are yet to be fully understood.

Much of the preclinical research into FLASH RT has used UHDR sources of electrons or photons. Such dose rates are not readily achievable with clinical linear accelerators (LINACs), and so laboratory-based research accelerators have been used. This makes the clinical translation of electron and photon FLASH RT challenging. Most contemporary clinical PBS-based PBT systems, however, are capable of delivering UHDR radiation, and so there is interest in the development of carefully designed clinical trials for proton FLASH RT. The first in-human proton FLASH clinical trial (FAST-01) was completed in 2023 at the University of Cincinnati Health Proton Therapy Center. This was a nonrandomised safety trial of proton FLASH RT to symptomatic extremity bone metastases. Transmission beams were used for this trial as technical limitations prevented controlling the depth of the

Bragg peak at FLASH dose rates. No adverse effects were observed, and the feasibility of delivering proton FLASH in a clinical setting was demonstrated. Preparation for the FAST-01 trial also provided the catalyst for developing procedures for accurate and traceable calibration of absolute dosimetry with UHDR proton beams. This is of paramount importance for future trials.

Proton FLASH RT is moving towards translation into clinical practice. However, there are a number of hurdles yet to be cleared. Well-designed clinical trials need to be developed; an international consensus on proton FLASH trial design is currently being sought. Technical delivery of UHDR proton beams that maintain the Bragg peak advantage along with treatment planning techniques maximising FLASH dose rates in normal tissue need to be optimised. Finally, further preclinical characterisation of the FLASH effect is required.

Proton Minibeam Radiotherapy

Proton minibeam radiotherapy (pMBRT) is a form of spatially fractionated PBT consisting of fields of submillimetre parallel beams. Dose profiles from each portal consist of peaks and valleys, similar in principle to photon-based 'GRID' RT. The rationale for spatially fractionated RT is that normal tissue tolerance has been shown to be higher for smaller beam sizes while maintaining curative intent. Several studies have reported reduced neurotoxicity with spatially fractionated RT in small animal models compared to standard RT.

Comparing the nanodosimetric characteristics of photon-based MBRT with pMBRT, it has been shown that pMBRT is more effective at sparing normal tissue due to less energy deposition with fewer DNA double strand breaks in the dose peaks and valleys. Furthermore, pMBRT causes an increase in complex DNA breaks and higher energy deposition in the tumour region owing to the characteristic Bragg peak. Prezado et al. (2018) have reported an increase in the therapeutic window with pMBRT for high-grade gliomas (HGGs) in rat brains.

These preclinical findings are of interest and have led to numerous groups around the world conducting research into pMBRT. However, much like with proton FLASH RT, the underlying biological mechanisms for the observations reported are not yet fully understood.

Proton Arc Therapy

Proton arc therapy (PAT) has been the focus of treatment planning studies for a few years. The technique is based on the rotation of the proton gantry during beam delivery akin to the delivery of volumetric modulated arc therapy (VMAT). The rationale for considering PAT is to reduce the impact of proton range uncertainty on conformity, improve plan robustness and optimise the deposition of higher LET to increased the RBE in the tumour.

Several treatment planning studies have demonstrated robust and acceptable dose distributions. However, the feasibility of clinical PAT delivery remains an important question. With contemporary PBS systems, the impact of proton energy layer switching time on continuous rotational delivery is complicated to solve. Multiple discrete gantry angles are more achievable than continuous gantry rotation. This remains an area of ongoing investigation.

Upright Patient Positioning

To democratise PBT and increase accessibility to a greater number of cancer patients who may benefit, costs associated with this technology need to be reduced. Furthermore, the cost-effectiveness of PBT may be further improved by increasing treatment efficiency.

One of the ways to reduce costs is to design PBT facilities without rotating gantries in treatment rooms. Rather than a gantry, a treatment room may be served by a single fixed horizontal beamline. To enable single fixed horizontal beamlines to be as versatile as conventional gantries, upright patient positioning systems are now becoming commercially available. These upright patient positioning systems allow for the immobilisation of patients, as with conventional horizontal patient positioners, 360-degree rotation about their vertical axis and an off-axis tilt to enable noncoplanar beams. To acquire CT imaging of the patient in the correct orientation, both for treatment planning and volumetric image guidance, these upright patient positioning systems incorporate a vertical axis–mounted CT scanning system (Fig. 37.6).

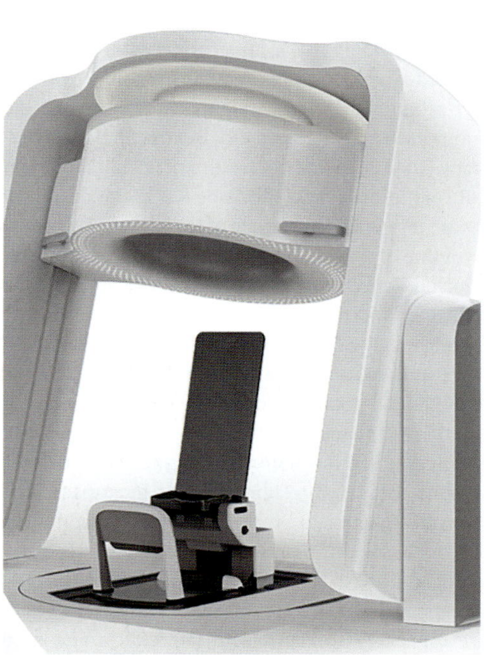

Fig. 37.6 An upright patient positioner with upright computed tomography scanner. (Courtesy LEO Cancer Care Ltd.)

Upright patient positioning may lead to significant cost savings in the development of PBT facilities. Not only do they potentially remove the need for rotating gantries, but they also reduce the footprint of each treatment room with associated reduction in cost for shielding materials required for room construction. Upright positioning may also improve treatment efficiency. Rotating patients to achieve multiple beam angles of incidence is likely faster than rotating larging gantries. A number of clinical PBT facilities are now testing these systems and clinical adoption seems inevitable.

PROTON BEAM THERAPY IN CHILDREN, TEENAGERS AND YOUNG ADULTS

Cancer in children, teenagers and young adults (TYA) remains relatively rare compared to the adult population. There were just over 1800 new cases of cancer diagnosed in children each year in the United Kingdom in the 2016 to 2018 period. There is a huge diversity and heterogeneity of tumour types seen. Leukaemia, central nervous system (CNS) tumours and lymphomas account for approximately two-thirds of tumours in children whereas in the TYA population, lymphomas are the most common tumour type. Survival from children's cancers continues to improve and has doubled in the past 40 years. Within the United Kingdom, approximately 84% of children now survive their disease for 5 years or more and 80% survive for 10 years or more. However, this success comes at a cost, with many studies showing the impact of treatments on the long-term health and quality of survivorship, especially for those treated for paediatric CNS tumours.

Improved understanding, including on a molecular level, has enabled patients to be increasingly risk stratified: intensifying treatment for those with a predicted worst outcome and deescalating treatment for those with a better prognosis. However, for many tumours, RT still forms an essential component of multimodality treatment alongside surgery and chemotherapy. The late toxicity of treatment is multifactorial, but RT has a significant role to play. Side effects of RT in the paediatric and TYA populations are influenced by the age of the patient, anatomical site, dose of RT and volume of normal tissue irradiated. The late complications of treatment include effects on growth and development, reproduction, neurocognitive, endocrine, vital organ function (cardiac, pulmonary, renal, gastrointestinal (GI)) and second malignancies.

Due to its unique beam characteristics, already described in this chapter, PBT has the potential to reduce the toxicity burden and also the secondary malignancy risk for paediatric and TYA oncology patients. Many studies have shown the superior dosimetric advantages of protons compared to photons. For most paediatric and TYA tumours, the effectiveness of protons is not expected to exceed that of photons as dose escalation is not being attempted. The advantages lie with the reduced dose to normal tissues both potentially in the acute setting but especially in the late effects setting. This young group of patients are especially susceptible to late effects and second malignancies. There is an increased risk of cancer when treating immature and developing tissues alongside the increased length of survival and potential development of second cancers compared to adults. Proton compared to photon techniques in modelling studies have been shown to reduce the risk of second malignancies. Sethi et al. (2014) performed a retrospective review of 55 retinoblastoma patients treated with protons and 31 treated with photons. The 10-year cumulative incidence of radiation-induced second malignancies was significantly different (proton 0% versus photon 14%; $p = 0.015$). In the United States and Canada, a large record linkage cohort of proton- and photon-treated patients is being used to compare subsequent cancer risks in paediatric patients, enabling a large-scale systematic comparison. The reduction in second malignancies is likely to be even greater with the adoption of PBS techniques as opposed to passive scattering.

There are no randomised controlled trials comparing photons with protons in the paediatric or TYA population, and there are very unlikely to be any in the future as they have been deemed both unethical and unfeasible. But purely on the improved dosimetric profile and the perceived benefit in toxicity and late effects burden, PBT is becoming the standard of care for many paediatric and TYA tumours. Delivering proton therapy to younger patients requires complex multidisciplinary management including anaesthetic support, play specialists and paediatric oncology support.

Worldwide, paediatric solid tumours are seen as a high priority for PBT. However, the proportion of patients receiving proton therapy will vary around the world. PBT still remains a limited resource worldwide, but many new centres are opening or in development. Some countries have had successful overseas proton therapy programs while establishing their own centres and have reported on the outcomes of these. However, there is worldwide inequity of access to proton therapy, usually related to geographical location or socioeconomic status. Many countries have produced recommended guidelines for the use of PBT in the paediatric and TYA populations. A consensus report from the Stockholm Pediatric Proton Therapy Conference was published in 2016 with agreement on the role of PBT for young children with curable tumours and the main indications. They did emphasise the important questions that remain in terms of patient prioritisation and magnitude of benefit.

Initially, most proton treatment for paediatric patients focused on brain and spinal tumours, but as we discuss in the following sections, more tumours and anatomical sites are now being treated. Early publications were mostly retrospective studies, often with early follow-up data comparing outcomes to historically published photon data. More prospective data with longer-term toxicity data are becoming available.

Central Nervous System Tumours

Focal and craniospinal RT form an important part of the curative treatment of childhood brain tumours with a range of late effects that could be potentially reduced with proton therapy including effect on neurocognition, endocrine effects, effects on hearing and risk of second malignancy. When using craniospinal treatment, the benefit of protons is in the reduced exit dose to the thoracic, abdominal and pelvic cavities, which may reduce acute and late effects. In the focal part of treatment, more benefits can be made in terms of, for example, neurocognition and hearing. One of the most devastating long-term effects of treatment for a childhood brain tumour is long-term neurocognitive effects. The potential to spare total brain, temporal lobe and hippocampal doses with proton therapy is starting to be translated into better neurocognitive outcomes.

Medulloblastoma

Medulloblastoma is the most common malignant brain tumour seen in children. Treatment is multimodal, with surgery, chemotherapy and RT all required. The RT component is in two phases: craniospinal RT and a boost to the posterior fossa tumour bed. The intensity of chemotherapy and the dose of craniospinal RT depend on the risk stratification by pathology and presence of metastases into standard or high-risk grouping. Subgrouping continues to evolve as the differing molecular subtypes and how they relate to outcome develop. Medulloblastoma survivors are known to be at significant risk of late effects including neurocognitive, hearing and endocrine effect, development of second cancers and effects, for example, on the heart, lungs and thyroid due to the craniospinal component of treatment. The younger the patient is at the time of treatment, the worse the late effects are likely to be.

Predictive dosimetric studies have shown a potential risk reduction for PBT in medulloblastoma for cardiac toxicities, premature ovarian failure, ototoxicity, neurocognition and second malignancy compared to photon-based techniques. Yock et al. (2016) have published a phase II single arm study of PBT in medulloblastoma. This was the first prospectively published study on the use of PBT for medulloblastoma, and outcomes in terms of disease control were similar to published photon data. There was less hearing loss compared to historically published photon data, but this comparison is imperfect as the boost volume has changed from whole posterior fossa to tumour bed only for standard-risk patients in this time frame. There was absence of cardiac, pulmonary and GI effects with a median follow-up of 7 years. Some have proposed the potential of vertebral sparing craniospinal treatment with protons, but this technique would require evaluation in a formal prospective clinical trial. Regarding pencil beam techniques for craniospinal irradiation (CSI) RT, there are early reports on outcomes with 2-year follow-up and low late toxicity rates.

Low-Grade Glioma

With regards to low-grade gliomas (LGGs), the most common subtype seen in paediatric patients is a pilocytic astrocytoma (WHO grade 1). Complete surgical excision if possible is the mainstay of treatment. In younger children with incomplete excision or progression, chemotherapy is used to delay the use of RT. Newer targeted molecular agents are an option for some who have progressed on chemotherapy. RT is an alternative, especially in older children and those who have progressed through chemotherapy and lines of targeted therapy. The 10-year overall survival in several studies is in excess of 90%. Children and TYA patients receiving RT for LGG are subject to a range of late effects depending on the age of the patient and the anatomical site of the tumour but include long-term effects on neurocognition, hearing, vasculature, endocrine and visual function as well as second malignancy risk. PBT therefore has the potential to reduce some of these effects.

An early study by Fuss et al. (1999) showed improved sparing of normal tissues with protons for optic pathway gliomas. A more recent retrospective comparison of conventional photon plans and proton plans in 74 patients with LGG showed superior sparing of structures involved in neurocognition, especially those on the contralateral side to the tumour. Of note, both of these studies have compared protons to conventional photon techniques and not newer IMRT techniques. The study with the longest follow-up for paediatric patients with LGG treated with PBT is from Greenberger et al. (2014). Their 8-year progression-free survival and overall survival rates are consistent with previously published photon data. For those patients in the study with serial neurocognitive testing, no significant declines in Full Scale Intelligence Quotient were seen compared to baseline. Within subgroup analysis, there were declines in those treated at an age of less than 7 years and those with significant dose to the left temporal lobe and left hippocampus. Indelicato et al. (2019) reported on 174 paediatric LGG patients treated with PBT with 5-year progression-free survival of 84%. Pseudoprogression was observed in 32% of patients. A small study of LGG paediatric patients with annual neurocognitive assessment following PBT did not show any significant changes in cognitive function.

Ependymoma

Ependymoma is the third most common primary brain tumour in children, representing approximately 10% of childhood CNS tumours. Two-thirds occur infratentoriarly and one-third in the supratentorium. The best reported outcomes have been with maximal tumour resection followed by postoperative RT to the tumour bed. They frequently present in children under age 4 years, and in the very young, postoperative chemotherapy has been employed to delay the use of RT. Late side effects of treatment in this group are of particular concern due to the usually young age of the patient and the proximity of tumours to critical structures. The potential to reduce the dose to the normal brain structures with protons could improve neurocognitive outcomes; have less long-term impact on endocrine function; reduce the dose to hearing apparatus; and reduce the risk of second malignancy. The literature on proton therapy for ependymoma has shown so far that outcomes are comparable with the published photon data in terms of tumour control. More recent studies have longer lengths of follow-up and maintain consistent outcomes.

Craniopharyngioma

Craniopharyngiomas are rare, benign tumours of epithelial origin arising in the suprasellar region from the remnant of Rathke pouch. Although benign, with excellent survival rates, they are complex to manage. There is often significant morbidity for patients in the long term from both the effects of the tumour and the treatments used. These include long-term toxicities related to visual impairment, pituitary and hypothalamic dysfunction, neurocognitive effects and vascular effects. Patients without a complete excision require postoperative RT either up front or at the time of progression. The combination of limited surgery and postoperative RT has been shown to reduce some of the toxicities of treatment related to the hypothalamus, pituitary and optic chiasm compared to radical surgery alone.

Planning studies have shown that compared to photon IMRT, proton therapy can reduce the dose to the cochlea, hypothalamus, supratentorial brain and temporal lobes in craniopharyngioma cases. Other studies have shown similar advantages for sparing other important structures such as the hippocampi and vasculature with PBT, especially with IMPT.

These tumours frequently have both solid and cystic components. The cystic component can potentially enlarge during PBT and this could impact significantly on target volume coverage and dosimetry. Therefore regular magnetic resonance imaging (MRI) scans to monitor the cyst should be performed during a course of PBT. Prospective outcome and toxicity data on the use of protons in craniopharyngiomas are now emerging, Merchant et al. (2023) have reported a 3-year progression-free survival (96.8%) and overall survival (100%) which is comparable to historical patients treated with photons. The most common grade 3 to 4 adverse events were headache (6%), seizure (5%) and vascular disorders (6%). They followed patients prospectively with neurocognitive assessments over 5 years and found a reduced risk for declines in intelligence and adaptive functioning following proton therapy compared to photons with a more than 10-Gy reduction in temporal lobe doses between the techniques.

There have been concerns that there may be an increased incidence of brainstem toxicity with PBT. A recent French study compared patients treated with either photons or protons for intracranial ependymoma. They found asymptomatic radiographic changes in 4.8% but no symptomatic brainstem injury and no correlation with dose or technique. Upadhyay et al. (2022) looked at 595 pediatric brain tumours receiving PBT. They found a low risk of symptomatic brain injury of 3.2%. The incidence was higher in those younger than age 3 years, female gender, atypical teratoid/rhabdoid tumour (AT/RT) histology and patients receiving high-dose chemotherapy and stem cell rescue.

Extracranial Tumours

Initially most paediatric and TYA patients receiving proton therapy for extracranial tumours were those with rhabdomyosarcoma or Ewing sarcoma. As discussed next, the number and variety of extracranial tumour types being treated are expanding.

Rhabdomyosarcoma

Rhabdomyosarcoma is the most common form of soft-tissue sarcoma seen in the paediatric and TYA populations. Patients are risk stratified in terms of prognosis and for treatment intensity depending on their pathology, site, surgical resectability, lymph node status, tumour size and age. Rhabdomyosarcomas can occur almost anywhere in the body, but the most common sites of primary tumour include parameningeal, bladder/prostate, orbit and extremities. Treatment requires a multimodality approach with systemic chemotherapy and surgery, RT or both. RT plays an important role in the local control of rhabdomyosarcoma for many patients. PBT can therefore offer a potential advantage in terms of toxicity for these patients depending on the particular anatomical site and age of the patient. An early study by Ladra et al. (2014) also compared proton and IMRT plans for patients enrolled on a phase II prospective study of patients with rhabdomyosarcoma and showed improved target normal tissue sparing in several anatomical sites with protons. The initial outcomes for these patients were published separately and were comparable to photon data, and late toxicity rates were favourable but require longer follow-up (Ladra et al., 2014). Childs et al. (2012) published the clinical outcome for a cohort of parameningeal rhabdomyosarcoma patients with 5-year outcome similar to historical photon cohorts but with improved functional results compared to photon studies. In terms of later musculoskeletal facial outcomes, Hol et al. (2023) found significantly less facial deformation in survivors with parameningeal rhabdomyosarcomas treated with protons compared to photon RT.

Ewing Sarcoma

Ewing sarcoma is the second most common childhood primary bone tumour after osteosarcoma, with a median age of presentation of 15 years. Eighty-five percent of Ewing sarcomas arise in the bones, but 15% can occur in the soft tissues. The most common primary site is extremity long bones (40%) followed by the pelvis (25%) and then the spine or ribs. RT forms an essential component of the local control strategy for Ewing sarcoma either alone or in combination with surgery (pre- or postoperatively). There is usually no role for PBT in extremity tumours. The potential benefit in terms of toxicity will be for those with large pelvic and chest wall tumours as well as spinal and the less common head and neck Ewing sarcomas. Data regarding early outcomes are now being published, with mainly early follow-up showing control rates similar to those seen with photons and reasonable toxicity rates.

Other Paediatric Tumours

Studies using proton therapy in abdominal neuroblastoma have been published with early follow-up and outcomes, but more prospective data in large clinical trials with longer-term data are required to fully understand its widespread role in this disease. Ensuring adequate tumour volume coverage with motion or bowel gas changes in these complex volumes is something to be considered when selecting these patients for proton therapy over modern photon-based techniques.

Published literature on the use of proton therapy for Wilms tumours is limited and mainly comprises dosimetric planning studies. For there to be a benefit in treating patients requiring postoperative flank RT, a more conformal approach to target volume delineation is required.

Hodgkin lymphoma is another disease with high cure rates and patients with long life expectancies where even low doses of radiation can have significant impacts on long-term health. Early studies showed potential benefit in terms of reducing doses to the heart, lung and breast. Significant reductions in heart, lung and breast doses have been achieved with proton therapy while treating patients with Hodgkin lymphomas, mainly with mediastinal disease, and show no grade 3 to 5 toxicities at 5 years follow-up, with 5-year progression-free survival of 90% and no marginal failures.

Whole lung radiotherapy (WLRT) is an important treatment for patients with lung metastases normally in the up-front setting of treatment of metastatic Wilms tumour, Ewing sarcoma and rhabdomyosarcoma. Delivering WLRT with protons has been shown to be feasible, with reduction in mean doses to the heart and thyroid, and merits further evaluation. Other indications such as reirradiation, for example, require evaluation within prospective clinical trials to establish its role and potential benefit.

Summary

PBT is likely to remain a limited resource, and the acceptance of cases with an expanding indications list is also likely to depend on other factors such as travel and limited capacity, and some prioritisation of appropriate cases will continue to be required. It is essential that good-quality outcomes and toxicity data are collected so that the full potential of PBT can be quantified. An amount of later follow-up data is starting to emerge.

In summary, proton therapy has the potential to significantly reduce the late effects of treatment for paediatric patients due to the reduction in dose to normal sensitive and growing tissues. However, it is essential that good-quality prospective outcome data collection occurs, and there are several collaborative groups around the world focusing on this.

PROTON BEAM THERAPY FOR ADULT CANCERS

As with the paediatric and TYA populations, the main advantage of PBT in adults is the ability to provide an effective therapeutic dose to tumours proximate to radiosensitive normal structures. The dose limitation depends on the tumour location to be irradiated but most notably includes the brainstem, spinal cord (and spinal nerve plexae), optic pathway, pituitary, cochleae, salivary glands, thyroid, lungs, heart, small bowel, liver, kidneys, large bowel and reproductive organs. Therefore there is potential benefit to most adult tumour sites.

In the adult population, using PBT to reduce dose to critical normal structures offers potential benefit in three separate scenarios:

- High likelihood of delivering desired dose without compromising planned dose to respect OAR tolerance
- Dose escalation not achievable with IMRT
- The opportunity for retreatment of previously irradiated sites in the setting of disease relapse

The further final benefit, which is irrespective of site, is the reduction in risk of secondary malignancy due to a smaller volume of tissue being irradiated.

To date, limited randomised controlled trials have been reported to underpin the rollout of PBT in a rapidly increasing number of international centres over the past decade. There are few studies which have made head-to-head comparisons of PBT with photon RT. Some of these have included three-dimensional conformal planning within their photon cohorts and passive scattering within their PBT cohorts, both arguably outdated in times of more conformal techniques such as IMRT and PBS PBT.

PBT use for multiple adult indications has nevertheless exponentially increased, which, in lieu of top-level randomised evidence, is based mainly on the solid but theoretical dosimetric advantage, small-scale randomised controlled trials, and outcomes from retrospective studies. Current indications for PBT are based on this limited body of evidence. These indications vary according to national or institutional commissioning practice. More recently, international bodies (e.g. PTCOG) have developed consensus documents for practice in multiple indications, reflecting an aim to reduce variation in global treatment regimens (Table 37.1).

However, the global variation in access to healthcare necessarily results in huge disparity in practice. Some wealthy nations will treat all patients in whom PBT is potentially indicated, while others that ration healthcare will restrict PBT candidates (e.g. under commissioning policy or by applying normal tissue complication probability modelling in real time). The majority of the global population lives in countries which are very unlikely to have ready access to PBT treatment for several decades to come. Developing a centre capable of delivering PBT is an enormous undertaking in terms of cost, time and complexity. PBT is a limited resource, even in developed countries, so it must be put to best use.

The need for proper evaluation of this potentially extremely valuable new RT tool is increasingly being recognised. In the United Kingdom, the service was both nationally commissioned to deliver PBT for approved indications and required to provide the robust and comprehensive collection of clinical outcome data to evaluate and demonstrate potential future benefit of PBT in the long term. Considerable resources have been invested in the UK NHS Proton Clinical Outcome Unit to ensure that findings will inform future practice. In the United Kingdom, the interlinked UK NCRI CTRad PBT Clinical Trial Strategy Group has been specifically established to encourage and support the development of UK-based prospective clinical trials in PBT. This is being echoed in other countries which have developed the infrastructure to deliver PBT to their populations. Eagerness to be early to deliver a new effective technique is now being accompanied by proactive engagement with research studies which can demonstrate this robustly.

Thus the rapidly increasing access to PBT, coupled with a scientific desire to elucidate its clinical benefits, means that development of new clinical trials is occurring at an exponential rate worldwide. Multiple randomised controlled trials evaluating PBT either are in the advanced

TABLE 37.1 Current Proton Beam Therapy Indications Guidelines for Adult Indications and Examples of Adoption by Selected Countries

	INTERNATIONAL GUIDELINES				INDIVIDUAL COUNTRY GUIDELINES		
	American Society for Radiation Oncology (ASTRO)[a]	Paul Scherrer Institute (PSI)/ Bundesamt für Gesundheit (BAG)	Particle Therapy Cooperative Group (PTCOG)	MedAustron	National Health Service (NHS) England	Denmark	Netherlands
Adult Indications							
Chordoma—base of skull/spinal	✓	✓	✓	✓	✓	✓	✓
Chondrosarcoma—base of skull	✓	✓	✓	✓	✓	✓	✓
Paraspinal/spinal sarcoma	✓	✓	✓	✓	✓		
Paranasal sinus/nasal cavity	✓	✓	✓	✓	✓		Potential
Other advanced/unresectable head and neck cancers	✓		Consider	Consider			
Ocular melanoma	✓	✓			✓	✓	
Intracranial arteriovenous malformation	✓			✓		✓	
Meningioma	✓	✓		✓		✓	✓
Low-grade glioma	✓	✓		✓		✓	
Acoustic neuroma	✓			✓			
Malignant and benign primary CNS tumours excluding IDH wild-type GBM, that are treated with curative intent and with potential for long-term prognosis	✓			Consider			
Primary and metastatic tumours requiring craniospinal irradiation	✓				✓		
Sarcomas	✓	✓	✓	✓	Selected	Selected	Potential
Hepatocellular carcinoma	✓			Consider			
Lymphoma	Mediastinal		Consider	Consider	Consider	✓	
Lung cancer	Group 2		Consider	Consider			
Mesothelioma	✓		Consider		Trial		
Oesophageal cancer	✓		✓				
Breast cancer	Group 2		Consider		Selected on trial		
Prostate cancer	Group 2		Consider				
Reirradiation	✓		Consider	✓		✓	Potential

Note: Three countries are shown as examples of adoption guidelines in practice from international guidelines, as shown in the first three columns.
[a]American Society for Radiation Oncology Group 2 tumours are those for which clinical evidence needs to be developed and comparative effectiveness analyses performed. Patients are currently suitable for treatment as part of a clinical trial or multiinstitutional patient registry.
CNS, Central nervous system; *GBM*, glioblastoma multiforme; *IDH*, isocitrate dehydrogenase.

stages of setup, are recruiting, were recently closed for analysis, are due to report or are due to open shortly. However, comparatively few such randomised studies have already reported. The forthcoming commentary describes the limited existing evidence (of various levels) for the adult indications of PBT and acknowledges future randomised controlled trials which will provide further vital high-quality evidence to influence future clinical practice.

Sarcoma/Connective Tissue Malignancy

Sarcomatous tumours can arise from any connective tissue and therefore have diverse histopathology with variable radio sensitivity. Historically, the preferred primary management of localised sarcoma has been surgical resection, where clear margins can be expected, regardless of histological subtype. However, since the advent of IMRT, a move towards a combined multimodal surgical and radiotherapeutic approach has afforded a better balance of disease control and optimisation of structure and function preservation.

Primary definitive radical irradiation of a tumour is usually reserved for when surgical resection at a particular tumour location would likely be incomplete and would threaten normal structure function. However, despite the improved dose distribution of IMRT as compared to three-dimensional chemoradiotherapy (CRT), the high doses typically required in the treatment of sarcomas remain limited by nearby OAR tolerance, even with IMRT. Hence the increasing interest in the use of proton beam RT to afford higher target-volume doses while sparing dose to neighbouring organs.

Sarcomas can be categorised by both location and histological subtype, specifically grouped by bone tumours (plus chordomas and chondrosarcomas) versus soft-tissue sarcomas. These are discussed in turn in the next section.

Chordoma and Chondrosarcoma

Chordomas are rare tumours originating from the remnant of the embryonic notochord. They most commonly occur in the skull base or sacrum, and standard treatment comprises maximal safe surgical resection followed by high-dose adjuvant RT.

Chondrosarcomas are rare, slow-growing tumours that arise from cartilage, typically affecting the pelvic bones. The management of chondrosarcomas has some similarities with the treatment of chordomas, consisting of primary surgery, where possible, with high-dose adjuvant RT to improve local control. However, when these tumours occur at the skull base, complete excision is often difficult due to their anatomical position. The infiltrative nature of these tumours into bone, along with the presence of residual tissue after surgery, means that local recurrence with surgery alone is high.

The delivery of adjuvant RT presents its own difficulties. Both chordomas and chondrosarcomas are relatively radioresistant and frequently occur in close proximity to the critical base of skull structures, such as the spinal cord and brainstem, which limit dose escalation with conventional RT. Historically, the compromised low doses associated with photon RT treatment volumes have resulted in poor outcomes (e.g. 5-year progression-free survival of 25%). Since 2015, global consensus recommends that in the treatment of chordomas, doses of at least 74 Gy should be delivered as postsurgical adjuvant treatment or following biopsy in inoperable patients. PBT therefore might have a particular benefit in these tumours by allowing dose to be escalated due to sharp dose falloff between tumour and critical organs.

An early series of 100 chordoma patients in the Proton Collaborative Group prospective registry (85 of whom had postoperative PBT and 15 of whom had primary PBT) was evaluated between 2010 and 2018. Over 3 years, local control, progression free survival and overall survival rates were 94%, 74% and 83%, respectively. Only 8% of patients had acute grade 3 PBT-related toxicities and none had grade 3 or higher PBT-related late toxicity.

Several further studies have found similar favourable disease control and toxicity rates. In the absence of randomised evidence, metaanalyses of retrospective research are informing practice. A 2022 systematic review which assessed PBT for base-of-skull chordomas (including 16 studies and a total of 752 patients) found 5-year local control, overall survival and progression-free survival rates of 76.6%, 79.6% and 89%; seemingly favourable compared to photon rates. Saito and colleagues' 2024 systematic review, which compared the two modalities in base-of-skull chordoma, found no statistically significant difference for overall survival (at 3 and 5 years), but 5-year progression-free survival rates for PBT versus photon RT were 67.8% versus 40.2% ($p = 0.0004$). This can be explained by the higher median dose in the PBT cohort than those receiving photons (65–78.4 Gy (RBE) versus 14.8–81 Gy (RBE)).

A retrospective analysis of 798 national registry patients confirmed that dosage greater than 6000 cGy was associated with increased overall survival (hazard ratio 0.51; $P = 0.038$), although it didn't find the RT modality to significantly influence survival measures. A recent metaanalysis of base-of-skull chondrosarcomas reported 3- and 5-year overall survival rates of 94.1% and 93.9%, respectively, and 3- and 5-year local control rates of 95.4% and 90.1%, respectively. PBT was significantly associated with improved 5-year overall survival.

Chordomas and chondrosarcomas equally affect the rest of the spine. Tumours of the mobile spine and sacrum involve a different set of toxicities and surgical challenges, with sacral-level disease being particularly likely to involve the cauda equina/exiting spinal nerves and proximate abdominopelvic organs including the bowel, bladder and gynaecological organs. As with more superior tumours, primary surgical resection may be accompanied by adjuvant RT, or this might be the definitive modality where effective surgery is not possible. High rates of local control in the pelvic area can be achieved with doses of 70.4 Gy, but the ability to achieve this is limited primarily by bowel toxicity. Series demonstrate that PBT can achieve higher doses, efficacy, acceptable toxicity and planning robustness.

Other Sarcomas

As relatively radioresistant tumours of the spinal axis, chordomas and chondrosarcomas were the first connective tissue tumours to be treated with PBT. However, the need for high doses combined with normal tissue sparing means that PBT has become commonplace in the treatment of multiple other types of sarcomas (including both primary bone and soft-tissue histologies), depending on location.

Typically, other sarcomas also require relatively high RT doses as a part of complex multimodality treatment plans, which often involve surgical resection and the concomitant uncertainty in RT margins postoperatively. They are not defined by any particular anatomical region and so any bone or soft-tissue sarcoma, proximate to a dose-limiting OAR, is worthy of consideration for treatment with PBT.

More recently, PBT is being used for sarcomas outside the craniospinal axis. In this situation the indication is not to just allow full-dose/dose escalation to the primary treatment site neighbouring a critical radiosensitive organ, but to maximally reduce dose to other nearby critical structures. Examples include sarcomas of the chest wall where the use of PBT reduces cardiac dose or retroperitoneal sarcomas where dose escalation is otherwise limited by the bowel, reproductive organs, liver or kidney tolerance. PBT plans for limb sarcomas may be more conformal and reduce dose to neighbouring uninvolved bone and soft tissue, potentially reducing late toxicity.

Head and Neck Tumours

Historically, the use of PBT in the treatment of head and neck cancers has been limited to a small subgroup of hard-to-manage tumours, such as those arising in the nasal cavity and paranasal sinuses. In these cases, primary treatment would typically be with surgery, where the tumour is small and amenable. But where local recurrence rates with surgery alone are high, adjuvant RT is also added to reduce this risk. Although some such tumours are resectable, their locations may make them inoperable and so RT is also used as the primary radical therapy.

Invasion of the skull base is a particular issue in this group of tumours; the close proximity of critical structures, such as the optic apparatus, brainstem, cranial nerves, cochlea and temporal lobes, limits the dose that can be safely delivered with RT. Surgical resection is also a limiting factor. Studies of PBT treatment for these head and neck indications and sarcomatous tumours of the skull base have provided evidence that the modality can deliver an effective radical dose treatment in the head and neck while ensuring safe dose to neighbouring structures.

Over the past decade, PBT has been increasingly used to treat a range of head and neck cancers, notably including the oropharynx, salivary glands, sinonasal cavity/nasopharynx and oral cavity. The Particle Therapy Co-operative Group (PTCOG) Head and Neck Subcommittee have developed a first set of consensus guidelines covering nasal, sinonasal, oropharyngeal and reirradiated tumours.

Given the extensiveness and complex geometry of head and neck target volumes and their anatomical proximity to multiple critical structures, the PTCOG guidelines advocate the use of the most advanced forms of proton planning and treatment delivery. Examples include the use of multifield IMPT versus single-field optimised planning to ensure clinical robustness and high-quality plans, and frequent verification imaging (e.g. daily cone beam CT) to ensure the early dynamic response needed for plan adaptation. These planning considerations are especially important in the planning of PBT treatment of tumours of the head and neck, where volume coverage is particularly susceptible to changes in external contour and sinus filling.

Nasal Cavity and Paranasal Sinuses

Only three or four decades ago, treatment of these tumours was delivered with direct-field/three-dimensional conformal RT and resulted in high rates of significant long-term toxicity. Forty-one percent of patients with paranasal sinus cancer developed blindness following conventional radiation therapy due to retinopathy or optic neuropathy. While the conformality IMRT offers has substantially reduced this effect, more recently PBT has further reduced the toxicity burden and delivered higher disease control rates. An early metaanalysis of 86 observational and 8 'in silico' studies demonstrated significantly higher 5-year local control rates with PBT than IMRT for paranasal and sinonasal cancers (86% versus 66%). A more recent retrospective review of patients with sinonasal cancer treated with PBT reports similar local control and low late toxicity rates. Complementary dosimetric studies confirm reduction of dose to nonadjacent OARs with IMPT versus IMRT, though potentially increased dose to abutting normal structures such as the eye.

Oropharyngeal Cancers

Oropharyngeal cancer, whose staging now reflects HPV status, affords a better prognosis than many other head and neck cancers. Given excellent survival outcomes, the use of PBT in this cohort has been specifically evaluated for its ability to spare long-term toxicity in addition to survival measures. Early studies of proton treatment postoperatively in patients with oropharyngeal cancer appear to show it to be superior to IMRT in terms of patient-reported outcomes, quality-of-life measures and CTCAE toxicities.

In a recent phase III trial from MD Anderson Cancer Center, 440 patients with locally advanced oropharyngeal cancer undergoing definitive CRT treatment to the bilateral neck with 70 Gy in 33 fractions were randomised between IMRT and IMPT. As per intention to treat, per protocol and as treated analysis, there was a statistically significant benefit of PBT over PFS. (In the intention-to-treat analysis, for example, the hazard ratio for disease progression at 3 years was 0.87 (95% CI 0.56, 1.35; $p = 0.006$). The benefit of PBT on overall survival was nonsignificant. Rates of nutrition-related toxicities including gastrostomy-tube dependence and weight loss were also significantly decreased with IMPT.

A further prospective phase III randomised trial, TORPEdO (TOxicity Reduction using Proton bEam therapy for Oropharyngeal cancer), run by the NHS, is underway. This randomly assigns definitive patients with oropharyngeal cancer to organ-preserving chemoradiation and bilateral neck treatment using IMRT versus IMPT, with primary outcome measures being late treatment-related toxicity but also includes a strong translational element, with the collection of imaging, physics and tissue/blood data to inform future patient selection. The outcomes of prospective trials such as this will guide future practice and inform future patient selection.

Other Head and Neck Cancers

Given the proximity of multiple critical head and neck organs, PBT is starting to be used in other tumours, with good local control and toxicity rates. These include nasopharyngeal, oral cavity, laryngeal and salivary gland tumours. The use of PBT for other head and neck tumours is likely to expand over the coming years.

Central Nervous System Tumours

Early use of PBT for CNS tumours predominantly began in the paediatric and TYA populations. The adult brain/CNS generally is thought to be somewhat less susceptible to radiation-related toxicity than children's brains. Irradiation of the adult CNS can nevertheless lead to significant temporary or permanent cortical neurocognitive functional deficits, endocrine dysfunction or cranial nerve impairment leading to visual/hearing problems. As such, any technique that improves conformality to treatment volume and consequent reduction in surrounding low dose bath and avoidance of critical structures may offer clinical benefit.

Following the paediatric indications, PBT treatment of adult CNS tumours has been rapidly adopted in tumours which affect the lower end of the adult age range (age 18 to 30 years). Evidence from the paediatric/TYA populations described earlier is echoed in the treatment practice of younger adults affected by medulloblastoma, ependymoma, craniopharyngioma and intracranial germ cell tumours, with excellent efficacy and toxicity profiles.

As with younger patients, PBT CSI in adults is advantageous relative to photon IMRT. It is noninferior for overall survival or progression-free survival compared to photon RT, but it significantly reduces rates of acute weight loss (16% versus 64%; $P = .004$), nausea and vomiting (26% versus 71%; $P = .004$), oesophagitis (57% versus 5%, $P < .001$) and myelosuppression (white blood cells 46% versus 55%, $P = .04$; hemoglobin 88% versus 97%, $P = .009$; platelets 48% versus 65%, $P = .05$).

PBT is now widely used in adults for the indications affecting the paediatric/TYA populations described earlier. However, it is also increasingly recognised as being beneficial in preserving adult cortical function. It has therefore become more widely used in multiple tumours.

Glial and Glial Neuronal Tumours

Over the past decade, PBT has become more frequently used in the treatment of adult glial tumours. The benefit of adjuvant RT in combination with appropriate chemotherapy following maximal safe resection of LGGs is underpinned by level 1 evidence (e.g. RTOG 9802, RTOG 9402, CANTON study). These patients have a prognosis of 10+ years and are likely to be affected by long-term neurocognitive deficits resulting from photon RT.

Better long-term neurocognitive outcomes with proton versus photon RT have been suggested by a small prospective study of 20 patients with LGG treated with PBT. After 5 years of follow-up, no decline in neurocognition was observed using a battery of cognitive tests. The NRG BN005 trial (NCT03180502), a phase II randomised trial assessing cognitive preservation in approximately 120 patients with isocitrate dehydrogenase (IDH) mutant, low-to-intermediate-grade gliomas randomised to proton versus photon RT closed to recruitment in spring 2024. The APPROACH trial (NIHR131082), a multicentre study run by NHS, is currently randomising 246 adults with oligodendroglioma 1:1 between PBT and photon adjuvant RT. The primary outcome is neurocognitive function at 5 years. In due course, such studies will provide valuable insight on the long-term cognitive benefit of PBT.

The standard of care for treating glioblastoma multiforme (GBM) (WHO grade 4) in fit patients includes maximal surgical resection and adjuvant CRT. A 2021 phase II prospective trial which randomised patients with newly diagnosed GBM to PBT versus IMRT aimed to establish whether PBT delayed time to cognitive dysfunction. The predicted difference was not found and there was no impact on survival outcomes, but there was a significant reduction in fatigue. Given the relative short prognosis of GBM and the limited benefit of PBT shown, it is unlikely that PBT will become the standard of care for GBM.

Meningioma

Management of meningiomas depends on grading and ranges from surveillance to definitive RT to surgical resection with or without postoperative RT.

Where appropriate, primary irradiation of grade 1 meningiomas achieves local control, at 5 to 10 years, in the range of 89% to 100% and low rates of late toxicity (0%–12%), with most studies reporting toxicity between 0% and 5% and being overwhelmingly low grade. Postoperative radiation for grade 2 (atypical) meningiomata improves progression-free survival, as evidenced by two prospective trials, a metaanalysis and a systemic review, which reviewed 24 studies comprising 3078 patients with atypical meningiomas and reported postoperative RT improved progression-free survival after either subtotal resection (hazard ratio 0.41) or gross total resection (hazard ratio 0.73). The benefit of RT in rarer grade 3 anaplastic meningiomata is less established, but they are typically treated as per grade 2 tumours, which some studies have grouped, but with treatment volume margins reflecting invasive behaviour.

Stereotactic RT offers targeted conformal RT and is in widespread use for benign grade 1 meningiomas. A large retrospective analysis of 4565 patients demonstrated 5- and 10-year progression-free survival rates of 95.2% and 88.6%, respectively. Several retrospective reviews of both conventionally and hypofractionated PBT in grade 1 meningiomas have demonstrated equivalent 5-year local control rates of 71% to 99%. A recent prospective study reported long-term results of 59 patients with 64 WHO grade 1 meningiomas treated with definitive or adjuvant PBT at a median dose of 50.4 Gy relative biological effectiveness (RBE) (range 48.6–61.2 Gy RBE), with median follow-up of 6.3 years, and found that the 5-year local progression rate was only 6% and the grade 3 + toxicity rate was 2%.

There are no randomised studies demonstrating the superiority of PBT in this setting, though NCT05895344 COG-PROTON-01, currently recruiting, assesses this in cavernous sinus meningioma. Nevertheless PBT is in widespread use and is of particular utility in challenging tumour locations where dose would otherwise be limited by OAR tolerance.

There is less evidence for PBT in grades 2 and 3, all of which is retrospective, but there appears to be comparable efficacy and toxicity profile. Given the dose-dependent response of these tumours, dose escalation with PBT is a promising avenue. The prospective PANAMA trial (NCT02978677) is evaluating this. As it stands, as with grade 1 meningiomas, PBT is used on a case-by-case basis.

Vestibular Schwannomas

PBT has also been used for the treatment of vestibular schwannomas, otherwise known as *acoustic neuromas*. A 2023 metaanalysis found a 95.4% rate of tumour control (both stability and decrease in volume). PBT was well tolerated, with preservation rates of 95.6% for trigeminal nerve function (absence of numbness), 93.7% for facial nerve function preservation and 40.6% for hearing .

Intraocular Melanoma

Treatment of ocular tumours was an early avenue in the use of PBT, with it becoming an alternative option to brachytherapy or enucleation. The role of PBT in the treatment of ocular melanoma has been extensively reported in historical series, with 95% local control rates and 90% eye retention rates. PBT has a particular benefit due to its small treatment volumes and the close proximity of critical structures such as the optic apparatus. Although PBT has not been directly compared, the only phase III trial comparing RT modalities to date reported local control for helium ion particle versus plaque brachytherapy of 100% versus 84% at 5 years and 98% versus 79% at 12 years, respectively. Additionally, the post-RT enucleation rate was lower after PBT: 11% versus 22% at 5 years and 17% versus 37% at 12 years. A 2016 systematic review [65] including 14 original studies and thousands of patients confirms the basis on which PBT has become standard treatment for this indication.

Breast Cancer

RT is a key component in the multimodality radical treatment of breast cancer. Given excellent survival, there has been recent focus on reducing long-term morbidity from treatment. As such, there has been rapid growth in PBT for breast cancer, and PTCOG has produced a consensus document evaluating the evidence for its use. PBT has two potential benefits over photon RT: better OAR dosimetry and improved target coverage, especially of the internal mammary chain lymph nodes which are frequently underdosed in IMRT plans to meet lung and heart tolerance.

These late toxicities which arise following RT for breast cancer include radiation-related heart disease, radiation pneumonitis/fibrosis, restriction of arm/shoulder function and secondary malignancy, including the contralateral breast.

A number of small prospective studies demonstrate disease control similar to the published literature, with lower toxicity rates. However, further randomised controlled evidence is needed to confirm improved outcomes with protons. Two forthcoming phase III clinical trials will provide this evidence in the future. The UK-led PARABLE trial randomises postoperative patients, with at least 2% estimated risk of cardiac disease, 1:1 between standard of care photon RT and PBT. The primary outcome measures are mean heart dose and patient-reported normal tissue toxicity. Secondary endpoints will assess survival outcomes, cardiac events and other toxicities. A similar multicentre US study, RADCOMP (NCT02603341), is also underway.

On the basis of the existing evidence, the PTCOG consensus statement acknowledges its use may be most beneficial for those with existing cardiothoracic disease, those with left-sided or right-sided medial tumours and those receiving regional nodal irradiation, and recommends enrolment of such patients in ongoing randomised controlled trials where appropriate to develop the future evidence base.

Gastrointestinal Malignancies

Oesophagus

Concurrent CRT is an important treatment option for inoperable oesophageal cancer, but it can cause serious late adverse effects including lung fibrosis, liver dysfunction, lymphopaenia and cardiac toxicity. The PTCOG consensus statement acknowledges multiple planning studies which have demonstrated effective thoracic organ sparing. For example, in one large real-world retrospective analysis of 727 patients with oesophageal cancer, IMRT demonstrated significantly lower radiation exposure to the whole heart and its substructures from PBT versus IMRT.

One retrospective analysis looking at survival outcomes has shown comparable rates (3-year overall survival, progression-free survival and local control were 59.2%, 56.3% and 69.8% respectively). In this series, there were no pleural or pericardial effusions, and 2 patients (4.3%) developed a radiation pneumonitis. A larger series demonstrated similarly low rates of toxicity, but a subgroup analysis by clinical stage also revealed considerably higher 5-year overall survival (34.6% versus 25.0%, $P = .038$) and progression-free survival rates (33.5% versus 13.2%, $P = .005$) in the PBT group for patients with stage 3 disease. A phase IIB trial which randomised 145 patients with locally advanced oesophageal cancer to IMRT versus PBT found that the overall treatment toxicity burden (TTB) was significantly lower in the PBT group but the 3-year progression-free survival (51.2% versus 50.8%) and overall survival (44.5% versus 44.5%) were equivalent between the groups.

Fortunately, currently recruiting randomised clinical trials aim to address this. NCT03801876, for example, a phase III multicentre trial analysing CRT using PBT compared to IMRT, has two coprimary endpoints: better overall survival with PBT and noninferior overall survival with reduced cardiopulmonary toxicity. Outcomes of these studies will better inform practice in the coming years. Currently, PTCOG recommends that PBT be *strongly* considered for patients with trimodality and nonoperative oesophageal cancer who could benefit from reduced toxicity rates and that clinicians actively enrol such patients in clinical trials.

Liver

Historically, the use of external beam radiotherapy (EBRT) in liver tumours has been limited by radiation-induced liver disease (RILD) Although the liver is considered a 'parallel' OAR, hepatocytes are susceptible to damage from low-to-medium-dose bath, and patients may well already have liver dysfunction. As techniques have become more sophisticated, IMRT, especially stereotactic body radiotherapy (SBRT), has become indicated as part of the treatment suite across all stages of hepatocellular carcinoma.

There are now multiple retrospective and some prospective studies and a recent prospective registry examining its use, which show good local control rates (93.3%–100% at 1 year, 86.5%–95% at 2 years) for liver tumours treated with PBT. PBT potentially offers an advantageous toxicity profile in large tumours which are challenging to treat with SBRT and those associated with venous thrombosis which increase risk in radiofrequency ablation (RFA).

There is no direct prospective trial comparison between photon SBRT and PBT. However, a recent dosimetric study showed the ability of PBT to spare dose to the liver by active-scanning PBT compared to CyberKnife stereotactic radiosurgery, VMAT-5 (V-MAT with 5-mm jaws flattening filter free) and VMAT-10 (V-MAT with 10-mm jaws with flattening filter). A national database study of outcomes for 918 patients receiving SBRT versus 71 patients receiving PBT reported 1-year survival of 64.3% versus 76.5% and 3-year survival of 30% versus 36.7%, respectively, despite the PBT cohort having prognostically poorer features such as larger tumour size and more significant comorbidities. In this study, a higher biologically effective dose (BED) (>100 Gy10) was independently associated with better outcomes. PBT can achieve these doses with plans being compromised to respect organ tolerance.

Forthcoming prospective work (e.g. NCT03186898) will distinguish the effects of photon RT, including photon SBRT, and PBT more clearly. It will also explore the benefit of hypofractionated stereotactic treatment delivered with proton beam RT and the integration of PBT within multimodality treatment regimens using targeted systemic anticancer therapy (e.g. NCT06133062). Future work will clarify the clinical scenarios in which PBT is particularly beneficial.

Lower Gastrointestinal

Standard definitive management of nonmetastatic rectal adenocarcinoma involves surgery, RT and chemotherapy, with 5-year local control and overall survival rates of 85% to 92% and 68% to 80%, respectively. Standard-of-care concurrent CRT for anal squamous cell carcinoma affords 5-year local control and overall survival rates of 68% to 87% and 65% to 74%. While advances in photon RT techniques such as IMRT versus three-dimensional conformal RT have reduced toxicity rates, the close proximity of the abdominopelvic organs means they remain susceptible to the effects of radiation.

To date, few studies have assessed the clinical application of PBT for lower GI/anal cancers. Eleven patients safely underwent short-course RT with PBS PBT for rectal cancer, with appreciably lower doses to normal structures in keeping with dose reduction from PBT in previous planning studies detailed in the PTCOG Gastrointestinal Subcommittee Lower Gastrointestinal Tract Malignancies Consensus Statement. This statement currently recommends careful patient selection based on tumour position relative to OARs but foresees the outcomes of prospective trials such as PRORECT (NCT04525989), which will directly randomise preoperative SCRT patients between protons and photons.

Definitive CRT for anal cancer, while effective, carries relatively high rates of both acute and late toxicity. RTOG 0529 found some reduction in OAR toxicity with IMRT as compared to conventional RT (though the primary endpoint was not met), but complication rates remained high. Despite a dosimetric study showing significant dose reduction to multiple local OARs, clinical studies to date have not consistently proven the translation of this to actual reduction in toxicity. Chuong et al. (2019) report a reduction in GI toxicity following PBT compared to IMRT, from the Proton Collaborative Group REG001-09 prospective multiinstitutional registry cohort. However, a large 2021 multicentre retrospective comparison failed to find any significant clinical benefits between those receiving IMPT versus IMRT, despite finding a significant low-dose reduction to both the bladder and bowel.

The evidence base for PBT irradiation of lower GI tumours is in its infancy, and pending further high-level evidence, it is not recommended routinely. However, PTCOG recommend that SCRT for rectal cancer could be considered for those at high risk of toxicity.

Prostate Cancer

IMRT already offers excellent local control rates with low rates of long-term GI and genitourinary (GU) dysfunction, so given that PBT is a limited resource, its use is somewhat controversial in the management of prostate cancer. While several prospective and large retrospective series have found disease control rates in line with modern IMRT rates, there is an absence of top-level evidence of improved disease-related outcomes. Nevertheless accumulating retrospective and prospective studies documenting a beneficial toxicity profile of PBT (evaluated in the 2021 PTCOG 2021 consensus statement) mean that it has become an established practice to deliver primary and postprostatectomy prostate irradiation.

Early comparative studies of proton with photon RT have shown a better toxicity profile: reduction in early but not late bowel and bladder symptoms, no difference, improved urinary toxicity and reduced bowel toxicity (though not universally). PBT may also offer the ability to improve outcomes in higher-risk patients with dose escalation not achievable by IMRT.

Earlier works have focused on conventionally fractionated definitive prostate cancer irradiation. In the salvage RT postprostatectomy setting, a case control–matched study of 307 males found that though PBT did reduce the low-medium OAR dose, there were no significant differences in GI or GU toxicity.

Ten-year outcomes from the CHHiP trial continue to show the noninferiority and low rates of late morbidity from hypofractionated (3 Gy per fraction) compared to normally fractionated. Single-site studies suggest PBT reflects this finding. Nakajima et al. (2018) found no difference between toxicity rates from 526 patients enrolled in phase II trials receiving PBT in either 2 Gy per fraction or 3 Gy per fraction.

A recently reporting systematic review reported significantly lower rates of grade ≥2 acute GI toxicity (2% versus 7%) and improved 5-year biochemical relapse-free survival (95% versus 91%) in the PBT arm compared to RT. The 5-year biochemical relapse-free survival improvement was maintained for the moderate hypofractionated arm ($p = 0.0122$) and intermediate -and low-risk patients ($p = <0.0001$ and 0.0368, respectively).

Enough existing evidence is available that prostate PBT is considered at least as safe and effective as IMRT. Several major current multiinstitutional trials are expected to report in the coming years (e.g. PARTIQoL (NCT01617161), COMPPARE trial (NCT03561220) and PAROS (NCT04083937)) and have the potential to further shape future use of PBT in prostate cancer.

Thoracic Malignancies

Tumours of the thorax are clearly a heterogeneous group, including primary lung cancers, mediastinal lymphomas and thymomas, among other, less commonly occurring tumours. Here, they are considered together on an anatomical rather than histological basis. The evidence base relating to the specific use of PBT in these tumours is less well developed than in many other primary tumour sites. Many of the relevant studies in the field apply due to the particular treatment delivery considerations involved in irradiation of the region. Effective RT for thoracic targets must account for respiration-related motion, associated changes in beam entry tissue density and evolving changes in target volume. Modern thoracic PBT plans include patient-related parameters, both pretreatment 4DCT acquisition and active motion management (breath-hold or gated breathing); planning solutions such as dose repainting, ensuring good beam angle separation and blurring of spot size; and systematic on-treatment imaging review to allow rescanning and adaptive planning.

Nonsmall cell lung cancers (NSCLCs) have typically had very poor outcomes relative to most other tumour types, despite widespread use of radical CRT for locally advanced patients who are well enough to be treated. In the past decade, two key findings have emerged from trial evidence to improve this. Consolidation durvalumab has significantly improved survival for those with locally advanced NSCLC, and RTOG 0617 found that increased mortality from dose escalation was due to cardiac effects. Given that smoking is the key common risk factor between lung cancer and cardiovascular/heart disease, and subsequent studies demonstrating the association between heart dose and significant cardiac events, cardiac dose reduction has become a priority in reducing morbidity from radical lung RT.

Planning studies have demonstrated substantial reduction in dose to critical structures. An early randomised controlled trial comparing the modalities (IMRT versus passively scattered PBT) found no difference in local failure rate, lung dosimetry or pneumonitis but did in heart dosimetry across all parameters. It also found significantly better outcomes in PBT patients treated later in the cohort, suggesting improvements in PBT planning techniques due to experience occurred over the trial period. There have been conflicting reports of the potential reduction in oesophageal and lung toxicity; with studies showing no difference versus improved toxicity rates in oesophagitis and lung toxicity.

The only phase III randomised controlled trial to address this to date has recently closed to accrual. RTOG 1308 (NCT01993810) randomised patients with inoperable NSCLC between photon and proton-based CRT with primary co-endpoints of overall survival, cardiac toxicity and lymphopaenia. Such studies will inform future patient selection for PBT.

The evidence for the use for protons in mediastinal lymphoma came first from planning studies, which demonstrated the theoretical ability to significantly reduce dose to the susceptible neighbouring organs, followed by retrospective studies comparing OAR dose between protons and photons, summarised by the PTCOG Lymphoma Subcommittee. Secondary cancers represent the most common cause of mortality among long-term survivors of lymphoma; breast cancer is the most common, followed by lung cancer (six times as likely in the neighbouring irradiated lung) and then upper GI cancers. Cardiac mortality (and morbidity) is the most common nonmalignant toxicity following lymphoma RT.

Patients with lymphoma are in the population most likely to benefit from PBT; they are young, they have relatively lower-dose RT, they have an excellent prognosis and radiation-related disease is likely to manifest decades after primary RT treatment. However, for those same reasons, there will likely never be randomised head-to-head trials comparing the toxicity benefit of protons versus photons in the treatment of lymphoma over the number of years which would be needed to evaluate it. Nevertheless there is a convincing body of nonrandomised evidence which points to at least comparative survival outcomes and potentially improved toxicity. For example, the biggest series to date included 80 patients over age 18 years who were diagnosed with Hodgkin lymphoma and were receiving consolidation PBT. The 3-year relapse-free survival rate was found to be similar to photon RT rates at 92%, and no grade 3 toxicities were reported in that time.

Mediastinal lymphoma patients overwhelmingly meet the criteria to indicate PBT treatment. Detailed long-term follow-up of such patients, vie either single-arm prospective trials or retrospective data collection under international registries, will influence RT practice for decades to come.

Thymic tumours are rare but share significant similarities with mediastinal lymphomas: young age at onset, potentially good prognosis and long natural history; and affected patients have the same potential to benefit from PBT dose-related reduction in long-term consequences to thoracic normal structures. Supported by retrospective evidence, thymomas have started to be treated, both definitively and postoperatively, with PBT, on this dosimetrically advantageous basis. The biggest study to date (70 patients from the Proton Collaborative Group registry, treated between 2011 and 2021) was favourable, with a 3-year overall survival rate of 82.6% for all (3-year overall survival was 94% for resected/adjuvant patients and 35.6% in the inoperable/definitive cohort) and three grade 3 adverse events but no grade 3 toxicities observed; this is in line with previously reported outcomes from smaller series. As with lymphoma, robust collection of decades-long follow-up, overseen by relevant international registries, will be required to determine the extent of reduction in long-term morbidity.

CONCLUSIONS AND FUTURE DIRECTIONS

PBT is rapidly evolving. Treatment delivery technology has advanced from passive scattering to pencil-beam scanning techniques and treatment planning expertise has become more sophisticated alongside it. The indications for the use of PBT, and the evidence base underpinning these, continue to grow. In the United Kingdom, as an example, there are now several times the number of indications which are the national standard of care for treatment as compared to when the service was commissioned. PBT use will increasingly widen to unexplored tumour types.

Current centres already providing PBT will continue to increase patient numbers, and many more centres will be opened worldwide. For developed nations, PBT has become a mainstream radiotherapeutic modality in certain settings. Development of these existing centres will focus on improvement of technical capabilities. Improved immobilisation, motion management and image capture with techniques such as 4DCT scanning, breathing modulation, abdominal compression and access to advanced MRI sequences will afford more precise target localisation and delineation. Further development of onset measures to track motion in real time will allow accuracy of treatment with tight margins.

Given the susceptibility of proton plans to changes in tissue separation and density, intensive involvement of an allied health professional multidisciplinary team is vital in ensuring reproducible setup (e.g. dietetic support for weight stability to ensure that body contours are maintained or physiotherapy support to ensure that a comfortable reproducible patient position is obtained). Despite such measures, frequent multidisciplinary team on-treat image review ensures that early reactive replanning can occur as quickly as possible when required.

There remains only a limited number of published randomised controlled trials directly comparing photons with protons. The adoption of PBT has been based on theoretical equivalent efficacy and perceived benefit in reducing late effects. However, there are now multiple trials assessing the potential benefits of PBT, which will report over the years to come. Result of these trials are awaited as they will shape future practice. Large-scale registry data will also continue to have a role. In the United Kingdom, the national Proton Clinical Outcomes Unit (PCOU) gathers detailed outcome data for patients who have undergone PBT at yearly intervals. Outcomes and toxicities are captured as per CT CAE for all UK patients to better understand the modality toxicity profile with a nationwide data set.

At present, PBT has been delivered in a manner analogous to conventionally fractionated IMRT. There have been some early explorations into hypofractionated PBT (e.g. in prostate cancer). This has yet to be widely investigated but is a likely focus in the coming years. Stereotactic photon RT and stereotactic radiosurgery share some similarities with IMPT in terms of dose conformality. Stereotactic proton therapy potentially enhances the effect. It might allow treatment of larger targets which would otherwise be precluded by low dose to OARs. However, uncertainty about RBE over the beam range may raise concerns about necrosis in the target. Reirradiation with protons is potentially risky for the same reasons, hence its tentative but widening use. FLASH RT, which delivers treatment at ultra-high dose rates (UHDRs), has the potential to spare normal tissue with minimal detriment to tumour kill. Proton FLASH is in its infancy but could further enhance this effect.

PBT will move increasingly into mainstream RT, and technical development will focus on reducing costs associated with setting up new facilities to enable it to become more widespread. Future research outcomes will fuel this need worldwide.

FURTHER READING

Aarhus University. *The danish national center for particle radiotherapy aarhus*. Denmark: Aarhus University; 2012. http://www.rm.dk/siteassets/om-os/a_udbud/dnu_partikelterapi/det-nationale-center-for-partikelterapi-2012.pdf

Aibe N, Demizu Y, Sulaiman NS, et al. Outcomes of patients with primary sacral chordoma treated with definitive proton beam therapy. *Int J Radiat Oncol Biol Phys*. 2018;100(4):972–979. https://doi.org/10.1016/j.ijrobp.2017.12.263

Aitkenhead AH, Bugg D, Rowbottom CG, Smith E, Mackay RI. Modelling the throughput capacity of a single-accelerator multitreatment room proton therapy centre. *Brit J Radiol*. 2012;85(1020):e1263–e1272.

Aleman BM, van den Belt-Dusebout AW, Klokman WJ, van't Veer MB, Bartelink H, van Leeuwen FE. Long-term cause-specific mortality of patients treated for Hodgkin's disease. *J Clin Oncol*. 2003;21(18):3431–3439. https://doi.org/10.1200/JCO.2003.07.131

ASTRO (American Society for Radiation Oncology). *Model policies: proton beam therapy (PBT)*. VA: Fairfax; 2022.

Atkins KM, Rawal B, Chaunzwa TL, et al. Cardiac radiation dose, cardiac disease, and mortality in patients with lung cancer. *J Am Coll Cardiol*. 2019;73(23):2976–2987. https://doi.org/10.1016/j.jacc.2019.03.500

Bagley AF, Grosshans DR, Philip NV, et al. Efficacy of proton therapy in children with high risk and locally recurrent neuroblastoma. *Pediatr Blood Cancer*. 2019;66(8):e27786.

Beddok A, Scher N, Alapetite C, et al. Proton therapy for adult craniopharyngioma: experience of a single institution in 91 consecutive patients. *Neuro Oncol*. 2023;25(4):710–719. https://doi.org/10.1093/neuonc/noac210

Beltran C, Roca M, Merchant TE. On the benefits and risks of proton therapy in pediatric craniopharyngioma. *Int J Radiat Oncol Biol Phys*. 2012;82(2):e281–e287.

Berrington de Gonzalez A, Gibson TM, Lee C, et al. The pediatric proton and photon therapy comparison cohort: study design for a multicenter retrospective cohort to investigate subsequent cancers after pediatric radiation therapy. *Adv Radiat Oncol*. 2023;8(6):101273.

Bhudia J, Thompson A, Mendes R, Gillies C, Carnell D. Precision delivery of adjuvant proton beam radiotherapy for olfactory neuroblastoma: the importance of perioperative management and sinus care. *J Neurolog Surg B Skull Base*. 2023;84(S01):S1–S344. https://doi.org/10.1055/s-0043-1762424

Bishop AJ, Greenfield B, Mahajan A, et al. Proton beam therapy versus conformal photon radiation therapy for childhood craniopharyngioma: multi-institutional analysis of outcomes, cyst dynamics, and toxicity. *Int J Radiat Oncol Biol Phys*. 2014;90(2):354–361.

Blanchard P, Garden AS, Gunn GB, et al. Intensity-modulated proton beam therapy (IMPT) versus intensity-modulated photon therapy (IMRT) for patients with oropharynx cancer—a case matched analysis. *Radiother Oncol*. 2016;120(1):48–55. https://doi.org/10.1016/j.radonc.2016.05.022

Boehling NS, Grosshans DR, Bluett JB, et al. Dosimetric comparison of three-dimensional conformal proton radiotherapy, intensity-modulated proton therapy, and intensity modulated radiotherapy for treatment of pediatric craniopharyngioma. *Int J Rad Onc Biol Phys*. 2012;2(2):643–652.

Bonù ML, Nicosia L, Turkaj A, et al. High dose proton and photon-based radiation therapy for 213 liver lesions: a multi-institutional dosimetric comparison with a clinical perspective. *Radiol Med*. 2023;129(3):497–506. https://doi.org/10.1007/s11547-024-01788-w

Boyce-Fappiano D, Nguyen Q-N, Chapman BV, et al. Single institution experience of proton and photon-based postoperative radiation therapy for non–small-cell lung cancer. *Clin Lung Cancer*. 2021;22(5):e745–e755. https://doi.org/10.1016/j.cllc.2021.02.002

Bradley JD, Paulus R, Komaki R, et al. Standard-dose versus high-dose conformal radiotherapy with concurrent and consolidation carboplatin plus paclitaxel with or without cetuximab for patients with stage IIIA or IIIB non-small-cell lung cancer (RTOG 0617): a randomised, two-by-two factorial phase 3 study. *Lancet Oncol*. 2015;16(2):187–199. https://doi.org/10.1016/S1470-2045(14)71207-0

Breen WG, Geno CS, Waddle MR, et al. Proton versus photon craniospinal irradiation for adult medulloblastoma: a dosimetric, toxicity, and exploratory cost analysis. *Neurooncol Adv*. 2024;6(1):vdae034. https://doi.org/10.1093/noajnl/vdae034

Brodin NP, Munck AF, Rosenschöld P, et al. Radiobiological risk estimates of adverse events and secondary cancer for proton and photon radiation therapy for pediatric medulloblastoma. *Acta Oncol.* 2011;50(6):806–816.

Brown AP, Barney CL, Grosshans DR, et al. Proton beam craniospinal irradiation reduces acute toxicity for adults with medulloblastoma. *Int J Radiat Oncol Biol Phys.* 2013;86(2):277–284. https://doi.org/10.1016/j.ijrobp.2013.01.014

Brown PD, Chung C, Liu DD, et al. A prospective phase II randomized trial of proton radiotherapy vs intensity-modulated radiotherapy for patients with newly diagnosed glioblastoma. *Neuro Oncol.* 2021;23(8):1337–1347. https://doi.org/10.1093/neuonc/noab040

Bryant CM, Henderson RH, Nichols RC, et al. Consensus statement on proton therapy for prostate cancer. *Int J Part Ther.* 2021;8(2): 1–16. https://doi.org/10.14338/IJPT-20-00031.1

Burnet NG, Mackay RI, Smith E, et al. Proton beam therapy: perspectives on the National Health Service England clinical service and research programme. *Br J Radiol.* 2020;93(1107):20190873. https://doi.org/10.1259/bjr.20190873

Cancer Research UK. Young people's cancers statistics. Accessed 26 June 2025. www.cancerresearchuk.org/health-professional/cancer-statistics/teenagers-and-young-adults-cancers

Carabe A, Karagounis I, Huynh K, et al. Radiobiological effectiveness difference of proton arc beams versus conventional proton and photon beams. *Phys Med Biol.* 2020;65(16):165002.

Catton C, O'Sullivan B, Bell R, et al. Chordoma: long-term follow-up after radical photon irradiation. *Radiother Oncol.* 1996;41(1): 67–72. https://doi.org/10.1016/S0167-8140(96)91805-8

Chan AW, Bernstein KD, Adams JA, Parambi RJ, Loeffler JS. Dose escalation with proton radiation therapy for high-grade meningiomas. *Technol Cancer Res Treat.* 2012;11(6):607–614. https://doi.org/10.7785/tcrt.2012.500267

Chang JY, Zhang X, Knopf A, et al. Consensus guidelines for implementing pencil-beam scanning proton therapy for thoracic malignancies on behalf of the PTCOG thoracic and lymphoma subcommittee. *Int J Radiat Oncol Biol Phys.* 2017;99(1):41–50. https://doi.org/10.1016/j.ijrobp.2017.05.014

Chang S, Liu G, Zhao L, et al. Feasibility study: spot-scanning proton arc (SPArc) for left-sided breast irradiation. *Radiat Oncol.* 2020;15:232.

Chang WH, Katsoulis M, Tan YY, Mueller SM, Green K, Lai AG. Late effects of cancer in children, teenagers and young adults: population-based study on the burden of 183 conditions, in-patient and critical care admissions and years of life lost. *Lancet Reg Health Eur.* 2022;12:100248.

Chhabra AM, Rice SR, Holtzman A, et al. Clinical outcomes and toxicities of 100 patients treated with proton therapy for chordoma on the proton collaborative group prospective registry. *Radiother Oncol.* 2023;183:109551. https://doi.org/10.1016/j.radonc.2023.109551

Chhabra AM, Snider JW, Kole AJ, et al. Proton therapy for spinal tumors: a consensus statement from the particle therapy cooperative group. *Int J Radiat Oncol Biol Phys.* 2024;120(4):1135–1148.

Childs SK, Kozak KR, Friedmann AM, et al. Proton radiotherapy for parameningeal rhabdomyosarcoma: clinical outcomes and late effects. *Int J Radiat Oncol Biol Phys.* 2012;82(2):635–642.

Choi JI, Wojcieszynski A, Amos RA, et al. PTCOG Gastrointestinal subcommittee lower gastrointestinal tract malignancies consensus statement. *Int J Part Ther.* 2024;11:100019. https://doi.org/10.1016/j.ijpt.2024.100019

Chowdhury T, Levitt GA. Late complications of cancer in childhood and adolescence. *Oncol Hematol Rev.* 2013;9:52–59.

Chung C, Trofimov A, Adams J, et al. Comparison of 3D conformal proton therapy, intensity-modulated proton therapy, and intensity-modulated photon therapy for retroperitoneal sarcoma. *Sarcoma.* 2022;2022:1–9. https://doi.org/10.1155/2022/5540615

Chuong MD, Kozarek J, Rubens M, et al. Reduced acute toxicity after proton versus photon chemoradiation for anal cancer: outcomes from the Proton Collaborative Group REG001-09 trial. *Int J Radiat Oncol Biol Phys.* 2019;105(1):S158. https://doi.org/10.1016/j.ijrobp.2019.06.173

Chuong MD, Hallemeier CL, Li H, et al. Executive summary of clinical and technical guidelines for esophageal cancer proton beam therapy from the Particle Therapy Co-Operative Group Thoracic and Gastrointestinal Subcommittees. *Front Oncol.* 2021;11. https://doi.org/10.3389/fonc.2021.748331

Coggins WS, Pham NK, Nguyen AV, et al. A systematic review of ion radiotherapy in maintaining local control regarding atypical and anaplastic meningiomas. *World Neurosurg.* 2019;132:282–291. https://doi.org/10.1016/j.wneu.2019.08.149

Corrao G, Marvaso G, Mastroleo F, et al. Photon vs proton hypofractionation in prostate cancer: a systematic review and meta-analysis. *Radiother Oncol.* 2024;195:110264. https://doi.org/10.1016/j.radonc.2024.110264

Cotterill SJ, Ahrens S, Paulussen M, et al. Prognostic factors in Ewing's tumor of bone: analysis of 975 patients from the European Intergroup Cooperative Ewing's Sarcoma study group. *J Clin Oncol.* 2000;18(17):3108–3114.

Cunningham DA, Breen WG, Johnson JE, et al. Proton whole-lung irradiation: Initial report of outcomes. *Int J Radiat Oncol Biol Phys.* 2023;115(4):866–872.

Dagan R, Uezono H, Bryant C, Holtzman AL, Morris CG, Mendenhall WM. Long-term outcomes from proton therapy for sinonasal cancers. *Int J Part Ther.* 2021;8(1):200–212. https://doi.org/10.14338/IJPT-20-00068.1

Dalmasso C, Alapetite C, Bolle S, et al. Brainstem toxicity after proton and photon therapy in children and young adults with localized intracranial ependymoma: a French retrospective study. *Radiother Oncol.* 2024;194:110157.

De Blank P, Bandopadhayay P, Haas-Kogan D, Fouladi M, Fangusaro J. Management of pediatric low-grade glioma. *Curr Opin Pediatr.* 2019;31(1):21–27.

Deman P, Vautrin M, Edouard M, et al. Monochromatic minibeams radiotherapy: from healthy tissue-sparing effect studies towards the first experimental glioma bearing rats therapy. *Int J Radiat Oncol Biol Phys.* 2012;82(4):E693–E700.

Dendale R, Lumbroso-Le Rouic L, Noel G, et al. Proton beam radiotherapy for uveal melanoma: results of Curie Institut–Orsay Proton Therapy Center (ICPO). *Int J Radiat Oncol Biol Phys.* 2006;65(3):780–787. https://doi.org/10.1016/j.ijrobp.2006.01.020

Dess RT, Sun Y, Matuszak MM, et al. Cardiac events after radiation therapy: combined analysis of prospective multicenter trials for locally advanced non–small-cell lung cancer. *J Clin Oncol.* 2017;35(13):1395–1402. https://doi.org/10.1200/JCO.2016.71.6142

Ding X, Li X, Zhang JM, Kabolizadeh P, Stevens C, Yan D. Spot-scanning proton arc (SPArc) therapy: the first robust and delivery-efficient spot-scanning proton arc therapy. *Int J Radiat Oncol Biol Phys.* 2016;96(5):1107–1116.

Ding X, Li X, Qin A, et al. Have we reached proton beam therapy dosimetric limitations? A novel robust, delivery-efficient and continuous spot-scanning proton arc (SPArc) therapy to improve the dosimetric outcome in treating prostate cancer. *Acta Oncol.* 2018;57(3):435–437.

Ding X, Zhou J, Li X, et al. Improving dosimetric outcome for hippocampus and cochlea sparing whole brain radiotherapy using spot-scanning proton arc therapy. *Acta Oncol.* 2019;58(4): 438–490.

Dos Santos M, Delorme R, Salmon R, Prezado Y. Minibeam radiation therapy: a micro- and nano-dosimetry Monte Carlo study. *Med Phys.* 2020;47(3):1379–1390.

Douw L, Klein M, Fagel SS, et al. Cognitive and radiological effects of radiotherapy in patients with low-grade glioma: long-term follow-up. *Lancet Neurol.* 2009;8(9):810–818. https://doi.org/10.1016/S1474-4422(09)70204-2

Eekers DBP, Zegers CML, Ahmed KA, et al. Controversies in neuro-oncology: focal proton versus photon radiation therapy for adult brain tumors. *Neurooncol Pract.* 2024;11(4):369–382. https://doi.org/10.1093/nop/npae040

Fang P, Mick R, Deville C, et al. A case-matched study of toxicity outcomes after proton therapy and intensity-modulated radiation therapy for prostate cancer. *Cancer.* 2015;121(7):1118–1127. https://doi.org/10.1002/cncr.29148

Farace P, Deidda MA, Amichetti M. Axillary irradiation omitting axillary dissection in breast cancer: is there a role for shoulder-sparing proton therapy? *Br J Radiol.* 2015;88(1054):20150274. https://doi.org/10.1259/bjr.20150274

Favaudon V, Caplier L, Monceau V, et al. Ultrahigh dose-rate flash irradiation increases the differential response between normal and tumor tissue in mice. *Sci Transl Med.* 2014;6(245):245ra93.

Fenwick J, Mayhew C, Jolly S, Amos RA, Hawkins MA. Navigating the straits: realizing the potential of proton flash through physics advances and further pre-clinical characterization. *Front Oncol.* 2024;14:1420337.

Frank SJ, Busse P, Rosenthal DI, et al. Phase III randomized trial of intensity-modulated proton therapy (IMPT) versus intensity-modulated photon therapy (IMRT) for the treatment of head and neck oropharyngeal carcinoma (OPC). *J Clin Oncol.* 2024;42(16_suppl):6006. https://doi.org/10.1200/JCO.2024.42.16_suppl.6006

Frisch S, Timmermann B. The evolving role of proton beam therapy for sarcomas. *Clin Oncol (R Coll Radiol).* 2017;29:500–506.

Fukumitsu N, Sugahara S, Nakayama H, et al. A prospective study of hypofractionated proton beam therapy for patients with hepatocellular carcinoma. *Int J Radiat Oncol Biol Phys.* 2009;74(3):831–836. https://doi.org/10.1016/j.ijrobp.2008.10.073

Fuss M, Hug EB, Schaefer RS, et al. Proton radiation therapy (PRY) for optic pathway gliomas: comparison with 3D planned conventional photons and a standard photon technique. *Int J Rad Onc Biol Phys.* 1999;45(5):1117–1126.

Gaito S, Hwang EJ, France A, et al. Outcomes of patients treated in the UK proton overseas programme: central nervous system group. *Clin Oncol (R Coll Radiol).* 2023;35(5):283–291.

Gaito S, Anzar MC, Burnet NG, et al. Assessing equity of access to proton beam therapy: a literature review. *Clin Oncol (R Coll Radiol).* 2023;35(9):e528–e536.

Geenen MM, Cardous-Ubbink MC, Kremer LC, et al. Medical assessment of adverse health outcomes in long-term survivors of childhood cancer. *JAMA.* 2007;297:2705–2715.

Gérard J-P, Conroy T, Bonnetain F, et al. Preoperative radiotherapy with or without concurrent fluorouracil and leucovorin in t3-4 rectal cancers: results of FFCD 9203. *J Clin Oncol.* 2006;24(28):4620–4625. https://doi.org/10.1200/JCO.2006.06.7629

Glynne-Jones R, Lim F. Anal cancer: an examination of radiotherapy strategies. *Int J Radiat Oncol Biol Phys.* 2011;79(5):1290–1301. https://doi.org/10.1016/j.ijrobp.2010.10.017

Gray PJ, Paly JJ, Yeap BY, et al. Patient-reported outcomes after 3-dimensional conformal, intensity-modulated, or proton beam radiotherapy for localized prostate cancer. *Cancer.* 2013;119(9):1729–1735. https://doi.org/10.1002/cncr.27956

Greenberger BA, Pulsifer MB, Ebb DH, et al. Clinical outcomes and late endocrine, neurocognitive, and visual profiles of proton radiation for pediatric low-grade gliomas. *Int J Rad Onc Biol Phys.* 2014;89(5):1060–1068.

Guardiola C, Prezado Y, Roulin C, Bergs JWJ. Effect of X-rat mini-beam radiation therapy on clonogenic survival of glioma cells. *Clin Transl Radiat Oncol.* 2018;13:7–13.

Hall EJ. Intensity-modulated radiation therapy, protons, and the risk of second cancers. *Int J Rad Onc Biol Phys.* 2006;65(1):1–7.

Harrabi SB, Bougatf N, Mohr A, et al. Dosimetric advantages of proton therapy over conventional radiotherapy with photons in young patients and adults with low-grade glioma. *Strahlenther Onkol.* 2016;192(11):759–769.

Hasan S, Abel S, Verma V, et al. Proton beam therapy versus stereotactic body radiotherapy for hepatocellular carcinoma: practice patterns, outcomes, and the effect of biologically effective dose escalation. *J Gastrointest Oncol.* 2019;10(5):999–1009. https://doi.org/10.21037/jgo.2019.08.03

He L, Zhang B, Zhang J, Guo Z, Shi F, Zeng Q. Effectiveness of post-operative adjuvant radiotherapy in atypical meningioma patients after gross total resection: a meta-analysis study. *Front Oncol.* 2021;10:556575. https://doi.org/10.3389/fonc.2020.556575

Health Council of the Netherlands. *De Gezondheidsraad.* Netherlands: The Hague; 2009. https://www.healthcouncil.nl.

Heitzer AM, Kahalley LS, Minard CG, et al. Treatment age and neurocognitive outcomes following proton beam radiotherapy for pediatric low and intermediate grade gliomas. *Pediatr Blood Cancer.* 2021;68(8):e29096.

Held T, Franke H, Lang K, et al. Intensity modulated proton therapy for early-stage glottic cancer: high-precision approach to laryngeal function preservation with exceptional treatment tolerability. *Radiat Oncol.* 2022;17(1):199. https://doi.org/10.1186/s13014-022-02144-w

Hol MLF, Indelicato D, Slater O, et al. Facial deformation following treatment for pediatric head and neck rhabdomyosarcoma: the difference between treatment modalities. Results of a trans-Atlantic, multicenter cross-sectional study. *Pediatr Blood Cancer.* 2023;70(8):e30412.

Holtzman AL, Rotondo RL, Rutenberg MS, et al. Clinical outcomes following dose-escalated proton therapy for skull-base chordoma. *Int J Part Ther.* 2021;8(1):179–188. https://doi.org/10.14338/IJPT-20-00066.1

Holtzman AL, Glassman GE, Dagan R, et al. Long-term outcomes of fractionated proton beam therapy for benign or radiographic intracranial meningioma. *J Neurooncol.* 2023;161(3):481–489. https://doi.org/10.1007/s11060-022-04207-0

Hoppe BS, Flampouri S, Su Z, et al. Effective dose reduction to cardiac structures using protons compared with 3DCST and IMRT in mediastinal Hodgkin lymphoma. *Int J Radiat Oncol Biol Phys.* 2012;84(2):449–455.

Hoppe BS, Michalski JM, Mendenhall NP, et al. Comparative effectiveness study of patient-reported outcomes after proton therapy or intensity-modulated radiotherapy for prostate cancer. *Cancer.* 2014;120(7):1076–1082. https://doi.org/10.1002/cncr.28536

Hoppe BS, Hill-Kayser CE, Tseng YD, et al. Consolidative proton therapy after chemotherapy for patients with Hodgkin lymphoma. *Ann Oncol.* 2017;28(9):2179–2184. https://doi.org/10.1093/annonc/mdx287

Horn S, Fourniwe-Bidoz N, Pernin V, et al. Comparison of passive-beam proton therapy, helical tomotherapy and 3D conformal radiation therapy in Hodgkin's lymphoma female patients receiving involved-field or involved site radiation therapy. *Cancer Radiother.* 2016;20(2):98–103.

Huynh-Le MP, Walker AJ, Burger PC, et al. Management of pediatric intracranial low-grade gliomas: long term follow-up after radiation therapy. *Childs Nerv Syst.* 2016;32(8):1425–1430.

Hwang E, Gaito S, France A, et al. Outcomes of patients treated in the UK proton overseas programme: non-central nervous system group. *Clin Oncol (R Coll Radiol).* 2023;35(5):292–300.

ICRU (International Commission on Radiation Units and Measurements). *Prescribing, recording, and reporting proton beam therapy.* Washington, DC: ICRU; 2007 ICRU Report No. 78.

Igaki H, Mizumoto M, Okumura T, Hasegawa K, Kokudo N, Sakurai H. A systematic review of publications on charged particle therapy for hepatocellular carcinoma. *Int J Clin Oncol.* 2018;23(3):423–433. https://doi.org/10.1007/s10147-017-1190-2

Indelicato DJ, Merchant T, Laperriere N, et al. Consensus report from the Stokholm pediatric proton therapy conference. *Int J Rad Onc Biol Phys.* 2016;96(2):387–392.

Indelicato DJ, Bradley JA, Rotondo RL, et al. Outcomes following proton therapy for pediatric ependymoma. *Acta Oncol.* 2017; 14:1–5.

Indelicato DJ, Rotondo RL, Uezono H, et al. Outcomes following proton therapy for pediatric low-grade glioma. *Int J Rad Oncol Biol Phys.* 2019;104(1):149–156.

Indelicato DJ, Mailhot Bega RB, Viviers E, et al. Modern therapy for chest wall Ewing sarcoma: an update of the University of Florida experience. *Int J Radiat Oncol Biol Phys.* 2022;113(2):345–354.

Iwata H, Ishikawa H, Takagi M, et al. Long-term outcomes of proton therapy for prostate cancer in Japan: a multi-institutional survey of the Japanese Radiation Oncology Study Group. *Cancer Med.* 2018;7(3):677–689. https://doi.org/10.1002/cam4.1350

Iwata H, Ogino H, Hattori Y, et al. A phase 2 study of image-guided proton therapy for operable or ablation-treatable primary hepatocellular carcinoma. *Int J Radiat Oncol Biol Phys.* 2021;111(1): 117–126. https://doi.org/10.1016/j.ijrobp.2021.03.049

Janssens GO, Melchior P, Mul J. The SIOP-Renal Tumour Study Group consensus statement on flank target volume delineation for highly conformal radiotherapy. *Lancet Child Adolesc Health.* 2020;4(11):846–852.

Jazmati D, Butzer S, Hero B, et al. Proton beam therapy for children with neuroblastoma: experiences from the prospective KiProReg registry. *Front Oncol.* 2021;10:617506.

Jeans EB, Jethwa KR, Harmsen WS, et al. Clinical implementation of preoperative short-course pencil beam scanning proton therapy for patients with rectal cancer. *Adv Radiat Oncol.* 2020;5(5):865–870. https://doi.org/10.1016/j.adro.2020.05.004

Jimenez RB, Hickey S, DePauw N, et al. Phase II study of proton beam radiation therapy for patients with breast cancer requiring regional nodal irradiation. *J Clin Oncol.* 2019;37(30):2778–2785. https://doi.org/10.1200/JCO.18.02366

Jones B, McMahon SJ, Prise KM. The radiobiology of proton therapy: challenges and opportunities around relative biological effectiveness. *Clin Oncol (R Coll Radiol).* 2018;30(5):285–292.

Kim D, Kim J-S. Current perspectives on radiotherapy in hepatocellular carcinoma management: a comprehensive review. *J Liver Cancer.* 2024;24(1):33–46. https://doi.org/10.17998/jlc.2024.02.26

Kim TH, Park J-W, Kim Y-J, et al. Phase I dose-escalation study of proton beam therapy for inoperable hepatocellular carcinoma. *Cancer Res Treat.* 2015;47(1):34–45. https://doi.org/10.4143/crt.2013.218

Klaver YLB, Hoogeman MS, Lu QR, Amos RA, Hawkins MA, Simone II CB. Requirements and study design for the next proton flash clinical trials: an international multidisciplinary Delphi consensus. *Int J Radiat Oncol Biol Phys.* 2024;120(2):S108–S109.

Kroesen M, Miladinovic V, Hutschemaekers SAJ, et al. Single-institution clinical experience using robust intensity modulated proton therapy in chordoma and chondrosarcoma of the mobile spine and sacrum: feasibility and need for plan adaptation. *Radiother Oncol.* 2022;166:58–64. https://doi.org/10.1016/j.radonc.2021.11.020

Ladra M, Edgington SK, Mahajan A, et al. A dosimetric comparison of proton and intensity modulated radiation therapy in pediatric rhabdomyosarcoma patients enrolled on a prospective phase II proton study. *Radiother Oncol.* 2014;113(1):77–83.

Ladra MM, Szymonifka JD, Mahajan A, et al. Preliminary results of a phase II trial of proton radiotherapy for pediatric rhabdomyosarcoma. *J Clin Oncol.* 2014;32(33):3762–3770.

Langendijk JA, Hoebers FJP, de Jong MA, et al. National protocol for model-based selection for proton therapy in head and neck cancer. *Int J Part Ther.* 2021;8(1):354–365. https://doi.org/10.14338/IJPT-20-00089.1

Laughlin BS, Golafshar M, Prince M, et al. Dosimetric comparison between proton beam therapy, intensity modulated radiation therapy, and 3D conformal therapy for soft tissue extremity sarcoma. *Acta Oncol (Madr).* 2023;62(5):473–479. https://doi.org/10.1080/0284186X.2023.2209267

Lawell MP, Indelicato DJ, Paulino AC, et al. An open invitation to join the pediatric proton/photon consortium registry to standardize data collection in pediatric radiation oncology. *Br J Radiol.* 2020;93(1107):20190673.

Le Mash, Kahalley LS, Okcu MF, et al. Superior verbal learning and memory in pediatric brain tumour survivors treated with proton versus photon radiotherapy. *Neuropsychology.* 2023;37(2):204–217.

Lee CT, Bilton SD, Famiglietti RM, et al. Treatment planning with protons for pediatric retinoblastoma, medulloblastoma and pelvic sarcoma: how do protons compare with other conformal techniques? *Int J Rad Onc Biol Phys.* 2005;63:362–372.

Lee E, Lourenço AM, Speth J, et al. Ultrahigh dose rate pencil beam scanning proton dosimetry using ion chambers and a calorimeter in support of first in-human flash clinical trial. *Med Phys.* 2022;49(9):6171–6182.

Lewis L, Kreinbrink P, Richardson M, et al. Intensity modulated proton therapy better spares non-adjacent organs and reduces the risk of secondary malignant neoplasms in the treatment of sinonasal cancers. *Med Dosim.* 2022;47(2):117–122. https://doi.org/10.1016/j.meddos.2021.11.002

Li X, Kabolizadeh P, Yan D, et al. Improve dosimetric outcome in stage III non-small-cell lung cancer treatment using spot-scanning proton arc (SPArc) therapy. *Radiat Oncol.* 2018;13(1): 1–9.

Liao Z, Lee JJ, Komaki R, et al. Bayesian adaptive randomization trial of passive scattering proton therapy and intensity-modulated photon radiotherapy for locally advanced non–small-cell lung cancer. *J Clin Oncol.* 2018;36(18):1813–1822. https://doi.org/10.1200/JCO.2017.74.0720

Lim PS, Pica A, Hrbacek J, et al. Pencil beam scanning proton therapy for paediatric neuroblastoma with motion mitigation strategy for moving target volumes. *Clin Oncol (R Coll Radiol).* 2020;32(7):467–476.

Lim PS, Tran S, Kroeze SGC, et al. Outcomes of adolescents and young adults treated for brain and skull base tumors with pencil beam scanning proton therapy. *Pediatr Blood Cancer.* 2020;67(12):e28664. https://doi.org/10.1002/pbc.28664

Lim PS, Rompokos V, Bizzocchi N, et al. Pencil beam scanning proton therapy case selection for paediatric abdominal neuroblastoma: effects of tumour location and bowel gas. *Clin Oncol (R Coll Radiol).* 2021;33(3):e132–e142.

Lin R, Hug EB, Schaefer RA, Miller DW, Slater JM, Slater JD. Conformal proton radiation therapy of the posterior fossa: a study comparing protons with three-dimensional planned photons in limiting dose to the auditory structures. *Int J Rad Onc Biol Phys*. 2000;48(4):1219–1226.

Lin A, Chang JHC, Grover RS, et al. PTCOG Head and Neck Subcommittee consensus guidelines on particle therapy for the management of head and neck tumors. *Int J Part Ther*. 2021;8(1):84–94. https://doi.org/10.14338/IJPT-20-00071.1

Lin SH, Hobbs BP, Verma V, et al. Randomized phase IIB trial of proton beam therapy versus intensity-modulated radiation therapy for locally advanced esophageal cancer. *J Clin Oncol*. 2020;38(14):1569–1579. https://doi.org/10.1200/JCO.19.02503

Liu G, Li X, Qin A, et al. Improve the dosimetric outcome in bilateral head and neck cancer (HNC) treatment using spot-scanning proton arc (SPArc) therapy: a feasibility study. *Radiat Oncol*. 2020;15(1):1–11.

Liu I-C, Holtzman AL, Rotondo RL, et al. Proton therapy for adult medulloblastoma: acute toxicity and disease control outcomes. *J Neurooncol*. 2021;153(3):467–476. https://doi.org/10.1007/s11060-021-03783-x

Lo AC, Hodgson D, Dang J, et al. Intracranial germ cell tumors in adolescents and young adults: a 40-year multi-institutional review of outcomes. *Int J Radiat Oncol Biol Phys*. 2020;106(2):269–278. https://doi.org/10.1016/j.ijrobp.2019.10.020

Lomax A. Physics of treatment planning using scanned beams. In: Paganetti H, ed. *Proton therapy physics*. CRC Press; 2012.

Louis DN, Perry A, Wesseling P, et al. The 2021 WHO classification of tumors of the central nervous system: a summary. *Neuro Oncol*. 2021;23(8):1231–1251.

Lourenço AM, Subiel A, Lee N, et al. Absolute dosimetry for flash proton pencil beam scanning radiotherapy. *Sci Rep*. 2023;13(1):2054.

Lowe M, Gosling A, Nicholas O, et al. Comparing proton to photon radiotherapy plans: UK consensus guidance for reporting under uncertainty for clinical trials. *Clin Oncol (R Coll Radiol)*. 2020;32(7):459–466.

MacDonald SM, Safai S, Trofimov A, et al. Proton radiotherapy for childhood ependymoma: initial clinical outcomes and dose comparisons. *Int J Radiat Oncol Biol Phys*. 2008;71(4):979–986.

MacEwan I, Chou B, Moretz J, Loredo L, Bush D, Slater JD. Effects of vertebral-body-sparing proton craniospinal irradiation on the spine of young pediatric patients with medulloblastoma. *Adv Radiat Oncol*. 2017;2(2):220–227.

Maclean J, Fersht N, Short S. Controversies in radiotherapy for meningioma. *Clin Oncol*. 2014;26(1):51–64. https://doi.org/10.1016/j.clon.2013.10.001

Mascia A, Daugherty E, Zhang Y, et al. Proton flash radiotherapy for the treatment of symptomatic bone metastases: the FAST-01 nonrandomized trial. *JAMA Oncol*. 2023;9(1):62–69.

Matloob SA, Nasir HA, Choi D. Proton beam therapy in the management of skull base chordomas: systematic review of indications, outcomes, and implications for neurosurgeons. *Br J Neurosurg*. 2016;30(4):382–387. https://doi.org/10.1080/02688697.2016.1181154

Mayo CS, Moran JM, Bosch W, et al. American Association of Physicists in Medicine Task Group 263: Standardizing nomenclatures in radiation oncology. *Int J Radiat Oncol Biol Phys*. 2018;100(4):1057–1066. https://doi.org/10.1016/j.ijrobp.2017.12.013

McDonald SM, Sethi R, Lavally B, et al. Proton radiotherapy for paediatric central nervous system ependymoma: clinical outcomes for 70 patients. *Neurooncology*. 2013;15(11):1552–1559.

MedAustron. Indications. Accessed 26 June 2025. https://www.medaustron.at/en/indications

Mendenhall NP, Hoppe BS, Nichols RC, et al. Five-year outcomes from 3 prospective trials of image-guided proton therapy for prostate cancer. *Int J Radiat Oncol Biol Phys*. 2014;88(3):596–602. https://doi.org/10.1016/j.ijrobp.2013.11.007

Mercado CE, Hartsell WF, Simone 2nd CB, et al. Proton therapy for thymic malignancies: multi-institutional patterns-of-care and early clinical outcomes from the proton collaborative group and the university of Florida prospective registries. *Acta Oncol (Madr)*. 2019;58(7):1036–1040. https://doi.org/10.1080/0284186X.2019.1575981

Merchant TE, Hua CH, Shukla H, Ying X, Nill S, Oelfke U. Proton versus photon radiotherapy for common pediatric brain tumors: comparison of models of dose characteristics and their relationship to cognitive function. *Pediatr Blood Cancer*. 2008;51(1):110–117.

Merchant TE, Li C, Xiong X, Kun LE, Boop FA, Sanford RA. Conformal radiotherapy after surgery for paediatric ependymoma: a prospective study. *Lancet Oncol*. 2009;10(3):258–266.

Merchant TE, Pollack IF, Loeffler JS. Brain tumors across the age spectrum: biology, therapy, and late effects. *Semin Radiat Oncol*. 2010;20(1):58–66. https://doi.org/10.1016/j.semradonc.2009.09.005

Merchant TE, Hoehn ME, Khan RB, et al. Proton therapy and limited surgery for paediatric and adolescent patients with craniopharyngioma (RT2CR): a single-arm, phase 2 study. *Lancet Oncol*. 2023;24:523–534.

Miralbell R, Lomax A, Cella L, Schneider U. Potential reduction of the incidence of radiation-induced second cancers by using proton beams in the treatment of pediatric tumors. *Int J Rad Onc Biol Phys*. 2002;54(3):824–829.

Mishra KK, Quivey JM, Daftari IK, et al. Long-term results of the UCSF-LBNL randomized trial: charged particle with helium ion versus iodine-125 plaque therapy for choroidal and ciliary body melanoma. *Int J Radiat Oncol Biol Phys*. 2015;92(2):376–383. https://doi.org/10.1016/j.ijrobp.2015.01.029

Mishra MV, Aggarwal S, Bentzen SM, Knight N, Mehta MP, Regine WF. Establishing evidence-based indications for proton therapy: an overview of current clinical trials. *Int J Radiat Oncol Biol Phys*. 2017;97(2):228–235.

Mohiuddin JJ, Jethwa KR, Grandhi N, et al. Multi-institutional comparison of intensity modulated photon versus proton radiation therapy in the management of squamous cell carcinoma of the anus. *Adv Radiat Oncol*. 2021;6(5):100744. https://doi.org/10.1016/j.adro.2021.100744

Morton LM, Gilbert ES, Stovall M, et al. Risk of esophageal cancer following radiotherapy for Hodgkin lymphoma. *Haematologica*. 2014;99(10):e193–e196. https://doi.org/10.3324/haematol.2014.108258

Moskowitz CS, Chou CF, Wolden SL, et al. Breast cancer after chest radiation therapy for childhood cancer. *J Clin Oncol*. 2014;32(21):2217–2223. https://doi.org/10.1200/JCO.2013.54.4601

Moyers MF, Miller DW. Range, range modulation, and field radius requirements for proton therapy of prostate cancer. *Technol Cancer Res Treat*. 2003;2(5):445–447.

Munzenrider JE, Gragoudas ES, Seddon JM, et al. Conservative treatment of uveal melanoma: probability of eye retention after proton treatment. *Int J Radiat Oncol Biol Phys*. 1988;15(3):553–558. https://doi.org/10.1016/0360-3016(88)90294-5

Munzenrider JE, Verhey LJ, Gragoudas ES, et al. Conservative treatment of uveal melanoma: local recurrence after proton beam therapy. *Int J Radiat Oncol Biol Phys.* 1989;17(3):493–498. https://doi.org/10.1016/0360-3016(89)90099-0

Mutter RW, Choi JI, Jimenez RB, et al. Proton therapy for breast cancer: a consensus statement from the Particle Therapy Cooperative Group Breast Cancer Subcommittee. *Int J Radiat Oncol Biol Phys.* 2021;111(2):337–359. https://doi.org/10.1016/j.ijrobp.2021.05.110

Nakajima K, Iwata H, Ogino H, et al. Acute toxicity of image-guided hypofractionated proton therapy for localized prostate cancer. *Int J Clin Oncol.* 2018;23(2):353–360. https://doi.org/10.1007/s10147-017-1209-8

Nakamura M, Mizumoto M, Saito T, et al. A systematic review and meta-analysis of radiotherapy and particle beam therapy for skull base chondrosarcoma: TRP-chondrosarcoma 2024. *Front Oncol.* 2024;14:1380716. https://doi.org/10.3389/fonc.2024.1380716

Nangia S, Gaikwad U, Noufal MP, et al. Proton therapy and oral mucositis in oral & oropharyngeal cancers: outcomes, dosimetric and NTCP benefit. *Radiat Oncol.* 2023;18(1):121. https://doi.org/10.1186/s13014-023-02317-1

Ng AK, Bernardo MP, Weller E, et al. Long-term survival and competing causes of death in patients with early-stage Hodgkin's disease treated at age 50 or younger. *J Clin Oncol.* 2002;20(8):2101–2108. https://doi.org/10.1200/JCO.2002.08.021

Ng WT, But B, Wong CHL, et al. Particle beam therapy for nasopharyngeal cancer: a systematic review and meta-analysis. *Clin Transl Radiat Oncol.* 2022;37:41–56. https://doi.org/10.1016/j.ctro.2022.08.011

NHS England. Proton beam therapy. Accessed 26 June 2025. https://www.england.nhs.uk/commissioning/spec-services/highly-spec-services/pbt/

Northcott PA, Buchhalter I, Morrissy AS, et al. The whole-genome landscape of medulloblastoma subtypes. *Nature.* 2017;547:311–317.

Nunna R, Patel S, Karuparti S, et al. Chordoma of the skull base: a national cancer database analysis of current practice patterns and outcomes. *World Neurosurg.* 2022;168:e260–e268. https://doi.org/10.1016/j.wneu.2022.09.102

Oeffinger KC, Mertens AC, Sklar CA, et al. Chronic health conditions in adult survivors of childhood cancer. *New Engl J Med.* 2006;355:1572–1582.

Ojerholm E, Kirk ML, Thompson RF, et al. Pencil-beam scanning proton therapy for anal cancer: a dosimetric comparison with intensity-modulated radiotherapy. *Acta Oncol (Madr).* 2015;54(8):1209–1217. https://doi.org/10.3109/0284186X.2014.1002570

Paganetti H, Niemierko A, Ancukiewicz M, et al. Relative biological effectiveness (RBE) values for proton beam therapy. *Int J Radiat Oncol Biol Phys.* 2002;53(2):407–421.

Paganetti H. Relative biological effectiveness (RBE) values for proton beam therapy. Variations as a function of biological endpoints, dose, and linear energy transfer. *Phys Med Biol.* 2014;59(22):R419.

Pahwa B, Medani K, Lu VM, Elarjani T. Proton beam therapy for skull base chordomas: a systematic review of tumor control rates and survival rates. *Neurosurg Rev.* 2022;45(6):3551–3563. https://doi.org/10.1007/s10143-022-01880-7

Pan HY, Jiang J, Hoffman KE, et al. Comparative toxicities and cost of intensity-modulated radiotherapy, proton radiation, and stereotactic body radiotherapy among younger men with prostate cancer. *J Clin Oncol.* 2018;36(18):1823–1830. https://doi.org/10.1200/JCO.2017.75.5371

Park PC, Zhu XR, Lee AK, et al. A beam-specific planning target volume (PTV) design for proton therapy to account for setup and range uncertainties. *Int J Radiat Oncol Biol Phys.* 2012;82(2):e329–e336.

Park S, Yoon WS. Rim CH. Indications of external radiotherapy for hepatocellular carcinoma from updated clinical guidelines: diverse global viewpoints. *World J Gastroenterol.* 2020;26(4):393–403. https://doi.org/10.3748/wjg.v26.i4.393

Particle Therapy Co-Operative Group. Statistics of patients treated in particle therapy facilities worldwide. https://www.ptcog.ch/index.php/ptcog-patient-statistics

Patterson BE, Baliga S, Bajaj BVM, et al. Clinical outcomes in a large pediatric cohort of patients with ependymoma treated with proton therapy. *Neuro Oncol.* 2021;23(1):156–166.

Pérez-Anúdjar A, Newhauser WD, Taddei PJ, Mahajan A, Howell RM. The predicted relative risk of premature ovarian failure for three radiotherapy modalities in a girl receiving craniospinal irradiation. *Phys Med Biol.* 2013;58(10):3107–3123.

Prezado Y, Jouvion G, Hardy D, et al. Proton minibeam radiation therapy spares normal rat brain: long-term clinical, radiobiological and histopathological analysis. *Sci Rep.* 2017;7(1):1–7.

Prezado Y, Jouvion G, Patriarca A, et al. Proton minibeam radiation therapy widens the therapeutic index for high-grade gliomas. *Sci Rep.* 2018;8(1):1–10.

PSI (Paul Scherrer Institute). Types of cancer we treat. Accessed 26 June 2025. https://www.psi.ch/en/protontherapy/types-of-cancer-we-treat

Ramaekers BLT, Pijls-Johannesma M, Joore MA, et al. Systematic review and meta-analysis of radiotherapy in various head and neck cancers: comparing photons, carbon-ions and protons. *Cancer Treat Rev.* 2011;37(3):185–201. https://doi.org/10.1016/j.ctrv.2010.08.004

RCR (Royal College of Radiologists). *Radiotherapy dose fractionation.* 4th ed.; 2024. https://www.rcr.ac.uk/our-services/all-our-publications/clinical-oncology-publications/radiotherapy-dose-fractionation-fourth-edition/

Remick JS, Schonewolf C, Gabriel P, et al. First clinical report of proton beam therapy for postoperative radiotherapy for non–small-cell lung cancer. *Clin Lung Cancer.* 2017;18(4):364–371. https://doi.org/10.1016/j.cllc.2016.12.009

Rogers L, Zhang P, Vogelbaum MA, et al. Intermediate-risk meningioma: Initial outcomes from NRG oncology RTOG 0539. *J Neurosurg.* 2018;129(1):35–47. https://doi.org/10.3171/2016.11.JNS161170

Rosenberg S, Tepper J, Glatstein E, Wesley R. The treatment of soft-tissue sarcomas of the extremities. *Ann Surg.* 1982;196(3):305–315. https://doi.org/10.1097/00000658-198209000-00009

Saito T, Mizumoto M, Oshiro Y, et al. Systematic review and meta-analysis of particle beam therapy versus photon radiotherapy for skull base chordoma: TRP-Chordoma 2024. *Cancers (Basel).* 2024;16(14):2569. https://doi.org/10.3390/cancers16142569

Santacroce A, Walier M, Régis J, et al. Long-term tumor control of benign intracranial meningiomas after radiosurgery in a series of 4565 patients. *Neurosurgery.* 2012;70(1):32–39. https://doi.org/10.1227/NEU.0b013e31822d408a

Santacroce A, Trandafirescu M-F, Levivier M, et al. Proton beam radiation therapy for vestibular schwannomas-tumor control and hearing preservation rates: a systematic review and meta-analysis. *Neurosurg Rev.* 2023;46(1):163. https://doi.org/10.1007/s10143-023-02060-x

Santos PMG, Barsky AR, Hwang W-T, et al. Comparative toxicity outcomes of proton-beam therapy versus intensity-modulated radiotherapy for prostate cancer in the postoperative setting. *Cancer.* 2019;125(23):4278–4293. https://doi.org/10.1002/cncr.32457

Sato M, Gunther JR, Mahajan A, et al. Progression-free survival of children with localized ependymoma treated with intensity-modulated radiation therapy or proton beam radiation therapy. *Cancer*. 2017;123(13):2570–2578.

Schulte F, Russell KB, Cullen P, et al. Systematic review and meta-analysis of health-related quality of life in pediatric CNS tumour survivors. *Pediatr Blood Cancer*. 2017;64(8). doi: 10.1002/pbc.26442

Sejpal S, Komaki R, Tsao A, et al. Early findings on toxicity of proton beam therapy with concurrent chemotherapy for nonsmall cell lung cancer. *Cancer*. 2011;117(13):3004–3013. https://doi.org/10.1002/cncr.25848

Sekino Y, Okumura T, Fukumitsu N, et al. Proton beam therapy for hepatocellular carcinoma associated with inferior vena cava tumor thrombus. *J Cancer Res Clin Oncol*. 2020;146(3):711–720. https://doi.org/10.1007/s00432-019-03096-7

Sethi RV, Shih HA, Yeap BY, et al. Second nonocular tumours among survivors of retinoblastoma treated with contemporary photon and proton therapy. *Cancer*. 2014;120(1):126–133.

Sharma S, Zhou O, Thompson R, et al. Quality of life of postoperative photon versus proton radiation therapy for oropharynx cancer. *Int J Part Ther*. 2018;5(2):11–17. https://doi.org/10.14338/IJPT-18-00032.1

Sherman JC, Colvin MK, Mancuso SM, et al. Neurocognitive effects of proton radiation therapy in adults with low-grade glioma. *J Neurooncol*. 2016;126(1):157–164. https://doi.org/10.1007/s11060-015-1952-5

Shiraishi Y, Xu C, Yang J, Komaki R, Lin SH. Dosimetric comparison to the heart and cardiac substructure in a large cohort of esophageal cancer patients treated with proton beam therapy or Intensity-modulated radiation therapy. *Radiother Oncol*. 2017;125(1):48–54. https://doi.org/10.1016/j.radonc.2017.07.034

Sienna J, Kahalley LS, Mabbott D, et al. Proton therapy mediates dose reductions to brain structures associated with cognition in children with medulloblastoma. *Int J Radiat Oncol Biol Phys*. 2023;30:S0360–S3016.

Snider JW, Schneider RA, Poelma-Tap D, et al. Long-term outcomes and prognostic factors after pencil-beam scanning proton radiation therapy for spinal chordomas: a large, single-institution cohort. *Int J Radiat Oncol Biol Phys*. 2018;101(1):226–233. https://doi.org/10.1016/j.ijrobp.2018.01.060

Song D, Xu D, Han H, et al. Postoperative adjuvant radiotherapy in atypical meningioma patients: a meta-analysis study. *Front Oncol*. 2021;11:787962. https://doi.org/10.3389/fonc.2021.787962

Spigel DR, Faivre-Finn C, Gray JE, et al. Five-year survival outcomes from the pacific trial: durvalumab after chemoradiotherapy in stage iii non–small-cell lung cancer. *J Clin Oncol*. 2022;40(12):1301–1311. https://doi.org/10.1200/JCO.21.01308

Stacchiotti S, Sommer J. Building a global consensus approach to chordoma: a position paper from the medical and patient community. *Lancet Oncol*. 2015;16(2):e71–e83. https://doi.org/10.1016/S1470-2045(14)71190-8

Stieb S, Snider 3rd JW, Placidi L, et al. Long-term clinical safety of high-dose proton radiation therapy delivered with pencil beam scanning technique for extracranial chordomas and chondrosarcomas in adult patients: clinical evidence of spinal cord tolerance. *Int J Radiat Oncol Biol Phys*. 2018;100(1):218–225. https://doi.org/10.1016/j.ijrobp.2017.08.037

Stross WC, Malouff TD, Waddle MR, Miller RC, Peterson J, Trifiletti DM. Proton beam therapy utilization in adults with primary brain tumors in the United States. *J Clin Neurosci*. 2020;75:112–116. https://doi.org/10.1016/j.jocn.2020.03.011

Stützer K, Lin A, Kirk M, Lin L. Superiority in robustness of multifield optimization over single-field optimization for pencil-beam proton therapy for oropharynx carcinoma: an enhanced robustness analysis. *Int J Radiat Oncol Biol Phys*. 2017;99(3):738–749. https://doi.org/10.1016/j.ijrobp.2017.06.017

Sugahara S, Oshiro Y, Nakayama H, et al. Proton beam therapy for large hepatocellular carcinoma. *Int J Radiat Oncol Biol Phys*. 2010;76(2):460–466. https://doi.org/10.1016/j.ijrobp.2009.02.030

Syndikus I, Griffin C, Philipps L, et al. 10-Year efficacy and co-morbidity outcomes of a phase III randomised trial of conventional vs. hypofractionated high dose intensity modulated radiotherapy for prostate cancer (CHHiP; CRUK/06/016). *J Clin Oncol*. 2023;41(6_suppl):304. https://doi.org/10.1200/JCO.2023.41.6_suppl.304

Takada A, Nakamura T, Takayama K, et al. Preliminary treatment results of proton beam therapy with chemoradiotherapy for stage I–III esophageal cancer. *Cancer Med*. 2016;5(3):506–515. https://doi.org/10.1002/cam4.607

Taylor C, Correa C, Duane FK, et al. Estimating the risks of breast cancer radiotherapy: evidence from modern radiation doses to the lungs and heart and from previous randomized trials. *J Clin Oncol*. 2017;35(15):1641–1649. https://doi.org/10.1200/JCO.2016.72.0722

Taylor S, Lim P, Ahmad R, et al. Risk of radiation-induced second malignant neoplasms from photon and proton radiotherapy in pediatric abdominal neuroblastoma. *Phys Imaging Radiat Oncol*. 2021;19:45–52.

Teoh S, Fiorini F, George B, Vallis KA. Van den Heuvel F. Proton vs photon: a model-based approach to patient selection for reduction of cardiac toxicity in locally advanced lung cancer. *Radiother Oncol*. 2020;152:151–162. https://doi.org/10.1016/j.radonc.2019.06.032

Thomson DJ, Teo B-K K, Ong A, et al. The impact of anatomic change on pencil beam scanning in the treatment of oropharynx cancer. *Int J Part Ther*. 2015;2(2):394–403. https://doi.org/10.14338/IJPT-15-00002.1

Thomson DJ, Cruickshank C, Baines H, et al. TORPEdO: a phase III trial of intensity-modulated proton beam therapy versus intensity-modulated radiotherapy for multi-toxicity reduction in oropharyngeal cancer. *Clin Transl Radiat Oncol*. 2023;38:147–154. https://doi.org/10.1016/j.ctro.2022.11.010

Tian S, McCook A, Choi IJ, et al. Treatment of thymoma and thymic carcinoma with proton beam therapy: outcomes from the Proton Collaborative Group prospective registry. *Int J Radiat Oncol Biol Phys*. 2023;117(2):e66. https://doi.org/10.1016/j.ijrobp.2023.06.792

Tiong SS, Dickie C, Haas RL, O'Sullivan B. The role of radiotherapy in the management of localized soft tissue sarcomas. *Cancer Biol Med*. 2016;13(3):373–383. https://doi.org/10.20892/j.issn.2095-3941.2016.0028

Travis LB, Gospodarowicz M, Curtis RE, et al. Lung cancer following chemotherapy and radiotherapy for Hodgkin's disease. *J Natl Cancer Inst*. 2002;94(3):182–192. https://doi.org/10.1093/jnci/94.3.182

Tringale KR, Modlin LA, Sine K, Forlenza CJ, Cahlon O, Wolden SL. Vital organ sparing with proton therapy for pediatric Hodgkin lymphoma: toxicity and outcomes in 50 patients. *Radiother Oncol*. 2022;168:46–52.

Tseng YD, Cutter DJ, Plastaras JP, et al. Evidence-based review on the use of proton therapy in lymphoma from the Particle Therapy Cooperative Group (PTCOG) Lymphoma Subcommittee. *Int J Radiat Oncol Biol Phys*. 2017;99(4):825–842. https://doi.org/10.1016/j.ijrobp.2017.05.004

Uezono H, Indelicato DJ, Rotondo RL, et al. Treatment outcomes after proton therapy for Ewing sarcoma of the pelvis. *Int J Radiat Oncol Biol Phys*. 2020;107(5):974–981.

Upadhyay R, Liao K, Grosshans D, et al. Quantifying the risk and dosimetric variables of symptomatic brainstem injury after proton radiation in pediatric brain tumours. *Neuro Oncol.* 2022;24(9):1571–1581.

Urie M, Goitein M, Wagner M. Compensating for heterogeneities in proton radiation therapy. *Phys Med Biol.* 1984;29(5):553–566.

Vazquez M, Bachmann N, Pica A, et al. Early outcome after craniospinal irradiation with pencil beam scanning proton therapy for children, adolescents and young adults with brain tumours. *Pediatr Blood Cancer.* 2023;70(2):e 30087.

Veiga C, Alshaikhi J, Amos R, et al. Cone beam computed tomography and deformable registration-based 'dose of the day' calculations for adaptive proton therapy. *Intl J Part Ther.* 2015;2(2):404–414.

Vennarini S, Colombo F, Mirandola A, et al. Clinical insight on proton therapy for paediatric rhabdomyosarcoma. *Cancer Manag Res.* 2023;15:1125–1139.

Verma V, Mehta MP. Clinical outcomes of proton radiotherapy for uveal melanoma. *Clin Oncol.* 2016;28(8):e17–e27. https://doi.org/10.1016/j.clon.2016.01.034

Vogel J, Berman AT, Lin L, et al. Prospective study of proton beam radiation therapy for adjuvant and definitive treatment of thymoma and thymic carcinoma: early response and toxicity assessment. *Radiother Oncol.* 2016;118(3):504–509. https://doi.org/10.1016/j.radonc.2016.02.003

Vogel J, Lin H, Both S, Tochner Z, Balis F, Hill-Kayser C. Pencil beam scanning proton therapy for treatment of the retroperitoneum after nephrectomy for Wilms tumor: a dosimetric comparison study. *Pediatr Blood Cancer.* 2017;64(1):39–45.

Waldron JN, O'Sullivan B, Warde P, et al. Ethmoid sinus cancer: twenty-nine cases managed with primary radiation therapy. *Int J Radiat Oncol Biol Phys.* 1998;41(2):361–369. https://doi.org/10.1016/S0360-3016(98)00018-2

Wang X, Amos RA, Zhang X, et al. External-beam accelerated partial breast irradiation using multiple proton beam configurations. *Int J Radiat Oncol Biol Phys.* 2011;80(5):1464–1472.

Weber DC, Ares C, Villa S, et al. Adjuvant postoperative high-dose radiotherapy for atypical and malignant meningioma: a phase-II parallel non-randomized and observation study (EORTC 22042-26042). *Radiother Oncol.* 2018;128(2):260–265. https://doi.org/10.1016/j.radonc.2018.06.018

Wenhua C, Khabazian A, Yepes P, et al. Linear energy transfer incorporated intensity modulated proton therapy optimization. *Phys Med Biol.* 2017;63(1):015013.

Wilson RR. Radiological use of fast protons. *Radiology.* 1946;47(5):487–491.

Woodward WA, Amos RA. Proton radiation biology considerations for radiation oncologists. *Int J Radiat Oncol Biol Phys.* 2016;95(1):59–61.

Xi M, Xu C, Liao T, et al. Comparative outcomes after definitive chemoradiotherapy using proton beam therapy versus intensity modulated radiation therapy for esophageal cancer: a retrospective, single-institutional analysis. *Int J Radiat Oncol Biol Phys.* 2017;99(3):667–676. https://doi.org/10.1016/j.ijrobp.2017.06.2450

Yang AH, Urrunaga NU, Siddiqui O, et al. Proton beam stereotactic body radiotherapy and hypofractionated therapy with pencil beam scanning is safe and effective for advanced hepatocellular carcinoma and intrahepatic cholangiocarcinoma: a single center experience. *J Radiosurg SBRT.* 2023;9(1):43–52.

Yang JC, Chang AE, Baker AR, et al. Randomized prospective study of the benefit of adjuvant radiation therapy in the treatment of soft tissue sarcomas of the extremity. *J Clin Oncol.* 1998;16(1):197–203. https://doi.org/10.1200/JCO.1998.16.1.197

Yang M, Zhu XR, Park PC, et al. Comprehensive analysis of proton range uncertainties related to patient stopping-power-ratio estimation using the stoichiometric calibration. *Phys Med Biol.* 2012;57(13):4095–4115.

Yegya-Raman N, Wang K, Kim S, et al. Dosimetric predictors of symptomatic cardiac events after conventional-dose chemoradiation therapy for inoperable NSCLC. *J Thorac Oncol.* 2018;13(10):1508–1518. https://doi.org/10.1016/j.jtho.2018.05.028

Yock T, Schneider R, Friedmann A, Adams J, Fullerton B, Tarbell N. Proton radiotherapy for orbital rhabdomyosarcoma: clinical outcome and a dosimetric comparison with photons. *Int J Rad Onc Biol Phys.* 2005;63:1161–1168.

Yock TI, Yeap BY, Ebb DH, et al. Long-term toxic effects of proton radiotherapy for paediatric medulloblastoma: a phase 2 single-arm study. *Lancet Oncol.* 2016;17(3):287–298.

Zakeri K, Wang H, Kang JJ, et al. Outcomes and prognostic factors of major salivary gland tumors treated with proton beam radiation therapy. *Head Neck.* 2021;43(4):1056–1062. https://doi.org/10.1002/hed.26563

Zeng C, Amos RA, Winey B, et al.. In: Lee NLJ, Cahlon O, Sine K, Jiang G, Lu J, Both S, eds. *Target volume delineation and treatment planning for particle therapy: practical guides in radiation oncology.* Springer; 2018:45–106.

Zhang R, Howell RM, Homann K, et al. Predicted risks of radiogenic cardiac toxicity in two pediatric patients undergoing photon or proton radiotherapy. *Radiat Oncol.* 2013;8(1):184.

Zietman AL, Bae K, Slater JD, et al. Randomized trial comparing conventional-dose with high-dose conformal radiation therapy in early-stage adenocarcinoma of the prostate: long-term results from Proton Radiation Oncology Group/American College of Radiology 95-09. *J Clin Oncol.* 2010;28(7):1106–1111. https://doi.org/10.1200/JCO.2009.25.8475

Zou Z, Bowen SR, Thomas HMT, Sasidharan BK, Rengan R, Zeng J. Scanning beam proton therapy versus photon IMRT for stage III lung cancer: comparison of dosimetry, toxicity, and outcomes. *Adv Radiat Oncol.* 2020;5(3):434–443. https://doi.org/10.1016/j.adro.2020.03.001

INDEX

Note: Page numbers followed by "*b*" indicate boxes, "*f*" indicate figures, and "*t*" indicate tables.

C

Q

V

W

X

Y